THE PHYSIOLOGIC BASIS OF GYNECOLOGY AND OBSTETRICS

THE PHYSIOLOGIC BASIS OF GYNECOLOGY AND OBSTETRICS

DAVID B. SEIFER, MD

Professor of Obstetrics, Gynecology and Reproductive Sciences
Department of Obstetrics, Gynecology and Reproductive Sciences
University of Medicine and Dentistry of New Jersey-
Robert Wood Johnson Medical School
New Brunswick, New Jersey

PHILIP SAMUELS, MD

Associate Professor of Obstetrics and Gynecology
Department of Obstetrics and Gynecology
The Ohio State University
Columbus, Ohio

DOUGLAS A. KNISS, PhD

Professor of Obstetrics and Gynecology
Department of Obstetrics and Gynecology
The Ohio State University
Columbus, Ohio

LIPPINCOTT WILLIAMS & WILKINS
A **Wolters Kluwer** Company
Philadelphia · Baltimore · New York · London
Buenos Aires · Hong Kong · Sydney · Tokyo

Acquisition Editor: Lisa McAllister
Developmental Editor: Raymond E. Reter
Production Editor: Rakesh Rampertab
Manufacturing Manager: Benjamin Rivera
Cover Designer: Tik Chuaviriya
Compositor: PRD Group
Printer: Edwards Brothers

Library of Congress Cataloging-in-Publication Data

The physiologic basis of gynecology and obstetrics / [edited by] David B. Seifer, Philip
Samuels, Douglas A. Kniss.
     p. ; cm.
     Includes bibliographical references and index.
     ISBN 0-683-30249-3
     1. Gynecology. 2. Obstetrics. 3. Generative organs, Female—
Pathophysiology. 4. Pregnancy—Physiological aspects. I. Seifer, David B., 1955– II.
Samuels, Philip, 1953– III. Kniss, Douglas. A.
     [DNLM: 1. Genital Diseases, Female—physiopathology. 2. Genitalia,
Female—physiology. 3. Pregnancy—physiology. 4. Pregnancy
Complications—physiopathology. WP 100 P578 2001]
RG103 .P48 2001
618—dc21
                                                                          00-051990

Care has been taken to confirm the accuracy of the information presented and to
describe generally accepted practices. However, the authors, editors, and publisher are
not responsible for errors or omissions or for any consequences from application of the
information in this book and make no warranty, expressed or implied, with respect to
the currency, completeness, or accuracy of the contents of the publication. Application
of this information in a particular situation remains the professional responsibility of
the practitioner.

The authors, editors, and publisher have exerted every effort to ensure that drug
selection and dosage set forth in this text are in accordance with current
recommendations and practice at the time of publication. However, in view of
ongoing research, changes in government regulations, and the constant flow of
information relating to drug therapy and drug reactions, the reader is urged to check
the package insert for each drug for any change in indications and dosage and for
added warnings and precautions. This is particularly important when the
recommended agent is a new or infrequently employed drug.

Some drugs and medical devices presented in this publication have Food and Drug
Administration (FDA) clearance for limited use in restricted research settings. It is the
responsibility of the health care provider to ascertain the FDA status of each drug or
device planned for use in their clinical practice.

10 9 8 7 6 5 4 3 2 1

To

our parents, families, and colleagues who have encouraged us to live intellectually rich lives,

those physician-scientists who persevere despite the inclement environment,

and our students who will improve upon the legacy of our knowledge.

CONTENTS

CONTRIBUTING AUTHORS

Deborah J. Anderson, PhD Fearing Laboratory, Brigham & Women's Hospital, Boston, Massachusetts

Laura K. Arbogast, MS Research Associate, Department of Obstetrics and Gynecology, Ohio State University, Columbus, Ohio

David E. Battaglia, PhD Associate Professor, Department of Obstetrics and Gynecology, University of Washington, Seattle, Washington; and Director, FEC Laboratory, University of Washington Medical Center, Seattle, Washington

William A. Bennett, PhD Assistant Professor, Department of Obstetrics and Gynecology, University of Mississippi Medical Center, Jackson, Mississippi

Joseph P. Bruner, MD Assistant Professor of Obstetrics and Gynecology, Division of Maternal and Fetal Medicine, Vanderbilt University Medical Center, Nashville, Tennessee

Patricia S. Choban, MD Assistant Professor of Clinical Surgery, Department of Surgery, Ohio State University, Columbus, Ohio

Bryan D. Cowan, MD Professor, Department of Obstetrics and Gynecology, University of Mississippi, Jackson, Mississippi

Lisa Dabney, MD Boston In Vitro Fertilization, Weston, Massachusetts

Douglas R. Danforth, PhD Associate Professor, Department of Obstetrics and Gynecology, Ohio State University, Columbus, Ohio

Louis Flancbaum, MD Associate Professor of Surgery, Department of Surgery, Ohio State University, Columbus, Ohio

Jodi Anne Flaws, PhD Assistant Professor, Department of Epidemiology and Preventive Medicine, University of Maryland, Baltimore, Maryland

Luis Miguel Garcia-Segura Instituto Cajal, C.S.I.C., Madrid, Spain

Debra K. Gardner, PharmD, RPh Assistant Clinical Professor, College of Pharmacy, Ohio State University; and Specialty Practice Pharmacist, Department of Pharmacy, Ohio State University Medical Center, Columbus, Ohio

Ernest M. Graham, MD Assistant Professor, Department of Obstetrics and Gynecology, Allegheny University of Health Sciences, Philadelphia, Pennsylvania

Geri D. Hewitt, MD Assistant Clinical Professor, Department of Obstetrics and Gynecology and Pediatrics, Ohio State University College of Medicine and School of Public Health, Columbus, Ohio; and Section Chief, Department of Gynecology, Columbus Children's Hospital, Columbus, Ohio

Joseph A. Hill, MD Associate Professor, Department of Obstetrics and Gynecology and Reproductive Biology, Harvard Medical School, Boston, Massachusetts; and Director of Reproductive Medicine, Department of Obstetrics and Gynecology and Reproductive Biology, Brigham and Women's Hospital, Boston, Massachusetts

Doreen L. Hock, MD Assistant Professor, Department of Obstetrics and Gynecology, University of Medicine and Dentistry of New Jersey-Robert Wood Johnson Medical School, New Brunswick, New Jersey; and Attending Physician, Department of Obstetrics and Gynecology, St. Peter's University Hospital, New Brunswick, New Jersey

Joseph W. Hogan, ScD Assistant Professor of Biostatistics, Department of Community Health, Center for Statistical Sciences, Brown University, Providence, Rhode Island, and Assistant Professor of Obstetrics and Gynecology, Department of Obstetrics and Gynecology, Women and Infant's Hospital of Rhode Island, Providence, Rhode Island

Carol J. Homko, PhD, RN Diabetes Nurse Specialist, Department of Obstetrics and Gynecology and Reproductive Sciences; and Nurse Manager, General Clinical Research Center, Temple University Hospital, Philadelphia, Pennsylvania

Tamas L. Horvath, PhD Associate Professor of Obstetrics and Gynecology, Department of Obstetrics and Gynecology, Yale University School of Medicine, New Haven, Connecticut

Brenda S. Houmard, MD, PhD Senior Fellow, Department of Obstetrics and Gynecology, University of Washington, Seattle, Washington

Jay D. Iams, MD   Frederick P. Zuspan Professor of Obstetrics and Gynecology, Department of Obstetrics and Gynecology, Ohio State University College of Medicine and Public Health; and Division Director and Vice-Chairman, Department of Obstetrics and Gynecology, Ohio State University Hospitals, Columbus, Ohio

Jeffrey R. Johnson, MD   Clinical Fellow, Department of Maternal-Fetal Medicines, Ohio State University College of Medicine and Public Health, Columbus, Ohio

Audrey H. Kang, MD   Assistant Professor, Department of Obstetrics and Gynecology, Vanderbilt University, Nashville, Tennessee; and Director, Maternal-Fetal Medicine, Baptiste Hospital, Nashville, Tennessee

Lisa M. Keder, MD   Assistant Professor, Department of Obstetrics and Gynecology, Ohio State University, Columbus, Ohio

Douglas A. Kniss, PhD   Professor of Obstetrics and Gynecology, Department of Obstetrics and Gynecology, Ohio State University, Columbus, Ohio

Neeraj Kohli, MD   Instructor, Department of Obstetrics and Gynecology, Harvard Medical School, Boston, Massachusetts; and Director, Division of Urogynecology, Mount Auburn Hospital, Cambridge, Massachusetts

Parul Krishnamurthy, MD, MRCOG   Chief Resident, Department of Obstetrics and Gynecology, the Reading Hospital & Medical Center, West Reading, Pennsylvania

Lawrence C. Layman, MD   Professor of Obstetrics and Gynecology, Chief, Section of Reproductive Endocrinology, Infertility, and Genetics, Department of Obstetrics and Gynecology, Medical College of Georgia, Augusta, Georgia

Mark Leondires, MD   5133 Fairglen Lane, Chevy Chase, Maryland

Andrew J. Levi, MD   Department of Obstetrics and Gynecology, Georgetown University Medical Center, Washington, D.C.

W. Michael Lin, MD   Senior Fellow, Division of Gynecologic Oncology, University of Texas Southwestern Medical Center, Dallas, Texas

David T. MacLaughlin, PhD   Associate Professor of Biochemistry, Department of Obstetrics and Gynecology, Harvard Medical School; and Associate Director of Pediatric Surgical Research Laboratory, Department of Pediatric Surgery, Massachusetts General Hospital, Boston, Massachusetts

John S. McDonald, MD   Professor, Department of Anesthesiology, UCLA School of Medicine, Los Angeles, California; and Chairman, Department of Anesthesiology, Harbor-UCLA Medical Center, Torrance California

David S. McKenna, MD   Wright Patterson Medical Center, 74th MDOS/SGOG, Wright Patterson Air Force Base, Dayton, Ohio

Jay E. Menitove, MD   Community Blood Center of Greater Kansas City, Kansas City, Missouri

Bradley T. Miller, MD   Reproductive Medicine Associates of New Jersey; and Attending Staff, Department of Obstetrics and Gynecology, Morristown Memorial Hospital, Morristown, New Jersey

David Scott Miller, MD   Professor and Director, Department of Obstetrics and Gynecology, University of Texas Southwestern Medical Center, Dallas, Texas; and Medical Director of Gynecologic Oncology, Department of Women's and Children's Services, Parkland Health and Hospital System, Dallas, Texas

Jay W. Moore, PHD, FFACMG   Director, Cytogenetics Laboratory, Genzyme Genetics, Santa Fe, New Mexico

Carolyn Y. Muller, MD   Assistant Professor, Department of Gynecology and Obstetrics, University of Texas Southwestern Medical Center, Dallas, Texas

Leslie Myatt, PhD   Professor, Department of Obstetrics and Gynecology, University of Cincinnati, College of Medicine, Cincinnati, Ohio

Frederick Naftolin, MD, DPhil   Professor of Obstetrics and Gynecology, Department of Obstetrics and Gynecology, Yale University School of Medicine, New Haven, Connecticut

A. George Neubert, MD   Clinical Assistant Professor, Department of Obstetrics and Gynecology, University of Pennsylvania School of Medicine, Philadelphia, Pennsylvania; and Director, Section of Maternal-Fetal Medicine, Department of Obstetrics and Gynecology, The Reading Hospital and Medical Center, West Reading, Pennsylvania

Errol R. Norwitz, MD, PhD   Assistant Professor, Department of Obstetrics and Gynecology, Harvard Medical School, Boston, Massachusetts; and Attending Perinatologist, Department of Obstetrics and Gynecology, Brigham and Women's Hospital, Boston, Massachusetts

Jeffrey F. Peipert, MD   Associate Professor, Department of Obstetrics and Gynecology, Women and Infants' Hospital, Brown University School of Medicine, Providence, Rhode Island

Alan S. Penzias, MD   Assistant Professor of Obstetrics, Gynecology and Reproductive Biology, Harvard Medical School, Boston, Massachusetts; and Surgical Director, Boston In Vitro Fertilization, Waltham, Massachusetts

Robin L. Perry, MD   69 Scenic View Drive, Sicklerville, New Jersey

E. Albert Reece, MD The Abraham Roth Professor and Chairman, Department of Obstetrics, Gynecology and Reproductive Sciences, Temple University School of Medicine, Philadelphia, Pennsylvania

Rosemary E. Reiss, MD Assistant Professor, Department of Obstetrics and Gynecology, Harvard Medical School, Brigham and Women's Hospital, Boston, Massachusetts

John T. Repke, MD Chair and Professor, Department of Obstetrics and Gynecology, University of Nebraska Medical Center, Omaha, Nebraska

Julian N. Robinson, MD, PhD Department of Obstetrics and Gynecology, Harvard Medical School, Boston, Massachusetts

John Rodis, MD Associate Professor of Obstetrics and Gynecology, Director of Residency Program, University of Connecticut Medical Center, Farmington, Connecticut

Philip Samuels, MD Associate Professor of Obstetrics and Gynecology, Department of Obstetrics and Gynecology, Ohio State University, Columbus, Ohio

Michael A. Saubolle, PhD Department of Pathology, Good Samaritan Regional Medical Center, Phoenix, Arizona

Peter A. Schwartz, MD Professor of Clinical Obstetrics and Gynecology, Department of Obstetrics and Gynecology, University of Pennsylvania, Philadelphia, Pennsylvania; and Chair, Department of Obstetrics and Gynecology, The Reading Hospital and Medical Center, Reading, Pennsylvania

Harish M. Sehdev, MD Assistant Professor, Department of Obstetrics and Gynecology, University of Pennsylvania, Philadelphia, Pennsylvania; and Assistant Professor, Department of Obstetrics and Gynecology, Pennsylvania Hospital, Philadelphia, Pennsylvania

David B. Seifer, MD Professor of Obstetrics, Gynecology and Reproductive Sciences, Director, Division of Reproductive Sciences and Infertility, Department of Obstetrics, Gynecology and Reproductive Sciences, University of Medicine and Dentistry of New Jersey-Robert Wood Johnson Medical School, New Brunswick, New Jersey

Fady I. Sharara, MD Director, Assisted Reproductive Technologies Program, The Fertility and Reproductive Health Center, Annandale, Virginia

Sandra R. Silva, MD Department of Obstetrics and Gynecology, Vanderbilt University Medical Center, Nashville, Tennessee

Joyce D. Steinfeld, MD Assistant Professor, Department of Obstetrics and Gynecology, Albert Einstein College of Medicine, Bronx, New York; and Attending Physician, Department of Obstetrics and Gynecology, Long Island Jewish Medical Center, New Hyde Park, New York

Joseph R. Wax, MD Associate Professor, Department of Obstetrics and Gynecology, University of Connecticut, Farmington, Connecticut; and Associate Director, Maternal Fetal Medicine, Department of Obstetrics and Gynecology, Hartford Hospital, Hartford, Connecticut

Eric A. Widra, MD Assistant Professor and Chief, Division of Reproductive Endocrinology and Infertility, Georgetown University Medical Center; and Shady Grove Fertility Reproductive Science Center, Washington, D.C.

Lisa D. Yee, MD Assistant Professor of Surgery, Department of Surgery, Ohio State University, Columbus, Ohio

Tony G. Zreik, MD Department of Obstetrics and Gynecology, Yale University School of Medicine, New Haven, Connecticut

FOREWORD

Basic science research is the foundation for important clinical advances in women's health. In turn, the many diseases that cause human suffering and are not yet "cured" create the context in which scientific discovery can provide the greatest value to society. The reciprocating cycle of bench to bedside and back again is a powerful dynamic that has accelerated the progress of women's health.

Most textbooks that deal with reproductive science and reproductive medicine focus either on the bench or the bedside, typically to the exclusion of the other. In this book, Drs. Seifer, Samuels, and Kniss blend the reproductive sciences with the common clinical problems seen in obstetrics and gynecology. It is organized into three parts. The first provides a thorough treatment of the reproductive sciences, including reproductive genetics, molecular and cell biology, developmental biology, neuroendocrinology, pharmacology, nutrition, wound healing and research design. The second and third portions of the text cover the fields of obstetrics and gynecology. The book provides a seamless journey through the advances in both reproductive science and reproductive medicine. Many chapters point out the vast potential for both reproductive science and reproductive medicine that exists at the interface of the bench and bedside.

This book achieves its goal of reviewing the scientific basis for our practice of obstetrics and gynecology, and helps to bridge the gap between basic science and clinical practice. It should be a memorable read for both reproductive scientists and reproductive medicine clinicians.

Robert L. Barbieri, M.D.
Kate Macy Ladd Professor of Obstetrics,
Gynecology and Reproductive Biology
Harvard Medical School
Boston, Massachusetts

PREFACE

"May the love of my art inspire me at all times . . ."

Maimonides

As practitioners of a fast-paced specialty, obstetricians/gynecologists must rely upon their knowledge and experience to make diagnoses, counsel patients, and perform complex procedures. The demands of office practice, however, often limit the time we have to review the basic science concepts that are an integral part of our daily activities. In addition, the rapid progress in molecular and cellular biology is accelerating our understanding of the pathogenesis of disease. The need to stay updated with this progress places ever-increasing demands on the clinician to remain current in the science relevant to women's health.

The purpose of this book is to review the physiological basis for our practice of obstetrics and gynecology—to assist in bridging the gap between basic science and clinical practice. Our intent is to provide a reference for residents, sub-specialty fellows and practitioners, and a source of clinical information for basic reproductive scientists. Many chapters are coauthored by clinicians and basic scientists to emphasize the most practical aspects of basic science as they apply to the practice of our specialty. This text should assist both new and veteran practitioners and investigators in their appreciation and understanding of the scientific foundation upon which our specialty is based.

D.B.S.
P.S.
D.A.K.

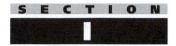

SECTION I

PRINCIPLES OF BASIC AND APPLIED SCIENCE

CELL AND MOLECULAR BIOLOGY FOR CLINICIANS

DAVID T. MACLAUGHLIN

It is axiomatic that biomedical research approaches assume a molecular basis of most diseases, and therefore experiments are designed to identify the molecule or molecules responsible. Also widely held is the hypothesis that the adverse health effects are caused by mutations of normal genes. These mutations produce the molecular "culprits" with either overactive, partially impaired, or completely inactive products. Furthermore, the most logical way to identify the abnormal, in this context, is to compare it with the normal. The systematic study of normal biologic processes, therefore, is the key to uncovering the causes of human disease. If we don't understand how things are supposed to be, how can we detect harmful changes? If we don't understand the molecular basis of disease how can rational treatments be designed? This admittedly simplistic description of biomedical research makes sense only if it is possible to actually study the more than 100,000 structural genes in the human genome. With the successful sequencing of the human genome, what was considered virtually impossible becomes a realistic goal and heralds what will be the next revolution in medicine. Namely, it will be possible to compare essentially the entire genome of patients to their controls and by the application of appropriate algorithms identify relevant genetic differences without isolating anything but some DNA or even having a well-defined experimental hypothesis. Until that time comes, however, we still need to study how cells function as well as to better understand the structure and expression of DNA, messenger RNA (mRNA), and proteins.

This chapter provides a brief overview of cell biology and some state-of-the-art methods for the clinician, who with increasing regularity is confronted by molecular biologic end points in the clinical literature.

This chapter discusses recent concepts in cell biology and current methods of molecular investigation. The chapter begins with a discussion of cell biology, focusing on the central dogma of biology because it provides a biologic framework for the review of the mammalian cell cycle, which includes the molecular mechanisms that control differentiated cell function, cell division, and programmed death. This is followed by a review of the structure and function of the biologic macromolecules DNA, mRNA, and proteins, and a primer on some state-of-the-art techniques employed to critically analyze these materials. Some illustrative cases of the application of these methods to successfully delineate the molecular pathophysiology of several all-too-common diseases are included to provide concrete examples of the progress possible with today's technology.

A glossary is provided at the end of the chapter.

This chapter is not a comprehensive review. There are extremely well-written, highly detailed basic texts available to the interested reader. The goal here is to provide a practical guide to help the reader better understand what follows in the rest of the chapters in this book.

THE CENTRAL DOGMA OF BIOLOGY

Ever since the discovery of DNA and the elaboration of the concept of genes, scientists have held a linear view of cell biology; namely, information flows downhill from structural genes through RNA intermediates to the final three-dimensional proteins and, often, the molecules they produce (Fig. 1.1). Structure, therefore, dictates function. Genes are perpetuated generation after generation by replication, but gene function is manifest in proteins. The biologic activity of these molecules is a function of their concentration, bioactivation, transport to a distant site of action, if necessary, and ultimately their deactivation by degradation or some other related process. In eukaryotes, DNA is sequestered in the nucleus away from sites of protein synthesis; thus, the mRNA intermediate is required. Transcription of genes into mRNA allows the information to pass from the nucleus to the cytoplasm for translation into protein. This pathway of transfer of information from nucleic acid (DNA) to nucleic acid (mRNA) all the way to protein is irreversible. There is no protein-to-protein or protein-to-nucleic acid transfer of primary structure information. The discovery of reverse transcriptase, however, revealed that RNA can serve as a template for DNA synthesis. This is the molecular basis for retroviral infection of host cells and for one of the most important tools in the laboratory today, namely reverse transcriptase—polymerase chain reaction (RT-PCR) methodology. Despite these revolutionary

REPLICATION

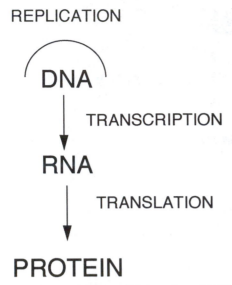

FIGURE 1.1. The central dogma of biology shows DNA duplicates via replication and its structural information transferred via transcription to RNA. Translation to protein encoded for by the gene is the ultimate result in this irreversible process.

new discoveries in biology, however, the central dogma remains intact.

This simple concept provides the rationale for many modern experimental protocols. For example, knowing the DNA sequence for a gene immediately reveals the amino acid sequence of its product. Therefore, without purifying a protein to homogeneity, it is possible to know its primary structure, and by deducing the mRNA sequence it is possible to design extremely specific reagents to detect and monitor its production. Furthermore, the theme of the central dogma explains how, if the genome is mutated by some accident of nature or environmental factor, the effects can be manifest at the level of proteins in the cell.

THE MAMMALIAN CELL LIFE CYCLE

One of the major scientific discoveries of the past 20 years is the finding that the molecular mechanisms whereby cells commit to and ultimately undergo cell division are remarkably conserved from single cell organisms to humans. The cell cycle proteins, as they are called, are nearly identical in yeast as in humans. In fact, studies of oncogenes, growth factors, hormones, and cytokines focus on how their activities affect those of the cell cycle proteins. Presented here is a representative array of cell cycle regulatory molecules that help illustrate how the cycle functions, but it is by no means a compete list.

The mammalian cell life cycle can be divided among several discrete stages including replicative, differentiated cellular function and finally programmed cell death. The

initiation and completion of these processes are precisely timed and controlled by auto- or paracrine stimuli provided by means of hormonal and other cytokine actions. Attempts to define the molecular pathophysiology of a disease, particularly of malignancies, often realize great advances by examining the control points for entry and/or exit from these phases of the life cycle for loss or gain of functions that can lead to the phenotype observed.

Cell replication is accomplished by completion of the cell cycle, a process that takes on the order of 18 to 24 hours, but the length of time it takes to progress through the cycle can be over 100 days. Some cells such as oocytes, neurons, red cells, and skeletal muscle cells never divide once fully differentiated. The cycle is divided into several discrete phases with each serving a different function (Fig. 1.2). Cells uncommitted to division are said to be in G0 (gap 0) and have not entered the cell cycle. Cells in G1 (gap 1), however, have responded to mitotic signals including certain nutrients, growth factors, hormones, and cytokines interacting with their receptors and are then transcribing genes that encode for DNA-synthesizing enzymes. The phase of the cell cycle most responsible for cell cycle length is G1, since, as a rule, the major difference between cells that divide rapidly and those that do so rarely is the length of time spent in this part of the cycle. DNA synthesis occurs in the S (synthesis) phase in which the full complement of cellular DNA is copied. The chemistry of this process is discussed in a later section of this chapter. Repair of the newly made DNA is done in G2 (gap 2) just before mitosis (M phase), wherein the copies of DNA are separated and two identical diploid daughter cells are produced. This cycle can be repeated immediately or cells may return to G0

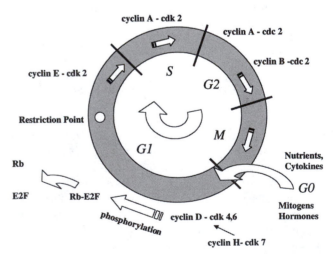

FIGURE 1.2. A representation of the cell cycle showing discrete phases G1, S, G2, and M as well as the location of several cyclins and cyclin-dependent kinases (CDKs). In addition, the position of one important tumor suppressor gene, Rb, is given as a reference for discussions later in this chapter.

for variable periods of time depending upon the cell type and function.

The transition from one phase to the next depends on the quantity and activity of at least six specific cyclin-dependent kinases (CDKs 2 to 4, 6, 7, and Cdc2) and five other proteins called cyclins (A, B, D, E, and H) with which they associate. Phosphorylation, therefore, can push the cell cycle forward, while dephosphorylation, on the other hand, can stop the cycle. Obviously, the relative activities of kinases and phosphatases is critical in directing cell division. Similarly, changes in the concentration of these proteins can alter cell cycle progression. Both of these phenomena have been shown to affect cell cycle rates. Activities of individual kinases and cyclins are found predominantly at specific transitions in the cell cycle (Fig. 1.2), and loss-of-function mutations of these complexes halt cell cycle progression. This is, in fact, how the function of these proteins was first identified in lower organisms. The most important control point for entry into the cell cycle in the so-called restriction site in the onset of G1, whose function it is to prevent progression through the cycle until conditions conducive to success are met. This is accomplished through the activities of two other regulatory proteins—retinoblastoma protein (Rb), and E2F, a nuclear transcription factor. When hypophosphorylated, Rb binds to E2F, preventing the latter from acting as a transcription factor that induces the synthesis of a wide variety of growth promoting gene transcripts including E2F-1, c-*myc*, cyclin A, and Cdc2. When phosphorylated by cyclin D/cdk 4/6 complexes, Rb releases E2F, thus overcoming the inhibition of cell cycle progression. This step is reversed by the CDK inhibitors (CDKIs), some of which are in fact phosphatases (Fig. 1.3). Inactive mutants of these inhibitors are implicated in a wide variety of cancers, not surprisingly, since loss of inhibition of cell

growth can be as disastrous as overstimulation by trophic factors. A more detailed discussion of this complicated process is beyond the scope of this chapter. See the Suggested Readings list at the end of the chapter for relevant recent reviews.

As important as the carefully orchestrated increase and maintenance of proper cell numbers in an organism is the orderly and controlled reduction in cell number or programmed cell death called apoptosis. In fact, even some unnatural inducers of cell death such as chemotherapeutic agents and hypoxia can cause apoptosis. Whether caused by withdrawal of hormones or other trophic stimuli as part of normal physiologic processes, or by infection by viruses or exposure to radiation, the induction of apoptosis is heralded by the morphologic changes in the nucleus that are the basis of the earliest definition of the process. It is now known that apoptosis requires energy and that genomic DNA is enzymatically cleaved such that a series of fragments of differing molecular weight are produced and readily visualized upon electrophoretic analysis as a "ladder" of discrete and sharp DNA bands. Nonapoptotic cell death also results in the degradation of nuclear DNA but in a random way that produces a smear under separation conditions with which one can see an apoptotic ladder. The molecular mechanisms producing apoptosis seem to vary with the cell type, and the complete story isn't known for any of them. There do seem to be several common themes, however. Namely, whether a cell undergoes apoptosis results from the balance of forces driving cell survival, cell division, and cell death. These three paths cross with the activities of three proteins, p53, bcl2, and bax2, factors that are associated with cell cycle arrest, cell survival, and cell death.

BIOCHEMISTRY OF BIOLOGIC MACROMOLECULES

Deoxyribonucleic Acid

Structure

Biologic information is passed from one generation to another in discrete units called genes that are organized in linear arrays of polymeric deoxyribonucleic acids (DNA). The DNA polymers of the nucleosides adenosine, guanosine, cytidine, and thymidine (Fig. 1.4) are held together by covalent phosphoester bonds between the 5 carbon ribose ring structures (Fig. 1.5). The numbering schema for nucleosides refers, by convention, to both the carbon and nitrogen atoms in the bases and carbons on the five-carbon ribose sugar. The "prime" designation is reserved for the sugar to avoid confusion with the numbering pattern of atoms in the purine or pyrimidine bases. Therefore, the 5' to 3' carbons in the phosphoesters always refer to the ribose molecule. Nucleosides are covalent complexes of a sugar

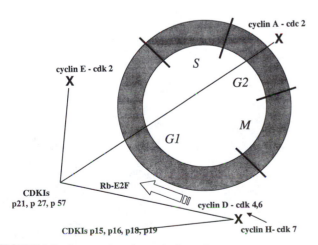

FIGURE 1.3. Progression through the cell cycle can be stopped (X) by the action of a number of inhibitors such as p15, 16, 18, 19, 27, and p57. These proteins are often among the gene products whose transcription or activation is regulated by endocrine and paracrine factors that block mitosis.

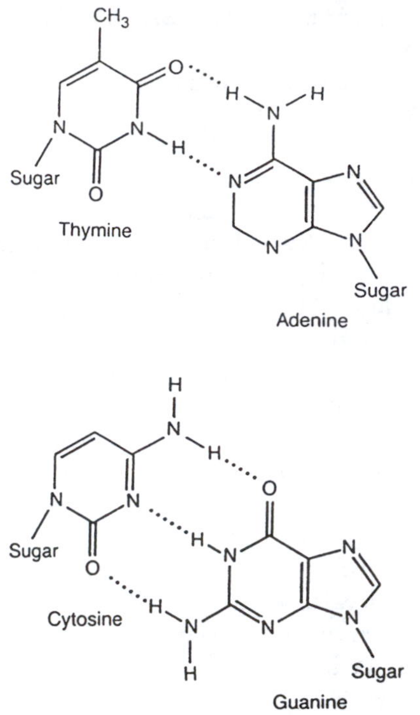

FIGURE 1.4. In DNA purines (adenine and guanine) hydrogen bonds to pyrimidines (thymine and cytosine) on opposite strands of the duplex structure. Note that guanine-cytosine pairs share three hydrogen bonds, making these interactions stronger than those of adenine and thymine.

directions (Fig. 1.6). The dimer is held together by the hydrogen bonds between complementary bases, two for adenine-thymine pairs and three for guanine and cytosine interactions. For each purine there is a pyrimidine, for every adenosine there is a thymidine, and for every guanosine there is a cytidine, a principle known as Chargaff's rule. In the DNA dimer, the bases are stacked on the inside of the resulting helical structure and the negatively charged phosphoester-linked deoxyribose backbone occupies the outer face of the dimer.

The majority of cellular DNA in the nondividing cell is in the nucleus and exists as chromatin, a complex in which the DNA is coated by proteins. The tendency of DNA to bind to proteins forms the basis for nature's solution to a rather difficult packaging problem. Namely, how can one fit a filament of DNA helix 1.8 m long (approximately 5 billion base pairs), the average length of the human genome, into a sphere, the average nucleus, that has a diameter 300,000 times smaller, i.e., 6 μm? The answer appears to be coiling and supercoiling of DNA-protein complexes called nucleosomes (Fig. 1.7), where the 200 base pairs of the DNA double helix wraps twice around an octamer of DNA-binding proteins called histones. The most common distribution of histones in these structures is two each of histones

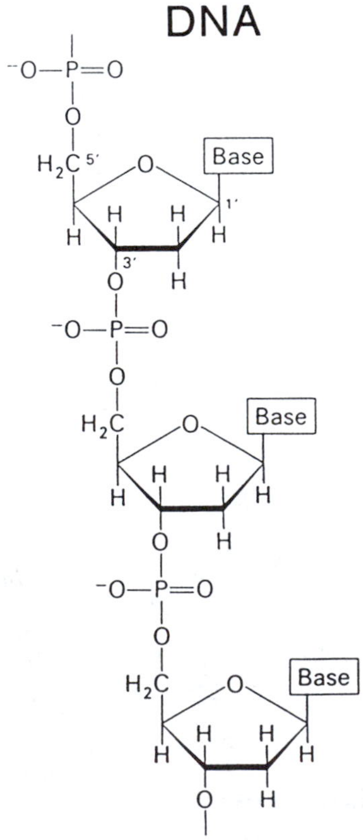

(deoxyribose) and a purine (adenine and guanine) or pyrimidine nitrogenous base (cytosine or thymine). There is a directionality to the oligonucleotide polymerization such that the phosphoester only forms between the hydroxyl group on the 3' carbon of a deoxyribose and the 5' carbon of the deoxyribose in the next nucleoside, thus, oligonucleotide chains are referred to as being oriented in the 5' to 3' direction or the 3' to 5' direction.

Chemically, DNA is among the most stabile of biologic macromolecules because it is highly resistant to hydrolysis at neutral pH in the absence of very sequence-specific enzymes. To have our genetic legacy encapsulated in nearly any other molecule would have disastrous results. Actually, it is the absence of the hydroxyl group at the 2' position on the ribose ring structure that eliminates the possibility of a nucleophilic attack on the phosphoester bond that would lead to breaks in the DNA chain and degradation of the genome (Fig. 1.5). Deoxyribonucleic acid gets its name because it lacks the 2' hydroxyl substituent. As described below, ribonucleic acid (RNA) has this 2' hydroxyl group and is much more susceptible to hydrolytic degradation as a result.

Under physiologic conditions DNA does not exist as a single oligonucleotide chain. Rather, it forms a noncovalent dimer with a complementary DNA molecule in an antiparallel fashion; thus, the DNA strands are oriented in opposite

FIGURE 1.5. This model of a single strand of DNA shows the 5' to 3' oriented phosphoester bond formed between the ring structure of adjacent riboses. Note that position 2' is not hydroxylated.

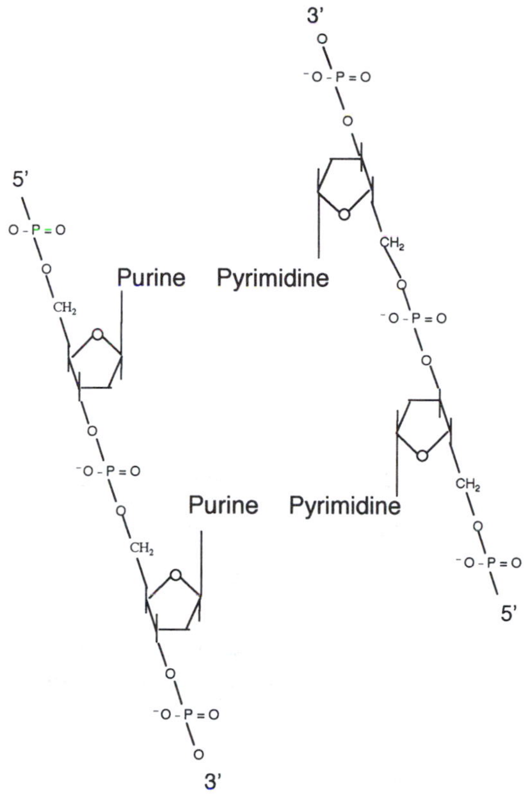

FIGURE 1.6. In the antiparallel orientation of double-stranded DNA, the bases stack in the central axis, and purines and pyrimidines must pair with one another to keep the radius of the helix constant.

H2, H2A, H3, and H4. The DNA wrapped around the histones have exposed surfaces that interact with other nuclear but nonhistone proteins that contribute to the packing phenomenon, as well as the specific regulation of gene transcription. Nucleosomes have a diameter of approximately 10 nm and appear at regular intervals along the entire linear sequence of DNA in the nucleus such that when chromatin is isolated from cell nuclei under mild denaturing conditions and examined by electron microscopy, they produce a beads-on-a-string appearance. A higher level of complexity is seen when nucleosomes are allowed to bind to histone H1 and form a coiled structure of six nucleosomes per turn and a diameter of nearly 30 nm. These coils can form even larger aggregates that all contribute to the dense packing of DNA that ultimately allows all of it to fit in the nucleus. DNA sequences that encode genes for proteins need to be transcribed into mRNA and need to be in loosely packed coils, called euchromatin, so that DNA transcription regulators and DNA-dependent RNA polymerases can envelop the DNA as a template. How the unfolding of the supercoiled DNA is regulated and influenced by transcription regulators remains the subject of intense investigation.

DNA Replication: The Sequence of One Strand Specifies the Sequence of the Other

Prior to cell division, the DNA content of cells needs to double by a process called replication. To accomplish this with high fidelity and sufficient speed to be completed in the S phase of the cell cycle, the DNA must be separated from proteins bound to it, and the hydrogen bond between the bases in the duplex structure must be broken so the helix can unwind, thus allowing the appropriate polymerizing enzymes to fit on the DNA template (Fig. 1.8). This is done simultaneously at discrete and relatively small (about 1,000 to 2,000 base pairs) regions along the genome. The considerable obstacle to unwinding presented by the plethora of interchain hydrogen bonds is overcome indirectly by the hydrolysis of adenosine triphosphate (ATP) due to the action of helicase, a DNA-binding enzyme that captures the 7 kcal/mol of energy derived from the cleavage of ATP to unwind the duplex. Helicase activity is enhanced by other DNA enzymes such as topoisomerase.

Spontaneous refolding is prevented by the association of the DNA with single-stranded (DNA) binding proteins (SSBs). These unwound stretches of DNA with DNA polymerases attached are called replication bubbles. The rules defining the origin of replication that each bubble represents are poorly defined at this time but they are the subject of intense investigation. The major determining factor in the essentially error-free process of making two polymers of 3 billion units each is the complementary base pairing just discussed for DNA duplex formation. Each strand of the old DNA serves as the template for a new strand. Thus, at the end of the replicative process each DNA duplex contains an old strand, which serves as the template, and a new strand. The DNA-dependent DNA polymerase enzyme (DNA POL I) only functions in the 5′–3′ direction and can extend the growing DNA oligomer at a rate of about 50 bases per second and requires a template to "copy" and a primer to initiate synthesis. The primer is a short stretch

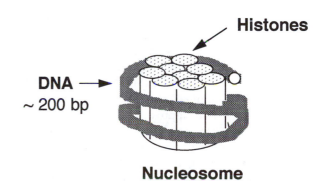

FIGURE 1.7. Nucleosomes are structures in which nucleic acid coils tightly around highly organized bundles of histone proteins. Specific surfaces of the DNA and histone proteins interact, leaving the remaining domains to interact with other nuclear proteins that are important for the regulation of gene transcription.

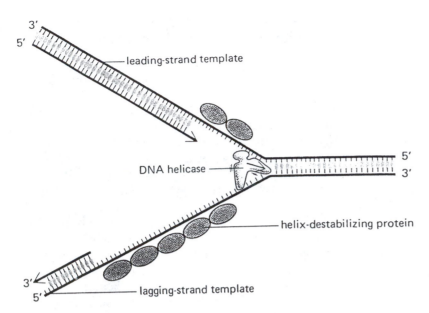

FIGURE 1.8. The replication fork of DNA synthesis directs the semiconservative synthesis of new DNA. The *arrows* indicate the direction of the chain elongation (5′–3′).

of RNA, actually, that forms a duplex needed for the polymerase to attach. ATP, thymidine triphosphate (TTP), cytidine triphosphate (CTP), and guanosine triphosphate (GTP) are the high-energy substrates used in the synthesis process, and the hydrolysis of these nucleotides provides the energetic driving force for the reactions. DNA polymerase copies one template into a new continuous, or "leading" 5′–3′ strand.

How is the synthesis of the antiparallel strand accomplished if the enzyme functions only in the 5′–3′ direction? The answer lies in the discovery of Okasaki fragments or short 100– to 200–base pair DNA oligomers each beginning with a small stretch of RNA. This finding predicted the existence of RNA primase enzymes that allow DNA polymerase to function and a ligase that would edit out the RNA and join the DNA segments together, thus elongating the new "lagging" strand of DNA. It is called "lagging" because it is formed on the antiparallel strand of DNA opposite the leading strand. DNA synthesis, therefore, is referred to as being "semiconservative" because each daughter strand consists of a new and an "old," or conserved, strand. Repairs of mismatched complementary bases are accomplished by endonucleases that recognize noncomplementary inserts and excise the incorrect base that is replaced by polymerase and ligase activity. Amazingly, synthesis mistakes occur at an infinitely small rate, about once every billion bases. If there are approximately 1 million births in the United States per year and the error rate in DNA replication were applied to the gestation, labor, and delivery process, it would be roughly analogous to having a serious, bad outcome every thousand years or so. DNA replication is a very efficient biologic process. In spite of this high-fidelity process, mistakes do occur. Spontaneous mutations can lead to heritable problems ranging from mild to life-threatening.

All of the genomic DNA replication processes take place in the nucleus, an intracellular membrane enclosed space occupying about 7% of the total cell volume. All of the enzymes and other DNA-binding proteins required are synthesized in the cytoplasm and transported via specific protein-targeting mechanisms through the nuclear membrane and into the inner nuclear space. Chemical energy in the form of the trinucleotides and the ATP for the helicase likewise are brought by appropriate carriers to the DNA synthesis machinery. Compartmentalization of cellular function as one mechanism whereby processes are controlled and regulated will be discussed in a subsequent section.

The property of base complementarity and the existence of highly sequence-specific and efficient DNA polymerases and nucleases are exploited for molecular biologic experiments. It is relatively easy to isolate DNA free of any adherent proteins and to make millions of copies of significantly large pieces for sequence analyses and evaluation. DNA is very stable and resistant to autohydrolysis.

Gene Structure

A primary role for DNA is to propagate heritable traits in the form of genes from generation to generation and to allow for the transcription of genes into mRNA that ultimately get translated into proteins and polypeptides needed for life-sustaining functions. In higher organisms it is generally true that approximately 1% of the entire genome ever gets transcribed and that only 3% to 5% of that is mRNA. Furthermore, genes are discontinuous and interrupted by sequences, called introns, or intervening sequences, that do not encode protein (Fig. 1.9). The gene segments that encode proteins are called exons. The gene for albumin, for example, the most abundant protein in serum, has seven

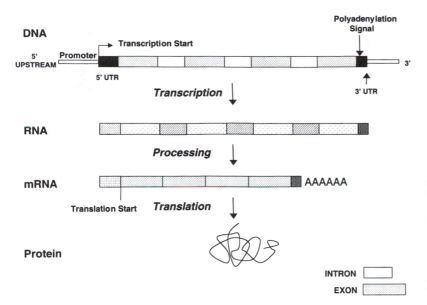

FIGURE 1.9. In DNA, exons, which contain the structural gene sequences, are separated by intervening sequences, called introns. Both of these types of domains get transcribed into RNA as do the 5' and 3' untranslated (UTR) regions. The promoter region upstream from the start site for transcription is a key site for interaction of nuclear transcription regulatory proteins with the DNA. Specific enzymes in the nucleus excise the introns and add a polyadenylate tail at the 3' end of the newly formed messenger RNA (mRNA) prior to transporting the message to the cytoplasm.

exons for a total of approximately 1,850 bases. Apart from the exons and introns, there are important sequences "upstream" (in the 5' direction) from the transcription start site and/or "downstream" (in the 3' direction) from the last exon that play a role in the control of gene transcription. These control sites are occupied by complexes of nuclear proteins that contribute to controlling the rate and duration of transcription. Many of these nuclear factors are part of the signaling cascades of hormones, cytokines, and growth factors.

mRNA

Structure

There are three important chemical differences between RNA and DNA. First, RNA has hydroxyl groups at both position 2' and 3' in the ribose ring (Fig. 1.10), a fact that contributes significantly to its instability and rapid rate of degradation *in vitro*. Second, RNA contains uracil instead of thymine as a nitrogenous base. Third, RNA doesn't form an double helix with another strand of RNA in an analogous manner to DNA. Helices are formed with RNA but these are largely due to the folding and looping of the single-stranded RNA as is seen in transfer RNA, for example. The secondary and tertiary structures of the different RNA species in the cell reflect their varied roles in the cell.

For example, if DNA is the repository of the blueprints of structural genes, RNA, among its other roles, is a messenger directing the translation of that information into protein. Thus, *translation,* a term synonymous with protein synthesis, requires mRNA. This species of RNA is formed by the action of DNA-dependent RNA polymerases that bind with other nuclear proteins that facilitate the formation of initiation complexes upstream (5') from the beginning of a gene.

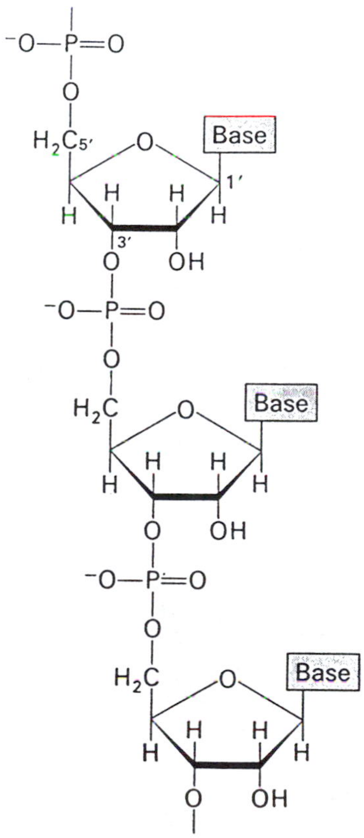

FIGURE 1.10. RNA, like DNA, is a polymer held together by phosphoester bonds. The hydroxyl group at position 2', however, contributes to the instability of RNA, owing to its ability to attack the adjacent 3' ester and hydrolyze the bond, thus fragmenting the RNA.

Amino-terminal residue ⟶ **Carboxyl-terminal residue**

FIGURE 1.11. This five amino acid polypeptide chain shows the side chains of each amino acid (R) projecting outward, away from the peptide bond backbone of the structure. (From Stryer L. *Biochemistry*, 3rd ed. New York: Freeman Press, 1988:22–28.)

Exons and introns are both copied from only one strand of the DNA called the sense strand because it bears the coding region for the protein. The completed RNA molecule needs to be further processed by nuclear enzymes that excise the introns and add a polyadenylate tail to the 3′ end of the RNA, thus allowing it to migrate to the cytoplasm as mRNA, ready to associate with ribosomal complexes that are part of the protein synthetic machinery of the cell. The regulation of where and when specific genes are transcribed is not fully understood, but it is clear that hormones, growth factors, cytokines, as well as other cell-signaling molecules stimulate the activity of nuclear proteins, which alter the activity of RNA synthetic complexes.

Proteins

Structure

Proteins are polymers of amino acids held together by peptide bonds (Fig. 1.11). Proteins have a much greater potential for diversity than the nucleic acids DNA and RNA because they are polymers of over 20 building blocks rather than four. The amino acid sequence of a protein is called its primary structure, while interactions between regions of this primary structure, such as helix and beta sheet formation, are referred to as secondary structures. Examples of these conformations are given in Figs. 1.12 and 1.13. In both these cases hydrogen bonds play a major role in stabilizing the structures, although they form the bonds in different ways. The hydrogen bonds in helices are between elements of adjacent residues, while the beta sheets interact more with distant amino acids. The result is different shapes with different functions. The forces responsible are those ionic and hydrophobic interactions of the amino acid side chains. Interactions between secondary structures produce tertiary structures, such as major regions of folding. When proteins interact with one another, the resulting quaternary structure often gains a biologic function such as the tetrameric hemoglobin molecule. Other factors that influence protein structure and function are posttranslational modifications such as glycosylation, lipidation, phosphorylation, activation by bond breaking by specific biosynthetic proteases, and association with prosthetic groups such as heme.

The sequence of a growing polypeptide chain can also direct its fate within the cell to some degree by containing signal sequences. These are specific amino acid sequences that recognize and bind to cytoplasmic proteins that shuttle the protein to specific areas within the cell, such as the nucleus, mitochondria, and other organelles like the Golgi apparatus for posttranslational modifications, or even out of the cell as a secretory molecule.

Protein Synthesis

A key feature of the translation process is the nature of the triplet code. Namely, each amino acid to be inserted into the growing peptide backbone is encoded by a very specific three-nucleotide sequence, the triplet code. For ex-

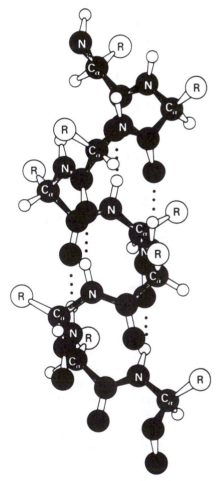

FIGURE 1.12. The protein α helix. The axis of the polypeptide is stabilized by the accumulation of hydrogen bonds between adjacent amino acids. (From Stryer L. *Biochemistry*, 3rd ed. New York: Freeman Press, 1988:22–28.)

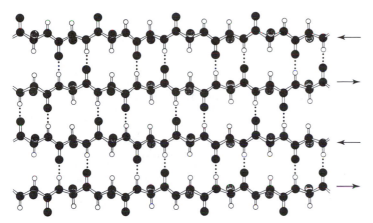

FIGURE 1.13. The beta pleated sheet structure found in some proteins is stabilized by hydrogen bonds, but, unlike the α helix, the residues interacting are not adjacent to one another, but are from distant domains of the protein. (From Stryer L. *Biochemistry*, 3rd ed. New York: Freeman Press, 1988:22–28.)

ample, the triplet GAG encodes for the amino acid glutamic acid. Each time a GAG appears in the mRNA, a glutamic acid and no other amino acid will be inserted into the protein. Each amino acid, however, has more than one triplet; some have as many as five or six. Glutamic acid, for example, has another valid triplet code. Both of the glutamic acid triplets begin with GA; therefore, only the third base varies between them. This is true of nearly all of the other amino acid codes as well, namely only one of the bases varies among the specific codes. The triplet code, therefore, is redundant but it is still very specific. This redundancy in the code is the reason why it is not possible to use the amino acid sequence of a protein to accurately predict the DNA exon sequences of its gene. To know with certainty a gene's sequence, it must be cloned.

A schematic outlining the process of protein synthesis is given in Fig. 1.14. This cytoplasmic process takes place in the endoplasmic reticulum, an organelle that sequesters the necessary cellular constituents such as the transfer RNA to shuttle the appropriate amino acid to the peptidyl-trans-ferase that forms the peptide bond and numerous other nucleic acid and polypeptide factors that are needed for the formation of the initiation complex depicted in an abbreviated way in Fig. 1.14. Amino acids are joined in order in a continuous string until the end of the mRNA is reached. The released peptide is then available for traffick-ing to other parts of the cell for modification or further biosynthetic steps.

The Control of Biologic Processes

The regulation of cell function must be considered to be the sum total of the activity of numerous stimulatory and inhibitory pathways. Most, as depicted in Fig. 1.15, arise from the high-affinity binding of hormones, growth factors, cytokines, and other factors with specific molecules in the cell membrane or nucleus. These molecules, called recep-tors, are the leading edge of intracellular cascades that lead to a biologic response such as inducing the transcription

of a gene. The activity of the new gene product can, in turn, alter the function of a cell. The induced biologic responses are dose dependent for both the receptor and the factor to which it binds. In addition, the biologic effects are quite cell specific; for example, only cells expressing the adrenocorticotropic hormone receptor will respond to the hormone. These cascades can involve enzymes, and there-

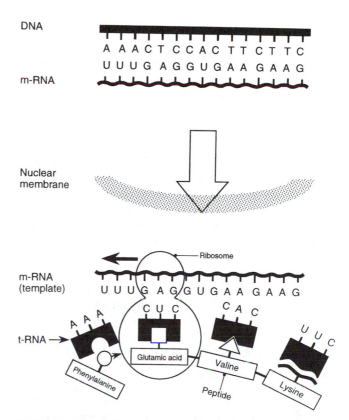

FIGURE 1.14. mRNA binds to a series of proteins and nucleic acids, the ribosomes, which bring together the necessary protein biosynthetic machinery in the cell. Transfer RNAs shuttle their specific amino acid to the site of peptide bond formation in the growing polypeptide chain. (From Mueller RF and Young ID, eds. *Emery's elements of medical genetics,* 3rd ed. Churchill Living-stone, 1998:18.)

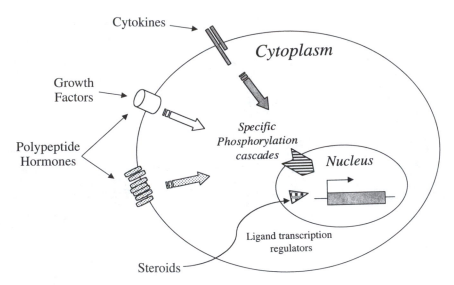

FIGURE 1.15. A schematic drawing of the types of signal transduction pathways that can function with a cell. Extracellular factors interact with specific receptors, each shaded in a different way. The specific phosphorylation pathways each stimulate a different set of substrates, and result often in the regulation of gene transcription or even cell division or cell death. Although only one *arrow* is shown flowing to the nucleus, each pathway alters its own set of genes. Steroids present a slightly different mechanism of altering gene transcription activity. Their receptors are actually transcription regulators themselves and receptor-steroid complexes go directly to the nucleus without intervening messenger molecules.

fore they can be catalytic, producing thousands of additional messengers in the cascade and thus producing exponential effects. Conversely, they can be simply the interaction of a few molecules, such as the steroid hormones binding their nuclear receptors, called ligand transcription regulators, to alter the transcription of their target genes. This process, by whatever mechanism it is accomplished, is referred to as signal transduction. These activities must be balanced, however, by counteracting processes, to avoid loss of control and the deleterious side effects resulting (see below). For example, when kinases begin a cascade, it is usually phosphatases that stop them; if gene transcription is a result, then usually another transcription regulator will interact with the transcription complexes to inhibit them; for every push there is a pull and vice versa. As discussed below for the congenital adrenal hyperplasia and retinoblastoma genes, loss of balance can have disastrous results. The uncoupling of the stimulatory and inhibitory signal transduction pathways can occur by a number of different mechanisms. Two of the most common are the deletion or loss of function of a critical molecule such as a receptor and mutations causing constitutively active molecules. The unregulated kinase activity of oncogenes associated with human malignancies is a fair example of the latter case.

PRIMER ON MOLECULAR TECHNIQUES

Purification of DNA

To conduct genetic analyses of human disease it is necessary to purify, to an appropriate degree of purity, sufficient amounts of DNA or RNA. This requires the investigator to harvest enough tissue or blood cells to have sufficient starting material. Furthermore, steps must be taken to ensure the purity of the samples and the maintenance of the quality of the material. DNA contamination of RNA

preparations, for example, is unacceptable if one is studying gene expression. DNA, given its length and high viscosity, is prone to damage by shearing forces that lead to fragmented specimens during centrifugation. RNA, on the other hand, is highly susceptible to hydrolytic cleavage of phosphoester bonds, thus producing mRNA of artificially lower molecular weight. These are particularly worrisome problems for the researcher because they can produce artifacts that confound the interpretation of results.

A brief look at the scientific literature including the documentation provided in commercially available kits reveals numerous different protocols for the purification of DNA. None is ideal but all strive to accomplish the same goal, namely, pure, intact (or as large as possible) double-stranded DNA free of adhering proteins or RNA. Common features of the methods include using freezing and pulverizing tissues or hypotonic solutions containing ionic detergents to break open the cells and their nuclei to liberate the DNA. Digestion of DNA with proteinase K to remove histones and other nucleic acid–binding proteins is followed by extraction of residual proteins with organic solvents and then precipitation of the DNA with alcohols for further analysis. Critical issues here are the speed of inactivating the degrading enzymes, which can be accomplished by rapid freezing in liquid nitrogen or mixing of lysates with denaturing buffers, and the control of fragmenting the DNA by shearing forces due to centrifugation.

The yields of DNA expected for these methods are on the order of 2 mg of DNA of at least 100 kilobase (kb) per gram of tissue, or 1 billion cells. This is an amount sufficient for most molecular analyses and cloning methods.

Purification of RNA

Depending on its ultimate use, purification protocols for RNA vary from extracting total RNA or limiting the isolation to mRNA from the cytoplasm. As with DNA collections, extreme care must be taken to prevent the degradation of the RNA by the virtually ever-present RNase enzymes or by simple hydrolysis of phosphoester bonds due to water in the buffers at modest temperatures. A very useful addition to any buffer used in RNA handling is diethylpyrocarbonate (DEPC). This compound is a potent inhibitor of RNases and it irreversibly blocks RNases that are on glassware and other surfaces due to contamination by laboratory personnel handling them without gloves. Once solutions are prepared, the DEPC must be inactivated by heating, usually by autoclaving, to prevent it from interacting with the nucleotide polymerases needed to replicate or transcribe the DNA and/or RNA templates. The lysis buffers used in the protocols denature cellular RNAses contained in the cells. Cells can be extracted with detergents and the extracts centrifuged to spin out nuclei, and, therefore, much of the DNA that might contaminate a sample. Tissue, on the other hand, can be homogenized with chaotropic salts such as guanidinium thiocyanate and the RNA precipitated from solution with organic buffers. Either way, one expects 30 to 100 μg of RNA per the equivalent of 10 million cells.

Reverse Transcriptase–Polymerase Chain Reaction

One of the most important technical advances in recent history is the RT-PCR method to create billions of copies of transcript-specific complementary DNA (cDNA) for cloning, sequencing, or any of a wide variety of other experimental end points. By copying the extremely small numbers of mRNA molecules into cDNA using enzymes that make DNA from RNA, it is possible to monitor transcription of specific genes, particularly when no other method exists to do so. It is an extremely sensitive method, able theoretically to detect a single copy of mRNA in a cell. The method begins with the RT step by using a microbial enzyme, a reverse transcriptase, of which there are many commercially available, to copy RNA to DNA. This requires a clean RNA template (see above); a mixture of deoxyribonucleotides; random primers, that is, nearly every combination and permutation of nucleic acid sequences possible within a six-membered oligonucleotide; slightly elevated temperature; and time, about 45 minutes. The resulting product is cDNA, which is complementary to the original RNA sample, but the reverse of transcription, hence the name. This material will not contain introns since we avoid nuclear products during the purification protocol; therefore, isolating a "gene" this way does not provide insight into the genomic sequences. Once sufficient cDNA has been made, PCR can begin. Figure 1.16 outlines the PCR portion of the method as it is usually conducted. The DNA has a tendency to form a duplex that must be denatured, a process called melting, by heating to high temperatures near to boiling. Next, the temperature is lowered and the single-

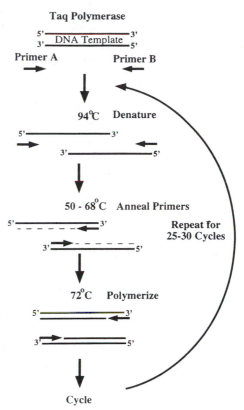

FIGURE 1.16. An outline of the polymerase chain reaction (PCR) technique as it is often performed. In this example, the DNA is made using Taq polymerase, and each cycle consists of melting double-stranded DNA at 94°C, annealing the primers to DNA at 50° to 68°C and polymerization reactions at 72°C. It is customary to have each incubation step be 1 minute long, the entire cycle repeated 25 to 30 times. (From Jameson LJ, ed. *Principles of molecular medicine.* Totowa, New Jersey: Humana Press, 1998: 15, with permission.)

stranded DNA complexes with primers, though now they are specific for a particular gene product. The primers are designed to copy both strands of the duplex; these are called forward, for the sense strand, for example, and backward for the antisense strand. Furthermore, the two primers will span a region of the DNA so that their products will overlap and form duplexes at low temperatures but usually not span the entire transcript from its 5′ to 3′ end. A heat-stable DNA-dependent DNA polymerase is then able to replicate the cDNA beginning with the primer. This process can be repeated over two dozen times to accumulate sufficient DNA for further use. This cycling approach is required to make enough cDNA. The cDNA products can be separated from the other components of the mixtures by agarose gel electrophoresis at neutral pH and visualized by light-sensitive DNA intercalating dyes such as ethidium bromide.

There is another method to examine cell extracts for gene transcripts in which the entire mRNA, rather than a portion of it is detected. These assays, called Northern analyses, begin with the purification of total cell RNA, in the case of abundant messages, or polyA, containing mRNA for rare messages. The RNAs are then separated by size by gel electrophoresis and then blotted onto a specialized oligonucleotide binding filter. Radiolabeled oligonucleotide probes specific for the mRNA of interest are incubated with the filter and then the filter is exposed to x-ray film. If the gene was transcribed, the probe will bind to it by base complementarity and the complex will be radiolabeled and therefore detected by autoradiography. Northern data complements the PCR approach because it can document the length of the message, confirming proper processing. In addition, deletion or truncation mutants are more easily identified by Northern analyses than by PCR.

cDNA Cloning

Cloning is the process of isolating a species of DNA and copying it in sufficient quantity for further study. It is simply not possible to isolate enough highly purified DNA from cells of tissue to be of much use in the laboratory; cloning is almost always a necessary step. The DNA can be a gene or any reasonably sized portion of the genome of interest to the investigator. Often cDNAs prepared by reverse transcriptase are cloned to study the proteins expressed in a particular tissue. This, by definition, keeps the size of the clone fairly small. If the goal is to clone a sequence of genomic DNA, the DNA is fragmented into manageable pieces, using combinations of restriction endonuclease enzymes. Cloning begins by inserting the DNA into a vector that can be put into bacterial cells where it and the DNA to be cloned are copied (Fig. 1.17). A vector can be a piece

of circular DNA such as a plasmid. These structures control their own replication within a cell and they are completely distinct from the bacterial host genome. Since this process is not 100% efficient, it is necessary to be able to distinguish between the bacteria that contain the vector and those that do not. The investigator needs what is called a selectable marker. This is accomplished by taking advantage of a special property of the vector, for example, conferring antibiotic resistance to the host bacterium. Successful uptake of the vector makes the bacterium, usually *Escherichia coli*, resistant to antibiotic treatment, while bacterium that did not take up the vector will die. When plated on agar dishes, surviving cells grow to visible colonies each the product of a single clone since only one plasmid is taken up by each bacterium. This combination of cloned DNA sequences is called a library. At this point it is necessary to screen the library for the clones that contain the sequence of interest. This is done by creating a replica of the agar dish by placing a nitrocellulose filter briefly on the plate to allow a sample of each clone to adhere to the filter. After incubating the filter with radioactive oligonucleotide probes specific to the sequence of interest, the clones that bind the probes can be detected by radiography. Positive clones are then harvested from the plate for further processing.

Plasmids are useful for segments of DNA up to about 10 kb but larger DNA species, on the order of 12 to 25 kb, are better cloned using a bacteriophage. A phage is a virus that infects the bacteria, and after a period of replication will lyse the host cell and spread to other bacteria. If the λ phage is spread onto a plate of bacteria, the lysis produces clear holes, called plaques on agar dishes. Even larger fragments of DNA approaching 200 kb can be cloned, but in these cases one needs to insert the DNA into bacterial artificial chromosomes (BACs) or, as was done for the human genome project, to clone 1,500- to 2,000-bp fragments in yeast using the yeast artificial chromosomes (YACs).

DNA Sequencing

There are a number of techniques available to sequence DNA, but the two most common approaches will be discussed briefly here. The first is the dideoxy-sequencing method in which DNA is copied in four separate reactions using DNA-dependent DNA polymerase. Each reaction contains the DNA template, an appropriate primer, a radiolabeled nucleotide building block for DNA such as ATP, and a mixture of the nonlabeled DNA deoxy (d) precursors dATP, dGTP, dCTP, dTTP. To complete the four reaction mixtures one of the dideoxynucleotides (dd)—ddATP, ddGTP, ddCTP, or ddTTP—is added so that the dideoxynucleotides are less than 1% of the total nucleotide composition. These precursors have no 3' hydroxyl group, and therefore they cannot make phosphoester bonds. Since the dideoxynucleotides block chain elongation, the synthesis reaction will continue until the dideoxynucleotide is

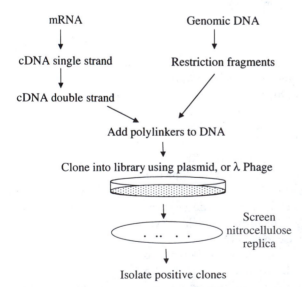

FIGURE 1.17. DNA cloning can be accomplished in a variety of ways. Two common strategies are outlined here. Fragments of genomic DNA or cDNA generated from mRNA are coupled to polylinkers so they may be inserted into a suitable cloning vector (a plasmid or λ phage). Clones containing transcripts of the DNA of interest are detected by hybridization with specific radiolabeled probes.

reached, stopping synthesis. The last base in the chain, therefore, will depend on the dideoxynucleotide in the reaction mixture, namely, it will be an A, G, C, or T. The products of each reaction are separated by size using polyacrylamide gel electrophoresis and visualized by radiography. Figure 1.18 is a schematic representation of this process showing how one manually reads a sequencing gel. The second method uses fluorescent precursors, gel electrophoresis, laser activated detection of DNA fragments, and automated computer analyses to complete the process.

DNA Microchip Array Technology

The impact of gene cloning and DNA-sequencing techniques on modern science is difficult to overstate. It is not unfair to say that nature can now be examined molecule by molecule. In the 25 years since the discovery of reverse transcriptase by David Baltimore and colleagues, an event that heralded the beginning of modern molecular biologic research, the study of complex biologic process has been able to focus on individual molecules at physiologically relevant concentrations. We have learned about the structure of normal and mutated mammalian genes, how they are transcribed and translated, how to mutate genes in the laboratory, and even how to make new organisms as tools to test biologic models. More recently, studies have begun to focus on the complex interactions of hundreds of membrane-bound, cytoplasmic, and nuclear factors that are responsible for cell replication, specialized function, and the programmed death of a cell. The majority of this work, however, was being accomplished by examining only a few genes at a time. It was just not practical for the average

laboratory to do otherwise with existing technology. That approach all changed recently with the advent of DNA microchip technology, however. This method combines the synthesis of specific oligonucleotide sequences on a microscale, laser-activated detection systems, and computer-assisted analysis of complex arrays organized on what resembles a computer chip. Each specific oligomer occupies a specific site in the array. This new device is used to screen biologic samples for hundreds to thousands of transcripts concurrently. These systems are tailor made for arrays of genes that are relevant to the test samples under study, all known growth factor signal transduction pathway genes, for example. The nucleic acid to be analyzed is isolated from tissues or cells amplified by reverse transcriptase, for example, and labeled with a fluorescent tag. The sample is incubated with the microarray to allow hybridization of transcripts to the DNA probes on the array, after which the array is scanned to detect the light-sensitive complexes. Since the position of each gene probe on the array is known, the identity of test transcripts producing positive signals is known. The beauty of this approach is the ability to examine essentially all of the relevant genes in a particular experiment, and rapidly, with great precision and complexity. What is limiting in this technology is the knowledge of sequences of the genes that are not yet cloned. The completion of the human genome project should solve that problem.

Examples of Molecular Pathophysiology

The three examples discussed below illustrate how the application of molecular pathophysiology to the definition, diagnosis, and treatment of disease can affect the practice of medicine by today's clinicians. Each of the cases involves cloning a disease-causing gene that, when fully characterized, turned out to be a mutant of a normally expressed gene. Furthermore, two of the examples, cytochrome P-450 21-hydroxylase (CYP21) and the cystic fibrosis transmembrane conductance regulator (CFTR) deficiencies, define monogenic diseases, which, paradoxically, present with a broad spectrum of phenotypes. The third, the retinoblastoma gene (Rb), although not sufficient, is required for the development of the cancer for which it is named. In each case the mutations cause a range of reduced activities from those barely different from normal to complete losses. Of course, disease phenotypes can arise also from gain of function mutations in genes, thereby producing more than the usual activity. As it happens, the examples cited here are loss of function types. The mutations range from the very subtle, such as single amino acid substitutions, to deletion of the entire protein. The magnitude of the mutation doesn't necessarily correlate with the severity of the phenotype, however. A substitution or deletion of a single amino acid can completely abolish activity, whereas deletions of entire exons can produce only modest changes in function. What matters is where within the protein do changes occur.

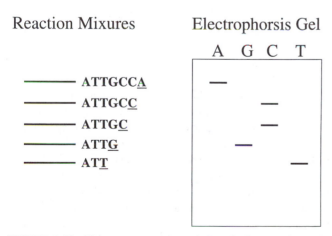

FIGURE 1.18. Dideoxy-sequencing of DNA is shown schematically. The polymerase products generated in the presence of dideoxynucleotides (*left*) and the resulting gel electrophoresis patterns (*right*) are shown. By reading the bases from bottom to top the sequence is determined.

Whether mutations occur in the domains of the protein critical to function is of prime importance. The resulting alteration in the activity of the protein is what counts in understanding the resulting phenotype. The concept that the more severe the loss of function the worse the phenotype is a logical assumption. Of course, there are always exceptions to this rule. For example, the most severe phenotypes in cystic fibrosis are expressed when the CFTR activity falls to only 10% of normal. In general though, the greater the loss (gain) of function the more severe the outcome.

Congenital Adrenal Hyperplasia (CAH)

When cytochrome P-450 21-hydroxylase, encoded for by the gene *CYP21,* is defective, congenital adrenal hyperplasia results. Affected individuals cannot make sufficient cortisol from the adrenal cortex; thus, adrenocorticotropic hormone (ACTH) secretion is stimulated, causing adrenal hyperplasia. Depending on the degree of loss of enzymatic activity, symptoms can be mild to severe. For example, in some cases steroid precursors of cortisol build up to high concentrations and are shuttled to other enzymes within the cortex and are converted to androgens. While not apparent in newborn boys, female embryos can be virilized at birth, often severely enough to require corrective surgery. In cases with a complete block in the 21-hydroxylase, aldosterone levels are reduced enough that patients cannot adequately control sodium reabsorption by the kidney, and therefore develop life-threatening salt wasting. Nearly two dozen different mutations have been identified and, within certain broad limits, many can be correlated with the severity of the phenotype including virilization, salt wasting, or even late-onset variants of CAH.

The 21-hydroxylase gene, *CYP21,* located on chromosome 6, actually exists as two isoforms, one of which if translated would produce a truncated, nonfunctional protein and is, therefore, a pseudogene, *CYP21P.* This gene contributes nearly all of the mutations to the functional allele leading to CAH. Misalignments during meiosis and segments of the pseudogene transferred to *CYP21* by gene conversion account for many of the important mutants isolated for this gene. Clinicians are now able to exploit this information for the benefit of their patients, particularly in prenatal diagnosis in pregnancies where CAH is suspected due to family history. DNA can be harvested from fetal cells by amniocentesis or chorionic villus sampling and tested by Southern analysis or by PCR using specific primer sets designed to identify relevant mutations. If mutations are detected, prenatal glucocorticoid treatment can be instituted to reduce ACTH secretion and, therefore, the overproduction of adrenal androgens minimizing the virilization of developing females. In this case the *CYP21* gene cloning can identify mutations that explain much of the phenotype of the patients as well as provide a molecular tool for early diagnosis and treatment.

Cystic Fibrosis

Cystic fibrosis is another monogenic disease for which cloning the gene responsible has provided much insight into the pathophysiology of the disease and an opportunity for early diagnosis, if not, as yet, a lifesaving therapy. In fact, it is possible to detect the defective gene in preimplantation embryos, thus presenting the option of terminating the gestation.

The gene responsible for cystic fibrosis, a 12-time membrane-spanning chloride channel protein called the cystic fibrosis transmembrane conductance regulator (CFTR), was cloned from affected individuals, hence its name. Cystic fibrosis is fairly common among whites (1 in 2,500 live births) and it is in fact the most common hereditary disease involving a single gene. Although hundreds of mutations have been described in the 27-exon gene, one accounts for over 70% of the cases identified. This mutation, a 3–base pair deletion eliminating a phenylalanine at position 508 in the translated protein, is called ΔF508, for change (loss) of phenylalanine (F, at position 508). The loss of one amino acid out of 1,480 total residues in CFTR can induce a change in ion transport function sufficiently to kill a patient. This finding is similar to the case of sickle cell anemia in which a single amino acid change, in this case a substitution of a valine for a glutamic acid, is sufficient to cause a life-threatening disease. The latter case was identified by classic biochemical means, not cloning. That is, enough of the affected hemoglobin beta globin chain had to be purified to homogeneity to create tryptic digests and complete peptide bond hydrolysis so individual residues could be examined. Two-dimensional amino acid chromatograms for comparison with normal beta globin chains similarly treated revealed that valine was substituted for glutamic acid. This approach, taken by Vernon Ingram and colleagues in the 1950s for hemoglobin S using a relatively abundant protein, is simply not possible with such a rare membrane-spanning protein like the CFTR. Without cloning, it would not be possible to know what is known about the CFTR.

Perhaps the most interesting finding about the most common CFTR mutant, ΔF508, is the wide variety of phenotypes encountered in patients. Cystic fibrosis presents a mixture of symptoms ranging from relatively mild conditions of excessive salt loss in sweat to the more severe pancreatic insufficiency contributing to impaired nutrition to life-threatening, recurring pulmonary infections. Any of these conditions can exist in isolation or in combination. ΔF508 is found in all of them; thus, a single mutation can produce symptoms in one patient that are entirely different from those in another patient with exactly the same mutation. If, as was discussed for *CYP21* above, the conductance activity of CFTR is measured in these patients, a clearer picture emerges. Namely, a normal phenotype is maintained with anything over 10% of maximal activity. The lower the activity becomes, the worse the symptoms. While adequate hydration and pancreatic enzyme therapy ameliorates the salt wasting and nutritional difficulties, treatments are less successful for the pulmonary infections. Lately, however, a gene therapy approach has begun that strives to deliver cDNA for the wild-type CFTR to bronchial airway epithelial cells of patients with pulmonary difficulties. Adenovirus vectors and liposomes are currently being used to transfer CFTR gene in small feasibility trials in humans.

Retinoblastoma Gene

Finally, recent studies on a relatively common childhood cancer, retinoblastoma, has revolutionized the field of cancer molecular pathophysiology. The discovery of the retinoblastoma gene (Rb) as a tumor suppressor, and not an oncogene in its native form, added a new dimension to the study of the ontogeny, treatment, and genetics of cancer. Rather than cancer resulting from an unregulated and overexpressed growth-stimulating factor pushing cells to grow uncontrollably, cancers can arise from the loss of growth inhibitors, or suppressors, the naturally occurring molecules whose normal function is to keep cells from dividing until it is appropriate to do so. Cancer biologists maintained that malignancies arise when a number of genetic changes converge on a cell to permit increased division, the production of factors that allow the cells to migrate and invade other tissues, to recruit a blood supply and to escape from apoptosis. It was generally assumed that oncogenes were, in large part, responsible for these events. Therefore, hyperstimulation of cells by growth factors was a necessary feature of the onset of cancer. The discovery of a cell cycle suppressor, Rb, changed all that. The concept that cells will divide unless Rb or other inhibitors tell them not to, for example, means that a new mechanism of carcinogenesis must be considered. Namely, the loss of the suppressor activity may have the same effect of hyperstimulation by trophic factors—carcinogenesis. Obviously, this is a gross oversimplification of very complex mechanisms, but the point to be made here is that molecular biologic research approaches to the study of cancer biology made this discovery possible. Although genetic testing will help identify people at risk for the Rb-associated malignancies, the development of new highly specific therapies targeting the restoration of Rb function and the control of events downstream of Rb will be the ultimate result of this discovery.

SUMMARY AND FUTURE DIRECTIONS

As stated at the beginning of this chapter, little progress in our understanding of any disease process can be made without understanding how things work in the absence of disease. This will always be a cornerstone of biomedical research. Never before in our history have so many scientists attacked these questions. Never before have so many incredibly powerful new technologies for *in vivo, in vitro,* and *ex vivo* experimentation been available. The questions remain the same but the method of scientific inquiry is changing dramatically. The result is an explosion of new information that, at one and the same time, provides answers for many important questions, and rather than simplifying concepts, these answers actually identify previously unsuspected layers of complexity that must now be explained. Fortunately, the same tools employed to create the new complexity will provide the solutions. Adding to the equation is the pending release of the results of the human genome cloning project. Disease-related genes will be decidedly easier to find, and their role in the disease process will be validated in animal studies using transgenic, knockout and knock-in mice to test the activity of wild-type and mutant genes whether naturally occurring or designed by investigators. The pace of discovery will also quicken dramatically. For example, cloning, transfection, and translation strategies for the study of protein structure and function will replace conventional, often laborious, and time-consuming biochemical purification protocols. Rational drug design, making new reagents that are tailored to be target specific, nontoxic, and easily delivered to counteract the effects of mutant or deleted genes will become more and more prevalent.

Gene therapy approaches to replace or repair aberrant genes, whether it occurs before fertilization, *in utero,* or in individuals manifesting problems after birth, are becoming more and more feasible. It is useful to think of this issue as a problem of delivery, namely, how does one replace a defective gene with a functional one and restore health to the individual? A direct approach is to transfect fully differentiated cells with vectors containing a normal gene, as described above for cystic fibrosis. This could produce a very local result, for example only in the lung or perhaps only transiently, but it could benefit the patient. More permanent benefits may come from more innovative approaches such as repairing the defect at the genomic level, thus affecting all cells, or even by creating new organs to replace diseased ones, a variant of the transplant approach.

The most common way to alter genomic sequences such as adding functional genes is by gene targeting of embryonic stem (ES) cells, as is done to produce transgenic mice. ES cells are the progenitors to all others and are thus totipotent. It is also possible with this approach to delete sequences from the genome, the so-called knockout animals. Transgenic and knockout mice are tremendously useful research tools to study gene function, but ES cell manipulations in other mammals including the human do not seem to work. Investigators have turned their interest to other cells, more differentiated than ES cells, called pluripotent cells (PCs). PCs are much more abundant than ES cells, and they are still capable of producing most, but not all, tissues. Three recent cloning experiments present several other possible solutions to this problem, including using a variant of somatic cell nuclear transfer (SCNT) to produce these cells (Kind et al.) and the collection of PCs from primordial gonadal tissue (Shamblott et al.) or inner cell mass cells from developing embryos (Thomson et al.).

Somatic cell nuclear transfer is the method employed to produce Dolly, the cloned sheep. The "cloned" animal was generated by isolating an egg, removing its nucleus, and placing the enucleated structure adjacent to a somatic cell so that the cells fuse. The new structure was able to develop a complete individual with the genetic composition of the somatic cell. The newest breakthrough with this method is the ability to alter a gene in the somatic cell nucleus before the SCNT is performed. Thus, gene targeting doesn't require ES cells as previously thought, and the realistic possibility of repairing the genome now exists. This advance greatly improves the chances of producing useful gene therapies in the future. Specific genes can now be inserted into mammalian genomes of embryos other than mice, and the efficacy of the process can be tested.

Pluripotent stem cells can also be harvested from two human sources that are becoming increasingly available to investigators, namely fetal tissues. Human embryos prepared by *in vitro* fertilization techniques are sometimes, for valid medical reasons and with the appropriate approvals, not implanted into the uterus. Pluripotent cells can be harvested from the inner cell mass of blastocyst stage of these nonimplanted embryos. The other source is from later-stage embryos made available through termination of pregnancies. Here the primordial gonad is the source of cells that still retain a pluripotent capacity. Although these cells are not the result of any genetic manipulation, they may, depending on how much can be learned about factors that control specific tissue organogensis, be directed to differentiate in an organ-specific manner. Thus, new sources of tissues for transplantation could be realized in the form of minitransplants of cells that continue organogenesis *in vivo*. Rather than focusing the treatment upon a single gene, replacing the affected organ may be a viable option. An added bonus could result if the patient were able to provide the somatic cell for the SCNT and thereby produce syngeneic pluripotent cells to eliminate the possibility of graft rejection.

Ultimately, individual patient-specific treatment strategies are envisioned where, rather than using a treatment based on phenotypic diagnoses, treatment will be tailored to best counteract the array of defective genes unique to the individual.

10 KEY POINTS

1. The central dogma of biology provides the rationale for the molecular biologic approach to the study of disease. The fact that one can use mRNA as a template to synthesize cDNA and deduce both the amino acid sequence of a protein and the nucleic acid of its gene (minus the introns) has changed the way research is conducted.

2. The differences in stability of RNA and DNA greatly influence, and sometimes limit, the design of experiments. Care must be taken to protect RNA from degradation prior to converting it to cDNA for cloning and other purposes. Failure to do so often creates artifacts that if not recognized lead to erroneous results.

3. The biochemical processes leading to cell division or cell death are highly conserved in nature. Hence, the study of cell cycle proteins in single cell organisms can provide valuable insights into the process in humans.

4. Virtually all biologic processes are subject to control by a specific feedback mechanism. Stimulatory signal transduction pathways are normally counterbalanced by inhibitory ones. Loss of this balance almost always has deleterious effects.

5. Cloning genes and gene fragments have become almost routine laboratory activities. It is not sufficient to identify the clone; rather, proof of the function must be established in a living biologic system.

6. It is particularly interesting that the genotype of monogenic diseases such as cystic fibrosis and congenital adrenal hyperplasia does not predict, except in the broadest of terms, with the resulting phenotype. For example, the same gene mutation may lead to mild symptoms in some patients and fatal outcomes in others. Clearly, the nature of the gene mutation is only part of the molecular definition of diseases.

7. The discovery of tumor suppressor genes led investigators to reconsider the idea that cells will divide unless they are inhibited from doing so. This fact revealed another possible mechanism of oncogenesis, that is, the loss of cell cycle arrest.

8. The invention of DNA chip technology holds great promise for the future study of biologic processes at the level of gene transcription. The ability to examine hundreds to thousands of genes simultaneously will dramatically accelerate the pace of discovery.

9. Gene defects associated with disease consist of either loss- or gain-of-function mutations. Analysis of the differences between the normal and abnormal gene products can lead to the rational design of new treatment strategies.

10. The success of somatic cell nuclear transfer (SCNT) opens the possibility of producing pluripotent cells to use for gene therapy and even the production of new organs to replace diseased ones. Implied in this methodologic breakthrough is the ability of cloning humans. Many in society today view this as a "when," not "if" issue. The ethical and moral implications of this possibility, however farfetched it may seem today, are staggering. This topic and the related issues of organogenesis warrant continued vigorous and open discussion across all levels of society around the world.

GLOSSARY

bacteriophage: (also abbreviated phage, e.g., λ phage) a virus that infects bacteria.

cDNA: DNA complementary to mRNA, the product of reverse transcriptase.

chromatin: protein-DNA complexes that make up chromosomes.

cytokines: any of the more than 100 proteins found in the blood. They are produced primarily by white blood cells, and they regulate various facets of cell growth and differentiation.

dephosphorylation: removal of phosphate esters by enzymatic or chemical means.

exons: portions of the coding region of a gene that are retained in processed mRNA after introns are removed.

introns: portions of the noncoding sequences of genes that exist between the exons.

kinase: an enzyme that catalyzes the transfer of phosphate from adenosine triphosphate (ATP) to an acceptor molecule including serine, threonine, and tyrosine residues of proteins.

knockout: the deletion of a gene from the genome by molecular biologic techniques.

ligand: a small organic molecule that can bind another molecule.

mRNA: messenger RNA, the species of RNA transcribed from DNA, carries the code for the amino acid sequence in protein from the gene to the cytoplasm.

nucleoside: a glycoside composed of a pentose sugar and a purine or pyrimidine base.

nucleotide: a phosphate ester of a nucleoside.

oncogene: a gene in a virus that can cause a cell to become malignant.

phosphatase: any enzyme that catalyzes the hydrolysis of phosphate esters.

phosphorylation: the process of combining phosphorus with an organic compound.

plasmid: a circular, double-stranded extrachromosomal genetic material into which DNA sequences may be inserted for infection of bacterial cells.

pluripotent cells: cells that are capable of giving rise to most tissues in an organism.

purine: an organic nitrogenous base consisting of two heterocyclic rings found in nucleic aids (e.g., adenine, guanine).

pyrimidine: an organic nitrogenous base consisting of one heterocyclic ring found in nucleic acids (e.g., cytosine, thymine, uracil).

receptor: a component of a cell that combines with another molecule to alter the function of a cell.

replication: the duplication process of genetic material.

reverse transcriptase: an enzyme that makes a copy of DNA from an mRNA template.

RNA polymerase: an enzyme that makes an RNA copy of an oligonucleotide template.

RT-PCR: reverse transcriptase–polymerase chain reaction.

somatic cell: any cell other than an egg or sperm.

stem cells: cells that can give rise to specialized cells.

totipotent cells: cells that are capable of developing into all tissues, including a complete organism.

transcription: the synthesis of mRNA from a genomic DNA template.

transgenic mice: a mouse to which the genetic material from another animal has been added.

translation: the synthesis of proteins from an mRNA template.

tumor suppressor: a gene product that counteracs the action of an oncogene, or one that block cell division.

SUGGESTED READINGS

Alberts B, Bray D, Lewis J, et al., eds. *Molecular biology of the cell.* New York: Garland, 1994.

Berne RM and Levy, MN, eds. *Physiology.* St. Louis: Mosby, 1998.

Cox TM, Sinclair J, eds. *Molecular biology in medicine.* Oxford, England; Malden, MA: Blackwell Science, 1997.

Harbour JW, Dean DC. Rb function in cell-cycle regulation and apoptosis. *Nat Cell Biol* 2000;2:E65–67.

Jameson LJ, ed. *Principles of molecular medicine.* Totowa, NJ: Humana Press, 1998:3–112.

McCreath KJ, Howcroft J, Campbell KH, et al. Production of gene-targeted sheep by nuclear transfer from cultured somatic cells. *Nature* 2000;405:1066–1069.

McDonald ER 3rd, El-Deiry WS. Cell cycle control as a basis for cancer drug development [review]. *Int J Oncol* 2000;16:871–886.

Shamblott MJ, Axelman J, Wang S, et al. Derivation of pluripotent stem cells from cultured human primordial germ cells. *Proc Natl Acad Sci USA* 1999;96:1162.

Thomson JA, Itskovitz-Eldor J, Shapiro SS, et al. Embryonic stem cell lines derived from human blastocysts. *Science* 1998;282:1827.

Zubay G, ed. *Biochemistry,* 4th ed. Dubuque, IA: Wm. C. Brown, 1998.

REPRODUCTIVE GENETICS

LAWRENCE C. LAYMAN

INHERITANCE PATTERNS OF HUMAN GENETIC DISEASE

Pedigrees in Clinical Medicine

For clinicians in any field of medicine, the taking of a good family history is of paramount importance (1). A family history of medical problems such as diabetes, hypertension, heart disease, stroke, and cancer should be obtained. For patients of reproductive age who might become pregnant, the clinician should ascertain a history of birth defects, mental retardation, Down syndrome, neural tube defects, and muscular dystrophy. In addition, more specific questions pertain to certain ethnic groups: cystic fibrosis in Caucasians, sickle cell anemia in persons of African descent, Tay-Sachs disease in Ashkenazi Jews and French Canadians, neural tube defects in individuals of English or Irish descent, and thalassemias in many different ethnic groups including those with Mediterranean or African descent. If a pedigree is not performed, important relevant family history may be missed (1).

The basic components needed to construct a pedigree are shown in Fig. 2.1. The proband, who is the person presenting to medical attention (affected or unaffected), is indicated with an arrow. If the proband is affected with the disease, he/she is the index case. First-degree relatives, such as parents, siblings, or offspring, share 50% of the proband's genes. Second-degree relatives, who share 25% of the genes, include the grandparents, aunts and uncles, nieces and nephews, and grandchildren. Pedigree analysis allows for the identification of potential genetic transmission, which may not be appreciated by family history alone.

Classic Genetic Disease

Classic genetic inheritance patterns include autosomal (the nonsex chromosomes 1 to 22) and X-linked diseases (2). For practical purposes, Y-linked inheritance is essentially unimportant, with the exception of sex-determining genes and possibly some spermatogenesis genes. If two copies of a mutant gene (one inherited from the maternal chromosome and one from the paternal chromosome) are required to produce the phenotype, the disorder is recessive; if only one copy results in a disorder, the inheritance is dominant. With autosomal-recessive inheritance (Fig. 2.2), affected individuals are homozygous (indicated by shading), and parents are heterozygous (half-shaded symbols). In some diseases, the affected individual has two different mutations, termed a compound heterozygote. The pedigree in Fig. 2.2 displays the characteristics of autosomal-recessive disease: (a) horizontal transmission (affected siblings); (b) equal distribution of affected males and females; (c) recurrence risk of 25% for each subsequent pregnancy for heterozygote couples; and (d) for normal-appearing offspring, two-thirds will be carriers and one-third will be homozygote normals (2). Examples of autosomal-recessive disorders include most enzyme defects (such as 21-hydroxylase deficiency), Tay-Sachs disease, cystic fibrosis, sickle cell anemia, thalassemias, and ataxia telangectasia. Disease is not usually manifested in heterozygotes because some normal protein, encoded by the normal allele, is present. If consanguinity occurs within a family, then there is an increased probability of rare autosomal-recessive diseases because of more frequent allele sharing.

For an autosomal-dominant disorder (Fig. 2.3), only a single copy of the mutant gene (i.e., the patient is heterozygous) is required to produce the phenotype. Occasionally, homozygosity may be observed, and this may increase disease severity in affected individuals, as has been demonstrated in patients with familial type 2 hyperlipoproteinemia, who have low-density lipoprotein (LDL) receptor mutations. Heterozygotes have an increased risk of heart disease during early middle age and have lipomas, but homozygotes have much more severe disease at an earlier age, commonly fatal heart disease in childhood. Important characteristics of autosomal-dominant diseases include (a) vertical transmission (parents to offspring), (b) a 50:50 sex ratio, and (c) a recurrence risk with each subsequent pregnancy of 50% (2). Examples of autosomal-dominant disease include neurofibromatosis, myotonic dystrophy, some forms of osteogenesis imperfecta, achodroplasia, Huntington disease, and some familial cancer syndromes such as Li-Fraumeni syndrome, retinoblastoma, and breast and ovarian cancer. Dominant mutations commonly cause disease when the protein encoded from the mutant allele interferes with the function of the protein product encoded by the normal allele. This mechanism of disease is sometimes called a dominant-negative effect. Dominant-negative effects are more likely to occur in genes that encode proteins that

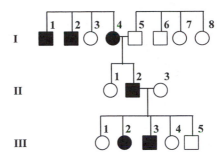

FIGURE 2.3. Autosomal-dominant inheritance in this pedigree.

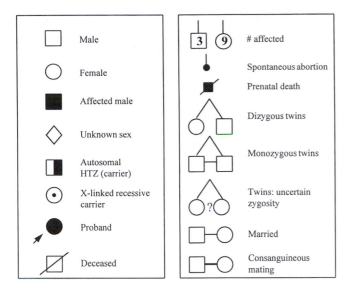

FIGURE 2.1. The more commonly used symbols for pedigree construction.

form multimers. When this occurs, the mutant protein may interfere with multimer formation and cause disease.

Several important features of autosomal-dominant disease are penetrance, variable expressivity, and anticipation (2). Penetrance is an all-or-none phenomenon that refers to whether or not the person who inherits a mutant gene manifests the disease. If reduced penetrance occurs for a particular disease, such as 70% penetrance, then only 70% of those who possess the mutation actually manifest the disease. Penetrance certainly complicates pedigree interpretation. Suppose that the affected male in Fig. 2.3 (II2) had the mutant gene, but did not manifest it (an unshaded square instead). He would be incorrectly counseled that his offspring would not be affected, when in fact they are at a 50% risk of inheriting the mutant gene and phenotype. Two

examples of incomplete penetrance in autosomal-dominant disease are retinoblastoma and split-hand deformity. Another factor complicating the interpretation of dominant diseases is variable expressivity. Variable expressivity refers to the variation in the manifestation of the disease, even within the same family. Neurofibromatosis type 1 is an autosomal-dominant disease of neuroectoderm, in which affected individuals manifest neurofibromas and café-au-lait spots. An apparently asymptomatic female with café-au-lait spots and a small number of neurofibromas may escape clinical detection unless a thorough exam is performed, but she still has a 50% risk of having an affected child, who could display more severe symptoms, such as central nervous system (CNS) neurofibromas and more disfiguring cutaneous neurofibromas. Marfan syndrome, an autosomal-dominant connective disorder affecting skeletal, cardiovascular, and ocular systems, also displays variable expressivity (1). Although not unique to autosomal-dominant disorders, some autosomal-dominant diseases increase in severity from one generation to the next, which is called anticipation. Myotonic dystrophy is a good example since a minimally affected woman with facial weakness may have a child with the severe congenital form of the disease with severe mental retardation and cardiac manifestations. Most diseases with anticipation have expansion of triplet repeats within the causative gene (discussed below) (3).

X-linked recessive disease occurs in males with mutations arising on one of their X chromosomes (Fig. 2.4) (2). The major clinical features of X-linked recessive diseases are the following: (a) disease is almost exclusively in males; (b) the trait is inherited from carrier females by half of her sons; (c) half of a female carrier's daughters will be carriers, who are at risk to pass it on to their sons; (d) the trait is never passed from an affected male to his son (since he gives a Y chromosome to all of his sons), but carrier status is passed to all of his daughters (from his affected X chromosome); and (e) the disease is transmitted through carrier females, so males in a pedigree will be related through females. Affected males are said to be hemizygous since they have one mutant X chromosome. Rarely, females may be affected with X-linked recessive diseases, and in this case, an abnormal X chromosome should be present. Women with a 45,X

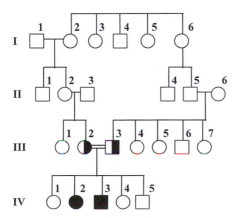

FIGURE 2.2. Autosomal-recessive inheritance. Consanguinity is demonstrated as a *double line*. Both parents of the affected male and female are heterozygotes (*half shaded*). Family members are labeled with a Roman numeral for each generation and an Arabic number within the generation.

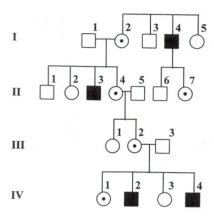

FIGURE 2.4. X-linked recessive inheritance. Carrier females (*dotted circles*) are identified.

karyotype or who have an X-autosome translocation are such examples, so chromosome analysis is warranted in any women who manifest an X-linked recessive disease. Examples of X-linked recessive disorders include Duchenne muscular dystrophy, Kallmann syndrome, hemophilia A and B, and androgen insensitivity syndrome.

X-linked dominant diseases (Fig. 2.5) are rare and may be difficult to distinguish from other patterns of inheritance since they have some characteristics of both autosomal-dominant and X-linked recessive diseases. Similar to autosomal-dominant disorders, the mutant gene in an X-linked dominant disorder exists on only one chromosome, and males and females can be affected (2). The prominent features of X-linked dominant inheritance are the following: (a) affected fathers with normal partners produce no affected sons (they do not give them an X) and 100% affected daughters (the X they have contains the mutant); (b) males or females born to a carrier female have a 50% chance of being affected with each pregnancy (carrier female can give

either normal or abnormal X); and (c) males and females are affected, but for rare diseases, affected females are about twice as common as affected males. Examples of X-linked dominant disorders include vitamin D–resistant (hypophosphatemic) rickets, the urea cycle defect ornithine transcarbamylase (OTC) deficiency, and Rett syndrome. Rett syndrome is a special example in which mental retardation occurs in females, but the disorder is lethal in males, so a pedigree may be seen with only living females. Fragile X syndrome is an X-linked dominant disease characterized by mental retardation and macro-orchidism. Fragile X syndrome displays incomplete penetrance since males with the mutation are usually affected, but about one-third do not manifest the disease.

Nonclassic Patterns of Inheritance

In addition to the classic modes of inheritance discussed above, some nonclassic modes of inheritance have been recognized, such as mitochondrial inheritance, uniparental disomy, genomic imprinting, and somatic cell and germline mosaicism. With mitochondrial inheritance (Fig. 2.6), females pass the disorder to all of their offspring, while males do not transmit the disease to any of their offspring (4). Disease is only transmitted from mother to all children because oocytes have several to 100,000 mitochondrial DNAs, while sperm contain several hundred. For practical purposes, when fertilization takes place, all of the mitochondrial DNA is maternal, which explains the inheritance (Fig. 2.6) (4). Diseases of mitochondrial DNA affect organs that expend high rates of energy, such as muscle, brain, CNS, heart, kidney, and endocrine organs such as the pancreas. Some examples of mitochondrial inheritance include Leber hereditary optic neuropathy (LHON), a form of adult-onset central blindness (peripheral vision may be spared), myoclonus epilepsy with ragged red fibers (MERRF), and mitochondrial encepholomyopathy, lactic acidosis, and stroke-like symptoms (MELAS) (4).

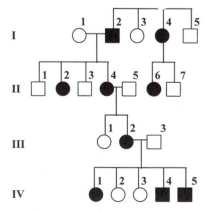

FIGURE 2.5. X-linked dominant inheritance. Although the pedigree resembles autosomal-dominant transmission, the lack of male-to-male transmission and the observation that all daughters of affected fathers have the disease makes X-linked dominant the likely mode of inheritance.

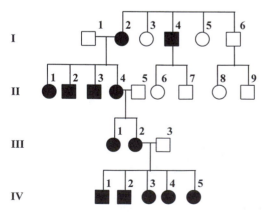

FIGURE 2.6. A pedigree of mitochondrial inheritance. Note that all offspring of affected females have the disease, while the affected male has no affected children.

Uniparental disomy (UDP) is a form of nonclassic genetic inheritance that can complicate pedigree interpretation (5). UPD refers to the observation that both chromosomes in a chromosome pair (for example, chromosome 7) are inherited from the same parent rather than one from each parent. Examples of UPD include Prader-Willi syndrome, Angelman syndrome, and cystic fibrosis (5). Cystic fibrosis is an autosomal-recessive disease, but in one family a puzzling situation was observed. One parent was heterozygous, while the other was homozygous normal for the cystic fibrosis transmembrane conductance regulator (*CFTR*) gene, yet they had a child affected with cystic fibrosis. Through DNA studies using polymorphic markers, it was demonstrated that both chromosomes 7 came from the same parent (mother). These findings demonstrate the importance of inheriting one set of chromosomes from the father and one from the mother.

Another nonclassic mode of inheritance is genomic imprinting, which is defined as the unequal expression of maternal and paternal alleles (5). Perhaps the most notable examples of genomic imprinting are Prader-Willi syndrome and Angelman syndrome, both of which are due to deletions of chromosome 15 q11q13 (5). Prader-Willi syndrome consists of hypotonia, poor sucking, developmental delay, characteristic facies with almond-shaped eyes, hypogonadotropic hypogonadism, and later hyperphagia. Angelman syndrome is characterized by severe mental retardation and seizures, and is often referred to as the happy puppet syndrome because of paroxysms of inappropriate laughter and movement. Prader-Willi syndrome occurs when the chromosome 15 deletion is paternal, but Angelman syndrome occurs when the deletion is maternal. Imprinting also underscores the importance of inheriting a maternal and paternal chromosome for each chromosome pair. These diseases are usually sporadic, so the recurrence risk is very small.

The recognition of germline mosaicism has solved previously unanswered questions in some cases of unexpected inheritance patterns (6). On occasion, phenotypically normal parents have a child with an autosomal-dominant disorder, or a noncarrier female has a son with an X-linked recessive disease. These cases were generally regarded to represent new mutations. Occasionally, however, a second affected individual was born with the disease to unaffected parents. Some of theses diseases were found to be caused by germline mosaicism, whereby the mutant allele is present within the gametes of the parent, but absent in other cells. An example of germline mosaicism is achondroplasia, the skeletal dysplasia manifesting extreme postnatal micromelia and frontal bossing due to mutations in the fibroblast growth factor receptor 3 gene. Another example of germline mosaicism is the X-linked disorder Duchenne muscular dystrophy occurring in the absence of a carrier female. The recurrence risks for these disorders with normal parents is usually in the range of several percent. Somatic cell mosaicism may also occur when mutations arise in some cells, but not all cells, of an organ (6). Benign neoplasms and cancers arise as somatic cell mutations, which then proliferate within the organ in which they arise.

Complex (Polygenic/Multifactorial) Disorders

Most human diseases do not follow obvious Mendelian patterns of inheritance, but probably result from the effects of a number of genes and environmental factors. The pedigree usually will contain no one with a history of the disease, or it might have one or two affected individuals. Examples include hypertension, diabetes mellitus (both types 1 and 2), cleft palate, schizophrenia, manic-depressive illness, neural tube defects, pyloric stenosis, and congenital heart anomalies. The recurrence risk is usually in the range of 1% to 4% depending on the type of disease, its prevalence, and the number of affected family members (2,7). For example, if a couple in the United States has had one prior child with a neural tube defect (NTD), the recurrence risk is about 2%. If they have two affected children, the recurrence risk is 4% to 6% (7). In the U.S. the prevalence of NTD is about 1/1,000 births, while in the United Kingdom it occurs in about 1/100 births. The recurrence risks in the U.K. are also higher, being 5% after one affected child and about 12% after two affected offspring (7). Some multifactorial disorders have markedly different male to female ratios, so the sex of the affected individual affects the recurrence risk. For example, congenital hip dislocation is five times as common in females. If a couple has one affected female with congenital hip dislocation, the recurrence risk is 2%. If the single prior affected child is a male (which is rarer), the recurrence risk is higher, on the order of 5% to 10% (7).

CHROMOSOME DISORDERS

Cytogenetics

Humans possess 23 pairs of chromosomes in the nucleus of all nucleated cells (Fig. 2.7). One pair consists of the sex chromosomes (X,Y in males and X,X in females), and the remaining 22 pairs of nonsex chromosomes are called autosomes (numbered 1 to 22). With the birth of cytogenetics in the early 1960s, the clinical diagnosis of chromosome disorders came into the realm of clinical medicine.

Chromosomes are composed of a short arm (denoted p) and a long arm (denoted q), which are connected by the centromere (8). They are numbered 1 to 22 with decreasing size (except 21, which is larger than 22), while the sex chromosomes size are separate, and by convention, are placed after the autosomes. The chromosome spread is displayed in a characteristic standardized pattern called a karyotype (Fig. 2.7). Chromosomes are also characterized by the position of the centromere, with metacentric chromosomes

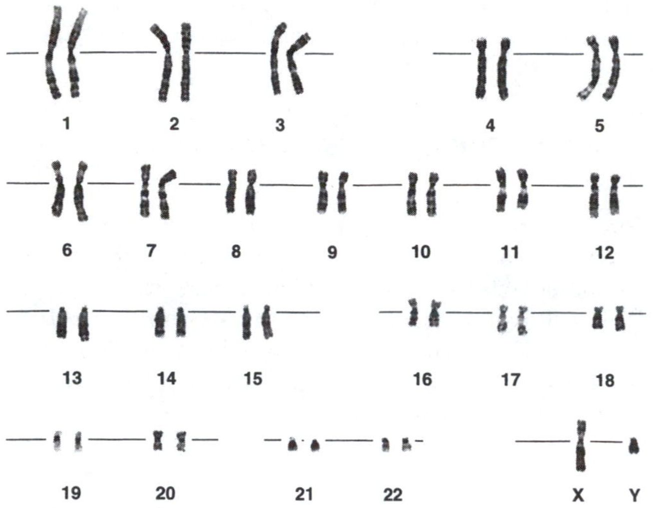

FIGURE 2.7. A 46,XY karyotype. (Courtesy of Dr. David Ledbetter, Genetics Laboratory, University of Chicago, IL.)

(chromosomes 1 to 5) having the centromere centrally placed so that the p and q arms are similar in size, submetacentric chromosomes (6 to 12, 16 to 18) having distinctly different sizes of the arms, and acrocentric chromosomes (13 to 15, 21, 22), in which the centromere is near the end of the chromosome (Fig. 2.7) (8).

To perform a karyotype, heparinized blood is drawn and white blood cells (WBCs) are isolated by centrifugation in a ficoll gradient (8). The WBCs obtained are incubated with a mitogen such as phytohemagglutinin, and grown in culture for about 72 hours at which time they are rapidly dividing. They are arrested in metaphase using agents such as colchicine, which inhibit spindle formation and delay centromere separation. After cell division is inhibited by colchicine, the cells are lysed using hypotonic solutions so that the chromosomes are released from the cells. The chromosomes are then fixed, spread onto slides, and stained with trypsin and Giemsa stain, which produce dark and light bands referred to as G banding (Fig. 2.7). Other methods are occasionally used, such as Q banding (quinacrine staining followed by fluorescence microscopy, producing bright Q bands, which correspond almost completely to dark G bands), and R banding (heat before Giemsa staining, which produces bands opposite of G banding). The standard metaphase karyotype produces about 400 bands, but if the cells are arrested at the prometaphase stage, 550 to 850 bands may be produced (extended banding karyotype) (8). The normal karyotype is written by standard nomenclature as 46,XY (males) and 46,XX (females).

The normal haploid number of chromosomes (23) in germ cells or an exact multiple of the haploid number of chromosomes (46, 69, etc.) is termed euploid. The diploid number of chromosomes (46) is observed in normal individuals. Although triploidy (3n) and tetraploidy (4n) are classified as euploid numbers, they do produce phenotypic abnor-

malities, usually resulting in spontaneous abortions, and, rarely, liveborns. The principal clinical utility of cytogenetics is to diagnose aneuploidy (an abnormal number of chromosomes that are not an exact multiple of the haploid number) and structural abnormalities, such as deletions, translocations, and inversions. Trisomy (three of a particular chromosome) and monosomy (one chromosome) represent the most common forms of aneuploidy.

Chromosomal abnormalities must be considered more likely in certain clinical situations. Well known is the association of advanced maternal age and the probability of having an affected fetus with a chromosome disorder (Table 2.1). The most common diagnoses, in decreasing frequency, are trisomy 21 (Down syndrome), trisomy 18, and trisomy 13. In addition to these autosomal trisomies, trisomy of the sex chromosomes may also occur, with Klinefelter syndrome (47,XXY) and 47,XXX being the most common. In general, derangements of autosomes result in more severe phenotypic abnormalities with mental retardation as one component

TABLE 2.1. WITH INCREASING MATERNAL AGE AT THE TIME OF DELIVERY, THE CHANCE OF A CHROMOSOMALLY ABNORMAL LIVEBORN INCREASE

Maternal Age	Risk of Down Syndrome	Total Risk of Chromosomal Abnormality
20	1/1,667	1/526
21	1/1,667	1/526
22	1/1,429	1/500
23	1/1,429	1/500
24	1/1,250	1/476
25	1/1,250	1/476
26	1/1,176	1/476
27	1/1,111	1/455
28	1/1,053	1/435
29	1/1,000	1/417
30	1/952	1/417
31	1/909	1/385
32	1/769	1/322
33	1/602	1/286
34	1/485	1/238
35	1/378	1/192
36	1/289	1/156
37	1/224	1/127
38	1/173	1/102
39	1/136	1/83
40	1/106	1/66
41	1/82	1/53
42	1/63	1/42
43	1/49	1/33
44	1/38	1/26
45	1/30	1/21
46	1/23	1/16
47	1/18	1/13
48	1/14	1/10
49	1/11	1/8

From Hook EB. Rates of chromosomal abnormalities of different maternal ages. *Obstet Gynecol* 1981;58:282, with permission.

than with sex chromosomes. The most common features for each of the trisomies are shown in Table 2.2 (9). An increased risk in trisomy does not appear to occur with increased paternal age, although the probability of autosomal dominant and X-linked recessive disorders increases with increasing paternal age. In general, if a couple has a child with a trisomy, the recurrence risk of trisomy in a subsequent pregnancy is about 1% (9).

Structural abnormalities such as chromosomal deletions and insertions may also be diagnosed using a karyotype. Since the human genome consists of 3 billion base pairs (bp) (3 million kilobases) per haploid genome, the average band is roughly 250,000 kilobases (kb). Deletions must be sufficiently large to be detectable by a karyotype, so single gene deletions are not detectable by cytogenetics. Often when a deletion is observed on karyotypic analysis, the region deleted is sufficiently large that several (or many) genes are absent, a so-called contiguous gene deletion syndrome. When this occurs on autosomes, a variety of somatic anomalies and mental retardation are commonly present. The deletion is written with particular attention to the deleted bands, such as with Prader-Willi syndrome, in which a deletion of the long arm of chromosome 15 is deleted between bands q11 to q13, written as del 15q11q13.

Cytogenetics has contributed to our understanding of reproductive fetal loss. Over half of all first trimester abortions that are karyotyped have a chromosomal abnormality (Table 2.3), and although the prevalence decreases with advancing gestation, risk is still significant in the second and third trimesters (Table 2.4) (10). When chromosomes

TABLE 2.3. KARYOTYPES OF FIRST TRIMESTER ABORTIONS

	Karyotype	%	Total %
Normal	Normal		54.5
Autosomal trisomy	T1	0	30.4
	T2	1.6	
	T3	0.3	
	T4	0.7	
	T5	0.1	
	T6	0.1	
	T7	1.3	
	T8	1.1	
	T9	1.1	
	T10	0.6	
	T11	0.1	
	T12	0.2	
	T13	1.5	
	T14	1.3	
	T15	2.4	
	T16	9.9	
	T17	0.2	
	T18	1.8	
	T19	0.1	
	T20	0.9	
	T21	2.6	
	T22	2.8	
Sex chromosome polysomy	47,XXX	0.2	0.7
	47,XXY	0.5	
Monosmy X	45,X		8.6
Triploidy	69,XXX	2.7	7.0
	69,XXY	4.0	
	69,XYY	0.2	
Tetraploidy	92,XXXX	1.9	2.6
	92,XXYY	0.7	
Structural abnormalities			1.5

From Simpson JL, Bombard A. Chromosomal abnormalities in spontaneous abortion: frequency, pathology, and genetic counselling. In: Bennett MJ, Edwards DK, eds. *Spontaneous and recurrent abortion.* Oxford, England: Blackwell Scientific, 1987;51–76, with permission.

TABLE 2.2. SOME OF THE MORE COMMON CHARACTERISTICS OF INDIVIDUALS AFFECTED WITH TRISOMY (T) 21, 18, AND 13

T21	T18	T13
1/800 LB	1/8,000 LB	1/20,000 LB
Mental retardation	Severe mental retardation	Severe mental retardation
Hypotonia	Clenched hand	Defects of eye, nose, lip, and forebrain of holoprosencephaly type
Flat facies	Short sternum	
Slanted palpebral fissures	Low arm dermal ridge pattern on fingertips	
Small ears		Polydactyly
Cardiac (40%)	Cardiac > 50%	Narrow hyperconvex fingernails
		Skin defects of posterior scalp
		Cardiac (80%)

LB, liveborn.
From Jones KL. *Smith's recognizable patterns of human malformation.* Philadelphia: WB Saunders, 1997, with permission.

TABLE 2.4. THE CHANCE OF A CHROMOSOMALLY ABNORMAL FETUS DECREASES WITH INCREASING GESTATION

Weeks Gestation	Chromosomal Abnormalities (%)
8–11	50
12–15	40
16–19	19
20–23	12
24–28	8
>28	5

From Simpson JL, Bombard A. Chromosomal abnormalities in spontaneous abortion: frequency, pathology, and genetic counselling. In: Bennett MJ, Edwards DK, eds. *Spontaneous and recurrent abortion.* Oxford, England: Blackwell Scientific, 1987;51–76, with permission.

are obtained from both members of couples with two or more spontaneous abortions or one spontaneous abortion and one malformed fetus, there is a tenfold increase in the detection of parental chromosomal rearrangements (Table 2.5). Instead of the baseline risk of 0.4%, the risk that either parent carries a balanced rearrangement is 4% to 5%. Most of the chromosomal rearrangements are translocations, which may be of two types: Robertsonian and reciprocal. Translocations may be balanced, which refers to a normal phenotype, and indicates that little or no chromosomal material was lost. An unbalanced translocation results in phenotypic effects, which often include mental retardation and various somatic anomalies.

Robertsonian translocations involve the acrocentric chromosomes (13 to 15, 21, 22), and occur when short arms from two acrocentric chromosomes are lost, and the long arm from one chromosome joins the long arm of the other chromosome (Fig. 2.8)

For the individual with a balanced Robertsonian translocation, the total chromosomal number is 45. If 46 chromosomes are present, a trisomy is present, so the patient has an unbalanced translocation. If the partial trisomy involves chromosome 21, the Down syndrome phenotype is present. Since 3% to 4% of all Down syndrome patients may have an unbalanced translocation, performing a karyotype is important in counseling the couple for recurrence risks. If the Robertsonian translocation is present in the mother, there is a 10% to 15% recurrence risk for a liveborn Down syndrome, but if it occurs in the father, the risk is less (0% to 2%). A reciprocal translocation occurs when two different chromosomes break, and exchange of material occurs between the two chromosomes (Fig. 2.8).

A reciprocal translocation occurs when two chromosomes break and exchange material (Fig. 2.8). With a balanced reciprocal translocation, the total number of chromo-

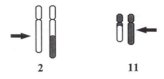

Reciprocal translocation

2   11

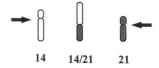

Robertsonian translocation

14   14/21   21

FIGURE 2.8. A: Reciprocal translocation. Breaks occur on two different chromosomes, and chromosomal material is exchanged between them. **B:** In a Robertsonian translocation, short arms are lost from two acrocentric chromosomes, and long arms from each join together to form one chromosome.

somes is 46, while in an unbalanced translocation, deletions/duplications can occur. With a reciprocal translocation, the recurrence risks of having an affected liveborn are similar whether carried by the mother or father, and are roughly 10% to 15% (8). Because translocations are expected to result in a mixed history of normal children, miscarriages, and abnormal liveborns, chromosomal analysis should be considered for such families.

Cytogenetic analysis should be considered in anyone with multiple somatic anomalies and mental retardation. Another instance in obstetrics and gynecology where a karyotype may be beneficial is in hypogonadism. In individuals with delayed puberty and elevated gonadotropins (hypergonadotropic hypogonadism), a karyotype should be performed to exclude chromosomal disorders (Table 2.6) (11). In females with primary amenorrhea and elevated gonadotropins, a 46,XY cell line should be excluded because of the increased risk of gonadoblastomas with a pure 46,XY

TABLE 2.5. PARENTAL KARYOTYPES OF COUPLES WITH EITHER RECURRENT ABORTION, DEFINED AS TWO OR MORE SPONTANEOUS ABORTIONS, OR WITH MULTIPLE REPRODUCTIVE LOSSES (AT LEAST ONE MALFORMED FETUS AND ONE LOSS)

	Recurrent Aborters		Multiple Reproductive Loss	
	F	M	F	M
Robertsonian translocation	2.2	0.9	2.4	1.1
Reciprocal translocation	0.6	0.3	0.6	0.3
Total	2.8	1.2	3.0	1.4

Note: sample size is 1,521 females and 1,490 males for the recurrent aborter group, and 1,589 females and 1,504 males for the multiple reproductive loss group.
From Warburton D, Strobino B. Recurrent spontaneous abortion. In: Bennett MJ, Edmonds DK, eds. *Spontaneous and recurrent abortion.* Oxford, England: Blackwell Scientific, 1987;193–213, with permission.

TABLE 2.6. THE PREVALENCE OF CHROMOSOMAL ABNORMALITIES IN WOMEN WITH OVARIAN FAILURE IS SHOWN AMONG GROUPS OF WOMEN WITH AMENORRHEA

	Amenorrhea (%)	
Hypogonadism	Primary	Secondary
Hypergonadotropic hypogonadism	43	11
Abnormal chromosomes	27	0.5
Normal chromosomes	16	10
Hypogonadotropic hypogonadism	31	42
Reversible	19	39
Irreversible	12	3
Eugonadism	26	46

karyotype (Swyer syndrome) and 45,X/46,XY (mixed gonadal dysgenesis, a form of Turner syndrome) (11). Although some degree of sexual ambiguity may be present in patients with a 45,X/46,XY karyotype, this feature may be absent. A 45,X cell line also must be excluded in women with primary or secondary amenorrhea since cardiac (40% to 50%) and renal (30%) anomalies commonly occur in these patients (11). It must be emphasized that the karyotype for Turner syndrome is written 45,X (not 45,XO as is often incorrectly indicated). The most consistent feature of 45,X individuals is short stature (usually 4'9"), while other anomalies such as shield chest, webbed neck, widely spaced nipples, etc., are much more variable (11). Approximately half of women with primary amenorrhea with hypergonadotropic hypogonadism have X chromosome abnormalities, and although less likely in women with secondary amenorrhea (a few percent), it is still wise to consider chromosome analysis, particularly in women with short stature (Table 2.6). Other potential abnormal karyotypes in women with ovarian failure include deletions of the p or q arms of the X chromosome, which are often associated with short stature (under 5'3") and primary or secondary amenorrhea, depending on the location of the deletion. Although these deletions do not carry the same serious consequences of medical complication as X chromosome monosomy, they can be inherited by half of the daughters, who are then at risk for premature ovarian failure (11).

Similarly, in males with hypergonadotropic hypogonadism, a karyotype will be useful for medical management (11). Abnormal chromosomes may occur in 5% to 15% of males with gonadal failure, with 47,XXY karyotype (Klinefelter syndrome) being most common and 46,XX (sex-reversed males) second (11). The most consistent finding in men with Klinefelter syndrome is testicular fibrosis and infertility, whereas mental retardation and behavioral disorders are less common. Since men with Klinefelter syndrome have an increased risk of testicular tumors, lymphoma, and diabetes, careful surveillance is important. Some authors have suggested obtaining karyotypes on all men with severe oligospermia (less than 5 million/cc) as the prevalence of chromosome anomalies is about 5% (12). Although portions of the Y chromosome may be deleted in some patients, such as the Yq12 region containing putative spermatogenesis genes [DAZ (deleted in azoospermia) and RBM (RNA-binding motif)], the more concerning abnormalities include translocations, which could be transmitted to offspring.

MOLECULAR MEDICAL GENETICS

With the advent of molecular genetic studies, finer detail of chromosomes down to the gene level is now possible (8,13,14). A basic knowledge of DNA structure is important in understanding the concepts for molecular biology techniques. DNA exists as a double-stranded helical structure within the nucleus of all living cells. Although it contains a sugar-phosphate backbone, the most important feature for its manipulation is the complementarity of the nitrogenous base pairs: adenine (A) pairs with thymine (T) via two hydrogen bonds, and guanine (G) joins with cytosine (C) via three hydrogen bonds (Fig. 2.9).

Several important terms facilitate the understanding of molecular genetics techniques. Denaturation is the separation of DNA into two single strands, and this is usually accomplished by either alkali (in Southern blots) or by heat [in polymerase chain reaction (PCR)]. When single strands of DNA join together, it is termed either hybridization (as in Southern blot analysis) or annealing (as in PCR). DNA will anneal or hybridize according to specific pairing of the nitrogenous bases. The principles of all molecular biology techniques rely on these features of nucleic acids.

Individual genes make up only a small percentage of the 3 billion bp, or 3 million kb, of nucleotides per haploid genome in humans (Fig. 2.9). Since human genomic DNA is large, but specific genes are small (several kilobases to rarely up to 1,000 kb), cutting DNA into smaller pieces greatly facilitates its study. Restriction enzymes (also called restriction endonucleases) present in bacteria cut (or digest) DNA into smaller pieces. Restriction enzymes recognize certain specific sequences, and they cut every time this particular array of bases is encountered (Fig. 2.10). They are named for the bacteria and the particular strain from which they were isolated. For example, EcoRI was isolated from *Escherichia coli*, strain R, and was the first enzyme characterized from this organism. EcoRI recognizes the bases GAATTC and cuts between the G and A (Fig. 2.10).

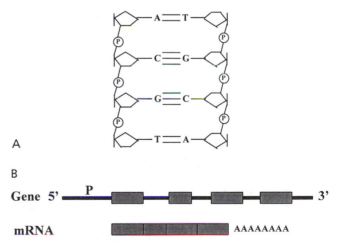

FIGURE 2.9. A: The basic structure of DNA, with the sugar (pentagon) and phosphate (P) backbone and inwardly directed nucleotide bases. Complementary base pairing occurs between adenine (A) and thymine (T) or between cytosine (C) and guanine (G). **B:** Basic gene structure is shown for a gene. By convention the 5' region (upstream) is on the *left* and the 3' region (downstream) is on the *right*. The four exons are shown as *boxes,* the three introns are shown between the exons, and the promoter (P) is the regulatory region.

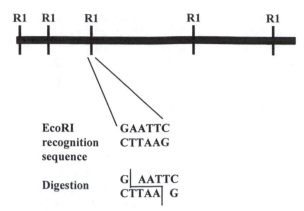

FIGURE 2.10. Restriction enzyme digestion with EcoRI. A fragment of DNA is shown, and EcoRI sites are indicated by *vertical lines* labeled with R1. The six base recognition site is shown, as is the location of digestion.

The discovery of these important enzymes allowed investigators to connect pieces of DNA cut with the same enzyme, a requirement to clone genes. These enzymes also constitute an important part of the generation of Southern blots.

DNA Techniques

Innumerable DNA techniques have now been described, but only some of those more commonly used in clinical diagnostics will be detailed. The principal types of molecular genetic tests include Southern blot analysis, PCR, PCR-based gene screening techniques, allele-specific oligonucleotide hybridization to dot blots, and fluorescent *in situ* hybridization (FISH). Although DNA sequencing, Northern blot analysis, and reverse transcriptase PCR are not commonly used clinically, basic concepts of these important techniques will also be reviewed.

Southern Blot Analysis

To study gene structure for large deletions or rearrangements, a Southern blot is used. Similar procedures are performed for the study of RNA (Northern blot) and proteins (Western blot) (13). A Southern blot contains single-stranded genomic DNA, which is immobilized on a nylon membrane. If we want to study an individual for a particular gene mutation, we can use that gene sequence as a DNA probe to detect any differences in gene in our patient (Fig. 2.11). DNA is first extracted from cells containing a nucleus (WBCs are most accessible), and is then digested with a restriction enzyme into smaller pieces. Next, the DNA is separated in an agarose gel, and the smaller pieces of DNA migrate faster and farther than larger ones. When the gel is stained with ethidium bromide and visualized with a UV light, the DNA can be observed (at this point, it looks like a smear, but is actually many overlapping fragments). The DNA is then denatured using alkali, such

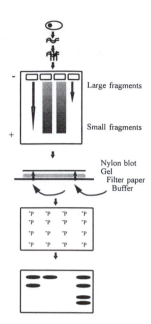

FIGURE 2.11. Construction of a Southern blot. A nucleated cell (*top*) has its DNA extracted (shown as *double-stranded line*), which is digested with a restriction enzyme (*vertical lines* through DNA). The DNA is then electrophoresed on an agarose gel from negative (−) to positive (+) as shown. The *arrow* indicates the direction of migration. The DNA is then transferred from the gel to a nylon membrane, which is then hybridized with a single-stranded labeled probe (*P). After washing off excess radioactivity and autoradiography, bands appear on the film when it is developed (*bottom*).

that it is now single stranded. The DNA from the gel is then transferred to a nylon membrane by capillary action, and baked to fix the DNA onto the gel. At this point, single-stranded DNA is spread out on the membrane so that it can be probed for mutations. A DNA probe is single stranded (or denatured to make it single stranded), then labeled with ^{32}P or a nonradioactive method. It is mixed with the membrane in a hybridization solution, so that complementary base pairing can occur. Excess radioactivity is washed off using dilute salt solutions at high temperature, and then the blot is placed next to a piece of x-ray film in a cassette, which is sealed and cooled to −70°C (autoradiography). The film is developed and bands are evaluated. If bands are missing, a deletion can be present (Fig. 2.12).

Many diseases are characterized by deletions, with some of the relevant ones for obstetricians/gynecologists including 21-hydroxylase gene in congenital adrenal hyperplasia, androgen receptor gene in androgen insensitivity, α-globin gene in α-thalassemia, dystrophin gene in Duchenne muscular dystrophy, and the cystic fibrosis transmembrane conductance regulator protein in cystic fibrosis. Unfortunately, not all individuals with a particular genetic disorder display the same deletion, so Southern analysis of deletions is not clinically useful for all diseases. Although there are a number of exceptions, about 5% to 10% of genetic diseases are characterized by gene deletions.

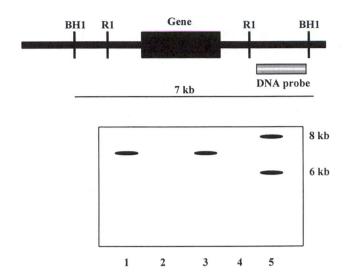

FIGURE 2.12. A gene deletion for patients in lanes 2 and 4, indicated by the absence of the 7-kb band. DNA was cut with BamHI, and a Southern blot was made. Note the location of the DNA probe, which detects the BamHI fragment, but would not detect the EcoRI fragment. Lane 5 is the molecular weight marker.

More common than gene deletions are the detection of benign sequence changes that alter a restriction cut site (Fig. 2.13), called restriction fragment length polymorphisms (RFLPs). Benign changes in genomic DNA termed polymorphisms occur every several hundred bases and produce no phenotypic effect. When the benign change segregates with a phenotype (Fig. 2.13), it may be used to diagnose the disorder even when the causative gene is unknown. For example, if two copies of the 9-kb fragment are seen only in patients with an autosomal-recessive disease such as β-thalassemia, and are not seen in any controls, then it is

highly likely that the causative gene is very close to this 9-kb marker, and it can be used for diagnosis. In this instance the polymorphism is informative, and so can be used to accurately predict who will be affected and who will not (Fig. 2.13). Note that both parents are heterozygous. If both parents were homozygous as is shown in Fig. 2.13B, then the polymorphism is not informative.

Direct gene analysis is the best method for mutation detection, and has largely replaced polymorphism analysis, but this technique remains useful in some diseases. Although β-thalassemia is caused by point mutations in the β-globin gene, most mutations are unique to each family, making generalized screening impractical. In this instance, if a polymorphism within the β-globin gene can be used, prediction of affected and unaffected individuals may be accomplished. The use of polymorphic DNA markers has been used extensively in gene mapping of unknown genes and in sequencing for the human genome mapping project.

Polymerase Chain Reaction (PCR)

Southern blot analysis is labor intensive, taking often 3 to 7 days, and generally requires 5 to 10 μg of DNA for analysis (13). Many of these problems have been obviated through the use of PCR. With PCR, smaller amounts of DNA are used (nanogram or even picogram quantities from a single cell), and results are generated within hours. In Southern blot analysis, a DNA probe is necessary to find a gene among the billions of bases of the genome. The basic idea of PCR is to create millions of copies of a piece of DNA to be analyzed, so DNA probes are not necessary.

The PCR procedure consists of three steps (Fig. 2.14). First, DNA is denatured (heated to 95°C to render it single

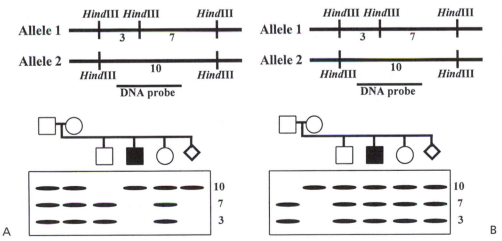

FIGURE 2.13. Restriction fragment length polymorphism (RFLP) analysis using an enzyme HindIII is shown. **A:** An informative polymorphism is shown in which the 10-kb fragment segregates with the disease. **B:** The polymorphism is not informative in this family since both parents are homozygous (either for allele number 1 with two copies of the 7- and 3-kb fragments or allele number 2 with two copies of the 10-kb fragment). All offspring will be heterozygotes whether they are affected or not.

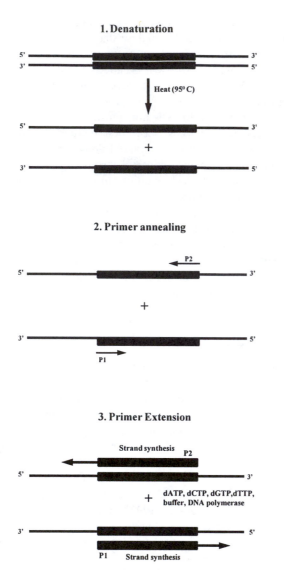

1. Denaturation

Heat (95° C)

+

2. Primer annealing

P2

+

P1

3. Primer Extension

Strand synthesis   P2

+   dATP, dCTP, dGTP, dTTP,
buffer, DNA polymerase

P1   Strand synthesis

FIGURE 2.14. One cycle of PCR, which consists of denaturation, primer annealing, and extension. After one cycle, the DNA content is doubled. The *thickened line* represents the sequence of interest: primers (P), and deoxynucleotide triphosphates (dNTPs) such as deoxynucleotide adenosine triphosphate (dATP), deoxynucleotide cytidine triphosphate (dCTP), deoxynucleotide guanosine triphosphate (dGTP), and deoxynucleotide thymidine triphosphate (dTTP).

stranded. Second, the temperature is lowered to 45° to 55°C, so that annealing will occur. However, the intent is not for the double-stranded DNA to anneal back to itself. Instead, specific primers, which are short pieces of DNA (called oligonucleotides) usually about 20 to 30 bp long, are exactly complementary to the ends of each piece of the double-stranded DNA to be amplified (Fig. 2.14), so they anneal to these regions. For this to occur, the sequence of at least part of the DNA template must be known. Third, the temperature is raised to about 72°C so that a heat-stable enzyme, such as Taq polymerase, can extend the fragment of DNA to the appropriate size so that the comple-

mentary strand of DNA will be completed. These three steps (denaturation, annealing of primers, and extension) compose a cycle of PCR. Typically, about 30 cycles are performed to achieve adequate amplification. A portion of the sample is then electrophoresed on a gel and stained with ethidium bromide to determine the presence or absence of a band (Fig. 2.15). Sometimes, five to nine different fragments of a gene can be analyzed simultaneously, as in multiplex PCR, which shortens the time required for diagnosis. Multiplex PCR has been used successfully in the diagnosis of Duchenne muscular dystrophy, in which gene deletions may compose up to 60% of all mutations. PCR can be used to detect polymorphisms, as described above for Southern blot analysis if the primers flank the polymorphic site.

Most mutations in genetic disease are not deletions, but are single base changes called point mutations. These point mutations cannot be detected by Southern blot analysis or electrophoresis of PCR products on agarose gels unless the point mutation happens to create or abolish a restriction enzyme recognition site. To determine the precise single base that has been altered, the PCR products must be directly sequenced (or cloned and sequenced). DNA sequencing is generally performed using the dideoxy chain termination reactions (Fig. 2.16). The exact bases can be read from DNA sequencing gels or by analyzing peaks on chromatographs from automated DNA sequencers. DNA sequencing is amenable to automation, which is becoming increasingly utilized by research laboratories. Automated DNA sequencing is absolutely mandatory for the success of the human genome mapping project. Although DNA

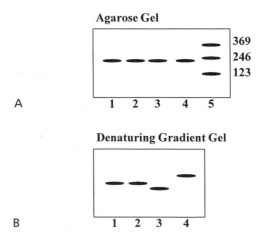

Agarose Gel

369
246
123

A   1   2   3   4   5

Denaturing Gradient Gel

B   1   2   3   4

FIGURE 2.15. **A:** Agarose gel electrophoresis in four individuals who each demonstrate the same-sized polymerase chain reaction (PCR) fragment (lanes 1 to 4), while a molecular weight marker is shown in lane 5. **B:** Denaturing gradient gel electrophoresis (DGGE) is shown for the same four fragments. Note that the fragments in lanes 1 and 2 migrate to the same location on the gel (these are wild-type), while lanes 3 and 4 both migrate differently due to differences in DNA sequence (these are the mutations). In DGGE, fragments migrate differently based on differences in melting temperature (due to the mutation).

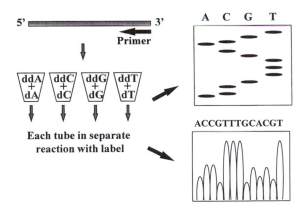

FIGURE 2.16. DNA sequencing. The fragment at the top of the figure is amplified using a primer, as shown. This reaction is divided into four separate reactions in the presence of one of the deoxynucleotide triphosphates (dNTPs), such as dATP, dCTP, dGTP, dTTP, as usually occurs. However, added into the reaction is a dideoxynucleotide triphosphate (ddNTP), such as ddATP, ddCTP, ddGTP, and ddTTP, which does not permit a new base to be added, so the reaction is terminated. For example, in the A tube, a mixture of dATP and ddATP is used so that fragments of differing lengths, but all ending in A, are produced. Each of the products from the A, C, G, and T reactions are labeled either with ^{35}S and electrophoresed in polyacrylamide gels, dried, and radiographs created **(A)**. The gel is read from the bottom toward the top, with the order being "ACCG," etc. If the label is fluorescin labeled and run in an automated DNA sequencer, a chromatogram **(B)** is produced.

sequencing has not generally been utilized very often by clinical labs, more recently automated DNA sequencing has been used by some clinical laboratories to sequence the entire *BRCA1* and *BRCA2* genes.

Gene-screening techniques may be used to determine if a certain sequence differs from another, and then DNA sequencing can be performed to identify the exact base change. These procedures obviate the need for DNA sequencing of a large number of samples, and necessitate sequencing only the fragments that differ from controls. There are a variety of gene-screening techniques that exploit certain characteristics of DNA. In denaturing gradient gel electrophoresis (DGGE), variant fragments are detected based on their differences in melting temperature. For example, if a 200-bp PCR fragment has a single base pair change in one patient, but is normal in another, the melting temperature of two fragments will differ when they are electrophoresed on a denaturing gradient gel (Fig. 2.15). In the most commonly employed screening method, single-strand conformation polymorphism (SSCP) analysis, the wild-type and mutant fragments are denatured into single-strand pieces of DNA and electrophoresed on nondenaturing cells. Since single-stranded DNA with a mutation will fold differently than the wild type, the two fragments will migrate differently in the gel. However, the exact DNA base pair change must be determined by DNA sequencing, a technique that is too laborious for common clinical use.

PCR is the most common technique used in clinical DNA diagnostics. There are many examples of diseases that can be diagnosed using PCR techniques. Examples include cystic fibrosis, fragile X syndrome, achondroplasia, Duchenne muscular dystrophy, and Huntington disease. Although not performed widely at the present time, analysis of PCR products performed on DNA from a single cell (such as a blastocyst), permits the diagnosis of certain disorders such as cystic fibrosis, β-thalassemia, hemophilia A, and α_1-antitrypsin deficiency.

Dot Blots and Allele-Specific Oligonucleotide Hybridization

Very often, diseases are composed of a variety of different mutations in different families, which makes clinical diagnosis difficult. In cystic fibrosis, it is now known that 32 different mutations compose over 90% of the mutations seen in patients in the United States. Each of these mutations can be tested for directly using PCR techniques. One important method to detect specific point mutations, without having to sequence them every time, is the creation of dot blots, which are probed by allele-specific oligonucleotide (ASO) probes. It must be stressed that this method tests only for the presence or absence of a specific mutation.

To perform ASO probing of dot blots, first the specific fragment of DNA is amplified by PCR. The DNA is denatured and spotted onto a nylon membrane (Fig. 2.17). The hybridization signal on the blot looks like a dot, hence the name dot blots. The probes are specifically designed so that they detect certain alleles—a particular mutant allele and the normal allele. One probe is complementary to the normal (or wild-type) allele and the other oligonucleotide probe is complementary to the mutant allele (Fig. 2.17). A homozygous normal individual hybridizes only to the normal oligonucleotide, and a homozygous mutant hybridizes only to the mutant probe. A heterozygote hybridizes to both the

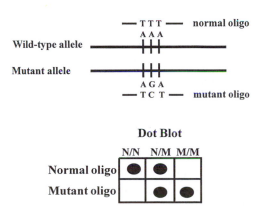

FIGURE 2.17. Allele specific oligonucleotide (ASO) probing of a dot blot. Note that the wild-type sequence (AAA) differs by one base from the mutant sequence (AGA). The wild-type probe and the mutant probe will only hybridize with the normal (N) or mutant (M) sequences, respectively.

mutant and wild-type oligonucleotides. This analysis can be repeated for each different mutation, so a panel of potential mutations can be tested for in a short period of time. This method of analysis is particularly suitable for sickle cell anemia where each affected individual has the same point mutation. The ASO technique is also amenable to automation, as large samples can be tested simultaneously.

Types of Mutations Present in Human Genetic Disease

The types of mutations present for genetic diseases depend on the specific disease and often the ethnic background. Deletions have been discussed, and though they are often detectable by Southern blot analysis, deletions generally compose only about 10% of all gene mutations. Some notable exceptions include steroid sulfatase deficiency (90% are due to whole gene deletions), Duchenne muscular dystrophy (DMD) (60% have deletions of a part of the dystrophin gene), cystic fibrosis (CF) (two-thirds have a 3-bp deletion of codon 508, the ΔF508). The deletions of steroid sulfatase deficiency may be detected by Southern blot analysis, while smaller deletions of DMD and CF may be detected using PCR techniques.

Point mutations compose the largest percentage of genetic mutations seen in human disease. Sickle cell anemia is the classic point mutation, in which a GAG (Glu) is changed to a GTG (Val) at codon 6 of β-globin. The sickle mutation is the same in every patient with sickle cell anemia, which makes diagnosis extremely easy and amenable to automation. However, the point mutations in β-thalassemia often differ in each family, which poses a significant diagnostic challenge. In many disorders, a certain number of mutations comprise most of the mutations, so these can be tested for in affected individuals. For example, 32 mutations in CF can be screened since they make up over 90% of all mutations in CF patients. DNA is obtained from the patient and the mutation battery is run to determine if any of these mutations are present. Important to remember with this type of testing is the individual with a negative test. Just because the patient does not have one of these 32 mutations, it does not mean he/she does not have CF. It merely means the individual does not have one of the mutations tested. A different mutation will be missed unless DNA sequencing of the entire gene is performed.

Point mutations may cause several different types of effects upon the protein. If the point mutation changes an amino acid, it is termed a missense mutation. Missense mutations may or may not affect the protein depending on the location of amino acid change or the specific amino acid. To prove that missense mutations cause the phenotype of a particular disease, they must be studied *in vitro* to determine if they affect protein function. Nonsense mutations are point mutations that cause a termination codon for translation so that the resulting protein is truncated and

dysfunctional. The three codons that signify the termination of translation in the ribosomes are TAA, TAG, and TGA. If a mutation changes a TAC to a TAG, for example, translation will not proceed beyond this point. Frameshift mutations are deletions or insertions of bases that are not an exact multiple of three, so the genetic code is altered. Amino acids downstream may be changed completely, and commonly a premature stop codon is produced. The following example demonstrates all three types of mutations in a single patient. A female presenting with delayed puberty was found to have isolated follicle-stimulating hormone (FSH) deficiency due to compound heterozygous mutations in the FSH-β gene (15). One mutation inherited from her father was a missense mutation in exon 3 changing a cysteine to a glycine, and the other was a 2-bp deletion in the same exon inherited from her mother. The 2-bp deletion caused a frameshift, altering all of the amino acids downstream to the mutation until a premature stop codon was created, truncating the carboxy terminus of the protein. Both the missense and frameshift mutations were shown to result in decreased immunoactive and bioactive FSH *in vitro*, confirming their involvement in the phenotype (15).

Commonly, ethnic background affects the prevalence of certain mutations. For example, in Tay-Sachs disease, three mutations make up over 90% of all identified mutations in the hexosaminidase A gene in autosomal-recessive disease common in Ashkenazi Jews. In non-Jews, these three mutations make up only about 20%, while other mutations make up the other 80%.

Another more recently recognized type of mutation is triplet repeat expansion (Table 2.7). Some genes normally have a certain number of copies of 3 bp, which are repeated. However, when these repeats increase in number, presumably by expansion in germ cells or early postmitotic events, a disease phenotype results. The classic example is fragile X syndrome, an X-linked dominant disease with reduced penetrance, which consists of mental retardation, macroorchidism, and somewhat subtle facial features (enlarged jaw and ears). The FMR-1 gene located at a fragile site on Xq27 normally contains 5 to 50 repeats of a CGG triplet repeat sequence. The disease is transmitted by carrier females, who possess an increased number of triplet repeats, called a premutation (50 to 200 repeats). These carrier females are more likely to have an expansion of the triplet repeat (greater than 200 and often over 1,000 repeats), and when this occurs, fragile X syndrome results. In fragile X syndrome, the increased number of repeats render the messenger RNA (mRNA) inactivated (due to methylation), so no protein is made. A number of other diseases are caused by the expansion of triplet repeat sequences (Table 2.7). Of interest, all of these disorders are neurologic diseases, and most are autosomal-dominant diseases. Notable exceptions are fragile X syndrome and Friedreich's ataxia (autosomal recessive).

Another notable feature of diseases caused by triplet

TABLE 2.7. TRIPLET REPEAT DISEASES, THE GENE NAME, THE SPECIFIC BASES OF THE TRIPLET REPEAT, AND THE MODE OF INHERITANCE ARE SHOWN

Triplet Repeat Diseases	Gene Name	Specific Bases	Mode of Inheritance
Fragile X syndrome	FMR-1	CGG	XLD
Myotonic dystrophy	Myotonin protein kinase	CTG	AD
Spinobulbar and muscular atrophy	Androgen receptor	CAG	XLR
Huntington disease	Huntington	CAG	AD
Spinocerebellar atrophy type 1	Ataxin-1	CAG	AD
Spinocerebellar atrophy type 2	Ataxin-2	CAG	AD
Machado-Joseph disease	Ataxin-3	CAG	AD
Friedreich ataxia	Frataxin	GAA	AR
Dentatorubral-palladoluysian atrophy	Atrophin-1	CAG	AD
Spinocerebellar ataxia type 6	CACNL1A4/Ca^{2+} channel	CAG	AD

XLD, X-linked dominant; XLR, X-linked recessive; AR, autosomal recessive; AD, autosomal dominant. From Caskey CT, Pizzuti A, Fu Y-H, et al. Triplet repeat mutations in human disease. *Science* 1992; 256:784–789; and Heintz N, Zoghbi H. α-Synuclein—a link between Parkinson and Alzheimer diseases? *Nat Genet* 1997;16:325–327, with permission.

repeat expansion explains a feature of autosomal diseases that is called anticipation. Anticipation refers to the observation that the severity of the disease increases with successive generations. The classic example is myotonic dystrophy, in which an affected female who is affected as an adult with facial muscle weakness may have an infant with myotonia congenita, who has severe cardiac disease and myotonia. Generally speaking, the greater the number of triplet repeats, the more severe the phenotype. This increased number of repeats is usually present in the more severe individuals.

Fluorescent In Situ Hybridization

Fluorescent *in situ* hybridization (FISH) is a technique that may be used in conjunction with karyotype analysis, but does not replace this technique. FISH bridges molecular genetics and cytogenetics. The principles of FISH, similar to other DNA techniques, rely upon the complementarity of the nitrogenous bases of nucleotides. DNA, RNA, tissue, cells, or chromosomes are fixed to a slide and denatured (Fig. 2.18). A fluorescently labeled single-stranded DNA or RNA probe is then hybridized with the sample, the nonspecific binding is removed, and the sample is observed under a fluorescence microscope. FISH can be used to diagnose trisomy, translocations, and gene deletions too small to be detected with cytogenetics. If probes to chromosomes 21, 18, 13, X, and Y are used, simultaneous screening for the most common chromosomal aneuploidies can be done. Because of the great sensitivity of FISH, chromosomes can be detected in interphase cells and even in a single cell (Fig. 2.18). Single-cell FISH has been used in preimplantation genetic diagnosis of sexing embryos (particularly in X-linked recessive disorders, to avoid a male who could be affected), and for the diagnosis of trisomies and monosomies.

Recently, FISH technology has expanded to include multiplex FISH (or multifluor FISH), a procedure in which each chromosome is able to be colored differently upon hybridization to FISH probes (16,17). Using six different fluors, a specialized filter set, and computer software, 27 different probes were able to be detected simultaneously, and give each chromosome a different color (17). Multiplex FISH offers many advantages over standard FISH, including easy identification of numerical abnormalities, translocations, and relatively large chromosomal deletions (16,17). However, at the present time, the cost and clinical utility are uncertain for this new procedure, which is likely to gain acceptance as more data are gathered. In general, FISH is a costly procedure for a laboratory, and well-defined criteria for performance have not been established. It seems unlikely that FISH techniques will replace standard karyotype analysis, but rather will augment it (16). For example, even if probes for chromosomes 21, 18, 13, X, and Y are used, most unbalanced translocations in liveborns will be detected, but up to 20% would be missed (16).

Techniques to Evaluate RNA

Ribonucleic acid (RNA) consists of three types—messenger RNA (mRNA), transfer RNA (tRNA), and ribosomal RNA (rRNA). DNA is transcribed by RNA polymerase in the nucleus to mRNA, which is then translated in the ribosomes to protein. Messenger RNA makes up only a few percent of total RNA. RNA is a single-stranded nucleic acid very similar to DNA except that the sugar is ribose instead of deoxyribose, and uracil (U) replaces thymine and is complementary to adenine. However, RNA is more difficult to analyze because of the ubiquitous presence of enzymes that degrade RNA (RNAses), so special care is required.

To determine the presence and size of a transcript, RNA can be electrophoresed on a gel (without restriction enzyme digestion) and transferred to a nylon membrane (Northern blot). The Northern blot can then be probed for the

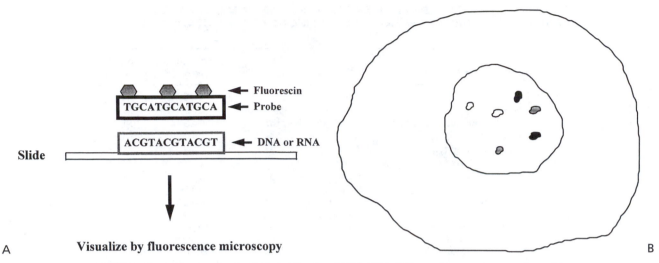

FIGURE 2.18. A: Fluorescent *in situ* hybridization (FISH). DNA, RNA, or chromosomes are immobilized on a slide, denatured, and hybridized with a single-stranded probe labeled with fluororescin. **B:** A schematic interphase cell is shown with two signals for chromosomes 21, 18, and 13.

transcript of interest similar to a Southern blot. Although DNA exists in every nucleated cell of the body, RNA is only expressed in certain tissues. For example, gonadotropin-releasing hormone (GnRH) is expressed in the hypothalamus and placenta, while FSH is expressed in the pituitary. If the gene is expressed in sufficient quantity, Northern blot analysis is able to detect expression. However, if the gene is expressed in only a small number of cells, such as the GnRH gene in neurons of the hypothalamus, Northern analysis may not easily detect its expression. In this instance, reverse transcriptase (RT)-PCR can be used to determine if expression occurs. RT-PCR has the sensitivity necessary to amplify small amounts of RNA within an organ. It even permits the detection of a low level of expression in peripheral WBCs, which do express most transcripts at low levels, so-called illegitimate transcription. With RT-PCR, RNA is first copied into complementary DNA (cDNA) using the enzyme reverse transcriptase. RT-PCR also takes advantage of mRNA, which normally has a poly-A tail placed on its 3′ end. To prime the synthesis of cDNA, a primer consisting of a string of complementary T sequence is often used. Following initial cDNA synthesis, primers specific for the transcript can then be used to amplify the cDNA. In addition to determining if expression occurs, RT-PCR may also be used clinically to determine if gene mutations affect RNA. As a general rule, RNA analysis is not usually used for clinical genetic analysis.

Genetic Basis of Cancer

Cancer results from genetic mutations, but overall only about 5% of cancers are familial. This is because most cancer is caused by an accumulation of mutations of many different genes over time, permitting increased cellular growth from normal cells to hyperplasia, to an adenoma, and then to a malignancy, which then may metastasize. These mutations are not usually in the germline (except in the 5% of familial cancers), but instead are in somatic cells, such as breast, ovary, prostate, etc. Since the mutations are not germline, they would not be expected to be inherited (18).

Among the first genetic mutations identified in cancer was the Philadelphia chromosome described in chronic myelogenous leukemia (CML). The Philadelphia chromosome was found to be a translocation between chromosomes 9 and 22, written as t(9;22)(q34;q11). A portion of the c-*Abl* proto-oncogene on 9q fuses with the BCR gene on chromosome 22. The resulting chimeric protein has tyrosine kinase activity and phosphorylating proteins, and causes uncontrolled cell growth. A number of translocations have been described in human leukemias, and other disorders (19). Recently, about 215 balanced and close to 1,600 unbalanced recurrent translocations were cataloged for 75 different neoplastic disorders including leukemias and tumors of the reproductive tract such as those of uterine, ovarian, or vaginal origin (19).

Presently, at least three types of cancer-causing genes are known: proto-oncogenes, tumor suppressor genes, and DNA repair genes. Proteins encoded by proto-oncogenes control normal cellular growth (18). When they acquire mutations in one allele, the proto-oncogene is converted to an oncogene and now uncontrolled cell growth may produce a malignancy. Examples include *ras*, *fos*, and *jun*, which may be mutant in somatic cells in a variety of sporadic cancers. The *RET* proto-oncogene is unique in that it causes an autosomal-dominant cancer in multiple endocrine neoplasia type 2 (MEN-2), consisting of three subtypes: MEN-2A [pheochromocytomas and medullary thyroid carcinoma

(MTC)]; MEN-2B (which has in addition skeletal abnormalities and ganglioneuromas of the gastrointestinal tract); and MEN-2C (MTC only) (20). However, in each of these three types of disease, mutations in the *RET* proto-oncogene, a gene encoding a protein containing a tyrosine kinase region, have been identified.

Tumor suppressor genes are genes that are effective in inhibiting tumor growth when both copies of each are present on a pair of chromosomes (such as the *BRCA1* gene on chromosome 17) (18,21). If both copies acquire mutations, rendering their suppression ineffective, uncontrolled tumor growth results. If an individual has inherited a mutation in one of these genes in the germline, one copy is nonfunctional from birth. If a second mutation occurs in a certain somatic cell such as the breast, both copies are now nonfunctional and breast cancer develops (Fig. 2.19). In this instance, disease tends to occur earlier in life (often in the 30s), is bilateral, and is transmitted in an autosomal-dominant fashion (Fig. 2.19). Examples include *BRCA1, BRCA2,* retinoblastoma, adenoma polyposis coli (APC), and Li-Fraumeni syndrome (18,21).

Two genes—*BRCA1* and *BRCA2*—account for the majority of familial breast cancers in humans (22). *BRCA1* mutations are more common than *BRCA2*, and cause breast and ovarian cancer in females, and prostate cancer in males. *BRCA2* mutations are more commonly associated with breast cancer–only families, and are more likely to be identified in families with affected males with breast cancer (22). Some familial cancer syndromes due to mutations in tumor suppressor genes can cause a variety of tumors, so pedigree analysis becomes extremely important. The Li-Fraumeni syndrome caused by mutations in the *p53* gene includes breast cancer, sarcomas, leukemia, brain, and adrenocortical tumors. This again, underscores the importance of obtaining a pedigree.

If no germline mutation of a tumor suppressor gene is

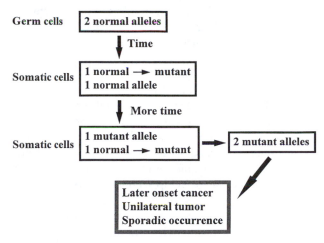

FIGURE 2.20. Sporadic cancer requires two hits to occur, so disease has later onset and is usually unilateral versus autosomal-dominant forms shown in Fig. 2.7.

present, it takes two "hits" to inactivate both copies of the tumor suppressor gene, which is much less likely. This causes sporadic cancer, of later onset, which is usually unilateral in location (Fig. 2.20).

Mutations in the DNA repair genes produce cancer in a similar pattern to tumor suppressor genes. Both copies need to contain mutations, and the probability is increased when a germline mutation exists. Normally, mutations continually occur in genomic DNA, but enzymes correct (or proofread) the mutant nitrogenous bases to their original sequence. The genes encoding these proteins, such as *MSH2, MLH1,* and others, may acquire mutations (germline or somatic) such that this proofreading activity is lost, and the sequences stay mutant. An example is hereditary nonpolyposis colon cancer (HNPCC), also termed Lynch type 2 syndrome due to *MLH1* and *MSH2* gene mutations (18). This autosomal-dominant disorder is characterized by the presence of colon cancer without precancerous polyps (unlike adenoma polyposis coli), but other cancers such as endometrial and breast cancer can also occur.

SUMMARY AND FUTURE DIRECTIONS

A basic understanding of clinical and molecular genetics is fundamental for clinicians of all specialties. To do proper counseling, the clinician must recognize potential patterns of inheritance in families. The construction of a pedigree greatly facilitates this process. The understanding of molecular genetic techniques is also important, as more and more DNA tests continue to be offered, and will eventually replace other methods of diagnosis. The human genome mapping project should be completed early in the 21st century, with the sequencing of the projected 100,000 human genes. The data from this project will lead to gene identification

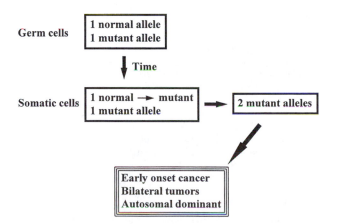

FIGURE 2.19. Autosomal-dominant cancer produces earlier, more severe disease since one mutant allele is present in the germline, so a second hit is much more likely to occur in somatic cells.

and diagnosis for an increasing number of human diseases. A better understanding of pathophysiology of disease will shortly follow, but ethics and treatment will lag behind gene discovery.

Newer automated techniques will render most currently used techniques obsolete. Multiplex FISH has recently been introduced into the research arena, and will likely gain clinical acceptance. FISH will be used to detect smaller and smaller areas of chromosomes, and already has been used to detect short repeated sequences of DNA. In the near future, FISH will probably permit the detection of single base changes. Automated chip technology will replace existing methods of gene screening (23). Chip technology has arisen from the interaction of the disciplines of synthetic oligonucleotide chemistry with photolithography used in the semiconductor industry (23). With these microchips, thousands of short oligonucleotide probes can be placed onto a small chip using photolithography. It has been estimated that up to 400,000 probes on a single chip may be resolved, which if 40 probes were used per gene, the entire genome could be screened using ten chips (23). Clearly, genetics will continue to advance at a rapid pace in the 21st century.

10 KEY POINTS

1. Pedigree construction provides additional information about family history that may not be obtained from a verbal history or written questionnaire.

2. Women should be rubella immune and take 0.4 mg of folic acid prior to conception to reduce the risks of birth defects (congenital rubella syndrome and neural tube defects, respectively).

3. The recurrence risk to offspring for a genetic disease depends upon its inheritance: autosomal dominant (50%), autosomal recessive (25%), X-linked recessive (50% males affected and 50% of females are carriers if the mother is a carrier), X-linked dominant (50% of males and 50% of females are affected if the mother is a carrier), and complex (usually 2%–4%).

4. Autosomal dominant diseases may have decreased penetrance (not all affected individuals have an abnormal phenotype) and variable expressivity (affected persons within the same family may have mild to severe symptoms), making their identification difficult.

5. Autosomal dominant diseases can be passed to offspring when neither parent is affected because of germline mosaicism, and the recurrence risk for future pregnancies is usually 2%–5%.

6. An individual with a balanced translocation has a chromosomal translocation, but is phenotypically normal; however, they are at risk of having a child with congenital anomalies with an unbalanced translocation.

7. A peripheral blood karyotype should be considered in patients with any of the following: recurrent abortion (two or more miscarriages or one miscarriage and one abnormal liveborn), gonadal failure (ovarian and testicular), and multiple congenital anomalies.

8. Most clinical genetic testing is performed by polymerase chain reaction (PCR) techniques with allele specific oligonucleotide probes, which test for specific mutations.

9. When the laboratory tests for gene mutations, it is important to know how many mutations are tested for, and if the results are negative, it only means that they are negative for the tested mutations (it is still possible a mutation not tested for is present).

10. Breast and ovarian cancer may occur in the same family in an autosomal dominant mode of inheritance due to *BRCA1* or *BRCA2* gene mutations.

REFERENCES

1. Layman LC. Pedigree analysis for the primary care physician. In: Sanfilippo JS, Smith RP, eds. *Primary care in obstetrics and gynecology: handbook for clinicians.* New York: Springer-Verlag, 1998:437–448.
2. Thompson MW, McInnes RR, Willard HF. Patterns of single gene inheritance. In: Thompson, Thompson, eds. *Genetics in medicine,* 5th ed. Philadelphia: WB Saunders, 1991:53–95.
3. Caskey CT, Pizzuti A, Fu Y-H, et al. Triplet repeat mutations in human disease. *Science* 1992;256:784–789.
4. Wallace DC. Diseases of the mitochondrial DNA. *Annu Rev Biochem* 1992;61:1175–1212.
5. Ledbetter DH, Engel E. Uniparental disomy in humans: development of an imprinting map and its implications in prenatal diagnosis. *Hum Mol Genet* 1995;4:1757–1764.
6. Hall JG. Somatic mosaicism: observations related to human genetics. *Am J Hum Genet* 1988;43:355–363.
7. Simpson JL, Golbus MS. Anatomical malformations inherited in polygenic/multifactorial fashion. In: Simpson JL, Golbus MS, eds. *Genetics in obstetrics and gynecology,* 2nd ed. Philadelphia: WB Saunders, 1992:79–92.
8. Gelehrter TD, Collins FS. Structure and behavior of genes and chromosomes. In: Gelehrter TD, Collins FS, eds. *Principles of medical genetics.* Baltimore: Williams & Wilkins, 1990:9–25.
9. Jones KL. *Smith's recognizable patterns of human malformation.* Philadelphia: WB Saunders, 1997.
10. Simpson JL, Bombard A. Chromosomal abnormalities in spontaneous abortion: frequency, pathology, and genetic counselling. In: Bennett MJ, Edmonds DK, eds. *Spontaneous and recurrent abortion.* Oxford, England: Blackwell Scientific, 1987:51–76.
11. Layman LC, Reindollar RH. The genetics of hypogonadism. *Infertil Reprod Med Clin North Am* 1994;5:53–68.
12. Micic M, Micic S, Diklic V. Hypospermiogenesis and chromosomal aberrations: a clinical study of azoospermia and oligospermic men with normal and abnormal karyotype. *Int J Androl* 1984;4:546–558.
13. Layman LC. Basic concepts of molecular biology as applied to pediatric and adolescent gynecology. *Obstet Gynecol Clin North Am* 1992;19:1–26.
14. Layman LC. Molecular biology in reproductive endocrinology. *Curr Opin Obstet Gynecol* 1995;7:328–339.
15. Layman LC, Lee EJ, Peak DB, et al. Delayed puberty and hypogonadism caused by a mutation in the follicle stimulating hormone beta-subunit gene. *N Engl J Med* 1997;337:607–611.

16. LeBeau M. One FISH, two FISH, red FISH, blue FISH. *Nat Genet* 1996;12:341–344.

17. Speicher MR, Ballard SG, Ward DC. Karyotyping human chromosomes by combinatorial multi-fluor FISH. *Nat Genet* 1996;12:368–375.

18. Weitzel JN. Cancer genetics. *Infertil Reprod Med Clin North Am* 1994;5:121–142.

19. Mitelman R, Mertens F, Johansson B. A breakpoint map of recurrent chromosomal rearrangements in human neoplasia. *Nat Genet* 1997;15:417–474.

20. van Heyningeny V. One gene-four syndromes. *Nature* 1994;367:319–320.

21. Haber D, Harlow E. Tumour-suppressor genes: evolving definitions in the genomic age. *Nat Genet* 1997;16:320–322.

22. Szabo CI, King M-C. Population genetics of BRCA1 and BRCA2. *Am J Hum Genet* 1997;60:1013–1020.

23. To affinity and beyond [editorial]. *Nat Genet* 1996;14:367–370.

24. Hook EB. Rates of chromosomal abnormalities of different maternal ages. *Obstet Gynecol* 1981;58:282.

25. Warburton D, Strobino B. Recurrent spontaneous abortion. In: Bennett MJ, Edmonds DK, eds. *Spontaneous and recurrent abortion.* Oxford, England: Blackwell Scientific, 1987:193–213.

26. Heintz N, Zoghbi H. α-Synuclein—a link between Parkinson and Alzheimer diseases? *Nat Genet* 1997;16:325–327.

3

IMMUNOBIOLOGY OF REPRODUCTION

JOSEPH A. HILL
DEBORAH J. ANDERSON

Immmunologic aspects of reproductive medicine have been the subject of many contemporary studies. Many of the immunologic theories proposed to be involved in reproduction have not withstood vigorous investigation. However, immunologic questions remain since the conceptus and spermatozoa must evade rejection in immunologically foreign hosts. This chapter reviews the basic immunologic principles and how they have been applied to reproductive biology.

IMMUNOLOGIC PRINCIPLES

The primary function of the immune system is to defend the host against non-self tissue (reviewed in refs. 1 and 2). Immune responses are either innate or acquired depending on prior exposure to antigen, acquired specificity of response, and immunologic memory. Innate immunity provides a rapid, nonspecific response such as occurs in inflammation. Inflammation is a localized protective response characterized by vascular dilatation, increased blood flow, and vascular permeability with protein exudation and diapedesis of white blood cells (WBCs). Soluble components of inflammation include complement proteins; eicosanoids, oxygen radicals, and platelet-activating factors; lysozyme and histamine; chemokines; other cytokine/growth factors; and defensins. These soluble factors are secreted by macrophages, other phagocytic cells, lymphocytes [including T cells, B cells, and natural killer (NK) cells], mast cells, basophils, platelets, fibroblasts, and epithelial and endothelial cells. Innate immunity also includes mechanical barriers such as the skin and mucosal epithelium, and effector cells such as phagocytes and NK cells. The innate immune response does not have memory and is similar in intensity whether it is a reaction to a first or a repeat pathogenic or antigenic exposure. Amplification of the innate immune response may occur through complement activation and cytokine-mediated gene activation.

The acquired immune response is a time-dependent, specific response relying on the differentiation of antigen-primed T and B lymphocytes. The first exposure (primary immune response) of these cells to an antigenic stimulus may sensitize these cells to become activated and to prolifer-

ate upon subsequent exposure (secondary immune response, "memory"). The magnitude of secondary immune responses may be different from initial exposure. Acquired immunity involves antigen-presenting cells (antibodies); CD4[+] and CD8[+] T lymphocytes; plasma cells, which secrete antigen-specific immunoglobulins and lymphocytes; and lymphocyte-derived cytokines.

Innate and acquired immunity are complementary in terms of timing and degree of specificity. Macrophages, important phagocytes in innate immune responses, also play a critical role in antigen presentation for acquired immunity, while antibodies, involved primarily in acquired immunity, may also participate in innate immunity by binding pathogens, which facilitate their phagocytosis by macrophages.

The source of antigens (substances capable of eliciting immunity) may be non-self (bacteria; virus; and potentially in the case of women, sperm, embryo, and trophoblast) or self (DNA, histones, phospholipids, and potentially in the case of women, oocytes, endometrium, decidua, and endometriosis tissue, or in the case of men, spermatozoa). An immune response against non-self tissue derived from a different member of the same species is termed allogenic immunity, while that against self is termed autoimmunity.

Immune responses are initiated by antigen-processing cells, which include macrophages, dendritic cells, fibroblasts, endothelial cells, Kupffer cells of the liver, Langerhans' cells of the skin, and Hofbauer cells of the placenta. Antigen-processing cells present antigens to T cells in association with surface protein molecules called major histocompatibility complex (MHC) determinants, grouped as either MHC class I [human leukocyte antigen (HLA)-A, -B, -C] molecules or MHC class II (HLA-DR, -DP, -DQ) molecules. Class I determinants are expressed on nearly all nucleated cells and normally bind peptides from endogenously processed antigens for presentation to CD8[+] cytotoxic T cells. Class II determinants are expressed primarily on antigen-processing cells where they bind peptides from exogenously derived antigens, and present them to CD4[+] helper T cells. In both CD4[+] and CD8[+] T cells, antigens presented with MHC molecules activate the T-cell receptor and trigger immunologic functions. In contrast, NK cells also recognize MHC allotypes, but in these cells MHC class I recognition inhibits their cytolytic function.

Whether an acquired immune response develops along a cellular or humoral pathway often depends on the differentiation pathway of CD4$^+$ T-helper (Th) cells. It is now clear that CD4$^+$ TH cells have at least two different profiles of cytokine production (TH1 and TH2). TH1 cytokines include interleukin-2 (IL-2), IL-12, interferon-γ (IFN-γ), tumor necrosis factor-β (TNF-β), and perhaps TNF-α. Th2 cytokines include IL-4, IL-5, IL-6, IL-10, IL-13, and perhaps IL-15. These cytokine patterns determine the type of response mediated by CD4$^+$ T-helper cells. Th1 cytokines activate cytotoxic, inflammatory, and delayed hypersensitivity reactions that underlie cellular immunity, while TH2 cytokines are associated with the stimulation of strong antibody and allergic responses. Cytokines from TH1 cells inhibit the action of TH2 cells and vice versa. Therefore, an immune response generally tends to settle into a TH1-type or TH2-type response. Factors that influence the differentiation of CD4$^+$ TH cells include (a) the local cytokine environment at the time of antigenic stimulation, (b) the antigen dose, (c) the antigen-presenting cells and the cytokines they produce, (d) the host genetic background, and (e) the activity of co-stimulatory molecules and hormones present in the local environment (3,4).

Cellular immunity is mediated by cytotoxic T cells and NK cells. The most important role of cellular immunity is the elimination of cells infected with virus. Cytotoxic T cells and NK cells use a variety of different mechanisms to kill their targets. These include direct cell–cell signaling via surface molecules and indirect signaling via cytokines. In addition, many CD8$^+$ cytotoxic T cells and NK cells have granules that contain several proteins, including perforin and granzyme, that damage target cell membranes. CD4$^+$ cytotoxic T cells can also mediate cytotoxicity via Fas or the TNF receptor on target cells.

Humoral immunity is mediated by immunoglobulins (Igs) that are produced by plasma cells in response to antigenic stimuli. Immunoglobulins can be classified into five isotypes: IgG, IgA, IgM, IgE, and IgD. IgD and IgE are primarily membrane associated, and play a role in β-cell maturation and allergic responses, respectively. IgA predominates in most mucosal secretions, whereas IgG predominates in serum. Immunoglobulins of the IgM isotype are produced early during the humoral immune response, and are often of lower affinity than other antibody isotypes.

Although there is clear operational evidence for the existence of antigen-specific suppressor (T^s) cells, it is unlikely that they represent a functionally separate T-cell subset. There is evidence that both CD4$^+$ and CD8$^+$ lymphocytes can suppress immune responses. This might operate through direct cytotoxicity of antigen-presenting T cells, negative regulation of signal transduction, or through "suppressive" cytokines such as transforming growth factor-β (TGF-β), which is inhibitory to virtually all immune functions, especially if present before cell activation.

IMMUNOLOGY AND REPRODUCTION
Female Genital Tract

Immunologic factors have been implicated in infertility and recurrent pregnancy loss. Reproductive processes may be affected adversely by cellular or antibody-mediated mechanisms either before or after fertilization or implantation. For reproductive processes to be affected immunologically, immune response cells and their secreted products must be present in reproductive tissues and secretions. WBCs of all lineages have been described in both male and female reproductive tissues (reviewed in refs. 5–7). These cells are capable of activation, proliferation, and secretion of a myriad of soluble cytokine and growth factor proteins. Thus, an anatomic basis exists for immunologic involvement in reproductive physiology and pathophysiology. However, very few B cells and antibody-secreting plasma cells are present in normal reproductive tissues except in the subepithelial layers of the endocervix, the ectocervix, the vagina, and the fallopian tubes. Approximately 70% of these plasma cells are IgA positive, and of these, 50% to 75% colabel for J-chain, indicating that the majority of local IgA synthesis is polymorphic. IgG present in human cervical mucus is thought to represent a serum transudate primarily. Plasma cells are rarely detected in the human ovary or uterus. Thus, an anatomic basis does not exist for local antibody involvement in uterine and ovarian events. This, however, does not preclude the possibility of systemic antibody-mediated mechanisms, as antigen trafficking into pelvic-draining lymph nodes may still enable antibody production and secretion leading to antibody localization in reproductive tissues. Local IgA production does occur normally in the cervical vaginal environment and is increased in cases of infection. Accumulation of antibody-secreting plasma cells also occurs in cases of endometritis and salpingitis.

Endometrium

Several cytokines have been localized in human endometrium throughout the menstrual cycle. The presence of immune cell–derived cytokines in the endometrium provides a mechanism for antigen recognition and immune responses, which facilitate host defense. These proteins may also affect local reproductive processes. Perturbations of the endocrine system, the immune system, or both, may lead to alterations of the normal implantation process resulting in reproductive failure. The presence of IL-1α, IL-1β, TGF-α, IL-6, and IL-1 receptor antagonist (IRAP) have been reported in human endometrium, and cells with morphologic features resembling macrophages contain IRAP. IL-6 localized to epithelial cells, while IL-1, IL-1α, and TGF-α localized to cells in the stroma and epithelium. TNF-α, colony-stimulating factor 1 (CSF-1), and IFN-γ have also been found in human endometrium. The presence of TNF-α and CSF-1 appear to be hormonally regulated as their concentrations vary with phase of the menstrual cycle. Granulocyte-macrophage CSF (GM-CSF) and CSF-1 stimulate the proliferation and differentiation of macrophage precursors and may be responsible for increased macrophage numbers in the endometrium during implantation.

Ovary

A growing body of evidence suggests that immunologic cytokines may have important direct modulatory roles within the ovary. TNF-α is found within the human corpus luteum. Follicular fluid and granulosa cell culture supernatants contain immunoreactive TNF-α by enzyme-linked immunosorbent assay (ELISA) with levels of 100 to 170 pg/mL and 145 to 806 pg TNF-α/500,000 cells, respectively. The cellular source of TNF-α may be granulosa cells and ovarian macrophages. TNF-α inhibits granulosa cell progesterone and estradiol synthesis *in vitro* (reviewed in ref. 8).

IL-1α and IL-1β, which are secreted by macrophages, T lymphocytes, and other cells, may also play important roles in ovarian physiology. Circulating levels of IL-1 peak after ovulation and have been proposed to be involved in the process of ovulation (8). IL-1β and IL-1α messenger RNA (mRNA) transcripts have been found in whole human ovary, and IL-1β mRNA expression has been detected in granulosa cell suspensions free of macrophages (9). IL-1 has been found to affect *in vitro* human luteinized granulosa cell estradiol but not progesterone production at concentrations of 1 to 50 ng/mL in some, but not all, studies.

IFN-γ has also been demonstrated in the human ovary. The cellular source of IFN-γ within the human ovary appears to be activated T lymphocytes. IFN-γ was found in highest concentrations in atretic follicles and regressing corpora lutea, suggesting that IFN-γ may be involved in follicular atresia and corpus luteum demise (10). Ovarian T-lymphocyte expression of IFN-γ is stimulated by TNF-α. IFN-γ has also been demonstrated in the follicular fluid (11) of women during *in vitro* fertilization (IVF) cycles at concentrations ranging from 5 to 35 IU/mL (0.25 to 1.75 ng/mL). IFN-γ has also been reported to inhibit estradiol and progesterone biosynthesis of human granulosa cells (12), and therefore may be an important intraovarian regulator of follicular atresia and corpus luteum regression.

Vaginal/Cervical Factors

Sexually active females are repeatedly exposed to allogenic sperm (several billion over the course of a lifetime), yet they usually do not develop sperm immunity that results in infertility. However, IgA and IgG immunoglobulins directed against sperm antigens are often found in cervicovaginal secretions of infertile women. Antibodies to sperm are present in approximately 5% of reproductive-age women. In one series, circulating cervical and vaginal antisperm antibodies were present in 13% and 8% of infertile women,

respectively (13). Several mechanisms have been postulated to explain antisperm antibody-mediated infertility including tail-directed antibodies that may impair motility and thus penetration of cervical mucus; antisperm antibodies may facilitate macrophage phagocytosis of sperm (sperm cytolysis is also facilitated through the complement pathway); or head-directed antibodies may impair oocyte penetration. Antisperm antibodies in animals and humans have been associated with impaired fertilization, and in cases where fertilization occurred, subsequent embryo development (reviewed in ref. 14). Head-directed antisperm antibodies have been associated with decreased fertilization of human oocytes *in vitro,* and antibodies to sperm heads have been reported in the sera of 66% of women who failed to fertilize, but in only 6% of women who achieved fertilization during IVF (15).

The integrity of mucosal surfaces of the reproductive tract, the number of partners, and the amount of exposure to sperm antigens may be important variables in determining who develops immunity to sperm. Lesions of the female genital tract including cervical cancer may also contribute to the development of antisperm antibodies. Immunosuppressive factors present in semen and vaginal fluids may prevent sensitization and protect spermatozoa from immunologic attack, but these factors have been reported to be absent or diminished in many males with antisperm antibody–positive partners (reviewed in ref. 16).

Given the unreliability of the postcoital test as a predictor of cervical factor infertility, and the fact that there is no difference in IVF–embryo transfer (ET) outcome between women with antisperm antibodies and women with tubal factor infertility (16), direct sperm and cervical mucus testing for sperm antibodies is considered by many to be a historic relic.

Cellular immunity to sperm antigens in women has been documented. However, the precise role that cellular immunity to sperm may play as a contributing factor to female infertility has yet to be determined. *In vivo,* it is possible that leukocytes, microorganisms, and other antigens present in seminal fluid may elicit immune responses that could impair normal reproduction through immune cell activation, culminating in the release of soluble factors detrimental to sperm viability or function. This theory is supported by evidence of increased leukocyte numbers in women with cervical factor infertility and unexplained infertility compared with controls (17). Further studies are needed to determine the contribution of cell-mediated immune responses originating in the cervix to infertility.

Uterine/Tubal Factor

Immunologic infertility at the level of the uterus and fallopian tube may occur as the result of cellular immune responses or antibody-mediated immune responses to pelvic infection, endometriosis, sperm, or other antigens. The presence of immune and inflammatory cells within reproductive tissues may contribute to reproductive difficulty through the secretion of Th1-type cytokines since IFN-γ can inhibit embryo development (18), implantation (19), and trophoblast proliferation (20) *in vitro*. While syncytiotrophoblasts appear to support local reproductive events through expression of IFN-γ at low concentrations (21), higher concentrations of local IFN-γ produced by large numbers of activated T lymphocytes may hinder reproduction (22).

Reproductive events taking place in the fallopian tube may be influenced in a similar fashion by the WBCs and cytokines present in peritoneal fluid. Direct actions of leukocyte-derived cytokines on gametes and embryos have been well documented. Supernatants from cultures of peripheral blood leukocytes decrease sperm motility (23). TNF-α and IFN-γ have adverse effects on sperm motion parameters *in vitro* (24) and may theoretically contribute to infertility. Cytokines secreted into the peritoneal fluid may impair fertilization as suggested by inhibited fertilization in the hamster egg penetration assay (25). Inhibition of *in vitro* sperm penetration has been attributed to peritoneal macrophages (26). Macrophages may also impair fertilization through phagocytosis of spermatozoa (27). Embryotoxicity may result from exposure of the embryo to peritoneal fluid of women with unexplained infertility and endometriosis containing high concentrations of TNF-α or IFN-γ. Similarly, high levels of complement, which have been reported in cases of endometriosis (28), impair sperm-egg binding (29). This could occur since both sperm and the oolemna of the egg express complement receptors, and complement has been proposed to be necessary for fertilization by facilitating sperm-egg interaction. Therefore, in cases where there is excess complement, the corresponding receptors may be saturated, which would prevent sperm-egg binding. Thus, WBCs and their secreted cytokines in peritoneal fluid, in some cases, may adversely affect normal reproductive processes.

Ovarian Factor

The immune system may be involved in ovarian physiology and pathophysiology through both cellular and antibody-mediated mechanisms. Resident macrophages and T lymphocytes in the ovary may inhibit estrogen and progesterone synthesis through the secretion of the cytokines IFN-γ, TNF-α, and IL-1. The presence of large numbers of activated macrophages and T lymphocytes in atretic follicles and regressing corpora lutea contribute to the process of follicular atresia and corpus luteum regression through the secretion of their cytokines. It is also possible that immunologic cytokines may inhibit estrogen production in the developing follicle, thereby thwarting folliculogenesis, leading to anovulation or oligoovulation. High local concentrations of these cytokines may also have direct effects on the oocyte, and thus interfere with fertilization or embryo development. Disease states such as endometriosis and pelvic infection,

which increase immune cell infiltration into reproductive tissues, increasing the local concentrations of immunologic cytokines, may also affect follicular development. Conversely, TNF-α and IFN-γ may facilitate normal luteal regression and follicular atresia when present at concentrations of >0.5 ng/mL, which are within the physiologic ranges found in follicular and peritoneal fluids. Alternatively, cytokine-induced impairment of normal follicular development or progesterone secretion in the luteal phase of the cycle may result in luteal phase insufficiency.

Cytokines secreted by activated WBCs within the peritoneal cavity may affect reproductive processes through local paracrine influences on adjacent reproductive organs such as the ovary. Increased concentrations of IL-1α (0.5 to 1.0 ng/mL) and TNF-α (>10 ng/mL) are found in peritoneal fluid samples of patients with primary infertility and endometriosis (30,31), and these cytokines may adversely affect follicular growth and corpus luteum viability at these concentrations.

Although B lymphocytes, plasma cells, and immunoglobulins are generally not present in the human ovary, premature ovarian failure (POF) may occur through cellular and antibody-mediated mechanisms. Cytokines such as IFN-γ may play a role in the pathogenesis of POF and unexplained infertility through the induction of MHC class II antigens on granulosa cells (32). IFN-γ–enhanced expression of MHC class II antigens in response to foreign antigens or genetic predisposition could trigger a humoral and cell-mediated immune response, allowing recognition of granulosa cells by immune response cells, culminating in disordered ovulation or ultimately to ovarian failure.

Autoantibodies in Female Reproductive Difficulty

Antiovarian antibodies have been reported in the sera of infertile women undergoing fertility treatments but not in fertile controls. In the small number of infertile women studied, the presence of these antibodies correlated with decreased fertilization rates, cleavage rates, and pregnancy rates (reviewed in ref. 33). While the stimulus for the production of antiovarian antibodies in this report was undetermined, viral antigens have been implicated as an antibody-mediated cause of ovarian failure in cases of mumps orchitis.

The concept that autoantibodies are an important cause of reproductive difficulty has been proposed historically. It has been speculated that antiphospholipid antibodies (APAs), which have been associated with recurrent pregnancy loss, may interfere with reproductive processes prior to implantation or after implantation, but prior to the detection of a clinical pregnancy. Some have suggested that polyclonal B-cell activation represents a basic immunologic abnormality associated with pregnancy loss and have speculated that this B-cell abnormality can also be operative in infertile patients with endometriosis, unexplained infertility, or failing repeated IVF-ET attempts (34). Testing for a variety of antismooth muscle, nuclear, and DNA antibodies in addition to antiphospholipid antibodies has been performed in an attempt to detect immunologic infertility. Unfortunately, none of the studies seeking to correlate autoantibodies with various infertility categories and pregnancy outcomes have been adequately controlled or have used standardized assays, which renders a definitive conclusion regarding causality problematic.

IgG, IgM, and IgA immunoglobulins against smooth muscle, nuclear, and phospholipid antigens have been compared between women with and without reproductive difficulty. The prevalence of autoantibodies to smooth muscle, nuclear, and phospholipid antigens was significantly greater in women with unexplained infertility compared to normal pregnant women (reviewed in ref. 35). The results of a battery of 33 separate autoantibody assays against a number of different antigens in women with unexplained infertility and unexplained recurrent pregnancy loss revealed that one test result was positive in 23 of 26 (88%) women with unexplained infertility, prompting the suggestion that women with unexplained infertility suffer from polyclonal B-cell activation with resultant production of autoantibodies (34). Unfortunately, fertile controls were not included in this study, rendering conclusions conjectural. Given the number of unstandardized assays performed on these individuals, it is likely that a positive result occurred by chance alone, especially when using greater than the 95th percentile as the definition of an abnormal test result. When this is done, the chance of finding an abnormal value in 21 such tests would be $1 - (0.95)^{21}$ or approximately 69%.

Studies correlating autoantibody status with reproductive outcome during IVF are conflicting with the majority of studies reporting no correlation. One study (36), in which serum was assayed from 105 randomly selected IVF patients with tubal factor and unexplained infertility, reported that IVF outcome including pregnancy rates and pregnancy loss did not correlate with a positive antibody status. While the results of this study were negative, adequate controls necessary to draw a meaningful conclusion were not included in this study. Nevertheless, these data do not support the theory that polyclonal B-cell activation is responsible for adverse reproductive outcome in couples exposed to assisted reproductive technologies. In another report (37) comparing autoantibody production with IVF outcome, 32% of women who failed to conceive were reported to be antibody positive compared with 0% of those who conceived. Treatment with prednisone and aspirin resulted in a 47% pregnancy rate in a subsequent cycle. Unfortunately, this report did not state when antibody status was assessed (before, during, or after pregnancy) and treatment was neither randomized nor effectively controlled. The pregnancy rates of those women not treated were also not given. Thus, couples may have done equally well in a subsequent cycle regardless of being treated with aspirin and prednisone.

Notwithstanding the lack of scientific data supporting the autoantibody theory for unexplained infertility, many individuals promote empiric treatments for autoantibodies in conjunction with IVF. It is beyond the scope of this text to explain all the reasons that this recommendation should go unheeded, except to say that at the present time there is little convincing data to support the concept of autoantibody-related infertility in couples with unexplained infertility.

In a study evaluating 498 infertile women, a positive antiphospholipid antibody test was found in 2% to 4% compared with 0% in 125 fertile women. Positive values were not found in women with unexplained infertility (n = 53), but were found in those with tubal factor (49%), male factor (2.7%), an ovulation disorder (1.7%), and in those with endometriosis (1.4%). Antiphospholipid antibodies were observed in only four of 40 women (three with tubal factor fertility and one with endometriosis) who had repeatedly failed to achieve a pregnancy following IVF-ET. A positive value was not found in any of the seven women with unexplained infertility who consistently failed to achieve a pregnancy following IVF-ET (38). The largest study published to date in 798 women having IVF-ET indicated that testing for APA was not clinically useful (39). Although many women may be autoantibody positive, especially when using poorly standardized assays, the presence of these autoantibodies was associated with neither the establishment nor the maintenance of successful pregnancy (39). The concept that autoimmunity is a cause of infertility is also unlikely since infertility is not a component of well-characterized autoimmune disorders such as systemic lupus erythematosus.

Additional studies would be needed to develop a scientific rational for a theory of autoantibody-mediated infertility, since no specific autoantibody has been identified that can consistently interfere with specific reproductive processes. Randomized, double-blind, placebo-controlled, clinical trials should provide the basis for broad-based treatment recommendations in couples with unexplained infertility rather than belief in efficacy based on inadequately designed observational studies.

Recurrent Pregnancy Loss as an Immune Disorder

A workup to rule out non-immunologic causes of recurrent pregnancy loss includes: hysterosalpingogram to exclude uterine anomalies, submucosal leiomyomata or Asherman's syndrome, hormonal evaluation (TSH, prolactin) to exclude hypothyroidism or hyperprolactinemia, karyotyping of the couple to exclude balanced translocation, and endometrial biopsy to exclude luteal phase defect. The workup may also include a day 3 FSH and estradiol to exclude diminished ovarian reserve and an examination for thrombophila as demonstrated by a deficiency of antithrombin 3, protein C, protein S, the presence of a Factor 5 Leiden mutation or hyperhomocysteinemia. In addition to these possible causes of recurrent pregnancy loss, a discussion of immunological etiology is appropriate.

The developing conceptus is immunologically foreign to the maternal immune system due to its paternally inherited gene products and tissue-specific differentiation antigens. Speculation has therefore arisen that pregnancy loss may be due to impaired maternal immune tolerance to the semiallogenic fetus (reviewed in ref. 40). Both autoimmune and alloimmune mechanisms have been proposed.

The autoimmune theory with the most validity regarding pregnancy loss involves the antiphospholipid antibody syndrome in which IgG and perhaps IgM antibodies against negatively changed phospholipid components of cell membranes lead to vascular thrombosis within the placental bed or inhibit trophoblast syncytial formation culminating in pregnancy loss. This condition usually manifests in fetal loss after 10 weeks of gestation (41). Whether antiphospholipid antibodies are causative, coincidental, or a consequence of pregnancy loss remains controversial. Similarly, which antiphospholipid antibodies are involved, the incidence of their occurrence and the precise mechanisms of how they mediate loss also remains controversial.

Most investigators would agree that testing for lupus anticoagulant with an activated partial thromboplastin time (aPTT) or the more informative Russell viper venom time, and the IgG and perhaps IgM isotypes of anticardiolipin and antiphosphatidyl serine antibodies, should be part of the clinical evaluation of recurrent pregnancy loss. Confirmation of positive results is mandatory as low levels or unsustained moderate levels are not clinically helpful. Determination of the IgA isotype for anticardiolipin and antiphosphatidyl serine or any of the isotypes of other antiphospholipid antibodies are not useful clinically (42).

Precisely how to treat the antiphospholipid syndrome is also a matter of controversy. Prophylactic anticoagulation with 81 mg aspirin and heparin (10,000 to 20,000 units daily) or low molecular weight heparin (2,500 to 5,000 units daily) appears to be the treatment of choice since placental damage due to thrombosis is thought to be the end result of phospholipid autoimmunity. Due to the inherent risks of anticoagulant therapy even with aspirin (2% risk of abruption), the empiric use of these therapies is not justified for women without evidence of the antiphospholipid syndrome. Initiating these therapies prior to conception is also potentially dangerous due to the risk of bleeding at the time of ovulation.

Other therapeutic approaches have been attempted, including plasmaphoresis and intravenous immunoglobulin (IVIG) infusions. These therapies are not justified due to the lack of definitive studies substantiating their use (43).

The most recent alloimmune hypothesis proposed for some cases of reproductive difficulty is that of immunodystrophism (44) involving TH1 immunity to trophoblast or other antigens (45). Currently, an ELISA is used (ETF-

L Assay, Sage Biopharma, CA) to assess the potential of peripheral blood mononuclear cells to secrete the potentially embryo and trophoblast toxic (46) TH1 cytokine, IFN-γ, in response to trophoblast stimulation (45). Modifications of this assay have been used in over 3,500 women with a history of recurrent pregnancy loss in the Center for Reproductive Medicine at Brigham and Women's Hospital since 1986. Depending on the series, approximately 20% of women with otherwise unexplained recurrent pregnancy loss produce IFN-γ in response to trophoblast stimulation.

Another alloimmune hypothesis for recurrent pregnancy loss that received attention historically was that involving "blocking antibodies." This hypothesis was based on the supposition that a maternal, antifetal, cellular immune response developed in all pregnancies unless it was blocked by a serum factor (presumed antibody), and in the absence of this antibody, fetal loss occurred (47). This theory has not fulfilled the criteria for causality largely because 40% of normal multigravid women do not make antibodies against paternal antigens (48). When they did occur, they usually did so following 28 weeks of gestation and they may disappear between normal pregnancies (49). The most compelling evidence disproving the blocking antibody hypothesis is that women incapable of antibody secretion nevertheless can achieve successful pregnancies (50).

Immunologic testing and therapies designed to address the blocking antibody hypothesis have been disputed repeatedly (reviewed in ref. 51). Nevertheless, these tests continue to be offered by some to couples experiencing reproductive difficulty. These include parental HLA typing, specifically HLA-DQα; antipaternal cytotoxic antibodies (leukocyte antibody detection assay); embryotoxicity and cytokine assessment of peripheral serum; and immune phenotype profiles (CD56 and CD16 positive cells) of peripheral blood.

Endometriosis as an Immune Disorder

Both innate and adaptive immunity have been proposed to be involved in the development and continuance of endometriosis and its sequalae (reviewed in ref. 52). Endometriosis has also been hypothesized to be an autoimmune disease (reviewed in ref. 53). According to these theories, abnormal immunologic defense results in the inability to clear retrograde menstrual debris from the peritoneal environment. Ectopic endometrium is believed to be phagocytosed by activated macrophages and presented to T cells. T cells are supposed to become activated by ectopic endometrial antigens presented by macrophages, which proliferate and differentiate into functional T-cell subsets with helper, suppressor, and cytotoxic properties. NK cells are also believed to participate in the clearance of endometrium that is shed retrograde into the peritoneal cavity during menses. The inability to remove autologous ectopic endometrium is theorized to prolong the accompanying inflammatory response leading to the elaboration of growth and other competence cytokine factors that facilitate ectopic endometrial implantation, maintenance, and growth. Cytokines produced in response to ectopic endometrial antigen activation are believed in turn to activate resting B cells, facilitating their differentiation into antibody-secreting plasma cells. Antibodies may then be produced against endometrial cell-derived phospholipids, histones, and nucleotides. These aberrant immunologic responses may then lead to the sequalae of endometriosis, including adhesion formation, infertility, and pelvic pain. Despite the many articles claiming the validity of these intriguing hypotheses very little rigorously derived data exists (reviewed in ref. 54).

Correlations between endometriosis and autoimmune diseases include the observation that they both normally occur in women and have a tendency to run in families. Autoimmune diseases, however, are associated with certain HLA alleles, so much so that it is now possible to estimate the relative risk of developing autoimmunity with every known HLA allele. Pelvic endometriosis affects women predominantly because only women menstruate and are thus at risk for disease development. A strong genetic component exists for developing endometriosis; however, no association with specific HLA haplotypes has been substantiated. To prove definitively that a particular disease is autoimmune in origin, demonstration of disease must be confirmed in normal animals following the adaptive transfer of immunoglobulin from the blood or affected tissues of individuals with the disease. Such adaptive antibody transfer studies have not been performed. There is also no proof that complement activation occurs specifically in the endometrium of women with endometriosis. Many studies have reported levels of immunoglobulin and complement in the peripheral circulation of women with and without endometriosis; however, these studies cannot be compared properly due to differences in study design and the methodologies used. Study design flaws have compromised most endometriosis studies, with imprecise definitions of patient populations and poorly standardized methodologies being the most common flaws.

The observation that cellular immunity to autologous endometrium was suppressed in rhesus monkeys with spontaneous endometriosis led to speculation that endometriosis developed only in women with altered cellular immunity (55). Cell-mediated immunity facilitates the removal of foreign antigens. However, the antigenicity of ectopic endometrium has never been proven. Ectopic endometrium has also never been shown to be a natural target for phagocytic or other antigen-presenting cells, and has never been shown to cause activation of any immune or inflammatory cell population. There are data that demonstrate, however, that endometriosis is associated with an inflammatory response, but this may simply be the effect of intraperitoneal bleeding. T-cell–mediated cytotoxicity to autologous, nonstandarized, endometrial tissue was reported to be significantly reduced in subfertile women with endometriosis compared to subfertile women without disease (reviewed in refs. 52–54). Studies

assessing cytotoxic T-lymphocyte (CTL) responses to nonautologous target cells are invalid because such responses require MHC self-recognition.

Defective NK cell activity has also been reported in women with endometriosis (52). *In vitro* studies indicate that the expression of MHC class I determinants on eutopic and ectopic endometrial cells modify the susceptibility to NK cell lysis, and that lysis mediated by CTL is inhibited by the HLA-B7 allele on endometrial cells. These data suggest that the resistance to lysis of endometrial cells is related to expression of surface HLA class I molecules, and that the HLA-B7 allele inhibiting the cytotoxic activity of CTL suggests that the growth of ectopic endometrial cells might be under genetic control, but as yet no association between individuals with endometriosis and particular HLA haplotypes has been observed. NK-cell–mediated lysis is non-MHC restricted. However, downregulation of MHC class I is known to modify NK cell lysis. Whether downregulation of endometrial expression of MHC class I can occur *in vivo* or is just an artifact of *in vitro* culturing remains to be determined. Both eutopic and ectopic endometrium express both MHC class I and class II determinants and similar profiles of immune and inflammatory cells, although relative numbers of these cells and their cytokines have been observed to be increased in ectopic compared to eutopic endometrial tissues.

Observations of reduced NK-cell activity only in individuals with advanced endometriosis compared to milder forms of disease challenge the concept that decreased NK-cell activity represents a primary etiologic factor in endometriosis development. Reports of aberrant NK-cell activity in women with endometriosis have also been challenged due to the low levels of percent lysis in both NK-cell and CTL cell assays and the overlapping standard deviations between controls and study participants. The biologic relevance of such data especially in light of the inappropriately used statistical tests (Student's t-test) applied to nonparametric, multiple groups has also been questioned. Data obtained from functional studies on peripheral lymphocytes must be carefully interpreted since the biologic activities of peripheral lymphocytes may not reflect the biologic activities of lymphocytes from specific tissue sites. Variability may also be related to target cell sensitivity or to donor-related variables such as medications, smoking, and exercise, resulting in high, medium, and low responses in NK cell and CTL assays. Lastly, it is hard to reconcile that ectopic endometrium, which is self-tissue, is antigenic and thus could serve as a target for NK cells or other activated killer cells.

Further evidence against altered NK cell and cytotoxic lymphocyte responsiveness being involved in the development of endometriosis comes from the baboon model for this disease. Using appropriately applied analyses and strict criteria correcting for the high spontaneous release of ^{51}Cr from labeled target cells, unlike what was done in human studies, no differences were observed in either lymphocyte-mediated cytotoxicity or NK-cell activity between animals with and without endometriosis (56). Similarly, immuno-suppression in animals with and without endometriosis caused neither disease development nor disease progression (57). Therefore, it is premature to conclude that either NK-cell or cytotoxic T-cell responses are etiologic factors in the development or progression of endometriosis. Potentially, more plausible hypotheses to propose are (a) the immuno-logic phenomena associated with endometriosis represent the effect of disease rather than its cause; and (b) immuno-logic mechanisms may facilitate the maintenance of endo-metriosis once it is established and contribute to disease sequalae (54).

Peritoneal macrophages are potentially the pivotal cells involved in the immunologic mechanisms contributing to the maintenance and progression of endometriosis (58). Macrophages and activated lymphocytes are increased in the peritoneal environment of subfertile women with endo-metriosis compared to fertile individuals without disease. However, peritoneal fluid (PF) macrophages are activated even in normal fertile women, with activation progressively increasing during the menstrual cycle. This activational sta-tus has been reported to be increased in women with endo-metriosis over normal controls. The ability of peritoneal macrophages from women with endometriosis to internalize MHC class II antigens and to cap fluorescent markers more readily than macrophages from control women provides fur-ther evidence that peritoneal macrophages from women with endometriosis have a higher basal activation status than mac-rophages from controls (59). Immune and inflammatory cells are attracted to the peritoneal cavity in women with endome-triosis, apparently in response to peritoneal irritation caused by retrograde menstruation. Many chemoattractants have been described in the peritoneal fluid and have been reported to be increased in women with endometriosis compared to samples from women without disease. These chemokines in-clude C3, RANTES (regulated upon activation, normal T expression, presumably secreted), (macrophage chemotactic peptide) MCP1-3 and IL-8. Once recruited, these cells can be further activated to secrete a wide variety of cytokines and growth factors that may influence the maintenance and pro-gression of endometriosis (54).

For endometriosis to develop, retrograde menstrual endo-metrium must adhere to peritoneal surfaces. Following ad-herence, enzymatic digestion must occur to disrupt perito-neal integrity. This in turn leads to invasion and ultimate growth, resulting in endometriosis. The eutopic endometrial cell responsible for endometriosis has never been identified. Endometrium from the functionalis layer is normally shed at menstruation. Therefore, how could functionalis endome-trium, which is a terminally differentiated tissue, grow and differentiate into the glands and stroma required for the diag-nosis of endometriosis? Perhaps it is not functionalis endome-trium that causes endometriosis, but rather fragments of bas-alis endometrium that is abnormally shed in women who develop endometriosis since basalis endometrium is not ter-minally differentiated but is the progenitor of both glandular

and stromal tissue. Therefore, our laboratory has proposed that endometriosis may arise from basalis endometrium that is shed inadvertently into the peritoneal cavity (60).

Precisely how endometriosis develops remains specula-tive. The macrophage-secreted cytokine, TNF-α, may facili-tate endometrial adhesion onto peritoneal mesothelium (61), which provides a potential mechanism for the initial event necessary for endometriosis development. Peritoneal fluid and conditioned media from peritoneal immune and inflammatory cell cultures from women with endometriosis are capable of promoting endometrial stromal cell prolifera-tion significantly more than similar cultures from women without endometriosis (62,63). Peritoneal fluid also con-tains angiogenic factors (64). Immune and inflammatory cytokines are capable of modulating the growth of endome-trial cells.

Aromatase is increased in endometriosis tissue compared to autologous eutopic endometrium, which is increased over levels demonstrable in eutopic endometrium from women without endometriosis, indicating that both eutopic endo-metrial tissues and ectopic endometrium are biochemically different from normal eutopic endometrium of disease-free women (65). These data suggest that the presence of aromatose expression in eutopic endometrium from women with endometriosis may be related to the peritoneal implan-tation capability of these tissues since estrogen production in these tissues could promote ectopic growth. Other cytokines/growth factors, such as epidermal growth factor (EGF), TGF, fibroblast growth factor (FGF), insulin-like growth factor (IGF), and platelet-derived growth factor (PDGF), may also facilitate the growth of endometrial cells *in vitro* (52) and may influence the growth of ectopic endo-metrium that has implanted within the peritoneal cavity.

MALE GENITAL TRACT

IgG, IgM, and IgA subclass antibodies have been detected in semen, prostatic fluid, and preejaculatory (urethral) fluid from healthy men (reviewed in ref. 66). Few plasma cells are detected in the normal human prostate, and recent evidence suggests that the penile urethra may be the primary source of secreted immunoglobulin A (sIgA) in semen from normal men.

T lymphocytes are not usually detected in the healthy human testis, but are observed in the rete testis, epididymis, vas deferens, and accessory glands, with CD8$^+$ cells within the epithelium and CD4$^+$ cells primarily in the stroma. T cells are also seen in the human urethra, with a predomi-nance of CD8$^+$ cells in the intraepithelial space, and a mixture of CD8$^+$ and CD4$^+$ cells in the stroma. T cells in the urethra are positive for the integrin $\alpha_E\beta_7$ (mucosal-associated antigen). Macrophages are abundant in the hu-man and primate urogenital tract—in the testicular intersti-tium, the epididymis, the epithelium and connective tissue of the excurrent ducts and accessory glands, and in the penile urethra. Unlike the female lower urogenital tract, Langerhans' cells are rarely detected in the penile urethra, but are abundant in the epithelium of the foreskin and the fossa navicularis. Unique innate defense mechanisms of the male reproductive tract include the presence of high concentrations of zinc, polyamines, and prostaglandins (reviewed in ref. 67).

REPRODUCTIVE DIFFICULTY IN MEN AS AN IMMUNE DISORDER

Leukocytospermia

Leukocytospermia is defined by the World Health Organization as a WBC concentration above 10^6/mL of semen. The prevalence of leukocytospermia in the infertile population varies between 10% and 20%. Conflicting data exist concerning the importance of leukocytospermia in infertility, as not all studies agree on the effects of leukocytospermia on the outcome of IVF-ET. However, when WBC counts were above 10^6 polymorphonuclear cells (PMNs)/mL of semen, IVF success rates were reported to be decreased (68). A potential reason for the discrepancies noted between studies has been the unreliability of earlier techniques to clearly delineate the difference between immune cells and immature germ cells in semen. Reports of round cell numbers in a semen analysis are not helpful in determining the numbers or types of leukocytes present in semen samples, since immature germ cells compose up to 90% of round cells in semen. Furthermore, different thresholds for WBC concentrations have been used to define leukocytospermia in various studies (reviewed in ref. 69).

Utilizing immunocytologic techniques, the major WBC population in semen is granulocytes (50% to 60%), followed by macrophages (20% to 30%), and T lymphocytes (2% to 5%). Therefore, the preponderance of the detrimental effects that seminal leukocytes might have on sperm function could be attributed to granulocytes since they are generally present in the highest concentration in semen. However, infertile men may present with a higher than normal proportion of specific subsets of leukocytes, such as T lymphocytes, which have been reported to be correlated with reduced sperm motility. A significant reduction in sperm motility has been reported when sperm were exposed to leukocyte supernatants. When further studies were performed using recombinant cytokines *in vitro* to determine which factors in the leukocyte supernatants might be responsible for decreasing sperm motility, the cytokines TNF-α and IFN-γ were found to independently decrease sperm motion parameters by some but not all investigators. Under similar conditions, IL-1, IL-2, and B-cell growth factor (IL-6) had no effect on sperm motility. TNF-α and IFN-γ have also been shown to inhibit fertilization in the zona-free hamster egg penetration test, providing further evidence that products of activated lymphocytes and macrophages

may contribute to infertility in leukocytospermic males. Similar observations were made using peripheral blood granulocytes to determine their effects on sperm. The addition of granulocytes to sperm *in vitro* significantly decreased hamster ovum penetration. Granulocytes also markedly reduced sperm motility at concentrations as low as 0.6×10^6 PMN/mL. These inhibitory effects may be mediated by the free radicals H_2O_2 and OH released by granulocytes and other cells (69).

Treatment of leukocytospermia is controversial since there is no clear, consistent association between infection and WBCs in semen. A prospective, randomized, controlled study to determine whether leukocytospermia would resolve with a 14-day course of either doxycycline 100 mg b.i.d. or trimethoprim 160 mg/sulfamethoxazole 800 mg b.i.d. revealed no difference between treated individuals and controls. This was largely due to spontaneous resolution of leukocytospermia, which occurred in 82% of untreated controls (70). Therefore, antibiotic therapy should be used only in cases of documented infection, as antibiotic therapy alone could lead to abnormal sperm function (reviewed in ref. 70).

Sperm Antibodies

The incidence of antisperm antibodies (ASAs) in cases of unexplained infertility differs between reports depending on the source used for antibody measurement (serum or cervical mucus in the female, and serum or semen in the male), the specific test chosen, and whether testing was performed only on couples with no other factor potentially explaining their infertility. ASAs have been reported in 46% and 57% of women with unexplained infertility and endometriosis, respectively. Others have detected ASAs in the sera of approximately 13% of women with unexplained infertility (14).

Although not all investigators concur that ASAs are associated with reduced pregnancy rates, antibodies to sperm antigens have been associated with infertility and reduced success rates following IVF-ET (14). Removing ASAs containing serum from the IVF insemination medium has been reported to improve fertilization rates (71). ASAs have been reported in the serum of 54% of women undergoing IVF who did not fertilize, 64% of women who fertilized <20% of their oocytes, and in 16% of women who fertilized >40% of their oocytes. Both IgG and IgA ASAs were found, but in contrast to most reports of clinically significant ASAs, the majority of the antibodies in this report were tail-directed. In the male partners of these individuals, serum ASAs were present in 8% whose partners did not fertilize, 36% of men whose partners fertilized <20% of oocytes, and in 0% of men whose partners fertilized >40% of oocytes (16).

Antisperm antibodies may impede sperm function by altering motility, cervical mucus penetration, fertilization, and possibly implantation (14). Treatment modalities have been directed at preventing the formation of ASAs and at treating the underlying mechanisms of ASA interference with sperm function. The use of corticosteroids in the past was popularized to reduce the concentration of ASAs, thereby improving sperm penetration through the cervical mucus to facilitate pregnancy. However, corticosteroids are not currently used for the treatment of infertility due to their potential for severe adverse side effects and their unproven efficacy. Intrauterine insemination has been attempted in cases of cervical mucus ASAs, but the potential remains that ASAs present in the uterus or fallopian tubes may affect the ability of sperm to achieve fertilization. Assisted reproductive technologies offer the ability to observe fertilization while removing the sperm from a potentially hostile environment. IVF is the current treatment of choice for clinically significant ASAs. ASA-containing serum should not be used in the fertilization medium. Other approaches include the use of proteases to cleave ASAs from sperm prior to use during IVF. Intracytoplasmic sperm injection has also been shown to be highly effective in treating couples with severe male immunologic infertility who otherwise responded poorly to conventional IVF.

SUMMARY

Human reproductive tissues are replete with immune and inflammatory cells capable of secreting soluble products that contribute to the host defense against pathogenic organisms and other antigens. Under normal conditions, these cells and their secretions may facilitate normal reproductive events. Perturbations in natural immunity involving cellular or antibody-mediated mechanisms are speculated to culminate in reproductive difficulty. Specific treatments for many potential immunologic causes of reproductive difficulty await a better understanding of the mechanisms potentially involved and the outcome of well-designed clinical trials.

Immunologic testing and therapy for reproductive difficulty has been advocated on the basis of many different hypotheses, very few of which have been substantiated adequately on the principles of evidence-based medicine. The utility of many of the immunologic tests advertised as being useful in the diagnosis of reproductive difficulty is doubtful. A definitive answer regarding the best and most effective way to evaluate and treat the couple experiencing reproductive difficulty must await cost-effective analyses based on outcome research.

The field of reproductive immunology is evolving. Investigating the potential molecular immunologic mechanisms involved in reproductive health and disease is important. Knowledge of the precise mechanisms involved together with definition of the inciting antigens may provide solutions to the major reproductive health problems facing humanity, including the sexual transmission of disease, unwanted fertility, infertility, endometriosis, and recurrent pregnancy loss.

10 KEY POINTS

1. An immune response against non-self tissue derived from a different member of the same species is termed allogenic immunity; while that against self is termed autoimmunity.

2. Cellular immunity is mediated by cytokine-directed cytotoxic T cells and Natural Killer cells; while humoral immunity is mediated by immunoglobulins produced by B-cell-derived plasma cells.

3. Reproductive processes may be adversely affected by cellular or antibody-mediated mechanisms either before or after fertilization or implantation.

4. Antibodies to sperm are present in approximately 5% of reproductive-age women and 10% of men and may adversely affect sperm motility, penetration of cervical mucus, and oocyte penetration.

5. Premature ovarian failure may occur through cellular (interferon-gamma induction of MHC class II antigens on granulosa cells) and antibody-mediated (anti-ovarian antibodies) mechanisms.

6. The concept that autoimmunity is a cause of infertility is unlikely since infertility is not a component of well-characterized autoimmune disorders such as systemic lupus erythematosus.

7. The autoimmune theory with the most validity regarding pregnancy loss involves the antiphospholipid antibody syndrome mediated by high titre IgG anticardiolipin antibody and potentially IgM antiphosphatidylserine antibody.

8. The most recent alloimmune hypothesis proposed for recurrent pregnancy loss involves Th1 immunity to trophoblast or other antigens.

9. There is no compelling data supportive of immunotherapy for reproductive dysfunction other than heparin and aspirin for the antiphospholipid syndrome.

10. Although immunologic mechanisms may be involved in the sequelae of endometriosis, there remains no substantive data indicating that endometriosis is caused by immune aberrancy.

REFERENCES

1. Janeway CA, Travers P. *Immunobiology: the immune system in health and disease.* New York: Garland, 1994.
2. Roitt I, Brostoff J, Male D. *Immunology,* 5th ed. London: Mosby International, 1998.
3. Grossman CJ. Interactions between the gonadal steroids and immune system. *Science* 1985;227:257–261.
4. Panvonen T. Hormonal regulation of immune responses. *Ann Med* 1994;26:255–258.
5. Hill JA, Anderson DJ. Evidence for the existence and significance of immune cells and their soluble products in reproductive tissues. *Immunol Allergy Clin North Am* 1990;10:1.
6. King A, Loke YW. Uterine large granular lymphocytes: a possible

role in embryonic implantation. *Am J Obstet Gynecol* 1990; 162:308–310.

7. Tabidzadeh S. Human endometrium: an active site of cytokine production and action. *Endocr Rev* 1991;92:272–290.

8. Adashi EY, Resnick CE, Croft CS, et al. Tumor necrosis factor-α inhibits gonadotropin hormonal action in nontransformed ovarian granulosa cells. *J Biol Chem* 1989;264:1591–1597.

9. Hurwitz A, Loukides J, Riciarelli E, et al. Human intraovarian interleukin-1 (IV-1) system: highly compartmentalized and hormonally dependent regulation of the genes encoding IL-1, its receptor, and its receptor antagonist. *J Clin Invest* 1992;89:1746–1754.

10. Best CL, McKinley D, Welch WR, et al. Interferon-gamma messenger ribonucleic acid expression and protein localization in human ovary. *Am J Obstet Gynecol* 1998.

11. Grasso G, Muscettola M, Traina V, et al. Presence of interferons in human follicular fluid after ovarian hyperstimulation for in vitro fertilization. *Med Sci Res* 1988;16:167–168.

12. Best CL, Griffin PM, Hill JA. Interferon gamma inhibits luteinized human granulosa cell steroid production in vitro. *Am J Obstet Gynecol* 1995;172:1505–1510.

13. Moghissi KS, Sacco AG, Barin K. Immunologic infertility. I. Cervical mucus antibodies and postcoital test. *Am J Obstet Gynecol* 1980;136:941–950.

14. Haas GG Jr, Bronson RA, D'Cruz DJ, et al. Antisperm antibodies and infertility. In: Bronson RA, Alexander NJ, Anderson DJ, et al., eds. *Reproductive immunology.* Cambridge, MA: Blackwell Science, 1996:171–211.

15. Mandelbaum SC, Diamond MP, DeCherney AH. Relationship of antisperm antibodies to oocyte fertilization in vitro fertilization embryo transfer. *Fertil Steril* 1987;47:644–651.

16. Moghissi KS, Sacco AG, Barin K. Immunologic infertility. I. Cervical mucus antibodies and postcoital test. *Am J Obstet Gynecol* 1980;136:941–950.

17. Wah R, Anderson DJ, Hill JA. Asymptomatic cervicovaginal leukocytosis in infertile women. *Fertil Steril* 1990;54:445–450.

18. Hill JA, Haimovici F, Anderson DJ. Products of activated lymphocytes and macrophages inhibit murine embryo development in vitro. *J Immunol* 1987;139:2250–2254.

19. Haimovici F, Hill JA, Anderson DJ. The effects of soluble products of activate lymphocytes and macrophages on blastocyst implantation events in vitro. *Biol Reprod* 1991;44:69–75.

20. Berkowitz RS, Hill JA, Kurtz CB, et al. Effects of products of activated leukocytes (lymphokines and monokines) on the growth of malignant trophoblast cells in vitro. *Am J Obstet Gynecol* 1988;158:199–203.

21. Bulmer JN, Morrison L, Johnson PM, et al. Immunohistochemical localization of interferon in human placental tissues in normal, ectopic and molar pregnancy. *Am J Reprod Immunol* 1990; 22:109–116.

22. Hill JA, Anderson DJ. Cell-mediated immune mechanisms in recurrent spontaneous abortion. In: Talwar GP, ed. *Contraceptive research for today and the nineties.* New York: Springer-Verlag, 1988:171–180.

23. Eisenman J, Register KB, Strickler RC, et al. The effects of tumor necrosis factor on human sperm motility in vitro. *J Androl* 1990;10:270–274.

24. Hill JA, Haimovici F, Politch JA, et al. Effects of soluble products of activated lymphocytes and macrophages (lymphokines and monokines) on human sperm motion parameters. *Fertil Steril* 1987;47:460–465.

25. Hill JA, Cohen J, Anderson DJ. The effects of lymphokines and monokines on human sperm fertilizing ability on the zona-free hamster egg penetration test. *Am J Obstet Gynecol* 1989;160: 1154–1159.

26. Chacho KJ, Chacho S, Andersen PJ, et al. Peritoneal fluid in patients with and without endometriosis: prostanoids and macrophages and their effect on the spermatozoa penetration assay. *Am J Obstet Gynecol* 1986;155:1290–1299.

27. Muscatto JJ, Haney AJ, Weinberg JB. Sperm phagocytosis by human peritoneal macrophages: a possible cause of infertility in endometriosis. *Am J Obstet Gynecol* 1982;144:503–510.

28. Isaacson KB, Coutifaris C, Garcia CR, et al. Production and secretion of complement component 3 by endometriotic tissue. *J Clin Endocrinol Metab* 1989;69:1003–1009.

29. Anderson DJ, Abbott AF, Jack RM. The role of complement component C3b and its receptors in sperm-oocyte interaction. *Proc Natl Acad Sci USA* 1993;90:10051–10053.

30. Eiserman J, Gast MJ, Pineda J, et al. Interleukin-1: a possible role in the infertility associated with endometriosis. *Fertil Steril* 1987;47:213–217.

31. Fakih H, Baggett B, Holtz G, et al. Interleukin-1: a possible role in the infertility associated with endometriosis. *Fertil Steril* 1987;47:213–217.

32. Hill JA, Welch WR, Faris HP, et al. Induction of class II major histocompatibility complex (MHC) antigen expression in human granulosa cells by gamma interferon: a potential mechanism of autoimmune ovarian failure. *Am J Obstet Gynecol* 1990;162: 534–540.

33. Navayanan M, Murphy PS, Munaf SA, et al. Antiovarian antibodies and their effects on the outcome of assisted reproduction. *J Assist Reprod Genet* 1995;12:599–605.

34. Gleicher N. Autoimmunity and reproductive failure. *Ann NY Acad Sci* 1991;626:537–544.

35. Taylor V, Campbell JM, Scott JS. Presence of autoantibodies in women with unexplained infertility. *Am J Obstet Gynecol* 1989; 161:377–379.

36. Gleicher N, Liu HC, Dudkiecz A, et al. Autoantibody profiles and immunoglobulin levels as predictors of in vitro fertilization success. *Am J Obstet Gynecol* 1994;170:1145–1149.

37. Birkenfeld A, Mukaida J, Minichiello L, et al. Incidence of autoimmune antibodies in failed embryo transfer cycles. *Am J Reprod Immunol* 1994;31:65–68.

38. Balasch J, Crews M, Fabreques F. Antiphospholipid antibodies in human reproductive failure. *Hum Reprod* 1996;11:2310–2315.

39. Denise AL, Guido M, Adler RD, et al. Antiphospholipid antibodies and pregnancy rates and outcome in in vitro fertilization patients. *Fertil Steril* 1997;67:1084–1090.

40. Hill JA. Immunologic factors in spontaneous abortion. In: Bronson RA, Alexander NJ, Anderson DJ, et al., eds. *Reproductive immunology.* Cambridge, MA: Blackwell Scientific, 1996:433–442.

41. ACOG Educational and Practice Bulletin, no. 244. Antisyndrome. February, 1998.

42. Branch DW, Silver RM, Dierangeli S, et al. Antiphospholipid antibodies other than lupus anticoagulant and anticardiolipin antibodies in women with recurrent pregnancy loss, fertile controls and antiphospholipid syndrome. *Obstet Gynecol* 1997;89: 549–555.

43. Hill JA. Immunotherapy for recurrent pregnancy loss: standard of care or buyer beware. *J Soc Gynecol Invest* 1997;4:267–273.

44. Hill JA. Implications of cytokines in male and female sterility. In: Chaouat G, Mowbray J, eds. *Cellular and molecular biology of the materno-fetal relationship.* London: John Libbey Eurotext, 1991:123–129.

45. Hill JA, Polgar K, Anderson DJ. T-helper 1-type cellular immunity to trophoblast antigens in women with recurrent spontaneous abortion. *JAMA* 1995;73:1933–1936.

46. Hill JA, Polgar K, Harlow BL, et al. Evidence of embryo- and trophoblast toxic cellular immune response(s) in women with recurrent spontaneous abortion. *Am J Obstet Gynecol* 1992; 166:1044–1052.

47. Rocklin RE, Kitzmiller JL, Carpenter CB, et al. Maternal-fetal relation: absence of an immunologic blocking factor from serum of women with chronic abortion. *N Engl J Med* 1976;295:12009.

48. Amos DB, Kostyn DD. HLA: a central immunological agency of man. *Adv Hum Genet* 1980;10:137–141.

49. Regan L, Brande PR, Hill DP. A prospective study of the incidence time appearance of antipaternal lymphocytotoxic antibodies in human pregnancy. *Hum Reprod* 1981;6:294–298.

50. Rodger C. Lack of a requirement for a maternal humoral immune response to establish and maintain successful allogenic pregnancy. *Transplant* 1985;40;372–375.

51. Hill JA. Recurrent pregnancy loss. In: Creasy R, Resnick RE, eds. *Maternal Fetal Medicine.* New York: WB Saunders, 1998;423–464.

52. D'Hooghe T, Hill JA. Immunobiology of endometriosis. In: Bronson R, ed. *Reproductive immunology.* Cambridge, MA: Blackwell Scientific, 1996:322–356.

53. D'Hooghe TD, Hill JA. Autoantibodies in endometriosis. In: Kurpisz M, Fernandez N, eds. *Immunology of human reproduction.* BIOS Scientific, Oxford, United Kingdom 1995:133–162.

54. Hill JA. Immunology and endometriosis: fact, artifact or epiphenomena? *Obstet Gynecol Clin North Am* 1997;24:291–306.

55. Dmowski WP, Steele RN, Baker GF. Deficient cellular immunity in endometriosis. *Am J Obstet Gynecol* 1981;141:377–383.

56. D'Hooghe TM, Scherlinck JP, Koninckx PR, et al. Antiendometrial lymphocytotoxicity and natural killer cell activity in baboons (*Papioanubis* and *Papis cynocephalus*) with endometriosis. *Hum Reprod* 1995;10:558–562.

57. D'Hooghe TM, Bambra CS, Raeymaekers BM, et al. The effects of immunosuppression on development and progression of endometriosis in baboons (*Papio anubis*). *Fertil Steril* 1995;64:172–178.

58. Halme J, Becker S, Haskill S. Altered maturation and function of peritoneal macrophages: possible role in pathogenesis of endometriosis. *Am J Obstet Gynecol* 1987;156:783–789.

59. Halme J, Becker S, Wing R. Accentuated cyclic activation of peritoneal macrophages in patients with endometriosis. *Am J Obstet Gynecol* 1984;148:85–90.

60. Chiang CM, Hill JA. Localization of T-cells, interferon-gamma and HLA-DR in eutopic and ectopic human endometrium. *Gynecol Obstet Invest* 1997;43:245–50.

61. Zhang R, Wild RA, Ojago JM. Effect of tumor necrosis factor-alpha on adhesion of human endometrial stromal cells to peritoneal mesothelial cells: an in vitro system. *Fertil Steril* 1993;59:1196–1201.

62. Halme J, White C, Kauma S, et al. Peritoneal macrophages from patients with endometriosis release growth factor activity in vitro. *J Clin Endocrinol Metab* 1988;66:1044–1049.

63. Olive DL, Mantoya I, Riehl RM, et al. Macrophage conditioned media enhance endometrial stromal cell proliferation in vitro. *Am J Obstet Gynecol* 1991;164:953–958.

64. Osterlynck DJ, Meuleman C, Sobig H, et al. Angiogenic activity of peritoneal fluid from women with endometriosis. *Fertil Steril* 1993;59:778–782.

65. Bulcum SE, Zeitoun KM, Takayama K, et al. Estrogen biosysthesis in endometriosis: molecular basis and clinical relevance. *J Mol Endocrinol* 2000;25:35–42.

66. Pudney J, Anderson DJ. Immunobiology and the penile urethra. *Am J Pathol* 1995;147:155–165.

67. Alexander N, Anderson JD.Immunology and semen. *Fertil Steril* 1987;47:192–205.

68. Deyerle KL, Sims JE, Power SK, et al. Peroxidase-positive round cells and microorganisms in human semen together with antibiotic treatment adversely influence the outcome of in vitro fertilization and embryo transfer. *Int J Androl* 1994;17:127–134.

69. Wolff H. The biologic significance of white blood cells in semen. *Fertil Steril* 1995;63:1143–1157.

70. Yanushpolsky EH, Politch JA, Hill JA, et al. Antibiotic therapy and leukocytospermia: a prospective randomized controlled study. *Fertil Steril* 1995;63:142–147.

71. De Almeida M, Henry M, Testart J, et al. Relation between antisperm antibodies and the rate of fertilization of human oocytes in vitro. *J Assist Reprod Genet* 1992;9:9–13.

CYTOKINES AND GROWTH FACTORS IN FEMALE REPRODUCTIVE BIOLOGY

DOUGLAS A. KNISS
DOREEN L. HOCK

Cytokines and polypeptide growth factors coordinate myriad cellular processes in the female reproductive tract. Several cytokines have been implicated in female reproductive events such as ovum–granulosa cell communication and regulation of ovarian steroidogenesis, embryo-uterine receptivity and implantation, immunologic tolerance of the conceptus, placental growth and differentiation, and the initiation and/or maintenance of parturition. Classically, cytokines were thought to govern immune cell behaviors such as proliferation and differentiation of T and B lymphocytes, activation of mononuclear phagocytes (monocytes and macrophages), chemotaxis of neutrophils, and degranulation of mast cells.

Growth factors, on the other hand, were envisaged to stimulate mitogenesis in nearly all cells with some cell-type specificity. More recently, however, the strict lines of demarcation between cytokines and growth factors have become blurred. Many cytokines are potent mitogenic stimuli, while several growth factors activate complex immune cell functions.

The most important property of cytokine/growth factors is their local site of synthesis and action in contrast to bona fide endocrine hormones such as steroids or insulin. Although some cytokines and growth factors can be measured in body fluids (e.g., plasma, amniotic fluid, semen, urine), it is highly unlikely that these mediators exert profound distal actions as they do intramurally. Several key principles should be considered when discussing cytokines and, perhaps to a lesser extent, growth factors. First, while a plethora of experimental data have elucidated several important roles of these polypeptides on cellular functions, simple *in vitro* models likely do not accurately represent the intricate interactions that occur between cytokines and growth factors and their target cells *in vivo*. That is, cytokines and growth factors rarely, if ever, act in isolation. Thus, their actions are highly context dependent. In addition, the order or timing in which they participate in various processes can dramatically alter the ways in which they modulate cell phenotype. Second, cytokines are highly redundant. For example, elimination of a particular cytokine by homologous recombination or knockout technology in mice often reveals only subtle or unexpected phenotypic changes. This is due to complementation of the loss of one cytokine by a close family member or a more distant cousin. Third, a given cytokine may exert different biologic actions upon several different cell types. Fourth, cytokines and growth factors can direct cellular events via autocrine mechanisms, or locally through paracrine or juxtacrine interactions.

The classification of cytokines and growth factors is frequently made on the basis of their receptor type, since defining them via their functional properties is complicated by redundancies. This chapter presents the biology of the individual cytokine and growth factors, and discusses their respective roles in select reproductive functions (e.g., ovarian and endometrial function, implantation, placentation, pregnancy, and parturition). Given the large number of mediators present in reproductive tissues, it is impractical to comprehensively describe every agent. The reader is directed to selected reviews for a more thorough treatment of many of the cytokines and polypeptide growth factors.

Before discussing the individual cytokines, it is important to consider a few issues about nomenclature. Historically, humoral mediators of immune cell functions were named for their specific biologic functions. Thus, a substance that participated in the elevation of basal body temperature during systemic infections was termed endogenous pyrogen (1). The terms *cachectin* and *tumor necrosis factor* (TNF) were coined to describe a factor that contributed to a wasting syndrome during chronic infections and malignancies (2). Interleukins were so named because it was thought at the time that these biomolecules governed leukocyte functions; they were then given a numerical designation based on the order in which they were first described.

Chemokines were defined as a general class of cytokines with some structural similarities. However, the predominant common feature of chemokines is their role in chemoattraction of leukocytes into sites of tissue inflammation. Finally, polypeptide growth factors were identified initially as mediators of cellular growth and proliferation. It is important to note that, as investigations of these biomediators has expanded, it is appreciated that significant overlap in function exists, such that some cytokines exert mitogenic activity, and certain traditional growth factors behave as cytokines, communicating intercellular biologic signals.

PROINFLAMMATORY CYTOKINES

Interleukin-1

Interleukin-1 (IL-1) is the central pleiotropic cytokine mediator of myriad inflammatory and physiologic events. The scope of cellular targets for IL-1 is vast and includes nearly every cell type. Because the potency of IL-1 is extremely high and so many biologic processes are affected by this cytokine, a very narrow threshold exists between potential therapeutic benefits and systemic toxicity (3). However, therapeutic agents that block or limit IL-1 actions are likely to be beneficial in some clinical settings.

There are three members of the IL-1 family, each encoded by separate structural genes (1,3). IL-1α and IL-1β serve as potent receptor agonists, while IL-1 receptor antagonist (IL-1RA) is a circulating endogenous IL-1 receptor blocker (3,4). Both IL-1α and IL-1β are synthesized as 31-kd precursors that must be proteolytically processed to mature 17-kd polypeptides (3).

IL-1α and IL-1β

IL-1α is a largely cell-associated isoform of IL-1 and is secreted into the extracellular milieu in minute amounts (3). During apoptotic or necrotic cell death, IL-1α can be released from dying cells and processed by extracellular Ca^{2+}-dependent cysteine proteases known as calpains (5). Initially, IL-1α is translated as a 31-kd propeptide that can be proteolytically cleaved via IL-1 converting enzyme (ICE) into the mature 17-kd form. However, unlike IL-1β, IL-1α is bioactive in the precursor form (3). An interesting feature of IL-1α biosynthesis is its association with microtubules in the cytoplasm rather than endoplasmic reticulum (6).

Since IL-1α lacks a leader sequence necessary for secretion from the cell, IL-1α acts largely intracellularly. In this way, IL-1α can act as an autocrine growth factor, especially in epithelial cells and differentiated keratinocytes. However, several differences exist between IL-1α and IL-1β, including control of transcriptional activity of the IL-1 genes, stability of nascent RNA transcripts, and posttranslational processing (7).

IL-1β was originally thought to be produced only by monocyte/macrophages in response to challenge with bacterial lipopolysaccharide. Research from a number of fields reveals that IL-1 likely plays the pivotal role in early inflammatory events leading to activated leukocytes, endothelium, parenchymal cells (e.g., heptocytes, uterine decidua and amnion/chorion cells, and placental trophoblast) (8–10). Within female reproductive biology, IL-1 exerts an array of important functions including ovarian regulation,

early embryogenesis and implantation, and parturition. In the ovary, IL-1 promotes granulosa cell proliferative activity and interrupts differentiation events (11,12). IL-1 induces cyclooxygenase-2 gene expression and prostaglandin release from granulosa cells, which has been implicated in ovum maturation and rupture of the ovarian follicle (13). During the luteal phase of the menstrual cycle, there is a sharp increase in the level of IL-1 within granulosa cells and circulating peripheral blood monocytes (14).

It has been suggested that IL-1 is produced by early blastocysts en route to implantation into the decidualizing endometrium. Simon and colleagues (15) demonstrated cyclical changes in IL-1 receptor abundance in the endometrium during the menstrual cycle, and showed that treatment of pregnant mice with the IL-1RA inhibited blastocyst implantation.

IL-1 plays a pivotal role in the initiation and/or maintenance of the inflammatory events that define labor. Nearly every intrauterine tissue (placenta, fetal membranes, decidua, and cervix) exhibits IL-1 receptors, responds to IL-1, and/or produces IL-1. Romero and co-workers (16,17) have written extensively on the presence of IL-1α and IL-1β in amniotic fluid in women with preterm labor, especially in the setting of intrauterine bacterial infection. In pregnant mice stimulated with bacterial endotoxin to initiate premature labor, IL-1 levels are elevated (18). Romero's group (19) has further shown that the decidua is the source of amniotic fluid IL-1. IL-1 is a very potent stimulator of prostaglandins (PGs) E_2 and $F_{2\alpha}$ biosynthesis in human amnion, chorion, endometrium and decidua, and placental trophoblast (9,20–25). This is due to the induction of the two central enzymes in the arachidonic acid cascade: cytosolic phospholipase A_2 and cyclooxygenase-2 (9,23,26,27). It has been postulated that local production of IL-1 within the decidua in response to chorioamnionitis or occult bacterial infection triggers the prostaglandin cascade. PGE_2 and $PGF_{2\alpha}$ produced following upregulation of cyclooxygenase-2 then stimulates myometrial contractions.

IL-1 also plays a role in cervical ripening and dilatation. Fibroblasts within the musculoelastic tissue of the cervix secrete PGE_2 and collagenase and other matrix metalloproteinases in response to IL-1 (28–30). Dissolution of the extracellular matrix then allows for the thinning and remodeling of the cervical canal in preparation for expulsion of the fetus.

IL-1 Receptors

Two genetically distinct receptors bind IL-1α and IL-1β with differential affinities (31). While both receptors are members of the immunoglobulin superfamily of cell surface proteins and share significant sequence homology with one another, they do exhibit subtle albeit important differences. The IL-1 receptor type I is composed of an 80-kd transmembrane glycoprotein that mediates most of the pleiotropic biologic effects of IL-1 (31). The number of type I receptors is exceedingly small on most primary cells and tissues (200 sites/cell), while some established cell lines express up to 5,000 receptor binding sites per cell (31). Interestingly, the signal transduction mechanisms coupled to the IL-1 type I receptor are highly efficient, and reports have suggested that as few as ten binding sites per cell may be sufficient to confer biologic effects (31).

In contrast to the type I IL-1 receptor, the type II receptor has a very short intracellular domain of 29 amino acids, which is insufficient to transduce signals (31). Both cell surface and soluble forms of the IL-1 type II receptor have been described as "decoy" receptors, since they bind ligand with high affinity, but do not activate downstream signaling pathways within cells (32). Since the IL-1 type II receptor preferentially binds IL-1β, it has been suggested that high-affinity binding of this cytokine by the type II receptor could lower the biologic efficacy of IL-1β (31,33). Both IL-1 receptors also exhibit in soluble form and circulate in plasma and other body fluids (e.g., synovial fluid and amniotic fluid) of healthy and diseased (e.g., septic) humans (31).

In addition to the binding domain of the IL-1 type I receptor, an IL-1 accessory protein (IL-1RAcP) appears to be absolutely required for transducing biologic signals in IL-1–responsive cells (33). No such interaction occurs between the type II IL-1 receptor and IL-1RAcP or the natural IL-1RA and IL-1RAcP (31). Upon binding of IL-1α or IL-1β to the type I IL-1 receptor and subsequent docking with the IL-1RAcP, intracellular phosphorylation cascades are initiated via the mitogen-activated protein (MAP) kinase signaling pathway that ultimately leads to the activation of nascent gene expression via the nuclear factor (NF)-κB transcription factor (34–37).

IL-1 receptor expression has been reported in the ovary, endometrium, and placental trophoblast (15, 38–40). Polan's group (38) demonstrated that within uterine endometrium, IL-1β was a potent inducer of type I IL-1 receptor gene expression. Moreover, this group has shown experimentally that administration of IL-1RA to pregnant mice blocks implantation of the conceptus, further implicating this cytokine as a critical paracrine factor in early maternal-fetal communication (41,42).

IL-1 Receptor Antagonist

In addition to the two IL-1 receptor agonists (IL-1α and IL-1β), there is also a naturally occurring IL-1 receptor antagonist (IL-1RA). The IL-1RA is encoded by a gene near the IL-1 locus (7). This molecule interacts with the IL-1 receptor type I and blocks the actions of IL-1α and IL-1β. However, IL-1RA has a low affinity for the type II IL-1 receptor. Thus, it has been postulated that IL-1RA serves to compete with IL-1α and/or IL-1β for binding to the cell-associated, fully functional IL-1 receptor. In turn, this may provide more IL-1 in solution for binding to the soluble decoy IL-1 receptor type II. This IL-1RA and the

soluble IL-1 type II receptor are analogous to other soluble cytokine receptors [e.g., soluble IL-6 (sIL-6) receptor, soluble tumor necrosis factor (sTNF) receptor].

Tumor Necrosis Factors

Tumor necrosis factors (TNFs) are a family of cytokines that play a central role in many forms of immunologic and inflammatory pathophysiologic disorders. TNF-α was originally discovered for its ability to cause regression of tumors in animal models (43,44). Later, it was shown that TNF-α exerted a variety of actions, including upregulation of intercellular adhesion molecule-1 (ICAM-1), on endothelial cells to allow transmigration of leukocytes into inflamed tissues, increased synthesis of other inflammatory cytokines and fatty acid-derived autocoids (e.g., prostaglandins and leukotrienes), and increased formation of reactive oxygen species (e.g., nitric oxide, superoxide, and peroxynitrite) (45).

One of the most fascinating activities of TNF-α is its ability to induce programmed cell death (apoptosis) (46). Apoptosis is a highly coordinated set of energy-requiring reactions within cells that are destined to die by a process characterized by activation of intracellular proteases, release of mitochrondrial enzymes, and condensation and fragmentation of genomic DNA (47,48).

In addition to TNF-α, there are two other members of the TNF family. TNF-β (lymphotoxin-α, LT-α) and lymphotoxin-β (LT-β) were discovered relatively recently and exert many of the same functions as TNF-α. There are two types of receptors that recognize TNF-α. A high-affinity TNF receptor I (TNF-RI) [molecular weight ratio (M_r) 55 to 60 kd] is chiefly responsible for mediating apoptosis. TNF-RII (M_r 75 to 80 kd) mediates most of the proinflammatory actions of TNF-α and TNF-β (49). Finally, LT-β has its own high-affinity receptor (50).

TNF-α appears to be intimately involved in several normal and abnormal aspects of pregnancy. Hunt and colleagues (51) have shown that TNF-α and its receptors are expressed in placental trophoblasts. Others have demonstrated that the TNF system is found in cells of the fetal membranes (amnion and chorion laeve) (52). Romero et al. (53) have shown that TNF-α accumulates in amniotic fluid in women experiencing preterm labor in the setting of intrauterine infection, and the most likely source of this cytokine is the maternal decidua. Using *in vitro* models, TNF-α has been shown to stimulate the production of PGs via induction of the cyclooxygenase-2 gene (54,55), and may thereby be an endogenous trigger of parturition in cases of intrauterine inflammation.

Interleukin-6

Few cytokines have been as extensively studied as IL-6. Within the network of proinflammatory cytokine actions, IL-6 occupies perhaps the central role in conveying local immune cell responses into more global consequences (e.g., production of acute-phase reactants, fever, lymphocyte activation). IL-6 produced locally by many different cell types including activated macrophages and tissue cells regulates the synthesis of acute-phase reactants (e.g., C-reactive protein, serum amyloid A), which are then released systemically (56).

Extensive studies of IL-6 in the setting of preterm labor have been conducted. Several laboratories have reported that elevation of IL-6 in maternal serum or amniotic fluid in the second trimester of pregnancy is highly predictive of subsequent preterm labor and delivery (57–60). *In vitro,* IL-6 is produced by a variety of intrauterine cells, i.e., chorion laeve trophoblasts, amnion cells, decidual cells, and placental trophoblasts (61–63).

Elevated levels of IL-6 have been noted in women presenting for endometriosis-induced infertility (64). Thus, IL-6 may have diagnostic value in managing gynecologic disorders of the pelvis that impact endometrial receptivity and fertility. However, the specificity of IL-6 in predicting the exact cause of pelvic or intrauterine inflammation is questionable. In many medical conditions, IL-6 is likely the earliest harbinger of occult inflammation, leading the clinician to continue diagnostic measures. However, the extreme sensitivity of this cytokine in the face of a plethora of host defense responses will likely lead to a relatively high false–positive rate. Thus, while IL-6 is considered by many to be a principal cytokine in identifying local or systemic inflammation, more thorough study is required to ascertain the clinical utility of this important biomediator in the diagnosis of specific disease.

ANTIINFLAMMATORY CYTOKINES

In addition to cytokines that mediate proinflammatory responses to exogenous insults, certain cytokines serve to dampen inflammation so as to limit the degree of local tissue damage. The three best-appreciated of the so-called antiinflammatory cytokines are IL-4, IL-10, and IL-13. In general, these cytokines are released from activated T helper (TH) lymphocytes of the TH2 lineage and serve to dampen or attenuate cellular immune responses. They also promote antibody-mediated immunity by augmenting the function of B lymphocytes and accessory cells.

IL-4 and IL-10

IL-4 is a 19-kd glycoprotein cytokine that is associated with CD4$^+$ T lymphocytes and has been described as the prototypic immunoregulatory cytokine (65). It is involved in immunoglobulin (Ig) class switching from IgG$_1$ to IgE (65,66). By virtue of its ability to stimulate resting murine B lymphocytes to proliferate, IL-4 was originally named B-cell growth factor (BCGF) (66).

IL-4 acts in an antagonistic manner with IL-2 to enhance the growth and function of so-called TH2 lymphocytes, while suppressing the same activities in TH1 lymphocytes (67). In this way, IL-2 and IL-4 are pivotal counterregulatory cytokines in T-cell networks. While the evidence presented thus far indicates that IL-4 is exclusively inhibitory toward IL-2-challenged cells [e.g., TH1 and natural killer (NK) cells], nonetheless IL-4 can also augment the mitogenesis and cytotoxic activities of NK cells that have been pretreated with IL-2 (68).

IL-4 may also exert influences on nonlymphoid cells such as monocytes and mast cells, and bone marrow stromal fibroblasts. Furthermore, the human uterine epithelium as well as the amnion basal lamina have been labeled with antibodies to IL-4 indicating local synthesis. Highly sensitive reverse transcriptase–polymerase chain reaction (RT-PCR) analysis has also revealed IL-4 transcripts in these same tissues. There is some preliminary evidence to indicate that IL-4 is also expressed within the human placental trophoblast (both cytotrophoblast and differentiated syncytiotrophoblast) (69,70). Bry and Lappalainen (71) reported that IL-4 increased production of IL-1RA within uterine decidual cells grown in culture and potentially led to resolution of proinflammatory responses. In addition to IL-4, two other cytokines (IL-10 and IL-13) exert significant antiinflammatory actions in a variety of cells, including immune cells and cells of the female reproductive tract.

IL-10 is an 18-kd protein expressed *in vivo* as a homodimer in monocyte/macrophages, T and B lymphocytes, mast cells, and keratinocytes. In general, the actions of IL-10 on immune effector cells are inhibitory, similar to those of IL-4 (72). IL-10 appears to be produced primarily, albeit not exclusively, by cells of the TH2 lineage, and exert inhibition over their TH1 cell counterparts. Some of these actions include the suppression of interferon-γ, TNF-α, and IL-6 production by activated TH1 cells (73). Interestingly, IL-10 also promotes the enhanced synthesis of IL-1RA, thus further reducing the magnitude of proinflammatory responses in cells responsive to IL-1 (71). The murine uterus (likely decidual stromal fibroblasts) is a rich source of IL-10 during mid-gestation, indicating an important role of this cytokine in pregnancy maintenance (73).

Thus, it appears that, as in other areas of systemic immunity, antiinflammatory cytokines as well as traditional proinflammatory cytokines (e.g., IL-1, TNF) exert a delicate balance over reproductive tissues and serve to orchestrate a controlled biologic response to immune effectors.

CHEMOATTRACTANT CYTOKINES

IL-8 and Related Chemokines

Chemokines are a somewhat recently discovered family of polypeptide immune cell modulators whose primary role is that of chemoattraction of cells to sites of inflammation or imminent immune recognition. This category of cytokines has become so extensive in recent years that is far beyond the scope of this chapter to cover them all.

Interleukin-8 was one of the earliest chemokines to be described and was originally named for its known function—neutrophil activating protein-1 (NAP-1). This chemokine has been shown to mediate the chemoattraction of activated neutrophils across capillary endothelium and into sites of tissue inflammation. Structurally, IL-8 is an 8- to 10-kd polypeptide derived from a gene localized to chromosome 4 (4q12-21) and physically close to other genes of the chemokine family ([growth-related oncogene] GROα, [platelet factor] PF-4, and IP-10) (74). The IL-8 peptide is a member of the subclass of chemokines designated CC to denote the fact that two disulfide linkages exist between cysteines 7 to 34 and 9 to 50. This CC designation differentiates IL-8 and related members from the CXC subclass of chemokines in which two cysteine residues are separated by another amino acid.

IL-8 is produced by a variety of cell types including mononuclear phagocytes, endothelial cells, tissue fibroblasts, keratinocytes, synovial cells, chondrocytes and a limited number of tumor cells (74). In addition, evidence indicates that neutrophils are also capable of releasing IL-8 and then responding to it in an autocrine manner (74). This is especially the case in neutrophils stimulated with lipopolysaccharide (75). IL-8 can be induced at the level of messenger RNA (mRNA) expression by proinflammatory cytokines IL-1α, IL-1β, and TNF-α. Phagocytes treated with endotoxin are also able to trigger IL-8 production.

Functionally, IL-8 elicits two chief biologic effects in target cells, especially granulocytes. First, this chemokine induces rapid and sustained chemotaxis toward sites of inflammation. Second, once granulocytes arrive at their site of action, they exhibit a robust degranulation response and a short-term respiratory burst (74).

Within the realm of reproductive biology, IL-8 has been extensively studied, and, as predicted, appears to mediate leukocyte chemotaxis and migration into tissues of the uterus and placenta during inflammatory episodes. The increase in chemokine (including IL-8) expression within human endometrium is highly associated with the accumulation of leukocytes (principally neutrophils and tissue macrophages) (76,77). Considerable research has shown that during term and preterm labor in women and animal models, IL-8 expression increases dramatically. Cherouny et al. (78) reported increased levels of IL-8 in association with clinically diagnosed chorioamnionitis and preterm labor in women. This observation was later substantiated in an expanded study by Mitchell's group (79).

IL-8 is likely to play an important role in attracting leukocytes into the uterus and cervix even during normal labor at term. Increases in neutrophil cell counts and IL-8 levels have been detected in human uterine lower segment biopsies following labor at term (80). In addition, using a rabbit model of pregnancy, IL-8 directly elicits biochemical changes that result in cervical ripening (81). Thus, IL-8 (and by extension, possibly other chemokines) clearly participates in the orchestrated cytokine response that characterizes inflammation within the uterine environment during preterm labor (especially in association with infection), and may even help to mediate the biochemical events of normal parturition.

POLYPEPTIDE GROWTH FACTORS

Epidermal Growth Factor/Transforming Growth Factor-α

Epidermal growth factor (EGF, urogastrone) is among the first polypeptide growth factors to be discovered that control cellular proliferation and differentiation (82). EGF was originally identified by its ability to promote the premature eruption of incisor teeth in neonatal mice (83). After this initial discovery, it was shown that this growth factor exhibited pleiotypic actions including control of cell proliferation and differentiation events in a variety of cell types (e.g., fibroblasts, mesenchymal cells, neural cells, and endothelial cells), not just epithelial cells.

The mRNA coding for EGF was originally cloned by Scott et al. (84) from a mouse submandibular gland complementary DNA (cDNA) library and was found to be a large transcript of >4,000 bases, yielding a prepro-EGF polypeptide of 1,217 amino acids. After several proteolytic processing steps, the mature peptide is 53 amino acids long (~6 kd). Subsequently, others demonstrated that EGF is synthesized in a variety of tissues, including kidney (85).

Increasing levels of EGF have been reported in amniotic fluid and fetal umbilical cord blood in association with advancing gestational age, leading to speculation that it is an important growth factor for fetal development (86,87). In this regard, ablation of the submandibular gland in pregnant mice leads to spontaneous abortion of fetuses, suggesting that EGF is required for successful pregnancy (88).

Reports by several researchers indicate that EGF may be a stimulus derived from the fetus that elicits prostaglandin biosynthesis in fetal membrane amnion cells, and may thus contribute to the onset of parturition. In this way, the maturation of fetal organ systems, especially the lung and kidney, could provide a communication pathway for controlling the timing of labor (89).

Recently, it has been demonstrated that transforming growth factor-α (TGF-α) is a polypeptide that binds to the EGF receptor with equal or greater affinity than EGF. Many or all of the actions of EGF are also exerted by TGF-α, including high-affinity binding and autophosphorylation of the EGF receptor, and stimulation of cell proliferation. Using Northern blot analysis and *in situ* hybridization Han's group (90,91) detected mRNA transcripts for TGF-α only in the uterine decidua adjacent to the embryo and not in the embryo proper or placenta. The nonpregnant uterus also did not express a TGF-α message, further indicating that an inductive force during pregnancy is responsible for upregulating TGF-α gene expression. Thus, the fetal origin of EGF and apparent maternal contribution of TGF-α suggests that this polypeptide growth factor family plays an important role in development and reproductive functions in the mammalian female.

Insulin and Insulin-Like Growth Factors

The insulin family of growth factors includes insulin synthesized by the endocrine pancreas, locally produced insulin-like growth factors I and II (IGF-I and IGF-II), as well as six IGF binding proteins (IGFBP-1 to -6), and two receptor types (I and II). A complete discussion of insulin structure and action is beyond this brief review, and the reader is referred to many endocrine texts for more thorough treatment of the subject. However, a brief review is in order here. Insulin is made almost exclusively in the endocrine pancreas (β-cells of the islets of Langerhans). In contrast, IGFs are produced in a variety of epithelial and mesenchymal tissues. The primary site of systemic IGF-I and IGF-II biosynthesis is the liver, where these growth factors are controlled by circulating levels of the anterior pituitary hormone, growth hormone (GH). In addition, IGF-I and IGF-II produced locally by myriad cell types within tissues provide paracrine signals without the need for direct regulation by GH.

Insulin is the most critical endocrine modulator of glucose uptake into insulin-sensitive tissues (i.e., adipose, and cardiac and skeletal muscle), and is the principal control system for carbohydrate utilization by tissues. Most tissues are not strictly insulin-sensitive and respond to changes in systemic insulin fluctuations with only minor metabolic alterations. In contrast, certain tissues (i.e., skeletal and cardiac muscle, and adipose tissue) take up glucose from the circulation with remarkably rapid kinetics when challenged with insulin. This is due to the presence of a highly sensitive pool of glucose transport proteins within the cytoplasm of skeletal and cardiac muscle cells and adipocytes (GLUT-4) that rapidly translocates to the plasma membrane of these cells in response to physiologic levels of insulin (92,93). The GLUT-4 glucose transport protein serves to rapidly transport glucose from the circulation into cells where it can be utilized for intermediary metabolism (muscle tissues) or storage as potential energy (adipocytes). Insulin also plays a critical role in the metabolism of fatty acids and proteins, but this subject is beyond the scope of this review. The reader is referred to an excellent review (94). IGFs are principally considered to be polypeptide growth factors that function to regulate cell cycle activity and prevent programmed cell death (95,96). They have less profound effects on cellular intermediary metabolism. These peptides derive their names (IGF-I and IGF-II) from their amino acid sequence homology (approximately 50%) to insulin, the parent hormone in the insulin family of polypeptides.

In general, IGF-I mediates cellular proliferation during postnatal development, while IGF-II is considered to be a fetal growth factor (97). During postnatal life, the synthesis and release of IGF-I from the liver are under the endocrine control of GH. Greater than 95% of the secreted IGF-I circulates in bound form complexed to IGF-binding proteins (IGFBP-1 to -5) (98). Thus, a great deal of the regulation of IGF-I action occurs at the level of IGFBP expression. In addition to the endocrine role of IGF-I, many cell types also produce IGF-I locally for paracrine or autocrine control of cellular growth. This paracrine mechanism is independent of GH.

The receptor for IGF-I is structurally quite similar to that for insulin. It is composed of a tetramer of two α (ligand binding) and two β (signal transducing) subunits (99). The β subunit carries within its structure an intrinsic tyrosine kinase motif that acts as the initial trigger in transducing binding events at the cell surface into intracellular signals for cellular responses. Subsequent cascades of phosphorylation then convey the signal from the cell surface to the interior of the cell for information concerning growth signals. In contrast, the receptor for IGF-II is structurally homologous (99%) to the mannose 6-phosphate receptor, and it is not clear at this time whether this receptor actually transduces useful signals to the cell (100). Instead, IGF-II may exert many of its actions through the IGF-I or even insulin receptors.

In addition to the IGFs and their receptors, IGFBPs also play an important role in the insulin growth factor system. IGFBPs bind to IGFs, prolong their half lives, and regulate their availability for receptor binding (101). IGF-I and -II produce mitogenic effects and augment steroidogenesis within the ovary. IGF-I stimulates the synthesis of DNA and basal (estradiol) E_2 levels in human granulosa cells (102, 103). It is synergistic with gonadotropins in increasing estradiol and progesterone production (104–106). Theca cell DNA and androgen synthesis are augmented by IGF-I, which is synergistic with luteinizing hormone (LH) in androstenedione production (107). *In vitro* maturation of human oocytes is enhanced by IGF-I (108). IGF-II stimulates granulosa cell production of estradiol and progesterone (109–111). Studies have shown that IGF-II is the major IGF functioning in the human ovary (112–114). IGFBPs appear to modulate the actions of IGFs, and, when elevated in androgen-dominant follicles, decrease the amount of bioavailable IGFs, thereby leading to arrested follicular development (101). The affinity of IGFBPs for the IGFs is affected by IGFBP proteases (115). IGFBP regulation is further influenced by gonadotropins, insulin-like peptides, and activin A.

IGF-I suppresses the increase in apoptotic DNA fragmentation of preovulatory and early antral follicles. This effect is neutralized by IGFBP-3. In addition, the suppressive effects of gonadotropins on follicular apoptosis are partially reversed by IGFBP-3, suggesting that IGF-I and other intrafollicular factors are involved in mediating the actions of gonadotropins on follicle survival (116).

The marked insulin resistance noted in obese women with polycystic ovarian syndrome (PCOS) may decrease hepatic production of IGFBP-1, which increases the bioavailability of IGF-I. IGF-I then stimulates thecal androgen production (117). Intraovarian aberrations in the IGF system may contribute to the inability of the PCOS ovary to generate a dominant follicle (118). Small, androgen-dominant follicles contain lower levels of IGF-II and IGFBP-4 protease and elevated levels of IGFBP-2 and IGFBP-4, as compared to estrogen-dominant follicles (119). Oral contraceptive pills increase circulating levels of IGFBP-1 and decrease total IGF-I levels in women with PCOS, which may aid in decreasing ovarian androgen production (120).

There have been numerous animal studies suggesting the presence of IGF-I and IGF-II as well as IGFBPs in the testes. However, it has been noted that men with isolated growth hormone deficiency have intact reproductive function (121).

IGF-I, IGF-II, both IGF receptors, as well as IGFBPs have been documented in mammalian oviductal cells and embryos (122,123). IGF-I has been found to stimulate mitogenic effects in some studies (124). Inhibition of IGF-II decreases the rate of progression to the blastocyst stage with reduced blastomere numbers in mouse embryos (125). In addition, IGFs are thought to promote endometrial cellular mitosis and differentiation with IGF-I, which is believed to be a mediator of estrogen action, and IGF-II, a mediator of progesterone action (126).

The IGF system may play a role in uterine leiomyomata. IGF-I, IGF-II, and the IGF-I receptor levels are higher in leiomyomata than normal myometrial cells (127,128). Levels of IGF-II receptors are similar in leiomyoma and myometrial tissue. Leiomyoma cells also produce IGFBPs (129).

Activin

Activin is a member of the TGF-β superfamily. It is a homodimeric glycoprotein consisting of two β-subunits. Two β-subunits, β_A and β_B, result in activins A (β_A, β_A), AB (β_A, β_B), and B (β_B, β_B). Activin is well known to be a potentiator of follicle-stimulating hormone (FSH) release. In the early follicular phase, activin A stimulates aromatase activity, FSH receptor expression, and inhibin production (130,131). In the late follicular phase, activin A inhibits progesterone and estradiol production (132,133). Activin suppresses apoptotic DNA fragmentation in early antral follicles. Coincubation with follistatin abolishes this suppressive effect (116).

Depending on the conditions, activin may stimulate or inhibit spermatogonial cell proliferation (134). Animals with insertional disruption of the activin receptor have decreased seminiferous tubule volume probably secondary to decreased Sertoli cell number (135).

Inhibin

Inhibin is also a member of the TGF-β superfamily. Inhibins are glycoproteins produced by the granulosa and theca cells of the ovary, by the Sertoli cells of the testis, and in lower proportions by some extragonadal tissues such as the bone marrow, brain, pituitary, liver, and adrenal gland. There are two active molecular forms of inhibin, inhibin A and inhibin B, which are heterodimers made by an α-subunit and either a β_A-subunit (inhibin A) or a β_B-subunit (inhibin B) (136).

Production of inhibin is stimulated by the gonadotropins, with levels rising throughout the menstrual cycle. Levels of inhibin A are low in the early follicular phase and rise from the late follicular phase to peak at midluteal phase. Inhibin B levels rise sharply from the early follicular phase, peak following the FSH rise, and progressively fall during the remainder of the follicular phase. A second peak occurs 2 days after midcycle LH peak with a subsequent rapid decrease during luteal involution (137). These patterns suggest that inhibin B is the major marker of follicular growth, and inhibin A is secreted mostly by the corpus luteum and may be involved in the negative feedback of FSH during the luteal-follicular transition (138).

The rise in FSH as a result of aging may be a consequence of lower levels of inhibin B by a declining number and quality of ovarian follicles. Levels of inhibin A are also reduced in aging women, and levels of both inhibins are nearly undetectable in postmenopausal women (139,140).

It has been shown that granulosa cells of patients with higher levels of cycle day 3 FSH produce lower levels of dimeric inhibin (141). These lower levels may be responsible for the higher levels of FSH seen in women with poor results on the clomiphene citrate challenge test (142). These data suggest that inhibin B is an early marker of ovarian aging and may be a useful tool with which to predict the response to assisted reproductive technology (143).

Inhibins have also been implicated to play a role in ovarian hyperstimulation syndrome (OHSS). Inhibin B levels have been noted to rise during gonadotropin stimulation in patients who later develop OHSS, and inhibin A levels are elevated after OHSS onset (144).

Levels of inhibins are reduced in women with premature ovarian failure (145). In women with PCOS, inhibin levels are elevated as a result of a persistent cohort of small follicles contributing to inhibin production (146). This elevation may lead to the relative deficit of FSH in women with PCOS. The paracrine action of inhibin stimulation of thecal cell androgen production may contribute to the hyperandrogenism (147).

Inhibins may play a role in the occurrence and detection of ovarian tumors. Knockout mice lacking the inhibin α-subunit gene are prone to develop gonadal stromal tumors (148). Women with ovarian cancer may have imbalanced levels of inhibin and activin (149,150). Some tumors, such as granulosa cell tumors, secrete inhibins into the circulation (151). Inhibins may be useful in identifying sex cord-stromal neoplasms (152,153). Elevated levels of inhibin in postmenopausal women may be useful as a tumor marker (154), and measurements of inhibin may be useful in the follow-up of women treated for ovarian cancer.

Inhibin A and B are also found in the human placenta, fetal membranes, decidua, and amniotic fluid (146). Levels of inhibin in these tissues are regulated by a number of hormones and growth factors. Inhibins may participate in placental hormone secretion, placental immune modulation, and control of cell growth and differentiation. Abnormally low serum levels of inhibin B are noted in pregnant women with chronic hypertension, intrauterine growth retardation, and preeclampsia. Serum levels of inhibin are elevated in pregnant women with a Down syndrome baby (146).

Follistatin

Follistatin is a high-affinity activin-binding protein. It has one binding site for the activin β-subunit and therefore can also bind to inhibin, but with 1,000-fold weaker affinity (155). It antagonizes activin in every system (156), including stimulation of FSH synthesis and secretion. Therefore, it has been implicated in the functional impairment of the FSH-granulosa cell axis in PCOS (157). The follistatin gene was demonstrated to have the strongest evidence of linkage and association with PCOS or hyperandrogenemia in 150 families (158). However, a follow-up analysis did not reveal a single mutation in the follistatin gene of women with PCOS (157).

Müllerian Inhibiting Substance (MIS)

MIS is a member of the TGF-β superfamily. It is produced by Sertoli cells and leads to resorption of the müllerian ducts, and the analgen of the female internal reproductive structures (uterus, oviducts, and the upper third of the vagina) of the male fetus (159). It has also been isolated in the ovary and inhibits the resumption of oocyte meiosis and granulosa cell mitosis (160). Serum levels of MIS in the male remain substantial after birth and are suppressed at puberty. Some studies suggest actions of MIS on spermatogenesis (161); however, currently the most clinically useful feature is measurement of serum levels to assess patients with disorders of sex differentiation and reproduction. Levels of MIS have been noted to fluctuate during the menstrual cycle, with levels peaking at midcycle and then decreasing in the midluteal phase (162).

Platelet-Derived Growth Factors

Platelet-derived growth factors (PDGFs) are proteins of 30 kd with two subunits (A and B) connected by disulfide bonds. The subunits can be combined interchangeably, resulting in three dimeric forms (AA, AB, and BB). The receptors belong to a family of tyrosine kinase receptors and also have a dimer of subunits, with each subunit (α and β) interacting with one of the subunits of the PDGF molecule. Type α binds to all PDGF dimers with high affinity, while type β only binds PDGF-BB (126). PDGFs have been identified in the mouse embryo (163) and in media from *in vitro* fertilization (IVF) human embryos at the blastocyst stage (164). It has also been identified in cow oviducts and human endometrium (126). PDGF has been noted to stimulate endometrial stromal cell proliferation *in vitro*. This effect is enhanced by estradiol. Macrophage in women with endometriosis release growth factor activity to a greater extent than those derived from women without endometriosis. This growth factor may be similar or identical to PDGF (165). Addition of PDGF to cultured myometrial or leiomyoma cells results in a threefold increase in DNA synthesis (166).

Vascular Endothelial Growth Factor

Vascular endothelial growth factor (VEGF) is a 45-kd heparin-binding angiogenic glycoprotein that enhances vascular permeability and vascular endothelial cell mitosis (167). It is a likely angiogenic factor in the ovary. Compelling evidence suggests that VEGF has a major role in the pathogenesis of OHSS and has been identified as the primary contributor to capillary permeability in OHSS (168). It is one of many angiogenic cytokines produced by granulosa cells and is believed to be involved in the microvascular remodeling noted during resumption of meiosis (169). Production of VEGF is stimulated by LH and human chorionic gonadotropin (hCG) and has also been demonstrated to be enhanced by hypoxia (170). The follicular fluid of older women has been noted to contain higher levels of VEGF (171). This may be a result of a more hypoxic environment within these aging follicles. Higher levels of VEGF in follicular fluid have been documented in women having poorer outcomes with assisted reproductive technology (172). VEGF also plays an angiogenic role in endometrial development. Levels of endometrial VEGF increase throughout the menstrual cycle and peak during the secretory phase and are stimulated by estradiol and medroxyprogesterone acetate (173). Women with moderate to severe endometriosis appear to have higher peritoneal levels of VEGF than those with minimal to mild endometriosis, or those without endometriosis. In lieu of these findings as well as the hypervascularization associated with endometriosis, VEGF may play a role in the pathogenesis of this disease.

10 KEY POINTS

1. Cytokines mediate proinflammatory and antiinflammatory actions in a variety of cell types and tissues.

2. Interleukins-1α and -1β mediate identical functions in target cells and have similar affinities for the IL-1 receptor.

3. The type IL-1 receptor mediates the biologic effects of IL-1α and IL-1β, while the type II receptor serves as a decoy receptor without signal transducing capacity.

4. IL-1 and tumor necrosis factor induce robust prostaglandin biosynthesis in gestational tissues.

5. Chemokines are cytokines that mediate chemotactic activities in granulocytes and other target cells.

6. EGF and TGF-α share a common receptor and elicit nearly identical biologic actions.

7. The marked insulin resistance noted in obese women with polycystic ovarian syndrome (PCOS) may decrease hepatic production of IGFBP-1, which increases the bioavailability of IGF-I. IGF-I then stimulates thecal androgen production.

8. Intraovarian aberrations in the IGF system may contribute to the inability of the PCOS ovary to generate a dominant follicle.

9. The rise in FSH as a result of aging may be a consequence of lower levels of inhibin B by a declining number and quality of ovarian follicles. Levels of inhibin A are also reduced in aging women, and levels of both inhibins are nearly undetectable in postmenopausal women.

10. Compelling evidence suggests that VEGF has a major role in the pathogenesis of ovarian hyperstimulation syndrome (OHSS).

REFERENCES

1. Dinarello CA. Role of interleukin-1 and tumor necrosis factor in systemic responses to infection and inflammation. In: Gallin JI, Goldstein IM, Snyderman R, eds. *Inflammation: basic principles and clinical correlates.* New York: Raven Press, 1992:211–232.

2. Beutler B, Cerami A. Cachectin: more than a tumor necrosis factor. *N Engl J Med* 1987;316:379–385.

3. Dinarello CA. Biological basis for interleukin-1 in disease. *Blood* 1996;87:2095–2147.

4. Eisenberg SP, Brewer MT, Verderber E, et al. Interleukin 1 receptor antagonist is a member of the interleukin 1 gene family: evolution of a cytokine control mechanism. *Proc Natl Acad Sci USA* 1991;88:5232–5236.

5. Kobayashi Y, Yamamoto K, Saido T, et al. Identification of calcium-activated neutral protease as a processing enzyme of human interleukin 1 alpha. *Proc Natl Acad Sci USA* 1990;87:5548–5552.

6. Hay DWP, Torphy TJ, Undem BJ. Cysteinyl leukotrienes in asthma: old mediators up to new tricks. *Trends Pharmacol Sci* 1995;16:304–309.

7. Dinarello CA. Interleukin-1 and interleukin-1 antagonism. *Blood* 1991;77:1627–1652.

8. Geller DA, Nussler AK, Di Silvio M, et al. Cytokines, endotoxin, and glucocorticoids regulate the expression of inducible nitric oxide synthase in hepatocytes. *Proc Natl Acad Sci USA* 1993;90:522–526.

9. Kennard EA, Zimmerman PD, Friedman CI, et al. Interleukin-1β induces cyclooxygenase-2 in cultured human decidual cells. *Am J Reprod Immunol* 1995;34:65–71.

10. Alnaif B, Benzie RJ, Gibb W. Studies on the action of interleukin-1 on term human fetal membranes and decidua. *Can J Physiol Pharmacol* 1994;72:133–139.

11. Vinatier D, Dufour P, Tordjeman-Rizzi N, et al. Immunological aspects of ovarian function: role of the cytokines. *Eur J Obstet Gynecol Reprod Biol* 1995;63:155–168.

12. Hurwitz A, Loukides J, Ricciarelli E, et al. Human intraovarian interleukin-1 (IL-1) system: highly compartmentalized and hormonally dependent regulation of the genes encoding IL-1, its receptor, and its receptor antagonist. *J Clin Invest* 1992;89:1746–1754.

13. Narko K, Ritvos O, Ristimaki A. Induction of cyclooxygenase-2 and prostaglandin $F_{2\alpha}$ receptor expression by interleukin-1β in cultured human granulosa-luteal cells. *Endocrinology* 1997;138:3638–3644.

14. Polan ML, Loukides JA, Honig J. Interleukin-1 in human ovarian cells and in peripheral blood monocytes increases during the luteal phase: evidence for a midcycle surge in the human. *Am J Obstet Gynecol* 1994;170:1000–1007.

15. Simon C, Piquette GN, Frances A, et al. Localization of interleukin-1 type I receptor and interleukin-1β in human endometrium throughout the menstrual cycle. *J Clin Endocrinol Metab* 1993;77:549–555.

16. Romero R, Mazor M, Brandt F, et al. Interleukin-1 alpha and interleukin-1 beta in preterm and term human parturition. *Am J Reprod Immunol* 1992;27:117–123.

17. Romero R, Brody DT, Oyarzun E, et al. Infection and labor. III. Interleukin-1: a signal for the onset of parturition. *Am J Obstet Gynecol* 1989;160:1117–1123.

18. Fidel PL, Romero R, Wolf N, et al. Systemic and local cytokine profiles in endotoxin-induced preterm parturition in mice. *Am J Obstet Gynecol* 1994;170:1467–1475.

19. Romero R, Wu YK, Brody DT, Oyarzun E, et al. Human decidua: a source of interleukin-1. *Obstet Gynecol* 1989;73:31–34.

20. Tabibzadeh S, Kaffka KL, Satyaswaroop PG, et al. Interleukin-1 (IL-1) regulation of human endometrial function: presence of IL-1 receptor correlates with IL-1-stimulated prostaglandin E_2 production. *J Clin Endocrinol Metab* 1990;70:1000–1006.

21. Mitchell MD, Edwin SS, Romero RJ. Prostaglandin biosynthesis by human decidual cells: effects of inflammatory mediators. *Prostaglandins Leukot Essent Fatty Acids* 1990;41:35–38.

22. Romero R, Durum S, Dinarello CA, et al. Interleukin-1 stimulates prostaglandin biosynthesis by human amnion. *Prostaglandins* 1989;37:13–22.

23. Albert TJ, Su H-C, Zimmerman PD, et al. Interleukin-1β regulates the inducible cyclooxygenase in amnion-derived WISH cells. *Prostaglandins* 1994;48:401–416.

24. Ishihara O, Khan H, Sullivan MHF, et al. Interleukin-1β stimulates decidual stromal cell cyclooxygenase enzyme and prostaglandin production. *Prostaglandins* 1992;44:43–52.

25. Ishihara O, Numari H, Saitoh M, et al. Prostaglandin E_2 production by endogenous secretion of interleukin-1 in decidual cells obtained before and after the labor. *Prostaglandins* 1996;52:199–208.

26. Lin L-L, Lin AY, DeWitt DL. Interleukin-1α induces the accumulation of cytosolic phospholipase A2 and the release of prostaglandin E$_2$ in human fibroblasts. *J Biol Chem* 1992;267:23451–23454.

27. Xue S, Slater DM, Bennett PR, et al. Induction of both cytosolic phospholipase A$_2$ and prostaglandin H synthase-2 by interleukin-1β in WISH cells is inhibited by dexamethasone. *Prostaglandins* 1996;51:107–124.

28. Imada K, Ito A, Sato T, et al. Hormonal regulation of matrix metalloproteinase 9/gelatinase B gene expression in rabbit uterine cervical fibroblasts. *Biol Reprod* 1997;56:575–580.

29. Rath W, Osmers R, Adelman-Grill BC, et al. Biochemical changes in human cervical connective tissue after intracervical application of prostaglandin E$_2$. *Prostaglandins* 1993;45:375–384.

30. Sennstrom MR, Granstrom LM, Lockwood CJ, et al. Cervical fetal fibronectin correlates to prostaglandin E$_2$-induced cervical ripening and can be identified in cervical tissue. *Am J Obstet Gynecol* 1998;173:540–545.

31. Dinarello CA. Interleukin-1. *Cytokine Growth Factor Rev* 1997; 8:253–265.

32. Colotta F, Re F, Muzio M, et al. Interleukin-1 type II receptor: a decoy target for IL-1 that is regulated by IL-4. *Science* 1993; 261:472–475.

33. Greenfelder SA, Nunes P, Kwee L. Molecular cloning and characterization of a second subunit of the interleukin-1 receptor complex. *J Biol Chem* 1995;270:13757–13765.

34. Guy GR, Chua SP, Wong NS, et al. Interleukin 1 and tumor necrosis factor activate common multiple protein kinases in human fibroblasts. *J Biol Chem* 1991;266:14343–14352.

35. Renard P, Zachary M-D, Bougelet C, et al. Effects of antioxidant enzyme modulations of interleukin-1-induced nuclear factor κB activation. *Biochem Pharmacol* 1997;53:149–160.

36. Mallinin NL, Boldin MP, Kovalenko AV, et al. MAP3K-related kinase involved in NF-κB induction by TNF, CD95 and IL-1. *Nature* 1997;385:540–544.

37. Wilmer WA, Tan LC, Dickerson JA, et al. Interleukin-1β induction of mitogen-activated protein kinases in human mesangial cells: role of oxidation. *J Biol Chem* 1997;272:10877–10881.

38. Simon C, Piquette GN, Frances A, et al. The effect of interleukin-1β (IL-1β) on the regulation of IL-1 receptor type I messenger ribonucleic acid and protein levels in cultured human endometrial stromal and glandular cells. *J Clin Endocrinol Metab* 1994;78:675–682.

39. Simon C, Piquette GN, Frances A, et al. Interleukin-1 type I receptor messenger ribonucleic acid expression in human endometrium throughout the menstrual cycle. *Fertil Steril* 1993; 59:791–796.

40. Kauma SW, Walsh SW, Nestler JE, et al. Interleukin-1 is induced in the human placenta by endotoxin and isolation procedures for trophoblasts. *J Clin Endocrinol Metab* 1992; 75:951–955.

41. Simon C, Frances A, Piquette GN, et al. Embryonic implantation in mice is blocked by interleukin-1 receptor antagonist. *Endocrinology* 1994;134:521–528.

42. Simon C, Frances A, Piquette GN, et al.Interleukin-1 system in the materno-trophoblast unit in human implantation: immunohistochemical evidence for autocrine/paracrine function. *J Clin Endocrinol Metab* 1994;78:847–854.

43. Old LJ. Tumor necrosis factor (TNF). *Science* 1985;230:630–632.

44. Strieter RM, Kunkel SL, Bone RC. Role of tumor necrosis factor-alpha in disease states and inflammation. *Crit Care Med* 1993;21:S447–463.

45. Meager A. Cytokine regulation of cellular adhesion molecule expression in inflammation. *Cytokine Growth Factor Rev* 1999; 10:27–39.

46. Larrick JW, Wright SC. Cytotoxic mechanism of tumor necrosis factor-α. *FASEB J* 1990;4:3215–3223.

47. Wallach D. Suicide by order: some open questions about the cell-killing activities of the TNF ligand and receptor families. *Growth Factor Cytokine Rev* 1996;7:211–221.

48. Jacobson MD, Weil M, Raff MC. Programmed cell death in animal development. *Cell* 1997;88:347–354.

49. Medvedev AE, Espevik T, Ranges G, et al. Distinct roles of the two tumor necrosis factor (TNF) receptors in modulating TNF and lymphotoxin α effects. *J Biol Chem* 1996;271:9778–9784.

50. Tartaglia LA, Weber RF, Figari IS, et al. Two different receptors for tumor necrosis factor mediate distinct cellular responses. *Proc Natl Acad Sci USA* 1991;88:9292–9296.

51. Hunt JS, Chen HL, Miller L. Tumor necrosis factors: pivotal components of pregnancy? *Biol Reprod* 1996;54:554–562.

52. Fortunato SJ, Menon R, Swan KF II. Expression of TNF-α and TNFR p55 in cultured amniochorion. *Am J Reprod Immunol* 1994;32:188–193.

53. Romero R, Mazor M, Manogue K. Human decidua: a source of tumor necrosis factor. *Eur J Obstet Gynecol Reprod Biol* 1991;41:123–127.

54. Imseis HM, Zimmerman PD, Samuels P, et al. Tumour necrosis factor-α induces cyclo-oxygenase-2 gene expression in first trimester trophoblasts: suppression by glucocorticoids and NSAIDs. *Placenta* 1997;18:521–526.

55. Perkins DJ, Kniss DA. Tumor necrosis factor-α promotes sustained cyclooxygenase-2 expression: attenuation by dexamethasone and NSAIDs. *Prostaglandins* 1997;54:727–743.

56. Heinrich PC, Castell JV, Andus T. Interleukin-6 and the acute phase response. *Biochem J* 1990;265:621–636.

57. Ghidini A, Jenkins CB, Spong CY, et al. Elevated amniotic fluid interleukin-6 levels during the early second trimester are associated with greater risk of subsequent preterm delivery. *Am J Reprod Immunol* 1997;37:227–231.

58. Greig PC, Ernest JM, Teot L, et al. Amniotic fluid interleukin-6 levels correlate with histologic chorioamnionitis and amniotic fluid cultures in patients in premature labor with intact membranes. *Am J Obstet Gynecol* 1993;169:1035–1044.

59. Hsu C-D, Meaddough E, Hong S-F, et al. Elevated amniotic fluid nitric oxide metabolites and interleukin-6 in intra-amniotic infection. *J Soc Gynecol Invest* 1998;5:21–24.

60. Wenstrom KD, Andrews WW, Hauth JC, et al. Elevated second-trimester amniotic fluid interleukin-6 levels predict preterm delivery. *Am J Obstet Gynecol* 1998;173:547–550.

61. Dudley DJ, Trautman MS, Edwin SS, et al. Biosynthesis of interleukin-6 by cultured human chorion laeve cells: regulation by cytokines. *J Clin Endocrinol Metab* 1992;75:1081–1086.

62. Mitchell MD, Dudley DJ, Edwin SS, et al. Interleukin-6 stimulates prostaglandin production by human amnion and decidual cells. *Br J Pharmacol* 1991;192:189–191.

63. Kameda T, Matsuzaki N, Sawal K, et al. Production of interleukin-6 by normal human trophoblasts. *Placenta* 1990;11:205–213.

64. Harada T, Yoshioka H, Yoshida S, et al. Increased interleukin-6 levels in peritoneal fluid of infertile patients with active endometriosis. *Am J Obstet Gynecol* 1997;176:593–597.

65. Paul WE. Interleukin-4: a prototypic immunoregulatory lymphokine. *Blood* 1991;77:1859–1870.

66. Howard M, Farrar J, Hilfiker M, et al. Identification of of a T-cell derived B-cell growth factor distinct from interleukin 2. *J Exp Med* 1982;155:159.

67. Kopf M, Le Gros G, Bachmann M, et al. Disruption of the

murine IL-4 gene blocks Th2 cytokine responses. *Nature* 1993; 362:245.

68. Lala PK, Scodras JM, Graham CH, et al. Activation of maternal killer cells in the pregnant uterus with chronic indomethacin therapy, IL-2 therapy, or a combination of therapy is associated with embryonic demise. *Cell Immunol* 1990;127:368–381.

69. Jones CA, Williams KA, Findlay-Jones JJ, et al. Interleukin-4 production by human amnion epithelial cells and regulation of its activity by glycosaminoglycan binding. *Biol Reprod* 1995.

70. Haynes MK, Jackson LG, Tuan RS, et al. Cytokine production in first trimester chorionic villi: detection of mRNAs and protein products in situ. *Cell Immunol* 1993;151:300–308.

71. Bry K, Lappalainen U. Interleukin-4 and transforming growth factor-β1 modulate the production of interleukin-1 receptor antagonist and of prostaglandin E$_2$ by decidual cells. *Am J Obstet Gynecol* 1994;170:1194–1198.

72. Moore KW, O'Garra A, de Waal Malefyt R, et al. Interleukin-10. *Annu Rev Immunol* 1993;11:165–190.

73. Robertson SA, Seamark RF, Guilbert LJ, et al. The role of cytokines in gestation. *Crit Rev Immunol* 1994;14:239–293.

74. Baggiolini M, Dewald B, Walz A. Interleukin-8 and related chemotactic cytokines. In: Gallin JI, Goldstein IM, Snyderman R, eds. *Inflammation: basic principles and clinical correlates.* New York: Raven Press, 1992:247–263.

75. Cassatella MA, Gasperini S, Calzetti F, et al. Lipopolysaccharide-induced interleukin-8 gene expression in human granulocytes: transcriptional inhibition by interferon-gamma. *Biochem J* 1995;310:751–755.

76. Jones RL, Kelly R, Critchley HOD. Chemokine and cyclooxygenase-2 expression in human endometrium coincides with leukocyte accumulation. *Hum Reprod* 1997;12:1300–1306.

77. Arici A, Head JR, MacDonald PC, et al. Regulation of interleukin-8 gene expression in human endometrial cells in culture. *Mol Cell Endocrinol* 1993;94:195–204.

78. Cherouny PH, Pankuch GA, Romero R, et al. Neutrophil attractant/activating peptide-1/interleukin-8: association with histologic chorioamnionitis, preterm delivery, and bioactive amniotic fluid leukoattractants. *Am J Obstet Gynecol* 1993;169: 1299–1303.

79. Keelan JA, Marvin KW, Sato TA, et al. Cytokine abundance in placental tissues: evidence of inflammatory activation in gestational membranes with term and preterm parturition. *Am J Obstet Gynecol* 1999;181:1530–1536.

80. Winkler M, Fischer D-C, Ruck P, et al. Parturition at term: parallel increases in interleukin-8 and proteinase concentrations and neutrophil count in the lower uterine segment. *Hum Reprod* 1999;14:1096–1100.

81. El Maradny E, Kanayama N, Halim A, et al. Interleukin-8 induces cervical ripening in rabbits. *Am J Obstet Gynecol* 1994; 171:77–83.

82. McAdam B, Keimowitz RM, Maher M, et al. Transdermal modification of platelet function: an aspirin patch system results in marked suppression of platelet cyclooxygenase. *J Pharmacol Exp Ther* 1996;277:559–564.

83. Carpenter G, Cohen S. Epidermal growth factor. *Annu Rev Biochem* 1979;48:193–216.

84. Scott J, Urdea M, Quiroga M, et al. Structure of a mouse maxillary messenger RNA encoding epidermal growth factor and seven related proteins. *Science* 1983;221:236–240.

85. Rall LR, Scott J, Bell GI. Mouse prepro-epidermal growth factor synthesis by the kidney and other tissues. *Nature* 1985;313: 228–231.

86. Ichiba H, Fujimura M, Takeuchi T. Levels of epidermal growth factor in human cord blood. *Biol Neonate* 1992;61:302–307.

87. Scott SM, Buenaflor GG, Orth DN. Immunoreactive human epidermal growth factor concentrations in amniotic fluid, um-

bilical artery and vein serum and placenta in full-term and preterm infants. *Biol Neonate* 1989;56:246–251.

88. Tsutsumi O, Oka T. Epidermal growth factor deficiency during pregnancy causes abortion in mice. *Am J Obstet Gynecol* 1987; 156:241–244.

89. Casey ML, Korte K, MacDonald PC. Epidermal growth factor stimulation of prostaglandin E$_2$ biosynthesis in amnion cells: induction of prostaglandin H$_2$ synthase. *J Biol Chem* 1988; 263:7846–7854.

90. Bonvissuto AC, Lala PK, Kennedy TG, et al. Induction of transforming growth factor-alpha gene expression in rat decidua is independent of the conceptus. *Biol Reprod* 1992;46:607–616.

91. Han VK, Hunter ES III, Pratt RM, et al. Expression of rat transforming growth factor alpha mRNA during development occurs predominantly in the maternal decidua. *Mol Cell Biol* 1987;7:2335–2343.

92. Klip A, Tsakiridis T, Marette A, et al. Regulation of expression of glucose transporters by glucose: a review of studies in vivo and in cell cultures. *FASEB J* 1994;8:43–53.

93. Kahn BB. Glucose transport: pivotal step in insulin action. *Diabetes* 1996;45:1644–1654.

94. Flakoll P, Carlson MG, Cherrington A. Physiologic action of insulin. In: LeRoith D, Taylor SI, Olefsky JM, eds. *Diabetes mellitus: a fundamental and clinical text.* Philadelphia: Lippincott-Raven, 1996:121–132.

95. Moise KJ, Huhta JC, Sharif DS, et al. Indomethacin treatment of premature labor. Effects on the fetal ductus arteriosus. *N Engl J Med* 1988;319:327–331.

96. Heemskerk VH, Daemen MARC, Buurman WA. Insulin-like growth factor-1 (IGF-1) and growth hormone (GH) in immunity and inflammation. *Cytokine Growth Factor Rev* 1999;10: 5–14.

97. D'Ercole AJ. Insulin-like growth factors and their receptors in growth. *Endocrinol Metab Clin North Am* 1996;25:573–590.

98. Clemmons DR. Insulin-like growth factor binding proteins. In: LeRoith D, ed. *Insulin-like growth factors: molecular and cellular aspects.* Boca Raton: CRC Press, 1991:151–179.

99. Cohick WS, Clemmons DR. The insulin-like growth factors. *Annu Rev Physiol* 1993;55:131–153.

100. Nissley P, Kiess W, Sklar MM. Insulin-like growth factor-II/ mannose 6-phosphate receptor. In: LeRoith D, ed. *Insulin-like growth factors: molecular and cellular aspects.* Boca Raton: CRC Press, 1991:111–150.

101. Guidice LC, Cataldo NA, van Dessel T, et al. Growth factors in normal ovarian follicle development. *Reprod Endocrinol* 1996; 14:179–196.

102. Olsson J-H, Carlsson B, Hillensjo T. Effect of insulin-like growth factor-1 on deoxyribonucleic acid synthesis in cultured human granulosa cells. *Fertil Steril* 1990;54:1052–1057.

103. Yong EL, Baird DT, Yates R, et al. Hormonal regulation of the growth and steroidogenic function of human granulosa cells. *J Clin Endocrinol Metab* 1992;74:842–850.

104. Erickson GF, Garzo VG, Magoffin DA. Insulin-like growth factor-1 regulates aromatase activity in human granulosa and granulosa-luteal cells. *J Clin Endocrinol* 1989;69:716–720.

105. Mason H, Margara R, Winston RML, et al. Insulin-like growth factor-I (IGF-I) inhibits production of IGF-binding protein-1 while stimulating estradiol secretion in granulosa cells from normal and polycystic human ovaries. *J Clin Endocrinol Metab* 1993;76:1275–1279.

106. Erickson GF, Garzo VG, Magoffin DA. Progesterone production by human granulosa cells cultured in serum free medium: effects of gonadotrophins and insulin-like growth factor-I (IGF-I). *Hum Reprod* 1991;6:1074–1081.

107. Hillier SG, Yong EL, Illingworth PJ, et al. Effect of recombinant

activin on androgen synthesis in cultured human thecal cells. *J Clin Endocrinol Metab* 1991;72:1206–1211.

108. Gomez E, Tarin JJ, Pellicer MD. Oocyte maturation in humans: the role of gonadotropins and growth factors. *Fertil Steril* 1993; 660:40–46.

109. Kamada S, Kubota T, Taguhi M, et al. Effects of insulin-like growth factor-2 on proliferation and differentiation of ovarian granulosa cells. *Horm Res* 1992;37:141–145.

110. Kubota T, Kamada S, Ohara M, et al. Insulin-like growth factor-2 in follicular fluid of the patients with in vitro fertilization and embryo transfer. *Fertil Steril* 1993;59:844–849.

111. Dor J, Ben-Shlomo I, Lunenfeld B, et al. Estradiol production by granulosa cells of normal and polycystic ovaries: relationship to menstrual cycle history and concentrations of gonadotropins and sex steroids in follicular fluid. *J Clin Endocrinol Metab* 1994;79:1355–1360.

112. Lunenfeld B, Menashe Y, Dor Y, et al. The effect of growth hormone, growth factors, and their binding globulins on ovarian responsiveness. *Contracept Fertil Sex* 1991;19:133–136.

113. Menashe Y, Sack J, Mashiach S. Spontaneous pregnancies in two women with Laron-type dwarfism: are growth hormone and circulating insulin-like growth factor mandatory for induction of ovulation? *Hum Reprod* 1991;6:670–671.

114. Dor J, Ben-Shlomo I, Lunenfeld B. Insulin-like growth factor-I (IGF-I) may not be essential for ovarian follicular development: evidence from IGF-I deficiency. *J Clin Endocrinol Metab* 1992; 74:539–542.

115. Chandrasekher YA, Giudice LC. Estrogen, but not androgen-dominant human ovarian follicular fluid contains an insulin-like growth factor binding protein-4 protease. *J Clin Endocrinol Metab* 1995;80:2734–2739.

116. Chun S-Y, Eisenhauer K, Minami S, et al. Growth factors in ovarian follicle atresia. *Reprod Endocrinol* 1996;14:197–202.

117. Poretsky L, Peiper B. Insulin resistance, hypersecretion of LH, and a dual-defect hypothesis for the pathogenesis of polycystic ovary syndrome. *Obstet Gynecol* 1994;84:613–621.

118. Giudice LC, Morales AJ, Yen SSSC. Growth factors and polycystic ovarian syndrome. *Reprod Endocrinol* 1996;14:203–208.

119. van Dessel HJHMT, Yap OW, Chandrasekher YA, et al. Ovarian follicular levels of insulin-like growth factor (IGF)-I, IGF-II, and IGF binding proteins-1 and -3 during the follicular phase of the normal menstrual cycle. *J Clin Endocrinol Metab* 1996;81:1224–1231.

120. Suikkari A-M, Tiitinen A, Stenman U-H, et al. Oral contraceptives increase insulin-like growth factor binding protein concentration in women with polycystic ovarian disease. *Fertil Steril* 1991;55:895–899.

121. Brinster RL, Zimmermann JW. Spermatogenesis following male germ-cell transplantation. *Proc Natl Acad Sci USA* 1994;91:11298–11302.

122. Carlsson B, Hillensjo T, Nilsson A, et al. Expression of insulin-like growth factor-I (IGF-I) in the rat fallopian tube: possible autocrine and paracrine action of fallopian tube-derived IGF-I on the fallopian tube and on the preimplantation embryo. *Endocrinology* 1993;133:2031–2039.

123. Watson AJ, Watson PH, Arcellana-Panlilio M, et al. A growth factor phenotype map for ovine preimplantation development. *Biol Reprod* 1994;50:725–733.

124. Kaye PL, Gardner HG, Harvey MB, et al. Insulin and insulin-like growth factors in mouse development: insulin as an embryonic growth factor. Organon Embryology Symposium, Canberra, Australia, 1989;12–15.

125. Rappolee DA, Strum KS, Behrendtsen O, et al. Insulin-like growth factor II acts through an endogenous growth pathway regulated by imprinting in early mouse embryos. *Genes Dev* 1992;6:939–952.

126. Tazuke SI, Giudice LC. Growth factors and cytokines in endometrium, embryonic development, and maternal:embryonic interactions. *Reprod Endocrinol* 1996;14:231–245.

127. Rein MS, Friedman AJ, Pandian MR, et al. The secretion of insulin-like growth factors I and II by explant cultures of fibroids and myometrium from women treated with a gonadotropin-releasing hormone agonist. *Obstet Gynecol* 1990;76:388–394.

128. Chandrasekhar Y, Heiner J, Osuamkpe C, et al. Insulin-like growth factor I and II binding in human myometrium and leiomyomas. *Am J Obstet Gynecol* 1992;166:64–69.

129. Giudice LC, Irwin JC, Dsupin BA. Insulin-like growth factor (IGF), IGF binding protein (IGFBP), and IGF receptor gene expression and IGFBP synthesis in human uterine leiomyomata. *Hum Reprod* 1993;8:1796–1806.

130. LaPolt PS, Aoro S, Au J-G. Activin stimulation of inhibin secretion and messenger RNA levels in cultured granulosa cells. *Mol Endocrinol* 1989;3:1666–1673.

131. Hillier SG, Miro F. Inhibin, activin, and follistatin: potential roles in ovarian physiology. *Ann NY Acad Sci* 1993;687:29–38.

132. Li W, Ho YB, Leung PCK. Inhibition of progestin accumulation by activin-A in human granulosa cells. *J Clin Endocrinol Metab* 1992;75:285–289.

133. Brannian JD, Woodruff TK, Mather JP, et al. Activin-A inhibits progesterone production by macaque luteal cells in culture. *J Clin Endocrinol Metab* 1992;75:756–761.

134. Mather JP, Attie KM, Woodruff TK, et al. Activin stimulates spermatogonial proliferation in germ-Sertoli cell cocultures from immature rat testis. *Endocrinology* 1990;127:3206–3214.

135. Matzuk MM, Kumar TR, Bradley A. Different phenotypes for mice deficient in either activins or activin receptor type II. *Nature* 1995;374:356–360.

136. Hayes FJ, Hall JE, Boepple PA, et al. Differential control of gonadotropin secretion in the human: endocrine role of inhibin. *J Clin Endocrinol Metab* 1998;83:1835–1841.

137. Groome NP, Illingworth PJ, O'Brien M, et al. Measurement of dimeric inhibin B throughout the human menstrual cycle. *J Clin Endocrinol Metab* 1996;81:1401–1405.

138. Welt C, Martin KA, Taylor AE, et al. Frequency modulation of follicle-stimulation hormone (FSH) during the luteal-follicular transition: evidence for FSH control of inhibin B in normal women. *J Clin Endocrinol Metab* 1997;82:2645–2652.

139. Danforth DR, Arbogast LK, Mroueh J, et al. Dimeric inhibin: a direct marker of ovarian aging. *Fertil Steril* 1998;70:119–123.

140. Burger HG, Cachir N, Robertson DM, et al. Serum inhibins A and B fall differentially as FSH rises in perimenopausal women. *Clin Endocrinol* 1998;48:809–813.

141. Seifer DB, Gardiner AC, Lambert Messerlian G, et al. Differential secretion of dimeric inhibin in cultured luteinized granulosa cells as a function of ovarian reserve. *J Clin Endocrinol Metab* 1996;81:736–739.

142. Hofmann GE, Danforth DR, Seifer DB. Inhibin-B: the physiologic basis of the clomiphene citrate challenge test for ovarian reserve screening. *Fertil Steril* 1998;69:474–477.

143. Seifer DB, Lambert-Messerlian GM, Hogan JW, et al. Day 3 serum inhibin-B is predictive of assisted reproductive technologies outcome. *Fertil Steril* 1997;67:101–104.

144. Enskog A, Nilsson L, Brannstrom M. Peripheral blood concentrations of inhibin B are elevated during gonadotrophin stimulation in patients who later develop ovarian OHSS and inhibin A concentrations are elevated after OHSS onset. *Hum Reprod* 2000;15:532–538.

145. Petraglia F, Hartmann B, Luisi S, et al. Low levels of serum inhibin A and inhibin B in women with hypergonadotropic amenorrhea and evidence of high levels of activin A in women with hyothalamic amenorrhea. *Fertil Steril* 1998;70:907–912.

146. Petraglia F, Zanin E, Faletti A, et al. Inhibins: paracrine and

endocrine effects in female reproductive function. *Reprod Endocrinol* 1999;11:241–247.

147. Pigny P, Desailloud R, Cortet Rudelli C, et al. Serum alpha-inhibin levels in polycystic ovary syndrome: relationship to the serum androstenedione level. *J Clin Endocrinol Metab* 1997;82:1939–1943.

148. Matzuk MM, Finegold MJ, Su JJ, et al. α-Inhibin is a tumour-suppressor gene with gonadal specificity in mice. *Nature* 1992;360:313–319.

149. Zheng W, Luo MP, Welt C, et al. Imbalanced expression of inhibin and activin subunits in primary epithelial ovarian cancer. *Gynecol Oncol* 1998;69:23–31.

150. Welt C, Lambert, Messerlian G, Zheng W, et al. Presence of activin, inhibin, and follistatin in epithelial ovarian carcinoma. *J Clin Endocrinol Metab* 1997;82:3720–3727.

151. Petraglia F, Luisi S, Pautier P, et al. Inhibin B is the major form of inhibin/activin family secreted by granulosa cell tumors. *J Clin Endocrinol Metab* 1998;83:1029–1032.

152. Hildebrandt RH, Rouse RV, Longacre TA. Value of inhibin in the identification of granulosa cell tumours of the ovary. *Hum Pathol* 1997;28:1387–1395.

153. Pelkey TJ, Frierson HF Jr, Mills SE, et al. The diagnostic utility of inhibin staining in ovarian neoplasms. *Int J Gynecol Pathol* 1998;17:97–105.

154. Burger HG, Baile A, Drummond AE, et al. Inhibin and ovarian cancer. *J Reprod Immunol* 1998;39:77–87.

155. Schneyer AL, Rzucidlo DA, Sluss PM, et al. Characterization of unique binding kinetics of follistatin and activin or inhibin in serum. *Endocrinology* 1994;135:667–674.

156. Cataldo NA, Fujimoto VY, Jaffe RB. Follistatin antagonizes the effects of activin-A on steroidogenesis in human luteinizing granulosa cells. *J Clin Endocrinol Metab* 1994;79:272–277.

157. Liao WX, Roy AC, Ng SC. Preliminary investigation of follistatin gene mutations in women with polycystic ovarian syndrome. *Mol Hum Reprod* 2000;6:587–590.

158. Urbanek M, Legro RS, Driscoll DA, et al. Thirty-seven candidate genes for polycystic ovarian syndrome: strongest evidence for linkage is with follistatin. *Proc Natl Acad Sci USA* 1999;96:8573–8578.

159. Lee MM, Donahoe PK. Müllerian inhibiting substance: a gonadal hormone with multiple functions. *Endocr Rev* 1993;14:152–164.

160. Kim JH, Seibel MM, MacLaughlin DT. The inhibitory effects of mullerian-inhibiting substance on epidermal growth factor induced proliferation and progesterone production of human granulosa-luteal cells. *Endocrinology* 1992;75:911–917.

161. Smith EP, Conti M. Growth factors and testicular function: relevance to disorders of spermatogenesis in humans. *Reprod Endocrinol* 1996;14:209–217.

162. Cook CL, Siow Y, Taylor S, et al. Serum mullerian-inhibiting substance levels during normal menstrual cycles. *Fertil Steril* 2000;73:859–861.

163. Palmieri SL, Payne J, Stiles CD, et al. Expression of mouse PDGF-A and PDGF α-receptor genes during pre- and post-implantation development: evidence for a developmental shift from an autocrine to a paracrine mode of action. *Mech Dev* 1992;39:181–191.

164. Svalander PC, Holmes PV, Olovsson M, et al. Platelet-derived growth factor is detected in human blastocyst culture medium but not in human follicular fluid—a preliminary report. *Fertil Steril* 1991;56:367–369.

165. Oral E, Arici A. Peritoneal growth factors and endometriosis. *Reprod Endocrinol* 1996;14:257–267.

166. Fayed YM, Tsibris JCM, Langengerg PW, et al. Human uterine leiomyoma cells: binding and growth responses to epidermal growth factor, platelet-derived growth factor and insulin. *Lab Invest* 1989;60:30–37.

167. Senger DR, van de Waer L, Brown LF. Vascular permeability factor (VPF, VEGF) in tumor biology. *Cancer Metastasis Rev* 1993;12:303–324.

168. Hock DL, Seifer DB. Ovarian hyperstimulation syndrome. *Infertil Clin Reprod Med North Am* 2000;11:399–417.

169. Koos RD. Increased expression of vascular endothelial growth/permeability factor in the rat ovary following an ovulatory gonadotropin stimulus: potential roles in follicle rupture. *Biol Reprod* 1995;52:1426–1435.

170. Goldberg MA, Schneider TJ. Similarities between the oxygen-sensing mechanisms regulating the expression of vascular endothelial growth factor and erythropoietin. *J Biol Chem* 1994;269:4355–4359.

171. Friedman CI, Danforth DR, Herbosa-Encarnacion C, et al. Follicular fluid vascular endothelial growth factor concentrations are elevated in women of advanced reproductive age undergoing ovulation induction. *Fertil Steril* 1997;68:607–612.

172. Friedman CI, Seifer DB, Kennard EA, et al. Elevated level of follicular vascular endothelial growth factor is a marker of diminished pregnancy potential. *Fertil Steril* 1998;70:836–839.

173. Shifren JL, Tseng JF, Zaloudek CJ, et al. Ovarian steroid regulation of vascular endothelial growth factor in the human endometrium: implications for angiogenesis during the menstrual cycle and in the pathogenesis of endometriosis. *J Clin Endocrinol Metab* 1996;81:3112–3117.

5

NEUROENDOCRINE CONTROL OF REPRODUCTION

FREDERICK NAFTOLIN
TONY G. ZREIK
LUIS MIGUEL GARCIA-SEGURA
TAMAS L. HORVATH

The neuroendocrine control of reproduction is only part of a larger enterprise, reproduction, which is most important for all animal species, maintaining the germline through the ages. This chapter discusses neuroendocrine aspects of reproduction, but they should not be seen in a vacuum. The central axis (the hypothalamus and pituitary) connects with the systemic circulation from which it receives cues about metabolic function, and for feedback from the gonads, etc. The central axis is also connected to the sensory system, which receives cues from the environment, and receives intrinsic connections from within the brain itself. Thus, sensory cues, systemic regulators, and intracerebral connections all funnel toward the hypothalamus. Although within the hypothalamus and pituitary gonadotropes, we have the elements of the reproductive neuroendocrine system, it is necessary to interpolate central function with other activities, especially feedback mediators from the gonads (Fig. 5.1). In addition to their neuroendocrine effects, these mediators are important in phenotypical development including appearance and behavioral responses (1).

GONADOTROPHIN-RELEASING HORMONE CELLS

The cells that are pivotal to neuroendocrine control of reproduction are the so-called gonadotrophin[1] releasing hormone (GnRH) cells (2). This relative handful of cells (estimated to be less than 10,000 per adult brain) is bilaterally distributed. In rodents, the GnRH cells are located in the anterior part of the hypothalamus, the so-called preoptic area, thus necessitating an internuclear neural connection with the controlling cells in the hypothalamic arcuate nu-

cleus. In primates, GnRH cells reside in the arcuate nucleus as well, and are controlled by interneurons. During development, this additional circuit in the rat brain, made up of internuclear connections, appears to confer immutable brain sexual differentiation with males failing to show an estrogen-induced gonadotrophin surge under any conditions. Male primates lack this characteristic (3). Because of these differences and other reasons mentioned below, we will focus on the GnRH cells and GnRH that we will be able to explain the neuroendocrine control of reproduction.

The GnRH cells are perhaps the most unusual cells in the entire body. First, even though they ultimately reside in the hypothalamus, to get there during development the GnRH cells migrate out from the nasal placode's sensory-fated cells into the brain; that is, they are actually cells that originated as precursor peripheral sensory neurons of the nasal epithelium but became neuroeffector cells in the brain. These cells begin their migration into the brain along the terminal nerve, into the central areas that will ultimately become the hypothalamus. This is the longest known migration of neurons within the brain (4,5). Today, it is still not known what triggers that migration, what induces GnRH expression or what limits the length of migration or distribution of these migrant cells in different species. Failure of the migration results in hypogonadotrophic hypogonadism with absent GnRH to stimulate the pituitary gonadotrophs (6).

The second remarkable thing about these cells is that they are apparently devoid of axonal connections with other neuronal networks. GnRH cells do, however, coexpress the stimulatory neuromodulator galanin and do receive both stimulatory and inhibitory connections from other neurons in, for example, the arcuate nucleus (7). In addition, GnRH cells also have recurrent GnRH axons that synapse on (other) GnRH cells (Fig. 5.2), raising the possibility of a self-regulating population of neurons with a microfeedback system (8,9). The GnRH cells direct their major axons into the median eminence, where they are apposed to the pituitary-portal vessels. GnRH is translated as a prohormone

---

[1] While a tropin merely turns on or off a switch, a trophin both turns a switch and nourishes its subject. Therefore, "gonadotropin" should properly be called "gonadotrophin," since it exercises both functions. Therefore "gonadotrophin" is the term used in this chapter context.

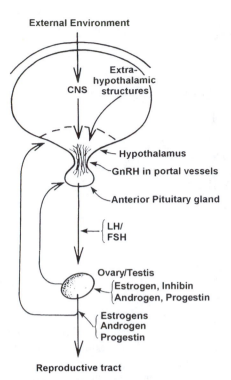

External Environment

Extra-
hypothalamic
structures

CNS

Hypothalamus

GnRH in portal vessels

Anterior Pituitary gland

LH/
FSH

Ovary/Testis

Estrogen, Inhibin
Androgen, Progestin

Estrogens
Androgen
Progestin

Reproductive tract

FIGURE 5.1. Schematic illustration of the interplay between central and peripheral components of the reproductive system. (From Harris GW, Naftolin F. The hypothalamus and control of ovulation. *Br Med Bull* 1970;26:3–9, with permission.)

and passed down axons to the median eminence by fast axon transport, indicating that in addition to being targeted by stimulating and inhibiting neurotransmitter systems, there may be cellular (metabolic) control of GnRH synthesis, processing, and release (1). Finally, since the branches of the pituitary-portal system are geographically bounded by glial foot processes, it has been suggested that the shifting

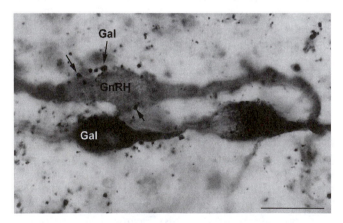

Gal

GnRH

Gal

FIGURE 5.2. Light micrograph taken of a hypothalamic section from an 85-year-old woman, double immunostained for galanin (*black*) and gonadotrophin-releasing hormone (GnRH) (*light brown*). A population of the hypothalamic GnRH cells produce the regulatory peptide galanin (Gal) that stimulates the activity of GnRH neurons, in part by synaptic inputs (*arrows* point to Gal-immunoreactive axon terminals in contact with the GnRH perikaryon). Scale bar represents 10 μm.

of these processes during changing hormonal conditions may control access of GnRH to the pituitary-portal vessels (10).

The next interesting thing about the GnRH cells is that they have a rhythmic intrinsic depolarization and secretory activity. Under all circumstances thus far tested, either *in vivo* or *in vitro,* GnRH cells or experimental surrogates appear to secrete in a self-generated pulsatile manner; they may be viewed as cells that are secreting constitutively in a pulsatile manner under the regulation of stimulatory and inhibitory synapses. It may be that this spontaneous GnRH cell(s) activity may actually be the hypothalamic "pulse generator" signal reported by Knobil (11) and studied by Horvath (12). If so, this could be a direct explanation of the pulsatile nature of GnRH secretion (13,14), which is subject to modulation by inputs from neurons targeting the GnRH cells. Under such a self-driven system it would be possible to control GnRH secretion merely by regulation of inhibitory circuits, such as an endorphin (8,15). However, since there are both inhibitory and stimulatory connections on the GnRH cells, it is likely that the GnRH secretion is regulated by both stimulatory and inhibitory inputs (see Fig. 5.6), the final output being the GnRH pulse frequency and amplitude.

The GnRH cells in humans and lower primates are largely in the hypothalamus, particularly the arcuate nucleus and the organum vasculosum lamina terminalis (OVLT). Since the GnRH processes from OVLT cells do not enter the median eminence (i.e., do not approach the portal vessels), it is assumed that the GnRH cells from the arcuate nucleus that target the portal circulation are the only source of GnRH in the portal vessels. To be sure, GnRH cells are present in other areas of the mammalian brain than the hypothalamus, and GnRH has been shown to have effects on maternal behavior. Such considerations, however, are beyond the scope of this chapter.

In terms of external regulation, during normal life (pre- and postpuberty and postmenopause) the GnRH cells are responsive to circulating sex steroids, especially estrogen (Fig. 5.1) (16,17). However, GnRH cells have not been shown to contain significant amounts of estrogen receptor or to bind radiolabeled estradiol (E_2) (18); therefore, it must be that estrogen-sensitive neurons that directly or indirectly target the GnRH cells regulate GnRH secretion with their stimulatory or inhibitory synapses. The neurons targeting the GnRH cells may or may not contain estrogen receptors (ERs). However, even ER-negative neurons connect with ER-positive neurons as they target the GnRH cells; therefore, an estrogen-sensitive network regulates the (ER-negative) GnRH cells. The brain areas that feed (target) the GnRH cells may include the inner hypothalamic nuclei where the GnRH cells are found, and receive interneurons (connections from cells in the same nucleus). In monkeys and humans this is localized in the arcuate nucleus (infundibular nucleus), and the interneurons include endorphin, γ-amino isobutyric acid (GABA), and glutamate neurons

(19,20). As described above, in other species, including rodents and sheep, GnRH cells that target the median eminence are limited to the preoptic area, which also has interneurons including GABA, catecholamines, and glutamate, in addition to connections from the arcuate nucleus, especially pro-opiomelanocortin (POMC) synapses from the arcuate nuclei (15). Other connections to the GnRH cells come from the zona inserta and from the septal area of the brain. Their significance for gonadotrophin control is unknown.

Formation of the Hypothalamus and Its Relationship to the Control of the Pituitary Gland

In the late 1930s, Geoffrey Harris proposed, on the basis of his animal experiments, that there is a chemical connection between the brain (the hypothalamus) and the anterior pituitary gland (1). The anterior pituitary is not part of the central nervous system. During development, a branchial pouch (Rathke's pouch) becomes apposed to the folding brain at the area that will become the diencephalon. Perhaps it is the adherence of Rathke's pouch to the forming hypothalamus that results in the pulling out of the median eminence of the hypothalamus during the folding of the neural tube and brain. The median eminence is supplied by the superior hypophyseal vessels, which send off branches to form the primary portal plexus. This pituitary-portal system links the hypothalamus and pituitary gland both anatomically and via GnRH and other regulating substances to the pituitary gland (Fig. 5.3).

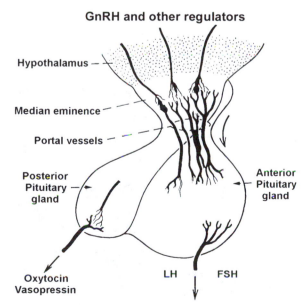

GnRH and other regulators

Hypothalamus —

Median eminence —

Portal vessels —

Posterior Pituitary gland —

Anterior Pituitary gland —

Oxytocin Vasopressin

LH   FSH

FIGURE 5.3. Schematic drawing illustrating the anatomic relationship between the hypothalamus and the pituitary. (From Harris GW, Naftolin F. The hypothalamus and control of ovulation. *Br Med Bull* 1970;26:3–9, with permission.)

The Pituitary-Portal System

The portal vessels themselves are branches of both the superior and inferior hypophyseal vessels. The superior hypophyseal vessels are twigs arising from the circle of Willis. This circle of arteries surrounds the hypothalamus, and indicates how critical the hypothalamus is for survival. That is, the hypothalamus is one of the areas of the body with a blood supply that has no end vessels, so that, in the event of a vascular occlusion, or loss of blood supply from one of the vessels, other vessels of the circle of Willis would continue to feed blood to the hypothalamus. This arrangement likely reflects the importance to the body of this area of the brain and is a fine example of Darwinian adaptation.

The portal vessels are like other endocrine vessels; they are made up largely of endothelium, with little muscularis. They also have gaps large enough to allow bulky molecules to pass between the endothelial cells. There is even evidence of pinocytosis in the portal vessels, indicating that large molecules can be phagocytosed and passed across into the portal bloodstream (1).

GnRH and the Anterior Pituitary Gonadotrophins

GnRH is a small (10 amino acid) peptide that is unusual because both its N- and C-terminals are blocked to enzymatic degradation. This resistance to classic enzymatic degradation analysis was the main stumbling block to decoding hypothalamic releasing hormones, including GnRH until the 1970s. Solution of this puzzle led to a Nobel Prize for Roger Guillemin and Andrew Schally (21).

GnRH binds to the pituitary gonadotrophs (Fig. 5.4). These cells secrete the gonadotrophins luteinizing hormone (LH) and follicle-stimulating hormone (FSH). They are called gonadotrophins because not only do they possess a tropic response (the turning on and turning off response), they also are trophic to the gonad (see earlier footnote). For example, when GnRH increases as following hemiovariectomy, the ovary that is left behind enlarges 50% or more as a result of the gonadotrophin effect of these pituitary hormones.

The pituitary gonadotrophs are glandular cells located in the bloodstream of the pituitary, where they are exposed to all passing hormones. GnRH is present in the pituitary bloodstream since it has not yet been degraded by peptidase digestion. But this endopeptidase is present in relatively large amounts and quickly removes it from the circulation, so that even jugular vein levels are decreased. The GnRH levels in the general circulation are not reliably measurable (22).

The Glycoprotein Family

The gonadotrophins are glycoproteins that are part of a family that includes LH, FSH, thyroid-stimulating hor-

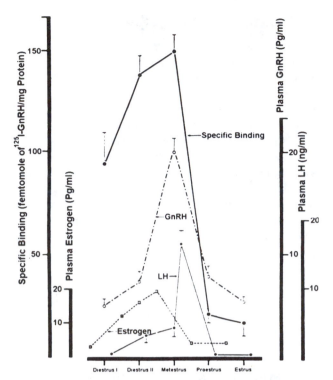

FIGURE 5.4. Temporal relationship between circulating estradiol and luteinizing hormone (LH) levels, GnRH release, and GnRH binding in the pituitary. (From Park KR, Saxena BB, Gandy HM. Specific binding of LH-RH to the anterior pituitary gland during the oestrous cycle in the rat. *Acta Endocrinol* 1976;82:62–70, with permission.)

mone (TSH), and human chorionic gonadotrophin (hCG). All are made up with two subunits: the common subunit is arbitrarily named the α subunit, while the other is the hormone-specific β subunit, which determines the biologic action of that hormone. This has given rise to one of the most important clinical aspects of our understanding of reproductive endocrinology. The subunit nature of the gonadotrophins allows the development of highly specific antisera that allow the precise measurement of LH, FSH, TSH, and hCG by immunoassays (RAs). Such assays have revolutionized reproductive endocrinology, making possible specific and sensitive clinical tests for hormone measurement, and making available data on which our understanding of human reproduction is based.

GnRH and LH/FSH Secretion; The Pituitary Gonadotroph as a Biologic Transducer and Amplifier

Because of the above-described rapid clearance by blood peptidases and the meager amount of GnRH secreted by the small number of GnRH cells, the effect of GnRH on the blood levels of LH and FSH is commonly used as an indicator of GnRH secretion. In this manner it has been inferred that in humans GnRH is secreted in a pulsatile manner (22), just as is the case in direct GnRH measurements in experimental animals (23,24). These pulses gener-

ally range between 30 and 90 minutes during the normal follicular phase. During the luteal phase the pulse interval stretches out even longer (25).

So then, how could reproduction be controlled by GnRH, if it is so rapidly cleared from the blood? The answer lies in the partnership between the hypothalamus (GnRH) and the anterior pituitary gonadotrophs, the latter acting to amplify the GnRH signal (Figs. 5.4, 5.5). The gonadotroph has GnRH receptors that, in binding their ligand, GnRH, trigger a group of mechanisms [3', 5'-cyclic adenosine monophosphate (cAMP), G protein, and calcium mediated] that are already present in the gonadotrope. These secondary messengers cause the already present and available LH and FSH granules to be extruded from the cell into the blood (26), powerfully amplifying the feeble GnRH signal. The LH and FSH are thus dispersed into the jugular veins and superior vena cava, to be mixed and distributed to the systemic circulation by the heart. LH and FSH have long $t_{1/2}$ and remain in the circulation (see below), further amplifying the feeble GnRH signal. Exposure of LH and FSH to the ovary, where they trigger gonadotrophic actions before they are cleared by the kidney via the urine. The anterior pituitary gonadotroph in this way amplifies the signals coming from the hypothalamus (see below). Thus, this transduction of the GnRH message to circulating gonadotrophin levels may be used as a surrogate indicator of GnRH secretion (22).

What Determines Circulatory Gonadotrophin Levels

Secretion from the pituitary and the kidney's clearance of the gonadotrophins form the balance that determines the levels of gonadotrophins in the blood at any moment. Dilutional volume is relatively constant, so it is not a practical factor in determining momentary blood levels. The reflection of pulse pattern of GnRH secretion is reflected in the pattern of LH and FSH in the blood in proportion to how rapidly the reservoir of LH or FSH is cleared from the blood between each pulse (22). Restated, unless there is

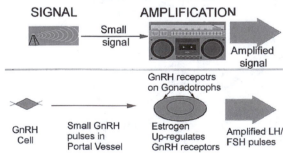

FIGURE 5.5. Schematic illustration depicting the analogy between an electronic amplifier, such as a radio receiver, and the hypothalamic-pituitary interaction regulating gonadotrophin secretion.

adequate time for LH/FSH clearance between pulses, it is not possible to recognize a direct ratio between GnRH- and -gonadotrophin pulses.

The clearance rate, total amounts in the blood, and hormonal action of individual gonadotrophins are determined by their chemical structure. Both gonadotrophins are glycopeptides whose sugars determine their biologic action in two ways: (a) they dictate their ability to act as ligands, triggering second messenger systems in the gonads; and (b) the sugar moieties determine the clearance rate by the kidney, which affects gonadotrophins' duration of action. LH is cleared with a half-time of about 30 minutes, whereas FSH has a half-time of about 300 minutes, ten times as long as LH (22). A pulse of LH occurring between 30 and 90 minutes in frequency will pass through more than one half-life and be cleared from the blood sufficiently to show a distinct pulsatile pattern. There is not much blood storage or reserve of LH. Therefore, blood LH is a good monitor of GnRH secretion patterns.

Conversely, the same frequency of FSH release will not be cleared, and FSH will accumulate in the circulation. Because of this large buildup or reserve, FSH pulses will be harder to distinguish than LH pulses. Perhaps this explains our finding in animal studies that the total amount of gonadotrophins present ("ramping up") is more important, with respect to ovarian function, than the frequency or amplitude of administered gonadotrophins (27).

Renal clearance of the gonadotrophins is relatively constant from hour to hour, but is affected by estrogen, which increases glycosylation of the gonadotrophins (13). Increased glycosylation of LH and FSH thus increases the $t_{1/2}$ and protracts the gonadal exposure to LH and FSH. This level of glycosylation is the basis of so-called "biologically active" hormone measures vs. "immunoreactive" hormone largely related to the peptide backbone of the subunits. Increased bioactivity results in greater activity on a molar basis probably because of delayed clearance of the more glycosylated hormones. In addition to estrogen's sensitization of pituitary gonadotrophins (see Figs. 5.4, 5.5, and below), this may play a secondary part in the midcycle increase in circulatory gonadotrophins by estrogen.

Control of the Biologic Amplifier Function of the Pituitary Gonadotrophs

The pituitary's gonadotroph's response to GnRH is typical of a membrane-bound receptor-mediated system (26). A pulse of GnRH causes changes in the intracellular calcium levels. The latter causes microtubules to eject LH/FSH from the cell. Thus, the release caused by individual molecules of GnRH is dependent on liganding a receptor. The more receptors on a cell, the greater the likelihood of release. Increasing the number of GnRH receptors is the main means of amplifying the effect of GnRH at the pituitary level (Fig. 5.5). The amplification of the GnRH signal is primarily under the control of GnRH and estrogen (11).

GnRH

Through a mechanism that is poorly understood, GnRH causes an increase in its own receptors and the production of LH/FSH by the pituitary cell (11,28). Thus GnRH is said to be self-priming or sensitizing to the pituitary gonadotrophs. This is particularly of importance during puberty and during the regression syndromes (29). However, when either pulse frequency or amplitude is excessive there is a downregulation of GnRH receptors, with an accompanying diminution of the sensitivity to GnRH. This characteristic is of great clinical importance. Increased GnRH pulses lay the basis for puberty and recovery from GnRH deficiency or regression syndromes (hypogonadotropic hypogonadism) (29). Administration of a pharmacologic amount of GnRH also causes hypogonadotrophic hypogonadism.

Effects on GnRH Pulses

Regulation of GnRH pulses may be changed to increase or decrease dose and frequency, with expected effects on circulating gonadotrophin levels.

REGRESSION SYNDROMES

Eating disorders and GnRH-induced menopause, respectively, are examples of each form of spontaneous and induced regression to puberty-like gonadotrophin control. In fact recent evidence indicates that the prepubertal state may be a form of hypogonadotrophic hypogonadism that reflects the inhibitory effect of the neurotransmitter GABA (30–33). Although implicated in some regression syndromes, the role of body weight is controversial (34).

Following puberty, once the baseline GnRH secretion of adults is present, circulating estrogens are very powerful regulators of pituitary sensitization via induction of GnRH receptors on the cell surface of the gonadotrophs (26). Estrogens can thereby cause massive biologic amplification of the GnRH signal: the more estrogen, the more receptor; and the more receptor, the more response, and so on. There seems to be no downregulation by excess estrogen, although progestins and androgens can cause downregulation by inhibiting production of estrogen receptors. In fact, this may be a mechanism for physiologic control of pituitary gonadotrophin release in men and androgenized women (polycystic ovary syndrome).

The Key Role of the Dual Action of Estrogen on Gonadotrophin Levels

During the menstrual cycle, estradiol determines circulating gonadotrophin levels (35). Estrogen has a dual action on gonadotrophin secretion: (a) Estrogen acts on the *pituitary gland*, sensitizing it, and increasing the release of LH and FSH by individual pulses of gonadotrophin-releasing hormone. (b) At the same time, the hypothalamus responds to estrogen with inhibition of GnRH release via decreased pulse amplitude of GnRH. We believe that this estrogen-regulated balance is the major determinant of normal feedback control of the pituitary gonadotrophins. The other steroids appear to have mitigating and long-term effects, and the activin-inhibin systems' effect appears to be limited to actions on FSH release at the pituitary level.

Androgens

Both women and men secrete androgens such as testosterone and androstenedione from their ovaries and testes, respectively. Besides serving as prohormones for estrogens or ring A reduced androgens, androgens appear to be long-term modulators rather than rapid, direct controllers of gonadotrophin secretion. This is exemplified in androgen insensitivity syndromes. Women who are carriers and therefore 50% insensitive have normal cycles and fertility. Men who have partial or complete androgen insensitivity have only slightly elevated gonadotrophins and can be caused by estrogen to show apparently normal feedback, including an estrogen-induced gonadotrophin surge (36). In the obverse, several studies have not shown ring A reduced androgens to be active in controlling gonadotrophin in men. Further, clomiphene, an estrogen antagonist, triggers a rise in gonadotrophins in normal men, despite the secondary rise in androgens attendant to clomiphene administration (37).

This evaluation is not to diminish the role of long-term exposure to androgens, particularly in blocking the estrogen-induced gonadotrophin surge in men or women. The latter appears to be a local, pituitary effect since castrated men eventually show a gonadotrophin surge following estrogen administration, while intact subjects do not (38).

Progesterone

The role of progesterone in gonadotrophin control remains enigmatic. In men there is little evidence. In animal models progesterone is inhibitory when the gonadotrophs are elevated. In females, there are two clinical instances when progesterone (progestins) clinically affect the gonadotrophins. During the final maturation of the ovarian follicle the ovary secretes progestin, primarily 17-hydroxyprogesterone. Although both descriptive and pharmacologic studies have indicated that this could either trigger or substantiate the midcycle gonadotrophin surge, the role of this action remains conjectural in physiology (39). More study has been given to the effect of progesterone in combination with estrogen, as seen during the luteal phase, pregnancy, and contraception. Under these conditions the addition of progesterone to estrogen results in a decreased frequency of gonadotrophin pulses (40). This appears to be a combined effect on the pituitary gonadotrophs and hypothalamus, since the response to administrative GnRH by the gonadotrophs is high and each pulse is usually large, further indicating that the hypothalamic pulses must be decreased during the initial phase. The role played by the pituitary under these circumstances is not clear since proper estrogen-blocking controls have not been reported.

Inhibin

Although the chief controlling steroid for gonadotrophin control in males and females is estrogen, inhibin is another feedback factor that is secreted by both ovary and testes (13). Inhibin is a protein that blocks FSH release at the pituitary gonadotroph level; this could explain why FSH dynamics are less obvious than LH's (see above). Because it is produced by ovarian granulosa cells, inhibin is a good indicator of ovarian reserve. No other neuroendocrine effects of inhibin are reported. The inhibin-activin family of peptides are important, but beyond the scope of this chapter.

Other Factors

There are many substances that at the hypothalamic level have been shown in animals or human pharmacologic studies to affect GnRH release [corticotrophin-releasing factor (CRF), leptin, narcotics, dopamine-agonists, prolactin, and melatonin, to name a few], but it is beyond the scope of this chapter to categorize or to conjecture about their sites of action.

A WORKING SUMMARY OF INDIVIDUAL FACTORS REGULATING GnRH GONADOTROPIN RELEASE

We have given a simplified description of gonadotrophin dynamics and hormonal control. The following discussion is an attempt to set all of these factors into action as is seen in physiologic gonadotrophin homeostasis represented as feedback during the ovarian cycle.

Feedback Control of the Gonadotrophins

The term *feedback* is nearly a century old and stems from attempts to use engineering terms that largely describe linear systems to describe complex, nonlinear biologic systems. The terms, therefore, are of value only when the biologic systems remain linear, as may be seen during reciprocal or negative feedback, but not when they become nonlinear during positive feedback, which is inhibition followed by disinhibition of GnRH/LH/FSH. We will use the terms *negative* (or *reciprocal*) *feedback* and *estrogen-induced gonado-*

trophin surge (or *biphasic feedback*). Since *positive feedback* is a misleading term, it will not be used.

Negative or Reciprocal Feedback Control of Gonadotrophins

About 90% of the time for cycling women, the control of the gonadotrophins, is via reciprocal or negative feedback, with estrogen and inhibin being the chief agents. Increased estrogen sensitizes the pituitary gland but lowers the GnRH reaching the pituitary. This results in a net fall of the LH and FSH levels in the blood. In normal (intact) men, negative feedback occurs 100% of the time. Since estrogen is also the primary steroidal regulator of gonadotrophins in men, a rise of estrogen will result in reciprocal or negative feedback, causing a net lowering of the gonadotrophins. Lowered estrogen does the reverse. In fact, the estrogen receptor blocker, clomiphene, given to a man, will cause his gonadotrophins to rise, despite a secondary rise of blood testosterone. Furthermore, the gonadotrophins will remain elevated despite a massive administration of testosterone (14). In men and male monkeys the failure of an estrogen-induced gonadotrophin surge is obviated by castration or blockade of androgen action (38). Thus, primates do not have brain sexual differentiation of gonadotrophin control as do rats, whose males never are triggered to release gonadotrophins by rising estrogen, even after castration (3).

At the level of the central nervous system, effects of estrogen predominate. Estrogen-sensitive interneurons that connect to the GnRH cells include endorphin, GABA, and the catecholamines (41)—all are inhibitory neurotransmitters. In concert they act on the GnRH neurons to suppress the pulsatile release of GnRH. Estrogen rise induces these neurotransmitters, causing a diminution of the release of GnRH (Figs. 5.6, 5.7). This apparently does not overcome the GnRH pulse generator (11) since it is the amplitude of the pulse, not the frequency, that is affected by estrogen alone. This fall in the pulse amplitude of GnRH release induced by estrogen leads to a decrease in the gonadotrophin levels, despite sensitization of the pituitary due to the rise in estrogen levels.

As the ovarian cycle progresses, estrogen continues to rise and the pituitary continues to be sensitized. LH and FSH fall as the latter part of the follicular phase is reached. The fall in FSH is partly due to inhibin from the developing granulosa cells. From the fall in gonadotrophin despite estrogen-induced pituitary sensitization, one can only infer that the GnRH must be falling. In confirmation, researchers at the Oregon Regional Primate Research Center (23), studying monkeys, have used push/pull hypothalamic cannulas to show that at midcycle the GnRH falls during physiologic cycles. This confirms data that have long been known in rats and previous work in monkeys, using direct measurements from portal vessels, showing that at midcycle

the GnRH falls. This suppression of GnRH and LH/FSH ends with the preovulatory surge of estrogen.

The Estrogen-Induced Gonadotrophin Surge or Biphasic Feedback

How could an estrogen surge cause the gonadotrophins to rise? In surgically prepared monkeys, Knobil's elegant pharmacologic studies showed that it is possible to administer estrogen to induce gonadotrophin suppression followed by gonadotrophin release in the presence of constant amounts of GnRH. However, the evidence suggests that in physiologic situations, GnRH actually does decrease as a result of the secretion of increased levels of estrogen from the maturing follicle before the gonadotrophin surge (12), and that there are neuroendocrine-driven changes in GnRH that underlie the estrogen-induced gonadotrophin surge (3).

We have already presented the evidence that the midcycle inhibition of the anterior pituitary gonadotrophs must be via diminution of GnRH, since the anterior pituitary gonadotrophs are actually sensitized by estrogen during this period. Estrogen can also induce expression of inhibitory neurotransmitters such as GABA and endorphin, to inhibit the GnRH cells (12).

Why, then, doesn't the continued rise of estrogen before ovulation simply suppress even further the release of GnRH and of LH and FSH? Many possibilities have previously been proposed (42). Among those proposed, stimulatory neurotransmitters may be secreted under the pressure of these high levels of estrogen, or the cells may convert from secreting inhibitory to stimulatory nerve transmitters, perhaps through coexpression. While all of this makes sense at an intellectual level, at this time the experiments that support this idea are pharmacologic, and may not have a basis in physiology (42).

How then could one explain biphasic (inhibition followed by disinhibition) feedback? Recently, it has become possible to study whether the inhibition of GnRH by estrogen via increasing inhibitory neurotransmitter tone in already present synapses is *abridged* by an estrogen-induced disconnection of the inhibitory synapses. This would allow the GnRH cells to pulse normally. With the increase of GnRH the massively sensitized pituitary gonadotrophs release greatly increased pulses of LH and FSH. This triggers the ovulatory process and the estrogen falls, allowing reconnection of the inhibitory synapses (12). We now have data in rats and monkeys that support this formulation. These data indicate that normally in midcycle, just before the preovulatory LH surge, there is a disengagement, or a synaptic retraction, of about half of the axosomatic and axodendritic synapses in the arcuate nucleus of rats and monkeys (43,44). The majority of these, if not all, are estrogen-sensitive synapses, that is, they represent neurotransmitter systems in which the cell bodies contain estrogen receptors. These synapses retract or are sheared off by the surrounding glial processes, when the level of estrogen exceeds about fivefold the normal basal levels. Prior to this, the rising estrogen suppresses or inhibits the gonadotrophin-releasing hormone and sensitizes the pituitary (Fig. 5.6).

The Integrated Choreography of the Ovarian Cycle (Fig. 5.7)

Now that we have described gonadotrophin control by the neuroendocrine axis, we can integrate what is known about neuroendocrine control of secretion by the ovary, and about maturation of the ovarian follicles.

The follicular phase begins when, for reasons that are still not understood, certain primordial oocytes are activated. In primates, of the 20 or so primordial follicles that are activated in any period, only one will become a dominant follicle, and thus primates are monotocous. On the other hand, in rodents, of the 20 or so primordial follicles that are activated, perhaps as many as 12 to 20 will form dominant follicles. The basis of this difference appears to be the relationship of the gonadotrophin levels to the development of the follicle at the beginning of the follicular phase; women who are normally monotocous become polytocous when given gonadotrophins.

As described elsewhere in this chapter, during follicle maturation the oocyte inside the follicle, which has been held at its first meiotic division, is triggered to begin its second meiotic division. This oocyte is also going to get larger by accumulating maternal RNA, glycogen, and other nutrients along with accumulation or proliferation of mitochondria, so that energy sources can be utilized by the oocyte when needed in its free-living existence prior to, during, and subsequent to its conception. All of this building-up of the oocyte is supported by the granulosa cells, and is mainly due to estrogen. The (theca cell) androgens are converted to estrogens by the granulosa cells of the follicle. Each granulosa cell of the follicle is a small estrogen factory, and in the presence of sufficient numbers of estrogen-producing cells, estrogen increases to a level that drives multiplication of the granulosa cells, since estrogen is a mitotic agent for granulosa cells, as it is for other tissues.

In contrast, under these conditions atresia may occur if there are not enough granulosa cells present to clear the androgen via aromatization when androgens are produced by the theca cells. This androgen–estrogen interaction is in response to gonadotrophin levels that are regulated by reciprocal feedback. If the rising androgen cannot be turned

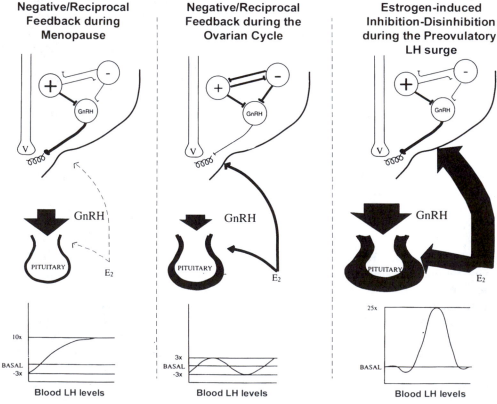

FIGURE 5.6. The significance and temporal relationship between circulating estradiol levels, the synaptology of GnRH-producing hypothalamic cells, and the sensitization of the pituitary to GnRH and circulating LH levels in three fundamental gonadotrophin feedback paradigms. The thickness of *lines* and *arrows* represent quantitative values.

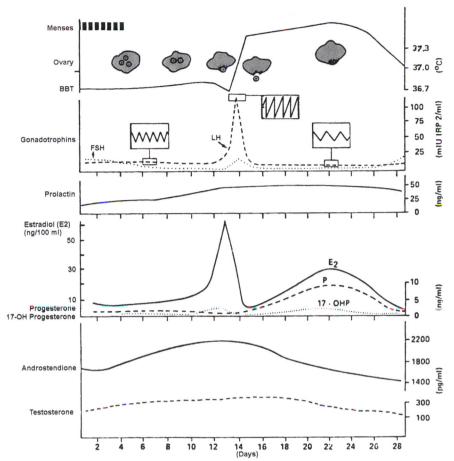

FIGURE 5.7. The normal ovarian cycle. Key hormone levels are noted. The gonadotrophin pulse frequency and amplitude are shown for each segment of the cycle (in *box*). Inhibin levels follow the course of follicle development.

into estrogen at a sufficiently rapid rate, the excess testosterone will be instead converted into dihydrotestosterone, which is a powerful antiestrogen. Dihydrotestosterone will inhibit the formation of estrogen receptors. This blocks estrogen-induced granulosa cell proliferation. These differentiated granulosa cells fail to proliferate, and ultimately the follicular fluid will compress the lining of differentiated granulosa cells, leading to an atretic follicle. Without the estrogen from growing granulosa cells, the ovum undergoes apoptosis.

If the granulosa cells are able to aromatize the androgen that is secreted from the theca cell, they will divide and will form gap junctions between themselves. Through these gap junctions messages are passed back and forth between granulosa cells, and to the so-called cumulus cells. At the same time, the granulosa cells are converting the androgen to estrogen in the dominant follicles. This process appears to be due to the level of gonadotrophins present during the first week of the cycle since administration of gonadotrophin at that time results in multiple dominant follicles.

The rising level of estrogen in the dominant follicle results in the export of estrogen into the blood. At some point there is enough estrogen production from the domi-

nant follicle, and follicle vascularization becomes sufficient to furnish estrogen for export into the general circulation, causing a rise in the circulating levels of estrogen. At the same time that estrogen is maturing the dominant follicle it is inducing progresses to the second meiotic division. However, if the second meiotic division occurs too early, there will be a hypermature oocyte ovulated, and if the meiotic division occurs too late, an immature oocyte. A mechanism has evolved to allow the second meiotic division to proceed only so far, not to the separation of chromosomes. Estrogen levels influence this sequence partly via gap junction formation between follicle cells and a miotic inhibitory substance, perhaps cAMP. Thus, rising estrogen levels mature the follicle arrest oocyte division and suppress GnRH while sensitizing the pituitary gonadotrophs.

This process has arisen evolutionarily to support the timely maturation of the oocyte for ovulation. The surge of estrogen levels exported by the developed follicle results in a rise in GnRH in part is due to the disengagement of GnRH-inhibiting arcuate (see above). The sensitized gonadotrophin release massively augments LH and FSH pulses. These gonadotrophin pulses entrain ovulation (a 12-hour process) and cause estrogen secretion to drop. The turning off of the estrogen surge closes the gap junctions, preventing cAMP from reaching the oocyte, and the second maturation division is completed. The oocyte is then ovulated because by now the wall of the follicle has been weakened by the effects of estrogen on the collagen/mucopolysaccharides in the wall. There also is a rise in follicle angiotensin (45), which causes contraction of the myofibrillar cells surrounding the follicles. A mature oocyte is thus ovulated.

This choreography takes about 12 hours, and that is why we refer to it as the "process" of ovulation. After ovulation is completed and the estrogen and gonadotrophin have fallen, there is a return to reciprocal or negative feedback, as the synaptic connections are reapplied and the normal number of synaptic connections is found, during the remainder of the cycle.

SUMMARY

The neuroendocrine control of the gonads is in the main led by a small group of cells, the GnRH cells, and the anterior pituitary gonadotrophins. GnRH is the signal that goes out from the brain to a massive biologic amplifier, the anterior pituitary gonadotrophins. The signal triggers the release of LH and FSH into the blood. The size of GnRH pulses and of gonadotrophin is controlled by estrogen; it is estrogen that turns up the sensitivity of the pituitary gonadotrophins while inhibiting GnRH secretion. With the rise of estrogen that occurs during oocyte maturation and development, there is a period of extended reciprocal feedback with an inhibition of GnRH and sensitization of the anterior pituitary gonadotrophs. At the end of this period, the mature follicle delivers a massive increase of estrogen into the bloodstream that exceeds by fivefold the normal baseline levels. This causes the disinhibition of GnRH secretion, in part through the release of inhibiting synapses that either directly or indirectly target the GnRH cells. The increased GnRH pulses trigger the highly sensitized gonadotrophs to induce the midcycle estrogen-induced gonadotrophin surge (the estrogen-induced gonadotrophin surge, formerly called "positive feedback"). Following the rise of LH, which blocks aromatase and shuts off the estrogen secretion and blood estrogen falls, triggering the completion of the second meiotic division in time for the extrusion of the mature oocyte. In the luteal phase, negative or reciprocal feedback predominates. Thus, the levels of gonadotrophin reached during that time are the lowest during the whole cycle, because while estrogen changes in pulse amplitude, progesterone plus estrogen decrease pulse frequency. Accordingly, when the frequency gets slower without change in the clearance time, the levels of gonadotrophin between pulses, particularly of LH, reach their lowest point.

10 KEY POINTS

1. GnRH is the peptide that regulates LH and FSH release from the anterior pituitary gland. In primates the GnRH cells reside in the arcuate nucleus, and their secretion is responsive to estrogen-sensitive neurons that synapse with the GnRH cells.

2. The anterior pituitary gonadotrophs secrete both LH and FSH. This is in response to the GnRH reaching them via the pituitary-portal vessels.

3. The concentration of GnRH receptors on the gonadotrophs is dependent on the levels of GnRH and estrogen that reach them via the blood (pituitary sensitization). This pituitary sensitization determines the response to pulses of GnRH in the pituitary-portal blood.

4. Circulating gonadotrophin levels are regulated in response to the secretion of estrogen from the gonad. This reciprocal/negative feedback controls the gonadotrophin levels about 24 days of the 28-day cycle.

5. During reciprocal feedback, increasing estrogen causes hypothalamic GnRH secretion to fall while at the same time the estrogen is also sensitizing the pituitary gonadotrophs.

6. At midcycle (days 11–12 through 14–15), there is a dramatic rise in estrogen, which further suppresses GnRH and sensitizes the pituitary gonadotrophs. Maximum GnRH/gonadotrophin inhibition occurs at the peak of follicular estrogen secretion. Shortly after the estrogen peaks there is a disinhibition of GnRH secretion, partly due to the retraction of inhibitory synapses in the GnRH delivery system [the estrogen-induced gonadotrophin surge (EIGS), or positive feedback]. The disinhibited GnRH pulses cause massive pulses of gonadotrophin release from the estrogen-sensitized pituitary gonadotrophs.

7. Inhibin is secreted by the granulosa cells of the ovarian follicle and has a reciprocal/negative feedback relationship with FSH secretion from the pituitary gonadotrophs. Inhibin has not been shown to affect GnRH secretion.

8. The levels of circulating LH and FSH reflect the balance of pituitary secretion, dilution into the blood volume, and continuous clearance by the kidney. Since GnRH is secreted into the pituitary-portal system in pulses, this explains the peaks of LH and FSH in the blood.

9. GnRH is secreted in pulses (peaks). Since the FSH clearance ($t_{1/2}$) is much slower than the frequency of GnRH peaks, FSH accumulates in large amounts in the blood and blood levels may obscure GnRH secretion. In contrast, LH with its shorter $t_{1/2}$ is markedly cleared between pulses of GnRH secretion and therefore faithfully reflects GnRH secretion dynamics.

10. Testosterone is also important in gonadotrophin regulation: (a) Testosterone is converted to estradiol in the ovary and elsewhere via the enzyme aromatase. It then has an indirect effect on GnRH/gonadotrophins. (b) Testosterone

also is reduced by 5-α reductase to form dihydrotestosterone (DHT). DHT is a powerful antiestrogen that can inhibit estrogen receptor expression and thereby block the estrogen-induced gonadotrophin surge (positive feedback). DHT may have other effects that remain to be demonstrated. In men, estrogen appears to be the regulator of GnRH, as is the case in women.

REFERENCES

1. Harris GW, Naftolin F. The hypothalamus and control of ovulation. *Br Med Bull* 1970;26:3–9.
2. Yen SS. Gonadotrophin-releasing hormone. *Annu Rev Med* 1975;26:403–417.
3. Naftolin F. Brain aromatization of androgens. *J Reprod Med* 1994;39:257–261.
4. Quanbeck C, Sherwood NM, Millar RP, et al. Two populations of luteinizing hormone-releasing hormone neurons in the forebrain of the rhesus macaque during embryonic development. *J Comp Neurol* 1997;380:293–309.
5. Schwanzel-Fukuda M, Zheng LM, Bergen H, et al. LHRH neurons: functions and development. *Prog Brain Res* 1992;93:189–201.
6. Shivers BD, Harlan RE, Morrell JI, et al. Absence of estradiol concentration in cell nuclei of LHRH-immunoreactive neurons. *Nature* 1983;304:345–347.
7. Merchenthaler I, Lennard DE, Lopez FJ, et al. Neonatal imprinting predetermines the sexually dimorphic, estrogen-dependent expression of galanin in luteinizing hormone-releasing hormone neurons. *Proc Natl Acad Sci USA* 1993;90:10479–10483.
8. Chen WP, Witkin JW, Silverman AJ. Beta-endorphin and gonadotrophin-releasing hormone synaptic input to gonadotrophin-releasing hormone neurosecretory cells in the male rat. *J Comp Neurol* 1989;286:85–95.
9. Leranth C, Garcia-Segura LM, Palkovits M, et al. The LH-RH containing neuronal network in the preoptic area of the rat: demonstration of LH-RH-containing nerve terminals in synaptic contact with LH-RH neurons. *Brain Res* 1985;345:332–336.
10. King JC, Williams TH, Gerall AA. Transformation of hypothalamic arcuate nucleus. I. Changes associated with stages of the estrous cycle. *Cell Tissue Res* 1974;153:497–515.
11. Knobil E. The neuroendocrine control of the menstrual cycle. *Recent Prog Horm Res* 1980;36:53–88.
12. Horvath TL, Leedom L, Lewis C, et al. Estrogen-induced hypothalamic synaptic plasticity and the regulation of gonadotrophins. *Curr Opin Endocrinol Diabetes* 1995;2:186–190.
13. De Kretzer DM, Philips DJ. Mechanisms of protein feedback on gonadotrophin secretion. *J Reprod Immunol* 1998;39:1–12.
14. Naftolin F, Yen SS, Tsai C. Rapid cycling of plasma gondotrophins in normal men as demonstrated by frequent sampling. *Nature New Biol* 1972;236:92–93.
15. Leranth C, MacLusky NJ, Shanabrough M, et al. Immunohistochemical evidence for synaptic connection between pro-opiomelanocortin-immunoreactive axons and LH-RH neurons in the preoptic area of the rat. *Brain Res* 1988;449:167–176.
16. Chongthammakun S, Claypool LE, Terasawa E. Ovariectomy increases in vivo luteinizing hormone-releasing hormone release in pubertal, but not prepubertal, female rhesus monkeys. *J Neuroendocrinol* 1993;5:41–50.
17. Jeppsson S, Rannevik G, Thorell JI, et al. Influence of LH/FSH releasing hormone (LRH) on the basal secretion of gonadotrophins in relation to plasma levels of oestradiol, progesterone and prolactin during the post-partum period in lactating and in non-lactating women. *Acta Endocrinol (Copenh)* 1977;84(4):713–728.
18. Garcia-Segura LM, Chowen JA, Naftolin F, et al. Steroid effects on brain plasticity: role of glial cells and trophic factors. In: Baulieu EE, Robel P, Schumacher M, eds. *Contemporary endocrinology: neurosteroids: a new regulatory function in the nervous system,* vol 15. Totowa, NJ: Humana Press, 1999:255–268.
19. Goldsmith PC, Thind KK, Perera AD, et al. Glutamate-immunoreactive neurons and their gonadotrophin-releasing hormone-neuronal interactions in the monkey hypothalamus. *Endocrinology* 1994;134(2):858–868.
20. Leranth C, MacLusky N, Brown T, et al. Transmitter content and afferent connections of estrogen-sensitive progestin receptor-containing neurons in the primate hypothalamus. *Neuroendocrinology* 1992;55:667–682.
21. Wade N. Guillemin and Schally: the three-lap race to Stockholm. *Science* 1978;200:411–415.
22. Rebar R, Perlman D, Naftolin F, et al. The estimation of pituitary luteinizing hormone secretion. *J Clin Endocrinol Metab* 1973;37:917–927.
23. Pau FKY, Berria M, Hess DL, et al. Preovulatory gonadotrophin-releasing hormone surge in ovarian-intact rhesus macaques. *Endocrinology* 1993;133:1650–1656.
24. Sarkar DK, Chiappa SA, Fink G, et al. Gonadotrophin-releasing hormone surge in pro-oestrous rats. *Nature* 1976;264:461–463.
25. Yen SS, Tsai C, Naftolin F, et al. Pulsatile patterns of gonadotrophin release in subjects with and without ovarian function. *J Clin Endocrinol Metab* 1972;34:671–675.
26. Stanislaus D, Pinter JH, Janovick JA, et al. Mechanisms mediating multiple physiological responses to gonadotrophin-releasing hormone. *Mol Cell Endocrinol* 1998;144:1–10.
27. Soendoro T, Diamond M, Pepperell J, et al. The in vitro perifused rat ovary: I. Steroid secretion in response to ramp and pulsatile stimulation with luteinizing hormone and follicle stimulating hormone. *Gynecol Endocrinol* 1992;6:229–238.
28. Naftolin F, Harris GW, Bobrow M. Effect of purified luteinizing hormone releasing factor on normal and hypogonadotrophic anosmic men. *Nature* 1971;232:496–497.
29. Golden NH, Shenker IR. Amenorrhea in anorexia nervosa. Neuroendocrine control of hypothalamic dysfunction. *Int J Eat Disord* 1994;16:53–60.
30. Mitsushima D, Hei DL, Terasawa E. Gamma-aminobutyric acid is an inhibitory neurotransmitter restricting the release of luteinizing hormone-releasing hormone before the onset of puberty. *Proc Natl Acad Sci USA* 1994;91:395–399.
31. Mitushima D, Marzban F, Luchansky LL, et al. Role of glutamic acid decarboxylase in the prepubertal inhibition of the luteinizing hormone-releasing hormone release in female rhesus monkeys. *J Neurosci* 1996;16:2563–2573.
32. Terasawa E. Control of luteinizing hormone-releasing hormone pulse generation in nonhuman primates. *Cell Mol Neurobiol* 1995;15:141–164.
33. Newmark S, Rossini A, Naftolin F, et al. Gonadotrophin profiles in fed and fasted obese women. *Am J Obstet Gynecol* 1979;133:75–80.
34. Cunningham MJ, Clifton DK, Steiner RA. Leptin's actions on the reproductive axis: perspectives and mechanisms. *Biol Reprod* 1999;60:216–222.
35. Corker CS, Naftolin F, Exley D. Interrelationship between plasma luteinizing hormone and oestradiol in the human menstrual cycle. *Nature* 1969;222:1063.
36. Naftolin F, Judd HL. Testicular feminization. In: Wynn RM, ed. *Obstetrics and gynecology annual, 1973*. New York: Appleton-Century-Crofts, 1972:25–53.

37. Naftolin F, Judd HL, Yen SS. Pulsatile patterns of gonadotrophins and testosterone in man: the effects of clomiphene, with and without testosterone. *J Clin Endocrinol Metab* 1973; 36:285–288.

38. Goh HH, Wong PC, Ratnam SS. Effects of sex steroids on the positive estrogen feedback mechanism in intact women and castrate men. *J Clin Endocrinol Metab* 1985;61:1158–1164.

39. Chang RJ, Jaffe RB. Progesterone effects on gonadotrophin release in women pretreated with estradiol. *J Clin Endocrinol Metab* 1978;47:119–25.

40. Hall JE, Schoenfeld DA, Martin KA, et al. Hypothalamic gonadotrophin-releasing hormone secretion and follicle-stimulating hormone dynamics during the luteal-follicular transition. *J Clin Endocrinol Metab* 1992;74:600–607.

41. Leranth C, McLusky NJ, Naftolin F. Interconnections between neurotransmitter- and neuropeptide-containing neurons involved in gonadotrophin release in the rat. In: Moody TW, ed. *Neural and endocrine peptides and receptors.* New York: Plenum Press, 1986:177–193.

42. Kalra SP. Mandatory neuropeptide-steroid signaling for the preovulatory luteinizing hormone-releasing hormone discharge. *Endocr Rev* 1993;14:507–538.

43. Horvath TL, Garcia-Segura LM, Naftolin F. Control of gonadotrophin feedback: The possible role of estrogen-induced hypothalamic plasticity. *Gynecol Endocrinol* 1997;11:139–143.

44. Zsarnovszky A, Horvath TL, Garcia-Segura LM, Horvath B, Naftolin F. Estrogen-induced changes in the synaptology of the monkey (Cercopithecus aethiops) arcuate nucleus. *J Neuroendocrinol* 2000;13:1–7.

45. Pepperell J, Nemeth G, Palumbo A, Naftolin F. In: Eli Adashi and Peter CK Keung, ed., *The ovary,* New York: Raven Press, 1993, pp. 363–381.

PHARMACOLOGY AND PHARMACOKINETICS

DEBRA K. GARDNER

Pharmacokinetics deals with the description of drug absorption, distribution, metabolism, and excretion and with the time course of the drug's pharmacologic effect in the body. During pregnancy the woman's body develops into a complex multicompartmental unit. Each compartment—the mother, placenta, fetus, and amniotic fluid—has very unique functions and contributions to drug distribution, metabolism, and excretion (Fig. 6.1). Not only is this physiologic unit very complex in itself, but it is constantly changing as pregnancy progresses, making drug therapy selection and dosing extremely difficult during pregnancy.

PHYSIOLOGIC AND PHARMACOKINETIC CHANGES DURING PREGNANCY

Absorption

Gastrointestinal (GI) absorption of drugs is affected by several physiologic factors including the composition and pH of gastric and intestinal secretions, the rate of gastric emptying, intestinal motility, and intestinal blood flow. The chemical properties of the drug, such as molecular weight, whether it is an acid or base, degree of ionization (pKa), and lipid solubility, affect where in the GI tract the drug will be absorbed and the rate and extent of its absorption.

Although absorption has not been well studied in pregnancy, several physiologic changes in the GI tract occur during pregnancy that may affect absorption of drugs. There is a 40% reduction in gastric acid secretion during pregnancy, reduced peptic acid activity, and a significant increase in mucus production (1). These changes cause the gastric pH to be higher and increase the buffer capacity of the stomach, which may alter drug dissolution and absorption. Gestational hormones, particularly progesterone, cause delayed gastric emptying and prolonged intestinal motility by as much as 30% to 50% (1–3). A high osmolality meal also slows gastric emptying and GI transit time. The bioavailability of slowly absorbed drugs such as digoxin may be increased by prolonged GI transit time, and readily absorbed drugs may have delayed peak plasma levels. Significant effects on drug absorption resulting from reduced GI motility are rare, however.

Cardiac output also increases during pregnancy. This would be expected to cause increased GI blood flow, which may result in an increase in the rate and extent of absorption of drugs for which blood flow and membrane transport are the rate-limiting steps (1).

Alterations in diet, such as increased intake of iron and calcium, which often occurs during pregnancy, can also alter drug bioavailability. These minerals can chelate or bind with certain medications such as phenytoin, limiting their absorption (2).

Distribution

Factors that affect drug distribution include plasma and tissue protein binding, plasma volume, cardiac output and its regional distribution to certain organs, and fat and body water composition. All of these factors undergo significant changes during pregnancy.

Plasma protein binding is an important factor in drug disposition since it controls the amount of free drug available to leave the vasculature and gain access to tissue receptors and sites of metabolism and excretion. In therapeutic drug monitoring (TDM), the total (free plus bound) drug is measured. In normal individuals the ratio of free drug to bound drug falls within a predictable range, so that the total drug concentration can be taken to represent the free drug concentration. However, when there is a significant alteration in protein binding, total drug concentrations will no longer be a valid measurement of free drug levels for use in drug dosage adjustments. Understanding the changes in protein binding that occur in pregnancy is valuable in predicting response and making dosage adjustments.

The level of albumin, the primary binding protein for acidic drugs, decreases during pregnancy from a mean nonpregnant value of 4 g/dL to 3.3 g/dL at term (4). It was originally thought that the decrease in albumin concentration during pregnancy was due to hemodilution resulting from an increase in plasma volume. However, the decrease in albumin concentration after the tenth week of gestation is too small to be solely the result of hemodilution. The rate of albumin synthesis and catabolism remains unchanged during pregnancy (4). It is thought that the net

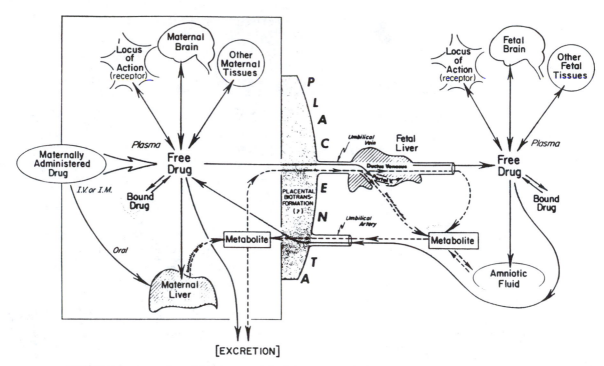

FIGURE 6.1. Drug disposition in a model of the maternal-placental-fetal unit. (From Mirkin BL. Drug distribution in pregnancy. In: Boreus LO, ed. *Fetal pharmacology.* New York: Raven Press, 1973, p. 22, with permission.)

increase in albumin is due to a rise in the rate of lymphatic return (4). The result of these factors is a gradual decrease in albumin plasma concentration throughout pregnancy and a reduction in binding sites for acidic drugs (Fig. 6.2). Drugs that are bound to albumin include valproic acid, phenytoin, and cloxacillin (4).

α_1-Acid glycoprotein (AAG) is a low-capacity, high-affinity protein that binds to a number of basic and neutral drugs such as carbamazepine and bupivacaine. Although it was thought to remain unchanged in pregnancy (1), more recent studies have found that after an initial increase in the first trimester, the concentration of AAG decreases with a 30% reduction at term (4) (Fig. 6.3). This results in an increased free fraction of certain basic drugs.

Free fatty acid concentrations increase during pregnancy to a value that is nearly double the normal value at term (4). Free fatty acids are known to be displacers of acidic drug binding to albumin and other proteins due to competitive inhibition (1). This is another factor causing increased free drug concentrations.

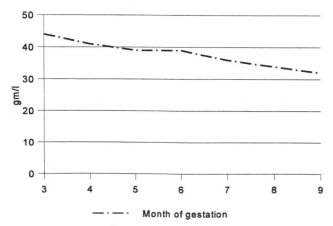

FIGURE 6.2. Albumin concentration during pregnancy. (From Notarianni LJ. Plasma protein binding of drugs in pregnancy and in neonates. *Clin Pharmacokinet* 1990;18:20–36, with permission.)

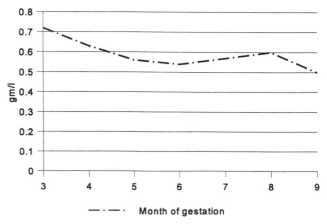

FIGURE 6.3. α_1-Acid glycoprotein (AAG) concentration during pregnancy. (From Notarianni LJ. Plasma protein binding of drugs in pregnancy and in neonates. *Clin Pharmacokinet* 1990;18:20–36, with permission.)

An increase in free fraction of drug results in a greater concentration of pharmacologically active drug. Therefore, for a given total drug concentration, the response will be greater. For instance, for a highly bound drug such as phenytoin, which is normally 90% protein bound (10% unbound) in the nonpregnant state, doubling the free concentration, which occurs in pregnancy, would produce a twofold increase in response at the same total drug concentration. Therefore, changes in protein binding make total drug concentrations difficult to interpret. For drugs that are restrictively cleared by the liver (not rate-limited by blood flow), an increase in the free fraction will also result in an increase in the amount of drug available to be cleared by the liver. Therefore, a decrease in serum protein binding can lower average steady-state serum concentrations of total drug while the concentration of free drug remains unchanged. Although the normal response to a decrease in total drug concentration would be to increase the dose, in this circumstance it would be inappropriate since the free, pharmacologically active concentration has not changed. Because we usually monitor total drug concentrations rather than free drug levels, changes in protein binding during pregnancy may lead to misinterpretation of assay results and inappropriate changes in drug dosages. Table 6.1 shows the effect of altered protein binding for certain drugs where a change in dosing may be required.

PLASMA VOLUME

There is a marked increase in blood and plasma volume during pregnancy (1–5). Total body water increases by as much as 8 L, of which 80% is extracellular and 20% is intracellular (1,4). Plasma volume increases by 50%, which increases normal plasma volume of 2.5 L by 1.2 L. This increase is even greater in multiple gestations. Increased body water allows a greater volume in which drugs are distributed, especially polar drugs that are confined to the extracellular space.

Hemodynamic Changes

Cardiac output increases by nearly 50% during pregnancy, with the maximum being reached between 30 and 34 weeks' gestation (1). The increase in output is brought about by an increase in resting heart rate and stroke volume. The increase in cardiac output is associated with changes in blood flow to individual organs that are characteristic of pregnancy. Uterine blood flow progressively increases almost tenfold, reaching a maximum of 700 mL/min at term; 80% perfuses the placenta and 20% perfuses the myometrium. Renal blood flow increases by about 50% by the end of the first trimester, which is associated with a corresponding increase in glomerular filtration rate (GFR) (6). Pulmonary blood flow increases by approximately 30%

TABLE 6.1. DRUGS WITH ALTERED PROTEIN BINDING IN PREGNANCY

Drug	Binding	Comment
Bupivacaine	Reduced in pregnancy	Bound to AAG
Diazepam	Decreases from 98% to 95% at term	Decreased binding due to decreased albumin concentration and displacement by FFA
Lidocaine	Reduced from 68% to 50%	Bound to AAG
Phenobarbital	Reduced from 49% to 42%	Bound to albumin
Phenytoin	Progressively decreases from 90% to 80%	Decreased binding due to decreased albumin concentration and displacement by endogenous substances
Propranolol	Decreased from 85% to 80% at term	Bound to AAG; displaced by endogenous substances
Salicylic acid	Reduced	Reduced binding due to reduction in association constant
Theophylline	Reduced from 41% to 32% at term	Kinetics altered as a result of increased V_d
Valproic acid	Reduced from 90% to 74% at term	Bound to albumin, displaced by FFA

AAG, α_1-acid glycoprotein; FFA, free fatty acid, V_d, volume of distribution.
From Notarianni LJ. Plasma protein binding of drugs in pregnancy and in neonates. *Clin Pharmacokinet* 1990;18:20–36, with permission.

(1). Hepatic blood flow does not appear to change significantly during pregnancy. Variable changes in cardiac output and its regional distribution occur during labor and with changes in body position.

Body Composition and Volume of Distribution

The apparent volume of distribution (V_d) of a drug is a value relating the plasma concentration to the amount of drug in the body. This volume does not necessarily correspond to a physiologic space, which is why it is referred to as "apparent." A large V_d implies wide distribution or extensive tissue uptake. A small V_d indicates limited distribution, usually the result of high plasma protein binding, which confines the drug mostly to the intravascular space with little tissue uptake. This relationship is represented by the following equation, where f_{up} stands for the fraction unbound to plasma proteins, f_{ut} stands for the fraction unbound to tissues, V_p is the plasma volume, V_t is the tissue volume, and V_{ss} is the volume of distribution at steady state:

$$V_{ss} = V_p + [V_t \times f_{up}/f_{ut}]$$

Body fat composition changes during pregnancy, with normal fat stores of 3 to 4 kg in the first two trimesters (2). Women who gain more than 12 kg have even larger fat stores. In studies using serial measurements of arm skinfold thickness, increases of 20% to 40% have been found (1). Increases in adipose tissue act as a reservoir for lipophilic drugs (7). Drugs that affect the central nervous system (CNS) are typically very lipophilic since this characteristic is required to cross the blood–brain barrier. Drugs such as benzodiazepines and barbiturates will be taken up by the larger adipose tissue stores and slowly released into the circulation where they will be metabolized and excreted. Therefore, the larger V_d for these agents results in prolonged half-lives and an extended duration of action (7).

Metabolism

The metabolism of drugs in the liver during pregnancy is influenced by increasing amounts of steroid hormones. High levels of progesterone stimulate hepatic microsomal enzyme activity (1,2). This results in enhanced metabolism of many drugs. Progesterone and estrogen have been shown to be competitive inhibitors of microsomal oxidases and may have a cholestatic effect (1). The net effect on enzyme activity may depend on the balance between the increasing hormone levels (2). The lower the estrogen/progesterone ratio, the greater the enzyme induction. Smoking, alcohol consumption, and many medications such as carbamazepine, phenobarbital, and rifampin are also potent enzyme inducers. Table 6.2 shows the changes in intrinsic clearance of certain drugs during pregnancy.

Drugs that are greater than 70% metabolized in their first pass through the liver have a high extraction ratio. For these drugs blood flow to the liver is the rate-limiting step in their metabolism, and protein binding does not affect their clearance. Drugs with a great disparity between the oral and intravenous dose are typically high extraction ratio drugs such as hydralazine, propranolol, labetolol, and meperidine. Since clearance for these drugs is dependent on blood flow, and liver blood flow does not change in preg-

nancy, the rate of elimination for these drugs does not change in pregnancy.

Restrictively cleared drugs have a low extraction ratio, usually less than 30%. For these drugs, systemic clearance depends on intrinsic liver enzyme activity, and the rate of elimination is proportional to or restricted by the free drug concentration. Restrictively cleared drugs include theophylline, phenytoin, and diazepam.

Placental Metabolism

The placenta contains most of the same enzyme systems as the liver, only at about half the level, so oxidation, reduction, hydrolysis, and conjugation of substances can occur in placental tissue (2). The placenta contains multiple forms of the P-450 enzyme system as well as large quantities of monoamine oxidases and catechol-O-methyltransferase, which are thought to limit the transfer of endogenous catecholamines (2). It is well established that some of the cytochrome P-450 enzymes bioactivate compounds to highly reactive, potentially toxic metabolites (8). Certain subgroups of these enzymes are inducible by maternal cigarette smoking. The contribution of placental enzymes to bioactivation and metabolism of drugs remains unclear (8).

Excretion

Of all the physiologic systems that are modified by pregnancy, renal function probably undergoes the greatest change. Renal plasma flow increases continuously until about 26 weeks, when values are 60% to 80% above normal, then decreases somewhat during the third trimester (6). GFR increases from about 100 to 170 mL/min by 15 weeks' gestation and remains at that value until 6 days postpartum when values do not differ significantly from the nonpregnant state (7). Figure 6.4 shows the pattern of change in

TABLE 6.2. CHANGES IN HEPATIC CLEARANCE OF CERTAIN DRUGS IN PREGNANCY

Increased Clearance	Decreased Clearance	Clearance Unchanged
Phenytoin	Caffeine	Lidocaine
Acetaminophen	Theophylline	Propranolol
Pancuronium	Diazepam	Meperidine
Metoprolol		Labetolol
Carbamazepine		Hydralazine

From Reynolds F, Knott C. Pharmacokinetics in pregnancy and placental drug transfer. *Oxf Rev Reprod Biol* 1989;11:389–449, with permission.

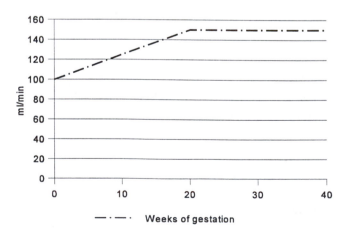

FIGURE 6.4. Changes in glomerular filtration rate (GFR) during pregnancy. (From Davison JM, Dunlop W. Changes in renal hemodynamics and tubular function induced by normal human pregnancy. *Semin Nephrol* 1984;4:198–207, with permission.)

GFR during pregnancy. These changes in GFR cause polar, water-soluble drugs such as penicillins, cephalosporins, aminoglycosides, and lithium, which are predominantly eliminated by renal excretion, to be more rapidly cleared during pregnancy and to have shorter half-lives (2).

Fetal Pharmacokinetics

The primary route of fetal absorption of drugs is from the placenta through the umbilical vein. The fetus can also absorb drugs from the GI tract after fetal swallowing of amniotic fluid develops around 8 to 11 weeks' gestation (9). Substances circulating in the amniotic fluid can also be absorbed through the fetal skin (9).

Drug distribution varies considerably as the fetus develops. Total body water decreases from 94% to 75% at term (9). Fat composition increases from 0.5% when the fetus weighs 300 g to 12% at term (9). Plasma protein levels are very low in the fetus, so the unbound fraction of drugs will be high. Because of these factors, the volume of distribution of drugs in the fetal circulation will be much higher than in the mother.

Fetal liver metabolizing enzymes develop at different rates. Metabolizing capacity during early development is extremely low. Four types of drug transformations were compared in liver biopsies from adults and fetuses of 9 to 22 weeks' gestation. The percentage of adult enzyme activity ranged from 2.4% for hydroxylases to 36.1% for oxidases (9). The contribution of fetal metabolism of drug is very minor compared to the main route of drug metabolism, which is via the mother's liver.

Glomerular and tubular function of the kidneys develop early in fetal life. Glomerulogenesis ends at around 32 to 34 weeks and glomerular function accelerates at this point, whereas tubular function develops more slowly (9). Fetal urine flow increases from about 2 mL/h at 22 weeks to 25 mL/h by term (9). Drugs excreted renally such as penicillins and cephalosporins enter the amniotic fluid where they circulate and are swallowed by the fetus. The fetus can swallow 200 to 450 mL of amniotic fluid per day at term (9). Drugs present in the amniotic fluid can be absorbed by the GI tract, prolonging drug exposure by the fetus.

PRINCIPLES OF DRUG TRANSFER ACROSS THE PLACENTA

Passive diffusion is the most common method of drug transfer, and in this case the placenta behaves like any lipid membrane (10). Passive diffusion requires no energy, and compounds move from a high concentration to a lower concentration until an equilibrium is established. The physical and chemical properties of the drug, such as molecular weight, lipid solubility, protein binding, and degree of ionization, determine the rate and extent of transfer. Water-soluble drugs will diffuse across the placenta easily only if their molecular weight is less than 100 (2). Hydrophilic compounds with higher molecular weights such as mannitol and neuromuscular blockers have very limited placental passage. Lipophilic drugs with molecular weights less than 600 that are unbound to plasma proteins such as ethanol and meperidine will readily cross the placenta. Nutrients and waste products are more polar and require specialized transport systems to cross the placenta. Drugs with molecular weights greater than 1,000, such as heparin, do not cross the placenta to any measurable degree (10).

Most drugs are either weak acids or weak bases and cross biologic membranes more readily in the un-ionized state than in the ionized state. Therefore, bases with high measures of acid strength (pKas) and acids with low pKas diffuse across all biologic membranes poorly. Ionized drugs will cross the placenta to a limited degree only if a sufficiently high maternal to fetal concentration gradient exists. When there is a difference in maternal and fetal blood pH, the ionization of a drug changes when it enters the fetus. For example, near term the mother's blood may be slightly alkalotic from hyperventilation and the fetus may be slightly acidotic. Therefore, a basic drug that is mainly un-ionized in the maternal circulation crosses the placenta and becomes ionized in the more acidic fetal blood. This results in higher fetal drug concentrations since the ionized form of the drug cannot readily diffuse back across the placenta. The opposite is true for weakly acidic drugs where fetal drug concentrations are lower than maternal drug concentrations.

The rate of blood flow to the placenta, and placental membrane surface area, thickness, and permeability are also factors in the amount of drug that reaches the fetus by simple diffusion (10). For un-ionized, lipophilic drugs, the rate-limiting step in placental drug transfer is blood flow to the placenta. Placental blood flow gradually increases during pregnancy to meet the growing demands of the fetus. This increase in delivery of nutrients and oxygen to the placenta also means delivery of drugs present in the maternal circulation. Drugs such as cocaine and sympathomimetic agents like amphetamine and pseudoephedrine can decrease placenta blood flow, and if used in high doses on a chronic basis, can cause intrauterine growth retardation (8).

Facilitated diffusion is a transport process that enables compounds to be transported down a concentration gradient faster than simple diffusion allows. No energy is required for facilitated diffusion, but it is selective, stereospecific, and saturable and susceptible to competition (10). This mechanism carries glucose to the fetus and waste products such as lactate away from the fetus (10). Theoretically, drugs that are similar to endogenous compounds could compete for transfer via this carrier-mediated system and reach higher peak concentrations in the fetus than by simple diffusion (10).

Active transport is a carrier-mediated system that requires energy to move compounds from a low concentration to a higher concentration. Amino acids, calcium, and magnesium are actively transported by the placenta (10). Only drugs that are analogues of endogenous compounds transported by this mechanism, such as methyldopa and 5-fluorouracil, can compete for carrier sites (8). This system is also stereospecific and saturable.

Pinocytosis is a process that involves invagination of the cell membrane to envelope and package macromolecules that are then transported to the opposite cell surface and released intact. Although pinocytosis has been postulated to be a method of transfer of the placenta, it is not thought to play a major role in drug transport (8). Immunoglobulin G may be taken up by the fetus by pinocytosis (2).

Drug transfer from mother to fetus is more limited in early gestation than it is in late gestation (11). This is partially due to increased placental surface area, decreased thickness of lipid membranes between placental capillaries, and increased blood flow to the placenta. A decrease in protein binding in late gestation also makes more free drug available for placental transfer.

FETAL DRUG THERAPY

Corticosteroid therapy to aid in accelerating fetal lung maturity is recommended for all women at risk of delivering prior to 34 weeks' gestation (12). Early studies found that administering betamethasone phosphate 6 mg with betamethasone acetate 6 mg (Celestone 12 mg) IM daily for two doses to the mother was effective in inducing surfactant synthesis and release in the fetus, and the incidence of respiratory distress syndrome in the neonate was reduced (13). Similar studies using cortisone and prednisolone were not effective (13). Hydrocortisone and prednisolone undergo rapid and extensive inactivation by the placenta. The placenta metabolizes 88% of a dose of prednisolone to its inactive form—prednisone (13). Prednisolone is structurally similar to endogenous corticosteroids, which are also inactivated by the placenta. Betamethasone and dexamethasone, the α-stereoisomer of betamethasone, are fluorinated corticosteroids that pass through the placenta nearly intact (13). Current recommendations by the National Institutes of Health (NIH) are for all women without chorioamnionitis at risk of delivery before 34 weeks' gestation to receive either Celestone 12 mg IM daily for two doses or dexamethasone 6 mg IM or IV every 12 hours for four doses (12).

With improvements in ultrasound technology, fetal cardiac arrhythmias, pericardial effusions, and congestive heart failure can be detected *in utero*. When fetal arrhythmias such as supraventricular tachycardia (SVT) are sustained, they can be life threatening. The most practical method of treating the fetus is by administering drug therapy to the mother. In this case the drug must cross the placenta efficiently and be relatively nontoxic to the mother. The most frequently used therapy for fetal SVT is digoxin. Digoxin

is a cardiac glycoside with a molecular weight of 780 and low protein binding (20% to 40%). Fetal serum concentrations of digoxin are equal to maternal levels within 30 minutes after intravenous administration to the mother (13). To maintain therapeutic levels in the fetus, high maternal doses and frequent dosing intervals must be used due to increased renal clearance and an expanded volume of distribution (13). Maternal serum level monitoring and fetal heart rate response should be employed to guide dosage. Some radioimmunoassay kits for digoxin may detect digoxin-like immunoreactive substances (DLIS) present in pregnancy, renal insufficiency, and congestive heart failure. This should be kept in mind when monitoring digoxin levels. Rarely, digoxin has been administered directly to the fetus via intraperitoneal, intramuscular, or intravenous injection (13). When digoxin alone is ineffective, it can be combined with other antiarrhythmic agents such as procainamide, quinidine, or verapamil.

MATERNAL DRUG THERAPY IN PREGNANCY

Antibiotics

Antibiotics are the most common therapeutic class of drugs prescribed in pregnancy. The site and nature of the infection and the physiologic and pharmacokinetic changes are the critical factors that determine the therapeutic options and dosing of antibiotics in pregnancy. Shorter half-lives, lower serum concentrations, and increased clearances have been reported for many antibiotics including penicillins and cephalosporins (5). This may be of little consequence if the site of infection is the urinary tract where drug excretion occurs and local drug concentrations are adequate to produce the desired therapeutic effect. However, if the infection requires high serum concentrations for therapeutic efficacy, such as pneumonia or endocarditis, higher doses and more frequent dosing intervals determined by serum concentration monitoring and dosage adjustment will be necessary. Whether or not the fetus is to be treated concurrently is another consideration in antibiotic selection. If only the mother is to be treated, the use of an antibiotic that does not cross the placenta well may be chosen. However, if both mother and fetus are infected, as in syphilis, the chosen agent must be both safe and effective and adequately cross the placenta. Penicillin remains the drug of choice for treating all stages of syphilis in pregnancy (14). In the treatment of chorioamnionitis, although penicillin and ampicillin achieve excellent maternal and fetal concentrations, peak amniotic fluid levels of antibiotic are delayed by 6 to 8 hours, making systemic therapy inadequate (15). Recommended antimicrobial therapy for common infections that occur in pregnancy are listed in Table 6.3.

The volume of distribution and clearance of ampicillin and amoxicillin are increased in pregnancy, and their half-

TABLE 6.3. ANTIBIOTIC REGIMENS FOR COMMON BACTERIAL INFECTIONS IN PREGNANCY

Infection (27)	First choice regimen	Alternative regimen
Urinary tract infection	Amoxicillin 500 mg TID × 7 days OR 3 g × 1 Cephalexin 500 mg QID for 7–10 days	Nitrofurantoin 100 mg PO QID for 7–10 days Trimethoprim/Sulfameth-oxazole BID × 5 days
Pyelonephritis	Cefazolin 1 g IV q8h Ceftizoxime 1 g IV q8h	Gentamicin 2 mg/kg × 1, 1.5 mg/kg q8h AND ampicillin 1 g q6h
Chlamydia	Azithromycin 1 g PO × 1	Erythromycin 500 mg PO QID × 7 days
Gonorrhea (14)	Cefixime 400 mg PO × 1 Ceftriaxone 125 mg IM × 1	Ceftizoxime 500 mg IM × 1 Cefotetan 1 g IM × 1
Syphilis (14), primary <1 year	Benzathine penicillin 2.4 MU IM	Penicillin allergic patients must be desensitized
Syphilis (14) >1 year	Benzathine penicillin 2.4 MU IM q week × 3	Penicillin allergic patients must be desensitized
Neurosyphilis (14)	Aqueous penicillin G 2–4 MU IV q4h × 10–14 days	Penicillin allergic patients must be desensitized
Group B beta streptococcus prophylaxis (28)	Penicillin 5 MU IV q6h	Ampicillin 2 g IV × 1, 1 g q4h Clindamycin 900 mg IV q8h
PROM (15)	Ampicillin 1 gm IV q4h Azithromycin 500 mg IV qd × 2, then 500 mg PO qd × 5 days	Clindamycin 900 mg IV q8h Erythromycin 500 mg IV q6h
Chorioamnionitis (15)	Ampicillin 2 GM IV × 1, 1 g q4h and Gentamicin 2 mg/kg × 1, 1.5 mg/kg q8h	Cefazolin 1 g IV q6h Gentamicin 2 mg/kg × 1, 1.5 mg/kg IV q8h Clindamycin 900 mg IV q8h
Postpartum endometritis (15)	Gentamicin 7 mg/kg IV qd and clindamycin 900 mg IV q8h Piperacillin/tazobactam 4.5 g IV q8h	Ampicillin 2 g IV × 1, 1 g q4h AND Gentamicin 2 mg/kg × 1, 1.5 mg/kg q8h Clindamycin 900 mg IV q8h OR ampicillin/sulbactam 3 g IV q6h and gentamicin 7 mg/kg IV qd
Bacterial vaginosis (29)	Clindamycin 300 mg PO BID × 7 days Clindamycin 2% to 5% vaginal cream × 7 days Metronidazole vaginal suppository 500 mg qd × 7 days	Amoxicillin/clavulanate 500 mg PO q8h × 7 days
Pelvic inflammatory disease (14) (inpatient, nonpregnant)	Gentamicin 7 mg/kg IV qd AND clindamycin 900 mg IV q8h OR azithromycin 500 mg IV qd × 2, then 500 mg PO × 5 days	Cefotetan 2 gm IV q12h AND doxycyline 100 mg IV/PO q12h

PROM, premature rupture of membrane.

lives are shorter than in nonpregnant women (5). Therefore, if normal doses are used in pregnancy, plasma concentrations are lower, often below the minimum inhibitory concentration (MIC) (2). When the standard dose of ceftazidime is administered to a pregnant woman, serum concentrations are half the level in a nonpregnant woman (2). A similar situation exists for aminoglycoside antibiotics. The average half-life of gentamicin is 93 minutes in pregnancy compared to 159 minutes in the nonpregnant state (2).

Most antibiotics cross the placenta by simple diffusion. Penicillins and cephalosporins are weak acids with relatively low pKas, making them highly ionized and hydrophilic (10). Their molecular weights range from 350 to 500 (10). Ampicillin is only 20% protein bound and rapidly crosses the placenta and peaks in fetal serum about 1 hour after administration to the mother (16). Ampicillin gradually accumulates in amniotic fluid via fetal renal excretion and peaks at 8 hours (16) (Fig. 6.5). Methicillin and dicloxacillin are protein bound to a greater extent in maternal plasma

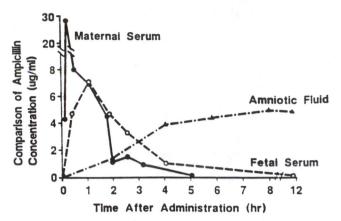

FIGURE 6.5. Maternal and fetal levels of ampicillin after administration of 0.5 g to the mother. (From Ledger WJ. Antibiotics in pregnancy. *Clin Obstet Gynecol* 1977;20:411–421, with permission.)

than ampicillin, about 40% and 96%, respectively (10). To illustrate the effect of protein binding on the extent of placental transfer, these two penicillins were compared. Methicillin levels in the fetus were 81% of maternal levels, and the amniotic fluid levels rose progressively, reaching 50% of peak fetal levels at 6 hours. Dicloxacillin fetal levels were only 7% of maternal levels and amniotic fluid levels were insignificant (2).

The aminoglycoside antibiotics are weak bases with pKas ranging from 7.5 to 8. They are poorly lipid soluble and less than 30% protein bound (10). Fetal gentamicin concentrations range from 21% to 37% of maternal plasma levels, and amniotic fluid levels are not detectable (10).

Antihypertensives

Antihypertensive agents are used to treat essential hypertension and pregnancy-induced hypertension. Beta-blockers, methyldopa, hydralazine, and calcium channel blockers are the most common agents used to treat hypertension in pregnancy. The angiotensin-converting enzyme inhibitors are contraindicated in pregnancy due to fetal and neonatal injury, including renal failure and skull hypoplasia (17).

Although the V_d is enlarged and the protein binding to AAG is decreased slightly, overall the pharmacokinetics of propranolol is unchanged in pregnancy (2). This is probably because propranolol is a high extraction drug and its clearance is dependent on liver blood flow. The kinetics of labetolol and atenolol are also unchanged in pregnancy (18).

Propranolol is a lipophilic base with a pKa of 9.5 and therefore it freely crosses the placenta and becomes more ionized in fetal circulation. This results in a fetal to maternal (F/M) concentration ratio of 1.39 (2). Propranolol is associated with intrauterine growth retardation and neonatal bradycardia and transient hypotension (2). Labetolol is less

lipid soluble than propranolol and average F/M ratios of 0.5 to 0.8 have been found (2). Mild neonatal bradycardia and hypotension have also been reported for atenolol and labetolol (2).

Hydralazine was used extensively for treatment of hypertension in pregnancy until the parenteral form was unavailable for a period of time in the early 1990s in the United States. It is a high hepatic extraction drug so its pharmacokinetics is not significantly changed in pregnancy. Hydralazine is a basic compound (pKa 7.4) with a molecular weight of 160. The F/M ratio of hydralazine is 1.9 (2). Hydralazine causes reflex tachycardia in the mother and can reduce placental perfusion resulting in fetal distress (18).

Nifedipine undergoes extensive first-pass metabolism and its half-life is shortened in pregnancy. Peak concentrations are slightly lower in pregnant women (19). It also freely crosses the placenta with a F/M ratio of 1.3 (19). No significant fetal or neonatal adverse effects are associated with the use of nifedipine.

Anticonvulsants

Although the anticonvulsants pose an increased risk of teratogenesis, particularly when multiple drug regimens are used, continuing therapy during pregnancy is recommended due to the risk to the fetus of anoxic damage, which may follow sustained seizures (20). Anticonvulsant serum concentrations frequently fall as pregnancy progresses and can be a reason for increased seizure frequency. This is due to altered pharmacokinetics, including decreased protein binding, increased hepatic metabolism, changes in plasma volume, and altered drug absorption (20). Protein binding is progressively reduced, particularly for the highly bound agents such as phenytoin and valproic acid (4). Because of the alterations in unbound phenytoin levels, total drug concentrations are difficult to assess. In certain circumstances, such as uncontrolled seizures, free phenytoin levels may need to be drawn. Dramatic increases in intrinsic clearance occur for phenytoin and valproic acid and to a lesser degree for carbamazepine, necessitating dosage adjustments in the second and third trimesters (2). Clearance of these agents declines rapidly postpartum, making frequent dosage reductions necessary to avoid toxicity. Table 6.4 lists commonly used anticonvulsants in pregnancy and their doses and characteristics.

All anticonvulsants interfere with the metabolism of folic acid. Folic acid deficiency has been associated with neural tube defects and other congenital malformations (20). Folic acid supplementation is recommended for all patients taking anticonvulsants both before and during pregnancy (20).

Several new anticonvulsants have been approved by the Food and Drug Administration (FDA) recently, including gabapentin (Neurontin), felbamate (Felbatol), and lamotrigine (Lamictal). Although little is known about these

TABLE 6.4. COMMONLY USED ANTICONVULSANTS IN PREGNANCY

Drug	$t_{1/2}$	Protein Binding	Nonpregnant Dose	Therapeutic Level
Carbamazepine	36 h (initially) 16 h (chronic)	75% to AAG	600–1,200 mg/day in 3–4 divided doses	4–12 mg/L
Phenobarbital	100 h	40% to 60%	90–180 mg/day in 2–3 divided doses	15–40 mg/L
Phenytoin	Average 24 h	90% nonpregnant; 80% to 85% pregnant	300–400 mg/day in single or divided doses	5–20 mg/L (free levels 1–2 mg/L)
Primidone	8 h	0	750–1,500 mg/day in 3 divided doses	5–15 mg/L
Valproic acid	13 h	80% to 94%	550–2,000 mg/day in 3–4 divided doses	50–150 mg/L

agents in pregnancy, occasionally a woman taking one of these agents may become pregnant. Gabapentin is used as adjunctive therapy for partial seizures. It has a molecular weight of 171 and is not bound to serum proteins (21). For these reasons, it is expected to cross the placenta freely (21). Gabapentin is excreted unchanged in the urine with a half-life of 6 hours (22). It is not appreciably metabolized. Gabapentin is structurally related to the neurotransmitter γ-aminobutyric acid (GABA), but it does not interact at GABA receptors and its mechanism is unknown (22). In animal studies it was shown to cause delayed ossification of bones of the skull, vertebrae, forelimbs, and hindlimbs (21). Hydroureter and/or hydronephrosis was observed in rats exposed to 1,500 mg/kg/day during organogenesis (21). Little is known about its effects in human pregnancy.

Lamotrigine is chemically unrelated to existing anticonvulsants and is used as adjunctive therapy for the treatment of partial seizures (22). Glaxo Wellcome, the manufacturer of lamotrigine, has maintained a pregnancy registry and published preliminary data in 1997. The prospective portion of the registry involved 125 pregnancies, the outcomes of which 86 were known. Among those exposed in the first trimester, there were five spontaneous abortions, 18 elective abortions, three infants with anomalies (all on polytherapy), and 58 infants without birth defects (21). The anomalies included one infant with an extra digit on one hand, an infant with bilateral talipes (mother also taking valproic acid), and an infant with skin tags on the left ear and no opening to the ear canal on the right ear (21). The limited animal and human data available do not appear to indicate a major risk for congenital malformations following exposure to lamotigine (21).

Felbamate was approved in 1993 for use as adjunctive therapy for partial seizures or generalized seizures. Soon after it was approved serious toxic effects began to surface. Aplastic anemia and serious hepatotoxic effects caused death in several patients (22). The FDA currently recommends that felbamate be given only to patients whose seizures are refractory to other treatments.

Methylxanthines

Both theophylline and caffeine are cleared progressively more slowly during pregnancy (23–25). This is due to

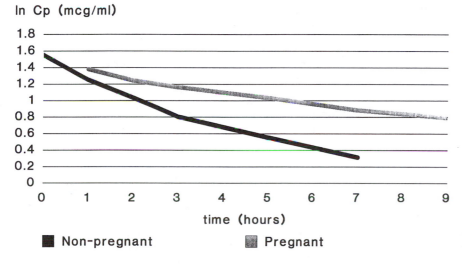

FIGURE 6.6. Caffeine plasma concentration-time curves in a pregnant and nonpregnant woman. (From Brazier JL, Ritter J, Berland M, et al. Pharmacokinetics of caffeine during and after pregnancy. *Dev Pharmacol Ther* 1983;6:315–322, with permission.)

reduced hepatic metabolism and an expanded volume of distribution. Both drugs are lipid soluble and distribute to enlarging adipose tissue stores, making less drug available to the liver. The half-life of caffeine is prolonged up to three times the half-life in a nonpregnant woman (25). Figure 6.6 shows the serum concentration time curves for caffeine in a pregnant and nonpregnant woman. The clearance of caffeine returns to prepregnancy values rapidly after delivery (25). Theophylline clearance is reduced nearly in half by the late second trimester (23). Women who are taking theophylline for asthma should have their dosage reduced to avoid toxicity. Serum levels of theophylline should be monitored in the second and third trimesters to guide dosage adjustments. Levels greater then 20 mg/L have been known to cause ventricular arrhythmias or seizures. Clearance returns to normal by 2 months postpartum (23).

The lipophilicity of the methylxanthines cause them to freely cross the placenta and enter fetal circulation. Maternal and fetal blood levels are similar (2). Amniotic fluid levels of theophylline are 76% of the cord serum levels (2). The neonate metabolizes the xanthines very slowly due to immaturity of oxidative enzymes.

10 KEY POINTS

1. All aspects of pharmacokinetics, absorption, distribution, metabolism, and excretion, are altered during pregnancy.

2. The serum concentrations of albumin and α_1-acid glycoprotein decrease in pregnancy resulting in increased free drug concentrations. The free or unbound drug is the pharmacologically active component.

3. The volume of distribution of most drugs is increased in pregnancy due to increases in total body water and plasma volume.

4. Increases in fat stores act as a reservoir for lipophilic drugs. The half-life of these agents is prolonged due to slow release from adipose tissue into the circulation where they are metabolized and excreted.

5. Drugs that undergo first-pass hepatic metabolism are considered high extraction ratio drugs. Since the clearance of these drugs is dependent on hepatic blood flow, their clearance remains unchanged in pregnancy.

6. Progesterone stimulates hepatic enzyme activity, which results in enhanced metabolism of many drugs.

7. Glomerular filtration rate increases from approximately 100 to 170 mL/min by 15 weeks' gestation. This results in increased excretion of renally eliminated drugs.

8. The primary method of drug transfer across the placenta is by passive diffusion. Lipophilic drugs with molecular weights less than 600 and hydrophilic drugs with molecular weights less than 100 readily cross the placenta.

9. Large molecules with molecular weights greater than 1,000 usually do not cross the placenta.

10. Fetal drug therapy requires that the agent cross the placenta intact. For example, betamethasone is effective for accelerating fetal lung maturity, whereas predisolone is not due to placental metabolism to an inactive form.

REFERENCES

1. Parker WA. Effects of pregnancy on pharmacokinetics. In: Benet LZ, ed. *Pharmacokinetic basis for drug treatment.* New York: Raven Press, 1984;249–268.
2. Reynolds F, Knott C. Pharmacokinetics in pregnancy and placental drug transfer. *Oxf Rev Reprod Biol* 1989;11:389–449.
3. Krauer B, Krauer F, Hytten FE. Drug disposition and pharmacokinetics in the maternal-placental-fetal unit. *Pharmacol Ther* 1980;10:301–328.
4. Notarianni LJ. Plasma protein binding of drugs in pregnancy and in neonates. *Clin Pharmacokinet* 1990;18:20–36.
5. Chow AW, Jewesson PJ. Pharmacokinetics and safety of antimicrobial agents during pregnancy.*Rev Infect Dis* 1985;7:287–313.
6. Davison JM, Dunlop W. Changes in renal hemodynamics and tubular function induced by normal human pregnancy. *Semin Nephrol* 1984;4:198–207.
7. Murray L, Seger D. Drug therapy during pregnancy and lactation. *Emerg Med Clin North Am* 1994;12:129–149.
8. Simone C, Lidia LO, Koren G. Drug transfer across the placenta. *Clin Perinatol* 1994;21:463–481.
9. Ward RM. Pharmacologic treatment of the fetus. *Clin Pharmacokinet* 1995;28:343–350.
10. Pacifici GM, Nottoli R. Placental transfer of drugs administered to the mother. *Clin Pharmacokinet* 1995;28:235–269.
11. Ward RM. Maternal-placental-fetal unit. Unique problems of pharmacologic study. *Clin Pharmacol* 1989;36:1075–1087.
12. NIH Consensus Conference. Effect of corticosteroids for fetal maturation on perinatal outcomes. *JAMA* 1995;273:413–418.
13. Ward RM. Drug therapy of the fetus. *J Clin Pharmacol* 1993;33:780–789.
14. Kraynak MA, Knodel LC. Sexually transmitted diseases: an update. *Am Pharm* 1995;NS35:41–47.
15. Newton ER. Chorioamnionitis and intraamniotic infection. *Clin Obstet Gynecol* 1993;36:795–808.
16. Ledger WJ. Antibiotics in pregnancy. *Clin Obstet Gynecol* 1977;20:411–421.
17. Barr M, Cohen MM. ACE inhibitor fetopathy and hypocalvaria: the kidney-skull connection. *Teratology* 1991;44:485–495.
18. Redman CWG. The treatment of hypertension in pregnancy: maternal and fetal implications. In: Krauer B, Krauer F, Hytten FE, et al., eds. *Drugs and pregnancy.* London: Academic Press 1984:151–176.
19. Levin AC, Doering PL, Hatton RC. Use of nifedipine in the hypertensive diseases of pregnancy. *Ann Pharmacother* 1994;28:1371–1378.
20. Samuels P. Seizure disorders in pregnancy. *ACOG Educational Bull* 1996;231:1–7.
21. Briggs GG, Freeman RK, Yaffe SJ.Gabapentin. *Update: Drugs in Pregnancy and Lactation.* 1997;10:2–3.
22. Dichter MA, Brodie MJ. New antiepileptic agents. *N Engl J Med* 1996;334:1583–1590.
23. Carter BL, Driscoll CE, Smith GD. Theophylline clearance during pregnancy. *Obstet Gyncol* 1986;68:555–559.
24. Gardner MJ, Schatz M, Cousins L, et al. Longitudinal effects of

pregnancy on the pharmacokinetics of theophylline. *Eur J Clin Pharmacol* 1987;31:289–295.

25. Brazier JL, Ritter J, Berland M, et al. Pharmacokinetics of caffeine during and after pregnancy. *Dev Pharmacol Ther* 1983;6: 315–322.

26. Mirkin BL. Drug distribution in pregnancy. In: Boreus LO, ed. *Fetal pharmacology.* New York: Raven Press, 1973, 22.

27. Lucas MJ, Cunningham FG. Urinary infection in pregnancy. *Clin Obstet Gynecol* 1993;36:855–868.

28. U.S. Department of Health and Human Services, Centers for Disease Control. Prevention of perinatal group B streptococcal disease: a public health perspective. *MMWR* 1996;45:1–24.

29. Hedstrom S, Martens MG. Antibiotics in pregnancy. *Clin Obstet Gynecol* 1993;36:886–892.

7

LABORATORY TECHNIQUES: BASIC ASSAY METHODOLOGY

LAURA L. ARBOGAST
DOUGLAS R. DANFORTH

The accurate measurement of biologic compounds is important to many scientific fields, including reproductive biology. Reproductive biology has made major advancements in the last several decades due in part to the development and enhancement of assay methodology. Of these methodologies, some of the most widely used in clinical practice and basic research are radioimmunoassay, enzyme-linked immunosorbent assay (ELISA), radioreceptor assay, and bioassay. These techniques have allowed for the rapid detection and measurement of minute quantities of biologic substances. Each of these techniques is discussed in this chapter.

RADIOIMMUNOASSAYS

The development of radioimmunoassay (RIA) provided the scientific community with a major advancement in measurement of substances of biologic interest. The technique was first described by Yalow and Berson (1) in 1959 as the competitive inhibition by unlabeled antigen of binding of radiolabeled antigen to its antibody. Yalow and Berson (2,3) described an assay to measure circulating insulin in human blood using an antisera to animal insulins produced in guinea pigs. At approximately the same time, Ekins (4) reported a similar method of competitive binding for the determination of thyroxine levels in human plasma. Since the 1960s, RIA has been applied to hundreds of substances of biologic importance since it provides the specificity and sensitivity required to measure the minute concentrations of these substances in circulation.

Among the first reproductive hormones to be measured using RIA were the polypeptide hormones, human chorionic gonadotropin (hCG) (5,6), and prolactin (7–9), followed later by luteinizing hormone (LH) (10,11) and follicle-stimulating hormone (FSH) (12). The inherent antigenicity of these protein hormones allowed for the production of specific antibodies that could identify and distinguish these hormones from the tremendous excess of other proteins in the circulation. In contrast, steroid and thyroid hormones are not inherently antigenic and must be coupled to carrier proteins or binding globulins for production of specific antibodies for use in RIA (13). Other substances of reproductive interest measured by RIA are the prostaglandins, in particular prostaglandin E_2, prostaglandin $F_{2\alpha}$, and prostacyclin (14,15).

Theory

In general, RIA can utilize either radiolabeled antigen or radiolabeled antibody, although most RIAs use radiolabeled antigen. The basic principle of radiolabeled antigen RIA depends on the ability of unlabeled antigen to competitively inhibit binding of radiolabeled antigen to its antibody (Fig. 7.1). The amounts of labeled antigen and antibody are controlled in this assay system. Thus, the more unlabeled antigen present in a sample, the fewer binding sites available for the radiolabeled antigen, and fewer radiolabeled antigen–antibody complexes will be formed. After separation of bound from free hormone, measurement of radioactivity indicates the amount of labeled antigen–antibody complexes and is inversely related to the amount of the hormone of interest in the sample.

RIA consists of three basic steps. The first step, referred to as the incubation step, consists of using varying amounts of a standard, the same as the unlabeled antigen, to generate a standard curve for use in determination of unknown amounts of unlabeled antigen in samples (16). A known amount of specific antibody and radiolabeled antigen are added to the standard curve tubes and to the unknown samples and allowed to reach equilibrium. The next step is the separation of bound complexes from free components. There are several methods to accomplish this separation including electrophoresis, gel filtration, adsorption, solid-phase systems, and double or second antibody (17). Electrophoresis was the first method described for separation (2), but along with gel filtration it is cumbersome and not routinely used. Adsorption with charcoal (18) was widely used for the adsorption of the free fraction but was found unsuitable for all systems since the charcoal can also bind bound antigen or even split the antigen antibody complex. Charcoal is still used for the separation step of

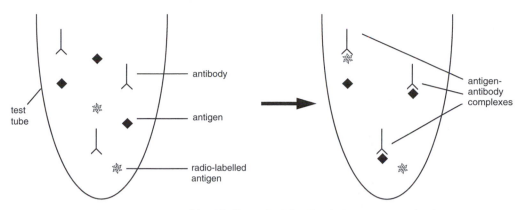

FIGURE 7.1. Competitive binding principle of radioimmunoassay (RIA).

some antigens, particularly prostaglandins and steroids. Adsorption has also been performed with silicates and ion exchange resins. Solid phase systems that are used in RIA include antibody attached to tubes, wells, glass beads, and magnetic particles (19). These types of systems are convenient, but may lack reproducibility. However, recent advances in solid phase coupling technology has resulted in highly reproducible and simple assay systems. An example is the Count-a-Count assays developed by DPC Corporation. These assays utilize primary antibody directly attached to polypropylene tubes. Thus, no secondary separation techniques are necessary. An unknown sample is added, along with radioactive tracer, to the antibody-coated tubes, and after incubation, the tubes are simply decanted to remove nonbound hormone. Utilizing highly specific antiserum, a variety of steroidal and nonsteroidal hormones can now be easily measured by this one-step method.

Aside from this coated tube technology, the most widely used separation system is the second or double antibody system. Basically, the double antibody system uses a second antibody generated in another species against the gamma globulin of the species of the first antibody (20). For example, if the first antibody was generated in the rabbit against luteinizing hormone, the second antibody could be generated in the goat against rabbit gamma globulin (Fig. 7.2). Binding of the second antibody results in precipitation of the antibody-antibody complexes. The primary antibody concentration in most RIAs is often not high enough for precipitation to occur, so addition of additional carrier proteins is usually required. Measurements using the double or second antibody method of separation are sensitive and reproducible, and have been optimized for a wide variety of hormones. Due to its relatively low cost, compared to coated tube assays, and its applicability to a wide variety of hormones from different species, it is the most widely used separation technique.

After separation of bound from free components, the final step in the RIA is the measurement of radioactivity. The gamma counter is used for those antigens labeled with

isotopes emitting gamma rays such as ^{125}I and ^{131}I. The liquid scintillation counter is used to count those isotopes emitting beta rays such as ^{3}H and ^{14}C. Gamma counting is simpler, allowing for sample counting directly without the addition of scintillation fluid, which is required for the beta emitters.

There are two assay methods utilizing radiolabeled antibodies. They are immunoradiometric assay (IRMA) and two-site IRMA. The IRMA method, first described by Miles and Hales (21) in 1968, combines antigen with soluble radiolabeled antibody (Fig. 7.3A). The unbound radioactive antibodies are then removed by binding to a solid phase antigen while the antigen-radiolabeled complex remains in solution. In this assay, the concentration of antigen is directly proportional to the amount of radioactivity in the solution. The two-site IRMA requires insolubilization of the antigen by binding to a solid phase antibody (22) (Fig. 7.3B). Radiolabeled antibody is then added forming an insoluble antigen-radiolabeled antigen complex. Unbound radiolabeled antibody can then be washed away. The concentration of antigen in this assay system is also proportional to the radioactivity.

Both RIA and IRMA offer the advantages of sensitivity, specificity, and convenience. Sensitivity refers to the minimum detectable quantity of a substance in an assay. The sensitivity of an RIA is dependent on the amount of tracer, the quality of tracer, the amount of antibody, incubation time, and the purity of the antibody. The sensitivity of IRMA, however, is not directly related to antibody affinity, and thus it may be a more sensitive method than RIA. Specificity refers to the ability to measure a single substance in a heterogeneous mixture. Interference in an RIA can be of specific or nonspecific origin. The specific interference refers to the identification and subsequent binding of substances similar to the antigen by the antibody. Nonspecific binding refers to unidentified components that interfere with the binding of antigen and antibody. In this aspect, IRMA is more specific than RIA since it requires binding of two specific antibodies. In addition, IRMA can produce

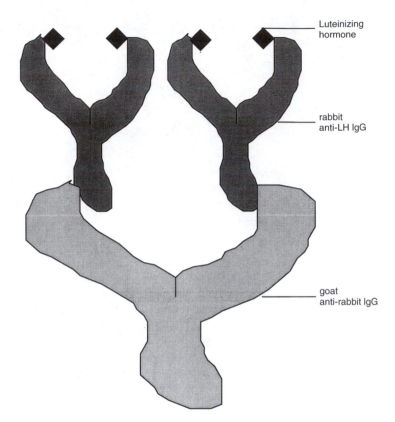

Luteinizing hormone

rabbit anti-LH IgG

goat anti-rabbit IgG

FIGURE 7.2. Second or double antibody technique for separation of bound antigen from free antigen.

results quite different from those of RIA. For example, Wheeler et al. (23) described an IRMA that gave LH values much lower than those from RIA. Another problem encountered with IRMA is the variation between kits or assays.

Regardless of the assay method used, it is important for the clinician to recognize that there is much potential variability in assay values among different assay techniques and even among different manufacturers using similar techniques. As an example, serum FSH levels are often used to assess the reproductive potential of the infertility patient, and an (RIA determined) FSH value of >15 mIU/mL is often considered to indicate an aging ovary (24). However, with a different assay using monoclonal instead of polyclonal antibodies, an FSH value of >9.5 mIU/mL is considered indicative of the aging ovary (25). Thus, not only the type of assay (ELISA versus RIA), but the assay manufacturer and type of antibody used (polyclonal versus monoclonal)

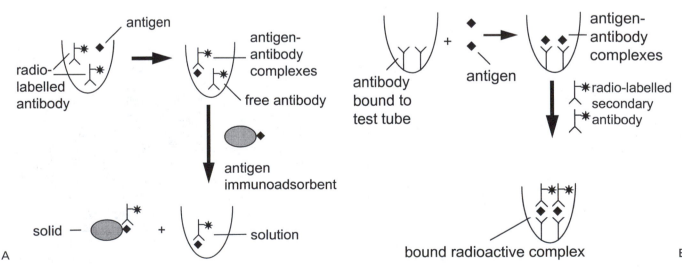

A

antigen

radio-labelled antibody

antigen-antibody complexes

free antibody

antigen immunoadsorbent

solid + solution

B

antibody bound to test tube

antigen

antigen-antibody complexes

radio-labelled secondary antibody

bound radioactive complex

FIGURE 7.3. **A:** Immunoradiometric assay (IRMA). **B:** Two-site IRMA.

can have a significant impact on the values obtained and the clinical decisions made.

Data Analysis

A wide variety of sophisticated techniques are available to analyze RIA-binding data. In general, data are transformed to linearize the sigmoidal dose-response relationship that is typical of most RIA and IRMA procedures. Initially this can consist of logarithmic transformation of standard curve dose and/or logit transformation of binding data. More sophisticated data reduction procedures such as four-parameter logistic regression (17) and weighted or un-weighted linear regression can also be used. It is beyond the scope of this chapter to review the multitude of data analysis techniques; there are several excellent reviews of this subject for the interested reader (17,26–28).

Although a detailed discussion of data analysis techniques will not be presented, there are several aspects of data interpretation that warrant mention. For example, many reproductive hormones are secreted in a pulsatile manner. Therefore, depending on the half-life of the hormone, serum levels may fluctuate widely depending on when the sample was obtained in relation to when the pulse of hormone secretion occurred. This is perhaps most evident with LH secretion where serum LH levels can vary over several orders of magnitude in a single day. Since ovarian steroids proges-terone (P) are stimulated by LH, the serum levels of these hormones may also vary significantly throughout the day; however, their longer half-lives and binding by serum pro-teins reduces the magnitude of the pulses observed.

Along these lines their clinician should never trust a single abnormal hormone value, as there are numerous factors that may contribute to the value obtained including hormone pulsatility, presence of serum-binding proteins, and even assay error. When an abnormal lab test (hormone value) is obtained, it is always advisable to either have the assay repeated or, better yet, get another sample and retest. Many if not most hormone assays only recognize "free" hormone. Remember that steroid hormones circulate in several forms including free, loosely bound (i.e., to albumin) and tightly bound (i.e., to specific binding proteins). De-pending on the extraction technique and antibody specific-ity, one or more of these forms may be detected in the assay. It is especially important to recognize this when con-sidering that certain conditions and treatments may offer the concentration of serum-binding proteins in the circula-tion as well as change the actual hormone concentration.

Finally, it is important to pay attention to the units of measure for various hormone assays. The busy clinician often memorizes "normal" values for the hormones they routinely deal with, without paying attention to the units associated with these values. This becomes especially impor-tant as scientific journals move to the International System of Units (SI) standard of reporting hormone values and as recombinant (pure) protein hormones become available. In the past, most protein hormone measurements were re-ported in international units (IU) due to the fact that pure preparations were not available for standards; thus, units based on mass (i.e., ng/mL) were not appropriate. As such, many if not most protein hormone units of measure are based on reference preparations that have been calibrated against international standards and thus are presented as IU. As recombinant proteins become available for hormone assay, there may be a shift toward expression of protein hormone values based on mass instead of relative units.

In summary, RIAs are frequently used in clinical medi-cine and research for their ability to measure minute quanti-ties of specific antigens in biologic fluids. The correct inter-pretation of clinical RIA data requires an awareness of the clinical picture and hormone physiology as well as an under-standing of the strengths and weaknesses of the assay being utilized. The primary disadvantage of RIAs is the generation and handling of radioactive waste products, which can add considerable time and expense to the laboratory using RIAs.

ENZYME-LINKED IMMUNOSORBENT ASSAY

Enzyme-linked immunosorbent assay (ELISA) is a general term referring to assay systems using enzymatically labeled antigen or antibody to determine the concentration of un-known substances. Most ELISA methods involve the bind-ing of either antigen or antibody (depending on which is the target of the assay) to a solid object, usually a microtiter plate. An indicator enzyme attached to the antibody or antigen is then allowed to bind to the target substance attached to the plate. A chromogenic substrate is added that will result in a color change in the presence of the target-enzyme complex. In 1971, Van Weemen and Schuurs (29) described an immunoassay for hCG in which an hCG-enzyme conjugate was designed and used to measure either antigen or antibody. In 1972, Engvall and Perlmann (30) used an immunoglobulin-enzyme conjugate to quantitate antibody concentrations. Substances of interest in reproduc-tive biology are increasingly being measured by ELISA methods due to convenience, speed, use of nonisotopic labels, sensitivity, and accuracy. The most prevalent ELISA methods in clinical use are the ovulation predictor kit and the pregnancy predictor kit, which detect the presence of urinary LH and hCG, respectively. Additionally, many of the cytokines and growth factors important to reproductive biology are currently measured using commercially available ELISA kits.

Theory

ELISAs are useful for measuring either antigen or antibody in samples. The most useful technique for measuring anti-gen concentrations is the two-antibody sandwich technique.

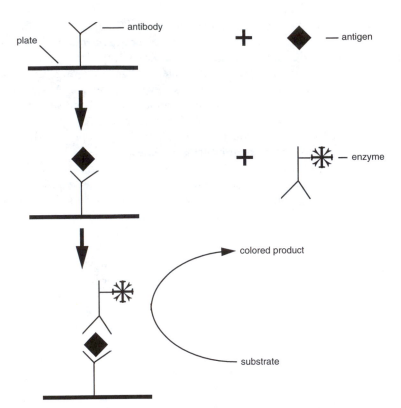

FIGURE 7.4. Two antibody sandwich technique for enzyme-linked immunosorbent assay (ELISA).

This technique requires two antibodies that bind to non-overlapping sites on the antigen. Briefly, the first antibody is bound to a solid phase. The antigen is then added and allowed to bind to the first antibody-forming an antigen-antibody complex bound to the solid phase. The unbound antigen is removed, and the labeled second antibody then binds to the antigen that is bound to the first antibody (Fig. 7.4). The second antibody is labeled with an enzyme that catalyzes the formation of a colored substrate that can be measured using a spectrophotometer. In this method, the more antigen in a sample, the more intense the color development. This method is rapid, easy, accurate, and very specific. The disadvantage of this method is the need for two antibodies that bind different sites of the antigen.

If two antibodies are not available for a particular antigen,

the next method of choice for quantitating antigens is competitive binding. In the case of antigen competition, the antibody is bound to the solid phase. A fixed amount of labeled antigen is added with the sample containing unlabeled antigen, allowing for a competition between the two for binding sites on the bound antibody (Fig. 7.5). The more unlabeled antigen in the sample, the less labeled antigen bound, and the less color development upon addition of substrate.

The simplest method of measuring antibodies in ELISA is the antibody capture assay. The antigen is bound to a solid phase, and antibody is allowed to bind. Antibody concentrations can be measured directly if the antibody is labeled, or indirectly by use of a second antibody such as antiimmunoglobulin (Fig. 7.6). This method can be used

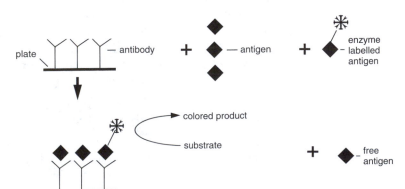

FIGURE 7.5. Quantitation of antigen by the competitive binding technique of ELISA.

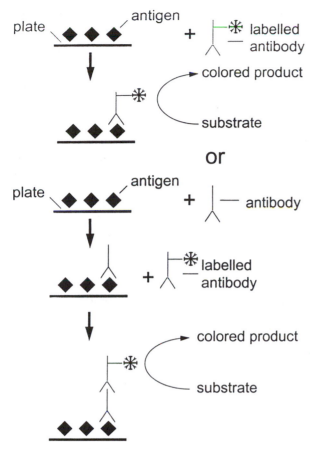

FIGURE 7.6. Antibody capture ELISA technique: a method for measuring antibodies with either a single labeled antibody or by the use of a labeled second antibody.

to titrate antibodies in a test solution and determine antibody titer.

ELISA systems rely on enzyme labels to convert a substrate into a colored product. The most commonly used enzymes in ELISA systems are alkaline phosphatase and horseradish peroxidase (31). The most widely used substrates for horseradish peroxidase in ELISA are ABTS [2,2'-azinobis(ethylbenzthiazoline-6-sulfonate)], OPD (O-phenylenediamine), and TMB (tetramethylbenzidine) in the presence of hydrogen peroxide. Of these, TMB is the preferred substrate due to low background, nonmutagenicity, and high absorbance values. The most commonly used alkaline phosphatase substrate is *p*-nitrophenyl phosphate. ELISAs using horseradish peroxidase labels are more sensitive by an order of magnitude in signal intensity than those using alkaline phosphatase.

For products having a weak signal causing difficulty in measurement due to high background, some ELISA systems use an amplification system whereby the enzyme acts on a substrate to create a product. This product is then converted by recycling enzymes, the amplifier, to another form and back again with a colored product being generated as the product of one of the side reactions of these recycling enzymes (Fig. 7.7).

The purity of the antibodies used in ELISA is very important. Antibodies can be polyclonal, monoclonal, or even recombinant. Polyclonal antibodies are usually generated in rabbits. Monoclonal antibodies are generated in mouse lymphocytes, which are immortalized by fusing with myeloma cells (32). Recombinant antibodies are basically generated through immortalization of the antibody genetic code (33).

In summary, ELISAs are excellent alternatives to tradi-

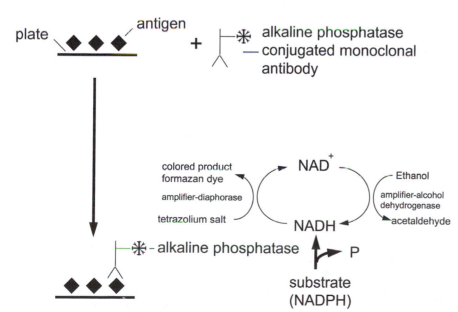

FIGURE 7.7. An example of ELISA amplification system.

tional RIAs for the measurement and detection of many hormones. The main advantages of ELISA systems are that they allow for quick results, are easy to perform, and have low limits of detection. Moreover, they do not involve use of radioactive materials, thereby eliminating the hazards and expense of dealing with reproductive waste. The primary disadvantages are the susceptibility to interference and the variation between assays.

RADIORECEPTOR ASSAYS

Although not as widely used as RIAs, ELISAs, or even bioassays, radioreceptor assays can sometimes be a useful tool for measuring various compounds in biologic fluids. Radioreceptor assays provide some of the benefits of RIAs such as relative ease of use and the ability to assay numerous samples, while also maintaining some of the usefulness of bioassays in that they identify the molecular forms of substances that are necessary to bind to receptors. Thus, while not measuring true biologic activity like a bioassay, radioreceptor assays may at least measure a more biologically relevant form of the compound than perhaps a traditional RIA or ELISA.

Theory

The theory behind radioreceptor assays is essentially the same as that for RIAs, except that a receptor preparation is used instead of monoclonal or polyclonal antibodies for detection of the hormones of interest. As with RIAs, the quality and specificity of a radioreceptor assay will be directly proportionate to the quality of the receptor preparation one uses. In addition, a large supply of a consistent and homogeneous preparation of receptors that maintain their ability to bind radioligand upon extended storage is also a critical feature in establishing a quality radioreceptor assay.

Among the reproductive hormones that have been successfully analyzed by radioreceptor assay are LH (34) and FSH (35,36), gonadotropin-releasing hormone (GnRH) and its analogues (37), and a variety of steroid hormones (38,39). Notably absent from this list are the inhibins, as the receptor for the inhibins has yet to be identified and purified.

Perhaps one of the most useful applications of radioreceptor assay technology has been in the detection of GnRH analogues in physiologic and pharmacokinetic studies (37). Since GnRH agonists and antagonists bind to the same GnRH receptor, development of a GnRH analogue radioreceptor assay obviates the need for preparation of specific antibodies for individual GnRH analogues. Once appropriate GnRH analogues have been identified with favorable pharmacokinetic or pharmacodynamic properties, then specific antisera can be generated to develop more sensitive and specific RIAs or ELISAs for the particular analogue of interest. However, the lack of discrimination of the receptor for the various GnRH analogues, which makes radioreceptor assays especially useful for screening a variety of chemically synthesized compounds, also limits its usefulness in screening naturally occurring hormones in the circulation. For example, the gonadotropins exist in a variety of different molecular forms with different glycosylation patterns that affect not only their pharmacokinetic clearance, but also their biologic activity. In many cases radioreceptor assays will not discriminate among the various molecular forms and thus may not yield a representative estimate of the biologically available hormone in the circulation under different physiologic circumstances.

Many of the factors one must take into consideration when designing an RIA also apply to the design of radioreceptor assays, including the preparation of a suitably labeled hormone that will bind to the receptor, and the development of a suitable detection system and a separation system for determining bound versus free hormone. Recognition of potential problems and pitfalls, such as interference by other substances in the fluid being tested, and issues of specificity and sensitivity of the assay are also paramount. Since radioreceptor assays are essentially identical to RIAs in that they are both competitive displacement type assays, the same data analysis procedures and standard curve algorithms that are appropriate for RIAs can be applied to most radioreceptor assay systems. In general, no special equipment is needed for radioreceptor assays above that which would already be available for RIA procedures.

In summary, radioreceptor assays can be a valuable tool in the hormone assay laboratory, especially in those instances where specific antibodies are not available for a certain compound or when one wishes to detect an entire class of compounds that interact with a biologic receptor. Radioreceptor assays have the advantage of detecting only molecular forms that interact with the receptor, and thus may give a clearer picture of biologically relevant substances than RIAs or ELISAs. However, since many hormones exist in multiple molecular forms that vary in biologic activity, but may maintain similar receptor-binding characteristics, radioreceptor assays may not provide as accurate an indication of biologic activity as would a true *in vitro* or *in vivo* bioassay. Nevertheless, in certain circumstances the radioreceptor assay may be the most appropriate tool for a specific hormone assay.

BIOASSAYS

In general, bioassays, whether *in vitro* or *in vivo*, represent the ultimate tool for measuring the physiologically relevant and biologically active forms of hormones and compounds in the circulation. Before the development of sophisticated immunoassay techniques, *in vitro* and *in vivo* bioassays were the mainstay of the hormone assay laboratory. During the early 1940s and 1950s, the establishment of bioassays for the ovarian steroids and gonadotropins provided some of the fundamental work for our understanding of the regulation of the hypothalamic pituitary gonadal axis. The pioneering work of Greep and Parlow in establishing the mouse uterine weight bioassay for estrogen (40), the testicular weight bioassay for determination of FSH (40), and the ovarian ascorbic acid depletion assay for LH (41) laid the groundwork for our understanding of the role of estrogen in a variety of reproductive tissues and the importance of LH and FSH in regulating ovarian and testicular function. With the development of the RIA by Berson and Yalow in the early 1960s, bioassays fell somewhat out of favor as most researchers focused on and utilized the newer techniques of RIA and eventually ELISA, which were much more sensitive and specific than the previous generation of *in vitro* bioassays. However, the utilization of the *in vitro* bioassay has enjoyed a resurgence in the last decade as we begin to understand and appreciate the variety of molecular forms of hormones that exist in the circulation and the widely differing biologic activities each of these forms may possess. Thus, the *in vitro* or *in vivo* bioassay often provides the ultimate analysis and perhaps confirmation of data obtained with other types of assays including immunoassays and receptor assays.

The Gonadotropin Bioassays

In reproductive medicine, *in vitro* bioassays for LH and FSH have proven especially useful since these gonadotropins exist in a variety of molecular isoforms, often with differing biologic activities. In recent years the development of sensitive and specific *in vitro* bioassays for LH and FSH has led to considerable advances in our understanding of the role of these gonadotropins in a variety of different species. One of the major advantages of the development of bioassays for the gonadotropins has been in their usefulness to detect biologically relevant LH and FSH in species for which we do not currently have suitable immunoassays available. A good example of this is the use of the LH bioassay to detect serum LH levels in nonhuman primates. The lack of a suitable immunoassay for detecting LH in cynomolgus and rhesus monkeys has hindered our progress toward understanding the regulation of gonadotropin secretion in primates. Use of a sensitive *in vitro* bioassay for LH in nonhuman primate studies has provided important insight, for example, into the regulation of the midcycle LH surge. The *in vitro* bioassay for LH is usually based on the production of testosterone by mouse Leydig cells. As initially developed by Van Damme et al. (42) in 1974, this assay is a relatively straightforward technique to quantitate circulating LH levels in biologic fluids. However, the original assay suffered from a relative lack of sensitivity, which limited its usefulness in many applications. Modifications by Ellinwood and Resko (43) in 1980 and Debertin and Pomerantz (44) in

1992 greatly enhanced the sensitivity of this bioassay such that circulating levels of biologically active LH can now be detected throughout the menstrual cycle in a variety of different species. Recent modification of that assay has improved the sensitivity over 30-fold, and circulating LH levels can now be detected in as little as 1 to 5 μL of serum.

An important consideration in the LH bioassay is the potential inhibitory effect of serum on Leydig cell testosterone production. Both Leydig cells (and Sertoli cells) are exquisitely sensitive to the effects of high concentrations of serum in the bioassays, and greater than 10 to 30 μL of serum will inhibit steroid production. Indeed, this interfering effect of serum has been a major obstacle in the development of sensitive bioassays for both LH and FSH.

The FSH bioassay is based on a similar principle to that of the LH bioassay, except that Sertoli cells instead of Leydig cells are used and estrogen production in the cell-conditioned media is analyzed instead of testosterone (45). The FSH bioassay has been more problematic in its development than the LH bioassay, in part due to the exquisite sensitivity of the FSH bioassay to the negative effects of serum in the assay. As with the LH bioassay, modifications to the standard procedure have improved the sensitivity of the FSH bioassay, and circulating FSH levels can be detected in 1 to 5 μL of serum or plasma. For a detailed description of the LH and FSH bioassays, the reader is referred to the appropriate references at the end of this chapter.

Inhibins

Another hormone that has benefited greatly from the development of the useful bioassay is the inhibin family. The isolation, purification, and sequencing of the ovarian inhibins was critically dependent on the development of a reliable and reproducible *in vitro* bioassay for inhibin that could be utilized throughout the purification process. However, the inhibin story dramatically points out both the strengths and weaknesses of the *in vitro* bioassay. Whereas the bioassay was essential for the identification and purification of the inhibins, development of a bioassay sensitive enough to detect inhibin throughout the menstrual cycle remains elusive. With the preparation of specific antibodies for inhibin, sensitive and specific assays were developed that have only recently revealed the complex nature of inhibin secretion throughout the menstrual cycle. Since the inhibins and activins exist in multiple molecular forms with different combinations of α and β subunits, and since the various forms are secreted by different cell types throughout the menstrual cycle, utilization of *in vitro* bioassays to measure these compounds may prove less useful than for the gonadotropins. Nevertheless, *in vitro* bioassays to assess the relative potency and physiologic importance of, for example, inhibin A versus inhibin B may provide additional insight into the physiologic regulation and function of this important class of hormones.

Data Analysis

The analysis of *in vitro* bioassays requires careful consideration. Since most *in vitro* bioassays do not discriminate among the various biologically active forms of a compound, it is important to recognize that the dose-response relationship obtained will represent an aggregate of all the biologically relevant compounds in the particular sample. A serum sample may contain a mixture of gonadotropins, for example, with different biologic activities. Moreover, there may be endogenous antagonists or inhibitors of biologic activity in the sample that would also contribute to the aggregate response detected. Thus, the major strength of the *in vitro* bioassay, that it measures biologically active substances, is also its major weakness, in that it lacks specificity for specific molecular isoforms of the hormone of interest. Perhaps one of the best examples of this is the pituitary cell bioassay for the detection of inhibin. Whereas the development of this assay was critical for the isolation and characterization of inhibin, this bioassay also detects a biologically similar but structurally distinct molecule called follistatin. Both the inhibins and follistatins inhibit FSH secretion and are detected in the pituitary cell bioassay, yet they are completely distinct hormones. During the course of these experiments another family of hormones was discovered, the activins, which have a biologic activity opposite that of the inhibins and follistatins. Thus, when using the pituitary cell bioassay one must remember that the observed biologic response is an aggregate of the inhibitory effects of inhibin and follistatin on FSH and the stimulatory effects of activins, which might also be present in the sample.

Another important feature to consider when analyzing bioassay data is that many bioassays are biphasic in their response to the appropriate ligand. Rather than a typical sigmoid curve, which is typical of radioreceptor and RIAs, in which the top end of the dose-response curve flattens out at saturation of the antibody or receptor, many bioassays exhibit a bell-shaped curve in which increasing the concen-

tration of ligand actually inhibits the biologic response (Fig. 7.8). This is often due to desensitization or downregulation of the cellular response. As such, when analyzing unknowns in an *in vitro* bioassay, one must utilize at minimum two or preferably three or more different concentrations of the unknown sample to determine where on the dose-response curve the individual sample lies. In other words, serial dilution of unknown samples when corrected for volume must yield similar results.

Numerous articles have been written on the appropriate analysis of *in vitro* bioassay data (46–48). The individual analysis chosen depends at least in part on the nature of the bioassay and its purpose. That is, is the bioassay being used to quantitate hormone levels in a particular sample or being used as a screening procedure to identify a particular biologic activity during a purification procedure? Different analytic methods may be appropriate in each of these circumstances. In general, however, it is sufficient to transform the data to obtain a linear dose-response relationship (up to some maximum) and then simply perform a straightforward weighted or unweighted linear regression on the values to obtain the equation for the regression line to be used for determining the unknown sample concentrations. With respect to the gonadotropin bioassays, this is often accomplished by plotting the log of the standard concentration versus the absolute value or the log of the steroid concentration. The goal in this situation is to obtain a linear regression with the best fit. Other more sophisticated data analysis procedures are also available (49).

In summary, *in vitro* bioassays provide the ultimate analysis of biologically important compounds in reproductive medicine. Since *in vitro* bioassays only measure the biologically relevant forms of the compounds, they are often the most applicable to understanding the physiology and biochemistry of reproductive hormones. However, since bioassays often do not measure individual molecular forms, and detect the aggregate of all biologically relevant species in a

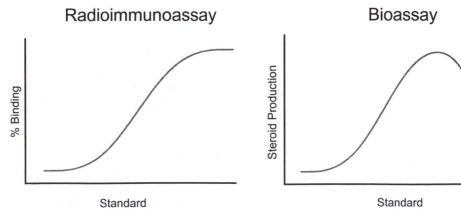

FIGURE 7.8. Typical dose-response curve for radioimmunoassays and the bell-shaped curve exhibited by many bioassays.

sample, the interpretation of *in vitro* bioassays can be difficult. Ultimately, it is often the combination of a variety of assay systems including *in vitro* bioassays and immunoassays that is used to fully understand the physiology and biochemistry of a particular hormone. Indeed, comparing the biologic to immunologic ratios of a variety of hormones has provided interesting insights into changes in molecular isoforms of secreted hormones that occur across the menstrual cycle and in various reproductive disorders.

10 KEY POINTS

1. Radioimmunoassay is described as the competitive inhibition by unlabeled antigen of binding of radiolabeled antigen to its antibody.

2. Radioimmunoassay consists of three basic steps: incubation, separation of bound complexes from free components, and measurement of radioactivity.

3. Immunoradiometric assay (IRMA) and two-site IRMA are radioassays that use radiolabeled antibodies.

4. Enzyme-linked immunosorbent assay (ELISA) refers to assay systems that use enzymatically labeled antigen or antibody to determine concentrations of antigens or antibodies in samples.

5. The most widely used ELISA techniques are the two-antibody sandwich, competitive binding, and antibody capture.

6. Radioreceptor assays identify the molecular forms of substances that are necessary to bind receptors.

7. Radioreceptor assays follow essentially the same principles as RIA, except that a receptor preparation that will bind the substance of interest is used instead of an antibody.

8. Bioassays measure physiologically relevant and biologically active forms of substances in circulation.

9. Bioassays can be useful for substances existing in multiple molecular forms, which often differ in biologic activity.

10. In vitro bioassays have been particularly useful for the gonadotropins especially in nonhuman primates and the inhibin family.

REFERENCES

1. Yalow RS, Berson SA. Assay of plasma insulin in human subjects by immunological methods. *Nature* 1959;184:1648–1649.
2. Yalow RS, Berson SA. Immunoassay of endogenous plasma insulin in man. *J Clin Invest* 1960;38:1157–1175.
3. Yalow RS, Berson SA. Remembrance project: origins of RIA. *Endocrinology* 1991;129:1694–1695.
4. Ekins RP. The estimation of thyroxine in human plasma by an electrophoretic technique. *Clin Chim Acta* 1960;5:453–459.
5. Paul WT, Odell WD. Radiation of the immunological and biological activities of human chorionic gonadotropin. *Nature* 1964;203:979–980.
6. Midgley AR Jr. Radioimmunoassay: a method for human chorionic gonadotropin and human luteinizing hormone. *Endocrinology* 1966;79:10–18.
7. Beck P, Parker ML, Daughaday WH. Radioimmunologic measurement of human placental lactogen in plasma by a doubling antibody method during normal and diabetic pregnancies. *J Clin Endocrinol* 1965;25:1457–1462.
8. Grumbach MM, Kaplan SL. On the placental origin and purification of chorionic "growth hormone-prolactin" and its immunoassay in pregnancy. *Trans NY Acad Sci* 1965;27:167–188.
9. Niswender GD, Chen CL, Midgley AR Jr, et al. Radioimmunoassay for rat prolactin. *Proc Soc Exp Bio Med* 1969;130:793–797.
10. Monroe SE, Parlow AF, Midgley AR Jr. Radioimmunoassay for rat luteinizing hormone. *Endocrinology* 1968;83:1004–1012.
11. Niswender GD, Reichert LE Jr, Midgley AR Jr, et al. Radioimmunoassay for bovine and ovine luteinizing hormone. *Endocrinology* 1969;84:1166–1173.
12. Midgley AR. Radioimmunoassay for human follicle-stimulating hormone. *J Clin Endocrinol Metab* 1967;27:295–299.
13. Midgley AR Jr, Niswender GD, Ram JS. Hapten-radioimmunoassay: a general procedure for the estimation of steroidal and other haptenic substances. *Steroids* 1969;13:731–737.
14. Dray F, Maron E, Tiloson SA, et al. Immunochemical detection of prostaglandins with prostaglandin-coated bacteriophage T4 and by radioimmunoassay. *Anal Biochem* 1972;50:399–408.
15. Cerini JC, Cain MD, Chamley WA, et al. Luteolysis in the ewe: a study using radioimmunoassay for prostaglandin F. *J Reprod Fertil* 1973;32:326–327.
16. Parker CW. *Radioimmunoassay of biologically active compounds.* Englewood Cliffs, NJ: Prentice-Hall, 1976.
17. Chard T. An introduction to radioimmunoassay and related techniques. In: Van Der Vliet PC, ed. *Laboratory techniques in biochemistry and molecular biology,* 5th ed. The Netherlands: Elsevier Science BV, 1995.
18. Herbert V, Lau KS, Gottlieb CW, et al. Coated charcoal immunoassay of insulin. *J Clin Endocrinol* 1965;25:1375–1384.
19. Berson SA, Yalow RS. Measurement of hormones—radioimmunoassay. In: *Peptide hormones.* New York: American Elsevier 1973:84–135.
20. Moss AJ, Dalrymple GV, Boyd CM, eds. *Practical radioimmunoassay.* St. Louis: CV Mosby, 1976.
21. Miles LE, Hales CN. Labeled antibodies and immunological assay systems. *Nature* 1968;219:186–189.
22. Miles LE. Immunoradiometric assay (IRMA) and two-site IRMA systems (assay of soluble antigens using labeled antibodies). In: Abraham GE, ed. *Handbook of radioimmunoassay.* New York: Marcel Dekker, 1977:131–177.
23. Wheeler MJ, D'Souza A, Horn AN. Evaluation of test kits for gonadotropins. *Lancet* 1989;2:616–617.
24. Ramey JW, Seltman HJ, Toner JP. Superior analytic characteristics of an immunometric assay for gonadotropins also provides useful clinical prediction of in vitro fertilization outcomes. *Fertil Steril* 1996;65:661–663.
25. Toner JP, Philput CB, Jones GS, et al. Basal follicle-stimulating hormone level is a better predictor of in vitro fertilization performances than age. *Fertil Steril* 1991;55:784–791.
26. Hunter OB Jr, ed. *Radioassay: clinical concepts.* Stokie, IL: Searle, 1974.
27. Rodbard D. Statistical quality control and routine data processing for radioimmunoassays and immunoradiometric assays. *Clin Chem* 1974;20:1255–1270.
28. Rodbard D. Mathematics and statistics of ligand assays: an illustrated guide. In: Langan J, Clapp JJ, eds. *Ligand assay: analysis of international developments on isotopic and nonisotopic immunoassay.* New York: Masson, 1981:45–101.
29. Van Weemen BK, Schuurs AHWM. Immunoassay using antigen-enzyme conjugates. *FEBS Lett* 1971;15:232–236.

30. Engvall E, Perlmann P. Enzyme-linked immunosorbent assay, ELISA III. Quantitation of specific antibodies by enzyme-labeled anti-immunoglobulin in antigen coated tubes. *J Immunol* 1972; 109:129–135.

31. Gosling JP, Basso LV, eds. *Immunoassay: laboratory analysis and clinical applications.* Newton, MA: Butterworth-Heineman, 1994.

32. Wild D, Davies C. Components. In: Wild D, ed. *The immunoassay handbook.* New York: Stockton Press, 1994, 49–82.

33. Chiswell D, McCafferty J. Phage antibodies. Will new coliclonal antibodies replace monoclonal antibodies? *Trends Biotechnol* 1991;10:80–84.

34. Booher CB, Prahalada S, Hendrickx AG. Use of a radioreceptorassay (RRA) for human luteinizing hormone/chorionic gonadotropin (hLH/CG) for detection of early pregnancy and estimation of time of ovulation in macaques. *Am J Primatol* 1983;4: 45–53.

35. Reichert LE Jr, Bhalla VK. A comparison of the properties of FSH from several species as determined by a rat testis tubule receptor assay. *Gen Comp Endocrinol* 1974;23(1):111–117.

36. Reichert LE Jr, Bhalla VK. Development of a radioligand tissue receptor assay for human follicle-stimulating hormone. *Endocrinology* 1974;94(2):483–491.

37. Danforth DR, Gordon K, Leal JA, et al. Extended presence of antide (NAL-LYS GnRH antagonist) in circulation: prolonged duration of gonadotropin inhibition may derive from antide binding to serum proteins. *J Clin Endocrinol Metab* 1990;70(2): 554–556.

38. Diczfalusy E, ed. Steroid assay by protein binding. *Acta Endocrinol Suppl* 1970.

39. Odell WD, Daughaday WH, eds. *Principles of competitive protein binding assays.* Philadelphia: JB Lippincott, 1971.

40. Greep RO, VanDyke HB, Chow BF. Gonadotropins of the swine pituitary. I. Various biological effects of purified thylakentrain (FSH) and pure metakentrin (ICSH). *Endocrinology* 1942;30: 635–649.

41. Parlow AF. In: Albert A, ed. *Human pituitary gonadotropins.* Springfield, IL: Charles C Thomas, 1961:300.

42. Van Damme MP, Robertson DM, Diczfalusy E. An improved in vitro bioassay method for measuring luteinizing hormone (LH) activity using mouse Leydig cell preparations. *Acta Endocrinol* 1974;77:655–671.

43. Ellinwood WE, Resko JA. Sex differences in biologically active and immunoreactive gonadotropins in the fetal circulation of rhesus monkeys. *Endocrinology* 1980;107:902–907.

44. Debertin WJ, Pomerantz DK. Improved sensitivity of the mouse interstitial cell testosterone assay with the addition of forskolin. *Can J Physiol Pharmacol* 1992;70:866–871.

45. Padmanabhan V, Chappel SC, Beitins IZ. An improved in vitro bioassay for follicle-stimulating hormone (FSH): suitable for measurement of FSH in unextracted human serum. *Endocrinology* 1987;121(3):1089–1098.

46. Finney DJ. *Statistical method in biological assay,* 2nd edition. London: Griffin, 1964.

47. Borth R, Diczfalusy E, Heinricks HD. Fundamentals of the statistical analysis of biological assays. *Arch Gynaekol* 1957;188: 497.

48. Sokal RR, Rohlf FJ. *Biometry,* 2nd ed. San Francisco: WH Freeman, 1981.

49. DeLean A, Munson PJ, Rodbard D. Simultaneous analysis of families of sigmoidal curves: application to bioassay, radioligand assay, and physiological dose-response curves. *Am J Physiol* 1978; 235(2):E97–E102.

8

PRINCIPLES OF LABOR AND DELIVERY ANALGESIA AND ANESTHESIA

JOHN S. McDONALD

This chapter discusses the basic principles of anesthesia as they pertain to labor and delivery. First, the general anesthetic techniques and agents are discussed in light of their utilization in one of several areas of labor and delivery care. Then regional anesthesia, local anesthesia, and systemic analgesia methods are discussed. In each instance, the current application of anesthesia is described as it is used to make both labor and delivery more pleasant and actually safer for both the mother and the newborn. The associated complications are also discussed.

This chapter provides a concise, abbreviated, up-to-date synthesis of labor and delivery anesthesia that will inform the practitioner of the serious considerations regarding the use of anesthetics in obstetrics. This information can assist the obstetrician in working with the anesthesiologist, who provides comfort and safety to the mother during various painful stages of labor and delivery, and an optimal environment for the newborn baby to safely enter the world.

GENERAL ANESTHESIA

Many techniques have been used for administration of inhalation analgesia (Table 8.1). Nitrous oxide can be administered either continuously or intermittently. Analgesia should be initiated with 35% nitrous oxide and 65% oxygen by face mask. The intermittent administration of nitrous oxide is more complicated. Nitrous oxide in oxygen is begun 20 to 30 seconds before the predicted time of the onset of each subsequent contraction. Life-threatening events for which general anesthesia may be required, such as severe fetal distress, cord prolapse, and shoulder dystocia, occur unpredictably. Thus, of fundamental importance is the maintenance of uteroplacental perfusion, incorporating both acute maternal intravascular volume expansion and avoidance of aortocaval compression, treatment with antacids to alter the pH of the mother's gastric contents to reduce the hazards of aspiration, and appropriate monitoring of the parturient and her fetus (1).

Modern general obstetric anesthesia is a combined technique utilizing an intravenous induction agent, a muscle relaxant, various mixtures of nitrous oxide and oxygen, endotracheal intubation, and prolonged maintenance with either narcotics or inhalation agents. Variations of this technique can be used to provide general anesthesia for cesarean section and difficult vaginal delivery, or to produce uterine relaxation for various obstetric maneuvers. This technique is reserved for situations where local, regional, or low-dose ketamine analgesia are not appropriate for vaginal delivery including fetal distress, where rapid vaginal delivery is necessary, in the case of a severely mentally retarded or extremely uncooperative patient who might injure herself or her fetus during delivery, and during situations requiring uterine relaxation, including intrauterine exploration, manual removal of a retained placenta, vaginal delivery of a second twin, delivery of an after-coming breech, and replacement of the inverted uterus (2).

Sodium thiopental (Pentothal) is the intravenous induction agent most frequently used in the United States (3). Sodium thiopental rapidly crosses the placenta, and fetal concentrations reach their peak between 2 and 4 minutes after maternal intravenous injection (3). Because it decreases uterine contractility, it is thought that uterine blood flow may be improved and placental intervillous perfusion increased by thiopental, as long as the maternal blood pressure is maintained (4). Thus, if used in appropriate doses, barbiturates are unlikely to compromise the fetus when the patient is otherwise healthy (5). Ketamine, a phencyclidine derivative, produces excellent analgesia, amnesia, and anesthesia by disassociation of the afferent pathways from cortical perception. Ketamine causes a release of catecholamines, which stimulate the cardiovascular system to increase heart rate, systemic and pulmonary vascular pressure, and cardiac output, and may therefore be useful in situations of maternal hypotension or hemorrhage (1). In the absence of further evidence, ketamine, as an induction agent, should be avoided throughout pregnancy, except when its advantages, such as blood pressure support, in the rare case of porphyria, or for a barbiturate allergy, outweigh the potential disadvantages (6).

Nitrous oxide also rapidly crosses the placenta. The fetal/maternal concentration ratio is 0.8 after just 3 minutes, and the umbilical artery/vein concentration ratio is almost 0.9 after 15 minutes of inhalation (7). Although nitrous

TABLE 8.1. ANESTHETIC AGENT SOLUBILITY COEFFICIENTS

Agent	MW	Solubility Coefficient Blood/Gas	% Inhaled
Nitrous oxide	44	0.47	50.00
Trichloroethylene	131	9.20	0.35 to 0.50
Methoxyflurane	165	13.00	0.35
Halothane	197	2.54	0.75
Isoflurane	185	1.38	0.50
Enflurane	185	1.90	0.50
Cyclopropane	42	0.42	5.00
Diethyl ether	74	12.10	1.00
Desflurane	168	0.42	3.00
Sevoflurane	200	0.68	0.75

MW, molecular weight.

oxide has little effect on uterine contractility (8), it is recommended to avoid nitrous oxide concentrations of greater than 50% (9). Halothane, enflurane, and isoflurane are considered to be complete analgesics because they provide amnesia, analgesia, and muscle relaxation. These agents can produce hypotension by lowering cardiac output via direct depression of the myocardium, or by vasodilation (10), and thus can lead to reduced placental blood flow. The new agents are desflurane and sevoflurane. Sevoflurane is another fluoronated ether with blood solubility so low as to rival nitrous oxide. Its immediate appeal as an induction agent is further enhanced by the fact that it does not have an offensive odor. Desflurane is also a fluoronated ether and is very similar to isoflurane, which currently is very popular. Its MAC is estimated to be 5.7%, compared to 1.7% for sevoflurane. Although increased blood loss due to anesthetic-induced uterine atony may occur at delivery (11), the use of oxytocin and rapid ventilation to blow off the anesthetic agent will allow normal uterine contractions and hemostasis to be achieved (12). The immediate uterine relaxation produced by these agents is an advantage in various intrapartum crises, such as shoulder dystocia, intrauterine manipulation, and vaginal delivery of breech or second twin, and in pelvic surgery during early pregnancy (10,13,14).

Since its first use in clinical anesthesia, the muscle relaxant succinylcholine has been the drug of choice in situations in which it is crucial to rapidly secure the airway, such as patients with a full stomach who are at high risk of regurgitation during induction of anesthesia (15,16). Whenever succinylcholine is used for tracheal intubation in the pregnant patient, cricoid pressure should be applied to prevent regurgitation (Fig. 8.1) (10). Succinylcholine has not been found in fetal umbilical cord blood unless the mother has received a bolus of 300 mg or more. Therefore, with the use of the usual clinical doses, succinylcholine will not cross the placental barrier in sufficient amounts to affect the Apgar score (17). Because of their high degree of ionization at a physiologic pH, all of the currently used muscle relaxants have insufficient placental transfer to cause any clinical effects in the neonate (18).

Aspiration associated with general anesthesia is an ever-present danger with all techniques. Every pregnant woman beyond the first trimester should be considered to have a full stomach. Therefore, when possible, these patients should have had no oral intake for at least 8 hours before general anesthesia (19). The most common cause of maternal death related to general anesthesia is aspiration pneumonia (20,21). It has been observed that raising the pH of the gastric contents reduces complications of aspiration (22–25). It has also been hypothesized that a volume of gastric contents of 25 mL or greater is a second etiology of aspiration pneumonia (23,26). These two etiologies constitute reasons for the commonplace usage of antacids, H_2-receptor blockers, and/or gastrointestinal tract stimulants as premedication for general obstetric anesthesia.

Once the gravid patient has been placed on the operating table, all monitoring devices should be applied. Similarly, the patient should have left lateral tilt or uterine displacement. Aortocaval compression has been observed to decrease uteroplacental perfusion through direct compression of the aorta, which reduces blood flow to the uterine arteries, and by decreased cardiac output secondary to impedance of venous return (27). Studies have confirmed that neonatal Apgar scores were improved when women were placed in left lateral tilt position during cesarean section rather than maintained in the supine position (28,29). Therefore, displacement of the uterus from the inferior vena cava and aorta is of prime importance in the conduct of both general and regional obstetric anesthesia (30).

Preoxygenation of the pregnant patient before induction of general anesthesia is very important. Oxygen consumption is increased and functional residual capacity is decreased during pregnancy, resulting in the susceptibility of the gravid patient to hypoxia during periods of induced apnea (31). Archer and Marx (32) determined arterial blood gas changes during 60 seconds of apnea in gravid and nongravid women undergoing surgery. Sellick (33) is credited with first describing the use of cricoid pressure in preventing regurgitation of stomach contents into the lungs during induction of general anesthesia. With the patient in slight

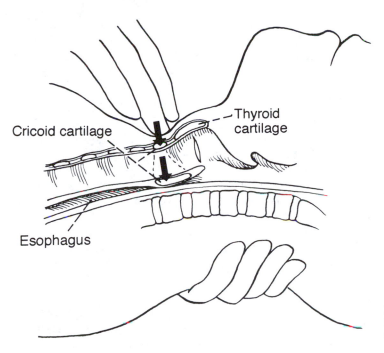

Cricoid cartilage

Thyroid cartilage

Esophagus

FIGURE 8.1. Regurgitation during induction is prevented by pressing the croicoid cartilage posteriorly against the sixth cervical vertebrae.

reverse Trendelenburg position during preoxygenation, the assistant identifies the thyroid cartilage prominence and gently places his/her thumb and second finger on either side of the cricoid cartilage, which is the first tracheal cartilage located one finger's width below this anatomic landmark. Cricoid pressure is continued until intubation is accomplished, the endotracheal tube cuff has been inflated, and tube placement has been verified by auscultation.

Thiopental (3 to 4 mg/kg) and ketamine (1 mg/kg) are the most commonly used agents for induction of general anesthesia. Thiopental crosses the placenta rapidly (3), making it impossible for the fetus not to be exposed to the drug before delivery. The peak concentration of thiopental is achieved in umbilical venous blood within 1 minute and in umbilical arterial blood in 2 to 3 minutes (34). Kosaka et al. (3) observed that 60% of neonatal Apgar scores were 7 or greater when a thiopental dose of 8 mg/kg was used for induction. Other investigators have demonstrated that thiopental in 4-mg/kg doses has no contribution to low Apgar scores (30,35). Similarly, Petrikovsky et al. (36) demonstrated that intravenous barbiturates and muscle relaxants administered during anesthesia induction were not associated with fetal heart rate changes. However, Jouppila et al. (37) demonstrated that thiopental, in conjunction with succinylcholine, lowered uterine blood flow by 35% during induction.

A new induction agent, propofol, is now becoming very popular as an intravenous anesthetic in many ambulatory settings because of its rapid central nervous system (CNS) depression/recovery cycle. Unconsciousness now can occur as rapidly as 30 to 60 seconds, yet return to consciousness can be as rapid as 5 to 15 minutes (38). The latter is due largely to an extremely fast blood–brain half-life of less than 3 minutes, a quick vascular distribution half-life of less than 4 minutes, and quick biotransformation and clearance rates. Its metabolism is hepatic and other extrahepatic sites (38). Etomidate, another induction agent with excellent characteristics suited for obstetrics, is a water-soluble agent that has minimal cardiovascular depression associated with its use. Its pharmacodynamic profile is such that it affects almost immediate (1-minute) unconsciousness. Its greatest potential contribution could be in those emerging hypovolemic situations that threaten the lives of both the mother and fetus, such as placenta previa, abruptio placenta, and uterine rupture. However, from the negative standpoint, the use in obstetrics most likely will come only after the concern about its potential suppression of the adrenals is ruled out (39).

Prior to intubation, intravenous administration of a muscle relaxant, such as succinylcholine (80 to 100 mg), offers optimal conditions to allow rapid endotracheal intubation. Although pregnancy reduces plasma cholinesterase activity (40), metabolization of a moderate succinylcholine dose is not usually prolonged (41). Because serum cholinesterase activity of a specific obstetric patient is generally unknown, return of the neuromuscular function should be monitored before the administration of another muscle relaxant (42). Maintenance of the muscle relaxation throughout a cesarean section operation is generally assured by administration of nondepolarizing muscle relaxants that are easily reversible and/or have a short duration of action (16). No neonatal adverse effects, as determined by Apgar scores, umbilical cord blood gases, or neonatal neurobehavioral scores, have been observed with moderate doses of these drugs (23,34).

The technique of tracheal intubation of the obstetric patient is no different from that for any other patient requiring general anesthesia. The use of a laryngoscope with either a Miller or MacIntosh blade is mandatory. These blades allow the direct observation of the endotracheal tube while it passes through the vocal cords. Pregnancy may present some unique problems for performing endotracheal intubation. Large and pendulous breasts can press against the laryngoscope handle, and mucosal edema of the larynx in the preeclamptic patient is also a challenge (43). Similarly, pulse oximetry has permitted continuous noninvasive analysis of arterial hemoglobin oxygen saturation, providing instantaneous warning of hypoxemia. This technology alerts the anesthesiologist when desaturation is occurring during repeated attempts at intubation.

The initial maneuver in the failed intubation drill is dependent on the obstetric indication for cesarean section. If the operation is elective, the patient can be awakened and a regional anesthetic performed. If a regional anesthetic is not possible, an awake blind oral or nasal intubation can be considered. Another alternative is bronchofiberscope-directed tracheal intubation (23,34,44,45). However, if the obstetrical indication for cesarean section is serious fetal distress, the next maneuver is dependent on the skill and experience of the anesthesiologist and his or her ability to easily ventilate the patient with bag and mask. If the patient is easily ventilated with a mask, emergency anesthesia may be maintained with nitrous oxide, oxygen, and halothane throughout the cesarean section. This technique of mask anesthesia with continuous cricoid pressure is not condoned except when both the obstetrician and the anesthesiologist are in full agreement that only this maneuver can save the life of the baby without serious jeopardy to the mother. Although mask anesthesia can often be administered successfully, the continuation of cricoid pressure along with adequate patient paralysis is extremely important in reducing the maternal risk of aspiration. For the hypertensive obstetrical patient, blood pressure must be well controlled before induction and laryngoscopy. The goal before intubation, in such a patient, is to decrease the diastolic blood pressure to 90 to 100 mm Hg. Various antihypertensive drugs have been used, such as hydralazine by intravenous bolus, or continuous infusions of trimethaphan, nitroprusside, nitroglycerin, or labetalol, to acutely decrease blood pressure and also to ablate the hypertensive response to endotracheal intubation (27). Trimethaphan has likewise been employed for this purpose. This drug has a high molecular weight (597 daltons), which somewhat limits its placental transmission. It also releases histamine and decreases cardiac output (46). Furthermore, prolonged respiratory paralysis may occur synergistically with succinyl-

choline administration (47). Trimethaphan acts more rapidly than hydralazine and reduces systemic arterial blood pressure without significantly affecting maternal cerebral blood flow (48). Sodium nitroprusside has also been employed to manage this condition. This agent has a very rapid onset of action and does not increase cerebral blood flow.

On occasion, however, preeclamptic patients may become significantly hypotensive, resulting in reduction of uteroplacental blood flow with consequent fetal distress (49). Labetalol is a nonselective β-adrenergic and selective α_1-adrenergic blocking agent with intrinsic β_2-agonist activity. In preeclampsia, labetalol lowers the blood pressure rapidly causing tachycardia, or increasing cerebrospinal fluid (CSF) pressure, but has only a moderate antihypertensive effect that is, nonetheless, sufficient to protect the maternal CNS from dangerously high blood pressure during intubation (50).

Maternal awareness under general anesthesia during cesarean section is a regrettable but sometimes necessary or unavoidable complication. In situations in which there is fetal compromise and urgency for delivery, it may be necessary to communicate frankly with the mother and make her aware that to save the baby's life she may have to undergo uncomfortable situations for a hastily performed emergency abdominal delivery. For example, it may be necessary not to use nitrous oxide so as to provide 100% oxygen concentration. All efforts should be undertaken to reduce the incidence of this phenomenon of maternal awareness.

There is virtually no place in modern obstetrics for inhalation anesthesia during abnormal vaginal delivery. Inhalation anesthesia today is usually part of the general anesthetic regimen that includes intravenous anesthetic induction agents, muscle relaxants, and endotracheal intubation. Patients with preterm labor are often delivered abdominally because of the higher incidence of breech presentations and multiple gestations. The preterm gestation will most like have received tocolysis with a β-adrenergic agent such as ritodrine hydrochloride. This produces uterine relaxation by increasing intracellular $3',5'$-cyclic adenosine monophosphate (cAMP), which can cause increased cardiac irritability. The perinatal team (pediatrician, obstetrician, and anesthesiologist) should be prepared to treat any neonatal anesthetic or drug exposure that might occur with maternal general anesthesia. The breech fetus presents three potential problems for obstetricians and anesthesiologists: (a) prematurity, (b) possible traumatic delivery, and (c) coexistent maternal illness or fetal anomaly. A major concern is the manner in which anesthesia may impact the delivery process. Umbilical cord prolapse occurs in 5% to 7% of all breech presentations (51). For this reason, the anesthesia team must be informed when a patient with a breech presentation is in labor, so that the team members may be prepared to administer general anesthesia should an emergency operation be required. Preparation should include a preanesthetic interview, assessment of the patient's risk status for anesthesia, and a discussion with the patient of the types of anesthesia and their complications. Communication is essential. Fetal distress of the breech presentation mandates rapid delivery, but not at the expense of maternal safety. Often, general anesthesia is most expedient; however, no single anesthetic technique is suitable for every patient. Both teams must be flexible and willing to alter the obstetric and anesthetic plans at a moment's notice.

There is no single "ideal" anesthetic method for cesarean section. The choice depends on the indications for delivery, the degree of urgency, maternal preference, and the experience and skill of the anesthesiologist. A successful anesthetic requires expert technical skills and a thorough understanding of maternal and fetal physiology and pharmacology. Because general anesthesia can be induced quickly, and support of the maternal cardiovascular system can be readily accomplished, this technique may be the method of choice for emergent situations such as fetal distress and maternal hemorrhage. However, the choice is less obvious for more common and less urgent indications, such as dystocia, repeat cesarean section, and breech presentation.

A brief discourse on the use of general anesthesia for cesarean section follows. Emergency cesarean sections are more likely to result in maternal mortality. Therefore, it would seem prudent for anesthetists to evaluate all patients admitted to the labor unit, regardless of the anticipated future need for anesthesia services. As with elective cesarean section, the choice of anesthesia for emergent cesarean section depends on the reason for the operation, the degree of urgency, the desires of the patient, and the judgment of the anesthesiologist. There is no single ideal method of anesthesia for cesarean section. The anesthesiologist must choose the method deemed safest and most comfortable for the mother, least depressant of the neonate, and conducive to optimal working conditions for the obstetrician (8).

General anesthesia has the theoretical advantages of a more rapid induction, less hypotension and cardiovascular instability, and better control of the airway and ventilation. Properly conducted general anesthesia for cesarean section provides protection for both fetus and mother. Fetal protective benefits include maintenance of normal uterine blood flow, increased fetal oxygenation, and limited anesthetic depression. Adequacy of oxygenation-ventilation, hemodynamic stability, muscle relaxation, and amnesia offer maternal protection (52). Although general anesthesia possesses these theoretical advantages, expeditious delivery is necessary to minimize neonatal depression. It is important for obstetricians, before they find themselves in emergency situations, to understand the capabilities and limitations of the available anesthesia personnel and, whenever possible, endeavor to use those most experienced and knowledgeable in obstetric anesthesia (53).

COMPLICATIONS OF GENERAL ANESTHESIA

Airway Obstruction

Difficult intubation scenarios must be protected against loss of airway by preoxygenation with 100% oxygen from a mask for several minutes, and by several deep breaths also with 100% oxygen. The lungs are thereby filled with oxygen because of the washout of nitrogen that usually is in an 80% ratio during air breathing. This provides a reservoir for a brief time when oxygen saturation can still be maintained. During general anesthesia induction, the loss of consciousness results very soon after the loss of control of the airway. Normally it is maintained by the tone of those same voluntary striated muscles that are rendered dysfunctional with induction. An obstructed airway can be rescued by extension of the head, by forcing the mandible forward, and by pulling the tongue out. Airway obstruction during induction sends a chill of terror through the anesthesiologist because it is appreciated that this complication is one of the greatest threats to the mother's life. Airway compromise must be approached with an aggressive and successful plan for reestablishment of the airway. During the time the anesthesiologist attempts to reestablish the airway with a mask to get positive oxygen pressure into the patient, an assistant helps by placing his or her fingers behind the mandible and raising it, pulling forward as forcibly as possible to get the tongue forward enough so to obtain an adequate airway. Mendelson described the classic aspiration syndrome associated with induction of anesthesia in the late 1940s. Despite many studies since, the incidence of nonfatal Mendelson's syndrome is essentially unknown even today. The stat cesarean because of fetal jeopardy in a heavy patient with unknown airway anatomy has been and still is one of the greatest health hazards in obstetric anesthesiology. The inability to determine which patients may be difficult to intubate means that any obstetric patient may be exposed to the hazard of acid aspiration syndrome or to asphyxia because endotracheal tube placement may not have occurred in a reasonable time. The primary anatomic causes of difficult intubation are

1. receding jaw
2. small mouth
3. high arched palate
4. prominent frontal incisors
5. short and thick neck
6. large tongue
7. large tonsils or other mass in the throat
8. reduced mobility of the mandible
9. reduced mobility of the cervical spine

Medical causes can include acromegaly, myxedema, goiter, Pierre Robin syndrome, Treacher Collins syndrome, and morbid obesity associated with pregnancy (54). Among the many complications of management of a difficult airway are soft tissue lacerations, swelling, and airway problems

TABLE 8.2. DIFFICULT INTUBATION SCENARIOS

Awake intubation
  Blind—nasal
  Direct laryngoscopy
    Nasal intubation
    Oral intubation
Fiberoptic endoscopy
Rigid optical stylet
Rigid bronchoscopy
Anterior commissure laryngoscopy
Retrograde translaryngeal intubation
Translaryngeal jet ventilation
Cricothyroidotomy
Tracheostomy
Mask ventilation

From Gupta B, McDonald JS. The difficult airway. *Hosp Physician* 1986;65:69–71,74, with permission.

including asphyxia, dislodged and broken teeth, atelectasis, and gastric content aspiration with pulmonary aspiration pneunomitis. Additional problems can include temporo-mandibular joint dislocation, C-spine injury subluxation, and hypoxia, resulting in brain damage, cardiac arrest, or even death.

Management of difficult intubation is not easy and perhaps the best management includes careful analysis at the time the patient enters the labor and delivery suite (Table 8.2). This is when the anesthesiologist can take the time to evaluate the patient thoroughly, including an evaluation of her airway (Figs. 8.2 and 8.3). This evaluation, combined with an evaluation of the patient's habitus, which might include morbid obesity, may dictate that the patient should be managed up front with a continuous spinal during labor with the ability to activate and elevate the patient's sensory level in case of a declared emergency. This is just one example of how preplanning can affect more favorable outcomes for the mother and the baby in such difficult scenar-

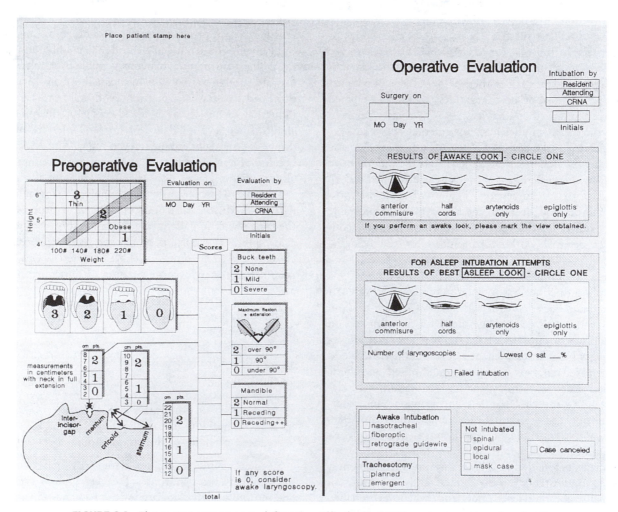

FIGURE 8.2. There are many ways to define the difficult airway. Here are examples of methods of evaluation for both preoperative and operative periods.

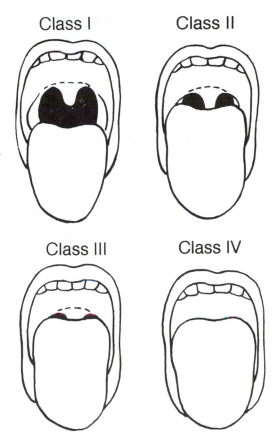

FIGURE 8.3. The four Mallampati classes. These views are generated by the patient sitting with mouth open and tongue extended to the maximum.

TABLE 8.3. FAILED INTUBATION DRILL

1. Ventilate by face mask with 100% O_2 maintaining cricoid pressure.
2. If no element of fetal distress is present, allow patient to awaken:
   a. If not contraindicated, use a regional technique.
   b. May attempt intubation using fiberoptic bronchoscope.
3. If surgery continues:
   a. Maintain mask ventilation with O_2 and 0.5 MAC halothane or isoflurane, continuing to apply cricoid pressure. Intravenous ketamine may also be administered.
   b. Decide whether to use further relaxants or to allow spontaneous ventilation to return.
   c. Following delivery of neonate, decide whether to make further attempts to intubate.
4. If mask ventilation fails:
   a. Perform cricothyrotomy using a cricothyrotomy cannula.
   b. A 12-gauge intravenous cannula with a 4.5-mm endotracheal tube adaptor suffices if specific cricothyrotomy cannulas are not available.

From Messeter KH. Endotracheal intubation with the fiberoptic bronchoscope. *Anaesthesia* 1980;35:294–298, with permission.

ios. If general anesthesia is the choice for a given patient, the anesthesiologist can still utilize different techniques that will improve the safety margin for the patient. Some of these include awake intubation, blind-nasal intubation, fiberoptic endoscopy using the oral approach, use of the rigid optical stylet, rigid bronchoscopy, retrograde translaryngeal intubation, cricothyroidotomy, and tracheostomy. Of course, one must not forget the possibility of management by mask ventilation with continuous cricoid pressure.

It is important to remember that a failed intubation can mean both maternal and/or fetal death. With such serious consequences one must view this challenge as a major one that demands superb preparation and an organized manner of approach by designing a carefully constructed failed intubation drill (Table 8.3). A competent team can handle these emergencies but the team must work together. In medicine, a bad outcome can occur in spite of a prepared and an experienced group (55).

Intubation by Fiberoptic Means

Oral fiberoptic intubation is the best choice because of the hazard of bleeding when airway tubes are passed via the nasal passage in pregnancy. The technique can be accomplished by one of three oral airways—Berman, Patel-Syracuse, and Williams. All of these are made to enable the passage of a fiberoptic bundle. This technique is accomplished by the passage of a fiberoptic scope via an endotracheal tube. It is important to secure good transtracheal analgesia in the mouth, base of the tongue, pharynx, and supraglottic area. The complete method can be reviewed in the Bonica and McDonald textbook, *Principles and Practice of Obstetric Analgesia and Anesthesia.*

Complications of Alternative Airway Methods

Nasal Bleeding

There is well-recognized hyperemia of the nasal mucosa during pregnancy. In addition, a specific mass may grow in the nasal area, referred to as nasal granuloma gravidarum, which is also a potential serious bleeding problem. It is not prudent to pass a nasotracheal tube or a nasogastric tube in a pregnant patient because of the nasal hyperemia. With the oral intubation methods available today, there is absolutely no need to place the patient at risk for major nasal bleeding (56).

Retropharyngeal Perforation

This is a rare but potentially lethal complication of nasotracheal intubation. It must be considered, though, when the end of the tube is not visualized in the retropharyngeal area during laryngoscopy.

Other Complications of Anesthesia

Hypertension

Induction of general anesthesia and intubation have resulted in a hypertensive response even in the rare and occasional normotensive patient. The hypertensive patient has a larger response. In extreme situations, it is possible to get some protection by the use of α-blockers, β-blockers, mask inhalation induction, deep anesthesia prior to intubation, or opioids (57–60). An ideal anesthetic to obviate this problem might be regional, and this is accepted if minimal fetal risk is present. In cases of fetal risk, the decision must be made between safety of the mother and safety of the baby. This decision can only be made after a discussion between the obstetrician and the anesthesiologist. General anesthesia with an opioid plus an effective β-blocker may be used to minimize the blood pressure fluctuations. With such a regimen, the cardiovascular response to tracheal intubation and the usual hypertension after laryngoscopy and intubation can be minimized by use of proper pharmacologic agents. Adverse responses can occur, however, decreasing uterine blood flow, (elevating pulmonary and systemic arterial pressure), and even precipitating pulmonary edema. The long-standing popular induction agent for cesarean section has been thiopental. However, thiopental can also be associated with adverse responses such as cardiac depression and hypotension or a hypertensive response to intubation.

Hypotension

It is well recognized that during regional anesthesia the pressure of the uterus on the vena cava and aorta worsens hypotension. The lateral tilt is used to help prevent its occurrence. Such a problem is ignored during general anesthesia to the great detriment of the patient.

Esophageal Intubation

The mistake of esophageal intubation must be ruled out by careful observation of chest movement, auscultation of the chest, and attention to a typical CO_2 waveform. This can be accomplished by noting a color change on an indicator or preferably by viewing the CO_2 waveform on a screen utilizing electronic detection methodology. A typical waveform confirms tracheal intubation. Unrecognized esophageal intubation is still one of the most common causes of death in general anesthesia, and such an error in the pregnant patient is more devastating because of more rapid desaturation causing reduced functional residual capacity and elevated metabolic rate (61). Add to this the complications of gastric distention, regurgitation, and aspiration, and it is apparent that esophageal intubation produces a major calamity.

Unintentional Awareness During Surgery

Maternal awareness during surgery was identified in the mid-1970s as a problem relating to the tendency to minimize the thiopental dosage during induction for a cesarean birth. Many of these cases also had N_2O concentration reduction from 70% to 50%. The incidence of awareness was significant, perhaps in the 20% to 25% range. One of the ways to counteract this phenomenon is by adding a small percentage of inhalation agent, such enflurane 0.8% or isoflurane 0.6% (62,63). The problem of maternal awareness is the result of inadequate analgesia or amnesia during general anesthesia, whereby the patient can have significant recall of the incision, the delivery, announcement of the sex of the baby, and the entire surgical closure. Such incidents can trigger malpractice suits against the anesthesiologist who really has little defense under such circumstances. It is wise to check the patient's pupils after delivery of the baby to note if they are widely dilated as a result of strong sympathetic stimulation related to poor analgesia. Other signs of inadequate anesthesia in a paralyzed patient may include increases in pulse rate and blood pressure, cardiac arrhythmias, sweating, tearing, and bronchospasm. In addition to recording pupil size, the anesthetist should record peak inspiratory pressure.

Embolism

Thrombotic pulmonary embolism occurs more frequently in pregnant women. Air embolism can and does occur as a complication at the time of delivery because torn uterine veins allow air to enter if a negative pressure should develop (64). This, of course, can occur when torn veins are placed at a level higher than the heart, as in the Trendelenburg position. Changing the posture immediately and occluding any open veins can rectify this situation. Amniotic fluid embolism may occur as a sudden, rapidly catastrophic event, manifested by cyanosis, dispense, hypotension, and other evidence of the adult respiratory distress syndrome, and has a high mortality rate. It may occur after a tumultuous labor or during or shortly after a cesarean operation. Frequently, there is confusion as to whether there was an anesthetic accident or an obstetric catastrophe. Definitive proof is the demonstration of lanugo hairs of fetal squames in the maternal pulmonary vessels (65).

Neurologic Disorders

The incidence of subarachnoid hemorrhage during pregnancy is 1 in every 10,000 patients, a rate five times higher than in nonpregnant women. Maternal mortality can vary considerably (from 0% to 14%), while fetal mortality is also considerable (from 10% to 28%). It is thought to be related primarily to less-than-adequate placental perfusion. An example of the ischemic cerebrovascular problem is a report of multiple cerebral infarcts in a young pregnant woman who has neurofibromatosis with thrombotic tendencies. One sobering statistic is that the risk of stroke in pregnant women is 13 times greater than in nonpregnant women of the same age. The major causes of stroke in pregnant women are arterial occlusion and cerebral venous thrombosis.

Cardiac Arrest

Cardiac arrest as a sequel of general anesthesia is caused almost exclusively by the problems discussed above in this chapter, namely, failed intubation and inability to establish an adequate airway. These result in rapid desaturation of the patient's blood because of her pregnant state. Asphyxia causes tachycardia, then bradycardia, and then arrhythmia, due to insufficient oxygenation of the myocardium. Complete cardiovascular collapse and arrest follow this within a few minutes. No greater calamity or emergency exists. The anesthesiologist must take direct and forceful control of the situation, and begin aggressive therapy, which is somewhat different from the management of cardiac arrest for a nonpregnant person. A woman at term has a distorted cardiac axis due to diaphragm elevation. This places the left ventricle outside the line between the sternum and the vertebral bodies. The effectiveness of closed cardiac resuscitation in nonpregnant patients is based on the ability to compress the ventricle between two bony structures, and produce a cardiac output. Because closed chest compression is ineffective for a woman at term, the anesthesiologist may need to call for open cardiac resuscitation, which is done by opening the chest and directly compressing the ventricles with the hand. The obstetrician should deliver the baby immediately, disregarding the resuscitation efforts with full attention given to a rapid delivery. This is important so that the mother's resuscitation can be started independently and so any vena caval obstruction is alleviated. Most important is that the mother's resuscitation can be more effective when the fetus is delivered.

Malignant Hyperthermia

This disease process is a potentially lethal complication of general anesthesia (mortality from less than 5% to 30%), regardless of whether or not a patient is pregnant. The disease process was described originally in the 1950s. Since then, there have been innumerable incidents of malignant hyperthermia reported, many of them culminating in death (66–70). The underlying mechanism is an alteration of calcium metabolism in muscle cells that causes phenomenal release of energy and heat. The patient suffers from both hyperthermia and muscle rigidity. The classic clinical features include hyperthermia, muscle rigidity, perspiration, cardiac arrhythmias, tachycardia, increased O_2 utilization, increased CO_2 production, hyperventilation, cyanosis, and

acidosis. Triggering agents can include anesthetic agents, muscle relaxants, and stress reactions. The absolute diagnosis depends on a skeletal muscle biopsy and a positive contracture test.

REGIONAL ANESTHESIA

First Stage of Labor

There is convincing evidence that the recent refinements in techniques for continuous epidural analgesia now have little or no effect on the progress of cervical dilation and the duration of the first stage of "normal" uncomplicated labor. Support of this statement requires several conditions:

1. Analgesia initiated at an appropriate time
2. A preload infusion of fluid to minimize maternal hypotension
3. Parturient in left or right lateral decubitus position during labor
4. Maternal blood pressure maintained throughout labor

Properly executed, continuous epidural analgesia is likely to enhance the progress of the first and second stage of labor in parturients with incoordinate uterine contractions and in those who are exhausted and in distress because of insufficient pain relief. In the latter circumstances, effective epidural analgesia allows maternal rest and composure while the uterus continues to contract with more vigor and more rhythmic patterns.

Second Stage of Labor

Primary elements for successful completion of the second stage of labor include uterine contractions, descent of the presenting part, and rotation of the presenting part; following the cardinal mechanisms of labor—internal flexion, internal rotation, and extension of the fetal head; and promptly after delivery—restitution, delivery of the shoulder, external rotation of the head, and finally delivery. Resistant forces consist of firm tone of the strong levator ani muscles. In some patients, the bony configuration of the pelvis restricts delivery by acting as an active impediment so that cesarean section may be indicated. For maximum efficiency of the resistant forces, the perineal muscles must retain their tone and strength dependent on the motor fibers of S2, S3, S4, and the anococcygeal nerve. Regional anesthesia achieved with low concentrations of local anesthetics alone or combined with opioids does not significantly influence the tone of the perineal muscle sling; however, regional anesthesia with high concentrations of local anesthetic produces motor block and interference with the basic second stage mechanisms noted above.

Continuous Epidural Infusion with Local Anesthetic

The advent of precise infusion pumps in the 1970s and the increase of the number of anesthesiologists interested in obstetric anesthesiology helped pave the way for the now-improved status of obstetric anesthesiology practices around the country. Many of the patients received very low dosage of local anesthetics for the first stage of labor and experienced good pain relief for the first stage with no negative impact upon labor. The patients did not have an increase in the frequency of malrotation or instrumental delivery, but did have lower rates (40% to 60%) of effective analgesia at the second and third stage of labor (71–81). When higher concentrations (e.g., 0.25% to 0.375% bupivacaine or 1% to 1.5% lidocaine) or quicker infusion rates (> 15 mL/h), or both, were used, perineal pain relief was good. Prolonged second stages were found, however, because of an increase in malrotation and eventual instrumental delivery (82–85).

Continuous Infusion of Local Anesthetics and/or Opioids

To solve the former problem of high instrumental delivery during the second stage, investigators began to carry out several randomized, double-blind, placebo-controlled studies to evaluate analgesic efficacy, as well as the effect on the second stage of labor (79,80,87,90). One was a continuous infusion of 0.75% lidocaine administered beyond 8 cm of cervical dilatation. This did not prolong the second stage (78). In contrast, continuous infusion of 0.125% bupivacaine provided excellent intrapartum analgesia but did prolong second stage and increased the incidence of instrumental delivery (79). A third study noted that continuous epidural infusion of 0.0625% bupivacaine with 0.0002% fentanyl (2 μ/mL) produced first-stage analgesia similar to that produced by continuous infusion of 0.125% bupivacaine. Several other groups have carried out double-blind randomized studies in an attempt to decrease the incidence of instrumental deliveries, most of which were mentioned in the previous section (83,88–95). The study by Vertommen and colleagues (95) deserves special mention because it is a multicenter study involving a large group of patients, and it was done in a randomized double-blind fashion. It revealed a reduction in instrumental deliveries.

Problems with Analgesia During Second Stage and Delivery

Perineal analgesia is a completely separate issue from first-stage uterine analgesia. Some obstetricians who believe it is important to maintain the bearing down reflex to expedite delivery do not want perineal analgesia. Others offer analgesia with lower concentrations of local anesthetics. Still others believe complete analgesia of the perineum is satisfactory for second stage. Some use either intermittent injection or continuous infusion of local anesthetics, which are given alone or in combination with opioids. Significant percentages (20% to 50%) of patients do not have adequate perineal analgesia during second stage. If perineal pain is experienced during the early part of the second stage, before flexion and internal rotation have taken place, 10 mL of an analgesic concentration of the local anesthetic and/or opioid can be injected with the patient in the semirecumbent position. This technique performed with the patient sitting usually enhances diffusion of the solution to the sacral segments.

REGIONAL ANALGESIA FOR OBSTETRICS OTHER THAN EPIDURAL

Four regional techniques can all be performed by the obstetrician (Figs. 8.4, 8.5, and 8.6):

1. pudendal block
2. local perineal anesthesia

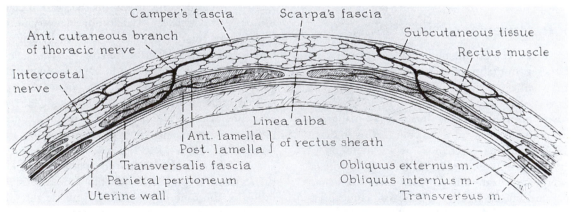

FIGURE 8.4. Nerve supply of abdominal wall is shown in cross section. Late in pregnancy, the uterine wall is right up against the abdominal wall muscles. Here it is possible to see how a nerve could be affected by the enlarging uterine organ.

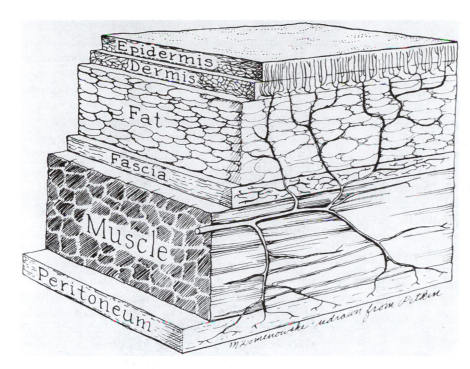

FIGURE 8.5. The distribution of the nerves in the layer of the skin. Note how the nerve manages to supply the peritoneum, muscle, fascia, fat, and skin layers.

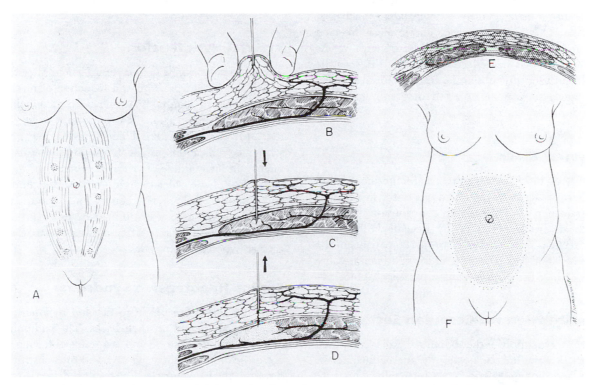

FIGURE 8.6. The method of abdominal wall anesthesia. **A:** Anterior view with eight local injection points identified. **B:** The method of skin pinch with needle puncture. **C:** Injection of local anesthetic deep in muscle. **D:** Needle retraction after local anesthetic deposition. **E:** The linea alba separating the rectus muscles in the midline. **F:** The local anesthetic field ideal for cesarean section (c/s) incision and delivery.

3. paracervical block
4. local infiltration for cesarean section

Pudendal Block

The pudendal nerve trunk divides into three main branches: the inferior hemorrhoidal nerve, the perineal nerve, and the dorsal nerve to the clitoris. Mueller of Germany was one of the first to describe the pudendal nerve block as used in obstetrics in 1907. The American contribution to pudendal nerve block was made by King (96) in 1916. Imagine the confusion by many who believed that a field block of the perineum would have to include the ilioinguinal nerve, the genital branch of the genitofemoral nerve, and the perineal branch of the posterior femoral cutaneous nerve. Thus, studies by Klink (97) and Zador et al. (98) established the standard of 10 mL of local anesthetic deposited at the ischial spines bilaterally to provide adequate perineal and vaginal analgesia for delivery and episiotomy.

Local Perineal Anesthesia

This technique can be used if a pudendal block has failed or if a pudendal block has not been done and delivery is imminent or actually occurring. It is best performed during maximum stretch of the perineum as the head of the fetus crowns. It can easily be performed with the use of a 1% lidocaine solution using a 10-ml syringe and a $1\frac{1}{2}$-inch, 25-gauge needle. The lidocaine can be continuously injected slowly along the line of the intended episiotomy site. As long as the needle is moved continuously, there is little danger of depositing any substantial amounts intravenously. Adequate analgesia can be expected in 5 minutes or so after injection.

Paracervical Block

The paracervical block affords pain relief for uterine contractions. Gellert of Germany published one of the first reports in the literature in 1926. American contributions began in 1945 with an article published by Rosenfeld (99), who reported excellent pain relief of labor in 100 patients in the first stage of labor. Currently, its use is restricted because of reports of bradycardia following a paracervical block.

Local Infiltration for Cesarean Section

The general nerve supply of the abdominal wall is composed of six of the lowest thoracic nerves, the ilioinguinal nerves bilaterally, and iliohypogastric nerves bilaterally. The three primary nerves that make up the sensory input from the abdomen all end as anterior cutaneous nerves in the abdominal wall. The iliohypogastric and the ilioinguinal nerves arise from the anterior primary division of the first lumbar

nerve. For emergency cases where a midline incision is necessary, one can use 1% lidocaine in a 10-mL syringe with a $3\frac{1}{2}$-inch, 25-gauge spinal needle and inject just under the skin from the umbilicus to near the symphysis pubis. The knife follows this line during incision and the patient should be very comfortable. This is the most rapid method for analgesia and delivery by cesarean section and is a logical choice in cases where anesthesia is not available or possible for a period of time. The remainder of the technique of local anesthesia for cesarean section can be gleaned from the Bonica and McDonald textbook referred to above.

COMPLICATIONS OF LOCAL ANALGESIA

Systemic toxic reaction from an overdose of local anesthetic solution has been the most frequent complication associated with local analgesia, and this is why an anesthesiologist should be consulted in regard to all the issues of analgesia and anesthesia mentioned in this chapter. The anesthesiologist who is qualified, certified, and well versed in the pharmacology and specifics of the various anesthetic agents should be called to assist with administration of all local anesthetic agents used in analgesia and anesthesia in appropriate situations. The reason for this is there are significant and numerous complications that can occur as a result of obstetric anesthesia, some of which are outlined briefly below.

Arterial Hypotension

Arterial hypotension is defined as a 20% to 30% reduction in baseline systolic pressure or a reduction of mean arterial pressure below 100 mm Hg, which is accepted as the general definition of hypotension. It is important to be cognizant that an acute fall in maternal blood pressure may precipitate serious complications in the fetus. In past years the frequency and magnitude of arterial hypotension, consequent to the use of the older techniques of subarachnoid block and epidural block, were frequent and serious in nature. Now the trend is to use minimal doses of an anesthetic agent along with various safety nets to protect the patient against hypotensive episodes.

Supine Hypotensive Syndrome

Certain mothers are prone to develop hypotension every time they are placed on their backs. The pathophysiology of this is well understood and is a result of having the large uterus lie on top of the vena cava and thus obstruct venous flow into the left ventricle. The result is decreased pumping pressure, decreased cardiac output, and decreased blood pressure. Many factors, however, aggravate the degree of hypotension in a parturient receiving subarachnoid or epidural block:

1. hypertension
2. hypovolemia
3. severe anemia
4. electrolyte imbalance
5. vasomotor tone disorder
6. depression of catecholamines
7. adrenocortical depression

Prevention of Supine Hypotensive Syndrome

Some decrease in blood pressure is to be expected with spinal or epidural anesthesia in obstetric patients. It is an important concept to prevent the severe hypotensive episodes by correcting hypovolemia, blood loss, and dehydration. All of these factors can be countered by adequate volume replacement. In some instances, central hemodynamic monitoring may be necessary and indicated to help assess a patient's volume status.

Intravenous Infusions

Experience has supported the infusion of 1,000 to 2,000 mL of a balanced nondextrose-containing solution within 30 minutes of a high spinal or epidural.

Lateral Uterine Displacement

The maintenance of continuous left lateral uterine displacement (LUD) cannot be overemphasized. Simply placing a wedge under the hip provides no guarantee of avoiding aortocaval compression. In some patients it is necessary to have active right uterine displacement.

Vasopressors

Some anesthesiologists use prophylactic vasopressors in obstetric anesthesiology. I do not, as ordinarily patients do well with administration of suitable vasopressors when indicated, e.g., during surgery.

Allergic/Hypersensitive Reactions

Many times allergic/hypersensitive reactions are due to subjective symptoms from intravenous injections of local anesthetic that contains high concentrations of epinephrine. True allergic reactions to local anesthetics are rare. The ones that do occur usually involve amino ester local anesthetics such as procaine, chloroprocaine, and tetracaine (100). This is not surprising, as these drugs are derivatives of *para*-aminobenzoic acid (PABA), which can act as a hapten and is known to be allergenic in nature. Allergic reactions to the amino amides such as lidocaine, bupivacaine, and mepivacaine are extremely rare, but have been reported (101).

Cardiac Arrest

Pregnant patient cardiac arrest is without doubt the most dramatic and frightening complication that can occur in obstetric anesthesia. This occurs when the heart ceases to function as an effective pump. In general, the cause is cardiac dysrhythmia, asystole, or electromechanical disassociation.

Prevention of Cardiac Arrest

It must be reemphasized that before initiating any regional procedure, all necessary equipment for proper airway management and resuscitation must be available for immediate use. This means that an intravenous infusion and appropriate monitors should be in place and shown to be working before starting the procedure. Proper patient positioning is important for any regional anesthetic procedure. Because of the reduction in sizes of the pregnant epidural and subarachnoid spaces, it behooves the practitioner to be aware of potentially decreased anesthetic requirements in the pregnant patient and to take a conservative dosing approach. Once the block is performed, one must remember to frequently check vital signs and progression of block, especially during the first 20 minutes.

For epidural anesthesia, an appropriate test dose of 30 to 60 mg lidocaine or 5 to 10 mg bupivacaine must be utilized to rule out subarachnoid needle or catheter placement. At least 3 to 5 minutes should elapse for a subarachnoid injection to manifest itself. The epidural block should be initiated slowly with incremental small doses to achieve the desired level and effect of analgesia.

Anesthetic Related Neuropathies

Neurologic injury due to regional anesthesia can be the result of a variety of causes:

1. direct needle trauma during the procedure
2. neurotoxicity from drugs or contaminants
3. infection
4. spinal hematoma
5. spinal cord ischemia due to vasoconstrictors
6. preexisting neurologic disease

LOCAL ANESTHESIA

There are two main groups of local anesthetics used in pregnancy: ester type and amide type. Their method of action, their metabolism, and their application to pregnancy are quite different.

Ester Anesthetics

An ester-type anesthetic is defined by its chemical configuration. Ester anesthetics are those local anesthetics that have an ester type of linkage between the lipophilic end and the amide end of the chemical structure of the compound. It is important to understand that the pattern of metabolism of the anesthetic is dependent on this very linkage between the two ends as described.

The pattern of metabolism of the ester local anesthetics is by hydrolysis via the enzyme pseudocholinesterase that is present in tissues and blood of the body. Of interest is the fact that this enzyme is also present in succinylcholine. Different ester anesthetics are metabolized at varying rates depending on the extent of change present in its aromatic ring. The fastest metabolized agent is 2-chloroprocaine. It is hydrolyzed four times faster than the older prototype local anesthetic, procaine. The slowest of the ester local anesthetics metabolized is tetracaine. To put it into perspective, 2-chloroprocaine's half-life in the normal adult is only about 30 seconds. Thus, there is no concern about the pharmacokinetic aspect of distribution, which is an issue when it comes to the amide-linked drugs. The reason for this, as mentioned above, is that metabolism of the esterase derivative drugs occurs in the blood by pseudocholinesterase, before tissue uptake can even occur.

The four universal basics of the foundation of drug metabolism are uptake, distribution, biotransformation, and excretion. The final pharmacologic effect or potency of any anesthetic is dependent on the relational aspect of these four mechanisms of drug metabolism. What if one of these four basics of metabolism is faulty? For example, suppose a given patient has an abnormal plasma pseudocholinesterase. In such a patient, the rate of ester anesthetic hydrolysis would be diminished, thus substantially prolonging the effectiveness of the anesthetic. In this case, we would conclude that the half-life or effective longevity of the anesthetic would be prolonged. This point is being made so that the obstetrician can appreciate that, although normally there is a built-in safety feature in using esterase local anesthetics, there can be this rare instance where because of an abnormal enzyme, the potential for toxicity can exist (102). If a 25% decrease in plasma pseudocholinesterase activity in the pregnant patient occurred, can this also be a cause for concern about toxicity in the esterase-based anesthetics? The answer is no. There is indeed a 25% reduction of pseudocholinesterase in pregnancy, but this is not clinically significant.

Amide Anesthetics

Since amide-linked local anesthetics are exclusively biotransferred by the liver, they must be transported there before biotransformation can occur. Of the four aforementioned mechanics of drug handling, it is biotransformation that largely controls a drug's effective potency, because without biotransformation, drugs could endlessly continue to circulate and be redistributed in the body without being excreted. Furthermore, any additional drug administered would tend to accumulate in a summation fashion. The latter could cause serious toxicity problems in every case. The amide anesthetics then more typify the ideal prototype of local anesthetic because they proceed through the four biotransformation stages in a stepwise fashion. Biotransformation of the amide local anesthetics cannot happen without adequate liver function and without effective liver blood flow. These are the two major factors operative in turnover of the amide-type drugs. Some of the medications that can reduce liver blood flow include some of the newer drugs such as calcium channel blockers, β-blockers, and the H_2-receptor blockers. If these drugs could reduce liver blood flow to a large enough degree, there could be an increase in the elimination half-life of amide local anesthetics. This too, then, could increase the potency of the amide local anesthetics by increasing blood levels. Other possibilities of diminishing effectiveness of hepatic function include liver damage and hypothermia, both of which negatively impact the effectiveness of the hepatic enzyme system responsible for accomplishing biotransformation of drugs.

We have now discussed the two most important aspects of biotransformation: blood flow to transport the drug to the hepatic cells for breakdown, as well as the health of the hepatic cells themselves. Under even normal disease conditions, neither of these significantly impacts the potency of the local anesthetics primarily because they just are not that far out of normal range.

MATERNAL FACTORS

The approach to pharmacology in obstetric anesthesiology is a bit more complicated because of the pregnancy state and the maternal-placental-fetal transfer dynamics. For example, we know all local anesthetics administered to the mother for the sake of producing analgesia for labor and delivery must traverse the placenta and are then taken up by the fetus. This is why it is necessary for us to understand the dynamics of drug transfer from the mother to the fetus. The transfer of drug from the mother to the fetus via the placenta is affected by both physical and biochemical barriers for the most part, so that only a small proportion of the amount of drug given to the mother ever really reaches the fetus. This is an important point to remember. Normally, only about 0.3 to 0.5 of the level of drug in the maternal circulation gets into the fetal circulation. This applies to systemic medications and local anesthetics alike. This reduction or "protective" effect is good, as it helps to protect the newborn by minimizing drug depression at the time of delivery. This, in turn, enables the newborn to breathe normally and react normally to its new environment. Despite this elaborate design, unfortunate iatrogenic injuries have occurred as the result of direct fetal brain local anesthetic injection during caudal analgesia. In addition, there have also been recorded fetal deaths after paracervical analgesia, due to the same accidental injection into the fetal head as the aforementioned caudal method, as well as because of rapid delivery, excessive uptake by uterine blood vessels, and rapid transfer to the fetus (103).

PLACENTAL FACTORS

Local anesthetics transfer through the placenta without difficulty; however, certain special factors influence this transfer. One example is the chemical makeup of the anesthetic. Is it fat soluble, ionized, or un-ionized? The transfer of drugs that are all three of these are measurably more rapid in transfer than drugs that are not. This does not mean that certain errors in administration cannot overcome this usual transfer rule. As noted above, certain disastrous direct anesthetic CNS injections have led to enormously elevated fetal local anesthetic blood levels. Again, we note that the amount of local anesthetic that ends up in the placenta is determined by the four basics of drug transfer (uptake, distribution, biotransformation, and excretion). Certain rules are operative for any drug given to the mother in regard to the amount that presents in the fetus/newborn. These operatives include:

1. Total dose impact. The larger the dose, the higher the maternal blood levels.
2. Delivery method. Direct intravenous injection will bypass all absorption barriers and produces the highest maternal blood levels.
3. Injection site vascularity. The higher the vascularity of the area injected, the higher the maternal blood levels may be because of rapid vascular absorption.
4. Vasoconstrictor use. The use of epinephrine will delay maternal blood levels due to a decrease in the immediate maternal blood level due to vasoconstriction.
5. Ionization. The less the ionization, the greater the tendency for rapid transfer across the placenta.
6. Protein binding. The less the protein binding, the greater the blood levels and the more available the drug is for placental transfer.
7. Fat solubility. The greater the fat solubility, the greater the potential for placental transfer.
8. Molecular weight. The smaller the molecular weight, the greater the potential for placental transfer.
9. Health of the placenta. The greater the placental blood flow pattern, the greater the transfer of the drug, and the healthier the placenta, the greater the potential for placental transfer.

FETAL FACTORS

The fetus acts as a passive reservoir since it is only directly linked to the mother via the intervillous space of the placenta. The important operative rules that impact the distribution of drugs to the fetus include:

1. Drug solubility
2. Amount of fetal blood in the intervillous space
3. Drug concentration in return from fetus
4. Fetal blood pH

In the days prior to neonatal intensive care units, it was imperative to deliver the fetus without any depression of the CNS. The reason for this was evident. Practical and fully integrated intensive care areas for these little patients were not available. Adult centers had nearly a decade of experience and favorable outcomes to bolster intensive care use in adult medicine. Thus, between the years 1968 and 1978, when neonatal intensive care units began to flourish, there were many transition possibilities that always erred on the side of minimal drug usage so the newborn could function as normally as possible at birth. Common consideration for drug depression was directed toward those who had general anesthetics, as it was understood that maternal blood levels were considerably lower following epidural, caudal, paracervical, or pudendal block as compared to drug levels following intravenous induction. Of all the regional methods, subarachnoid block was known to have the lowest blood levels in the fetus after maternal administration, because all local anesthetic was deposited into the subarachnoid compartment that did not communicate with the vascular system of the mother. Thus, all drugs deposited were compartmentalized and not available for transfer because the uptake from the spinal space was negligible.

In all the aforementioned regional nerve blocks, there was concern about reducing fetal absorption levels as much as possible. Thus, vasoconstrictors, the most popular being epinephrine, were used to reduce absorption of local anesthetics. This is accomplished by local vasoconstriction that in turn obstructs systemic absorption and results in lower maternal and fetal blood levels (104). For the newer lipid-soluble drugs such as bupivacaine and etidocaine, the local phenomenon of binding to epidural fat is significant and thus plays a greater role in blood levels than blood flow. Therefore, vasoconstrictors that are effective for lidocaine and mepivacaine are not as effective for these types of drugs.

Considering cardiac distribution, it is a fact that 10% of maternal cardiac output is diverted to the uterus and supplies the low-resistance placenta in pregnancy. Since intervillous blood flow is pressure dependent, an episode of maternal hypotension can impact placental blood flow and thus affect fetal blood drug levels. Since uterine blood supply is dependent on both cardiac distribution and uterine vascular resistance, the latter can also impact the final amount of uterine blood flow. This is significant because some of the amide local anesthetics used in *in vitro* experiments caused uterine artery vasoconstriction. This translates into an increase in vascular resistance and a resultant decrease in uterine blood flow. Fortunately, subsequent animal *in vivo* experiments in sheep using lidocaine, bupivacaine, and even the newer local anesthetic ropivacaine, did not reveal any significant effects on uterine blood flow and fetal condition (105,106). Epinephrine, the best-known vasoconstrictor used clinically, also did not affect uterine blood flow adversely when used in low doses of less than 100 μg (107).

Local anesthetics equilibrate across the placenta in an uncharged or base form. Differences between maternal and fetal blood pH cause variations of an ionized drug (charged drug) in equilibrium with the base form (uncharged drug) in the mother as opposed to the fetus. Charged particles (ionized drugs) do not traverse the placenta, making it possible for free local anesthetic concentration (base form) to be higher in the fetus than that in the mother. Normal fetal pH is 7.3, and somewhat acidotic compared to the mother. This effect is exaggerated further as the gradient between the fetus and mother increases. This is known as "ion trapping" (108). This situation of ion trapping and acidosis associated with fetal asphyxia increases anesthetic concentration in the brain, heart, liver, lungs, and kidneys (109).

The difference between drug levels in the fetus as compared to the mother is referred to as the fetal/maternal ratio. Certain drugs such as bupivacaine are more highly protein bound and make the fetal/maternal ratios appear even more favorable than those for lidocaine. The latter is of little clinical significance because it is the amount of free drug that is clinically significant. It is the unbound form that rapidly equilibrates across the placenta and other compartments in the fetus. Recall that the higher the maternal concentrations, the higher the drug levels to which the fetus will be exposed will be. Protein binding of local anesthetics is decreased in the fetus and newborn. This is due to a decreased level of α_1-acid glycoprotein that is age related; α_1-acid glycoprotein levels in the premature baby are half those of a term newborn, and newborn levels are three to four times lower than those in adults (110,111).

COMPLICATIONS OF LOCAL ANESTHESIA

Both major and minor complications can occur with the use of local anesthetics. Unfortunately, the major complications are life threatening and possibly fatal. High drug blood levels in either the CNS or the heart cause these complications. Because high drug blood levels can occur any time a drug is injected, one must be carefully trained and disciplined to identify, diagnose, and treat such complications. The maximum safe dosage of lidocaine in a single injection is 7 mg/kg. This ordinarily produces blood lidocaine levels of less than 3 mg/mL. Systemic symptoms of a metallic taste, ringing in the ears, and numbness of the lips occur at levels of around 5 mg/ml. CNS toxicity manifested by actual seizures can occur at blood levels of 10 to 12 mg/mL for lidocaine and 4 to 6 mg/mL for bupivacaine.

Premonitory signs and symptoms include slow speech, jerky movements, tremors, and hallucinations.

Local anesthetics also have triphasic brain effects. This means that there are three common effects on the brain depending on the level of local anesthetic. At low blood levels, it can have an anticonvulsant action. At slightly higher blood levels, seizure activity can occur. At very high blood levels, global CNS depression and seizures again can occur. At these higher blood levels, cardiotoxicity with subsequent heart damage and irreversible effects on the brain can ensue (112). Pregnancy does not increase the risk of CNS toxicity in association with high plasma levels of local anesthetics. In two studies performed in rats and sheep, there were no differences in blood or brain concentrations of lidocaine in pregnant versus nonpregnant animals. Thus, there does not appear to be a downward shift of the seizure threshold in pregnancy (113,114).

Treatment of local anesthetic seizures consists primarily of preventing the bad effects of hypoxia. During the seizure oxygen is administered and the airway is protected. A seizure is often such a dramatic event that observers are taken by the impressive motions of the moment and are frozen in an observant pose. But as each minute goes by the patient suffers from more and more hypoxia due to lack of an airway or ventilation or both. Thus, quick thinking and ventilation with 100% oxygen must be established. During this time the airway should also be protected with cricoid pressure, and at the same time the tongue protected so that it is not bitten or aspirated into the airway. Additionally, suppression of seizures can be achieved by administration of thiopental in a 50- to 100-mg bolus, or diazepam in a 5- to 10-mg bolus, or midazolam in a 1- to 2-mg bolus. Fortunately, there is an increase in cardiac output and cerebral blood flow, which help to quickly reduce the elevated levels of local anesthetic in the brain. In some instances, there may be such high levels of anesthetic that significant cardiac toxicity may occur. Often the patient can rapidly clear the toxic levels of the local anesthetic and no medications are needed because after 30 to 40 seconds the seizure may stop and the patient may regain normal ventilation and even awaken within a short period of time. It is important to use good judgment in such cases because the use of thiopental to treat seizures in the situation of cardiac toxicity is dangerous, as it adds another cardiac depressant on top of an already-depressed myocardium. Some patients with very severe signs of toxicity on the other hand may need to have tracheal intubation and succinylcholine to help terminate further seizures and continued tonic and clonic muscle activity. It must be recalled that prolonged seizures can lead to severe acidosis and further complication of the already-tenuous metabolic state of the patient. It must also be recalled that succinylcholine does not effect cessation of neuronal seizure activity. Since this is a time of increased metabolic activity and concurrent decreased oxygen supply, it is also a time when delivery of oxygen must be maintained. This is especially true in cases of paralyzed patients when protecting the CNS.

SYSTEMIC ANALGESIA

Labor Management

Like other optimum aspects of obstetric care, optimal sedation-analgesia requires a well-coordinated plan that should be initiated or completed by the obstetric anesthesiologist when one is available or by the attending obstetrician who has primary responsibility for care of the patient. Morgan et al. (115) surveyed 1,000 patients undergoing vaginal delivery and discovered that only 8% of parturients received no analgesia.

Unfortunately, today many centers still do not have full-time obstetric anesthesia coverage or have coverage only for operative cases. In these centers, systemic analgesics are still the primary method used for pain relief, and are provided by obstetricians (116).

The American College of Obstetricians and Gynecologists (ACOG) Committee on Obstetrics (117) recently recommended that a minimum effective analgesia/anesthesia plan—either regional or parenteral—should be available for laboring patients. When analgesia is required, the method is highly individualized depending not just on the patient's needs, but also on the skill of the person performing the analgesia. Parenteral analgesia can be given via either the intramuscular or intravascular route. In general, incremental intravenous doses of meperidine (25 mg) or butorphanol (1 mg) with or without promethazine (25 mg), promazine (20 mg), or hydroxine (50 mg intramuscular) should suffice in providing adequate analgesia.

Medications

Meperidine hydrochloride is preferable to morphine because it decreases nausea and lowers the result of depression in the neonate (118). It is approved and recommended by all manufacturers for obstetric analgesia. The drug is Food and Drug Administration (FDA) approved for oral (PO), intramuscular (IM), subcutaneous (SC), intermittent intravenous (IV), and continuous IV use. After an IM injection, the onset of action occurs in 15 minutes, with peak action taking place in 40 to 60 minutes. The duration of action is 2 to 4 hours. The half-life distribution of meperidine occurs 7.6 minutes following intravenous administration. Sixty percent of meperidine is plasma protein bound in the mother and 28% in the fetus and neonate (119). The drug exerts little if any effect on uterine activity (120). The principal metabolites of meperidine include normeperidine, meperidinic acid, normeperidinic acid, and meperidine N-oxide. It is important to be aware that some of the metabolites are also depressive to the neonate postpartum.

Intravenous meperidine in small dosages to obtain the desired effect is recommended during labor. Fetal equilibrium is reached 6 minutes following intravenous administration to the mother (121).

Butorphanol (Stadol) is a synthetic parenteral analgesic that has agonist and antagonist properties. It is newer than morphine and demerol, as it was first introduced in 1978. It is available in solutions containing either 1 or 2 mg/mL. Butorphanol's potency is five times that of morphine, and 40 times that of meperidine. Butorphanol is 80% protein bound in the mother. The onset of action of the drug occurs 10 minutes following intravenous injection and its action persists for 3 to 4 hours with a half-life of elimination of 2.7 hours. Butorphanol is metabolized predominantly in the liver by dealkylation and hydroxylation followed by conjugation to inactive metabolites. Excretion of the drug occurs mainly via the kidney by glomerular filtration with a small contribution by the biliary system. The respiratory-depression effects of 2 mg of butorphanol are similar to 10 mg of morphine. Both the respiratory and narcotic effects of butorphanol are reversed with naloxone. Butorphanol rapidly crosses the placenta. The umbilical venous to maternal venous ratio is 0.85 following equilibration $1\frac{1}{2}$ hours after administration to the mother (122). Quilligan et al. (123) compared meperidine and butorphanol for relief of pain occurring during labor and found that butorphanol provided superior analgesia. Hodgkinson et al. (124) noted that butorphanol provided excellent analgesia for labor with no neurobehavioral effects on the neonate. Many consider butorphanol to be the analgesic of choice for the parturient, and this drug is rapidly gaining in popularity. The drug is an excellent, potent analgesic, its metabolites are inactive, there is minimal risk of maternal respiratory depression, and no demonstrable neonatal neurobehavioral effects have been observed.

Nalbuphine (Nubain) was first introduced in 1979. There have been very few studies evaluating this drug as an obstetric analgesic, and it has failed to gain popularity for this indication (125). The drug is available in 10- or 20-mg/mL solutions. Nalbuphine is a synthetic agonist-antagonist with pharmacologic properties similar to pentazocine and butorphanol. Its potency is equivalent to morphine on a milligram basis. The onset of action of the drug following intravenous injection is 2 to 3 minutes with action duration of 5 to 6 hours, and its half-life of elimination is 5 hours. Similarly to butorphanol, nalbuphine has a plateau effect for respiratory depression reached when 30 mg of the drug has been administered. It is metabolized predominantly by the liver and excreted by the kidney. Naloxone reverses the respiratory depression that occurs secondary to nalbuphine.

Pentazocine (Talwin) is a synthetic analgesic with both opioid agonist and weak antagonist properties. Analgesia occurs 2 to 3 minutes following intravenous injection. There is extensive variation in metabolism of the drug by various individuals. Sixty percent of the drug is excreted predominantly as metabolites in the urine within 24 hours of administration. Doses in excess of 60 mg may be associated with psychomimetic effects, such as hallucinations and nightmares. Advantages claimed for pentazocine include less nausea, emesis, and postural hypotension than meperidine (126). Less placental transfer of pentazocine than meperidine occurs; however, the incidence of neonatal depression appears equal with equipotent dosages of the two drugs (127). The respiratory-depressant effects of Talwin also appear to plateau as compared to morphine. Pentazocine has failed to gain popularity as an obstetric analgesic because it lacks clear advantages and has psychomimetic effects. Naloxone reverses the respiratory depression that can occur secondary to this drug.

Fentanyl has been used successfully in labor as an analgesic by itself via the intravenous route and has been well received to date. One hundred patients with uncomplicated term pregnancies had either 50 to 100 μg of IV fentanyl or 1 to 2 mg of butorphanol for labor pain relief. Patients rated butorphanol higher as an analgesic and requested less repeat doses in comparison to fentanyl. However, both were effective as a first-stage analgesic medication for labor pain relief (128). A fentanyl patient-controlled analgesia (PCA) technique for pain relief during labor was used in a patient who had a documented platelet dysfunction that contraindicated use of epidural analgesia. A loading dose of 50 μg followed by intermittent 20-μg boluses by self-administration according to pain was effective in control of the first stage of labor pain over a 3-hour period (129).

SUMMARY

The choice of anesthesia for labor and delivery and for operative cesarean section is made by the anesthesiologist, who considers the needs of the patient and the needs and preferences of the obstetrician when deciding on the specific anesthetic technique and agent. In most cases today, regional anesthesia is chosen because of the very significant advantages for all concerned. Because of significant advances made over the last decade in regard to minimizing the anesthetic concentration and dosage, patients are now able to enjoy labor, as women in the past never were able to experience. Improved consciousness and participation of the mother reflect this with improved feeling in her legs and mobility of her body, as well as minimal, if any, motor blockade associated with her sensory level of anesthesia.

10 KEY POINTS

1. Important safety aspects for both the mother and baby of general anesthesia is the maintenance of uteroplacental perfusion, incorporating both acute maternal intravascular volume expansion and avoidance of aortocaval compression, treatment with antacids to alter the pH of her gastric contents to reduce the hazards of aspiration, and appropriate monitoring of the parturient and her fetus.

2. Aspiration associated with general anesthesia is an ever present danger with all techniques. Every pregnant woman beyond the first trimester should be considered to have a full stomach. Therefore, prevention steps consist of usage of antacids, H$_2$ receptor blockers, and/or gastrointestinal tract stimulants as pre-medication for general obstetric anesthesia.

3. Maternal awareness under general anesthesia during cesarean section is a regrettable but sometimes necessary or unavoidable complication. It may be necessary to communicate frankly with the mother and make her aware that to save the baby's life she may have to undergo uncomfortable situations for a hastily performed emergency abdominal delivery.

4. The breech fetus presents three potential problems for obstetricians and anesthesiologists: (1) prematurity, (2) possible traumatic delivery, and (3) coexistent maternal illness or fetal anomaly.

5. There is no single "ideal" anesthetic method for cesarean section. The choice depends upon the indications for delivery, the degree of urgency, maternal preference, and the experience and skill of the anesthesiologist.

6. It is not prudent to pass a nasotracheal tube or a nasogastric tube in a pregnant patient because of the nasal hyperemia. With the oral intubation methods available today, there is absolutely no need to place the patient at risk for major nasal bleeding.

7. There is convincing evidence that the recent refinements in techniques for continuous epidural analgesia now pose little or no effect on the progress of cervical dilation and the duration of the first stage of "normal" uncomplicated labor.

8. Regional anesthesia achieved with low concentrations of local anesthetics alone or combined with opioids does not significantly influence the tone of the perineal muscle sling and therefore should not affect adversely the second stage of labor; however, regional anesthesia with high concentrations of local anesthetic and high sensory levels can produce motor block and cause interference with certain basic second stage mechanisms and result in necessary instrumental delivery.

9. The study by Vertommen and colleagues (95) deserves special mention because it is a multicenter study involving a large group of patients who had continuous infusion of local anesthetic with opioid, and it was done in a randomized double-blind fashion. It revealed a reduction in instrumental deliveries.

10. If regional anesthesia is not available and a pudendal block has failed or not been done and delivery is imminent or actually occurring, one can perform a local analgesic perineal block during maximum stretch of the perineum as

the head of the fetus crowns. It can easily be performed with the use of a 1% lidocaine solution using a 10 ml syringe and a 25-gauge 1 1/2-inch needle.

REFERENCES

1. Gooding JM, Dimick AR, Tavakoli M. A physiologic analysis of cardiopulmonary responses to ketamine anesthesia in noncardiac patients. *Anesth Analg* 1977;56:813.
2. Dooley JR, Mazze RI, Rice SA, et al. Is enflurane defluorination inducible in man? *Anesthesiology* 1979;50:213.
3. Kosaka Y, Takahashi T, Mark LC. Intravenous thiobarbiturate anesthesia for cesarean section. *Anesthesiology* 1969;31:489–506.
4. White PF. Propofol: pharmacokinetics and pharmacodynamics. *Semin Anesth* 1988;7:4.
5. Crawford ME, Carl P, Bach V, et al. A randomized comparison between midazolam and thiopental for elective cesarean section anesthesia. I. Mothers. *Anesth Analg* 1989;68:229–233.
6. Dich-Nielsen J, Holasek J. Ketamine as induction agent for cesarean section. *Acta Anesthesiol Scand* 1982;26:139–142.
7. Marx, GF, Joshi CW, Orkin LR. Placental transmission of nitrous oxide. *Anesthesiology* 1970;2:429–432.
8. Heyman JH, Barton JJ. Safety of local versus general anesthesia for second-trimester dilatation and evacuation abortion. *Obstet Gynecol* 1986;68:877–878.
9. Delaney AG. Anesthesia in the pregnant woman. *Clin Obstet Gynecol* 1983;26:795–800.
10. Gaba DM, Baden JM. Physiological effects of drugs used in anesthesia. In: Baden JM, Broadsky JB, eds. *The pregnant surgical patient.* Mt. Kisco, NY: Futura, 1985:105–132.
11. Soyannwo OA, Elegbe EO, Odugbesan CO. Effect of flunitrazepam (Rohypol) on awareness during anesthesia for cesarean section. *Afr J Med Sci* 1988;17:23–26.
12. Hutson JM, Petrie RH. Drug effects on uterine activity and labor. *Clin Obstet Gynecol* 1982;25:189–201.
13. McDonald JS. Anesthesia and the high-risk fetus. In: Deep R, Eschenbach DA, Sciarra JJ, eds. *Gynecology and obstetrics,* vol 3. Philadelphia: JB Lippincott, 1988:1–16.
14. Robie GF, Payne GG Jr, Morgan MA. Selective delivery of an acardiac acephalic twin. *N Engl J Med* 1989;320:512–513.
15. Stirrat GM, Thomas TA. Prescribing for labour. *Clin Obstet Gynecol* 1986;13:215–229.
16. Famewo CE. Conditions for endotracheal intubation after atracurium and suxamethonium. *Middle East J Anesthesiol* 1986;8:371–377.
17. Zagorzycki MT. General anesthesia in cesarean section: effect on mother and neonate. *Obstet Gynecol Surv* 1986;39:134–137.
18. Biehl D, Palahniuk RJ. Update on obstetrical anesthesia. *Can Anaesth Soc J* 1986;33:238–245.
19. Blouw R, Scantliff J, Craig PB, et al. Gastric volume and pH in postpartum patients. *Anesthesiology* 1976;45:456–457.
20. Moir DD. Maternal mortality and anaesthesia. *Br J Anaesth* 1980;52:1–3.
21. Spielman FJ, Corke BC. Anesthesiologists' practice of obstetric anesthesiology. *J Reprod Med* 1984;29:683–685.
22. Shnider SM. Obstetric anesthesia coverage: problems and solutions. *Obstet Gynecol* 1969;34:615–620.
23. Ramanathan S. Anesthesia for cesarean section. In: *Obstetric anesthesia.* Philadelphia: Lea & Febiger, 1988:132–148.
24. Medelson CL. Aspiration of stomach contents into the lungs during obstetric anesthesia. *Am J Obstet Gynecol* 1946;52:191–205.
25. Burgess GE. Antacids for obstetric patients. *Am J Obstet Gynecol* 1975;123:577–579.
26. James CF, Gibbs CP, Banner T. Postpartum perioperative risk of aspiration pneumonia. *Anesthesiology* 1984;61:756–759.
27. Malinow AM, Ostheimer GW. Anesthesia for the high-risk parturient. *Obstet Gynecol* 1987;69:951–964.
28. Crawford JS, Burton M, Davies P. Time and lateral tilt at ceasarean section. *Br J Anaesth* 1972;44:477–484.
29. A comparison of general anesthesia and lumbar epidural analgesia for elective cesarean section. *Anesth Analg* 1977;56:228–235.
30. Zagorzycki MT, Brinkman CR. The effect of general and epidural anesthesia upon neonatal apgar scores in repeat cesarean section. *Surg Gynecol Obstet* 1982;155:641–645.
31. Maduska AL. Inhalation analgesia and general anesthesia. *Clin Obstet Gynecol* 1981;24:619–633.
32. Archer GW Jr, Marx GF. Arterial oxygen tension during apnea in parturient women. *Br J Anaesth* 1974;46:358–360.
33. Sellick BA. Cricoid pressure to control regurgitation of stomach contents during induction of anaesthesia. *Lancet* 1961;2:404–406.
34. Shnider SM, Levinson G. *Anesthesia for cesarean section,* 2nd ed. Baltimore: Williams & Wilkins, 1987:159–178.
35. Finster M, Poppers PJ. Safety of thiopental used for induction of general anesthesia in elective cesarean section. *Anesthesiology* 1968;29:190–191.
36. Petrikovsky B, Cohen M, Fastman D, et al. Electronic fetal heart rate monitoring during cesarean section. *Int J Gynecol Obstet* 1988;26:203–207.
37. Jouppila P, Kuikka J, Jouppila R, et al. Effect of induction of general anesthesia for cesarean section on intervillous blood flow. *Acta Obstet Gynecol Scand* 1979;58:249–253.
38. Shafer A, Doze VA, Shafer SL, et al. Pharmacokinetics and pharmacodynamics of propofol infusions during general anesthesia. *Anesthesiology* 1988;69:348–356.
39. Reddy BK, Pizer B, Bull PT. Neonatal serum cortisol suppression by etomidate compared with thiopentone for elective cesarean section. *Eur J Anaesth* 1988;5:171–176.
40. Shnider SM. Serum cholinesterase activity during pregnancy, labor, and puerperium. *Anesthesiology* 1965;26:335–339.
41. Blitt CD, Petty WC, Alberternst EE, et al. Correlations of plasma cholinesterase activity and duration of action of succinylcholine during pregnancy. *Anesth Anlg* 1977;56:78–83.
42. Baraka A. Neuromuscular blockade of atracurium versus succinylcholine in a patient with complete absence of plasma cholinesterase activity. *Anesthesiology* 1987;66:80–81.
43. Heller PJ, Scheider EP, Marx GF. Pharyngolaryngeal edema as a presenting symptom in preeclampsia. *Obstet Gynecol* 1983;62:523–524.
44. American College of Obstetricians and Gynecologists. *Anesthesia for cesarean section.* Technical bulletin 112. Washington, DC: ACOG, 1982.
45. Tunstall ME, Geddes C. Failed intubation in obstetric anesthesia. An indication for the use of the "esophageal gastric tube airway." *Br J Anaesth* 1984;56:659–661.
46. Goodman LS, Gillman AG. *Goodman and Gilman's the pharmacological basis of therapeutics,* 8th ed. New York: Pergamon Press, 1990.
47. Poulton TJ, James FM III, Lockridge O. Prolonged apnea following trimethaphan and succinylcholine. *Anesthesiology* 1979;50:54–56.
48. Fahmy NR, Soter NA. Effects of trimethaphan on arterial blood histamine and systemic hemodynamics in humans. *Anesthesiology* 1985;62:562–566.
49. Stempel JE, O'Grady JP, Morton MJ, Johnson KA. Use of sodium nitroprusside in complications of gestational hypertension. *Obstet Gynecol* 1982;60(4):533–538.

50. Macpherson M, Broughton PF, Rutter N. The effect of maternal labetalol on the newborn infant. *Br J Obstet Gynaecol* 1986; 93:539–542.
51. Collea JV. Current management of breech presentation. *Clin Obstet Gynecol* 1980;23:525.
52. McDonald JS, Mateo CV, Reed EC. Modified nitrous oxide or ketamine hydrochloride for cesarean section. *Anesth Anagl* 1972;51:975–985.
53. Shaw DB, Wheeler AS. Anesthesia for obstetric emergencies. *Clin Obstet Gynecol* 1984;27:112–124.
54. Cormack RS, Lehane J. Difficult tracheal intubation in obstetrics. *Anesthesia* 1984;39:1105–1111.
55. James FM, Wheeler AS, Dewan DM. *Obstetric anesthesia: the complicated patient.* Philadelphia: FH Davis, 1988:113.
56. Skau NK, Pilgaard P, Neilsen G. Granuloma gravidarum of the nasal mucous membrane. *J Laryngol Otol* 1987;101:1286–1288.
57. Fenakel K, Fenakel G, Appelman Z, et al. Nifedipine in the treatment of severe pre-eclampsia. *Obstet Gynecol* 1991;77:331–337.
58. Ludlow SW, Davies N, Davey DA, et al. The effect of sublingual nifedipine on uteroplacental blood flow in hypertensive pregnancy. *Br J Obstet Gynaecol* 1988;95:1276–1281.
59. Lurie S, Fenakel K, Friedman A. Effect of nifedipine on fetal heart rate in the treatment of severe pregnancy-induced hypertension. *Am J Perinatol* 1990;7:285–286.
60. Vink GJ, Moodley J, Philpott RH. Effects of dihydralazine on the fetus in the treatment of maternal hypertension. *Obstet Gynecol* 1980;55:519–522.
61. Archer GW Jr, Marx GF. Arterial oxygen tension during apnoea in parturient women. *Br J Anaesth* 1974;46:358–360.
62. Warren TM, Datta S, Ostheimer GW, et al. Comparison of the maternal and neonatal effects of halothane, enflurane and isoflurane for cesarean delivery. *Anesth Analg* 1963;62:516–520.
63. Wilson J, Turner DJ. Awareness during cesarean section under general anesthesia. *Br Med J* 1969;1:280–283.
64. Handler JS, Bromage PR. Venous air embolism during cesarean delivery. *Reg Anaesth* 1990;15:170–173.
65. Clark SL, Montz FJ, Phelan JP. Hemodynamic alterations associated with amniotic fluid embolism: a reappraisal. *Am J Obstet Gynecol* 1985;151:617–621.
66. Britt BA. Recent advances in malignant hyperthermia. *Anesth Anagl* 1972;51:841–850.
67. Brown RC. Hyperpyrexia and anesthesia. *Br Med J* 1954;1526–1527.
68. Editorial. Cause of death: malignant hyperpyrexia. *Br Med J* 1971;3(5772):441–442.
69. Saidman LJ, Harvard ES, Eger EJ II. Hyperthermia during anesthesia. *JAMA* 1964;90:1029–1032.
70. Morison DH. Placental transfer of dantrolen. *Anesthesiology* 1983;59:265.
71. Crawford JS. *Principles and practice of obstetric anaesthesia,* 2nd ed. London: Blackwell Scientific, 1965.
72. Crawford JS. Lumbar epidural block in labour: a clinical analysis. *Br J Anaesth* 1972;44:66–74.
73. Matouskova A, Dottori O, Forssman L, et al. An improved method of epidural analgesia with reduced instrumental delivery rate. *Acta Obstet Gynecol Scand* 1975;54:231–235.
74. Vanderick G, Doud TK, Khoo SS, et al. Bupivacaine 0.125% in epidural block analgesia during childbirth: clinical evaluation. *Br J Anaesth* 1974;46:838.
75. Glover DJ. Continuous epidural analgesia in the obstetric patient: a feasibility study using a mechanical infusion pump. *Anaesthesia* 1977;32:499–503.
76. Evans KRL, Carrie LES. Continuous epidural infusion of bupivacaine in labour: a simple method. *Anaesthesia* 1979;34:310.
77. Nadeau S, Elliott RD. Continuous bupivacaine infusion during labour: effects on analgesia and delivery. *Can Anaesth Soc J* 1985;32:S70.
78. Chestnut DH, Bates JN, Choi WW. Continuous infusion epidural analgesia with lidocaine: efficacy and influence during the second stage of labor. *Obstet Gynecol* 1987;69:323–327.
79. Chestnut DH, Vandewalker GE, Owen CL, et al. The influence of continuous epidural bupivacaine analgesia on the second stage of labor and method of delivery in nulliparous women. *Anesthesiology* 1987;66:774–780.
80. Gaylard DG, Wilson IH, Balmer HGR. Forum. An epidural infusion technique for labour. *Anaesthesia* 1987;42:1098–1101.
81. Hicks JA, Jenkins JG, Newton MC, et al. Continuous epidural infusion of 0.075% bupivacaine for pain relief in labour. *Anaesthesia* 1988;43:289.
82. Morison DH, Smedstad KG. Continuous infusion epidurals for obstetric analgesia [editorial]. *Can Anaesth Soc J* 1985;32:101–104.
83. Li DF, Rees GAD, Rosen M. Continuous extradural infusion of 0.0625% or 0.125% bupivacaine for pain relief in primigravid labour. *Br J Anaesth* 1985;57:264.
84. Rosenblatt R, Wright R, Benson D, et al. Continuous epidural infusion for obstetric analgesia. *Reg Anesth* 1983;8:10–14.
85. Ewen A, McLeod DD, MacLeod DM, et al. Continuous infusion epidural analgesia in obstetrics: a comparison of 0.08% and 0.25% bupivacaine. *Anaesthesia* 1986;42:143–147.
86. Chestnut DH, Laszewski LJ, Pollack KL, et al. Continuous epidural infusion of 0.0625% bupivacaine–0.0002% fentanyl during the second stage of labor. *Anesthesiology* 1990;72:613–618.
87. Chestnut DH, Owen CL, Bates JN, et al. Continuous infusion epidural analgesia during labor: a randomized double-blind comparison of 0.0625% bupivacaine/0.0002% fentanyl versus 0.125% bupivacaine. *Anesthesiology* 1988;68:754–759.
88. Youngstrom P, Eastwood D, Patel H, et al. Epidural fentanyl and bupivacaine in labor: double-blind study. *Anesthesiology* 1984;61:A414.
89. Van Steenberge A, Debroux HC, Noorduin H. Extradural bupivacaine with sufentanil for vaginal delivery. A double-blind trial. *Br J Anaesth* 1987;59:1518–1522.
90. Celleno D, Capogna G. Epidural fentanyl plus bupivacaine 0.125% for labor: analgesic effects. *Can J Anaesth* 1988;35:375–378.
91. Jones G, Paul DL, Elton RA, et al. Comparison of bupivacaine and bupivacaine with fentanyl in continuous extradural analgesia during labor. *Br J Anaesth* 1989;63:254.
92. Abboud TK, Afrasiabi A, Zhu J, et al. Epidural morphine or butorphanol augments bupivacaine analgesia during labor. *Reg Anaesth* 1989;14:115–120.
93. Abboud TK, Afrasiabi A, Zhu J, et al. Bupivacaine/butorphanol/epinephrine for epidural anesthesia in obstetrics: maternal and neonatal effects. *Reg Anaesth* 1989;14:219–224.
94. Rodriguez J, Payne M, Afrasiabi A, et al. Continuous infusion epidural anesthesia during labor: a randomized, double-blind comparison of 0.0625% bupivacaine/0.002% butorphanol and 0.125% bupivacaine. *Reg Anaesth* 1990;15:300–302.
95. Vertommen JD, Vandermeulen E, Van Aken H, et al. The effects of the addition of sufentanil to 0.125% bupivacaine on the quality of analgesia during labor and on the incidence of instrumental deliveries. *Anesthesiology* 1991;74:809–814.
96. King R. Perineal anesthesia in labor. *Surg Gynecol Obstet* 1916;23:615.
97. Klink EW. Perineal nerve block: an anatomic and clinical study in the female. *Obstet Gynecol* 1953;1:137.
98. Zador G, Lindmark G, Nilsson BA. Pudendal block in normal vaginal deliveries. Clinical efficacy, lidocaine concentrations, in maternal and foetal blood, foetal and maternal, acid-base values

and influences, on uterine activity. *Acta Obstet Gynecol Scand Suppl* 1974;34:51–64.

99. Rosenfeld SS. Paracervical anesthesia for the relief of labor pains. *Am J Obstet Gynecol* 1945;50:527.

100. Aldrete JA, Johnson DA. Allergy to local anesthetics. *JAMA* 1969;207:354–357.

101. Brown DT, Beamish D, Wildsmith JAW. Allergic reactions to an amide local anesthetic. *Br J Anaesth* 1981;53:435–437.

102. Smith AR, Hur D, Resano F. Grand mal seizures after 2-chloroprocaine epidural anesthesia in a patient with plasma cholinesterase deficiency. *Anesth Anagl* 1987;66:667–668.

103. Rosefsky JB, Petersiel ME. Perinatal deaths associated with mepivacaine paracervical-block anesthesia in labor. *N Engl J Med* 1968;278:530.

104. Abboud TK, David S, Nagappala A, et al. Maternal, fetal and neonatal effects of lidocaine with and without epinephrine for epidural anesthesia in obstetrics. *Anesth Anagl* 1984;63:973.

105. Biehl D, Schnider SM, Levinson G, et al. The direct effects of circulating lidocaine on uterine blood flow and foetal well-being in the pregnant ewe. *Can Anaesth Soc J* 1977;24:445.

106. Santos AC, Arthur GR, Roberts DJ, et al. Effect of ropivacaine and bupivacaine on uterine blood flow in pregnant ewes. *Anesth Anagl* 1992;74:62.

107. Albright GA, Jouppila R, Hollmen AL, et al. Epinephrine does not alter human intervillous blood flow during epidural anesthesia. *Anesthesiology* 1981;54:131.

108. Diehl D, Shnider SM, Levinson G, et al. Placental transfer of lidocaine: effects of fetal acidosis. *Anesthesiology* 1978;48:409.

109. Morishima HO, Covino BG. Toxicity and distribution of lidocaine in nonasphyxiated and asphyxiated baboon fetuses. *Anesthesiology* 1981;54:182.

110. Coyle DE, Denson DD, Essell SK, et al. The effect of nonesterified fatty acids and progesterone on bupivacaine protein binding. *Clin Pharmacol Ther* 1986;39:559.

111. Lerman J, Strong HA, LeDez KM, et al. Effects of age on the serum concentration of alpha-1-acid glycoprotein and the binding of lidocaine in pediatric patients. *Clin Pharmacol Ther* 1989;46:219.

112. Modica PA, Templehoff R, White PF. Pro- and anticonvulsant effects of anesthetics (part II). *Anesth Anagl* 1990;70:422.

113. Bucklin BA, Warner DS, Choi WW, et al. Pregnancy does not alter the threshold for lidocaine-induced seizures in the rat. *Anesth Anagl* 1992;74:57–61.

114. Morishima HO, Finster M, Arthur GR, et al. Pregnancy does not alter lidocaine toxicity. *Am J Obstet Gynecol* 1990;162:1320.

115. Morgan B, Bulpitt CJ, Clifton P, et al. Effectiveness of pain relief in labour: survey of 1000 mothers. *Br Med J* 1982;285:689–690.

116. Gibbs CP, Krischer J, Peckham BM, et al. Obstetric anesthesia: a national survey. *Anesthesiology* 1986;65:298–306.

117. American College of Obstetricians and Gynecologists. *Obstetric anesthesia and analgesia.* Technical bulletin 112. Washington, DC: ACOG.

118. Weitz CJ, Faull KF, Goldstein A. Synthesis of the skeleton of the morphine molecule by mammalian liver. *Nature* 1987;330:674–677.

119. Weitz CJ, Lowney LI, Feistner G, et al. Morphine and codeine from mammalian brain. *Proc Natl Acad Sci USA* 1986;83:9784–9788.

120. Herz A, Teschemacher H. Activities and site of antinociceptive action of morphine-like analgesics and kinetics of distribution following intravenous, intracerebral and intraventricular application. *Adv Drug Res* 1971;6:79–119.

121. Duggan AW, North RA. Electrophysiology of opioids. *Pharmacol Rev* 1983;35:219–282.

122. Maduska AL, Hajghassemali M. A double-blind comparison of butorphanol and meperidine in labor: maternal pain relief and effect on the newborn. *Can Anaesth Soc J* 1978;25:398–404.

123. Quilligan EJ, Keegan KA, Donahue MJ. Double-blind comparison of intravenously inject butorphanol and meperidine in parturients. *Int J Obstet Gynaecol* 1980;18:363–367.

124. Hodgkinson R, Huff RW, Hayashi RH, et al. Double-blind comparison of maternal analgesia and neonatal neurobehavior following intravenous butorphanol and meperidine. *J Int Med Res* 1979;7:224.

125. Henderson SK, Cohen H. Nalbuphine augmentation of analgesia and reversal of side effects following epidural hydromorphone. *Anesthesiology* 1986;65:216–218.

126. Moore J, Ball HG. A sequential study of intravenous analgesic treatment during labour. *Br J Anaesth* 1974;46:365.

127. Refstad SO, Lindbaek E. Ventilatory depression of the newborn of women receiving pethidine or pentazocine. *Br J Anaesth* 1980;52:265.

128. Atkinson BD, Truitt LJ, Rayburn WF, et al. Double-blind comparison of intravenous butorphanol (Stadol) and fentanyl (Sublimaze) for analgesia during labor. *Am J Obstet Gynecol* 1994;171(4):993–998.

129. Kleinman SJ, Wiesel S, Tessler MJ. Patient-controlled analgesia (PCA) using fentanyl in a parturient with a platelet function abnormality. *Can J Anaesth* 1991;38 (4 pt 1):489–491.

BASIC NUTRITIONAL REQUIREMENTS AND METABOLISM IN THE SURGICAL PATIENT

PATRICIA S. CHOBAN
LOUIS FLANCBAUM

INCIDENCE AND SCOPE OF MALNUTRITION

The identification, prevention, and treatment of malnutrition in patients remains a common problem. The incidence of malnutrition in hospitalized patients varies widely depending on the parameters used to diagnose malnutrition and the population studied.

Most research in this area has been conducted in populations of trauma and surgical patients, but it is relevant to and has broad application in obstetric and gynecologic patients. Gynecologic oncology patients with curable disease often undergo major surgery and may require prolonged hospitalization. They are often malnourished preoperatively and frequently become so after surgery. Yet a preoperative nutritional assessment is lacking in the vast majority of these patients. Furthermore, gynecologic oncology patients who undergo radiation therapy may develop some degree of radiation enteritis and may benefit from nutritional support.

In the obstetrics arena, the patient with hyperemesis gravidarum often undergoes inappropriate parenteral nutrition, and just as frequently the patient who needs nutritional supplementation may receive none. Also, patients placed on complete bed rest at home or in the hospital for 12 weeks with preterm labor or incompetent cervix might have a deficient diet and experience muscle wasting, but they rarely undergo a nutritional consultation. These problems can also be exacerbated if they are receiving weekly glucocorticoids, which are catabolic steroids.

In a group of surgical patients, the fraction considered malnourished varied from 15%, defining malnutrition as a serum albumin <3.5 g/dL, to 33% to 38% when it was defined as a serum prealbumin <20 mg/dL or a triceps skinfold <70% (1). Similarly, in medical patients, the incidence was 16%, based on >10% weight loss over the preceding 6 months, to 44%, using serum prealbumin <16 mg/dL (2). Three other studies using various other indices of malnutrition found the prevalence of mild malnutrition to be 48% and severe malnutrition to be 31% (3–5).

In 1994, a group in Scotland (6) reported a series of 500 patients admitted to the hospital of which 112 (22%) were hospitalized for at least a week and were reassessed at the time of discharge. They found that 200 patients (40%) were undernourished [body mass index (BMI) <20 kg/m²] on admission and only 96 had any nutritional information documented in their medical records. The mean weight loss in the group assessed at discharge was 5.4%, and 78% deteriorated nutritionally during hospitalization. Only ten of the initial 500 patients were referred for nutrition support.

These studies document that malnutrition is both highly prevalent and seriously underrecognized in hospitalized patients. The majority of hospitalized patients have other diseases, besides malnutrition, that have led to their hospitalization. Treatment is further complicated because it is often the response to the metabolic and physiologic stress imposed by these other illnesses that prevents the normal hypometabolic response to caloric deprivation.

METABOLIC RESPONSES TO STARVATION AND STRESS

Energy deprivation or starvation is a condition to which the body accommodates on a daily basis. This process of accommodation is designed to maximally protect lean body mass, which is that metabolically active portion of the body necessary for normal functioning. This usually includes the body's organs and muscles, and excludes fat. During brief periods of starvation, such as between meals or during an overnight fast, carbohydrates, in the form of hepatic glycogen, serve as the primary fuel source. The body can rapidly mobilize to glucose the 150 g of glycogen normally stored in the liver. In addition to glycogen, precursors of gluconeogenesis are derived from amino acids that have been shunted to the liver from skeletal muscle, primarily via alanine. A small contribution to gluconeogenesis is also derived from stored adipose tissue in the form of fatty acids and glycerol.

Further adaptation to starvation occurs after 7 to 10 days when the predominant fuel source changes from glucose to

TABLE 9.1. THE METABOLIC IMPACT OF STARVATION VERSUS STRESS

	Early Starvation	Late Starvation	Stress
Energy Expenditure	Slight decrease	Decrease	Increase
Mediator activation	None	None	++
Metabolic Responsiveness	Intact	Intact	Abnormal
Primary fuel	Carbohydrate	Ketone bodies	"Mixed"
Protein catabolism	Slight increase	Slight increase	Large increase
UUN excretion	Slight increase	Slight increase	Large increase
Malnutrition	Slow	Slow	Rapid

UUN, urinary urea nitrogen.

fat, in the form of ketone bodies. The ketone bodies become the primary energy source for metabolically active organs such as the brain, kidney, and heart. Reduction in the level of circulating insulin and a concomitant increase in circulating glucagon make free fatty acids more available as a source of fuel. These metabolic alterations result in a marked decrease in muscle protein breakdown, a fall in urinary excretion of nitrogen, and a decrease in the rate of metabolic expenditure. The sum of this adaptation is a marked diminution in the rate at which the vital metabolically active portion of the body, the lean body mass, is lost. This adaptation results in the ability to survive for approximately 60 to 70 days under conditions of complete starvation.

Provision of a small amount of glucose each day can reverse these adaptive mechanisms. This is the basis for the current clinical practice of providing 100 g of intravenous glucose each day [2 L of dextrose 5% in water (D_5W)] to hospitalized patients in order to achieve "protein sparing."

With illness, trauma, or other physiologic stress, numerous mediators are produced that alter the hormonal milieu and result in an adaptive state that differs significantly from the "conservative" metabolic state seen with starvation. These mediators include cytokines and eicosanoids, as well as changes in insulin and the "counterregulatory" hormones

glucagon, cortisol, growth hormone, and epinephrine. The elevation of insulin and the counterregulatory hormones leads to increased gluconeogenesis, hyperglycemia, and suppression of lipid mobilization (lipolysis). These changes commit the organism to a protein- or "mixed fuel"–based economy. In addition to the inability to utilize fat as the primary fuel source, as in starvation, the rate of fuel consumption increases substantially. This increase generally parallels the degree of stress. The characteristics of the metabolic response to starvation and stress are summarized in Table 9.1.

The stress or hypermetabolic response results in a rapid mobilization and loss of lean body mass as the body may "autocannibalize." This response is characterized by an increase in oxygen consumption and carbon dioxide production, which reflects the overall increase in energy expenditure. Additionally, the destruction of lean body protein to provide substrate for gluconeogenesis results in a marked increase in nitrogenous waste, manifested by an increase in urinary nitrogen excretion or elevations in blood urea nitrogen if the kidneys are unable to keep up (Fig. 9.1).

FUEL SUBSTRATES

The human body requires basic nutrients in the form of carbohydrate, fat, protein, vitamins, and water for maintenance. Energy exists in the form of adenosine triphosphate (ATP) and may be derived from carbohydrate, fat, or protein. It is derived most efficiently from carbohydrate (glucose and glycogen) followed by protein and fat. Protein plays a unique role as the basic structural component of all the significant biochemical, metabolic, and immunologic machinery of the body. Protein, fat, vitamins, minerals, and water provide substrates for the structural and functional (hormones, enzymes) proteins of the body.

As nutrients are utilized, varying amounts of carbon dioxide are produced for each oxygen molecule consumed. The relationship of CO_2 produced/O_2 consumed is called

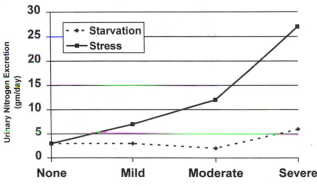

FIGURE 9.1. Urinary nitrogen excretion.

the respiratory quotient (RQ) and reflects the primary fuel being used by the body (normal RQ = 0.8). The RQ may be measured by using indirect calorimetry, which is available in many hospitals and may facilitate alimentation in many cases. An RQ of 1 reflects carbohydrate utilization, while pure fat utilization results in an RQ of 0.7. When a stressed patient is obligated to mixed fuel utilization, an RQ between 0.75 and 0.85 is usually seen. If the RQ is >1, it suggests that lipogenesis (fat production) is occurring and the individual is being overfed total calories, and carbohydrate calories in particular. An RQ <0.7 can occasionally be seen when patients are ketotic.

Energy

Carbohydrates and fats are the most efficient energy sources for humans. Carbohydrates (CHO) are stored as glycogen. This bulky hydrated molecule resides in liver or muscle. About 150 g, or 600 kcal (1 g CHO = 4 kcal when consumed enterally and 3.4 kcal when administered parenterally) can be stored in the liver, a reserve expended in the first 24 hours of starvation. Little contribution is actually made by muscle glycogen as it cannot be readily transferred into the general circulation.

Glucose remains the obligate fuel for the central nervous system, red blood cells, white blood cells, bone marrow, and adrenal medulla, even late into starvation. Though muscle, heart, and kidney adapt to the use of ketone bodies quite well, the utilization of glucose cannot be reduced to zero. Because fat cannot be converted to glucose, these requirements must be met from protein that is derived from the breakdown of viscera and skeletal muscle.

The majority of energy in the body is stored as fat; a healthy 70-kg man has about 60,000 kcal stored as fat. While an impressive reserve, the inability of all organs to utilize ketone bodies, the only source of energy available from fat, prevents the body from totally converting to energy derived from fat. Dietary fat is a highly concentrated source of energy (9 kcal/g when taken/consumed and 10 kcal/g in parenteral preparations because of the glycerol) as well as the fat-soluble vitamins A, D, E, and K. There are fatty acids that cannot be synthesized by humans and must be obtained from dietary sources; hence, they are deemed *essential fatty acids*. Linoleic acid is the predominant essential fatty acid, and linolenic the major nonessential fatty acid.

Protein

Proteins are composed of combinations of the 20 amino acids. An amino acid is composed of a keto acid and an amino group. The keto group is unique to each amino acid. The amino group, though the same for all amino acids, cannot be synthesized de novo, but can be transferred to existing keto acids by transamination, and in this way permits new amino acids to be derived from existing amino

acids. It is the amino group that contains the nitrogen moiety. The body can synthesize 12 of the keto acids (nonessential amino acids), leaving eight that are essential. Under certain conditions, such as during early childhood and following major trauma or surgery, when there are markedly increased requirements for protein synthesis, the body may be unable to synthesize sufficient quantities of certain amino acids, such as arginine and histidine; hence, they are considered conditionally essential amino acids (Table 9.2).

Proteins are degraded to small groups of amino acids known as peptides for absorption through the intestinal mucosa. They are then broken down to free amino acids, which can pass into the portal circulation. The liver extracts three fourths of the circulating amino acids for the synthesis of proteins, which are then released by the liver. A small amount of protein synthesis occurs at other sites, such as skeletal muscle. In fact, branch chain amino acids (leucine, isoleucine, and valine) are preferentially metabolized by skeletal muscle rather than the liver.

All 20 of the amino acids must be present in sufficient quantity for protein synthesis to occur. Deficiencies in even one of the essential amino acids can halt protein synthesis. The concentration of essential amino acids in particular foods determines the biologic quality. Animal foods, such as meat, milk, and eggs, contain proteins of high biologic quality, whereas vegetable proteins are more often low or deficient in one or more essential amino acids, and are therefore of less biologic quality. The preparations of amino acids for parenteral administration are specifically formulated to contain abundant amounts of the essential amino acids.

Amino acids are not only important for protein synthesis, they also play a central role in the catabolic reactions leading to the production of ATP, the transformation of keto acids to glucose or fat, the conversion of nitrogen to urea, and the use of nitrogen in the production of nonessential amino acids as well as purines and pyrimidines.

As energy needs increase with increasing degrees of stress, so do protein requirements. Protein quantities may be expressed in terms of the nitrogen content, and the terms may be used interchangeably. Most proteins contain approximately 16% nitrogen; therefore, a conversion factor of 6.25

TABLE 9.2. AMINO ACIDS

Essential Amino Acids	Conditionally Essential Amino Acids
Isoleucine (branch chain)	Histidine
Leucine (branch chain)	Alanine
Lysine	Arganine
Methionine	
Phenylalanine	
Valine (branch chain)	
Threonine	
Tryptophan	

TABLE 9.3. PHYSIOLOGIC STRESS AND THE EFFECT ON PROTEIN AND ENERGY REQUIREMENTS

	Impact on Resting Energy Expenditure	Protein (g/kg/day)	Energy (kcal/kg/day)
Normal to minimal stress	REE × 1.2	0.8	25–30
Mild stress	REE × 1.3	0.8–1.2	30–32
Moderate stress	REE × 1.5	1.3–1.5	32–36
Severe stress	REE × 2	1.5–2.0	36–40+

REE, resting energy expenditure (Harris Benedict equation):

$$males = 66 + [(13.7 \times wt\ in\ kg) + (5 \times ht\ in\ cm) - (6.8 \times age)]$$
$$females = 665 + [(9.6 \times wt\ in\ kg) + (1.7 \times ht\ in\ cm) - (4.7 \times age)]$$

Conditions that may produce a given degree of stress:
   Mild stress: Elective surgical procedures, e.g., hysterectomy, open cholecystectomy, colectomy minor burns <10% body surface area (BSA).
   Moderate stress: Urgent operative procedures, splenectomy after trauma moderate burns 10–30%, pneumonia, contained intraabdominal abscess.
   Severe stress: Multiple organ trauma including numerous long bone fractures, severe burns >50% BSA, intraabdominal infection with systemic sepsis.

is used [N (in grams) × 6.25 = protein (in grams)]. A balance between protein in and protein out is the goal in normal nutrition (nitrogen balance or nitrogen equilibrium). Urinary nitrogen excretion (urine urea nitrogen, UUN) can be measured over a 24-hour period. This accounts for the vast majority of nitrogen excreted, but there are other sites of loss (skin, gastrointestinal tract, wounds) and other forms of nitrogen (ammonia) that make up a small fraction of the total nitrogen excreted. The amount of nitrogen taken in as protein is determined and nitrogen balance can be calculated. In a normal healthy adult, 0.8 g/kg/day is adequate to maintain nitrogen equilibrium, or 0 nitrogen balance. In stressed patients, protein needs increase commonly to 1.2 to 1.5 g/kg/day and rarely as high as 2.0 g/kg/day or more. Table 9.3 lists several forms of physiologic stress commonly encountered and their approximate effect on protein and energy requirements.

The relationship between the amount of energy in a nutrient source and the amount of protein is described by the nonprotein calorie to nitrogen ratio (NPCal:N). In hospitalized patients, a ratio of 100–150:1 is usually used. For very highly stressed patients—trauma, sepsis, burns—the preferred ratio may be less than 100:1, whereas in situations that mandate protein restriction, such as renal or hepatic dysfunction, the ratio may be higher (>150:1).

Minerals and Vitamins

New dietary guidelines have been developed regarding vitamin requirements. They have focused on three levels for each vitamin: the dose to prevent deficiency, the dose that is recommended in a healthy diet, and the dose that should not be exceeded. These guidelines may not, however, be applicable to hospitalized patients. The vitamins and minerals that are most worrisome in stressed patients are vitamins A, B_6, C, folate, thiamine, iron, and zinc.

NUTRITION ASSESSMENT OF HOSPITALIZED PATIENTS

Nutrition assessment is a general term for the process by which one looks at the various body compartments, their composition individually, and the sum of their parts. It provides important objective data for classifying a patient as adequately nourished or malnourished. Malnourished may mean over- or undernourished. The goals of assessment are the early diagnosis of malnutrition, determination of the amount and type of therapy needed, assessment of the effectiveness of therapy on similar groups of patients, and correlation with the clinical course. Table 9.4 outlines some "red flags" that suggest an individual may be at increased risk of having protein-calorie malnutrition and warrants a nutrition assessment.

The diagnosis of malnutrition remains primarily clinical. As with many diseases, there is no single test available to

TABLE 9.4. WARNING SIGNS OF PROTEIN-CALORIE MALNUTRITION

Recent weight loss
Serum albumin <3.5 g/dL
Anticipated ICU stay >3 days
Associated chronic illness (DM, CHF, COPD, ASCVD, etc.)
Major surgery, illness, or injury
Obesity
Nonhealing wound or decubitus
Prolonged infection
Prolonged use of steroids, chemotherapy, or immunosuppressant
IV fluid support for >5 days
<10% of ideal body weight
Psychological problems (death of spouse, nursing home, ETOH abuse, etc.)

ASCVD, arteriosclerotic/atherosclerotic cardiovascular disease; CHF, congestive heart failure; COPD, chronic obstructive pulmonary disease; DM, diabetes mellitus; ETOH, ethyl alcohol.

establish the diagnosis; rather, it is diagnosed following interpretation of history, physical, and laboratory parameters. In a global sense, malnutrition represents a disturbance between dietary intake and an individual's needs. Contributing factors may be decreased dietary intake, increased energy requirements, and the altered utilization of nutrients. Although patients can end up with a number of selective nutritional deficiencies, protein-energy malnutrition remains the most prevalent form of malnutrition in hospitalized patients (2).

The ideal parameter for assessing nutritional status would be a simple noninvasive measurement that would delineate nutritional reserve consistently in an individual patient and reliably predict complications and outcome. Unfortunately, this ideal does not exist, so numerous methods have been devised to try to increase the overall accuracy of diagnosis. The primary goal remains the diagnosis of malnutrition when it is associated with adverse clinical outcomes, and the correction of the condition reduces the risk of nutrition-related complications. This has been defined by Mullens' group (7) as "clinically relevant malnutrition."

Anthropometric Measurements

Undoubtedly, the most common method used to diagnose malnutrition is a clinical assessment based on body weight and changes in body weight. To use body weight as a useful parameter in this regard, it is necessary to have a height and weight recorded in the medical record. In Butterworth's (8) retrospective review of patients hospitalized for 2 weeks or more, height was not recorded in 56% of the cases and weight was not recorded in 23% of the cases. In a 1990 review of blunt trauma victims at a level one trauma center, only 184 of 351 (52%) charts contained both height and weight (9). Static assessment of nutritional status provides a single data point for a patient at an isolated point in time, which may be repeated over time to establish a trend for an individual. The most obvious anthropometric measurement is patient weight. One may look at weight as a percentage of the ideal body weight based on the Metropolitan Life Insurance tables. This method is easy to use, but may not be terribly sensitive for the individual patient as the range of normality varies a great deal. Height and weight may also be used to calculate BMI (kg/m^2): weight (lbs) ×

$703/[height (inches)]^2$. A healthy BMI range is 20 to 27 kg/m^2. Values less than 19 kg/m^2 are consistent with malnutrition and over 27 kg/m^2 with obesity.

The lack of both weight and height in many patient charts significantly limits retrospective analyses of records to determine the incidence of malnutrition in hospitalized patients. One may use weight change for an individual patient, which may give slightly more reliable data. Difficulties arise using this method for a patient who is unable to give a reliable weight before the onset of his/her disease. Nevertheless, weight loss remains an important predictor of malnutrition and adverse clinical outcomes. It is likely, however, that it is associated with a substantial margin of error, and utilizing weight loss based on a recalled weight may miss a third of patients with a 10-kg weight loss, and 25% of patients would be erroneously counted as having had this weight loss (10). In general, a 10% weight loss over the preceding 6 months should raise great concern.

Weight loss was correlated with increased postoperative mortality by Studley in 1936. Since that time, it has repeatedly been correlated with an increase in surgical complications and mortality in both benign and malignant diseases. It has also been demonstrated to correlate with a decrease in median survival and response to chemotherapy in nonsurgical oncology patients. Table 9.5 summarizes the degree of malnutrition related to body weight.

There has been a widespread search for a single indicator for the diagnosis of malnutrition and for defining the risk posed by the major nutritional deficiency to hospitalized patients. Albumin, total lymphocyte count, transferrin, retinol-binding protein, and prealbumin are but a few that have been proposed and studied. Unfortunately, while each of these has some predictive power regarding complications or death, all are confounded by other clinical variables, such as the state of hydration, presence of concurrent liver disease, and infusion of albumin.

Body Compartments

Weight loss as a single parameter for predicting clinically significant malnutrition may lack sensitivity because of abnormalities of water and electrolyte balance; hospitalized patients may have an increase in total body water. The resultant edema may mask significant attrition of visceral

TABLE 9.5. DEGREE OF MALNUTRITION BASED ON BODY WEIGHT PARAMETERS

	None	Mild	Moderate	Severe
% IBW		80–90%	70–80%	<70%
BMI	20–25		19–20	<19
% weight change (1 mol/6 mo)			5%/10%	>5%/>10%

IBW, ideal body weight; BMI, body mass index.

proteins. Other anthropometric measurements can be utilized to try to define specific compartments more accurately. These include triceps skinfold (TSF) (normal: males, 12.5 mm; females, 16.5 mm; <35% malnutrition), which reflects subcutaneous fat stores, and the midarm muscle circumference (MAMC) (normal: males, 25.3 cm; females, 23.2 cm, <35% malnutrition), which reflects the skeletal muscle compartments. TSF is a simple measurement utilizing calipers, and the MAMC is calculated by measuring the midarm circumference at the same point the TSF is measured and subtracting the TSF times one tenth pi [MAMC = (midarm circumference − TSF) 0.31416]. These tests are noninvasive and inexpensive. Unfortunately, they are not consistently reliable in individual patients. The published standards vary between populations due to racial differences, so while they are applicable to epidemiologic studies, individual clinical use is limited.

Biochemical Parameters

Biochemical parameters have been advocated to provide assessment of various nutritional reserves. The creatinine : height index (CHI) has been utilized to reflect the state of the skeletal muscle mass, as there is a correlation of creatinine excretion and muscle mass. The formula is as follows: CHI = 24-hour urine Cr × 100 ideal body weight (IBW) (kg) for height. Protein calorie malnutrition is associated with a value <80% of normal; normal for males is 23 mg/kg IBW and for females 18 mg/kg IBW. CHI is a better predictor in chronically malnourished patients because it loses accuracy in stressed, injured, or septic patients. It requires collection of a 24-hour urine specimen and, therefore, is affected by changes in renal function and can be altered by dietary meats.

Visceral Proteins

Visceral proteins are commonly used as markers of malnutrition. In 1944, Cannon noted that hypoproteinemic patients had an increase in infections. In 1955, Rhoads documented an increase in postoperative complications in patients with decreased serum proteins. There are a variety of proteins that can be used in nutritional assessment. They vary in their half-lives, and therefore in the rapidity and accuracy with which they reflect change.

Albumin

Albumin is the major protein constituent of serum. It is synthesized in the liver and an alteration in nutritional status is the primary factor that decreases its production. It has a half-life of 17 days. It fluctuates significantly with the state of stress and hydration, and therefore is a better marker for chronic states than for acute ones. Several studies have

shown correlation with increased morbidity and mortality when values are less than 3 g/dL.

Transferrin

Transferrin is a serum β-globulin that binds and transports iron. It has a half-life of 8 days, and therefore is a more sensitive indicator of protein-calorie malnutrition than albumin. It may be significantly altered in the presence of coexisting iron deficiency. Significant increases in morbidity and mortality have been correlated with values less than 1.7 g/L. In addition, increases in transferrin levels with metabolic support have been correlated with improved survival.

Retinol-Binding Protein and Prealbumin

Retinol-binding protein and prealbumin have half-lives of 12 hours and 2 days, respectively. They are synthesized in the liver and hence may be decreased in liver disease. They reflect protein-calorie malnutrition, and nutritional repletion normalizes these parameters more rapidly than albumin and transferrin. Measurement of these proteins may or may not be easily available at all hospitals, and if it is a test that must be sent out to a commercial laboratory, it may not be cost-effective or clinically useful.

These are all parameters that show reasonable correlations in large populations. The influence of factors exclusive of nutritional status, however, can limit their sensitivity and specificity in any individual patient.

Immunologic Profile

Since an increase in septic complications is one of the risks of malnutrition, attempts have been made to use changes in immune function to diagnose malnutrition.

Total Lymphocyte Count

In malnutrition, the primary lymphoid structure of the immune system, the thymus, as well as secondary structures such as the spleen and lymph nodes, are altered in size, weight, and cellular components. A simple measurement of nutritional status is a blood total lymphocyte count (TLC), calculated as the white blood cell (WBC) count multiplied by the percent of lymphocytes (normal is >1,500 cells/mm^3, and malnutrition is <900 cells/mm^3). This decrease affects T lymphocytes, with B-lymphocyte numbers remaining normal or increased. It is also affected by other disease states, such as uremia, lymphoma, or medications such as immunosuppressants or chemotherapy.

Delayed Hypersensitivity Skin Tests

Response to delayed hypersensitivity skin testing has been utilized to demonstrate qualitative changes in immune function. Normal response would be induration to three or more of five skin antigens. While this may not reflect a specific defect in the immune system, anergy has been correlated with increased septic complications and mortality.

Global Assessments

Attempts to provide a more accurate diagnosis have resulted in multifactorial scores that combine several nutritional parameters in order to increase sensitivity, specificity, and accuracy. A well-studied score and the one used in the Veterans Affairs (VA) cooperative study of preoperative total parenteral nutrition is the prognostic nutritional index (PNI) (3):

$$
\begin{aligned}
\text{PNI (\%)} = 158\% &- 166 \text{ (albumin in g/L)} \\
&- 0.78 \text{ (TSF in mm)} \\
&- 2.0 \text{ (transferrin in mg/L)} \\
&- 5.8 \text{ (delayed hypersensitivity skin test scored} \\
&\quad \text{as } 0 = \text{nonreactive, } 1 = <\text{5-mm} \\
&\quad \text{induration, } 2 = \geq\text{5-mm induration)}
\end{aligned}
$$

High risk is a PNI $\geq$50%, intermediate risk is 40% to 49%, and low risk is <40%.

All of the anthropometric parameters and biochemical values have not eliminated the need for individual patient assessment and applying clinical judgment. A clinical evaluation method termed subjective global assessment (SGA) (11) looks at the following factors and findings:

Historical Factors	*Physical Findings*
Weight change	Loss of subcutaneous fat
Dietary intake change	Muscle wasting
GI symptoms of >2-weeks' duration	Ankle Edema
Functional capacity	Sacral Edema
Underlying disease	Ascites
Metabolic stress	

Based on these parameters, patients are classified as well nourished, moderately malnourished, or severely malnourished. This method has been shown to be reproducible between examiners with training and an interest in nutrition. It correlates well with future complications, with 42%, 9%, and 5% of patients in the severely malnourished, moderately malnourished, and well-nourished groups, respectively, developing postoperative complications.

NUTRITION SUPPORT

Once a patient has been classified as malnourished or at significant risk of developing malnutrition, intervention in the form of nutrition support should be considered. This may range from simple efforts, such as patient education

and assistance in picking menus that include foods the patient finds palatable, to providing all of the patients nutritional needs via total parenteral or enteral nutrition. Energy and protein requirements for an individual may be measured using indirect calorimetry and urinary nitrogen excretion, respectively. Generally, however these are estimated, using formulas such as in Table 9.3 or guidelines based upon population norms (Table 9.6). Usually, energy is provided in the form of dextrose and lipid, with 20% to 30% of calories provided as lipid. Because of the low RQ of lipid, patients exhibiting CO_2 retention and chronic obstructive pulmonary disease are occasionally provided high fat formulations, but rarely are >50% of calories provided as lipid.

Special Populations

Patients with renal or hepatic dysfunction cannot utilize protein optimally or are unable to clear the nitrogenous waste products provided. In these populations protein is restricted to between 0.6 g/kg/day and 1.2 g/kg/day in renal failure patients receiving renal replacement therapies such as hemodialysis. Energy should still be provided at doses appropriate for the degree of stress, often resulting in formulations with a high calorie to nitrogen ratio exceeding 150 : 1. Virtually all commercially available sources of parenteral or enteral protein are enriched with essential amino acids, so there is no indication to use other disease specific formulations, such as those enriched with branch chain amino acids. These have not been demonstrated to alter outcome in clinical trials and can be quite expensive.

Obesity is a chronic disease that affects over one third of the adult population and 30% to 40% of the hospitalized adult population, if defined as a BMI >27 kg/m². With progressive obesity, fat mass increases disproportionately to lean body mass, which makes formulas that estimate energy needs much less accurate in this population. In this group of patients, a strategy that provides protein at a rate of 2 g/kg of ideal body weight and restricts energy to encourage patients to mobilize excessive energy stores has been successful. These patients achieve positive nitrogen balance and are at a reduced risk of being overfed, with the attendant problems of hyperglycemia, hyperinsulinemia, etc. Energy is provided at 20 to 25 kcal/kg IBW (12).

TABLE 9.6. GUIDELINES BASED UPON POPULATION NORMS

	Protein (g/kg/day)	Energy (kcal/kg/day)
Normal to minimal stress	0.8	25
Mild stress	1.0	30
Moderate stress	1.5	35
Severe stress	2.0	40

Populations with increased growth requirements, such as children and pregnant women, require special consideration. In addition to needs for organ maintenance and disease-related stress, energy and protein substrates to permit growth must be included. It is estimated that an additional 250 to 300 kcal/day (3 to 5 kcal/kg/day) above baseline are needed to supply maternal and fetal tissues and to cover the elevated basal metabolic rate. The increase in daily protein needs for pregnancy is estimated to be about 10 g. The risk factors for malnutrition are the same as in the general population, and the selection of route for nutrition support is similar to that of the general population. The pregnant adolescent is of special concern, as this group is already at increased risk for malnutrition, and both mother and fetus have additional needs for growth above basal requirements (13).

Of particular interest are patients undergoing major surgery who may benefit from nutritional support in the perioperative period. Normally nourished individuals can tolerate elective surgery without nutritional intake for a period of 5 to 7 days. The results of the VA cooperative trial (14) and a subsequent study by Brennan et al. (15) in patients undergoing pancreatic surgery demonstrated that routine use of parenteral support in the perioperative period resulted in an increase in infectious complications in patients who were not severely malnourished.

Route of Nutrition Support

Once a patient has been identified as requiring nutritional intervention and the formulation of substrates determined, the route, enteral or parenteral, must be determined. The preferred route of nutrition support has been studied in several prospective series in humans and animals. These studies have repeatedly demonstrated that enteral feedings are associated with a reduced risk of septic complications.

The reasons for the apparent benefit of enteral nutrition are likely multifactorial. In animals, the initial effect was attributed to a reduction in the incidence of gut bacterial translocation due to maintenance of improved mucosal integrity. Several studies have documented reductions in villous height and mucosal thickness in animals maintained on parenteral nutrition. However, human studies have not shown the increase in the incidence of bacterial translocation in trauma patients to account for the increased incidence of pneumonia, intraabdominal abscesses, or other infections.

It is possible that the gut-associated lymphoid tissue (GALT) may be a mediator of this improved outcome. In addition to changes in morphology of the gut, bacterial translocation has been associated with bacterial overgrowth in the gastrointestinal tract as well as diminished levels of immunoglobulin A (IgA). The GALT has an arm that responds to antigenic challenge, with B cells being sensitized in the Peyer's patches. These activated B cells then travel through the thoracic duct to reach the lamina propria and assist in mucosal defense by the production of IgA. These cells are not confined to the lamina propria of the gastrointestinal tract; rather, they may be found within the lamina propria of the nasopharynx, bronchus, and bronchioles. This mechanism could possibly explain why the route of feeding could impact GALT, and therefore generalized mucosal immunity provide at nonintestinal sites (16,17).

In addition to these benefits of the enteral route, it appears that there are some potential problems with parenteral support. Fatty liver, hyperglycemia, and CO_2 retention have all been associated with overfeeding. It is much easier to deliver all of estimated needs to a patient parenterally; however, at times, this may result in overfeeding. Hyperglycemia, serum glucose >220 mg%, has been associated with infectious complications. Parenteral lipid emulsions have been implicated in having immunosuppressive effects as well. Finally, there are numerous mechanical and infectious complications associated with the need for a central venous catheter in order to provide parenteral nutrition (Table 9.7).

Because of the many physiologic and economic advantages of enteral nutrition support, parenteral support should be reserved for those patients in whom enteral support is impossible because of surgical absence of properly functioning gastrointestinal tract (massive small bowel resection, enterocutaneous fistulae, paralytic ileus) or for patients who have failed attempts at enteral support because of malabsorption or intolerance.

SUMMARY

Malnutrition remains a prevalent problem in the hospitalized patient. Perioperative complications occur with increased frequency in patients with moderate to severe malnutrition. Accurate clinical assessment can allow accurate estimation of nutrition-related risk and identify those patients who will benefit from early aggressive nutrition intervention. Nutrition support has become a highly sophisticated therapy allowing individualization of therapy to optimize benefit and minimize risk for the individual patient.

10 KEY POINTS

1. Malnutrition in hospitalized patients remains a common problem, with almost half of the patients suffering from mild malnutrition and a third with severe malnutrition.

2. The body has a very sophisticated response to starvation that decreases energy expenditure and conserves lean body mass. With stress, this ability to autoregulate may be lost, leading to a rapid loss in lean body mass.

3. Providing 100 g of intravenous glucose each day (2 L of D$_5$W) to hospitalized fasting patients can achieve maximal protein sparing, though nitrogen loss is never zero.

TABLE 9.7. COMPLICATIONS OF NUTRITION SUPPORT

	Either	Enteral	Parenteral
Metabolic	Hypo-/hyperglycemia Hypophosphatemia Hypo-/hyperkalemia Hypo-/hypernatremia Acid/base balance abnormalities Liver function abnormalities	Diarrhea Nausea/vomiting	Fatty acid deficiency Bone disease GI atrophy
Mechanical		Nasopharyngeal erosion Esophagitis Intestinal obstruction Aspiration pneumonia Otitis media Esophageal perforation Transtracheal tube placement w/wo pneumothorax GI tract perforation/erosion Ileus/abdominal distention	CVL site bleeding hematoma Pneumothorax Hemothorax Chylothorax Hydrothorax Arterial injury Brachial plexus injury Air embolus Catheter embolus Failure of cannulation Bacteremia/fungemia

4. The stress mediators include cytokines and eicosanoids, as well as changes in insulin and the counterregulatory hormones glucagon, cortisol, growth hormone, and epinephrine. The elevation of insulin and the counterregulatory hormones leads to increased gluconeogenesis, hyperglycemia, and suppression of lipid mobilization (lipolysis), effectively thwarting the "starvation response."

5. The diagnosis of malnutrition remains primarily clinical. Nutritional assessment should be prompted by a high index of clinical suspicion.

6. Nutrition support should be considered in the previously normally nourished individual after 5 to 7 days and in the severely catabolic or previously malnourished individual within 1 to 2 days of hospitalization.

7. If the gut is present, an initial attempt should be made to provide nutrition support via the enteral route.

8. Nutrition support has associated complications, and these need to be prevented when possible, and recognized promptly and treated appropriately when they occur.

9. Nutritional requirements in stress states and illness can be markedly increased in comparison to normal.

10. Concurrent illnesses, such as renal, hepatic, or respiratory failure, may limit the amount of protein and other nutrients that patients may be able to tolerate. These limitations must be considered when devising the appropriate nutritional formula.

REFERENCES

1. Buzby GP, Williford WO, Peterson OL, et al. A randomized clinical trial of total parenteral nutrition in malnourished surgical patients: the rationale and impact of previous clinical trials and pilot study on protocol design. *Am J Clin Nutr* 1988;47:357–365.

2. Kinosian B, Hooper F, al-Ibrahim M. Assessing the risk of malnutrition-associated complications among elderly medical inpatients. *Nutrition* 1994;10:481.

3. Bistrian BR, Blackburn GL, Vitale J, et al. Prevalence of malnutrition in general medical patients. *JAMA* 1976;235:1567.

4. Bistrian BR, Blackburn GL, Hallowell E, et al. Protein status of general surgical patients. *JAMA* 1974;230:858.

5. Hill GL, Blackett RL, Pickford I, et al. Malnutrition in surgical patients: an unrecognized problem. *Lancet* 1977;1:689.

6. McWhirter JP, Pennington CR. Incidence and recognition on malnutrition in hospital. *Br Med J* 1994;308:945.

7. Buzby GP, Mullen JL, Matthews DC, et al. Prognostic nutritional index in gastrointestinal surgery. *Am J Surg* 1980;139:160.

8. Butterworth CE. The skeleton in the hospital closet. *Nutr Today* 1974;2:4–8. (Reprinted as a nutrition/metabolism classic in *Nutrition* 1994;10:435–441.)

9. Choban PS, Weireter LJ, Maynes C. Obesity and increased mortality in the blunt trauma victim. *J Trauma* 1991;31:1253–1257.

10. Morgan DB, Hill GL, Burkinshaw L. The assessment of weight loss from a single measurement of body weight: problems and limitations. *Am J Clin Nutr* 1980;33:2101.

11. Baker JP, Detsky AS, Wesson DE, et al. Nutritional assessment. a comparison of clinical judgment and objective measurements. *N Engl J Med* 1982;306:969.

12. Choban PS, Burge JC, Flancbaum L. Nutrition support of obese hospitalized patients. *Nutr Clin Pract* 1997;12:149–154.

13. Wolk RA, Rayburn WF. Parenteral nutrition in obstetric patients. *Nutr Clin Pract* 1990;5:139–152.

14. The VA TPN Cooperative Study Group. Perioperative total parenteral nutrition in surgical patients. *N Engl J Med* 1991;325:525–532.

15. Brennan MF, Pisters PWT, Posner M, et al. A prospective randomized trial of TPN after major pancreatic malignancy for malignancy. Ann Surg 1994;220:436–444.

16. Janu P, Li J, Renegar KB, et al. Recovery of gut-associated lymphoid tissue and upper respiratory tract immunity after parenteral nutrition. *Ann Surg* 1997;225:707–715.

17. Kudsk KA, Li J, Renegar KB. Loss of upper respiratory tract immunity with parenteral feeding. *Ann Surg* 1996;223:629–635.

THE SURGICAL PRINCIPLES OF WOUND HEALING

LISA D. YEE

GENERAL ASPECTS

Wound healing is a complex and highly regulated process involving a series of diverse cellular and molecular interactions. As in embryogenesis, development, regeneration, and malignant progression and metastasis, the processes of cell migration, proliferation, and proteolytic degradation are integral to wound healing. Conceptually, wound healing represents a progression through three overlapping phases: inflammation, proliferation, and maturation (Fig. 10.1). During the inflammatory phase, hemostasis is followed by an influx of neutrophils and macrophages. The proliferative phase is marked by the migration of fibroblasts to the wound, with elaboration of interstitial matrix and collagen. Collagen remodeling occurs over years during the maturation phase. Cellular activity is regulated by factors secreted by a cell itself or its neighbors, in an autocrine or paracrine fashion, respectively (Table 10.1). Aberrant cellular signals or responses can lead to significant morbidity.

INFLAMMATORY PHASE

Wounding leads to disruption of blood vessels, followed by coagulation of blood at the site of injury (1–4). This clot consists of a meshwork of fibrin and platelets, with rapid infiltration by neutrophils and macrophages. Vasodilation and increased vascular permeability occur at the wound site.

Coagulation

The disruption of blood vessels during tissue injury is followed rapidly by transient vasoconstriction. Exposed to subendothelial collagen, platelets aggregate and secrete the vasoconstrictors serotonin and thromboxane. Within minutes, however, vasodilation occurs, in response to histamine released from platelets, which facilitates the subsequent entrance of cells and of cytokines and other soluble factors to the wound.

Coagulation is initiated with the platelet plug, which serves as the substrate for the intrinsic coagulation pathway.

Exposed collagen at the injured site activates Hageman factor (factor XII), which in the presence of high molecular weight kininogen and prekallikrein activates factor XI. Activated Hageman factor also converts prekallikrein to kallikrein, with kallikrein stimulating the continued activation of Hageman factor. Activated factor XI leads to the activation of factor IX. The cascade continues with activated factor IX triggering the activation of factor VIII, both of which then combine with platelet phospholipids to activate factor X.

Activation of factor X in the extrinsic pathway results from the release of tissue thromboplastin, namely phospholipids and glycoproteins, from injured tissue. Tissue thromboplastin in the presence of calcium ions activates factor VII, which then activates factor X.

The extrinsic and intrinsic pathways converge with the activation of factor X, with this activated factor cleaving prothrombin to thrombin in conjunction with activated factor V, calcium, platelets, and phospholipids. Thrombin enzymatically removes fibrinopeptides A and B to yield fibrin, which polymerizes in a meshed network. Thrombin itself can convert prothrombin to thrombin by activating factor XIII. This factor facilitates the polymerization of fibrin monomers and the formation of a stable clot. Contact with thrombin as well as exposed collagen leads to persistent platelet activation with the resultant release of alpha granules containing inflammatory mediators such as transforming growth factor-β (TGF-β) and adhesive proteins such as fibronectin.

Kinins and Complement

In addition to the intrinsic clotting pathway, activated Hageman factor initiates the kinin and complement cascades. Kinins are endogenous peptides that effect vasodilation and increased vascular permeability, whereas complement comprises multiple proteins that combine in various sequences and participate in such activities as cell lysis, anaphylaxis, and phagocytosis. The protease kallikrein, activated by Hageman factor in the intrinsic pathway, converts kininogen to bradykinin. Bradykinin effects vasodilation and increased vascular permeability, augmenting the hista-

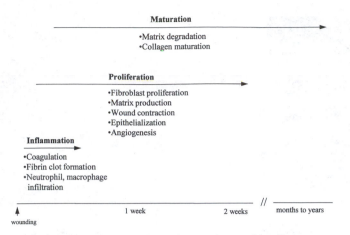

FIGURE 10.1. The three phases of wound healing.

mine-induced vasodilation associated with platelet degranulation at the onset of wounding. Kallikrein also promotes the activation and aggregation of neutrophils. Leukocyte lysosomal enzymes acting on plasma proteins lead to the production of leukokinins, which also increase vascular permeability. Plasmin formed in response to activated Hageman factor takes part in the complement cascade, activating early component C1 and cleaving C3 to create the anaphylatoxin C3a. C3a acts to increase histamine release from mast cells and basophils. Lysosomal enzymes can also activate C1 and cleave C5 to the anaphylatoxin C5a, which induces vasodilation, leukocyte chemotaxis, and histamine release.

In addition to activation by Hageman factor, the generation of C5a and C3a can also be triggered by devitalized tissue, proteases released by neutrophils, and platelet-bound thrombin. Although C3a is generally in greater abundance, C5a is the more potent of the two anaphylatoxins by two to three orders of magnitude. C5a is the major chemoattractant of neutrophils to the wound site. It also promotes neutrophil adhesion to endothelial cells.

Arachidonic Acid

Arachidonic acid is a 20-carbon fatty acid derived from phospholipids in the cell membrane, produced by the action of cellular phospholipases stimulated by tissue injury, complement component C5a, and various other factors. The metabolites of arachidonic acid include prostaglandins, thromboxane A_2, leukotrienes, and chemotactic lipids. Cyclooxygenation of arachidonic acid yields the endoperoxides prostaglandin (PG) G_2 and H_2, which undergo further modification to either thromboxanes or prostaglandins. Platelets exposed to collagen or thrombin convert the endoperoxides to thromboxane A_2, which induces platelet aggregation and vasoconstriction. Endothelial cells convert the endoperoxides to prostacyclin, an inhibitor of platelet aggregation that also increases vasodilation and tissue edema. Also derived from endoperoxides, PGE_1 and PGE_2 are potent vasodilators that augment the tissue edema generated by bradykinin and histamine.

TABLE 10.1. WOUND HEALING: CELLS AND SECRETED FACTORS

Cell Type	Product	Major Effects
Platelets	Serotonin	Vasoconstriction
	Thromboxane	Vasoconstriction, platelet aggregation
	Histamine	
	PDGF	Macrophage, neutrophil, fibroblast chemotaxis, fibroblast proliferation
	TGF-β	Macrophage, neutrophil, fibroblast chemotaxis, stimulation of collagen synthesis
Neutrophils	Lysosomal enzymes	Increased tissue and vascular permeability, release of leukokinins, activation of complements C1, C3, C5
	Nitric oxide	Cytotoxin, signaling molecule
Macrophages	TGF-β	Macrophage, neutrophil, fibroblast chemotaxis, stimulation of collagen synthesis
	PDGF	Macrophage, neutrophil, fibroblast chemotaxis, fibroblast proliferation
	TGF-α	Growth of endothelial cells and fibroblasts
	TNF-α	Stimulation of endothelial cell migration, capillary formation
	FGF	Endothelial cell, fibroblast, smooth muscle cell mitogen
	Proteases	Matrix degradation
Fibroblasts	Hyaluronic acid	Fibroblast and macrophage migration
	Proteases	Matrix degradation
	Nitric oxide	Cytotoxin, signaling molecule
Keratinocytes	Proteases	Epithelial cell migration

FGF, fibroblast growth factor; PDGF, platelet-derived growth factor; TGF, transforming growth factor; TNF, tumor necrosis factor.

Inflammatory cells such as neutrophils and macrophages activate the 5-lipoxygenase pathway of arachidonic acid metabolism, which leads to the production of leukotrienes; 5-lipoxygenase degrades arachidonic acid to 5-hydroperoxy-eicosatetraeonic acid (5-HETE). 5-HETE is an unstable compound and spontaneously breaks down into 5-hydroxy-eicosatetraenoic acid (5-HETE) or leukotriene A4 (LTA4); the latter is converted to other leukotrienes. Leukotrienes induce leukocyte granule secretion, neutrophil migration, and increased vascular permeability.

Neutrophils

Numerous chemoattractants are present at the wound site to promote the entry of neutrophils early in the healing process. Neutrophils must bind to endothelium at the wound area, pass between cells in the venule wall, and migrate into the injured tissue or clot matrix. As mentioned above, C5a is a potent chemoattractant for neutrophils. Additionally, leukotrienes and fibrin degradation products attract neutrophils to the wound. C5a also increases neutrophil adhesion to endothelium. Formyl methionyl peptides released by bacteria also attract neutrophils to the wound. Certain factors, such as interleukin-1 (IL-1) and tumor necrosis factor (TNF), may also enhance the ability of endothelium to bind neutrophils.

Although nonessential to wound healing, neutrophils are associated with lower rates of wound infection. Additionally, less tissue edema is present in wounds depleted of neutrophils. Neutrophils release microbicidal and inflammatory factors. These cells destroy bacteria by phagocytosis and by releasing oxygen free radicals. The reactive product nitric oxide (NO) results from the metabolism of arginine by nitric oxide synthase in neutrophils (5,6). NO causes the death and lysis of microbial contaminants as well as neutrophils. Free radicals also inflict endothelial damage. Armed with a number of lysosomal enzymes, neutrophils secrete a variety of proteases, elastases, and collagenases to promote tissue infiltration. As noted above, these lysosomal enzymes also act on plasma proteins to produce leukokinins, which enhance vascular permeability. Arachidonic acid metabolites generated by neutrophils contribute to platelet aggregation, increased vascular permeability, and leukocyte chemotaxis.

Macrophages

The macrophage performs vital regulatory functions in wound healing (7). By the third or fourth day after injury, macrophages replace neutrophils as the dominant cell population of the wound. Matrix components such as collagen, fibronectin, and elastin may serve to attract circulating monocytes and tissue macrophages. C5a, thrombin, and fibrin degradation products also function as chemoattractants. TGF-β is chemotactic for macrophages, released by the macrophage itself as well as by platelets and lympho-

cytes. Macrophages also secrete platelet-derived growth factor (PDGF), which amplifies the inflammatory response by attracting macrophages and neutrophils. Upon exiting the vascular system, monocytes differentiate into activated macrophages in response to fibronectin and other components of the clot matrix. In addition to removing bacteria, expended neutrophils and other cellular debris, the wound macrophage regulates fibroblast proliferation, angiogenesis, and tissue remodeling by producing a variety of enzymes, growth factors, and cytokines.

The many macrophage-secreted products include PDGF, TGF-α, TGF-β, acidic and basic fibroblast growth factors (aFGF, bFGF), IL-1, and TNF. Macrophages also secrete NO, which in addition to cytotoxicity, has numerous functions as a regulatory and signaling molecule (8,9). PDGF is chemotactic for macrophages, neutrophils, and fibroblasts, and stimulates fibroblast proliferation. In addition to inducing macrophage, neutrophil, and fibroblast chemotaxis, TGF-β also promotes collagen and matrix synthesis. TGF-α stimulates the growth of endothelial cells, fibroblasts, and epithelial cells. FGF is mitogenic for a variety of different cell types, including vascular endothelial cells, fibroblasts, and smooth muscle cells. TNF-α is an angiogenesis factor, inducing endothelial cell migration and capillary formation.

Macrophages promote degradative processes by secreting several matrix-degrading enzymes such as plasminogen activator, collagenases, and elastase. Interstitial collagenase, also known as matrix metalloproteinase-1 (MMP-1), degrades collagen, and gelatinase (MMP-9) breaks down degraded or cleaved collagen. Fibroblast collagenase production is stimulated by IL-1. TGF-β modulates this degradative activity by blocking the synthesis of collagenases and upregulating the production of metalloproteinase inhibitors.

PROLIFERATIVE PHASE

The inflammatory phase merges into the proliferative phase of wound repair. The clot matrix evolves into a more complex network, synthesized by fibroblasts under the direction of macrophages. The inflammatory response subsides as a result of decreased production of the various mediators of inflammation, enzymatic degradation, and macrophage scavenging. The proliferative phase is distinguished by fibroblast proliferation, extracellular matrix (ECM) production, wound contraction, epithelialization, and angiogenesis. Numerous cytokines are secreted by macrophages, fibroblasts, and endothelial cells, with paracrine and autocrine stimulation of mitogenic, motogenic, and synthetic activities.

Fibroblasts

Fibroblasts are drawn to the wounded area by a variety of chemotactic factors, becoming the major cell population of the wounded site by the fifth day. PDGF is a fibroblast chemoattractant secreted primarily by platelets (10). Hyaluronic acid is a glycosaminoglycan secreted by fibroblasts into the wound matrix that facilitates the migration of fibroblasts and macrophages expressing hyaluronan receptors, such as the lymphocyte receptor CD44 (11). Fibronectin induces fibroblast infiltration of the clot matrix (12); collagen also appears to stimulate fibroblast migration.

The migration of fibroblasts, as well as other cells in wound healing, involves the expression of cell surface receptors known as integrins, which bind fibronectin and other components of the ECM (13). Integrins are heterodimeric proteins composed of an α chain and a β chain, which confer specific binding affinities and distinct cellular functions (14). For example, $\alpha_2\beta_1$ binds certain collagens and laminin, and $\alpha_5\beta_1$ interacts with fibronectin (15,16). As a process of adhesion and de-adhesion, migration may require the differential expression of integrin subtypes for release from one substrate with subsequent attachment and movement to a new site. PDGF upregulates the expression of the α_5 integrin subunit in fibroblasts, which might facilitate attachment to fibronectin rich substrates such as the initial fibrin clot matrix (17). Type I collagen and TGF-β also modulate the expression of different integrins (15,18). Integrin expression thus appears to be modulated by both ECM and growth factor signals (19). Entry of cells to the injured site is facilitated by the localized breakdown of matrix components by means of proteases and collagenases released by wound macrophages and fibroblasts.

Resident and newly migrated fibroblast populations are stimulated to proliferate and secrete collagen by numerous growth factors including PDGF, FGF, TGF-β (20), and epidermal growth factor (EGF). Macrophages, platelets, and fibroblasts are responsible for the release of these mitogens. Platelets release their stores of PDGF and TGF-β upon aggregation during clot formation. Injured endothelial cells also secrete these factors as well as others to promote proliferation and matrix deposition.

Fibroblasts secrete new matrix material consisting of structural and adhesive components. One such adhesive component, fibronectin, is a glycoprotein composed of two nearly identical subunits containing binding domains for cell–cell and cell–matrix attachments; it is produced by macrophages and endothelial cells in addition to fibroblasts. It is an early matrix constituent; collagens appear several days later (21). Levels of fibronectin decline as wound healing progresses, whereas collagen becomes organized in bundles. Types I to IV are the most common collagens produced by fibroblasts, with the fibrillar types I to III differing structurally from type IV, a primary constituent of basal lamina. Type III collagen is prevalent in the early phases of wound healing, replaced later by type I to form scar. Elastin is another structural protein secreted by fibroblasts. Whereas collagen is organized into cross-linked fibrils (types I–III) or sheets (type IV), elastin is secreted into the matrix

as random coils. The matrix also contains glycosaminoglycans and proteoglycans, such as hyaluronic acid and heparin sulfate, that regulate cell adhesion, migration, and proliferation (22). A large hydrophilic molecule, hyaluronic acid, controls the diffusion of substances through the matrix and facilitates cell locomotion and migration (11). Hyaluronic acid may modulate cell proliferation by the binding of growth factors. Heparan sulfate and other proteoglycans also regulate the activation of growth factor receptors, as in the case of fibroblast growth factors and their receptors (23–25).

Unlike normal dermal fibroblasts, wound fibroblasts synthesize NO, a highly reactive lipophilic molecule that may function as a signaling molecule as well as a cytotoxin (26). Collagen deposition appears related to the production of NO by macrophages and fibroblasts; although the mechanism for the effect of NO requires elucidation, it is possibly at the posttranslational level (27). Impaired wound healing correlates with decreased NO levels (28,29).

Contraction

As fibroblasts migrate through the wound matrix, pulling themselves alongside collagen fibrils, tractional forces are exerted. In response to the mechanical forces resisting contraction and in the presence of TGF-β, certain fibroblasts differentiate into myofibroblasts. These granulation tissue fibroblasts are specialized to express contractile proteins such as the alpha smooth muscle actin, the actin isoform found in vascular smooth muscle cells. The expression of alpha smooth muscle actin is induced by TGF-β (30,31). Myofibroblasts also have massive microfilament bundles with dense bodies, similar to those identified in smooth muscle cells (32). Signals relating to the tensional status of the wound may be transmitted via integrin receptors, to facilitate coordination of cell–cell and cell–matrix interactions during contraction (33). Thus equipped, myofibroblasts may help exert forces needed for wound contraction (34,35). Lamellipodial extension appears to be the main mode of wound closure; closure via purse-string–like contraction of wound edges along an actin filament, as noted in fetal healing, does not seem to occur in nonfetal tissue (36,37). The mechanisms responsible for wound contraction require further elucidation.

Epithelialization

Re-epithelialization begins within hours of wounding an overlying epithelial layer. Epithelial cells migrate across the wound matrix, resurfacing the site of injury. Proliferation of cells at the wound edges occurs within the next 1 to 2 days. In cutaneous wounds, the leading edges of the epithelial layer move toward one another via lamellopodial movements. This sheet-like progression proceeds from the edges of the wound area or residual epidermal structures such as hair follicles. Fibronectin in the clot and matrix promote this migration (38–40). Prostaglandins may induce epithelial proliferation and migration in mucosal injury (41,42). The ubiquitous cellular signal NO is also involved in promoting epithelial cell migration during wound healing (43). Acidic fibroblast growth factor, TGF-α, and EGF appear to stimulate epithelial proliferation and migration (44–47).

In embryos, re-epithelialization occurs via a purse-string contraction along an actin cable formed at the wound periphery (48). The free epidermal edges are gathered together such that the opening closes. Lamellipodia used by adult epidermal cells during re-epithelialization are not present.

In cutaneous wounds, keratinocytes express increased levels of the protease urokinase-type plasminogen activator (uPA) and its receptor, which allows for localized proteolysis to facilitate migration through the matrix as well as alterations in cell–cell and cell–matrix attachments (49–51). uPA expression is localized to the leading edge of migrating keratinocytes (51,52). uPA may also be associated with keratinocyte proliferation (53), but migration and re-epithelialization can occur in the absence of proliferation (52). Other degradative enzymes are also required for epithelialization, including gelatinases and collagenases (54–56).

Angiogenesis

The growth of blood vessels into the avascular wound matrix requires endothelial cell proliferation and migration. In small vessels adjacent to the wound, stimulated endothelial cells migrate through the basal lamina of the vessel wall, to proliferate in the perivascular space. Vacuoles in adjoining cells coalesce and create a lumen. These small offshoots grow and fuse with other capillary buds and tubes to form an interlacing vascular network. Granulation tissue, the connective tissue filling the wound space, is characterized by prominent vascular sprouts in the fibroblast- and macrophage-generated matrix.

Soluble factors and other components of the ECM stimulate angiogenesis (57,58). Proteases allow localized proteolysis at the basal lamina and subsequent cell transit to the perivascular space. Angiogenic factors stored in the ECM can also be released by matrix-degrading enzymes. Endothelial proliferation is induced by factors such as aFGF, bFGF, TGF-α, TGF-β, vascular endothelial growth factor (VEGF), and TNF-α. aFGF and bFGF stimulate endothelial cell growth and migration. For example, bFGF induces endothelial cell expression of uPA and its receptor (uPAR), facilitating the breakdown of ECM and basement membrane barriers to migration (59). VEGF is specifically mitogenic for endothelial cells. TGF-α directly stimulates endothelial cell proliferation, whereas TGF-β is chemotactic for macrophages and thus indirectly enhances the release of angiogenic factors (60). TNF-α promotes the migration of endothelial cells and subsequent formation of tubules. Fibrin and fibrin degradation products may serve as indirect

angiogenic agents. In addition, endothelial cells themselves modulate their environment by secreting basement membrane proteins upon entry and migration through the matrix (61). Integrin $\alpha_v\beta_3$ promotes endothelial cell proliferation, migration, and survival during neovascularization (62,63). Cytokine stimulation of angiogenesis may be mediated by different vascular cell integrins, as the effects of FGF and VEGF require expression of $\alpha_v\beta_3$ and $\alpha_v\beta_5$, respectively (64).

Angiogenesis is regulated by inhibitory as well as stimulatory molecules. Angiostatin is a paracrine or endocrine inhibitor of endothelial cell proliferation (65). As tissue hypoxia stimulates macrophage expression of angiogenesis factors, capillary proliferation in the previously avascular wound space may decline with increased oxygen tension (66).

MATURATION PHASE

Wound maturation occurs over a period of years. The process of remodeling involves the opposing processes of matrix synthesis and degradation. The wound is initially well vascularized, but this regresses over time. The wound matrix proteoglycan composition also changes such that wound water content decreases. Reorganization of collagen fibers leads to strengthening of the wound.

Matrix Degradation

Plasminogen activators cleave plasminogen to plasmin, a protease with a broad range of substrates. As detailed previously, uPA is secreted by various cell types in the wound, including neutrophils, fibroblasts, keratinocytes, and endothelial cells. Tissue-type plasminogen activator (tPA) does not appear to be involved significantly in wound healing. In the early stages of wound healing, the proteolytic action of uPA leads to the breakdown of fibrin, fibronectin, and laminin, which facilitates cell migration by providing passageways as well as chemotactic degradation products. uPA activity is regulated by numerous growth factors and cytokines. Plasmin also activates other enzymes vital to the remodeling process, such as collagenases and elastases. Enzymatic activity is additionally regulated by inhibitors, such as the type 1 and type 2 inhibitors (PAI-1, PAI-2) of uPA (50,53) or the tissue inhibitors of matrix metalloproteinases (TIMPs).

Neutrophils, macrophages, and fibroblasts release procollagenases, which are converted to active enzymes extracellularly by various proteases. Collagenases are specific for certain types of collagen. Dermal fibroblasts secrete collagenase against types I to III, and macrophages produce collagenase directed against type IV. PDGF, TGF-β, and EGF are among the growth factors stimulating fibroblast production of collagenase.

Collagen Maturation

Although collagen deposition and accumulation ends at about 21 days postwounding, the breaking strength of the wound continues to increase. Breaking strength increases most rapidly between the second and sixth weeks. The strength of healed wounds is approximately 80% that of unwounded skin, attained at about 3 months (67). Wounds continue to strengthen over months to years, with collagen synthesis and degradation in dynamic equilibrium (68). This increased strength presumably results from the reorganization of collagen fibers in a linear arrangement, with additional cross-linking between and among fibrils. The diameter of the collagen fibers also increases (69). Most of the type III collagen is replaced with type I.

FETAL WOUND HEALING

Wound healing in the embryo is rapid and scarless (48,70). Only toward the late stages of fetal development is there evidence of scar formation. The inflammatory response appears muted. Early in embryogenesis, neutrophils and macrophages are not recruited to wound sites. Whereas injured tissues in adults are remarkable for prolonged elevation of TGF-β levels, fetal wounds demonstrate only transient expression of lower levels of TGF-β (71). The absence or short-lived appearance of TGF-β in fetal wounds may account for the lack of scar tissue, as TGF-β appears to induce fibrosis and scarring (72). The lack of neovascularization in fetal wounds may result from reduced levels of growth factors such as TGF-β and FGF (73).

Differences in the ECM are evident (70,74). Collagen synthesis appears to occur more rapidly in the fetus, with increased type III collagen content in comparison to adult wounds (75). Fetal wounds are also remarkable for a rapid and increased deposition of fibronectin (76). Higher levels of hyaluronic acid are found in fetal wounds, with a decrease to adult-like levels at late gestation (74,77–79). An increased amount of this large hydrated molecule may enhance cell motility and migration. Hyaluronic acid may also affect the organization of wound collagen.

The transition to an adult healing response most likely occurs over the gestational period, completed before birth in the late second or early third trimester. This transition may be related to the state of differentiation of the tissue rather than strict gestational age (48).

Abnormal Healing Response

Coordination of the processes of cellular proliferation, substrate degradation and synthesis, and cell migration is required throughout the healing of a wound. Abnormal stimulation or inhibition of any of these processes can lead to improper wound healing.

Dermal Fibroproliferative Disorders

The two types of excessive scarring, hypertrophic scars and keloids, result from an imbalance in the synthesis and degradation of wound matrix. Excessive production of ECM proteins, coupled with deficient matrix degradation and remodeling, may generate the raised, erythematous, fibrous welts characteristic of hypertrophic scars and keloids. Whereas hypertrophic scars remain within the original wound margins and may regress over time, keloids expand beyond the wound boundaries and rarely regress. Hypertrophic scars can also cause contractures. Keloids are composed of thick, large collagen fibers, while hypertrophic scars have nodules of fibroblasts and randomly oriented, thin collagen fibers (80). The tendency toward keloid formation appears hereditary. Hypertrophic scarring is typically associated with severe burns or other deep dermal injuries.

The mechanisms underlying abnormal scar formation require further delineation. Fibroblasts in keloid and hypertrophic scars may have decreased and/or deficient collagenase activity (81). Alterations in proteoglycan content are noted, with attendant changes in wound water content and collagen organization (82–84). Excessive or prolonged exposure to certain growth factors or cytokines, such as TGF-β and histamine, appears to enhance fibrosis (72,85). Fibroblasts in hypertrophic scars may produce increased amounts of collagen, in response to TGF-β (86,87).

At present, treatment of dermal fibroproliferative disorders includes pressure therapy, intralesional corticosteroids, simple surgical excision, and radiation therapy. With pressure therapy for burn scar management, custom-made pressure garments are worn continuously from the time of epithelialization until scar maturation. By occluding vessels in the hypertrophic scar, pressure therapy may generate a relatively hypoxic environment and thus prevent excessive fibroblast proliferation and collagen deposition (88). However, the exact mechanism of action of pressure is as yet unknown. Topical silicone gel sheeting is also utilized for the prevention and treatment of hypertrophic scars (89). The application of silicone gel or non–silicone gel dressings may stimulate collagenolysis, resulting in decreased scar development (90). Local injections of corticosteroids can lead to flattening of the scarred area (91). Surgical excision is generally accompanied by recurrence rates of over 50%, but improved results can be obtained by such measures as the removal of all inflamed tissues, reduction of wound tension, and postoperative corticosteroid injections into the wound edges or radiation therapy (92).

Adhesions

Postsurgical adhesions following intraabdominal operations can result in intestinal obstruction, infertility, and pelvic pain (93–95). Even laparoscopic procedures utilizing microsurgical technique lead to the formation of pelvic adhesions (96). Peritoneal repair following surgery proceeds rapidly, with the apposition of damaged areas of peritoneum leading to the formation of adhesions. The balance of fibrin deposition and fibrinolysis affects the development and character of these adhesions.

The peritoneum is a delicate membrane composed of a superficial mesothelial cell lining, with underlying layers of elastin and collagen and a rich vascular network. Interspersed among the connective tissue proteins are undifferentiated fibroblast-like cells capable of mesothelial differentiation. Following injury, the peritoneal surface is completely repaired within 1 week (97). Re-epithelialization proceeds predominantly from islands of mesothelial cells that migrate throughout the wounded areas. After the initial step of coagulation, a fibrin wound matrix forms over the injured site; apposition of two such wound surfaces leads to the formation of a connecting band. Continued deposition of fibrin is counteracted by the action of tPA, which degrades fibrin to nonadhesiogenic fibrin split products (98). Fibrinolytic activity is also influenced by the presence of plasminogen activator inhibitors, such as PAI-1 and PAI-2. Inadequate fibrinolysis leads to residual fibrin, which undergoes organization into permanent adhesions. Macrophages and fibroblasts migrate to the site, with subsequent matrix deposition and neovascularization (99). Adhesions may evolve into acellular fibrous bands or well-defined structures with mesothelium, blood vessels, and collagen and elastin fibers.

Numerous factors influence the development of adhesions. Adhesion formation is associated with peritoneal trauma sustained during surgery, including abrasion, desiccation, overheating, ischemia, or exposure to irritants such as starch, talc, or gastrointestinal fluid (97,100,101). The use of sponges in the peritoneal cavity and talc dispersed from surgical gloves induce adhesions, presumably by inducing an exaggerated inflammatory response (101). Downregulation of plasminogen activators or upregulation of PA inhibitors may be induced by inflammation and ischemia (102). Hypoxia also appears to decrease fibrinolysis (100). Peritoneal closure when closing an abdominal incision does not influence wound integrity or healing, but can generate adhesions (103). Nonetheless, even careful attention to surgical technique and tissue handling cannot fully offset the formation of adhesions.

Antiadhesion research has focused on the development of agents to prevent the apposition of wounded peritoneal surfaces (104,105). Instillation of crystalloid or dextran solutions fails to reduce adhesion formation. Antiinflammatory agents such as nonsteroidal antiinflammatory drugs or steroids appear to lack clinical efficacy against adhesions; such drugs may in fact impair other aspects of wound healing. Several adhesion prevention adjuvants demonstrate efficacy in reducing the formation of adhesions, forming a gelatinous coating that when applied to wound or deperitonealized surfaces is ultimately resorbed (106–109). Adding a fibrinolytic agent to these gels, such as tPA, may increase the antiadhesive effect (98). As TGF-β stimulates the development of adhesions, blockade of this growth factor by means of neutralizing antibody against the protein or antisense oligonucleotides to TGF-β mRNA may prove useful in adhesion prevention (110).

Nonhealing Wounds

Chronic or poorly healing wounds generally occur in the setting of another disease state, such as infection, poor nutritional status, diabetes mellitus, immunosuppression, and ischemia. Delayed healing in diabetic wounds is associated with impaired cellular infiltration during the inflammatory phase. Topical application of growth factors such as PDGF, TGF-α, FGF, and insulin-like growth factor (IGF) may accelerate closure of diabetic wounds (111–113). TGF-β appears to reverse steroid-induced impairment of wound healing (114). Nonhealing wounds in cachectic cancer patients, who may be both malnourished and immunosuppressed, appear to respond to topical granulocyte-macrophage colony-stimulating factor (GM-CSF) (115). In addition to correction of the underlying disease process, the use of exogenous cytokines or other factors may also offset deficiencies in the wound healing response.

SUMMARY

The response to tissue injury involves a highly regulated and integrated series of cellular and molecular interactions. The processes of cell migration, proliferation, and matrix synthesis and degradation are common to the different phases of wound healing. Further understanding of these processes and regulatory mechanisms will allow for the development of novel therapies to address problems of impaired and abnormal wound healing.

10 KEY POINTS

1. The wound healing process involves three interwoven phases of inflammation, proliferation, and maturation.

2. The processes of cell migration, proliferation, and proteolytic degradation are repeated throughout the different phases of wound healing.

3. The inflammatory phase of wound healing is initiated with platelet plug formation, with subsequent recruitment of neutrophils and macrophages.

4. Fibroblast proliferation, extracellular matrix deposition, wound contraction, epithelialization, and angiogenesis characterize the proliferative phase of wound healing.

5. Numerous growth factors, including platelet derived growth factor (PDGF), fibroblast growth factor (FGF), transforming growth factor beta (TGF-β) and epidermal

growth factor (EGF) are produced locally by macrophages, platelets, and fibroblasts during the proliferative phase.

6. Angiogenesis involves endothelial cell proliferation and migration, as well as the production of growth factors and extracellular matrix proteases.

7. Wound maturation is a long-term process that occurs over a period of years.

8. Wound remodeling represents a balance of matrix synthesis and degradation.

9. Abnormal healing responses represent aberrations in the balance of the synthetic and degradative processes of wound healing.

10. Nonhealing wounds can result from local or systemic disease processes such as infection, ischemia, and diabetes mellitus.

REFERENCES

1. Lind SE. The hemostatic system. In: Handin RI, Stossel TP, Lux SE, eds. *Blood: principles and practice of hematology.* Philadelphia: JB Lippincott, 1995:949–960.
2. Jesty J, Nemerson Y. The pathways of blood coagulation. In: Beutlers E, Lichtman M, Coller BS, et al., eds, *Williams' hematology,* 5th ed. New York: McGraw-Hill, 1995:1227–1238.
3. Furie B, Furie BC. The molecular basis of coagulation. *Cell* 1988;53:505–518.
4. Vaporciyan AA, Ward PA. The inflammatory response. In: Beutlers E, Lichtman M, Coller BS, et al., eds. *Williams' hematology,* 5th ed. New York: McGraw-Hill 1995:48–57.
5. Shearer JD, Richards JR, Mills CD, et al. Differential regulation of macrophage arginine metabolism: a proposed role in wound healing. *Am J Physiol* 1997;272:E181–190.
6. Nathan C. Nitric oxide as a secretory product of mammalian cells. *FASEB J* 1992;6:3051–3064.
7. Riches DWH. Macrophage involvement in wound repair, remodeling, and fibrosis. In: Clark RAF, ed. *The molecular and cellular biology of wound repair,* 2nd ed. New York: Plenum Press, 1996:95–141.
8. Nathan C, Xie Q. Nitric oxide synthases: roles, tolls, and controls. *Cell* 1994;78:915–918.
9. Schmidt HHHW, Walter U. NO at work. *Cell* 1994;78:919–925.
10. Seppa H, Grotendorst G, Seppa S, et al. Platelet-derived growth factor is chemotactic for fibroblasts. *J Cell Biol* 1982;92(2):584–588.
11. Laurent TC, Fraser JRE. Hyaluronan. *FASEB J* 1992;6:2397–2404.
12. Knox P, Crooks S, Rimmer CS. Role of fibronectin in the migration of fibroblasts into plasma clots. *J Cell Biol* 1986;102:2318–2323.
13. Hynes RO. Integrins: versatility, modulation, and signaling in cell adhesion. *Cell* 1992;69:11–25.
14. Chan BMC, Kassner PD, Schiro JA, et al. Distinct cellular functions mediated by different VLA integrin alpha subunit cytoplasmic domains. *Cell* 1992;68:1051–1060.
15. Klein CE, Dressel D, Steinmayer T, et al. Integrin alpha2beta1 is upregulated in fibroblasts and highly aggressive melanoma cells in three-dimensional collagen lattices and mediates the reorganization of collagen I fibrils. *J Cell Biol* 1991;115(5):1427–1436.
16. Schiro JA, Chan BM, Roswit WT, et al. Integrin alpha 2 beta 1 (VLA-2) mediates reorganization and contraction of collagen matrices by human cells. *Cell* 1991;67:403–410.
17. Gailit J, Xu J, Bueller H, et al. Platelet-derived growth factor and inflammatory cytokines have differential effects on the expression of integrins $alpha_1beta_1$ and $alpha_5beta_1$ by human dermal fibroblasts in vitro. *J Cell Physiol* 1996;169:281–289.
18. Heino J, Ignotz RA, Hemler ME, et al. Regulation of cell adhesion receptors by transforming growth factor-beta. *J Biol Chem* 1989;264:380–388.
19. Xu J, Clark RAF. Extracellular matrix alters PDGF regulation of fibroblast integrins. *J Cell Biol* 1996;132:239–249.
20. Mustoe TA, Pierce GF, Thomason A, et al. Accelerated healing of incisional wounds in rats induced by transforming growth factor-beta. *Science* 1987;237:1333–1336.
21. Kurkinen M, Vaheri A, Roberts PJ, et al. Sequential appearance of fibronectin and collagen in experimental granulation tissue. *Lab Invest* 1980;43:47–51.
22. Wight TN, Kinsella MG, Qwarnstroem EE. The role of proteoglycans in cell adhesion, migration and proliferation. *Curr Opin Cell Biol* 1992;4:793–801.
23. Mason IJ. The ins and outs of fibroblast growth factors. *Cell* 1994;78:547–552.
24. Schlessinger J, Lax I, Lemmon M. Regulation of growth factor activation by proteoglycans: what is the role of the low affinity receptors? *Cell* 1995;83:357–360.
25. Aviezer D, Hecht D, Safran M, et al. Perlecan, basal lamina proteoglycan, promotes basic fibroblast growth factor-receptor binding, mitogenesis, and angiogenesis. *Cell* 1994;79:1005–1013.
26. Murad F. Signal transduction using nitric oxide and cyclic guanosine monophosphate. *JAMA* 1996;276:1189–1192.
27. Schaeffer MR, Tantry U, Gross SS, et al. Nitric oxide regulates wound healing. *J Surg Res* 1996;63:237–240.
28. Schaeffer MR, Tantry U, Efron PA, et al. Diabetes-impaired healing and reduced wound nitric oxide synthesis: a possible pathophysiologic correlation. *Surgery* 1997;121:513–519.
29. Schaeffer MR, Efron PA, Thornton FJ, et al. Nitric oxide, an autocrine regulator of wound fibroblast synthetic function. *J Immunol* 1997;158:2375–2381.
30. Sporn MB, Roberts AB. Peptide growth factors and inflammation, tissue repair, and cancer. *J Clin Invest* 1986;78:329–332.
31. Desmouliere A, Geinoz A, Gabbiani F, et al. Transforming growth factor-beta1 induces alpha-smooth muscle actin expression in granulation tissue myofibroblasts and in quiescent and growing cultured fibroblasts. *J Cell Biol* 1993;122:103–111.
32. Ryan GB, Cliff WJ, Gabbiani G, et al. Myofibroblasts in human granulation tissue. *Hum Pathol* 1974;5:55–67.
33. Stephens P, Genever PG, Wood EJ, et al. Integrin receptor involvement in actin cable formation in an in vitro model of events associated with wound contraction. *Int J Biochem Cell Biol* 1997;29:121–128.
34. Welch MP, Odland GF, Clark RAF. Temporal relationships of F-actin bundle formation, collagen and fibronectin matrix assembly, and fibronectin receptor expression to wound contraction. *J Cell Biol* 1990;110:133–145.
35. Grinnell F. Fibroblasts, myofibroblasts, and wound contraction. *J Cell Biol* 1994;124:401–404.
36. Bement WM, Forscher P, Mooseker MS. A novel cytoskeletal structure involved in purse string wound closure and cell polarity maintenance. *J Cell Biol* 1993;121:565–578.
37. Martin P, Lewis J. Actin cables and epidermal movement in embryonic wound healing. *Nature* 1992;360:179–183.
38. Donaldson DJ, Mahan JT. Keratinocyte migration and the extracellular matrix. *J Invest Dermatol* 1988;90:623–628.
39. Clark RAF, Lanigan JM, DellaPelle P, et al. Fibronectin and fibrin provide a provisional matrix for epidermal cell migration

during wound reepithelialization. *J Invest Dermatol* 1982;79:264–269.

40. Couchman JR, Austria MR, Woods A. Fibronectin-cell interactions. *J Invest Dermatol* 1990;94:7S-14S.

41. Mizuno H, Kakamoto C, Matsuda K, et al. Induction of cyclooxygenase 2 in gastric mucosal lesions and its inhibition by the specific antagonist delays healing in mice. *Gastroenterology* 1997;112:387–397.

42. Uribe A, Alam M, Midtvedt T. E₂ prostaglandins modulate cell proliferation in the small intestinal epithelium of the rat. *Digestion* 1992;52:157–164.

43. Goligorsky MS, Noiri E, Peresleni T, et al. Role of nitric oxide in cell adhesion and locomotion. *Exp Nephrol* 1996;4(6):314–321.

44. Coffey RJ, Derynck R, Wilcox JN, et al. Production and autoinduction of transforming growth factor-alpha in human keratinocytes. *Nature* 1987;328:817–820.

45. Sun L, Xu L, Chang H, et al. Transfection with aFGF cDNA improves wound healing. *J Invest Dermatol* 1997;108:313–318.

46. O'Keefe EJ, Chiu ML, Payne RE. Stimulation of growth of keratinocytes by basic fibroblast growth factor. *J Invest Dermatol* 1988;90:767–769.

47. Barrandon Y, Green H. Cell migration is essential for sustained growth of keratinocyte colonies: the roles of transforming growth factor-alpha and epidermal growth factor. *Cell* 1987;50:1131–1137.

48. Martin P. Mechanisms of wound healing in the embryo and fetus. *Curr Top Dev Biol* 1996;32:175–203.

49. Groendahl-Hansen J, Lund LR, Ralfkiaer E, et al. Urokinase- and tissue-type plasminogen activators in keratinocytes during wound reepithelialization in vivo. *J Invest Dermatol* 1988;90:790–795.

50. Roemer J, Lund LR, Eriksen J, et al. Differential expression of urokinase-type plasminogen activator and its type-1 inhibitor during healing of mouse skin wounds. *J Invest Dermatol* 1991;97:803–811.

51. Roemer J, Lund LR, Eriksen J, et al. The receptor for urokinase-type plasminogen activator is expressed by keratinocytes at the leading edge during re-epithelialization of mouse skin wounds. *J Invest Dermatol* 1994;102:519–522.

52. Morioka S, Lazarus GS, Baird JL, et al. Migrating keratinocytes express urokinase-type plasminogen activator. *J Invest Dermatol* 1987;88:418–423.

53. Jensen PJ, Lavker RM. Modulation of the plasminogen activator cascade during enhanced epidermal proliferation in vivo. *Cell Growth Differentiation* 1996;7:1793–1804.

54. Woodley DT, Kalebec T, Banes AJ, et al. Adult human keratinocytes migrating over nonviable dermal collagen produce collagenolytic enzymes that degrade type I and type IV collagen. *J Invest Dermatol* 1986;86:418–423.

55. Salo T, Makela M, Kylmaniemi M, et al. Expression of matrix metalloproteinase-2 and -9 during early human wound healing. *Lab Invest* 1994;70:176–182.

56. Stricklin GP, Li L, Jancic V, et al. Localization of mRNAs representing collagenase and TIMP in sections of healing human burn wounds. *Am J Pathol* 1993;143:1657–1666.

57. Folkman J, Shing Y. Angiogenesis. *J Biol Chem* 1992;267:10931–10934.

58. Folkman J. Clinical applications of research on angiogenesis. *N Engl J Med* 1995;333:1757–1763.

59. Pepper MS, Sappino A-P, Stoecklin R, et al. Upregulation of urokinase receptor expression on migrating endothelial cells. *J Cell Biol* 1993;122:673–684.

60. Folkman J, Klagsbrun M. Angiogenic factors. *Science* 1987;235:442–447.

61. Sephel GC, Kennedy R, Kudravi S. Expression of capillary basement membrane components during sequential phases of wound angiogenesis. *Matrix Biol* 1996;15:263–279.

62. Brooks PC, Montgomery AMP, Rosenfeld M, et al. Integrin alpha v beta 3 antagonists promote tumor regression by inducing apoptosis of angiogenic blood vessels. *Cell* 1994;79:1157–1164.

63. Brooks PC, Clark RAF, Cheresh DA. Requirement of vascular integrin alpha v beta 3 for angiogenesis. *Science* 1994;264:569–571.

64. Friedlander M, Brooks PC, Shaffer RW, et al. Definition of two angiogenic pathways by distinct alpha_v integrins. *Science* 1995;270:1500–1502.

65. O'Reilly MS, Holmgren L, Shing Y, et al. Angiostatin: a novel angiogenesis inhibitor that mediates the suppression of metastases by a Lewis lung carcinoma. *Cell* 1994;79:315–328.

66. Knighton D, Hunt TK, Scheuenstuhl H, et al. Oxygen tension regulates the expression of angiogenesis factor by macrophages. *Science* 1983;221:1283–1285.

67. Levenson SM, Geever EF, Crowley LV, et al. The healing of rat skin wounds. *Ann Surg* 1965;161:293–308.

68. Madden JW, Peacock EE. Studies on the biology of collagen during wound healing: III. Dynamic metabolism of scar collagen and remodeling of dermal wounds. *Ann Surg* 1971;174:511–520.

69. Doillon CJ, Dunn MG, Bender E, et al. Collagen fiber formation in repair tissue: development of strength and toughness. *Collag Relat Res* 1985;5:481–492.

70. Dostal GH, Gamelli RL. Fetal wound healing. *Surg Gynecol Obstet* 1993;176:299–306.

71. Martin P, Dickson MC, Millan FA, et al. Rapid induction and clearance of TGF beta1 is an early response to wounding in the mouse embryo. *Dev Genet* 1993;14:225–238.

72. Shah M, Foreman DM, Ferguson MWJ. Control of scarring in adult wounds by neutralising antibody to transforming growth factor beta. *Lancet* 1992;339:213–214.

73. Whitby DJ, Ferguson MWJ. Immunohistochemical localization of growth factors in fetal wound healing. *Dev Biol* 1991;147:207–215.

74. Estes JM, Adzick NS, Harrison MR, et al. Hyaluronate metabolism undergoes an ontogenic transition during fetal development: implications for scar-free wound healing. *J Pediatr Surg* 1993;28:1227–1231.

75. Smith LT, Holbrook KA, Madri JA. Collagen types I,III, and V in human embryonic and fetal skin. *Am J Anat* 1986;175:507–521.

76. Longaker MT, Whitby DJ, Ferguson MWJ, et al. Studies in fetal wound healing: III. Early deposition of fibronectin distinguishes fetal from adult wound healing. *J Pediatr Surg* 1989;24(8):799–805.

77. Longaker MT, Chiu ES, Adzick NS, et al. Studies in fetal wound healing. *Ann Surg* 1991;213:292–296.

78. Longaker MT, Harrison MR, Crombleholme TM, et al. Studies in fetal wound healing: I. A factor in fetal serum that stimulates deposition of hyaluronic acid. *J Pediatr Surg* 1989;24:789–792.

79. Adzick NS, Longaker MT. Scarless fetal healing. *Ann Surg* 1992;215:3–7.

80. Ehrlich HP, Desmouliere A, Diegelmann RF, et al. Morphological and immunochemical differences between keloid and hypertrophic scar. *Am J Pathol* 1994;145:105–113.

81. Arakawa M, Hatamochi A, Mori Y, et al. Reduced collagenase gene expression in fibroblasts from hypertrophic scar tissue. *Br J Dermatol* 1996;134:863–868.

82. Swann DA, Garg HG, Jung W, et al. Studies on human scar tissue proteoglycans. *J Invest Dermatol* 1985;84:527–531.

83. Scott PG, Dodd CM, Tredget EE, et al. Chemical characterization and quantification of proteoglycans in human post-burn hypertrophic and mature scars. *Clin Sci* 1996;90:417–425.

84. Garg HG, Siebert JW, Garg A, et al. Inseparable iduronic acid-containing proteoglycan PG(IdoA) preparations of human skin and post-burn scar tissues. *Carbohydr Res* 1996;284:223–228.

85. Ghahary A, Shen YJ, Scott PG, et al. Immunolocalization of TGF-beta1 in human hypertrophic scar and normal dermal tissues. *Cytokine* 1995;7:184–190.

86. Ghahary A, Shen YJ, Scott PG, et al. Enhanced expression of mRNA for transforming growth factor-beta, type I and type III procollagen in human post-burn scar tissues. *J Lab Clin Med* 1993;122:465–473.

87. Zhang K, Garner W, Cohen L, et al. Increased types I and III collagen and transforming growth factor-beta 1 mRNA and protein in hypertrophic burn scar. *J Invest Dermatol* 1995; 104:750–754.

88. Kischer CW, Shetlar MR, Shetlar CL. Alteration of hypertrophic scars induced by mechanical pressure. *Arch Dermatol* 1975;111:60–64.

89. Ahn ST, Monafo WW, Mustoe TA. Topical silicone gel: a new treatment for hypertrophic scars. *Surgery* 1989;106:781–786.

90. Ricketts CH, Martin L, Faria DT, et al. Cytokine mRNA changes during the treatment of hypertrophic scars with silicone and nonsilicone gel dressings. *Dermatol Surg* 1996;22:955–959.

91. Kill J. Keloids treated with topical injections of triamcinolone acetonide (Kenalog). *Scand J Plast Reconstr Surg* 1977;11: 169–172.

92. Berman B, Bieley HC. Adjunct therapies to surgical management of keloids. *Dermatol Surg* 1996;22:126–130.

93. Stricker B, Blanco J, Fox HE. The gynecologic contribution to intestinal obstruction in females. *J Am Coll Surg* 1994; 178:617–620.

94. Peters AAW, Trimbos-Kemper GCM, Admiraal C, et al. A randomized clinical trial on the benefit of adhesiolysis in patients with intraperitoneal adhesions and chronic pelvic pain. *Br J Obstet Gynaecol* 1992;99:59–62.

95. Diamond E. Lysis of postoperative pelvic adhesions in infertility. *Fertil Steril* 1979;31:287–295.

96. diZerega GS. Biochemical events in peritoneal tissue repair. *Eur J Surg Suppl* 1997;577:10–16.

97. Ellis H. The aetiology of post-operative abdominal adhesion: an experimental study. *Br J Surg* 1962;50:10–16.

98. Holmdahl L. The role of fibrinolysis in adhesion formation. *Eur J Surg Suppl* 1997;577:24–31.

99. Milligan DW, Raftery AT. Observations on the pathogenesis of peritoneal adhesions: a light and electron microscopical study. *Br J Surg* 1974;61:274–280.

100. Raftery AT. Effect of peritoneal trauma on peritoneal fibrinolytic activity and intraperitoneal adhesion formation: an experimental study in the rat. *Eur Surg Res* 1981;13:397–401.

101. Ellis H. The hazards of surgical glove dusting powders. *Surg Gynecol Obstet* 1990;171:521–527.

102. Thompson JN, Paterson-Brown S, Harbourne T, et al. Reduced human peritoneal plasminogen activating activity: possible mechanism of adhesion formation. *Br J Surg* 1989;76:382–384.

103. Duffy DM, diZerega GS. Is peritoneal closure necessary? *Obstet Gynecol Surv* 1994;49:817–822.

104. Risberg B. Adhesions: preventive strategies. *Eur J Surg Suppl* 1997;577:32–39.

105. DeCherney AH, diZerega GS. Clinical problem of intraperitoneal postsurgical adhesion formation following general surgery and the use of adhesion prevention barriers. *Surg Clin North Am* 1997;77:671–688.

106. Burns JW, Skinner K, Colt MJ, et al. A hyaluronate based gel for the prevention of postsurgical adhesions: evaluation in two animal species. *Fertil Steril* 1996;66:814–821.

107. Rehman IU. Biodegradable polyurethanes: biodegradable low adherence films for the prevention of adhesions after surgery. *J Biomater Appl* 1996;11:182–257.

108. Costain DJ, Kennedy R, Ciona C, et al. Prevention of postsurgical adhesions with N,O-carboxymethyl chitosan: examination of the most efficacious preparation and the effect of N,O-carboxymethyl chitosan on postsurgical healing. *Surgery* 1997;121:314–319.

109. Diamond MP. Reduction of adhesions after uterine myomectomy by Seprafilm membrane (HAL-F): a blinded, prospective, randomized, multicenter clinical study. *Fertil Steril* 1996; 66:904–910.

110. Chegini N. The role of growth factors in peritoneal healing: transforming growth factor beta. *Eur J Surg Suppl* 1997; 577:17–23.

111. Greenhalgh DG, Sprugel KH, Murray MJ, et al. PDGF and FGF stimulate wound healing in the genetically diabetic mouse. *Am J Pathol* 1990;136:1235–1246.

112. Brown RL, Breeden MP, Greenhalgh DG. PDGF and TGF-alpha act synergistically to improve wound healing in the genetically diabetic mouse. *J Surg Res* 1994;56:562–570.

113. Brown DL, Kao WW, Greenhalgh DG. Apoptosis down-regulates inflammation under the advancing epithelial wound edge: delayed patterns in diabetes and improvement with topical growth factors. *Surgery* 1997;121:372–380.

114. Pierce GF, Mustoe TA, Lingelbach J, et al. Transforming growth factor beta reverses the glucocorticoid-induced wound-healing deficit in rats: possible regulation in macrophages by platelet-derived growth factor. *Proc Natl Acad Sci USA* 1989;86:2229–2233.

115. Raderer M, Kornek G, Hejna M, et al. Topical granulocyte-macrophage colony-stimulating factor in patients with cancer and impaired wound healing. *J Natl Cancer Inst* 1997;89(3):263.

11

RESEARCH DESIGN AND FUNDAMENTAL BIOSTATISTICS

JEFFREY F. PEIPERT
JOSEPH W. HOGAN

Reproductive health researchers and providers should have a common knowledge base regarding research design and fundamental biostatistics in order to critically review papers in the reproductive health literature and to plan and appropriately perform research projects. A basic knowledge of clinical epidemiology and biostatistics is indispensable as one plans and conducts reproductive research and analyzes results of research reports.

As the emphasis on evidence-based medicine increases (1), it is becoming more important to be able to evaluate the quality of medical evidence available. The U.S. Preventive Services Task Force (2) has adopted the criteria outlined in Table 11.1 to evaluate the quality of evidence (3). Some basic knowledge about research methodologies and their advantages and disadvantages is necessary to interpret studies and to evaluate evidence in the medical literature.

This chapter reviews the various types of clinical research design and discusses the essential principles of biostatistical methods. The first section provides a brief overview of various types of research design including the randomized controlled trial; observational studies such as cohort, case-control, and cross-sectional studies; and descriptive reports. We also provide a brief overview of systematic reviews of medical evidence including meta-analysis, decision analysis, and cost-effectiveness analysis. The second section provides an overview of fundamental biostatistics, including basic analytic methodology, regression models, and statistical aspects of study design.

Entire textbooks and courses of study are devoted to each of the topics introduced in this brief chapter. In the limited space allotted, we cannot provide the detail that is essential for properly conducted research and analyses. The reader is encouraged to pursue each topic in greater depth through the references provided. Researchers should not hesitate to consult with colleagues in epidemiology or statistical sciences when planning and performing research projects. Their expertise will only strengthen the scientific foundation upon which the research is based.

RESEARCH DESIGN

Overview of Research Methods

Research studies can be divided into two broad categories: experimental studies and observational studies. In experimental studies, the researcher controls the exposure to an agent or intervention. The randomized controlled trial (RCT) is the epitome of an experimental study. The RCT is considered the "gold standard" of clinical research designs. If performed with sufficient methodologic rigor, it is the study design that is least likely to be susceptible to serious biases.

The second broad category of research studies is observational studies. Cohort, case-control, and cross-sectional studies are common observational studies used in reproductive health. Since the exposure or intervention is observed rather than controlled by the researcher, these methods are more susceptible to multiple types of bias that can be introduced and can distort the researcher's results.

Both experimental and observational studies are sometimes described as "analytic" studies, as a comparison and analysis is carried out to determine associations. Descriptive studies, however, are also "observational," but no comparisons or statistical analyses are necessary. Descriptive studies include case series and case reports. These studies are often interesting clinical vignettes but have limited scientific merit.

The following subsections review the basic components of these studies and their advantages, disadvantages, and limitations. Examples of these methods in reproductive health literature are provided to illustrate important concepts in reproductive research.

The Randomized Controlled Trial

In the history of medicine and the scientific method, historians will surely regard RCTs as one of the main scientific advances in methods of clinical research in the twentieth

TABLE 11.1. STRENGTH OF RECOMMENDATIONS AS SUGGESTED BY THE CANADIAN TASK FORCE ON THE PERIODIC HEALTH EXAMINATION

Strength of recommendations

A. There is good evidence to support the recommendation that the condition be specifically considered in a periodic health examination.

B. There is fair evidence to support the recommendation that the condition be specifically considered in a periodic health examination.

C. There is poor evidence regarding the inclusion of the condition in the periodic health examination, but recommendations may be made on other grounds.

D. There is fair evidence to support the recommendation that the condition be excluded from consideration in a periodic health examination.

E. There is good evidence to support the recommendation that the condition be excluded from consideration in a periodic health examination.

Quality of evidence

I. Evidence obtained from at least one properly designed randomized controlled trial.

II-1. Evidence obtained from well-designed controlled trials without randomization.

II-2. Evidence obtained from well-designed cohort of case-control studies, preferably from more than one center or research group.

II-3. Evidence obtained from multiple time series with or without the intervention. Dramatic results in uncontrolled experiments (such as the results of the introduction of penicillin treatment in the 1940s) could also be regarded as this type of evidence.

III. Opinions of respected authorities, based on clinical experience, descriptive studies, or reports of expert committees.

From Canadian Task Force on the Periodic Health Examination. The periodic health examination. *Can Med Assoc J* 1979;121: 1193–1254, with permission.

century (4). The idea of doing controlled trials, however, is not new. In the Bible, Daniel proposed a trial in which youths would eat either royal cuisine or a "kosher" collection of leguminous plants and water, and the "health" of the two groups would then be compared (5). R. A. Fisher and W. A. Mackenzie (6) proposed the concept of assigning treatment by randomization in 1923 for application in agricultural research.

The RCT is the criterion standard upon which other research methodologies are compared and by which medical interventions should be evaluated (7). The major advantage of the experimental design over observational studies is the strength of causal inference it offers. The major advantage of an RCT is its ability to control for the influence of known and unknown confounding variables (8).

The design of an RCT is based on five major steps:

1. Assemble the population of interest or the study population.

2. Evaluate the population's baseline characteristics.

3. Randomly assign participants to two or more study groups.

4. Apply treatment/intervention or placebo, preferably in a blinded fashion.

5. Follow the groups over time and measure outcome variables (blindly, if possible) (8).

A number of methodologic issues must be addressed in a properly performed RCT. The author must clearly list inclusion and exclusion criteria that are appropriate to the research question. Potential subjects with a contraindication to the intervention must be excluded. It is important to measure baseline characteristics that are known or potential predictors of the outcome. The effect of confounding variables should be considered. An adequate sample size should be determined a priori, and plans for recruitment and retention should be consistent with these calculations.

It is important to allocate patients in a truly random fashion, such as with a random number table or computer-generated random assignment, rather than by hospital number or day of the week. Concealing the assignment such as with opaque envelopes is necessary to avoid knowledge of treatment assignment (9). The investigator is therefore less likely to influence or "game" the randomization scheme to get patients into the preferred treatment group. It is important to blind the investigator and the subject to the group assignment (double-blind approach), if possible. This assures that the subject's follow-up and evaluation of the outcome will be performed in a strictly objective manner, and is uninfluenced by group assignment.

There are a number of important principles to keep in mind when analyzing the results of the RCT. One is the concept "once randomize, analyze." If many of the patients have been dropped from the analysis, the research should be carefully scrutinized, and the results may be subject to investigator bias.

There are many advantages to a properly performed RCT. The experimental method provides the greatest strength of causal inference and is the highest level of evidence to test the efficacy of treatment programs. If performed properly, randomization protects against selection bias and confounding if sample size is adequate. In addition, the possibility of ascertainment bias, diagnostic suspicion bias, and detection bias can be minimized with blinding of the participant and the evaluator.

The disadvantages of a randomized trial include expense, feasibility, and whether it is ethical to randomize patients to intervention or placebo. As an example, how can we randomize patients to a specific contraceptive method, smoking, or a specific risk factor for ovarian cancer? RCTs also may not be generalizable to the general population due to the strict inclusion and exclusion criteria of the trial, and the fact that patients who consent to participate may be different from nonparticipants. For these reasons, we often must turn to observational studies for answers to many clinical questions.

Observational Studies

Cohort Studies

Since RCTs cannot always be performed because of ethical and feasibility considerations, observational studies are often necessary. There are two major groups of observational studies: cohort (longitudinal or follow-up) and case-control. A cohort study is carried out by assembling a group of individuals who have been "exposed" to a medication, risk factor, or some agent and comparing this group to a control group of patients who have not been exposed. These two groups are followed longitudinally (over time) and evaluated for a specific outcome of interest (Fig. 11.1).

One classic example of a cohort study in the reproductive health literature is the Nurses' Health Study (10,11), one of the most comprehensive cohort studies ever performed. Thousands of nurses are followed over time with comprehensive interviews and medical record reviews to evaluate various risk factors (e.g., oral contraceptive use or estrogen replacement therapy) and the development of a disease (e.g., breast cancer or cardiovascular disease). A second recent example is the U.S. Collaborative Review of Sterilization (CREST) study (12), which followed over 10,000 women for 8 to 14 years to determine the long-term failure rates of tubal sterilization. This study helped to redefine rates of method failure that we quote to our patients.

One major advantage of cohort studies is increased "generalizability," that is, the likelihood that the findings of the study are representative of the population of interest. Since patients do not need to accept randomization and are not excluded due to the very rigorous (and sometimes limiting) exclusion criteria of an RCT, a wider range of patients with varying characteristics can be included and studied. A second major advantage is the opportunity to study agents or interventions that are not amenable to randomization. Cigarette smoking, for example, cannot be studied in an RCT as we cannot ethically and realistically randomize subjects to smoking! Therefore, a cohort study or some form of observational study must be utilized.

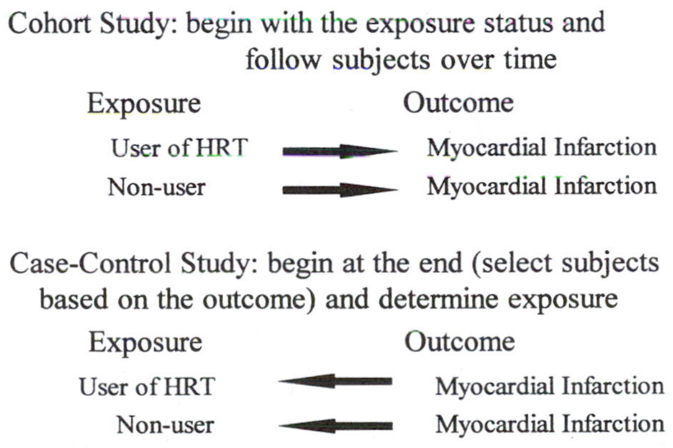

There are two main reasons why cohort studies are much weaker than RCTs in establishing causation. Since a clinician's decision to recommend a specific therapy and a patient's choice to accept therapy are clearly nonrandom decisions, we have lost one of the major strengths of an experimental method (randomization), which helped assure that the two groups are equal at baseline. Consider the example of oral contraceptive use. Women who use oral contraceptives may have very different baseline characteristics from women who use other forms of contraception or no contraception. These characteristics may be related to the outcome of interest. The second major limitation of cohort studies is that women receiving an intervention or medication may be cared for or evaluated differently from women who do not. Again, using the oral contraceptive example, women on oral contraceptives are more likely to be seen on a regular basis than women using an over-the-counter contraceptive. As a result, there is an increased chance of detecting an abnormality. This is called "diagnostic access" or "diagnostic suspicion" bias. Well-done cohort studies will attempt to control for differences in baseline characteristics and confounding variables through stratification and multivariate analysis. However, it is impossible to control for unknown or unmeasured confounding variables. As a result, cohort studies cannot provide the strength of association as evidence of causation that randomized trials can provide.

Case-Control Study

The case-control study is the second major class of observational studies. While the cohort study begins with an exposed and an unexposed group, the case-control study "begins at the end" by choosing subjects based on the outcome (Fig. 11.1) (13). Patients with a disease (cases) are compared to individuals without the disease (controls) to determine whether the exposure and the disease are associated. Since case-control studies select individuals based on the outcome or disease, they can only study one outcome but may evaluate several exposures. The Cancer and Steroid Hormone (CASH) Study, which evaluated the association of cancer (the disease) and the exposure (hormones), is a classic example of a case-control study (14).

One major advantage of case-control studies is that they are highly efficient. They often require the fewest number of patients (compared to an RCT or cohort study) to demonstrate an association and can be done in less time and with less money, especially when the disease in question is rare or takes years to develop. For example, consider how long it would take to evaluate a cohort of women using oral contraceptives (usually at a relatively young age) for the development of ovarian cancer.

Case-control studies, however, are easy to do poorly and are prone to numerous biases (13). As an example, the Women's Health Study was a multicenter case-control study

Cohort Study: begin with the exposure status and follow subjects over time

Exposure	Outcome
User of HRT	Myocardial Infarction
Non-user	Myocardial Infarction

Case-Control Study: begin at the end (select subjects based on the outcome) and determine exposure

Exposure	Outcome
User of HRT	Myocardial Infarction
Non-user	Myocardial Infarction

FIGURE 11.1. Study design of cohort and case-control studies.

to evaluate the relationship between pelvic inflammatory disease (PID) and the intrauterine device. As a result of a poor choice of control group (condom users), the study reported an inflated estimate of the relationship between the intrauterine device and PID, since condoms are known to protect against sexually transmitted diseases (15). As a general rule, the control group should be representative of persons at risk of the disease and should have the same opportunity for exposure as the cases. Therefore, the choice of control group is critical in these studies.

Cross-Sectional Studies

The cross-sectional studies fall somewhere in between observational studies, which can test hypotheses, and purely descriptive studies. Cross-sectional studies can be thought of as a "snapshot" of a group of individuals, some of whom have the disease (outcome) and exposure and some of whom do not. Associations between disease and exposure can be evaluated in cross-sectional studies; however, the temporal relationship between the two cannot be established. Consider the following example: a large group of young women, some of whom are using oral contraceptives (exposure) and some of whom are not, are assembled and we obtain prolactin levels in all the women. In this cross-sectional study, we may discover that there is an association between oral contraceptives and elevated prolactin levels. We cannot conclude from this finding that oral contraceptives "cause" elevations in prolactin, since we cannot be sure that oral contraceptives were administered before the elevation in prolactin. It is possible that women with elevated levels (and more irregular bleeding) are more likely to be prescribed oral contraceptives.

Cross-sectional studies are also called prevalent studies since they commonly use prevalent cases rather than incident cases (newly discovered cases during a period of follow-up). As a result, a temporal relationship usually cannot be established, and the information provided can be misleading.

Descriptive Studies

Case reports and case series are called descriptive studies. They represent the least sophisticated of study designs. The purpose of such studies is to assess and describe a finding in a case or group of cases. In descriptive studies, inferences regarding causal relationships cannot be drawn. However, these studies serve a role as the basis for future observational studies and clinical trials (hypothesis generation).

Descriptive studies have some advantages, despite their major limitations. Data are often already collected or relatively easy to obtain. Sources of information include hospital records, laboratory reports, morbidity and mortality documents and surveys, and questionnaires. It is usually unnecessary to perform statistical analyses; descriptive findings such

as percentages are all that is necessary. The cost of the study is low, and ethical problems are minimal.

These studies, on the other hand, are flawed by the lack of a comparison group and by the potential biases of the investigators. It is not possible to determine cause and effect in these studies. As an example, Caillouette and Koehler's (16) report of seven women who developed functional ovarian cysts while on phasic contraceptive pills represents a descriptive study. The authors' assertion that "phasic contraceptive pills may be a threat to patient health and safety" was later further investigated and refuted (17).

Screening and Diagnostic Tests

Cross-sectional studies are typically utilized to evaluate screening and diagnostic tests. The reader must first understand the concepts of reproducibility and validity to interpret and apply the results of screening and diagnostic tests. A test should consistently give the same result upon retesting (reproducibility). It should also closely correlate with the gold standard test for the presence of a particular disease or, if such a standard is not available, it should correlate with another objective measure of predictive ability (validity).

The other important concepts that the reader should understand include the diagnostic indices: sensitivity, specificity, and predictive value. A test's validity depends on its ability to correctly identify those with the outcome of interest (sensitivity or the proportion of patients with the disease who will have a positive test) and those without the outcome of interest (specificity or the proportion of nondiseased individuals who will have a negative test).

Figure 11.2 is a 2 $\times$ 2 table that illustrates the possible combinations of test results and presence or absence of a condition. Sensitivity is calculated as the number of patients with both a positive test and the presence of a condition (true positives) divided by the total number of patients with the condition regardless of the test results (true positives + false negatives). Specificity is calculated by dividing the number of patients with both a negative test result and the absence of the condition (true negatives) by the total number

| | Disease Status | |
Test Result	Present	Absent
Positive	TP	FP
Negative	FN	TN

Sensitivity = TP / (TP + FN)
Specificity = TN / (TN + FP)
PPV = TP / (TP + FP)
NPV = TN / (TN + FN)

FIGURE 11.2. Table for the calculation of sensitivity, specificity, and predictive values.

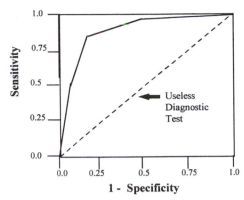

FIGURE 11.3. Receiver operating characteristic curve.

of patients without the condition (true negatives + false positives). Good screening or diagnostic tests should possess both high sensitivity and specificity and be reliable in clinical practice. When assessing the clinical applicability of a test, a broad spectrum of patients both with and without the condition under study must be tested (18,19).

It is often difficult to find a test with both high sensitivity and specificity. Choosing a cutoff for a screening or diagnostic test, then, will depend on the circumstances for the evaluation. When screening for malignancies, for example, high sensitivity (few false-negatives) is clearly the aim. On the other hand, a screening test for a less serious condition may benefit from high specificity (few false-positives).

When choosing a cutoff value for a diagnostic test, the receiver operating characteristic (ROC) curve is essential. The ROC curve allows the researcher to see the relationship between sensitivity (plotted on the y-axis) and 1 − specificity (plotted on the x-axis). Cutoff points can then be chosen along the generated curve that best correlate with the desired characteristics of the test being studied (Fig. 11.3).

More useful to the clinician than sensitivity and specificity are predictive values. Predictive values are based on the test's ability to predict the presence or absence of the disease given a positive or negative test. Using the 2 × 2 table (Fig. 11.2), the positive predictive value is expressed as the number of true positives divided by the number of patients with a positive test (true positives + false positives). The negative predictive value is calculated as the number of true negatives divided by the number of individuals with a negative test (true negatives + false negatives).

Bayes' theorem is another means of determining predictive values based on the known sensitivity and specificity of the test and the prevalence of the disease in the population. The formulas for calculating predictive values are below:

Positive predictive value
= (sensitivity × prevalence)/
[(sensitivity × prevalence)
+ (1 − specificity) × (1 − prevalence)]

Negative predictive value
= (specificity) × (1 − prevalence)/
[(specificity × (1 − prevalence)
+ (1 − sensitivity) × (prevalence)]

Systematic Reviews of Medical Evidence

Clinicians and researchers are often asked to summarize the evidence regarding a specific clinical issue or research question. Systematic reviews of medical evidence are published with increasing frequency in the literature on reproduction (20). Three types of systematic reviews—meta-analysis, decision analysis, and economic analysis—should be familiar to practicing clinicians and researchers. A brief overview of each of these methods is provided.

Meta-Analysis

The technique of meta-analysis is a method of combining data from several studies to produce a summary measure of the effect of a treatment, an intervention, or a risk factor for a specific outcome. Meta-analysis has been used to summarize both experimental (21) and nonexperimental data (22), and is becoming an increasingly popular method of summarizing a body of literature (20). This method is particularly useful when the outcome of interest is rare, when available studies are not large enough to show significant differences, or when different studies of the same question give conflicting results. Meta-analysis is also useful to define deficiencies in the medical literature in a specific area, and to define methodologic issues that may improve the study of a particular question. The discipline of obstetrics and gynecology has been a leader in the development and dissemination of meta-analyses (21).

There is considerable controversy about the validity of meta-analysis, especially when it is applied to nonexperimental data (23). All readers of the medical literature should have some familiarity with the elements of a good meta-analysis in order to evaluate the validity, quality, and clinical usefulness of reports of meta-analysis. It should be emphasized that meta-analytic techniques cannot overcome flaws in the design and execution of individual studies. The results of a meta-analysis are only as good as the studies that it contains (the "garbage in, garbage out" phenomenon).

There are several important differences between meta-analysis and traditional literature reviews. Meta-analyses and all systematic reviews are intended to reduce the subjectivity inherent in an unstructured review. Meta-analysis uses a systematic means of finding all the studies available on a particular topic usually using computer literature searches. Search terms used by the investigators should be specified so that the method of finding the studies is explicit and reproducible. It is often necessary to supplement computer searches with hand searches of bibliographies of relevant textbooks and journals since computer literature searches often fail to identify pertinent studies (24). In addition, experts in the field are often contacted to inquire about studies that the authors may have missed. Authors should explicitly state what methods of literature search were used. These methods are designed to ensure that all the available evidence on a subject is obtained.

Inclusion and exclusion criteria for the relevant articles in the meta-analysis are then developed. Criteria might include particular dates or languages of publication, or they may pertain to study design (e.g., only randomized trials) or study outcomes. Studies found in the literature search are then subjected to the established criteria, and studies are selected based on specified inclusion and exclusion criteria.

Once studies are selected, data on study design, exposure variables, outcomes, and important covariates are systematically collected. The purpose of meta-analysis is to combine data from studies in similar populations, which have examined the same relationship between the exposure (intervention) and outcome. All studies of a particular question are not alike. Therefore, once data on the measure of effect, such as an odds ratio or relative risk (risk ratio), are available from each study, statistical procedures are used to evaluate heterogeneity between studies. Testing for heterogeneity assesses whether there are very divergent results between studies or very different effects of a particular exposure on an outcome. If significant heterogeneity between studies is found, it suggests that the study populations or study designs were different. If significant heterogeneity is found, it may not be appropriate to combine results into a summary of the effect. Statistical methods to deal with such heterogeneity should be used in reported meta-analyses. If not, studies may be inappropriately combined, and summary results may be invalid.

Once heterogeneity has been addressed and excluded, study results can be combined. A summary measure of effect (such as an odds ratio) is typically calculated, which describes the overall effect found in the included studies. Traditional literature reviews can describe, in qualitative terms, the findings of a body of literature. Meta-analysis provides a method for quantitatively summarizing the results of several studies and producing a quantified summary measure of effect.

While meta-analysis is an attractive method of summarizing data, one should be cautious not to overinterpret the results. Meta-analysis cannot overcome flaws in the design or execution of the studies that are contained in it. The technique of weighting studies with a quality score has been proposed by some meta-analysts so that high-quality studies receive more weight in the summary statistic (25). An alternative strategy is to use measures of study quality, such as blinding or adequate randomization methods, in the inclusion criteria when selecting studies at the outset. The

effect of quality can also be explored by doing analyses with and without studies of low quality, and examining the effect on the overall summary statistic. Whichever method is chosen, some attention to the quality of the studies contained in the meta-analysis is essential for the reader to understand the overall quality of the meta-analysis itself.

Decision Analysis and Economic Analysis

Decision analysis and economic analyses are additional methods of combining information and systematically reviewing data to arrive at a summary conclusion. Decision analysis uses a quantitative approach to assess the relative values of different management options. The process is initiated by systematically breaking down a clinical problem into its components and creating an algorithm or "decision tree" to represent the components (parameters) and decision options. After a careful review of the literature and consultation with expert opinion, a range of probability values for each of these parameters is determined. Analysis of the decision tree is carried out using statistically based methods, and a net value of the different decision options in relation to each other is determined (26). Sensitivity analysis is a technique used to test how variations in these probabilities can affect the conclusions of the decision analysis.

Economic analyses, such as cost, cost-benefit, and cost-effectiveness analysis, are similar to decision analysis, but focus on monetary cost. Once a decision analysis is performed, data on costs of various management options are collected, and costs of the options are compared. The major difference between cost-benefit analysis and cost-effectiveness analysis is that the latter method values some of the consequences of the decision options in nonmonetary terms, such as years of life saved or disability avoided (26).

Health Services Research

The field of health services research is applied research that often combines the work of many disciplines to study an aspect of medical care delivery. Health services research studies can be methodologic, descriptive, analytic, or experimental (27). While there is considerable overlap between health services and what is considered traditional clinical research, health services research studies demonstrate how health care delivery systems, health policies, payment structure, and provider-patient interactions affect health. Health services methodologies can be used to study traditional clinical topics, such as the effect of a particular disease or treatment on health. However, it is often distinct from clinical research in the way that health and disease outcomes are measured and defined. In addition, health services research often uses methodologies such as meta-analysis, decision analysis, and cost-benefit analysis to synthesize data and compare different treatment strategies.

The variation in health care utilization is one area of health services research that examines differences in utilization between different geographic areas. These studies, called "small area variation studies," show that there is wide variation in the use of particular procedures and in hospitalization rates for certain diagnoses between geographic areas (28–30). This finding led to speculation about overuse or underuse of particular procedures in some areas, and spawned the development of methodologies to examine the appropriateness of medical care (31).

One specific method used in health services research is the creation of clinical scenarios in which procedures are deemed appropriate, equivocal, or inappropriate, as rated by expert panels, and then comparing these scenarios to actual practice. Appropriateness of carotid endarterectomy (32), coronary artery bypass graft surgery (33), and hysterectomy (34) are a few examples of what has been studied in this way. Significant levels of inappropriate use of procedures were found in each case. As an outgrowth of studies documenting the wide variation in health care utilization and possible inappropriate use of some procedures, guideline development and dissemination has become another important area of health services research (27).

Outcomes Research

The focus of health services research is measuring the health outcomes of medical interventions and services. Outcomes research attempts to define the effectiveness of medical interventions, and uses a broader definition of outcomes than traditional clinical studies. Outcomes research considers patients' subjective assessment of their own health—an important measure of the effectiveness of medical care. Methodologies from psychology and other social sciences have been used to devise and refine measures of functional status, psychological well-being, social functioning, general well-being, and other patient-rated domains. Several of these assessment tools have proven to be reliable and valid methods for assessing the results of care (35).

Outcomes research emphasizes the "real-world" situation, rather than the somewhat artificial conditions of the RCT. Randomized trials usually occur in academic institutions with highly trained physicians and with patients who fit stringent inclusion criteria. Outcomes research attempts to study the outcomes of care provided by regular doctors to regular patients. This is sometimes referred to as the study of effectiveness of care, as opposed to the study of "efficacy," which is the study of care under ideal conditions. The observational nature of outcomes research is both a strength and a limitation. A comparison of outcomes of different treatment options in nonrandomized populations requires detailed data on covariates, comorbidities, and confounding variables in order to properly control for a mixing of effects. Large administrative data sets are often used to do outcomes research. These data sets, however, are often limited in the availability of important covariates.

These above-mentioned studies are just a few examples of health services research. They share the common thread of studying the effects of the structure and process of medical care on the health outcomes of individuals and populations.

Interpreting the Medical Literature

Epidemiologic studies cannot prove causation. However, they can be used to determine the likelihood of causation. Some criteria to consider to determine a cause-and-effect relationship include:

Strength of the association: the stronger the association, the more likely it is to be real.

Consistency of the study findings over numerous reports.

Temporal relationship: Does the cause precede the effect?

Biologic plausibility: Does the relationship make biologic sense?

Biologic gradient: Is there a dose-response relationship?

Is there experimental evidence to support or refute the association?

A skilled and critical reader of the medical literature should be able to characterize the methodology of a research study and recognize its scientific value. When interpreting the medical literature, however, the reader should consider not only the methodology (e.g., randomized trial, observational study, etc.), but also the quality of the study. Critical reviewers of the literature should no longer accept the "gospel of the expert." Opinions of authorities and reports of expert committees are no longer acceptable as sound evidence. An astute reader will evaluate the evidence available from quality studies in the medical literature and recognize when evidence to support a specific practice or association is weak and in need of further study.

FUNDAMENTALS OF BIOSTATISTICS: OVERVIEW

We now review fundamental concepts and implementations of biostatistical methods, which encompass summarizing data, drawing basic inferences, interpreting and reporting results, and considering the statistics of study design (such as power and sample size). There are many study designs and data structures that are not easily handled with basic methodology, and which unfortunately cannot be given full treatment in this chapter. These are mentioned briefly.

We base our discussion of biostatistical methods on several published and ongoing studies in obstetrics and gynecology. Abbreviated analyses and interpretations are presented, with particular attention to identifying the most appropriate analysis and interpretation. Wherever possible, we highlight similarities and differences between clinical and statistical interpretations, and the relevance of each. Our goal is to assist the reader in choosing an analytic method and understanding the results of an analysis. Computational formulas are not given, primarily because they can be found in any introductory text in biostatistics. All analytic methods discussed here can be carried out on reasonably equipped statistical software platforms.

This section is divided into three parts: basic analytic methodology, regression models, and statistical aspects of study design. In our discussion of basic methods, we focus on tools for measuring association and making two-group comparisons; topics in this section include the *t*-test, rank sum test, correlation, 2-by-2 tables, odds and risk ratios, and survival estimation. The discussion of regression models demonstrates that most of the basic methods can be generalized to multivariable situations; for example, the *t*-test can be formulated as a least squares regression, from which point the effects of other explanatory variables can be investigated simultaneously. The discussion of regression outlines and illustrates least squares, logistic, and proportional hazards regression models. Finally, we discuss several statistical issues related to study design, such as power and sample size. We provide a checklist of considerations for calculating an appropriate and realistic sample size, and we illustrate with an example.

Many studies in clinical medicine and public health require design and analysis well beyond the basics. To name a few, these include complex observational studies with multiple sources of confounding and bias, multicenter randomized trials, and long-term longitudinal studies with survival end points or repeatedly measured outcomes. In most circumstances, handling design, analysis, and inference for complicated or very large studies such as these require enlisting the collaborative efforts of an experienced biostatistician or epidemiologist. We close with some discussion of the evolving collaborative relationship between medical and statistical investigators.

BASIC ANALYTIC METHODS

Continuous Response Variables

Example 1: A Randomized Clinical Trial Comparing Staples and Sutures for Wound Closure Following Cesarean Section

The data that we use to describe a wide variety of analytic tools for continuous outcomes are taken from a study of pain in 50 women who underwent cesarean section (36). Each woman was randomly assigned to have her wound closed by either staples ($n = 25$) or subcutaneous suture ($n = 25$), and afterward reported the number of pain pills taken in the hospital following surgery. Figure 11.4 shows a histogram of the number of pain pills taken in each group, and appears to indicate that, on balance, those in the suture group took fewer pain pills.

Before discussing numerical summaries, it is important to distinguish between statistics, which are calculated from a sample of data, and parameters, which refer to underlying but unobservable features of a population. In this example, the true mean of the number of pain pills taken by all women who have their wound closed by suture is unknown. We use the sample mean, which is a statistic calculated from the 25 women in the suture group, to estimate the true mean, which is the parameter referring to all women who receive sutures. Very often, the distinction between parameters, which are unknown quantities, and statistics, which are calculated from data, is not made explicit; however, it is important to understand the difference when interpreting confidence intervals (CIs) and *p*-values.

Summary Measures

Table 11.2 lists, for each group, the sample mean, the sample standard deviation, the standard error of the mean, and a 95% CI for each mean. Standard deviation is a measure of variability among the observed data, and can be roughly interpreted as the average absolute difference

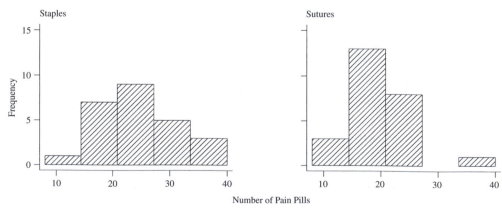

FIGURE 11.4. Pain pill histogram.

TABLE 11.2. SUMMARY STATISTICS FOR NUMBER OF PAIN PILLS TAKEN BY WOMEN WHO HAD C-SECTION WOUNDS CLOSED BY SUTURE AND STAPLES

Closure Method	n	Mean	Standard Deviation	Standard Error	95% Confidence Interval
Staples	25	24.6	6.9	1.4	(21.8, 27.4)
Sutures	25	19.7	6.2	1.2	(17.2, 22.3)
Difference		4.9	—	1.8	(1.2, 8.6)

between one observation and the sample mean. Among patients receiving sutures, the mean number of pain pills is 19.7 and the standard deviation is 6.2. Some women's pill counts are near 19.7 and some are far from it; on average, pill counts deviate by about 6 from 19.7. Standard deviation tells us how tightly observations cluster around the mean. In the staples group, the standard deviation is 6.9, indicating slightly more variation in the pill counts; this is evident in the histogram.

Because the sample mean is calculated from data, it is, like all other statistics, a random quantity. It does not represent the true mean, but rather an estimate of the true mean. If we drew a second sample of 25 women who underwent C-section, closed their wounds with sutures, and counted the number of pain pills taken in the hospital, surely we would get a different estimate of the population mean. Each new sample would yield a new estimate of the population mean. The standard error of the mean (or simply, standard error) refers to the variability of the sample mean; it estimates the standard deviation of all the sample means we could calculate from new groups of women. For the 25 women in the suture group, the standard error of the mean pill count is 1.2; thus, for samples of 25 women, the estimated mean will typically differ from the true mean by 1.2 pills. All statistics have an associated standard error, not just the sample mean.

Standard error is the usual quantity with which precision of an estimate is measured. In the case of the sample mean, standard error is found by dividing the standard deviation by the square root of the sample size: $SE = SD/\sqrt{n}$. From this equation, we see that increasing sample size decreases standard error and hence increases precision. If our sample size in the suture group was 50 instead of 25, the standard error would be $6.2/\sqrt{50}$.

The last summary elements in Table 11.2 are the respective 95% CIs for each mean. CIs are calculated by invoking a property of the normal distribution (or bell-shaped curve). Starting at the center of a bell-shaped curve, 95% of the area under the curve is covered by moving about 2 standard deviations in each direction. Recall that the standard error is the standard deviation of the sample mean. The bounds of a 95% CI for the mean are found by starting with the sample mean, and then adding and subtracting 1.96 ×

(standard error). A 95% CI is said to contain the true value of the parameter—in this case, the mean—with 95% probability.

Comparing Means

The primary question in this study is whether the two means differ. To answer this question formally using the data, we form a hypothesis to be tested. Typically, statistical hypotheses are statements of no difference (referred to as the null hypothesis), and the evidence against the "no difference" scenario is measured. Although the approach is somewhat counterintuitive, it can be thought of in the same terms as "innocent until proven guilty." Thus, answering the question of whether the means differ is done by weighing the evidence against the hypothesis that the true difference is zero. For continuous data, the most common test used to compare means is the two-sample t-test, which requires calculation of two important quantities: the difference of the sample means, and the standard error of this difference. The t statistic is simply the difference divided by the standard error of the difference; larger t statistics are regarded as stronger evidence against no difference.

The evidence against the null hypothesis is quantified in a p-value, which is a probability; formally, it is the probability of realizing the observed difference—or one more extreme—under the assumption that the null hypothesis is true. P-values are commonly misinterpreted as the probability that the null hypothesis is true. What is important to understand conceptually about a p-value is that it is a direct statement about your data and not about the null hypothesis. This notion is explained more fully below.

Returning to the example, p-values for t statistics can either be looked up in a table or calculated from a standard software package. Our sample gives a difference of 4.9 with standard error 1.8, so $T = 4.9/1.8 = 2.7$, with $p = .011$. We conclude that observing a difference of 4.9 or more pills would occur in only about 1.1% of samples of 50 women in which the true difference in mean number of pills is zero. This is strong evidence against the null hypothesis.

In carrying out a t-test, we are able not only to test whether the difference in the number of pain pills is zero, but also to calculate a CI for the difference. Like a p-value, a CI can indicate whether the difference is significant at the 5% level; unlike a p-value, however, it aids in the clinical interpretation of our finding. From our sample, we estimate that women whose wounds are closed with staples take 4.9 fewer pain pills on average; the 95% CI for the difference is (1.2, 8.6); this interval contains the true difference with 95% probability.

There is a duality between CIs and hypothesis tests; if a 95% CI excludes zero, then the p-value from the corresponding hypothesis test of no difference is less than .05. From a clinical point of view, we can further use CIs as an indication of a range of differences consistent with our observed data. This is most useful in distinguishing purely statistical differences from those that are clinically meaningful. Suppose for example that the CI for pill count difference was (1,2). This interval excludes zero, so we conclude that $p < .05$; however, the upper limit of the CI is 2 pills, hardly a clinically important difference. If a clinically meaningful difference is not contained in the CI but $p < .05$, chances are that the "significance" of our finding is purely statistical. By contrast, consider the situation where the CI is $(-1, 10)$. Here, the difference is not statistically significant but the observed data are consistent with true differences up to 10 pills, a clinically important difference! In these situations, it is likely that a large standard error is making the CI too wide, and that more subjects are needed to draw more precise conclusions.

In carrying out the *t*-test, we are making two assumptions about the nature of the responses. First, we assume that they follow a normal distribution; second, we assume that the standard deviations in the two groups are equal. In practice, the normality assumption rarely is met; however, the *t*-test has a robustness property such that correct inference about differences in means can be made in moderate-size to large samples (e.g., more than 30 per group) even when normality does not hold. Correct inference in smaller samples relies more heavily on the normality assumption being correct. In samples of any size, the assumption of equal standard deviations is somewhat more critical to making correct inference. Fortunately, most software packages calculate a modified *t*-test that allows for unequal standard deviations. Perhaps the most important consideration when using a *t*-test, however, is whether comparing the means—rather than another measure like the medians—is appropriate in the first place!

Summaries and Comparisons Using Percentiles

Consider another variable in this study—length of hospital stay measured in days. Histograms are given in Fig. 11.5, and clearly the distributions are skewed such that most stays are less than 5 days. For skewed distributions, the mean and standard deviation often are not appropriate summary measures because they can be unduly influenced by outlying observations; instead, points that define quartiles of the observations are used. These are the 25th, 50th, and 75th percentiles; together, they indicate central location (the 50th percentile is the median) and dispersion (the 25th and 75th percentiles indicate spread from the center on either side). Table 11.3 lists the percentiles together with the mean and standard deviation for length of stay. Although the mean length of stay differs by 0.6, the medians are identical. Furthermore, the 25th, 50th, and 75th percentiles in the suture group are all equal, which indicates that more than half of the patients stayed for exactly 3 days; in the staples group, more than half stayed for 3 or 4 days. Comparing means may lead us to believe that those in the suture group had slightly shorter length of stay, but this is an artifact of one woman staying for 11 days; otherwise, the length of stay is nearly identical in the two groups.

For comparing medians, the Wilcoxon rank sum statistic (also known as the Mann Whitney U-statistic) is appropriate. To form the statistic, all the observations are ranked without regard to group membership. In situations where the sample size is the same in both groups, the null hypothesis of equal medians implies that the sum of ranks in each group should be equal; in other situations, the sum of ranks should differ only in proportion to the sample size ratio. The rank sum test compares the observed sum of ranks in each group to the sum that corresponds to equal group medians. In comparing length of stay, we rank 50 observations; the sum of the ranks is $1 + 2 + 3 + \cdots + 49 + 50 = 1,275$. Under equal medians, each group rank sum should be $1275/2 = 637.5$. The rank sum in the suture group is 603.5 (there are some ties), slightly less than expected, indicating lower length of stay; however, $p = .836$. Incidentally, the *t*-test for comparing means gives $p = .160$, not significant but more nearly so than the median comparison.

Means and Standard Deviations or Percentiles?

We have reviewed two methods for comparing the distribution of a continuous variable between two groups: the

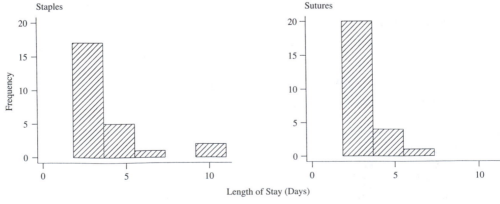

FIGURE 11.5. Length of stay histogram.

TABLE 11.3. SUMMARY STATISTICS FOR LENGTH OF STAY IN DAYS BY WOMEN WHO HAD C-SECTION WOUNDS CLOSED BY SUTURE AND STAPLES

Closure Method	n	Mean	Standard Deviation	Percentiles		
				25	50	75
Staples	25	3.9	2.1	3	3	4
Sutures	25	3.3	0.7	3	3	3
Difference		0.6		0	0	1

t-test and the rank sum test. The *t*-test compares means and should be used only when comparison of the means is of direct interest. Proper inference relies on the observations being normally distributed (although this is less important in large samples) and the group standard deviations being equal. Adjustment can be made when the variances are not equal. In highly skewed data, the *t*-test will usually give valid inference about the mean, but a comparison of the mean may not be appropriate. The data should be summarized using quartiles rather than the mean and standard deviation, and the Wilcoxon rank sum test used to test equality of medians.

Example 2: Insulin Resistance and Hypertension in Pregnancy

Although studies designed for group comparisons are common in clinical research, many times there is reason for quantifying association between two continuous variables. Consider a recent study of pregnancy-induced hypertension and insulin resistance conducted by Yasuhi et al. (37). In this study, 330 normotensive, healthy pregnant women were enrolled in their second trimester and followed prospectively for the remainder of the pregnancy. One of the primary research questions concerned the relationship between mean arterial pressure (MAP) and insulin resistance

(fasting immunoreactive insulin) at the second trimester. The two-way scatterplots of insulin versus MAP are shown in Fig. 11.6; insulin is graphed in its original scale on the left, and in the log scale on the right. Although both plots exhibit a positive relationship, the one that uses log-insulin makes the relationship more linear; furthermore, there are fewer outlying observations.

These relationships can be quantified in a variety of ways, but perhaps the most common is correlation. The Pearson (or product moment) correlation is a unitless measure ranging from −1 to 1; it indicates the direction of the relationship and also, in the squared correlation, the degree to which variation in one outcome is explained by the other. In our example, the Pearson correlation between MAP and log insulin is 0.28, indicating a positive relationship. Squaring the correlation gives 0.08, meaning that 8% of the variation in MAP is explained by variations in insulin. The correlation between MAP and insulin is only slightly lower, 0.25. The similarity highlights an important limitation of using correlations. While the Pearson correlation has the advantage of giving a quick characterization of the relationship between two variables, it has no direct clinical interpretability. In our example, we measured insulin on the original scale and on the log scale, and yet the correlations are almost identical.

Statistical significance tests on correlation coefficients should be applied and reported with caution if the primary interest is drawing clinical conclusions. In large samples, even very small nonzero correlations can turn up statistically significant; in small samples, outlying observations can substantially influence the Pearson correlation coefficient. An important assumption required for valid inference about correlation is that the two variables have a linear relationship; as with the normality assumption in the *t*-test, meeting this assumption is particularly important in small to moderate-sized samples.

If sensitivity to outliers is problematic, a useful alternative is the Spearman correlation, which is the Pearson correlation

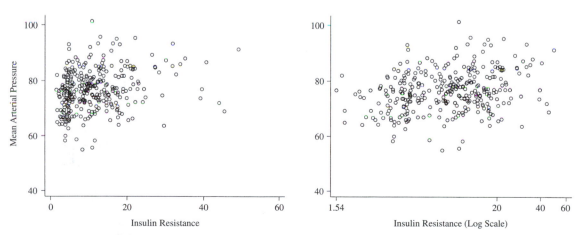

FIGURE 11.6. Two-way scatterplots of insulin versus mean arterial pressure (MAP).

applied to the ranks of the observations rather than to the observations themselves. One property of the Spearman correlation is invariance to certain transformations of the data such as log and square root. To illustrate how even one outlier can influence the correlation, consider from example 1, above, the number of pain pills versus length of stay among the 25 women receiving sutures in the C-section example. A graph of pain pills vs. length of stay appears in Fig. 11.7. With the exception of the woman who took 40 pain pills during her 6-day stay, there appears to be no relationship between these outcomes. The Pearson correlation is 0.34; without the outlier, it turns negative, to −0.26. The Spearman correlations for the same comparisons are 0.07 and −0.12; their signs are opposite but their difference is far smaller, indicating less sensitivity to the outlier.

Analyzing Rates and Proportions

Example 3: A Randomized Clinical Trial of Calcium to Prevent Preeclampsia

The role of aspirin and calcium in preventing preeclampsia has been widely studied and hotly debated in recent years. Part of the reason for the controversy is that preeclampsia is a relatively rare event, occurring in only 5% to 10% of pregnancies of healthy women in the United States; therefore, any study of preeclampsia will require large numbers of women simply to observe enough events for meaningful inferences.

Most recently, Levine et al. (38) conducted a multicenter clinical trial to study the association between calcium supplements during pregnancy and the development of preeclampsia. In this trial, 4,589 health nulliparous women were randomly assigned to receive calcium (2,295) or placebo (2,294) during pregnancy. The women were followed through pregnancy, and preeclampsia status (yes/no) was noted at term. This is an example of a study with a binary (two-level) response, which is the simplest kind of categorical response. During the study, 158 (6.9%) on calcium and 168 (7.3%) on placebo developed preeclampsia. Through brief analyses, we illustrate methods for testing the hypothesis that the rates are equal and for measuring the treatment effect (or association between calcium therapy and eventual development of preeclampsia).

Testing for Differences in Proportions

The most common methods for testing hypotheses about proportions are Fisher's exact test and Pearson's chi-square test, both of which are most easily understood in terms of cross-tabulations of the outcomes. In general, these tests may be applied to cross-classified data with arbitrary numbers of categories; here, our focus is on 2-by-2 tables. The outcomes from the calcium trial can be tabulated as follows:

	Preeclampsia?		
Treatment	*No*	*Yes*	*Total*
Placebo	2,126	168	2,294
Calcium	2,137	158	2,295
Total	4,263	326	4,589

In cross-classified data, the null hypothesis of no association states that the row effects (treatment) are independent of the column effects (preeclampsia); in a table with two rows, this is equivalent to the hypothesis that the row proportions (rates of preeclampsia) are equal. Fisher's exact test considers all possible tables that have the same row totals as the observed table, and calculates the probability of each table under the "no difference" hypothesis (i.e., tables corresponding to large differences have small probabilities under the "no difference" hypothesis). The *p*-value is the total probability of all tables that have rate differences equal to or larger than the observed rate difference. The *p*-value from Fisher's exact test is valid regardless of sample size, but it has traditionally been applied only to smaller samples because of the computational burden of enumerating all possible tables; however, the widespread availability of high-speed computers and efficient algorithms has made it routine to apply Fisher's exact test even in large samples. For the calcium data, Fisher's exact test gives *p* = .566.

Pearson's chi-square test is based on differences between cell counts that are observed and cell counts that would have been observed had the proportions been equal (or more generally, if the row effects were perfectly independent of the column effects). If the differences are relatively and consistently large, the test statistic is large (indicating evidence against the null hypothesis). Unlike Fisher's exact test, which is valid for any sample size, chi-square tests based on Pearson's statistic are only valid in large samples. One rule of thumb states that the expected count of cell

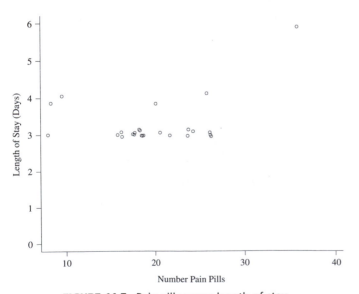

FIGURE 11.7. Pain pills versus length of stay.

in a table should exceed 5. In the calcium data, Pearson's statistic is 0.33, with $p = .563$ (compare to Fisher's exact p-value above).

Measuring Effect Size

Neither Fisher's exact test nor Pearson's chi-square test can be used to measure the degree of association or the difference in rates. For two-group comparisons of proportion, association can be measured in one of three ways: odds ratio, rate (or risk) ratio, or risk difference. Let p_0 represent the proportion with preeclampsia in the placebo arm, and p_1 the proportion in the calcium arm. The rate ratio is $RR = p_1/p_0$, and measures the relative increase or reduction in risk associated with taking calcium. In our example, the risk ratio is estimated by

$$\frac{158/2295}{168/2294} = \frac{0.069}{0.073} = 0.945,$$

indicating that calcium reduces risk of preeclampsia by about 5.5%.

Rather than using rates, the odds ratio measures association using relative odds of preeclapsia. The odds of an event with rate p is just $p/(1 - p)$, or the chances of event divided by the chances of no event. For rare events like preeclampsia, the odds and the rate are nearly identical; in the placebo arm, where the rate is 0.073, the odds of preeclampsia is $0.073/(1 - 0.073) = 0.073/0.927 = 0.079$. Because of this similarity, the odds ratio is a good approximation to the risk ratio for rare events. The odds ratio here is

$$\frac{0.069/(1 - 0.069)}{0.073/(1 - 0.073)} = \frac{0.074}{0.079} = 0.937$$

meaning that calcium reduced the odds of preeclampsia by about 6.3%, a figure very close to that found using the risk ratio.

Despite their similarities, odds ratios and risk ratios have important differences. A risk ratio is defined only in studies designed to measure risk (or prevalence) of an event within groups. Many prospective designs, such as randomized clinical trials, are designed precisely for this purpose; for situations where underlying risk can be estimated, both risk ratios and odds ratios are appropriate measures of association. A notable design in which underlying risks cannot be measured is the case of case–control study; risk ratios are not defined, but odds ratios are valid measures of association, and indeed are valid estimates of relative risk for rare events.

Odd ratios have a direct correspondence to coefficients in the logistic regression model, a widely popular tool for analyzing binary data (see below).

Like the risk ratio, the risk difference, which measures absolute change in risk, can only be used in situations where group-specific risks can be estimated. The choice between risk difference and risk ratio depends largely on the goals of the study. Consider a comparison of two large populations, one of which is exposed to a carcinogen. Cancer rate in the exposed group is in 10,000 (0.0004), and in the unexposed group 4 in 10,000 (0.0001). Exposure increases risk by a factor of 4 (the risk ratio), quite an impressive association. However, one can also conclude that it increases the probability of cancer by 0.0003 (the risk difference). To an individual, the likelihood of getting cancer appears equally remote in either population; however, to a regulatory agency viewing the populations as a whole, a fourfold increase on cancer rate is likely to be alarming, even if the underlying rates are low.

In large samples, results of testing equivalent hypotheses will usually agree. The null hypothesis of no association between calcium and preclampsia can be stated three ways: risk ratio = 1, odds ratio = 1, or risk difference = 0. Table 11.4 gives estimates and 95% CIs for each measure. Each of the CIs contains the value corresponding to the null hypothesis, so we can conclude that $p > .05$ regardless of which measure is used.

Clinically speaking, can we reasonably conclude that calcium has no beneficial effect? A nonsignificant p-value by itself gives no indication. One way to answer the question is to see whether all clinically meaningful differences are excluded from the CI. The CI for the risk ratio runs from 0.76 to 1.16; this suggests, for example, that 24% reduction in the risk of preeclampsia as a result of taking calcium cannot be ruled out by this clinical trial. The lower bound of the CI for risk difference is −0.019 (or 1.9%), meaning that a reduction in rate of preeclampsia from 7.3% to 5.4% as a result of taking calcium is not ruled out by these data.

Analyzing Time to Event Data

Many studies of medical intervention use time to event as a primary outcome; examples include time to tumor recurrence, disease progression, or death. Unlike other continuous outcomes in which means or medians serve as adequate summaries, perhaps the most useful characterization

TABLE 11.4. ESTIMATES AND 95% CONFIDENCE INTERVALS FOR THREE MEASURES OF ASSOCIATION IN THE CALCIUM CLINICAL TRIAL: RATE OF PREECLAMPSIA

Placebo	Calcium	Risk Difference	Risk Ratio	Odds Ratio
168/2,294 (7.3%)	158/2,295 (6.9%)	−0.0044 (−0.019, 0.010)	0.94 (0.76, 1.16)	0.94 (0.75, 1.17)

of an event time distribution is its survival curve, in which the probability of surviving (or remaining event-free) beyond time t is plotted as a function of t. This curve is also called the survivor function, and is denoted as $S(t)$. In many studies, the goal is to estimate $S(t)$ and possibly to compare it between groups.

Example 4: Clinical Symptoms in Patients with Ovarian Cancer

In a study of clinical symptoms in ovarian cancer patients, DiSilvestro et al. (39) compared the distribution of survival time in months among 137 patients at three stages of clinical symptomatology: asymptomatic, simple, and complex. Patients were followed for up to 5 years. A complication in analyzing data from this study, and one that is common in analysis of survival data, is that not all event times are observed. Many patients simply had not experienced the event within the 5-year time frame; others may have dropped out of the study for a variety of reasons, such as moving away or refusing further participation. When the survival time is not observed, we say it is censored. Analyzing data in which some end points are censored requires specialized methods, which we illustrate through an analysis of the ovarian cancer data.

A common estimate of $S(t)$, and one that is available in nearly every statistical software package, is the Kaplan-Meier (or product-limit) estimator (40). The Kaplan-Meier estimator gives an estimate of $S(t)$ only at the times where end points are observed, but makes use of all individuals in the sample. Consider the group with simple symptomatology; at time zero, 77 women begin observation. The probability of surviving beyond time 0, or $S(0)$, is equal to 1. The first death occurs at month 1, where all 77 women are still being followed (i.e., there has been no censoring). Because 76 of the women survive beyond month 1, $\hat{S}(1) = 76/77 = 0.987$. The subset of women "at risk" is reduced to 76; survival probability remains at 0.987 until the next death time, which is month 4 (one woman dies here). The probability of survival beyond month 4 is the proportion still surviving up to month 4 (0.987) times the proportion of those women surviving past month 4 (75/76 = 0.987), which gives $\hat{S}(4) = 0.987 \times 0.986 = 0.974$. This calculation is made at each observed death time; only women who have not yet died or been censored are included in the denominator (Table 11.5). Women who are censored contribute to the survival estimator only for times at which they remain in the sample.

The Kaplan-Meier estimator is nonparametric, meaning that no parametric distribution is assumed for the survival times; however, to obtain valid estimates, censoring must be unrelated to the survival process, or noninformative. In the ovarian cancer study, suppose that the sickest patients were moved to hospice care outside the hospital shortly before death and thus lost to follow-up; this is informative censoring because the act of being removed from the study is directly related to the eventual outcome. Applying the Kaplan-Meier estimator here is likely to result in an upwardly biased estimate of survival at each time. The plausibility of noninformative censoring should always be addressed when analyzing survival data, especially where censoring is moderate to heavy (for example, more than 15% to 20%).

Figure 11.8 shows the Kaplan-Meier estimates of $S(t)$ for patients in the simple and complex symptom categories. The Kaplan-Meier estimator is a step function, taking steps down at each time where subjects are observed to die; the plus (+) signs on the curve indicate times at which patients

TABLE 11.5. CALCULATION OF THE KAPLAN MEIER ESTIMATOR FOR SURVIVAL DATA

Time (t)	No. at Risk	No. Died	No. Censored	No. Remaining	Survival Estimator
0	77	0	0	77	1.0
1[a]	77	1	0	76	1.0 × (76/77) = 0.987
4[a]	76	1	0	75	0.987 × (75/76) = 0.974
5[a]	75	1	0	74	0.974 × (74/75) = 0.961
.	.	.	.	.	.
.	.	.	.	.	.
23[a]	60	4	0	56	0.779 × (56/60) = 0.727
25[b]	56	0	1	55	0.727
26[a]	55	1	0	54	0.727 × (54/55) = 0.714
.	.	.	.	.	.
46[c]	39	1	1	37	0.644 × (38/39) = 0.628
.	.	.	.	.	.
.	.	.	.	.	.

[a]Times at which only deaths occur.
[b]Times at which only censoring occurs; survival estimate remains unchanged.
[c]Times at which both death and censoring occur; survival estimate is updated using only the observed deaths.

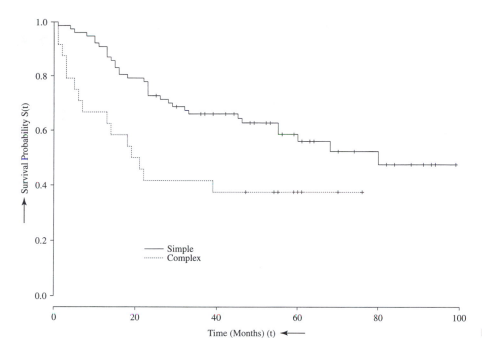

FIGURE 11.8. Kaplan-Meier curves.

are censored. Notice that the Kaplan-Meier curve cannot estimate survival beyond the last data point; it is possible, but not typically advisable except in special circumstances, to use model-based extrapolations (41).

A natural question to ask is whether the survival curves are statistically different from each other. The log rank statistic is used expressly for this purpose; it tests the null hypothesis that the two survival curves are equal. In the ovarian cancer example, the log rank statistic uses a cumulation of cross-tabulations of symptom status vs. death at each time where any death occurs; in that respect, it is calculated from a collection of chi-square statistics for many 2-by-2 tables. If, on average, the death rates are substantially different from what would be expected under equal survival at points along the time axis, then the null hypothesis of equal survival rates is rejected. The log rank statistic can be applied to any number of survival curves, but is most effective in situations where the survival curves are ordered (Fig. 11.8). For the ovarian cancer data, the log rank statistic gives $p = .014$, which together with the Kaplan-Meier curve suggests that survival rates among those presenting with complex symptoms are much lower.

REGRESSION METHODS

Up to now our focus has been on relating a response variable to a single independent variable (such as type of closure for C-section, type of prevention for preeclampsia, and symptom stage in ovarian cancer). In many studies, particularly observational studies, several variables need to be considered collectively. Regression models provide one means

for doing so. A regression model is used to describe some characteristic of a response variable, such as its mean or the probability of positive response, in terms of one or more explanatory variables, called covariates. The choice of model depends on the type of outcome; here we briefly discuss three particular regression models: the linear least squares model (for continuous response), the logistic regression model (for binary response), and the proportional hazards regression model (for event time data).

Linear Regression Model for Continuous Response

In example 2, above, we calculated a correlation coefficient to measure association between insulin resistance and MAP. We might think that MAP is functionally related to insulin resistance. For cases where the functional relationship is linear (or can be made so by transformations), linear regression provides a way to model it. If we use μ to represent the mean MAP, and x to represent insulin resistance, a linear model for mean MAP as a function if insulin resistance is

$$\mu = \beta_0 + \beta_1 x,$$

which states that for every unit increase in insulin resistance (x), MAP is expected to increase by β_1 units. The parameters β_0 and β_1 are called regression coefficients, and can be estimated using any statistical software package. For the MAP-insulin model, we find that measuring insulin resistance in the log scale provides a good linear relationship (so that x represents log insulin in the model above); the estimate of β_1 is 2.9, indicating that each log-unit increase in insulin resistance is associated with an increase of 2.9

points in MAP. The fitted line and the data are shown in Fig. 11.9.

In this particular example, several other factors may be related to MAP; one is body mass index (BMI). In some sense this is a nuisance variable because the relationship between BMI and MAP is not of direct interest. It may even be a confounding variable because it is related both to MAP and to insulin. The regression model allows us to examine the MAP-insulin relationship while controlling for the effects of BMI by simply adding it into the model. The expanded model, called a multiple linear regression model (due to multiple explanatory variables), is

$$\mu = \beta_0 + \beta_1 x_1 + \beta_2 x_2,$$

where now x_1 is log-insulin and x_2 is BMI. The coefficient β_1 is the change in MAP associated with a log-unit increase in insulin, for any fixed value of BMI. Conceptually, this conditional or partial effect of log-insulin is calculated by stratifying on levels of BMI and finding the average insulin effect across the various levels; this is in contrast to the unconditional insulin effect, in which the comparisons are not stratified on BMI at all. From the multiple linear regression, $\hat{\beta}_1 = 2.1$, indicating that conditional on BMI, log-unit differences in insulin are associated with only 2.1 unit increases in MAP. BMI is positively correlated with both MAP and with insulin, which is reflected in the decreased insulin effect from the first to the second model.

There is an important connection between t tests and linear regression. Recall example 1, where we studied consumption of pain pills in women undergoing C-section. Consider the regression model where μ is the mean number of pain pills, and x is a binary indicator of whether the wound is closed with staples ($x = 1$) or sutures ($x = 0$). The model

$$\mu = \beta_0 + \beta_1 x,$$

indicates the following: (a) the mean number of pain pills in the suture group is β_0, (b) the mean in the staples group is $\beta_0 + \beta_1$, and (c) the difference in means is β_1. In the linear least squares regression model, the hypothesis test for $\beta_1 = 0$ is exactly the t-test for equal means. This connection between t-tests and regression indicates two ways in which regression models generalize simple comparisons of group means: first, the group comparison can be adjusted for other variables by adding those variables into the regression model; second, several groups can be compared in the same model by adding the appropriate indicator variables. This second extension provides the basis for analysis of variance (ANOVA), which is used to test hypotheses about variations in the mean across several groups. ANOVA is just a particular formulation of least squares regression, and the t-test corresponds to ANOVA for two groups.

The analyst is making several assumptions when fitting a regression model, and care must be taken to examine the appropriateness of the chosen model. This is particularly true when using continuous explanatory variables such as BMI. In least squares regression, two important assumptions (among several) are linearity (whether the response and explanatory variables have a linear relationship) and homoscedasticity (constant variance among the residuals). A residual is the difference between observed and predicted response; many graphical and analytic checks of model assumptions can be made from the residuals [see Hamilton (42) for examples]. Severe violations of model assumptions indicate that the model does not accurately describe the data and often lead to erroneous inferences. Most regression textbooks delineate methods for model diagnostics; an excellent reference is Hamilton (42).

Logistic Regression Models for Binary Response

The logistic regression is an analogue to the linear regression for binary data. The mean of a binary response is the probability p of positive outcome (i.e., probability that the response is equal to 1). Logistic regression specifies the log odds of a positive response, or $\log [p/(1 - p)]$, as a linear function of explanatory variables. The log odds may seem like a peculiar function to model, but it lends two important properties to logistic regression: the regression coefficients have odds ratio interpretations, and predicted probabilities are constrained between 0 and 1.

Consider a study of the likelihood of pregnancy in women with tubal disease treated by *in vitro* fertilization (IVF) (42). The primary research question is whether women with hydrosalpinx have a reduced likelihood of pregnancy. Among women undergoing a first IVF cycle, 21 of 90 with hydrosalpinx (23.3%) and 51 of 229 without hydrosalpinx (22.3%) delivered at least one child; the odds ratio is 1.06 (log odds ratio = 0.06), indicating little if any difference in odds of delivering a baby. The log odds ratio also can be estimated—and adjusted for other factors—

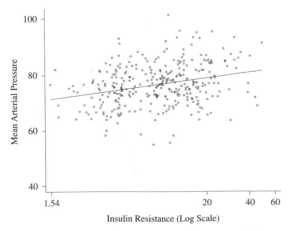

FIGURE 11.9. Regression of insulin and mean arterial pressure (MAP).

using a logistic regression model. Using p to represent probability of delivery, and x to indicate hydrosalpinx status ($x = 1$ if hydrosalpinx and $= 0$ otherwise), we have the model

$$\log \left(\frac{p}{1 - p} \right) = \beta_0 + \beta_1 x.$$

The log odds ratio is exactly β_1, making the odds ratio e^{β_1}. The null hypothesis of no association (or odds ratio = 1) is equivalent to $\beta_1 = 0$.

A potential confounding variable here is age, which certainly is related to the likelihood of a delivery. By entering age as the covariate, we can use a logistic regression to calculate the age-adjusted effect of hydrosalpinx:

$$\log \left(\frac{p}{1 - p} \right) = \beta_0 + \beta_1 x_1 + \beta_2 x_2.$$

The estimate of β_1, the conditional effect of hydrosalpinx, is 0.031; this gives a conditional (or age-adjusted) odds ratio of $e^{0.031} = 1.03$. Comparing to the unadjusted odds ratio, we see that age has little if any effect on the relationship between delivery and hydrosalpinx; this is because even though age is related to delivery probability, there exists little association between age and presence of hydrosalpinges. The age effect is $\hat{\beta}_2 = -0.073$, with 95% CI ($-0.138, -0.007$), which indicates that age has a significant negative effect on delivery probability. The estimated odds ratio for age is $e^{\hat{\beta}_2} = 0.930$, meaning that a 1-year increase in age is associated with a 7% reduction in the odds of delivery. Another interpretation is that for two randomly selected women with a 1-year age difference, the older woman's odds of delivery are 93% of the younger woman's. As in linear regression, model diagnostics for the logistic regression are a necessary step in any model fitting process (41,43,44).

Proportional Hazards Regression for Time to Event Response

We turn finally to the proportional hazards regression model for event time data, which is often called a Cox model because one popular formulation was developed by British statistician D. R. Cox (45). In this regression, we model the hazard of failure at time t using explanatory variables. The hazard measures likelihood of failure for the group of subjects still remaining at time t; it has a direct correspondence to the survival function, so proportional hazards regression can be viewed as a model for the survival curve. We illustrate using the ovarian cancer data from example 4, except we add International Federation of Gynecology and Obstetrics (FIGO) tumor stage and age as explanatory variables. Consider first a simple model in which the symptom status is denoted by x ($= 0$ if simple, $= 1$ if complex). The Cox model takes the form

$$h(t) = h_0(t) \times e^{\beta x},$$

where $h(t)$ is the hazard at time t. For those with simple symptoms ($x = 0$) the hazard function is $h_0(t)$; for those with complex symptoms the hazard is changed by a factor of e^{β_1}, making the symptom-specific hazards proportional to each other. This factor by which they differ is called the hazard ratio, a measure with interpretation very similar to the risk ratio. It measures the relative risk of death at time t among all patients who have survived up to time t. In the ovarian cancer data, $\hat{\beta}_1 = 0.75$, which implies a hazard ratio of $e^{0.75} = 2.1$; thus, among a group of survivors at any time point, those with complex symptoms are at twice the risk for death. Furthermore, the log rank test of equal survival distributions corresponds to testing whether the hazard ratio is equal to 1, or whether $\beta_1 = 0$.

Because risk of death and possibly symptom status also are related to age and tumor stage, our second analysis adds these to the model as predictors x_2 and x_3, respectively. The expanded Cox model is

$$h(t) = h_0(t) \times e^{\beta_1 x_1 + \beta_2 x_2 + \beta_3 x_3}.$$

Applying this model, we find the adjusted hazard ratio $e^{\beta_1} = e^{0.88} = 2.4$, implying that even if we hold tumor stage and age constant when comparing symptomatology, those with complex symptoms are still at more than twice the risk of death (actually 2.4) when compared to those with simple symptoms. This clinically dramatic effect is also statistically significant ($p = .006$). From the same model, we find also that tumor stage and age also significantly impact survival rate. Most notably, holding age and symptomatology constant, a one-stage increase in tumor classification is associated with a nearly three-fold increase in the risk of death ($e^{\beta_2} = e^{1.03} = 2.8$).

A Final Word on p-Values

The careful reader will notice that emphasis has been placed on understanding methods and interpreting analytic results rather than on making determinations of statistical significance. It is the opinion of a majority of statisticians (46) and a growing number of medical investigators (39) that in clinical and public health investigations (indeed, nearly all investigations involving data analysis), far too much emphasis is placed on evaluating statistical significance and far too little on determining clinical relevance. The preoccupation with a 5% cutoff value is so firmly ingrained in our decision making that we are sometimes led to believe (irrationally so) that $p = .04$ is somehow much stronger evidence of a "real" effect than $p = .06$. In addition, many investigators feel compelled to report p-values for numerous irrelevant comparisons in a study; in extreme cases, this can result in published papers containing as many p-values as subjects in the study!

Judiciously applied in properly designed studies, p-values are valuable for weighing evidence against a null hypothesis; however, they always should be reported in conjunction with a measure and interpretation of effect (such as the odds ratio, the hazard ratio, the difference in means, or whatever measure is appropriate), preferably with a CI. *P*-values alone give no indication of clinical or public health implications of the research, and even highly significant *p*-values can correspond to clinical effects that are too small to be meaningful.

DESIGN AND SAMPLE SIZE

It is difficult to overstate the importance of choosing an appropriate and realistic study design when undertaking scientific research, especially research on individuals. Every researcher who has been involved in a study, even of seemingly small proportions, has some understanding of the effort, cost, and inconvenience to both the investigators and the study subjects. In most cases, a well-designed and properly implemented study is worth the effort and expense. No amount of statistical effort or sophistication can be used to draw valid conclusions from a poorly designed study. Our foregoing discussion of statistical methods assumes that data have been collected from a properly and carefully designed study.

In almost any study where conclusions will be drawn from data, the investigator is confronted with the issue of sample size. Several factors are considered before arriving at a target sample: budgetary constraints, availability of patients or cases, type of study design (e.g., case control, randomized controlled trial), characteristics of the population under study, and the method of data analysis. Sample size calculations can serve as useful guides to what can and cannot be accomplished in a study with a given amount of resources. In the hypertension study outlined in example 2, above, the investigators proposed a prospective cohort study. Preliminary sample size calculations indicated that approximately 350 patients would be needed to ensure a high likelihood of finding an effect with clinical meaning. A decision was made to take advantage of the large prenatal population at their hospital and to allocate resources to the study; at a smaller hospital, the sample size calculation would likely have dissuaded investigators from spending time and money for naught.

Some Guidelines

Several pieces of information are required to carry out a meaningful sample size calculation. Fortunately, many software packages are available for crunching numbers through the necessary formulas; therefore, we concentrate here on qualitative issues regarding sample size. The investigative team should answer these questions to help themselves set up the calculations.

1. What are the primary outcomes? Initial sample size determinations should be based on these.
2. On what scale will the outcome be recorded? Binary (yes/no), ordinal categorical, and continuous are examples. In a study of hypertension, one might record actual diastolic blood pressure or simply indicate whether it is greater than 90. Categorizing a continuous outcome usually results in a loss of information and thus power, requiring larger sample sizes.
3. How variable is this outcome in the population to be measured? For continuous data, this usually can be captured by standard deviation; higher standard deviation is associated with larger sample size. With binary data, variability is directly related to the proportion of "positives" in some baseline category (e.g., proportion of women delivering in the group with no hydrosalpinx). Small pilot studies, chart reviews, and reviews of existing studies using the same outcome variable are useful for obtaining indicators of variability.
4. What defines a relevant effect size (e.g., difference in means, odds ratio, hazard ratio, etc.) in the context of the study? This is perhaps the most challenging question, and its answer often relies on subjective information. It takes more subjects to detect a smaller effect; decreasing an effect size can drastically increase sample size requirements.
5. What summary measure or statistic will be used to draw conclusions from the data collected?
6. What is the desired power and type I error rate? Power is the probability of finding a statistically significant effect under the circumstance that an effect truly exists. Type I error (or alpha) is the probability of declaring significance when there really is no effect at all. More power requires more subjects; likewise, a lower type I error rate requires more subjects.
7. If this is an observational study, are there any variables for which we need to adjust? Typically, adjusting for confounders and other factors increases sample size requirements.
8. Are the outcomes clustered in any way? Two examples are multisite studies or situations that call for repeated measurements on the same subject. Clustering induces correlation between responses, and situations such as this sometimes require a two-tiered sample size calculation: one for the number of subjects (or clusters), and another for the number of measurements per subject (or cluster).

An Example

At the beginning of a study, it is wise to calculate sample size under a wide variety of scenarios; after all, specifying features of the population in a sample size calculation is a process of making educated guesses. We illustrate the pro-

TABLE 11.6. SAMPLE SIZE REQUIREMENTS, PER ARM, FOR A RANDOMIZED CLINICAL TRIAL WITH TYPE I ERROR RATE (ALPHA) EQUAL TO 5%, FOR VARIOUS COMBINATIONS OF EFFECT SIZE AND STANDARD DEVIATION

Effect Size (cm)	Power	Standard Deviation (cm)		
		0.8	0.9	1.0
0.4	80%	63	80	99
	90%	85	107	132
0.6	80%	28	36	44
	90%	38	48	59
0.8	80%	16	20	25
	90%	22	27	33

From Frishman G, Schwartz, Hogan JW. Closure of Pfannenstiel skin incisions. Staples vs. subcuticular suture. *J Reprod Med* 1997;42: 627–630, with permission.

cess using the randomized trial on closure after C-section (example 1) as an example. The original design of this study was based on comparing patient reports of pain from a 10-cm visual analogue scale. The investigators found from a previous study using the same scale that standard deviation was 0.9 cm. Defining a relevant effect size is difficult here; one can rely on previous studies (another study of closure after laparotomy observed a 0.7-cm difference on an identical scale) or on expert opinion. It is highly unlikely that data from one study will mimic that from another, which is further reason to construct a table in which several scenarios are considered.

Table 11.6 shows sample size calculations—based on a *t*-test for comparing means—where power ranges from 80% to 90%, the effect size from 0.4 to 0.8 cm, and the standard deviation from 0.8 to 1.0. Tables like this are useful in understanding the potential of a study to uncover relationships. For example, if budgetary constraints limit the number of patients to be recruited to 70, then hoping to detect a difference in mean pain scale of 0.4 cm—even if that is the true difference—is unrealistic; however, if the true difference is 0.6 cm, then finding a significant effect is more likely with the 70 patients. Particularly noteworthy is that sample size requirements increase at a faster rate as the desired detectable effect decreases; for example, assuming 80% power and standard deviation 0.8, 16 patients per arm would be needed to detect an effect of 0.8, 28 patients for an effect of 0.6, and 63 patients for an effect of 0.4! Small changes in effect size can lead to large changes in sample size requirements.

SUMMARY

We have presented basic methods for evaluating data collected under an appropriate design. Brief discussions such as this can provide the reader with only a starting point from which to pursue the topics in more detail. Furthermore, in practice, study design and data analysis rarely fall squarely within the boundaries of basic methodology. Situations that require design and analysis expertise beyond the basics include (but are not limited to) longitudinal studies with repeated measurements, observational studies with multiple sources of confounding and bias, and studies with significant amounts of missing data. In larger studies with considerable investment of resources, it is highly advisable (and often necessary) to include, from the beginning of the design stage, a biostatistician and/or an epidemiologist as a primary investigator. Even smaller studies are likely to realize enormous benefit if a qualified epidemiologist or biostatistician is included as a collaborator. In carrying out research, it is disastrous to realize after data are collected that you have chosen a faulty design, failed to identify an important source of bias, or miscalculated sample size; often, prevention lies in consulting a qualified expert at the beginning.

Choosing Software

The number of choices of statistical software grows regularly. Here are some quick assessments of software we have used in our research.

SAS is a comprehensive package for statistical software that requires a fair degree of programming ability, although menu-driven versions are now available for the PC. SAS is capable of implementing nearly any conceivable statistical method and has extremely powerful data management facility; however, graphics are difficult to produce. Documentation is thorough but dense. SAS is very expensive commercially but often available at deep discounts for academics.

Stata offers an enormous range of analytic tools, is driven by an interactive command line, and has easy-to-implement graphics. An impressive feature of the regression modules in Stata is the wide array of model diagnostic tools. Data management in Stata is somewhat more tedious than in SAS. Documentation is clear and full of examples. Stata is far less expensive than SAS.

Epi-Info 6.0 is a series of microcomputer programs produced by the Centers for Disease Control and Prevention (CDC) for handling epidemiologic data. It is a handy tool for questionnaire design, data entry, data analysis, and sample size calculations. The best feature of Epi-Info 6.0 is its price. Unlike commercial programs, Epi-Info may be copied and given to colleagues. It is also available by downloading the software from the CDC's Web site on the Internet at www.cdc.gov.

DBMSCOPY and Stat/Transfer allow conversion of data sets used on different platforms; for example, data entered on an Excel spreadsheet can be converted to a SAS data set, and vice versa. Each is easy to use and supports a wide array of statistical software platforms.

10 KEY POINTS

1. When properly performed, randomized trials provide the highest level of evidence for the efficacy of a therapeutic agent.

2. Observational studies are necessary to evaluate the many clinical questions that are not amenable to a clinical trial.

3. Observational studies such as cohort and case-control studies are prone to systematic error such as selection bias and information bias.

4. Meta-analysis, decision analysis, and economic analysis are examples of systematic reviews of medical evidence.

5. Criteria to consider when evaluating the evidence for causation include strength of association, consistency of the findings, dose-response, temporal relationship, experimental evidence, and biologic plausibility.

6. An exploratory analysis of data, including histograms, numerical summaries, and cross-tabulations is necessary before proceeding to confirmatory analyses (estimation and hypothesis testing).

7. A *p*-value gives no indication of the clinical or public health relevance of an effect, even if it is "statistically significant." In confirmatory analyses, measures of effect (such as odds ratios and differences in means), together with appropriate CIs, are more informative than tests of effect alone.

8. The first and most important ingredient in any successful study is proper; no amount of sophistication in the statistical analysis can salvage a poorly designed study.

9. Regression models are effective ways to summarize multivariate relationships, but their usefulness is limited by the extent to which various assumptions are met; therefore, it is necessary to carry out and report diagnostics that help assess the appropriateness and goodness of fit of a given model for the data.

10. For difficult or nonstandard designs such as repeated measure studies or studies that give rise to considerable amounts of missing data, enlist the collaborative efforts of a biostatistician or epidemiologist at the design stage.

REFERENCES

1. Grimes DA. Introducing evidence-based medicine into a department of obstetrics and gynecology. *Obstet Gynecol* 1995;86:451–457.
2. U.S. Preventive Services Task Force. *Guide to clinical preventive services,* 2nd ed. Baltimore: Williams & Wilkins, 1996.
3. Canadian Task Force on the Periodic Health Examination. The periodic health examination. *Can Med Assoc J* 1979;121:1193–1254.
4. Feinstein AR. *Clinical epidemiology: the architecture of clinical research.* Philadelphia: WB Saunders, 1985:684.
5. Sigerist HS. *The university at the crossroads.* New York: H. Shumann, 1946.
6. Fisher RA, Mackenzie WA. Studies in crop variation: II. The manurial response to different potato varieties. *J Agric Sci* 1923; 13:315.
7. Grimes DA. Randomized controlled trials: "It Ain't Necessarily So." *Obstet Gynecol* 1991;78:703–704.
8. Hulley SB, Cummings SR. *Designing clinical research: an epidemiologic approach.* Baltimore: Williams & Wilkins, 1988.
9. Schulz KF, Chalmers I, Grimes DA, et al. Assessing the quality of randomization from reports of controlled trials published in obstetrics and gynecology journals. *JAMA* 1994;272:125–128.
10. Colditz GA, Hankinson SE, Hunter DJ, et al. The use of estrogens and progestins and the risk of breast cancer in postmenopausal women. *N Engl J Med* 1995;332:1589–1593.
11. Grodstein F, Stampfer MJ, Manson JE, et al. Postmenopausal estrogen and progestin use and the risk of cardiovascular disease. *N Engl J Med* 1996;335:453–461.
12. Peterson HB, Xia Z, Hughes JM, et al., The risk of pregnancy after tubal sterilization: finding from the U.S. Collaborative Review of Sterilization. *Am J Obstet Gynecol* 1996;174:1161–1170.
13. Peipert JF, Grimes DA. The case-control study: a primer for the obstetrician-gynecologist. *Obstet Gynecol* 1994;84:140–145.
14. The Centers for Disease Control Cancer and Steroid Hormone Study. Oral contraceptive use and the risk of endometrial cancer. *JAMA* 1983;249:1600–1604.
15. Burkman RT. Association between intrauterine device and pelvic inflammatory disease. *Obstet Gynecol* 1981;57:269–276.
16. Caillouette JC, Koehler AL. Phasic contraceptive pills and functional ovarian cysts. *Am J Obstet Gynecol* 1987;156:1538–1542.
17. Grimes DA, Godwin AJ, Rubin A, et al. Ovulation and follicular development associated with three low-dose oral contraceptives: a randomized controlled trial. *Obstet Gynecol* 83:1994;29–34.
18. Peipert and Sweeney. Diagnostic testing in obstetrics and gynecology: a clinician's guide. *Obstet Gynecol* 82:1993;619–623.
19. Ransohoff DF, Feinstein AR. Problems of spectrum and bias in evaluating the efficacy of diagnostic tests. *N Engl J Med* 1978; 199:926–930.
20. Peipert JF, Bracken MB. Systematic reviews of medical evidence. The use of meta-analysis in obstetrics and gynecology. *Obstet Gynecol* 1997;89:628–633.
21. Enkin M, Keirse MJ, Chalmers I. *Effective care in pregnancy and childbirth.* New York: Oxford University Press, 1969.
22. Longnecker MP, Berlin JA, Orza MJ, et al. A meta-analysis of alcohol consumption in relation to risk of breast cancer. *JAMA* 1988;260:652–656.
23. Shapiro S. Meta-analysis/Shmeta-analysis. *Am J Epidemiol* 1994; 140(9):771–778.
24. Kirpalani H, Schmidt B, McKibbon KA, et al. Searching MEDLINE for randomized clinical trials involving care of the newborn. *Pediatrics* 1988;83:543–547.
25. L'Abbe KA, Detshy AS, O'Rourke K. Meta-analysis in clinical research. *Ann Intern Med* 1987;107:224–233.
26. Pettiti DB. *Meta-analysis, decision analysis, and cost-effectiveness analysis: methods for quantitative synthesis in* Medicine. New York: Oxford University Press, 1994:5–6.
27. Brook RH. Health services research: Is it good for you and me? *Acad Med* 1989;64:124–130.
28. Wennberg J, Gittelsohn A. Small are variations in health care delivery. *Science* 1973;182:1102–1108.
29. Wennberg JE, Freeman JL, Shelton RM, et al. Hospital use and mortality among Medicare beneficiaries in Boston and New Haven. *N Engl J Med* 1989;321:1168–1173.
30. Wennberg JE, Freeman JL, Culp WJ. Are hospital services rationed in New Haven or over-utilized in Boston? *Lancet* 1987;1: 1185–1189.
31. Chassin MR, Kosecoff J, Park RE, et al. Does inappropriate use explain geographic variations in the use of health care services? A study of three procedures. *JAMA* 1987;258:2533–2537.

32. Brook RH, Park RE, Chassin MR, et al. Predicting the appropriate use of carotid endarterectomy, upper gastrointestinal endoscopy and coronary angiography. *N Engl J Med* 1990;323:1173–1177.

33. Winslow CM, Kosecoff JB, Chassin M, et al. The appropriateness of performing coronary artery bypass surgery. *JAMA* 1988;260:505–509.

34. Bernstein SJ, McGlyn EA, Siu AL, et al. The appropriateness of hysterectomy: a comparison of care in seven health plans. *JAMA* 1993;269:2398–2402.

35. National Institutes of Health. Quality of life assessment: practice, problems and promise. Proceedings of a workshop, 1990.

36. Frishman G, Schwartz T, Hogan JW. Closure of pfannenstiel skin incisions: staples vs. subcuticular suture. *J Reprod Med* 1997;42:627–630.

37. Yasuhi I, Hogan JW, Canick JA, et al. Mid-pregnancy elevated C-peptide concentration and subsequent pregnancy-induced hypertension. Abstract presented at meetings of the American Diabetes Association, Boston, 1998.

38. Levine RJ, Hauth JC, Curet LB, et al. Trial of calcium to prevent preeclampsia. *N Engl J Med* 1997;337:69–76.

39. DiSilvestro P, Peipert JF, Hogan JW, et al. Prognostic value of clinical variables in ovarian cancer. *J Clin Epidemiol* 1997;50:501–505.

40. Kaplan EL, Meier P. Nonparametric estimation from incomplete observations. *J Am Stat Assoc* 1956;53: 457–481.

41. Hamilton LC. *Regression with graphics: a second course in applied statistics.* Duxbury Press, Pacific Grove, California, 1991.

42. Blazar AS, Hogan JW, Seifer DB, et al. The impact of hydrosalpinx on successful pregnancy in tubal factor infertility treatment by in vitro fertilization. *Fertil Steril* 1997;67:517–520.

43. Hosmer DW, Taber S, Lemeshow S. The importance of assessing the fit of logistic regression models: a case study. *Am J Public Health* 1991;81:1630–1635.

44. Lemeshow S, Hosmer DW. A review of goodness of fit statistics for use in the development of logistic regression models. *Am J Epidemiol* 1982;115:92–106.

45. Cox DR. Regression models and life tables. *J R Stat Soc* 1972;B34:187–220.

46. Freedman D, Pisani R, Purves R, et al. *Statistics,* 2nd ed. New York: Norton, 1991.

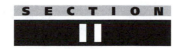

SECTION
II

GYNECOLOGY

FEMALE GROWTH AND DEVELOPMENT: NORMAL AND ABNORMAL

GERI D. HEWITT

Puberty is a time of profound psychologic and somatic growth as well as sexual maturation. These dramatic changes occur because of the awakening and coordinated interaction of the gonadotropic (gonadotropin-releasing hormone [GnRH], luteinizing hormone [LH], follicle-stimulating hormone [FSH], sex steroids, and glycoproteins) and somatotropic (growth hormone [GH], and insulin-like growth factor I [IGF-I], and its binding proteins) axes. *Adrenarche,* the increased adrenal androgen synthesis responsible for pubic and axillary hair growth occurs independently. Whereas the temporal order of puberty—thelarche, linear growth spurt, adrenarche, gonarche, and menarche—has been well described, not all aspects of the neuroendocrinologic events that are responsible for this coordinated effort have been clearly elucidated. Aberration in this process may lead to *precocious puberty,* defined as the onset of pubertal milestones before the age of 8 years, or *delayed puberty,* which is the absence of breast development by age 13.5 or menarche by age 16 years.

NORMAL GROWTH AND DEVELOPMENT

The human pubertal process involves rapid and coordinated growth including increases in linear bone growth, bone density, body mass, differentiated sex organ development, and psychosocial development. Although these endocrinologically controlled events are often related to chronologic age, they show a more direct correlation with Tanner pubertal stage or bone age. The secondary sexual characteristics are a result of androgen production from the adrenal glands in both sexes (*adrenarche*) and testosterone from the testes in the male and estrogens from the ovaries in females (*gonadarche*) (1).

The development of breast buds or *thelarche* heralds the onset of puberty in girls and is a direct result of the increasing levels of estrogen on the estrogen-sensitive breast tissue. This increase in estrogen production also leads to estrogenization of the vaginal mucosa as well as lengthening of the vagina and enlargement of the uterine corpus. In girls in the United States, this process normally begins between 8 and 13 years of age. Breast bud formation before the age of 8 years and the absence of breast bud formation after the age of 13.5 years are both considered abnormal and warrant investigation. The pubertal process then continues with rapid linear growth secondary to sex steroid and GH production and variable manifestations of adrenarche such as pubic and axillary hair growth, stimulated by the rising production of the weakly androgenic adrenal steroids dehydroepiandrosterone (DHEA) and its sulfate (DHEAS). Menarche occurs with further maturation of the gonadotropic axis and occurs between 1 and 5 years after thelarche (2).

Gonadotropic Axis

Awakening, or most likely a disinhibition, of the gonadotropic axis is the first biochemical marker of puberty. Hypothalamic GnRH is released into the hypothalamic-pituitary portal system in a pulsatile fashion stimulating the pulsatile release of gonadotropins from the pituitary, which, in turn, stimulate sex steroid production in the gonads (Fig. 12.1). Production of sex steroids stimulates the development of secondary sex characteristics as well as eventually, menarche. This pulsatile nature of the GnRH release is important in the regulation of gonadotropin production. If the gonadotropes are exposed to continuous rather than pulsatile stimulation from GnRH, gonadotrope GnRH receptors decrease in number and ultimately develop a reversible postreceptor defect leading to a decrease in production of sex steroid hormones (3). Some evidence suggests that the pulse generator for the GnRH release may reside in the GnRH-producing neurons themselves. Immortalized hypothalamic cells develop a labyrinth of interconnections in the culture dish that, when monitored in flow chambers, release GnRH in a pulsatile, coordinated manner (4).

The first endocrinologic event of puberty is the increase in amplitude and mass of the gonadotropin (LH) pulses secreted at night, a process that is stimulated by the hypothalamic GnRH (5). Although GnRH is responsible for this increased gonadotropin production, the mechanism by which it operates, whether increased GnRH pulse frequency, increased GNRH pulse amplitude, or increased gonadotrope sensitivity, is not clear (6).

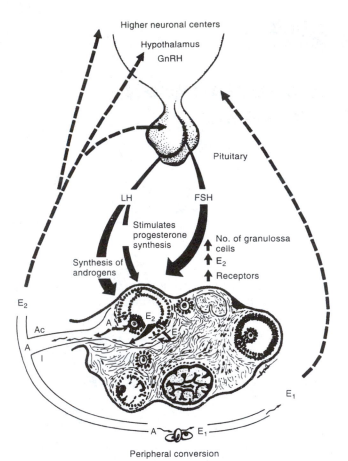

FIGURE 12.1. Hypothalamic-pituitary-ovarian axis interaction in the regulation of follicular maturation and steroid biosynthesis. A, androstenedione; Ac, activin; E1, estrone; E2, estradiol; FSH, follicle-stimulating hormone; GnRH, gonadotropin-releasing hormone; I, inhibin; LH, luteinizing hormone. The ovary shows the various stages of growth of the follicle and the formation and regression of the corpus luteum.

As mentioned before, the rate-limiting step in activating the onset of puberty in higher mammals is the pulse generator activity of the GnRH neurons in the hypothalamus (6). Factors that affect the GnRH pulse generator, in turn, have an impact on the onset and progression of normal and abnormal puberty. Many clinical situations illustrate this point. Hypothalamic hamartomas and gangliocytomas secreting GnRH or triggering GnRH secretion can lead to precocious puberty (7). Conditions interfering with the migration or loss of GnRH neurons result in hypogonadotropic hypogonadism and partial or complete pubertal arrest (8). Pulsatile administration of synthetic GnRH to a patient with absence of endogenous GnRH secretion leads to the onset and progression of the normal pubertal process (7). The putative central nervous system (CNS) processes responsible for declaring the onset of puberty must reside within pathways and networks whose output ultimately (directly or indirectly) affects GnRH neuronal activity (6).

Gonadotropin production is influenced by numerous other peptides and neurotransmitters besides GnRH including neuropeptide-Y, galanin, excitatory amino acids, opiates, dopamine, norepinephrine, serotonin, γ-aminobutyric acid, and sex steroids (7). Sex steroid hormones are major regulators of gonadotropin production both before and after puberty. Estrogen, at varying concentrations, either stimulates or inhibits gonadotropin production at the level of the pituitary; estrogen also inhibits the hypothalamic GnRH pulse generator. The enhancing effect of estrogen on gonadotropin production is illustrated in patients who are functionally agonadal; LH production in response to GnRH stimulation is increased in these patients when they receive exogenous estrogens (9). Sex steroid hormones also exert negative feedback on gonadotropin production. This is clinically apparent in patients with ovarian failure who have diminished estrogen levels, loss of the negative inhibition, and markedly elevated levels of gonadotropins (10). Additionally, estrogen can directly or indirectly affect the frequency of the hypothalamic GnRH pulse generator (10). The mechanism by which sex steroids exert a negative effect on the GnRH pulse generator is not clearly understood; however, investigators have suggested that the endogenous opioid receptors may be involved (7).

Adrenarche

Adrenarche occurs within months to 1.5 years of the onset of puberty (6). Increasing levels of the mildly androgenic adrenal steroids DHEA and DHEAS result in axillary and pubic hair growth. The exact neuroendocrinologic mechanisms that cause adrenal zona fasciculata reticularis cells to increase androgen secretion has not been elucidated. No pituitary-derived adrenal steroidogenesis-stimulating factor has yet been sequenced and cloned (6).

Although temporally related, adrenarche and gonadarche are physiologically two distinct events with independent mechanisms for pubertal awakening (Fig. 12.2). Clinical illustrations include girls with decreased or absent sex steroid hormone production who still experience a normally timed adrenarche (11,12), as well as patients with Addison's disease or isolated adrenocorticotropic hormone (ACTH) deficiency who still experience a normally timed gonadarche (6).

The activation of the adrenal gland during puberty is selective for androgen production. Evaluation of cortisol production in boys shows no change in pulsatile secretion or overnight production rates during puberty (13). Adrenal androgen production then decreases to prepubertal levels throughout the fifth through eighth decades of life.

Growth Hormone

The actions of both the somatotropic and gonadotropic axes are intimately related during the pubertal process (Fig.

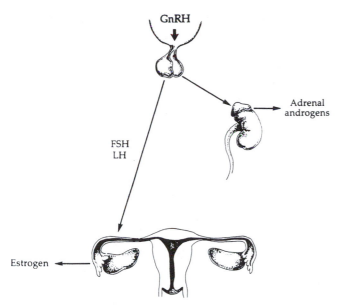

FIGURE 12.2. Hormones responsible for the onset of puberty. FSH, follicle-stimulating hormone; GnRH, gonadotropin-releasing hormone; LH, luteinizing hormone. The stimulus for the rise in adrenal androgens is unclear.

12.3). GH is secreted by the somatotrope cells, which are located in the anterior pituitary, in response to stimulation from hypothalamic GH-releasing hormone (GHRH). GH is a single-chain polypeptide that circulates in both a free form and a protein-bound form. GH secretion is pulsatile, with most secretion occurring during phases 3 and 4 of sleep (14). The pulsatile secretion of GH is regulated by many factors, but GHRH and the GH inhibitor, somatostatin, seem to be the most important; both factors are secreted by the hypothalamus (15). The amount of GHRH released influences the amplitude of the GH produced, whereas the somatostatin influences the frequency and duration of GH-secretory episodes (16). GH secretion is also under the influence of metabolic and hormonal signals from the periphery (including glucocorticoid, thyroid hormones,

and sex steroids), which may modulate somatotroph function either directly or through the hypothalamus (17). IGF-I, produced in response to GH, inhibits GH secretion through a negative feedback mechanism, possibly by binding to specific receptors on the pituitary (18).

GH has multiple end-organ effects, but its primary biologic actions are the stimulation of epiphyseal cartilage growth and other specific actions on carbohydrate, lipid, and mineral metabolism. At the cartilage level, GH stimulates differentiation of the progenitor cells located in the proximal zone of the epiphyseal growth plate, which then undergo clonal expansion in response to IGF-I action with resulting skeletal growth (17). GH also stimulates the production of IGF-I by the liver and other tissues. The metabolic effects of GH and IGF-I include stimulation of lipolysis, increased circulating free fatty acid and serum phosphorus concentrations, increased urinary excretion of calcium, and antagonism of insulin action (19).

GH secretion increases during spontaneous puberty in both boys and girls, particularly at night (17,20). This increase in GH production seems to be the result of increased pulse amplitude rather than increased pulse frequency (21). Rising estrogen and testosterone levels, in response to the maturing gonadotropic axis, stimulate an increased production of GH that, in turn, leads to a pubertal rise in IGF-I (22,23). The gonadal steroid hormones strongly regulate growth and GH secretion at puberty (1). This pubertal rise of GH occurs in both boys and girls, during spontaneous puberty as well as in puberty that is the result of stimulation by exogenous estrogens, androgens, and GnRH (24). Although both androgens and estrogens stimulate GH secretion, the effects of testosterone are believed to be mediated by estradiol after aromatization, because of the inability of dihydrotestosterone or oxandrolone, both nonaromatizable androgens, to affect GH secretion in boys (25,26) (Fig. 12.4).

Several clinical examples illustrate the dynamic interaction of the gonadotropic and somatotropic axes during pubertal development. The crucial role of GH in the pubertal process is illustrated in patients with isolated GH deficiency, who, in addition to having short stature and truncal obesity, may have delayed puberty and occasionally experience primary amenorrhea (15). Children with central preco-

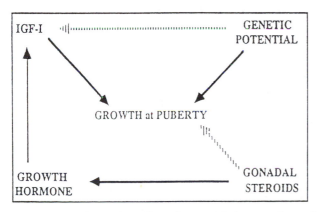

FIGURE 12.3. Schematic outline of some of the genetic nutritional and hormonal factors permitting growth at puberty.

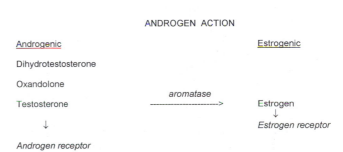

FIGURE 12.4. Possible mechanisms of androgen action.

cious puberty, which is associated with elevated levels of sex steroids, also have elevated GH and IGF-I, which then decrease with the therapeutic suppression of sex steroids with GnRH agonist treatment (27). Administration of sex steroids or pulsatile GnRH, which stimulates the production of sex steroids, to patients with hypothalamic hypogonadism results in increased production of GH and IGF-I and an increase in growth velocity (28). Finally, patients with hypopituitarism, who lack both GH and gonadotropins, will not undergo their growth spurt with the GH supplementation alone, but require additionally the presence of appropriate amounts of sex steroids (29). The exact mechanisms by which sex steroids influence GH secretion are unknown, but it is most likely at the level of the hypothalamus (30).

As mentioned previously, the increasing production of gonadal sex steroids at the time of puberty stimulates an increased secretion of GH. Conversely, evidence is accumulating that GH may have an important role in gonadal maturation and ovarian physiology. Numerous studies have illustrated that GH treatment can increase ovarian response to gonadotropins through a modulation of the local concentration of IGF-I (31). IGF-I acts as a co-gonadotropin, by increasing the ovarian response to FSH, enhancing differentiation of the granulosa cells, and inducing LH receptors (32).

Skeletal Physiology

Rapid linear growth is an integral part of the pubertal process. During childhood, the rate of linear growth is approximately 5.5 cm per year (1). Linear growth rate accelerates markedly to reach a peak during midadolescence and then diminishes to zero once the bony epiphyses fuse (1). This peak growth occurs in girls at an average age of 11 to 12 years and in boys at 13 to 14 years (19). The rapid growth occurs because of the rising levels of the gonadal steroid hormones, and it is also mediated by GH and the IGF (1). It appears that the concerted activation of the gonadal axis and augmented GH secretion are required for optimal growth at puberty (1). After epiphyseal closure, the serum testosterone levels continue to be elevated in adult men; however, GH levels return to prepubertal levels (33), a finding indicating that once the linear growth is completed, sex steroids may no longer stimulate the production of GH, and some independent mechanism must be responsible for the diminishing GH levels (1).

The relative importance of the somatomedins versus the sex steroids on the linear growth spurt is debated (19), but generally, GH and IGF seem to be most important (1). Several clinical situations illustrate the role both play in linear growth. GH is argued to have a pivotal role in the growth spurt, as illustrated by the suboptimal pubertal growth seen in children with GH deficiency. In one study (34), children with GH deficiency and hypogonadism were treated either with androgen alone or with androgen in combination with GH. Those patients treated with only androgen had insufficient growth velocities. A sustained augmentation of height velocity was observed only when androgens were administered in combination with GH.

However, evidence also supports a role for direct sex steroid effect on linear growth without stimulation of the GH axis as a mediator. Pubertal growth can be stimulated in boys by administering nonaromatizable androgens such as oxandrolone and dihydrotestosterone, without activating the somatotropic axis (25,26). In addition, the treatment of growth delay or delayed puberty with either testosterone or oxandrolone in boys with isolated GH deficiency on a constant GH dose regimen can induce a growth spurt despite this constant GH dose regimen (35). Studies in children with GH deficiency and sexual precocity provide additional evidence of an important role for the gonadal steroid hormones in promoting adolescent growth independent of GH action (36). In addition, sex steroids have direct effects on bone and cartilage *in vitro* (37).

Interesting questions remain regarding the relative roles of estrogen and androgens on pubertal growth and skeletal physiology. Patients with androgen insensitivity syndrome have disruptive mutations in the androgen receptor; the only functional sex steroid receptor is that for estrogen (38). These patients undergo a pubertal growth spurt that is appropriate in timing and peak height velocity when compared with physiologically normal girls (39). Patients with androgen insensitivity syndrome have a final stature that is closer to normal male adult height, a finding suggesting that factors linked to the Y chromosome may contribute to the taller stature of men than women (40). From the normal pubertal growth in persons with complete androgen insensitivity syndrome, it is clear that estrogen alone, in the absence of androgen action, is sufficient to support normal pubertal skeletal growth (41).

It is well known that increases in androgen levels in prepubertal children, whether endogenously or exogenously derived, result in accelerated growth and epiphyseal maturation (41). The question arises whether these effects are directly mediated by the androgen receptor or whether the effects are secondary to aromatization of androgen to estrogen and hence are estrogen-receptor mediated. Nonaromatizable androgens have been shown to have growth-promoting effects that are not mediated by the GH/IGF-I axis (25,26). Other clinical evidence that the growth-promoting effects of testosterone are not all mediated through aromatization to estrogen is that boys with familial male precocious puberty who are treated with an aromatize inhibitor do not revert to the normal prepubertal growth rate (42).

Puberty is associated with accelerated bone mineralization, especially trabecular bone (lumbar spine and femoral neck). Most bone mass is accumulated by the end of the second decade of life (43). Only slight increases occur in bone mineral density after 2 years beyond menarche (43).

There are multiple requirements to optimize bone mineralization in adolescent girls. Sex steroids are thought to be of major importance in initiating and maintaining bone mineralization, as illustrated by the decreased bone mineral density seen in amenorrheic athletes and postmenopausal women. Other requirements include calcium intake and exercise. Normal bone mineralization requires optimal calcium intake through childhood, adolescence, and adulthood (44). Weight-bearing and non–weight-bearing exercise promote bone mineralization; new bone formation occurs proportional to the stress applied across that bone (45).

Ample evidence indicates that estrogen is essential for normal pubertal epiphyseal maturation as well as skeletal mineralization (41). A case report of a man with estrogen resistance caused by a disruptive mutation in the estrogen receptor gene illustrates estrogen's crucial role in epiphyseal closure (46). This man had normal prepubertal growth and normal timing of onset of secondary sexual characteristics. However, epiphyseal fusion has not occurred, and he continues to grow at a growth velocity of 1 cm per year with a bone age of 15 years and a chronologic age of 28 years.

ABNORMAL GROWTH AND DEVELOPMENT
Precocious Thelarche

Precocious thelarche is unilateral or bilateral breast bud formation before 8 years of age without additional signs of puberty, accelerated growth, or bone maturation. It is most commonly seen in girls less than 2 years old and is a benign condition that usually spontaneously resolves within 6 months to 6 years of diagnosis (47). Premature thelarche requires no treatment, but the patient should be followed every 3 to 6 months to monitor for additional signs of pubertal changes or advancement of bone age that would suggest a diagnosis of precocious puberty. Occasionally, girls with precocious thelarche go on to develop precocious puberty (48). Obtaining a left wrist and hand radiograph for bone age is helpful to distinguish between premature thelarche, in which bone age is equal to chronologic age, and precocious puberty, in which bone age is advanced. Pelvic ultrasound examination may help to differentiate the two disorders; patients with precocious puberty often have multiple ovarian cysts (more than 6 cysts 4 mm in diameter or greater) (49) and a uterus length that is greater than the upper limit of normal in the prepubertal state (3.5 cm) (50). Girls with precocious thelarche have fewer than three ovarian cysts (49) and a uterine length that is similar to that of age-matched controls (51).

Thelarche variant is a condition clinically intermediate between premature thelarche and precocious puberty. Patients with thelarche variant have premature breast bud formation as well as accelerated growth and advancement of bone age, yet they do not develop precocious puberty (50). Unlike in premature thelarche, spontaneous breast bud resolution is uncommon; as in premature thelarche, patients with thelarche variant should be followed periodically to watch for signs of precocious puberty.

Premature Adrenarche

Premature adrenarche is isolated appearance of pubic and occasionally axillary hair before the age of 8 years without other signs of pubertal development or advancement of bone age. The cause of premature adrenarche is unknown; adrenal steroid biosynthesis appears to mature prematurely compared with the rest of the pubertal process. The mediator for the increased synthesis of steroids from the adrenal gland during either an appropriately timed pubertal process or with premature adrenarche is unknown. Premature adrenarche is more common among African-American and Latino girls as well as among obese boys and girls.

Evaluation of patients with premature adrenarche should include a left wrist and hand bone age to exclude precocious puberty, in which bone age is advanced. Some patients with premature adrenarche have defects in adrenal steroid biosynthesis; these enzyme abnormalities are more common in Ashkenazi Jews, Latinos, and Italians. At the minimum, girls should be screened for adrenal steroid abnormalities by obtaining a DHEAS level and a morning 17-OH progesterone level. If these results are abnormal, an ACTH stimulation test should be performed. Some authors advocate ACTH stimulation testing on all patients with premature adrenarche to rule out nonclassic adrenal hyperplasia (52), which is present in approximately 5% to 10% of patients with premature adrenarche (53).

Girls with premature adrenarche need follow-up every 3 to 6 months to rule out evidence of precocious puberty (growth spurt, increasing bone age, evidence of estrogenization) or virilization (rapidly growing pubic hair or clitorimegaly). Patients with virilization need to be evaluated for congenital adrenal hyperplasia and ovarian or adrenal tumors. Precocious adrenarche is considered a benign condition, and patients should anticipate an otherwise normal pubertal process compared with their age mates. However, some girls with premature adrenarche may experience hirsutism and irregular menstrual periods as adolescents (54).

Precocious Puberty

Precocious puberty in girls is the onset of pubertal changes before 8 years of age. Precocious puberty is more common in girls than in boys and usually follows the same pattern as normally timed puberty, with breast bud formation heralding the onset of changes, followed by pubic hair development, linear growth spurt, and finally menarche. Increased gonadal sex steroid production leads to increased height velocity, somatic development, and rate of skeletal maturation. Patients have a paradoxically tall stature in childhood and then, because of premature epiphyseal fusion, an adult height that is shorter than their genetic potential. Most clinicians believe that the compromised adult height is the most serious long-term sequela of precocious puberty.

Gonadotropin-Dependent Precocious Puberty

Gonadotropin-dependent precocious puberty (GDPP; complete isosexual precocious puberty, central precocious puberty, or true precocious puberty) is caused by a premature disinhibition of the hypothalamic-pituitary-gonadal axis and subsequent rising gonadal sex steroid production. In GDPP, the pubertal process often occurs more rapidly compared with normally timed puberty. The potential causes of GDPP include any lesion that impedes on the neural pathways that inhibit the GnRH pulse generator (Table 12.1). Hypothalamic tumors, most commonly hamartomas, as well as other CNS lesions such as hydrocephalus, head trauma, encephalitis, and optic gliomas, can all cause GDPP. Therapeutic interventions for CNS lesions such as surgery or radiation can also lead to GDPP (47). Idiopathic GDPP, accounting for the majority of cases in girls and for fewer than 10% of cases in boys, is a diagnosis of exclusion (55). Patients with GDPP have a normal pubertal response to GnRH stimulation testing.

Gonadotropin-Independent Precocious Puberty

Gonadotropin-independent precocious puberty (GIPP; incomplete isosexual precocious puberty, or peripheral precocious

TABLE 12.1. DIFFERENTIAL DIAGNOSIS OF PRECOCIOUS PUBERTY

Gonadotropin-dependent precocious puberty
  Idiopathic
  Hypothalamic tumors
    Hamartomas
    Astrocytomas
    Ependymomas
    Gliomas (often associated with neurofibromatosis)
    Neuroblastomas
  Other central nervous system lesions
    Hydrocephalus
    Granulomas
    Head trauma
    Infections (encephalitis, meningitis, and brain abscesses)
    Empty sella syndrome
    Opic gliomas
    Third ventricular cysts
  Secondary to gonadotropin-independent causes
Gonadotropin-independent precocious puberty
  Exposure to exogenous estrogens
  Adrenal conditions
    21-Hydroxylase deficiency
    11-Hydroxylase deficiency
    Tumor
  Ovary
    Follicular cysts
    McCune-Albright syndrome
    Tumor
  Severe hypothyroidism

puberty) involves sex steroid production that occurs independently without activation of the hypothalamic-pituitary-ovarian axis. LH and FSH levels are in the prepubertal range, and response to a GnRH stimulation test is suppressed (52). Long-term exposure to the elevated sex steroids, however, can lead to premature activation of the hypothalamic-pituitary-gonadal axis and secondary GDPP. Therefore, the presence of GDPP does not eliminate the possibility of an underlying gonadotropin-independent form of precocious puberty that needs to be identified and treated (52). GIPP can result from multiple causes including exposure to exogenous estrogen, production of sex steroids from adrenal hyperplasia and ovarian and adrenal tumors, and severe hypothyroidism (Table 12.1). The pathophysiology of hypothyroidism is uncertain; however, investigators have suggested that the extremely high levels of TSH have some intrinsic FSH activity (56). The puberty associated with hypothyroidism involves delayed growth and skeletal maturation and is reversible with thyroid hormone administration.

McCune-Albright Syndrome

McCune-Albright syndrome is a form of GIPP that characteristically also involves irregularly shaped hyperpigmented macules (*café-au-lait* spots) and a slowly progressive bone disorder (polyostotic fibrous dysplasia) (57). The syndrome is much more common in girls than boys, and it often first presents with vaginal bleeding (57). Several related endocrinopathies have been reported to occur with McCune-Albright syndrome including hyperthyroidism (57), excessive GH secretion (58), hyperprolactinemia (59), and Cushing's syndrome (60).

Patients with McCune-Albright syndrome have autonomous gonadal activity resulting in the production of pubertal levels of sex steroids and suppressed gonadotropin levels during childhood (61). Initially, the LH response to the GnRH testing is prepubertal. Later, as sex steroid levels remain elevated, the GnRH pulse generator becomes operative and results in ovulatory cycles as the patient makes a transition from GIPP to GDPP (47). The pathogenesis of the McCune-Albright syndrome has been related to the constitutive activation of the LH receptor and therefore the production of sex steroids (Fig. 12.5). A single-base substitution on the Gs protein portion of the receptor causes adenylyl cyclase activation resulting in cyclic adenosine monophosphate production, which then functions as a second messenger binding to specific regulatory regions on DNA to regulate gene transcription and expression (62).

Diagnosis and Evaluation of Precocious Puberty

Any child presenting with evidence of pubertal development, that is, breast bud formation, axillary or pubic hair growth, or suspected menarche, before the age of 8 years warrants clinical investigation. Evaluation should begin with a detailed history and physical examination (Fig. 12.6).

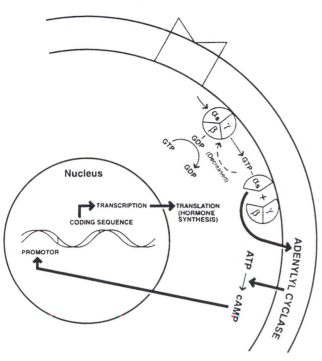

FIGURE 12.5. Mechanism of gonadotropin-independent sex steroid synthesis in McCune-Albright syndrome. In this syndrome, the Gsα subunit of the G protein is mutated at position 201 (histidine or cysteine substitution for arginine), which results in a reduction in intrinsic guanosine triphosphatase activity. This causes chronic activation of adrenylyl cyclase and constitutive cyclic adenosine monophosphate production (cAMP) resulting in precocious steroid production.

Important historical information includes chronology of the pubertal events such as thelarche, pubarche, growth spurt, and the onset of menarche. The presence or absence of axillary hair, odor, acne, and behavioral changes should be included. A family history of pubertal timing and abnormalities is also clinically relevant. Physical examination should begin with height, weight, and growth velocity assessment with the aid of appropriate growth charts. Examination of breast development and pubic and axillary hair growth is essential, as well as examining the vaginal mucosa for evidence of estrogenization or any vaginal discharge or bleeding. Abdominal examination should be performed to look for masses, such as ovarian or adrenal tumors, which could be potential sources for hormone production. A skin examination should be performed to look for any *café-au-lait* spots, and a neurologic evaluation should be performed to assess for any evidence of CNS disease.

The most important initial diagnostic test in a patient with suspected precocious pubertal development is the radiograph of the left hand to determine bone age. A bone age consistent with chronologic age is more consistent with premature thelarche or adrenarche. Parental reassurance and patient follow-up are sufficient. Some authors do suggest ACTH stimulation testing on all patients with premature adrenarche to rule out nonclassic adrenal hyperplasia (52). Further investigation is warranted if the bone age is ad-

vanced more than 2 standard deviations (SD) above chronologic age. Further evaluation is then guided by the patient's individual history and physical features.

In patients with advanced bone age, GnRH stimulation testing is important to determine whether there has been activation of the hypothalamic-pituitary-ovarian axis, to help to distinguish between GDPP and GIPP. Patients are given GnRH (100 μg) intravenously, and LH and FSH levels are obtained 30 and 60 minutes later. A pubertal response, as seen in GDPP, includes an LH-predominate rise in response to the GnRH. In GIPP, a prepubertal response is seen, with no significant rise in LH or FSH in response to GnRH stimulation. Patients with a pubertal response to the GnRH stimulation testing may have either a gonadotropin-dependent source of their precocious puberty or an underlying gonadotropin-independent source that has secondarily disinhibited the hypothalamic-pituitary axis. Therefore, all patients with a pubertal response to GnRH testing should be evaluated for both gonadotropin-dependent and gonadotropin-independent causes.

Various radiologic studies are helpful in the evaluation of the child with precocious puberty. Magnetic resonance imaging or computed tomography of the head is indicated in patients with a pubertal response to GnRH testing to rule out CNS lesions such as hamartomas. As mentioned earlier, pelvic ultrasound with examination of the uterus and ovaries is useful not only to rule out sex steroid–producing ovarian tumors or cysts, but also to look for evidence of pubertal changes in the uterus in response to estrogen production. Adrenal ultrasound can be used to rule out adrenal tumors; bone scans may be indicated in patients suspected of having McCune-Albright syndrome, to look for the classic skeletal changes.

The laboratory tests ordered should be individualized to the patient's presentation. Patients with virilization should be screened for adrenal and ovarian sources of hormone production with serum testosterone, DHEAS, and 17-OH progesterone levels. Patients with short stature, delayed bone age, or any other signs of hypothyroidism should be screened for thyroid disease with TSH.

Treatment of Precocious Puberty

GnRH agonist therapy is the mainstay of treatment for GDPP. GnRH administered in a continuous fashion suppresses pulsatile LH and FSH release and gonadal steroid output and therefore slows the pubertal process (3). Suppression initially results from downregulation and loss of GnRH receptors, but later receptor levels return to normal and suppression results from uncoupling of the receptors from the intracellular signaling effector pathway (63). Leuprolide acetate is the only depot GnRH agonist preparation that may be given every 4 weeks that is approved by the United States Food and Drug Administration, and it has been proven to be efficacious and safe for the treatment of GDPP (64).

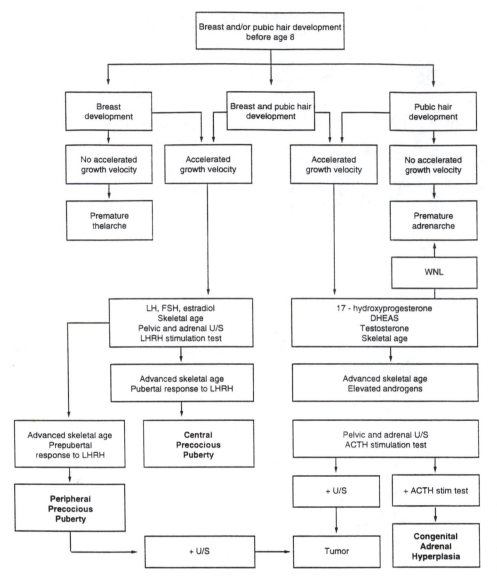

FIGURE 12.6. Schematic evaluation of precocious puberty. (From Meyers-Seifer C and Seifer DB. *Clinical reproductive medicine,* eds., Cowan BD and Seifer BD. Philadelphia: Lippincott-Raven, 1997, with permission.)

Although the safety and efficacy of GnRH agonist therapy are clearly established, controversy exists regarding which patients will potentially benefit from therapy. The decision to treat precocious puberty is based on several factors, including the child's age, the emotional impact of experiencing early puberty, and the predicted height (52).

Patients with GIPP should have interventions tailored to the specific cause of the sex steroid production. This may include medical therapy for patients with congenital adrenal hyperplasia or hypothyroidism or surgical therapy for patients with ovarian tumors.

Delayed Puberty

Puberty is *delayed* when there is no breast development by age 13.5 or the absence of menarche by age 16. These figures represent the mean +3 SD and describe the upper time limit for 99% of the female population in North America. Generally, the pubertal process from its onset with thelarche to its conclusion with menarche is usually completed within 5 years. Boys more commonly seek medical care for delayed growth or pubertal development than do girls, most likely because of the increased social and behavioral problems boys experience with this clinical situation. The actual incidence of delayed puberty does not differ markedly by gender (2). The disorders of delayed puberty can be classified into three major diagnostic categories: hypogonadotropic hypogonadism, hypergonadotropic hypogonadism, and eugonadotropic conditions (Table 12.2).

Hypogonadotropic Hypogonadism

Hypogonadotropic pubertal delay results from an absent or delayed secretion of pituitary gonadotropins with a broad

TABLE 12.2. DIFFERENTIAL DIAGNOSIS OF DELAYED PUBERTY

Hypogonadotropic hypogonadism
  Constitutional delay
  Hypothyroidism
  Anorexia nervosa
  Excessive physical training
  Malabsorption
  Prolactinoma
  Kallman's syndrome
  Chronic illness
  Cushing's syndrome
  Craniopharyngioma
  Idiopathic or secondary hypopituitarism
Hypergonadotropic hypogonadism
  Gonadal dysgenesis
  Premature ovarian failure
  Secondary ovarian failure
    Surgery
    Trauma
    Irradiation
  17-Hydroxylase deficiency
Eugonadotropic conditions
  Müllerian agenesis
  Transverse vaginal septum
  Imperforate hymen
  Androgen-resistant syndrome

range of causes including constitutional delay, systemic disease, and CNS lesions. Constitutional delay of puberty, the most common form of hypogonadotropic delay, is a variant of the pubertal process in which puberty, although initiated and completed at a later age, otherwise occurs normally with no long-term negative sequelae. Patients with constitutional delay have no endocrinologic abnormalities and present with serum gonadotropin levels that are appropriate for their stage of pubertal development. It is often difficult to differentiate between constitutional delay and other more serious causes of hypogonadotropic hypogonadism based on laboratory testing. Attempts to differentiate constitutional delay from other conditions have included using GnRH priming or superagonist GnRH to elicit an increased response of gonadotropin secretion in patients with constitutional delay compared with other forms of hypogonadotropic hypogonadism. Other studies have investigated measuring bioactive gonadotropin response to GnRH testing, with the assumption that patients with constitutional delay would have an increased response. Currently, no practical and reliable endocrinologic test is available to differentiate constitutional delay from other more serious causes of hypogonadotropic hypogonadism. Constitutional delay remains a diagnosis of exclusion that is confirmed retrospectively as the patient completes the pubertal process albeit at a later age than the norm.

In *Kallman's syndrome,* the most common form of hypogonadotropic hypogonadism, gonadotropin secretion is permanently absent. Patients with Kallman's syndrome have

decreased GnRH activity combined with an impairment in the sense of smell. Normally, GnRH neurons initiate outside the CNS in the olfactory placode and, by 19 weeks of gestation, migrate to the mediobasal hypothalamus, where they can communicate with and stimulate the pituitary. In patients with Kallman's syndrome, this migration does not occur, and GnRH neurons are found outside the CNS, in the nasal septum, in the cribriform plate, and within the dural layers of the meninges of the forebrain (65). The genetic basis for Kallman's syndrome has been determined; the lack of production of adhesion molecules necessary for the neuronal migration is coded by the *KAL* gene located at Xp22.3 (65).

Other CNS abnormalities responsible for hypogonadotropic hypogonadism include tumors such as craniopharyngioma, a slow-growing tumor arising from the squamous cells at the junction of the anterior and posterior pituitary, which through compression on the pituitary gland may decrease gonadotropin production. Iatrogenic causes such as radiation or trauma may also cause secondary panhypopituitarism and may lead to pubertal delay.

Many chronic diseases including Cushing's syndrome, hypothyroidism, prolactinomas, anorexia nervosa, renal insufficiency, and bowel disease may cause pubertal delay. Clinical improvement in these medical conditions usually results in catch-up growth and pubertal progress. Excessive physical activity such as ballet dancing may also cause delayed puberty. In dance, each year of intense training before menarche can result in a 5-month delay in menarche (66). Factors such as a favorable psychosocial environment and nutrition can also play a permissive role in normal growth and pubertal development.

Hypergonadotropic Hypogonadism

Most forms of *hypergonadotropic hypogonadism* involve a gonadal disorder with decreased production of estrogen and a secondary rise in the level of gonadotropins. The most common cause of hypergonadotropic hypogonadism is gonadal dysgenesis including Turner's syndrome and Swyer's syndrome. Ovarian failure in *Turner's syndrome* results from the accelerated atresia of the primordial follicles in the 45,XO germ cells. Mosaic forms of Turner's syndrome have been identified and have similar ovarian pathophysiology. The most common type of Turner's mosaicism is 45,X/46,XX. Buccal smears are unable to detect Turner's mosaicism. Lymphocytes from peripheral blood should be used for karyotype determination to avoid missing patients with mosaicism, particularly patients with the potentially carcinogenic types containing a Y chromosome in whom gonadectomy is warranted.

Patients with *Swyer's syndrome* have a 46,XY karyotype and streak gonads that fail to secrete müllerian-inhibiting substance (MIS) or testosterone. The absence of MIS results in complete development of the müllerian system; the absence of testosterone results in the lack of male sexual differentiation, stimulation of wolffian structures, or virilization. The end result is a phenotypic female with sexual immaturity, low levels of testosterone production, and elevated gonadotropins.

Premature ovarian failure is amenorrhea with elevated gonadotropins in a woman less than 35 years old and is another potential cause of hypergonadotropic pubertal delay. If premature ovarian failure occurs before the age of 30 years, a karyotype should be obtained to rule out the previously mentioned chromosomal causes, Turner's syndrome or Swyer's syndrome. Other causes of premature ovarian failure include iatrogenic damage to the ovaries from chemotherapy or radiation and pituitary tumors. Autoimmune diseases causing multiple gland failure can also cause premature ovarian failure. Other abnormalities presenting with the ovarian failure secondary to autoimmune disease can include thyroid disease, hypoparathyroidism, diabetes, adrenal insufficiency, myasthenia gravis, pernicious anemia, celiac disease, vitiligo, and alopecia.

A rare cause of hypergonadotropic pubertal delay is *congenital adrenal hyperplasia* resulting from a deficiency of 17α-hydroxylase. Impairment in the hydroxylation of progesterone and pregnenolone result in deficiencies in cortisol, estrogen, and androgens. Patients have diminished levels of estrogens and androgens that result in sexual immaturity and elevated gonadotropins. Patients also have hypertension resulting from the elevated production of mineralocorticoids.

Eugonadism

Most patients with *eugonadotropic conditions* present with primary amenorrhea resulting from the abnormal development of müllerian structures. Müllerian agenesis is the most common form of primary amenorrhea in adolescent girls with normal secondary sexual characteristics. Girls with müllerian agenesis have a 46,XX karyotype, ovaries, and normal estrogen production and gonadotropin levels, yet they fail to experience menarche because of the developmental absence of the upper vagina and uterus. Patients with a transverse vaginal septum and an imperforate hymen are unable to have egress of menstrual flow and therefore may present with primary amenorrhea and cyclic abdominal or pelvic pain with normal secondary sexual characteristics. Patients with a transverse vaginal septum may also have other associated müllerian developmental abnormalities.

Patients with androgen insensitivity are phenotypically female with a 46,XY karyotype. The presence of the testes determining factor (TDF) on the Y chromosome leads to the development of testes and normal male levels of MIS, testosterone, and gonadotropins. MIS production results in absence of müllerian structures and a blind-ending vagina. Although circulating levels of testosterone are at the normal male range, an androgen receptor defect inhibits a physiologic response to the testosterone that results in the absence

of male sexual differentiation, wolffian duct stimulation, or virilization. Patients have sparse pubic and axillary hair because of the androgen receptor defect. In some patients, the expression of the androgen receptor defect is incomplete and can result in varying degrees of masculinization. Peripheral aromatization of androgens to estrogens results in breast development. Androgen insensitivity is an X-linked recessive trait; a family history of infertility in female relatives may suggest this disorder. Androgen insensitivity results from a variety of genetic defects in the androgen receptor gene including a point mutation, a large deletion in the androgen-binding domain of the receptor gene, aberrant splicing, and a premature termination codon in messenger RNA (67).

Diagnosis and Evaluation of Delayed Puberty

Evaluation of a child with delayed puberty should begin with a careful history, noting in particular the patient's growth, history of chronic illnesses, age of onset of breast buds or pubic hair, and family history of pubertal development (Fig. 12.7). Physical examination should include the patient's height and weight, sense of smell, size of thyroid, axillary or pubic hair, breast contour, and evidence of galactorrhea. Pelvic examination with confirmation of a patent vagina and palpable uterus are particularly important in girls who present with mature secondary sexual characteristics and primary amenorrhea, to rule out eugonadotropic causes of pubertal delay.

Delayed or absent secondary sexual characteristics warrant obtaining serum FSH and LH levels to distinguish between hypogonadotropic and hypergonadotropic forms of pubertal delay. Patients with elevated gonadotropins require a karyotype from peripheral lymphocytes to rule out chromosomal abnormalities such as Turner's syndrome (including Turner's mosaicism) or Swyer's syndrome. A normal 46,XX karyotype could be consistent with pure gonadal dysgenesis or an autoimmune form of ovarian failure.

Patient's with low FSH and LH levels need additional laboratory work to rule out other chronic medical conditions or endocrinopathies that could be responsible for the pubertal delay including electrolytes, blood urea nitrogen, creatinine, thyroid-stimulating hormone, and prolactin. Bone age, which is delayed in constitutional delay, may be useful in suggesting that diagnosis. Magnetic resonance imaging may be required to rule out CNS lesions such as craniopharyngioma.

Treatment of Delayed Puberty

The treatment of pubertal delay depends on the underlying cause. For patients with constitutional delay, the primary arguments for treatment over observation are for psychosocial or behavioral reasons as well as to increase bone density. The psychologic effects of pubertal delay are varied and are more common in boys, but they can include depression, oppositional behavior, psychosomatic complaints, low self-

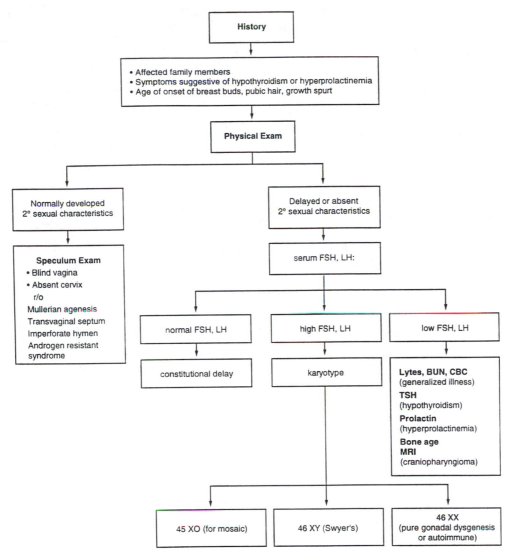

FIGURE 12.7. Schematic evaluation of delayed puberty. (From Meyers-Seifer C and Seifer DB. *Clinical reproductive medicine,* eds., Cowan BD and Seifer BD. Philadelphia: Lippincott-Raven, 1997, with permission.)

esteem, poor school performance, reduced peer contact, aggression toward peers, immature goals age, and general social immaturity (68). Because peak bone mass is accrued during the second decade of life, it seems reasonable to normalize the estrogen milieu during this critical period to avoid the risk of diminished adult bone density. Exogenous estrogen can be used in patients with constitutional delay to initiate or hasten development of secondary sexual characteristics and to facilitate bone mass accrual. Low levels of exogenous steroids are used to try to avoid skeletal maturation beyond chronologic age, premature epiphyseal closure, and shortened adult height. The amount of estrogen used can be slowly increased at 3 monthly intermittent sequences; eventually, these patients will require cyclic progestin as well. Oral contraceptive pills are an alternative form of therapy once secondary sexual characteristics have been established. Patients with permanent hypogonadism require estrogen replacement therapy for both development of sec-

ondary sexual characteristics and for bone mass accrual. Patients with hypogonadism secondary to chronic medical conditions or endocrinopathies usually experience catch-up growth and pubertal advancement with treatment of the underlying medical condition. Müllerian developmental anomalies may require surgical intervention for menstrual egress and sexual function. Patients identified with Y chromosomes need gonadectomy to protect them from an increased risk of forming dysgerminomas and gonadoblastomas.

10 KEY POINTS

1. The pubertal process, with rapid linear growth and sexual maturation, is controlled by the closely linked interaction of the gonadotropin and somatomedin axes as well as independent adrenal androgen production.

2. Gonadarche, or maturation of the GnRH, FSH/LH, sex steroid axis is important in the develop of secondary sexual characteristics, menarche, and eventually ovulatory menstrual cycles.

3. Adrenarche occurs independently of gonadarche and is responsible for axillary and pubic hair growth through rising levels of weakly androgenic adrenal hormones, DHEA and DHEAS.

4. GH is secreted from the anterior pituitary; its secretion is stimulated by GHRH produced from the hypothalamus and is inhibited by somatostatin production from the hypothalamus. GH secretion is also regulated by sex steroids, IGF-I, glucocorticoids, and thyroid hormones.

5. The pubertal linear growth spurt results from the concomitant rising levels of gonadal sex steroids that contribute the increased secretion of GH and IGF, all of which appear to have key roles in attaining maximum adult height.

6. Premature thelarche and premature adrenarche both have normal bone ages, are benign conditions with no negative long-term sequelae, and require long-term follow-up to monitor for evidence of precocious puberty.

7. Precocious puberty is more common in girls than boys, and it may be either gonadotropin dependent or gonadotropin independent. The mainstay of therapy in GDPP is the use of GnRH analogues; the mainstay of therapy in GIPP lesions is treatment, either medical or surgical, of the underlying cause.

8. McCune-Albright syndrome, more common in girls than boys, involves *café-au-lait* spots, polyostotic fibrous dysplasia, and GIPP; it is caused by a stimulatory defect in the Gs protein of the LH receptor.

9. Delayed puberty is defined by the absence of breast development by 13.5 years or the absence of menarche by 16 years.

10. Disorders of pubertal delay are generally classified as hypogonadotropic hypogonadism (constitutional delay, chronic illness, CNS lesions), hypergonadotropic hypogonadism (gonadal dysgenesis, ovarian failure, 17α-hydroxylase deficiency), and eugonadism (developmental abnormalities in the müllerian system, androgen resistance syndrome).

REFERENCES

1. Rogol A. Growth at puberty: interaction of androgens and growth hormone. *Med Sci Sports Exerc* 1994;26:767–770.
2. Kulin HE, Muller J. The biological aspects of puberty. *Pediatr Rev* 1996;17:75–86.
3. Belchetz PE, Plant TM, Nakai Y, et al. Hypophyseal responses to continuous and intermittent delivery of hypothalamic gonadotropin-releasing hormone. *Science* 1978;202:631–633.
4. Mellon PL, Windle JJ, Goldsmith PC, et al. Immortalization of hypothalamic GnRH neurons by genetically targeted tumorigenesis. *Neuron* 1990;5:1–10.
5. Styne DM. Physiology of puberty. *Horm Res* 1994;41[Suppl 2]:3–6.
6. Veldhuis JD. Neuroendocrine mechanisms mediating awakening of the human gonadotropic axis in puberty. *Pediatr Nephrol* 1996;10:304–317.
7. Veldhuis JD. The hypothalamic pituitary-testicular axis. In: Yen SSC, Jaffe RB, eds. *Reproductive endocrinology*, 3rd ed. Philadelphia: WB Saunders, 1991.
8. Fukuda M, Gick D, Pfaff DW. Luteinizing hormone–releasing hormone (LHRH) cells do not migrate normally in an inherited hypogonadal (Kallmann) syndrome. *Mol Brain Res* 1989; 6:311–326.
9. Wu FCW, Butler GE, Kelnar CJH, et al. Patterns of pulsatile luteinizing hormone secretion from childhood to adulthood in the human male: a study using deconvolution analysis and an ultrasenstive immunofluorometric assay. *J Clin Endocrinol Metab* 1995;81:1798–1805.
10. Veldhuis JD, Rogol AD, Perez-Palacios G, et al. Actions of estradiol on discrete attributes of the luteinizing hormone pulse signal in man: studies in postmenopausal women treated with pure estradiol. *J Clin Invest* 1987;79:769–776.
11. Blizzard RM, Thompson RG, Baghdassarian A. The interrelationship of steroids, growth hormone and other hormones in pubertal growth. In: Grumbach MN, Grave JD, Mayer FE, eds. *The control of the onset of puberty*. New York: Wiley, 1974.
12. Wierman ME, Beardsworth DE, Crawford JD, et al. Adrenarche and skeletal maturation during luteinizing hormone–releasing hormone analogue suppression of gonadarche. *J Clin Invest* 1986;77:121–126.
13. Kerrigan JR, Veldhuis JD, Leyo SA, et al. Estimation of daily cortisol production and clearance rates in normal pubertal males by deconvolution analysis. *J Clin Endocrinol Metab* 1993; 76:1505–1510.
14. Takahashi Y, Kipnis DM, Daughaday WH. Growth hormone secretion during sleep. *J Clin Invest* 1968;47:2079–2090.
15. Sharara FI, Giudice LC. Role of growth hormone in ovarian physiology and onset of puberty. *J Soc Gynecol Invest* 1997; 4:1–7.
16. Dracier J, Sheppard MS, Lake J, et al. Effect of withdrawal of somatostatin and growth hormone (GH)–releasing factor on GH release *in vitro*. *Endocrinology* 1985;117:2208–2216.
17. Isaksson OPG, Isgaard J, Nilson A, et al. Direct action of GH. In: Bercu BB, ed. *Basic and clinical aspects of growth hormone*. New York: Plenum, 1988:198–211.
18. Yamashita S, Weiss M, Melmed S. IGF-I regulates growth hormone secretion and mRNA levels in human pituitary tumor cells. *J Clin Endocrinol Metab* 1986;63:513–518.
19. Loche S, Casini MR, Faedda A. The GH/IGF-I axis in puberty. *BJCP* 1996;85:1–4.
20. Mauras N, Blizzard RM, Link K, et al. Augmentation of growth hormone secretion during puberty: evidence for a pulse amplitude modulated phenomenon. *J Clin Endocrinol Metab* 1972;35: 596–601.
21. Rose SR, Muicchi G, Barnes KM, et al. Spontaneous growth hormone secretion increases during puberty in normal girls and boys. *J Clin Endocrinol Metab* 1991;73:428–435.
22. Ross JL, Pescovitz OH, Barnes KM, et al. Growth hormone secretory dynamics in children with precocious puberty. *J Pediatr* 1987;110:369–372.
23. Furnaletto RW, Cara JF. Somatomedin-C/insulin-like growth factor-I as a modulator of growth during childhood and adolescence. *Horm Res* 1986;24:177–184.
24. Kerrigan JR, Rogol AD. The impact of gonadal steroid hormone action on growth hormone secretion during childhood and adolescence. *Endocrinol Rev* 1992;13:281–298.
25. Malhotra A, Poon E, Tse WY, et al. The effects of oxandrolone on the growth hormone and gonadal axes in boys with constitutional delay of growth and puberty. *Clin Endocrinol* 1993;38:393–398.
26. Keenan BS, Richards GE, Ponder SW. Androgen-stimulated pubertal growth: the effects of testosterone and dihydrotestoster

one on growth hormone and insulin-like growth factor-I in the treatment of short stature and delayed puberty. *J Clin Endocrinol Metab* 1993;76:996–1001.

27. Mansfield MJ, Rudlin CR, Crigler JF, et al. Changes in growth and serum growth hormone and plasma somatomedin-C levels during suppression of gonadal sex steroid secretion in girls with central precocious puberty. *J Clin Endocrinol Metab* 1988; 66:3–9.

28. Stanhope R, Pringle PJ, Brook CGD. The mechanism of the adolescent growth spurt induced by low dose pulsatile GnRH treatment. *Clin Endocrinol* 1988;28:83–91.

29. Tanner JM, Whitehouse RH, Hughes PCR, et al. Relative importance of growth hormone and sex steroids for the growth at puberty of trunk length, limb length, and muscle width in growth hormone–deficient children. *J Pediatr* 1976;89:1000–1008.

30. Wehrenberg WB, Giustina A. Basic counterpoint: mechanisms and pathways of gonadal steroid modulation of growth hormone secretion. *Endocrinol Rev* 1992;13:299–308.

31. Albanese A, Stanhope R. Growth hormone, growth factors and the gonad. *Horm Res* 1995;44[Suppl 3]:15–17.

32. Adashi EY, Resnick CE, Svobota ME, et al. Somatomedin C synergizes with FSH in the acquisition of projection of biosynthetic capacity by altered rat granulosa cells. *Endocrinology* 1985;116:2315–2342.

33. Ho KY, Evans WS, Blizzard RM, et al. Effects of sex and age on the 24-hr secretory profile of GH secretion in man: importance of endogenous estradiol concentrations. *J Clin Endocrinol Metab* 1987;64:51–58.

34. Aynsley-Green A, Zachman M, Prader A. Interrelation of the therapeutic effects of growth hormone and testosterone on growth in hypopituitarism. *J Pediatr* 1976;89:992–999.

35. Albanese A, Stanhope R. Treatment of growth delay in boys with isolated growth hormone deficiency. *J Eur Endocrinol* 1994;130:65–69.

36. Attie CM, Ramirez NR, Conte FA, et al. The pubertal growth spurt in eight patients with true precocious puberty and growth hormone deficiency: evidence for a direct role of sex steroids. *J Clin Endocrinol Metab* 1990;71:975–983.

37. Kasperk CH, Wergedal JE, Farley JR, et al. Androgens directly stimulate proliferation of bone cells *in vitro*. *Endocrinology* 1989;124:1576–1578.

38. Brown TR, Lubahn DB, Wilson EM, et al. Functional characterization of naturally occurring mutant androgen receptors from subjects with complete androgen insensitivity. *Mol Endocrinol* 1990;4:1759–1772.

39. Zachmann M, Prader A, Sobel EH, et al. Indirect evidence for the importance of estrogens in pubertal gowth of girls. *J Pediatr* 1986;108:694–697.

40. Pescovitz OH. The endocrinology of the pubertal growth spurt. *Acta Paediatr Scand* 1990;367[Suppl]:119–125.

41. Frank GR. The role of estrogen in pubertal skeletal physiology: epiphyseal maturation and mineralization of the skeleton. *Acta Paediatr* 1995;84:627–630.

42. Laue L, Kenigsberg D, Pexcovitz OH, et al. Treatment of familial male precocious puberty with spironolactone and testolatone. *N Engl J Med* 1989;320:496–502.

43. Theintz G, Buchs D, Rizzoli R, et al. Longitudinal monitoring of bone mass accumulation in healthy adolescents: evidence for marked reduction after 16 years of age at the levels of lumbar spine and femoral neck in female subjects. *J Clin Endocrinol Metab* 1992;75:1060–1065.

44. Hergenroeder AC. Bone mineralization, hypothalamic amenorrhea, and sex steroid therapy in female adolescents and young adults. *J Pediatr* 1995;126:683–689.

45. Donaldson CL, Hulley SB, Vogel JM, et al. Effects of prolonged bed rest on bone mineral. *Metabolism* 1970;19:1071–1084.

46. Smith EP, Boyd J, Frank GR, et al. Estrogen resistance caused by a mutation in the estrogen-receptor gene in a man. *N Engl J Med* 1994;331:1056–1061.

47. Styne D. New aspects in the diagnosis and treatment of pubertal disorders. *Pediatr Clin North Am* 1997;44:505–529.

48. Pasquino AM, Pucarelli I, Passeri F, et al. Progression of premature thelarche to precocious puberty. *J Pediatr* 1995;126:11–14.

49. Stanhope R, Brook CCD. Thelarche variant: a new syndrome of precocious sexual maturation? *Acta Endocrinol* 1990;123: 481–486.

50. Ivarsson SA, Nilsson KO, Persson PH. Ultrasonography of the pelvic organs in the prepubertal and postpubertal girls. *Arch Dis Child* 1983;58:352–354.

51. Haber HP, Wollmann HA, Ranke MB. Pelvic ultrasonography: early differentiation between isolated premature thelarche and central precocious puberty. *Eur J Pediatr* 1995;154:182–186.

52. Merke DP, Cutler GB. Evaluation and management of precocious puberty. *Arch Dis Child* 1996;75:269–271.

53. Balducci R, Boscherini B, Mangiantini A, et al. Isolated precocious pubarche: an approach. *J Clin Endocrinol Metab* 1994; 79:582–589.

54. Ibanez L, Potau N, Saenger P, et al. Postpubertal outcome in girls diagnosed of premature pubarche during childhood: increased frequency of functional ovarian hyperandrogenism. *J Clin Endocrinol Metab* 1993;76:1599–1603.

55. Pescovitz OH, Comite F, Hench K, et al. The NIH experience with precocious puberty: diagnostic subgroups and response to short-term luteinizing hormone releasing hormone analogue therapy. *J Pediatr* 1986;108:47–54.

56. Anasti JN, Flack MR, Froehlich J, et al. A potential novel mechanism for precocious puberty in juvenile hypothyroidism. *J Clin Endocrinol Metab* 1995;80:276–279.

57. Lee PA, Van Dop C, Migeon CJ. McCune-Albright syndrome: long term follow up. *JAMA* 1986;256:2980–2984.

58. Moran A, Pescovitz OH. Long-term treatment of gigantism with combination octreotide and bromocriptine in a child with McCune-Albright syndrome. *J Endocrinol* 1994;2:111–113.

59. Cuttler L, Jackson JA, Saeed uz-Zafer M, et al. Hypersecretion of growth horone and prolactin in McCune-Albright syndrome. *J Clin Endocrinol Metab* 1989;68:1148–1154.

60. Danson M, Robboy SJ, Kim S, et al. Cushing syndrome, sexual precocity and polystotic fibrous dysplasia (Albright syndrome) in infancy. *J Pediatr* 1975;87:917– 921.

61. Shanker RR, Pescovitz OH. Precocious puberty. *Adv Endocrinol Metab* 1995;6:55–89.

62. Weinstein LS, Shenker A, Gejman PV, et al. Activating mutations of the stimulatory G protein in the McCune-Albright syndrome. *N Engl J Med* 1991;325:1688–1695.

63. Conn PM, Crowley WF. Gonadotropin-releasing hormone and it analogs. *Annu Rev Med* 1994;45:391–405.

64. Carel JC, Lahlou N, Guazzarotti L, et al. Treatment of central precocious puberty with depot leuprorelin: French Leuprorelin Trial Group. *Eur J Endocrinol* 1995;120:709–715.

65. Schwanzel-Fukuda M, Bick D, Pfaff DW. Luteinizing hormone releasing hormone (LHRH)–expressing cells do not migrate normally in an inherited hypogonadal (Kallman) syndrome. *Mol Brain Res* 1989;6:311–326.

66. Albanese A, Stanhope R. Investigation of delayed puberty. *Clin Endocrinol* 1995;43:105–110.

67. Gustafson M, Donahoe P. Male sex determination: current concepts of male sexual differentiation. *Annu Rev Med* 1994;45: 505–524.

68. Kulin H. Extensive personal experience: delayed puberty. *J Clin Endocrinol Metab* 1996;81:3460–3464.

69. Meyers-Seifer C, Seifer DB. *Clinical reproductive medicine*, eds., Cowan BD and Seifer BD. Philadelphia: Lippincott-Raven, 1997.

FEMALE REPRODUCTIVE AGING

BRENDA S. HOUMARD
DAVID E. BATTAGLIA
DAVID B. SEIFER

The impact of reproductive aging on the health and well-being of modern women is great, with influences ranging from fertility and childbearing to menopausal health and diseases (Table 13.1). The aim of this chapter is to review the scope of clinical problems associated with reproductive aging, the physiologic mechanisms that result in reproductive aging, and the clinical management of health issues related to aging of the female reproductive system.

The effects of reproductive aging are clinically evident long before the menstrual irregularities of the perimenopause and the cessation of menses at menopause. Investigators have long known that fertility declines with age, particularly after the age of 35 years (1,2). In addition, spontaneous abortion rates increase with age (3,4), as does the incidence of chromosomal abnormalities in ongoing pregnancies (5).

As women in our society delay childbearing to their late 30s and 40s, these procreative issues resulting from reproductive age become increasingly important. With aging of the Baby Boom generation, the number of women aged 35 to 45 years is estimated to increase from 13 million in 1980 to 18.5 million in 2010 (6). Furthermore, these women are delaying childbearing, as reflected by an increase in the percentage of first births to women 30 to 34 years of age from 3% in 1970 to 12% in 1986 (7). The age-related infertility that some of these women may experience is not easily alleviated with current medical treatment. Although more than one-sixth of assisted reproductive technology (ART) in the United States is performed on women older than 39 years, the pregnancy rates are markedly lower in this age group. Whereas women less than 35 years old achieved a 25% to 27% delivery rate per oocyte retrieval during *in vitro* fertilization (IVF) cycles, women more than 39 years old experienced a much lower delivery rate (6% to 10%) (8). These lower delivery rates reflect both decreased conception rates and increased spontaneous abortion rates in the older women. Thus, the clinical impact of ovarian aging on fertility is substantial and occurs as early as the fourth decade of life.

The scope of clinical issues related to ovarian aging also extends beyond procreative issues. The impact of the menopausal state on the risks and progression of certain chronic diseases has become increasingly apparent. Menopause is an important risk factor for coronary artery disease and its associated risk factors (obesity, hypertension, and hyperlipidemia), as well as for osteoporosis and joint disease, urogenital dysfunction, Alzheimer's disease, and depression (9). In addition to altered risks for these debilitating and life-threatening diseases, perimenopausal women sometimes experience significant discomfort and distress from psychosocial and "hot flush" symptoms as well as from irregular uterine bleeding.

Understanding and addressing the impact of the menopause on women's health will become increasingly important as the 21st century advances. Population projections indicate that the number of postmenopausal women will increase from 467 million in 1990 to 1.2 billion by the year 2030, at which time approximately 47 million women will be entering menopause each year (10). Women in developed countries will spend approximately one-third of their lives in the postmenopausal state (11).

PHYSIOLOGIC BASIS OF REPRODUCTIVE AGING

Reproductive aging precedes aging in other organs and tissues. Other endocrine systems, such as the thyroid, adrenal, pituitary, and pancreas, also show age-related changes in function (12). However, these changes are typically observed in the sixth to seventh decade of life, which is much later than that observed in the female reproductive system.

Clinical success with oocyte donation programs, which alleviate age-related infertility in older women by using oocytes collected from younger women, support the notion that reproductive aging in women is primarily the result of diminished ovarian function and oocyte quality rather than uterine factors (13). The underlying physiologic basis for ovarian aging appears to involve attrition in follicle numbers in the ovary as well as qualitative changes in follicular function and oocyte characteristics.

TABLE 13.1. IMPACT OF REPRODUCTIVE AGING ON WOMEN'S HEALTH

Procreative issues
  Infertility
  Spontaneous abortion
  Incidence of aneuploidy
Menopausal issues
  Perimenopausal/Menopausal Symptoms
    Hot flushes
    Menstrual cycle irregularities
    Menorrhagia
    Vaginal dryness and atrophy
    Urinary incontinence
    Mood changes
  Risk of chronic diseases
    Coronary artery disease
    Osteoporosis
    Alzheimer's disease
    Colon cancer
    Macular degeneration

A thorough understanding of ovarian development and age-related changes in the germ cell (oocyte) and somatic components (granulosa cells, theca cells) of the ovary is essential to the elucidation of the physiologic basis of reproductive senescence.

Ovarian Follicle Number and the Reproductive Axis from Birth to Menopause

Fetal Ovarian Development

Early development of the human ovary is a complex process that requires coordinated differentiation of the primordial germ cells and the indifferent gonad (14). Primordial germ cells, which begin to differentiate in the blastocyst at about 4 to 5 days of life, migrate from the endoderm of the yolk sac into the gonadal ridge. At 5 to 6 weeks of gestation, the indifferent gonad consists of primordial germ cells, the mesenchyme of the gonadal ridge, and cells derived from the coelomic epithelium. During the latter half of the first trimester, these primordial germ cells localize to the cortex of the developing ovary and begin to multiply as oogonia by the process of mitosis. By 16 to 20 weeks of gestation, the peak number of germ cells is reached. Oogonia are converted to oocytes as the first meiotic division begins. Oogonia begin to enter meiosis at about 11 to 12 weeks gestation in the human ovary, and all are arrested in the diplotene stage of prophase I shortly after birth. As these primary oocytes are entering meiosis, they become associated with precursors to granulosa cells and form primordial follicles. They remain arrested in this stage of meiosis until the time of ovulation.

Follicle Numbers from the Fetal Period to Menopause

Attrition in follicle numbers during the latter portion of fetal development and throughout the remainder of a woman's reproductive life (Fig. 13.1) is now considered to represent the physiologic basis of reproductive aging. Peak numbers of germ cells (6 to 7 million) are found in the fetal ovary during the fifth month of gestation (15). Through the process of atresia, this population is reduced to approximately 2 million at birth. Studies of follicular numbers during childhood and puberty, which are limited to examinations of less than 20 prepubertal ovaries (15,16) and 5 pubertal ovaries (16), reveal that only 300,000 to 400,000 follicles are present in the ovaries when a woman becomes reproductively competent.

The numbers of primordial follicles steadily decline throughout the reproductive years (16,17). This decline appears to be biexponential (18,19), with an accelerated loss of primordial follicles occurring after the age of 38 years (17). Although primordial follicles have been reported to be present in the postmenopausal ovary (20), these data are difficult to interpret because the number of patients, their ages, the number of tissue sections examined, and the number of follicles present per ovary are not reported. A more recent quantitative study of follicle numbers during the perimenopausal transition revealed marked depletion of the follicle pool as menopause approaches (21). In women of similar ages, primordial follicle numbers were markedly reduced in women with perimenopausal menstrual patterns (about 140 primordial follicles per ovary) as compared with regularly menstruating women (about 1,400 primordial follicles per ovary). In the 4 postmenopausal ovaries examined in this study, only a single follicle was found. Thus, these findings support the hypothesis that reproductive aging results from depletion of the follicular reserve, and this reserve nears exhaustion at menopause.

Follicular Function during the Menopausal Transition

A review of follicular growth and atresia and the regulatory mechanisms that control these processes is helpful in understanding ovarian senescence. Gougeon elegantly described the various stages of follicular development in the human ovary (22). During the 85-day period that it takes a preantral follicle to reach ovulatory size, the follicle grows from 0.2 to 20 mm, and the number of granulosa cells increases markedly from 3,000 to 5,000 to about 60 million. This follicular growth is a complex process that results from interactions among the ovary, the pituitary gland, and the hypothalamus.

It is well known that the pituitary gonadotropins, luteinizing hormone (LH) and follicle-stimulating hormone (FSH), play a key role in stimulating both follicular growth

Primordial Follicle Numbers

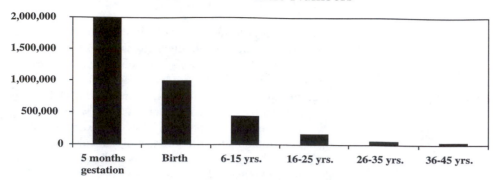

FIGURE 13.1. Numbers of primordial follicles of the ovary during the female life span. (From Soules MR, Bremner WJ. The menopause and climacteric: endocrinologic basis and associated symptomatology. *J Am Soc Geriatr* 1982;30:547–561, with permission.)

and ovarian secretion of various steroid and protein hormones. The principal ovarian steroid hormones, estradiol and progesterone, in turn, regulate gonadotropin production and release through feedback on both the hypothalamus and the pituitary. In addition, FSH synthesis and release are influenced by several peptide hormones (inhibin, activin, and follistatin) produced by granulosa cells. Evidence suggests that the depletion of follicular numbers during the menopausal transition is associated with diminished function of the granulosa cell compartment of the ovary and subsequent loss of feedback to the pituitary. At menopause, when follicular stores approach zero and ovarian secretory products decline, circulating levels of gonadotropins rise because of the loss of negative feedback.

One of the earliest and most consistent endocrine changes marking the onset of the perimenopause is the monotropic rise in FSH (23–27). Some early studies found this elevation in FSH to be associated with decreased levels of ovarian secretory products, such as estradiol (24,28,29) and inhibin (28–31). Other studies have shown no significant change in estradiol levels (25,26) or elevated estrogen levels (32–34) during the earliest stages of the menopausal transition. These conflicting data possibly arise from variations in the timing of sampling during the perimenopause. Perhaps the initial rise in FSH during the earliest stages of the perimenopause results in a compensatory increase in ovarian estradiol production. Later in the perimenopausal transition, estradiol levels may then decline when the aging ovary is no longer capable of responding to the heightened FSH stimulation. Thus, other secretory products of the granulosa cell, such as inhibin, may play an important role in the initiation of the monotropic rise in FSH.

Inhibin has received considerable attention for its potential role in the reproductive aging of women (35). Inhibin was first described as a gonadal product (from the testis or ovary) that inhibited FSH secretion from the pituitary (36). Investigators now know that two types of inhibin exist: inhibin A and B. These are dimeric glycoproteins consisting of an α subunit combined with either a β_A or a β_B subunit. Inhibin A and inhibin B show markedly different patterns of secretion over the menstrual cycle. The level of inhibin A is low during the early follicular phase, rises as ovulation nears, and peaks in the luteal phase of the menstrual cycle (37,38). In contrast, levels of inhibin B are highest during the midfollicular phase, display a transient peak at the time of the LH surge, and are low during the luteal phase (38). Evidence in the monkey confirmed that the major stimulus for ovarian inhibin secretion is follicular phase FSH (39).

Investigators have proposed that changes in inhibin production by the ovary may mediate the earliest sign of ovarian aging—the monotropic rise in FSH (35). Initial studies using a polyclonal antibody to the α subunit of inhibin (Monash assay) failed to show any significant change in circulating inhibin levels during the menopausal transition (32,40,41). However, when specific assays for inhibin A and B were developed, it became evident that the monotropic rise in FSH is closely associated with decreased levels of inhibin B (42–47). Other factors that may further contribute to the isolated follicular increase in FSH may include an increase in activin A (45,47) and a subsequent decline in inhibin A levels (44,46,47). Most recently, investigators have found that inhibin B levels may decline before an increase in FSH in women developing diminished ovarian reserve (48). If confirmed, this finding will provide evidence of a temporal sequence of endocrine, paracrine, or autocrine signal alterations that occur with follicular aging.

In summary, the ovarian theory of reproductive aging (35,49) asserts that a deficiency in inhibin B results from both diminished follicular stores and qualitative changes in granulosa cell function. These decreased inhibin levels lead to the monotropic rise in FSH, which represents the earliest sign of ovarian aging. As ovarian aging continues and follicular stores become further depleted, inhibin A and estradiol levels fall, further contributing to the rise in FSH. During this time, the menstrual irregularities of the perimenopause emerge and finally culminate in cessation of menses at menopause. It is useful to examine the age-related changes that occur in the ovary. The granulosa cell compartment displays both quantitative and qualitative changes during the ovarian aging process. It has also become apparent that important age-related changes in the oocyte likely contribute to the increased incidence of infertility, spontaneous abortion, and aneuploidy in women of advanced reproductive age.

Age-Related Changes in the Ovary

Granulosa Cell Function

Granulosa cells provide critical metabolic support and participate in vital intrafollicular communication with their enclosed oocyte. The life cycle of a granulosa cell is composed of periods of proliferation and differentiation followed by quiescence, senescence, or apoptosis. During this life cycle, granulosa cells produce many bioactive substances, including steroids, glycoproteins and other macromolecules yet to be discovered. Changes in these life cycle and secretory processes may reflect age-related changes in human granulosa cell competence that are concomitant with a decline in female fecundity.

Our understanding of granulosa cells has been greatly advanced by the availability of these cells from women undergoing ART. Access to granulosa cells have allowed investigators to probe some of the mechanisms and processes involved in female reproductive aging. Investigators have demonstrated that as a woman ages, her estradiol response to ovulation induction, the number of oocytes retrieved, and implantation and pregnancy rates decrease. In addition, there may be an increase in the resistance of follicles to exogenous gonadotropins, as demonstrated by a decreased ovarian response to an increased amount of gonadotropin stimulation with advancing age. This decrease in ovarian responsiveness has been termed *diminished ovarian reserve* and can be predicted by elevated basal (day 3) levels of FSH. Furthermore, as age increases, so does the incidence of spontaneous abortions, which occurs in more than 40% of pregnancies in women older than 40 years of age (3).

These clinical observations seem to parallel specific physiologic endocrine alterations of the aging ovary. With advancing reproductive age there is a decrease in the intermenstrual interval, with characteristic shortening of the follicular phase. This change is accompanied by higher early follicular estradiol and rising FSH levels as well as a premature rise in progesterone, leading to an earlier LH surge and ovulation. Although it is well accepted that quantitative follicular changes occur within the aging human ovary, we are recently beginning to understand that the remaining follicles demonstrate changes in quality as well. These qualitative changes may, in fact, support the concept of an aging follicular apparatus composed of compromised oocytes (germ cells) and their accompanying granulosa cells (somatic cells).

Granulosa Cell Number

Diminished ovarian function or reserve may be accompanied by granulosa cell compromise. The ovaries of women with diminished ovarian reserve not only have fewer developing follicles, but each follicle also contains fewer granulosa cells. These findings have been elucidated by the study of granulosa cells from women with normal (day 3 FSH less than 6 mIU/mL) and diminished ovarian reserve (day 3 FSH greater than 10 mIU/mL) who were undergoing superovulation for ART (50). As compared with women with normal ovarian reserve, women with diminished ovarian reserve have fewer luteinized granulosa cells. This is associated with a fourfold increase in the percentage of these granulosa cells undergoing apoptosis, rather than changes in the percentage of proliferating cells. Thus, these changes account for a 25% to 30% reduction in the number of luteinized granulosa cells in the follicles of older women, a change contributing to the development of a dysfunctional follicular apparatus in these women.

Secretory Capacity of the Granulosa Cell

In addition to the changes in granulosa cell number that occur with aging, various secretory functions of the granulosa cell have been shown to be diminished during the process of ovarian aging. These have included substances thought to be granulosa cell survival factors, such as insulin-like growth factor I (IGF-I), epidermal growth factor, and progesterone. These products have been termed *granulosa cell survival factors* because each has been shown to act directly on granulosa cells to inhibit them from becoming apoptotic (51,52). In addition, diminished secretion of other granulosa cell products, such as inhibin, occurs with the earliest stages of ovarian aging.

Of the proposed granulosa cell survival factors, both progesterone and IGF-I production by the granulosa cells appear to decline as women age. Pellicer and others examined progesterone secretion *in vivo* and *in vitro* in two populations of women of different ages (mean age, 40 years versus 32 years) who were preparing for ART (53). Both basal and gonadotropin-stimulated progesterone production by granulosa cells *in vitro* was significantly diminished in the group of older women as compared with the younger women. Other studies have shown that both follicular fluid (32) and serum levels (32,54) of IGF-I are lower in older women (aged 40 to 45 years) with ovulatory cycles as compared with normal young women (aged 20 to 25 years). These data suggest that granulosa cells from older women have reduced capacity to produce putative granulosa cell survival factors.

Given the key role inhibin is thought to play in mediating the monotropic rise in FSH during ovarian aging, it is important to evaluate changes in granulosa cell production of inhibin during this process. In one study, α-subunit inhibin (total inhibin) secretion by luteinized granulosa cells cultured *in vitro* was lower in older women undergoing

ART cycles as compared with younger women (mean age 40 versus 32 years) (53). This study was confounded by the absence of information regarding ovarian reserve because it is known that women of different chronologic age may have similar ovarian reserve and variability exists in age of onset of this diminished ovarian reserve. One investigation examined total and dimeric inhibin production by cultured luteinized granulosa cells from two groups of women of similar age but significantly different ovarian reserve as reflected by day 3 serum FSH levels (55). Both total and dimeric inhibin concentrations in the culture media were approximately twice as high in the low day 3 FSH group than in the high day 3 FSH group. These data suggest that a quantitative decline in immunoreactive and bioactive inhibin produced by granulosa cells is associated with declining ovarian reserve. Perhaps the monotropic rise of FSH during the early follicular phase is an indirect bioassay of declining bioactive inhibin production at the granulosa cell level. Furthermore, it is speculated that day 3 serum FSH may be partly determined by preceding luteal concentration of dimeric inhibin A.

Cell Cycle in Granulosa Cells

Studies of granulosa cells have examined aging in the context of alterations in secretory function of the cell, including the changes in steroidogenesis, glycoprotein, and growth factor production outlined earlier. It is also important to examine how the granulosa cell cycle may be altered with reproductive aging. The cell cycle is of particular interest because it represents the reproductive life span of the individual cell itself. The *cell cycle* can be defined as a sequence of events that begins with the completion of mitosis in the parent cell and ends with the subsequent mitosis that occurs in the daughter cell. Its purpose is to maintain DNA constancy from parent to daughter cell. When investigators examined apoptosis in the follicle, they found 70% of the apoptotic cells to be in the proliferative phase of the cell cycle (50). This observation suggests that most of the cells destined to become apoptotic have entered the cell cycle. It is generally believed that under normal conditions, cells are stimulated to undergo mitosis in the presence of both mitogens and other survival factors. Under optimal conditions, cells complete the cell cycle, and the population doubles. If cells are stimulated to traverse the cell cycle in the absence of survival factors, mitosis is then blocked, and the cells become apoptotic (56,57). Because cells isolated from women with elevated basal FSH levels show a fourfold increase in the percentage of apoptotic cells, it is likely that many follicles within the ovaries of these women are deficient in granulosa cell survival factors. This correlates the findings of the previously mentioned studies and also corroborates work in cell cycle research.

Investigators have examined the *proliferative index*— defined as the sum of the percentage of cells in the synthetic, postsynthetic, and mitotic growth phases (G_2M)—of lutein-

ized granulosa cells as a function of chronologic age and ovarian reserve. Despite large differences in ages (mean age, 28 years versus 41 years), chronologic age did not have a significant independent influence on the proliferative index in women with similar follicular phase serum FSH levels (58). However, in studying two groups of women undergoing ART cycles whose ages were similar (mean age, 32 years) but whose day 3 serum FSH values were different (mean serum FSH, 4.8 IU/L versus 25 IU/L), marked differences in the proliferative index of granulosa cells were noted. Luteinized granulosa cells from preovulatory follicles from women with higher day 3 serum FSH had a 25% lower proliferative index as compared with luteinized granulosa cells from women with normal day 3 serum FSH (59). This finding suggests that women with diminished ovarian reserve have a smaller percentage of their luteinized granulosa cells in the proliferative portion of the cell cycle as compared with women with uncompromised ovarian reserve. This finding may explain in part the more favorable response to ovulation induction protocols that younger women demonstrate compared with women of more advanced reproductive age.

Luteinized granulosa cells from women with diminished ovarian reserve appear to display significant changes with regard to their proliferative index and their secretion of steroids, glycoproteins, and growth factors. Compromised endocrine, paracrine, and autocrine signals from ovarian follicles of decreasing competence likely lead to altered interaction between the principal components of the follicular apparatus—granulosa cells and oocytes.

Maternal Aging and the Oocyte

The relationship between *maternal age* and the functional disposition of the human oocyte has been recognized for many years. Despite this recognition, the precise avenues whereby aging may affect oocyte behavior are poorly understood. The most obvious problem exhibited by oocytes is an increasingly high incidence of meiotic nondisjunction as a woman approaches menopause (5). Significant evidence indicates that this problem may be attributed directly to the functional and structural qualities of the oocyte (13,60). However, whether this dysfunction results from intrinsic abnormalities of the oocytes or is a consequence of the changing (i.e., aging) ovarian environment is unclear.

Chromosome mismanagement, leading to aneuploidy, may occur during either meiotic division. Many investigations have shown that most nondisjunction occurs during the first meiotic division in the oocyte, but it may also appear during the second division (61,62). Investigators have suggested that errors during the first division may actually be responsible for some of the errors previously attributed to the second division (63). Regardless of whether these errors in chromosome management occur in the first or second meiotic division, it is important to define the cellular mechanisms responsible for this problem, which plagues women in the latter stages of reproductive life.

Meiosis

Meiosis is an extremely protracted process, particularly in the human oocyte. This process begins during a woman's prenatal period, when all her oocytes are becoming organized into primordial follicles. During the fetal period, the oogonia cease mitotic activity and become committed to enter meiosis. The population of oocytes present at birth is arrested in meiotic prophase I and remains at this stage of meiosis until ovulation. Although most of these follicles are lost as a result of atresia, some are recruited to grow and mature in each menstrual cycle throughout a woman's reproductive life span. Thus, prophase arrest may last 40 to 50 years before meiosis resumes and chromosome segregation occurs. As reviewed earlier in this chapter, alterations in serum and follicular fluid hormones occur during the late reproductive years and may reflect a suboptimal follicular environment for the oocyte. Whether late recruitment and follicular stress are directly responsible for the higher incidence of aneuploidy has not been determined. However, it is certain that the oocyte that matures in the aging ovary is often poorly prepared for chromosome segregation, in contrast to oocytes that are recruited during prime reproductive years.

Meiosis is composed of two successive cell divisions that result in the reduction in chromosome content of the oocyte to the haploid state. As described earlier, the oocytes are arrested in prophase I before the time of birth and remain in maturational arrest until they are stimulated to ovulate. Near the time of ovulation, the prophase arrest is released, and the first meiotic division is rapidly completed (*first polar body release.*) The oocyte then quickly progresses to and becomes arrested at metaphase of the second division (MII). The arrest at the MII is released only if the oocyte becomes fertilized. With fertilization, the second meiotic division is completed, and the oocyte releases the second polar body to achieve a haploid state. Dysfunction in either division can result in the incomplete segregation of chromosomes, characteristic of aneuploidy.

Meiotic Apparatus. The biologic motor that physically drives the segregation of the chromosomes during meiosis is the *meiotic spindle* (64). This is a complex organelle with a distinct barrel-shaped cage of microtubules that encompasses the condensed chromosomes in metaphase. The coordination of polymerization of the microtubules in the spindle and kinesinlike protein activity is responsible for the motive force that segregates chromatin during meiosis. At metaphase of both divisions, the chromosomes are organized into a disc-shaped array (*the metaphase plate*) that is confined within the spindle. Correct placement of the chromatin into the metaphase plate appears to be essential for normal chromosome segregation.

The morphology of the human oocyte and its relationship with maternal age have been of interest for decades. Because of the stable (arrested) nature of the MII spindle, it is easier to observe this phase of maturation. Consequently, most examinations of human oocytes have been conducted during the MII phase. Early studies of the MII stage of meiosis in the human oocyte revealed that the longitudinal axis of the meiotic spindle is oriented perpendicularly to the cell surface, as in most mammalian oocytes (65,66). An extensive study of its ultrastructure confirmed these observations in finer detail (67). Non-spindle-associated microtubules can also be found in the cortex of the human oocyte (68), but whether they have any influence on meiosis is unknown. In these early studies, the age of the individuals from whom the oocytes were obtained was not clearly documented. Thus, the effect of maternal age on the assembly of these meiotic spindles was not initially appreciated. However, it has become clear that advanced maternal age is associated with distinctly abnormal assembly of the meiotic spindle. By comparing the oocytes obtained in natural menstrual cycles in women 40 to 45 years old and in women 20 to 25 years of age, Battaglia et al. revealed that 79% of the oocytes from the older women exhibited significant spindle disruption and chromosome disarray at MII (69). A few oocytes (17%) from the younger group were abnormal. These observations have been confirmed in *in vitro* matured oocytes from women of varying age groups (70). Interestingly, the incidence of abnormal spindle structure in the older groups reflects the high rate of aneuploidy described in oocytes from older women (63). The low incidence of abnormal spindles and chromosome displacement in the younger women also corresponds with the low incidence of aneuploidy in oocytes from women 35 years of age or younger (71).

Spindle abnormalities have also been noted in a specific strain of mice that display aneuploidy with advanced maternal age (60,72). Investigators have postulated that the key regulatory phases of meiosis may be altered in these older animals and may lead to irregular spindle assembly and incomplete chromosome segregation (60,73,74). Humans experience a far greater incidence of age-related aneuploidy than that observed in any animal model (75). Nevertheless, the data from both the animal model and human studies suggest that the regulatory mechanisms responsible for meiotic spindle assembly are altered during the process of ovarian aging. That the structural anomalies are coincident with errors in chromosome segregation provides compelling evidence that spindle assembly may be a target of age-related dysfunction.

Meiotic Spindle Assembly. One of the major components of the meiotic spindle is a polarized and highly organized matrix of microtubules. Polymerization of the protein tubulin is needed to create this structure and must occur at an appropriate time and location within the cell to ensure normal chromosome segregation by the meiotic spindle. Tubulin polymerization is directly linked to the biology of the centrosome, a complex biochemical domain in all dividing cells that orchestrates microtubule assembly. Animal studies have shown that once meiosis resumes, numerous microtubule-organizing centers (MTOC) appear and become part of the functionally complete centrosome near the prophase nucleus (76,77). Compelling evidence from the mouse oocyte even suggests that the appearance of MTOC foci near the nucleus depends on the meiotic competency of the cell (78). The role of MTOCs in meiotic spindle assembly remains unclear, and age-related changes in the MTOCs have not been studied.

The role of MTOC in human oocyte function is poorly understood. Unlike in studies in animal eggs, Pickering et al. failed to observe discrete MTOC-like structures in human oocytes treated with paclitaxel (Taxol), a microtubule-stabilizing drug conventionally used to examine MTOC domains (68). Thus, these investigators concluded that the human oocyte may not rely on MTOC activity during meiosis. In contrast, more recent data suggest that the human oocyte may recruit MTOC domains during meiosis. With the aid of paclitaxel treatment, numerous MTOCs have been shown to appear during meiotic maturation, many of which are adjacent to the prophase nucleus as meiosis progresses (79). Moreover, it appears that the MTOC domains located at the poles of the spindle may be responding to the influence of paclitaxel in an age-dependent manner (D.E. Battaglia, unpublished data, 1998). These data suggest that the biochemistry of spindle assembly may be altered as maternal age progresses, thus eventually influencing chromosome segregation.

Most data on the disposition of the meiotic spindle in the human oocyte have been obtained at MII of meiosis. The reason is that the first metaphase (MI) is transient and often is completed before ovulation, whereas the MII phase is more stable (up to the time of fertilization). However, the disposition of the MI spindle is certainly of great interest, considering the prevalence of nondisjunctional events seen during this phase of meiosis (63). By observing a limited number of *in vitro* matured oocytes at MI, Volarcik et al. noted spindle assembly abnormalities at this stage (70). Thus, we may be tempted to assume that the assembly mechanisms of the spindles at MI and MII are similar and that the data obtained at MII reflect events during MI. However, further study of the MI meiotic spindle is needed to confirm this hypothesis.

The biochemistry of the centrosome is complex and, as yet, poorly understood. The centrosome is composed of numerous molecular elements, including the proteins pericentrin and γ-tubulin. Pericentrin is integral to the formation and organization of microtubules in both *Xenopus* and mouse oocytes (80). It is highly conserved across species and may play an important role in the early stages of meiosis in the human oocyte. γ-Tubulin has been shown to modu-

late spindle assembly in animal cells and has been shown to be localized at the poles of the meiotic spindle in the human oocyte (81). Identification of more of the elements within the oocyte centrosome will aid our understanding of where age-related lesions may occur.

Because the phases of the cell cycle of both meiotic divisions are protracted in the oocyte, the mechanisms that regulate each phase have attracted much interest. Ample evidence demonstrates that a family of molecules, collectively called *maturation-promoting factor* (MPF), are the primary regulators of meiosis. Investigators have postulated that MPF may regulate the assembly of the meiotic spindle through its association with MTOCs (77,82). The two main components of MPF are the cyclins (regulatory proteins) and a family of cyclin-dependent protein kinases. Of particular importance is cdc2, a 34-kd protein kinase that is abundant in most animal oocytes. Through its interaction with microtubule-associated structures and the cyclins, cdc2 may be an important regulator of the assembly of the meiotic spindle (77,82). Moreover, evidence indicates that cyclin-cdc2 binding may modulate the microtubule-nucleating activity of MTOCs in oocytes (83). The activity of MPF in mouse oocytes declines with maternal age (84), a finding that lends further credence to the idea that the cyclins, MTOCs, and related molecules are compromised with advancing age.

Proteolytic modification of a cytostatic factor, c-*mos,* has been postulated as an important trigger for the transition from metaphase to anaphase in cell divisions (85). Because the disposition of microtubules is influenced by c-*mos* phosphorylation and the human oocyte expresses this proto-oncogene, it is likely that c-*mos* is linked to MPF activity in the human oocyte (86). A possible connection of c-*mos* activity to age-related aneuploidy is supported by the observation that the oocytes from c-*mos*–deficient mice exhibit abnormal meiotic spindle assembly (87). Evidence also suggests that c-*mos* is involved with the regulation of the kinesinlike molecule, CENP E, in the kinetochores of mouse oocytes (88). It is conceivable that such interactions are responsible for regulatory control of meiotic maturation and that aging may affect the efficiency of this control.

Extrinsic Versus Intrinsic Factors

To delineate the causes of age-related oocyte dysfunction, it is important to maintain a perspective on the entire biology of oocyte maturation. The ovarian follicle in the aging ovary may exert significant influence on the biologic machinery that is attendant to chromosome segregation in the oocyte. Research data have yet to confirm whether a suboptimal follicular environment directly affects the oocytes that are recruited for ovulation late in reproductive life. Conversely, the oocytes themselves may be dysfunctional, and that may be why they are recruited late.

As reviewed earlier, the quality of the follicular environment has been considered by many investigators to be altered with advanced maternal age. The significant rise in basal FSH levels and decreased serum levels of inhibin B that are evident in older women clearly coincide with abnormal meiotic spindle assembly and chromosome displacement in oocytes from these older women (69,70). Based on studies of *in vitro* matured human oocytes, Volarcik et al. believed that degradation in oocyte quality with advancing maternal age may be based at the somatic level (70). If this is true, then high-quality culture systems for immature oocytes may be able to overcome age-related dysfunction in the egg. Some support for the concept that reproductive aging begins in somatic cells comes from data from mouse experiments in which the normal atresia of ovarian follicles is prevented by a deficiency in the *Bax* gene, a key regulator of apoptosis. As these animals reach the typical age of reproductive senescence, their ovaries remain endowed with ample follicle reserve (89). Interestingly, despite an adequate number of ovarian follicles, these aged mice do not display normal reproductive function. With superovulation and IVF, mature MII oocytes, which can support early embryo development, can be obtained from these *Bax*-deficient animals. The lack of natural fertility in these aged mice with persistent follicular endowment likely reflects the decline in hypothalamic-hypophyseal function known to occur in rodents during reproductive senescence. Although reproductive senescence at this level does not occur in humans, these data do suggest that an atretic environment in the ovary is associated with the age-related depletion of follicular stores.

The possibility that intrinsic properties of older oocytes are the root cause of meiotic problems is interesting. The chromosomes themselves may play an important and direct role in the development of aneuploidy. Hunt et al. provided compelling evidence that the kinetochore-chromosome complex has a profound influence on meiotic maturation and chromosome segregation in the mouse oocyte (90). However, whether these relationships have a direct effect on meiotic spindle assembly remains unclear. It is also unclear whether oocytes from aging women possess significantly altered chromosome structure.

Further study is necessary to clarify whether meiotic nondisjunction arises directly from the follicular environment of the aging ovary or is intrinsic to the oocytes that are recruited during the later reproductive years. However, subtle changes in meiotic spindle assembly are clearly responsible for microtubule abnormalities and probable chromosome displacement in oocytes from older individuals. The precise molecular pathways that are perturbed by aging have yet to be identified, but changes are likely occurring in both the somatic cells (granulosa cells) and the oocyte.

Mechanisms of Ovarian Aging

The precise mechanisms that mediate the age-related changes in the granulosa cells and oocyte have not been extensively studied. However, mechanisms of aging in other cells, tissues, and organs may play a role in ovarian senescence. Proposed mechanisms of aging have included genetic influences (heritable conditions and activation of aging genes), programmed cell death (apoptosis), oxidative damage through the production of free radicals, and alterations in organ blood flow resulting in hypoxia.

A *genetic basis* for ovarian aging is supported by several familial observations. Age of maternal menopause appears to significantly correlate with the menopausal age of a woman's daughters (91–94). For example, a woman whose mother underwent menopause before the age of 46 years is five to six times more likely to experience an early menopause herself (92,94). Similarly, age at menopause correlates among siblings (92). In fact, a classic twin study of 275 monozygotic and 353 dizygotic twins estimated that about 45% of the variance in menopausal age resulted from genetic contributions (95). Several case reports also documented deletional abnormalities in the long arm of the X chromosome in families of women with premature ovarian failure (96,97). Additional evidence of a genetic basis for ovarian aging is derived from observations of genetic aging syndromes, such as Werner's syndrome and ataxia telangiectasia. These patients are either infertile or experience menopause at an early age (98,99).

Aging of the human ovary is likely to be regulated at the DNA level, in both granulosa cells and the oocyte, by alterations in the expression of various genes. Cellular senescence in other tissue types has been shown to be associated with changes in expression patterns of numerous genes. These include the genes for telomerase (100), IGF-binding proteins (101,102), manganese superoxide dismutase (101), fibronectin (103), c-*fos* (104), and numerous transcription factors such as E2F proteins (105), cdc2, and cyclin A and B (106). In fact, many of the other mechanisms of aging, such as apoptosis and free-radical damage, may result from alterations in gene expression. The expression patterns of these senescence genes have not been studied during the aging process of the human ovary but offer an interesting area for study.

Apoptosis, often called programmed cell death, is a common death mechanism induced in cells when they are damaged, unnecessary to the body, or dangerous to it. During apoptosis, condensation and fragmentation of DNA by endonucleases occur and are followed by phagocytosis by macrophages. Apoptosis has been identified as the principal mechanism responsible for prenatal loss of the oogonia as well as prenatal and postnatal follicular atresia (107). As previously mentioned, granulosa cells from women with diminished ovarian reserve show marked increases in the percentage of cells undergoing apoptosis. In addition, apoptotic lesions have been demonstrated in the chromosomes of oocytes from aging mice (108). Further studies are necessary to determine whether apoptosis plays a significant role in the poor oocyte quality observed in older women. It is likely, however, that apoptosis plays a major role in mediating quantitative changes in granulosa cell number and follicular reserve during aging of the human ovary.

Another proposed aging mechanism is *oxidative damage* caused by liberation of free radicals during oxidative metabolism within cells. The action of free radicals, such as peroxide and superoxide, is countered by antioxidants, such as vitamins A, C, and E, and by enzymes such as superoxide dismutase, catalase, glutathione peroxidase, and glutathione reductase. Thus, a decrease in these enzymes or antioxidants or an increase in free-radical production can lead to damage to cellular proteins, nucleic acids, and membranes. Oxidative damage appears to accumulate with age, and antioxidant mechanisms are more robust in long-lived species as compared with those with shorter life spans (109,110). Evidence in an animal model suggests that inhibitors of oxidative stress block *in vitro* apoptosis in granulosa cells (111). Furthermore, superoxide dismutase and glutathione peroxidase activities in the human ovary decrease with aging (112). Investigators have also shown that oxidative stress as related to mitochondrial function influences oocyte quality (113), and that an increase of free-radical damage to the oocyte may result in the age-associated increase in aneuploidy (114). Although further study is indicated, an increase in free-radical exposure may mediate age-related changes in both granulosa cells and the oocyte.

Another area ripe for research is the examination of the role of altered blood flow and *hypoxia* in the process of ovarian aging. The oocyte has no direct vascular supply and depends on oxygen diffusion through the follicular fluid from the granulosa cells. At the time of the LH surge, there is an increase in microvascular remodeling in the follicle. Investigators have proposed that, as women age, their developing follicles are surrounded by a deficient microcirculation that may be related to errors in meiosis (115). It has also been reported that chromosomal scattering is increased in oocytes obtained from follicles with reduced oxygen content (116). Vascular endothelial growth factor (VEGF) is one of many angiogenic cytokines secreted by granulosa cells that are undergoing microvascular remodeling during the resumption of meiosis. Investigators measured VEGF production by follicles from women broadly categorized by age. They found increased VEGF levels in follicular fluid from women of advanced age (117; D.E. Battaglia and J. Van Blerkom, unpublished data). This finding supports the hypothesis that follicles from aging women may be in a relatively hypoxic environment. VEGF, oxygen tension in the follicular fluid, and aneuploidy in the oocyte appear to be related (118), thus providing evidence that the follicular environment is affected by maternal age and may directly affect oocyte competency through oxidative stress. Thus, accumulating data from several perspectives suggest that as the ovary ages it may experience a relatively hypoxic state, which may further lead to important functional and structural changes in both granulosa cells and the oocyte.

Several of the foregoing mechanisms may participate in any given aging process, including reproductive senescence. Many of these mechanisms are interrelated, and activation of a cascade of events is likely to lead to the quantitative and functional changes observed in follicles and oocytes as the ovary makes the transition to a menopausal state.

CLINICAL SPECTRUM OF REPRODUCTIVE AGING AND ITS MANAGEMENT ISSUES

The clinical spectrum of reproductive aging ranges from procreative to menopausal issues. Procreative concerns include the decline in fertility and the increased rates of spontaneous abortion and aneuploidy that occur as women progress through the fourth and fifth decades of life (119). Perimenopausal and menopausal issues of reproductive aging include management of climacteric symptoms, alterations in the risk for chronic diseases brought about by the menopausal state, and weighing the risks and benefits of a wide variety of hormonal replacement regimens for each individual patient. The remainder of this chapter focuses on the diagnosis and treatment of the clinical manifestations of reproductive aging.

Procreative Issues

The transition into menopause represents a continuum that is first manifested by the decline in fertility evident in the fourth decade of life. With increasing age, women experience diminished responsiveness to ovulation induction (120–123), a decline in the number of oocytes retrieved during IVF (121,123–125), and overall lower pregnancy rates in treatment cycles (120,121,123,124,126–128). Often, this occurs without any detectable changes in the menstrual pattern. The concept of ovarian reserve has been introduced as a more accurate predictor of this decreased fertility than chronologic age (129). Diminished ovarian reserve, as assessed by elevated day 3 FSH levels (121,130), is associated with decreased success of ovulation induction (131) and IVF (121,132).

Diagnosis of Diminished Ovarian Reserve

Given the physical, emotional, and financial investments made with advanced fertility treatment, it is clinically useful to identify those women who are likely to respond poorly to therapy. Many endocrinologic tests (Table 13.2) have been proposed to be useful predictors of diminished ovarian reserve (133). The most widely used tests involve the measurement of *FSH*, under basal conditions (usually day 3) or after stimulation with clomiphene citrate or gonadotropin-releasing hormone (GnRH). Other proposed predictors include FSH:LH ratios and basal levels of estradiol and inhibin B.

The use of basal gonadotropin levels to predict ovarian

TABLE 13.2. ENDOCRINE TESTS FOR DETECTING DIMINISHED OVARIAN RESERVE

Basal tests (measured on day 3 of the menstrual cycle)
  Follicle-stimulating hormone (FSH) level
  Estradiol level
  Inhibin-B level
  Follicle-stimulating hormone: luteinizing hormone
    (FSH:LH) ratio
Stimulated tests
  Clomiphene citrate challenge test
  Gonadotropin-releasing hormone (GnRH) stimulation test
  Exogenous follicle stimulating hormone ovarian reserve
    test (EFORT)

---

responsiveness to gonadotropins and success with IVF was first described in 1988 (134). A subsequent and larger study confirmed that women with low basal (day 3) FSH levels had a significantly greater number of follicles per retrieval, increased recovery of preovulatory oocytes, and higher peak estradiol levels than women with elevated day 3 FSH levels (132). Furthermore, the ongoing pregnancy rates were four to five times greater in the women with low basal FSH (less than 15 mIU/mL) as compared with women with elevated day 3 FSH levels (greater than 25 mIU/mL). Additional studies have confirmed that basal FSH levels are more useful for predicting success with IVF therapy than patient age alone (121,135). Combining basal FSH determination with patient age further improves prognostic accuracy. Because considerable variation in normal basal FSH levels exists among laboratories, each institution needs to establish guidelines for normal and elevated basal FSH levels based on individual laboratory results. Although most studies describe measurement of FSH on day 3 of the cycle, serum FSH concentrations are similar on days 2 to 5 (41,136).

Some women display significant intercycle variability in basal FSH levels (137,138). Intercycle variability is greater in women who have had elevated basal FSH levels than in those with normal basal FSH levels (137). Furthermore, women who have had an elevated FSH in any prior cycle respond poorly in IVF cycles, even if their basal FSH is normal in the current cycle (137,138). A recent study even suggested that an elevated basal FSH may be associated with increased fetal aneuploidy (139). Thus, many clinicians recommend that women with elevated basal FSH levels be discouraged from pursuing further IVF cycles with their own eggs, regardless of whether FSH levels are persistently or variably elevated.

Although demonstration of an elevated basal FSH level is highly predictive of poor performance in IVF cycles, a normal day 3 FSH does not exclude patients who will be low responders to ovulation induction. Thus, other tests, such as the clomiphene citrate challenge test (129), have been sought in an effort to enhance detection of diminished ovarian reserve. The *clomiphene citrate challenge test* consists of measuring FSH levels on cycle days 3 and 10 with the administration of 100 mg of clomiphene citrate on days 5 to 9 of the cycle. An abnormal result is defined as elevation of either the day 3 or day 10 FSH level. It is theorized that normal recruitment of a cohort of follicles leads to increased feedback on the hypothalamic-pituitary axis to suppress FSH levels by day 10. Evidence suggests that this normal feedback mechanism may be mediated by inhibin B (43). An abnormal test result occurs when the ovary, because of diminished ovarian reserve, is unable to respond to the elevated FSH induced by clomiphene citrate. The lack of normal feedback from the ovary then leads to elevated FSH levels on day 10. Thus, the clomiphene citrate challenge test represents a provocative test used to improve detection of diminished ovarian reserve in women with a normal basal FSH level.

In the original study of the clomiphene citrate challenge test (129), women with diminished ovarian reserve, as defined by an abnormal day 10 FSH during the clomiphene citrate test, had a 6% pregnancy rate during their 1- to 2-year period of infertility treatment. In contrast, women with a normal clomiphene citrate challenge test experienced a 42% pregnancy rate over this same period. All these women were demographically similar and had normal basal FSH levels. The validity of this test for prediction of outcomes in ART protocols was confirmed by several subsequent studies (140–142). The specificity of this test is high; a 100% positive predictive value for failure to achieve pregnancy is typically found (141,142). The clomiphene citrate challenge test identifies about twice as many patients with diminished ovarian reserve as compared with the day 3 FSH level alone (142).

The clomiphene citrate challenge test has been used in the evaluation of the general infertility population (143). Abnormal clomiphene citrate challenge tests are found in about 10% of this population. The incidence of an abnormal test increases with age, from 3% in women less than 30 years old to 26% in women older than 39 years. As seen in patients undergoing advanced ART procedures, an abnormal result predicted significantly lower pregnancy rates (9%) than did a normal result (43%). The incidence of unexplained infertility is higher in patients with an abnormal clomiphene citrate challenge test (52% versus 9% in those patients with a normal test). Thus, diminished ovarian reserve may be a distinct cause of infertility in some patients previously labeled with unexplained infertility. Although an abnormal clomiphene citrate challenge test predicts poor pregnancy rates independent of age, patients of advancing age who have a normal clomiphene citrate challenge test still experience decreased pregnancy rates as compared with their younger counterparts (144). In other words, the clomiphene citrate challenge test has a high positive predictive value, but the negative predictive value remains suboptimal for detecting diminished ovarian reserve.

Several other endocrinologic tests have been examined for their ability to predict ovarian reserve. These have included measurement of basal FSH:LH ratios (134,145), the GnRH agonist stimulation test (146,147), and the exogenous FSH ovarian reserve test (EFORT) (148). Markedly diminished estradiol responses, oocyte recoveries, and pregnancy rates are seen in women with elevated day 3 FSH:LH ratios (134,145). The GnRH agonist stimulation test consists of administration of 1 mg of leuprolide acetate on cycle day 2, followed by analysis of the change in estradiol levels over the subsequent day. The peak estradiol levels after this stimulation were reported to correlate with the number of mature oocytes, the number of embryos, and the pregnancy rates better than either basal FSH levels or age (146). The change in estradiol levels also correlates with the number of follicles 15 mm or larger that were recruited during ovarian stimulation for IVF (147). EFORT considers both the basal FSH level and the change in estradiol levels from day 3 to 4 after administration of 300 IU of purified FSH. Ninety percent of women whose EFORT was normal (basal FSH up to 11 mIU/mL and change in estradiol of 30 pg/mL or more) had adequate responses to ovarian stimulation, whereas 81% of women with an abnormal EFORT (basal FSH greater than 11 mIU/mL and change in estradiol of less than 30 pg/mL) had poor responses to ovarian stimulation for IVF (148). Further studies are necessary to confirm the clinical usefulness of these stimulated tests.

Two other endocrine parameters have been proposed as predictors of ovarian reserve: day 3 levels of estradiol and inhibin B. Early studies failed to show any advantage of basal estradiol levels over day 3 FSH levels in the prediction of ovarian reserve (132). More recent examination of basal estradiol levels demonstrated that patients with elevated day 3 estradiol (80 pg/mL or greater) had a higher cancellation rate (18.5% versus 0.4%) and a lower pregnancy rate (15% versus 39%) than women with basal estradiol levels less than 80 pg/mL (149). This association was independent of the FSH level. Licciardi et al. also showed that elevated day 3 estradiol levels were associated with a poor response and pregnancy rate in ART cycles (150). The association was not independent of basal FSH levels in this latter study. However, prediction of ART performance was improved by using the day 3 estradiol and FSH level together compared with using the basal FSH level alone. Thus, an elevated estradiol level at day 3, alone or in combination with an elevated basal FSH level, is a useful clinical predictor of diminished ovarian reserve.

Given that inhibin B has been implicated as a possible regulator of the monotropic rise in FSH that occurs in the perimenopause, it is logical to suspect that inhibin B may be useful in predicting ovarian reserve. Investigators have demonstrated that women with day 3 serum inhibin B levels lower than 45 pg/mL perform poorly in ART cycles (151). The prognostic value of the day 3 inhibin B level for the number of oocytes retrieved and clinical pregnancy rate was independent of age as well as basal FSH and

estradiol levels. The odds ratio of clinical pregnancy was 6.8 for those women with inhibin B levels 45 pg/mL or higher as compared to those with inhibin B levels lower than 45 pg/mL. A recent study indicated that day 3 inhibin B levels may even decline before the rise in basal FSH is evident in women developing diminished ovarian reserve (48). Thus, with further clinical study, measurement of serum inhibin B levels may become a useful tool for assessing ovarian reserve. After the diagnosis of diminished ovarian reserve by one of the foregoing methods, patients and their physicians face limited treatment options to attain fertility.

Fertility Treatment in the Setting of Diminished Ovarian Reserve

As noted earlier, women who are older or who display diminished ovarian reserve have dramatically less success with standard fertility therapies, including IVF. Unfortunately, no current treatments exist to prevent or reverse the effects of aging on the ovary. Women undergoing treatment in this situation should be made aware of the diminished pregnancy rates with standard therapies and should be given the opportunity to evaluate other alternatives. These include adoption, remaining childless, and donor egg programs.

The availability of *donor oocytes* has provided a reasonable option for childbearing for many women unable to conceive with their own eggs. Pregnancy rates are remarkably higher with donor egg cycles as compared with standard IVF in older women. The most recent statistics available from the Society for Assisted Reproductive Technology Registry reveal that in women over the age of 39 years, live birth rates are only 9% using fresh embryos from nondonor eggs. However, donor egg cycles result in a live birth rate of 39% in this age group (152). Thus, oocyte donation represents a viable option for childbearing in women who would otherwise experience minimal success with traditional infertility treatments. The success with oocyte donation programs also further supports the notion that the principal determinant of reproductive senescence resides in the ovary.

Investigational techniques, cytoplasmic transfer and nuclear transfer, have been discussed as alternatives to oocyte donation. *Cytoplasmic transfer* involves placement of ooplasm from donor eggs at MII into patient eggs at the same stage of meiosis. The rationale behind this investigational technique is that the ability of oocytes to support normal embryo development may be related to cytoplasmic factors that are deficient in patients who display poor egg and embryo quality in IVF. Two techniques have been described for transfer of the ooplasm: electrofusion of an ooplasmic donor fragment into patient eggs and direct injection of a small amount of ooplasm from a donor egg into patient eggs (153). Preliminary results show more promise for the injection technique. However, this concept remains highly experimental. This technique has not been shown to cause a human pregnancy that otherwise would not have occurred. Further study is necessary before the efficacy and safety of these techniques can be determined. *Nuclear transfer* is even less well studied in this setting. Some investigators have hypothesized that egg and embryo quality may be improved by transferring the nucleus of a patient oocyte into an enucleated donor egg. Again, this hypothesis has yet to be proven. These techniques currently have no role in the clinical treatment of age-related infertility, but they remain interesting research questions.

Perimenopausal and Menopausal Issues

As women continue through the menopausal transition and procreative concerns are resolved, other significant issues related to reproductive senescence emerge. Perimenopausal women can sometimes experience significant debilitation from the changes in their menstrual cycles and the symptoms of hypoestrogenism that occur during this time. In addition, the menopausal state is a risk factor for a variety of chronic diseases, which can significantly affect the life expectancy and health of the growing population of postmenopausal women. In treating these symptoms and conditions, women and their physicians are faced with a variety of decisions. First, the risks and benefits of hormone replacement therapy (HRT) must be evaluated for each individual woman. Then, one must choose from a myriad of options in hormonal replacement, including nonhormonal alternatives.

Perimenopausal Symptoms

Symptoms during the climacteric can be absent, minimal, or distressing and debilitating. The most common symptoms include hot flushes, menstrual cycle irregularities and menorrhagia, mood changes, vaginal dryness, and urinary incontinence.

Hot flushes occur to some degree in most women during the menopausal transition. The hot flush is typically described as a sudden feeling of intense heat in the face, neck, and chest, often accompanied by flushing of the skin in those areas and profuse sweating. These episodes are usually brief (seconds to minutes), but they can recur frequently. The frequency of flushes seems to increase at night and during periods of stress. Although the underlying mechanism responsible for the hot flush appears to be related to a decline in estrogen, flushes have also been reported in 15% of premenopausal women and as a psychosomatic symptom. The incidence of hot flushes peaks just before the last menses and declines significantly by 4 years after menopause (154). Estrogen therapy is effective in treating these vasomotor symptoms in most cases.

Women often experience *changes in their menstrual patterns* several months to years before the last menses of menopause. One of the first cycle changes noted during the process of ovarian aging is shortening of intermenstrual length (155,156). This is followed by a period of increased cycle irregularity (155,157) and finally cessation of menses. *Menorrhagia* is common during this menopausal transition. Although possible pathologic causes such as fibroids, polyps, hyperplasia, and endometrial cancer need to be excluded, most cases of menorrhagia in this age group can be attributed to dysfunctional uterine bleeding. Disturbances in normal ovarian function during the perimenopause, such as sporadic anovulation and transient elevations in estrogen levels (32–34), may underlie this dysfunctional uterine bleeding. Therapies that exert control over the menstrual cycle, such as low-dose oral contraceptives, are often useful in treating both the menorrhagia and the intermittent hypoestrogenism that may occur during this period of ebb and flow in ovarian function.

Popular thinking has often attributed various *psychologic symptoms,* such as depression, insomnia, fatigue, irritability, and diminished ability to concentrate, to the hormonal changes occurring during the menopausal transition. Clearly, many women traverse the menopausal period without significant mood disturbances. Nevertheless, estrogen can influence mood (158). It is difficult, however, to separate whether perimenopausal mood changes result from fluctuations in estrogen levels, are secondary to poor sleep from nighttime hot flushes, or develop in response to various life changes and stressors that can occur at this time in a woman's life.

The mucosal tissues of the vagina, urethra and bladder are targets for estrogen action and can be adversely affected by the hypoestrogenism of menopause. Symptoms such as *vaginal dryness, dyspareunia, vaginal irritation from atrophic vaginitis,* and *urinary incontinence* are common in the postmenopausal population. Estrogen has been shown to be effective in treating these conditions (159).

In conclusion, these early signs and symptoms of the climacteric and the menopause can cause significant discomfort and distress and are a common reason that perimenopausal women seek advice from their physicians (160). HRT is efficacious for these problems and is often used transiently by women during the menopausal transition. However, the impact of long-term loss of estrogen poses the greatest risk to a woman's overall health and life span. One of the main goals of HRT is to prevent or reduce the risk of many conditions and diseases that afflict postmenopausal women.

Chronic Diseases: The Role of Menopause and Hormone Replacement Therapy

The menopausal state is a significant risk factor for many chronic diseases and conditions that can significantly limit the ability of the growing population of older women to enjoy a healthy, productive, and long life (9). These include cardiovascular disease, osteoporosis and hip fracture, Alzheimer's disease, colon cancer, and macular degeneration.

Coronary artery disease is the most common cause of

death in women age 50 years or older (161,162), and the mortality rate from cardiovascular disease is on the rise in women (163). Investigators have postulated that the later onset of cardiovascular disease in women results from pre-menopausal estrogen. After menopause, rates of coronary artery disease begin to increase in women and reach the male incidence at around age 75 years (164). Many epidemiologic studies have observed a reduction in relative risk of heart disease in women who use HRT. Estrogen users have been shown to have a relative risk ratio for coronary heart disease and events near 0.5 to 0.6 (165–170). The main criticism of these observational studies has been the potential for selection bias (i.e., women who choose to take HRT are healthier than their cohorts).

Most clinical trials of hormone therapy for the prevention of coronary artery disease to date have been limited in patient number and length of follow-up (171). The HERS study (Heart and Estrogen/Progestin Replacement Study) is a large, randomized, placebo-controlled trial of estrogen plus progestin for the secondary prevention of coronary artery disease in postmenopausal women (172). In this population of women with established heart disease, hormonal therapy did not reduce the overall rate of secondary cardiovascular events during the 4-year follow-up period. In fact, an increased rate of early events was noted. However, a more favorable pattern of cardiovascular events was noted several years after hormonal therapy was initiated. The results of this trial do not support the previous observational data suggesting a beneficial role of hormonal therapy in secondary prevention for women with established coronary artery disease. However, further data are needed to evaluate the role of estrogen in primary prevention of cardiovascular disease. Other randomized trials currently under way, the Women's Health Initiative (173) and the Women's International Study of Long-Duration Oestrogen after Menopause, are designed to address these important questions.

Despite the current lack of definitive data from clinical trials, the evidence for a cardioprotective effect of estrogen remains strong. Atherosclerosis appears to result from complex alterations in metabolic parameters (increased low-density lipoprotein, decreased high-density lipoprotein, hyperinsulinemia), endothelial function, vascular tone, thrombus formation, and fibrinolysis. Estrogen has been shown to exert beneficial effects on the lipid profile by increasing high-density lipoprotein and decreasing low-density lipoprotein (166,174). Fasting glucose levels are also lower in women taking estrogen (174). HRT also reduces thrombus formation and stabilization by decreasing fibrinogen levels (174) and by reducing plasminogen activator inhibitor type 1 and, thus, increasing fibrinolysis (175). In addition, administration of estrogen improves endothelial cell function and vascular tone by a variety of mechanisms (176). Thus, estrogen therapy influences cardiovascular risk in many ways and represents one of the principal long-term benefits of HRT.

Another area of women's health that can be significantly improved with the use of hormonal therapy is *osteoporosis* and osteoporotic fractures. Osteoporosis is estimated to affect 30% of white women (177). Many of these women will experience a *hip fracture,* the most common complication of osteoporosis, during their lifetimes. Significant morbidity and mortality are associated with hip fractures. In fact, up to 27% of patients die in the first year after fracture, and only 50% regain their preinjury ambulatory state (178). The direct treatment costs for osteoporotic fractures were estimated to be about $13.8 billion in 1995 (179). Thus, any measure to prevent and treat osteoporosis can significantly improve the health and well-being of postmenopausal women.

Risk factors for osteoporosis include family history, lean body habitus, smoking, reduced physical activity, poor life-long intake of calcium, and use of various medications (diuretics, anticonvulsants, glucocorticoids, lithium, and excessive thyroid hormone). Hypoestrogenism, resulting from premature ovarian failure, hypothalamic amenorrhea, use of GnRH agonists, or natural menopause, can significantly increase bone loss and lead to osteoporosis. HRT has been shown to be effective in increasing bone mineral density (180,181) and in preventing hip fractures (182–184). Thus, HRT is useful in the primary prevention of osteoporosis. In addition, all women should be counseled to ensure adequate calcium and vitamin D intake, to exercise regularly, to avoid tobacco and alcohol, and to use medications that contribute to bone loss judiciously. HRT also plays a significant role in the treatment of women with established osteoporosis (185). It may also be used in conjunction with other osteoporosis therapies, such as bisphosphonates, calcitonin, fluoride, and calcitriol.

In addition to the effects on cardiovascular disease and osteoporosis, evidence has suggested that estrogen therapy during menopause may lead to reduced relative risks of other significant diseases common in elderly women: Alzheimer's disease (186–190), colon cancer (191–193), and macular degeneration (194). Certainly, further research in the form of clinical trials is necessary to substantiate these potential benefits.

Overall, the most serious consequences of reproductive aging for women are the increased risks for these debilitating and often fatal chronic diseases that accompany menopause. Fortunately, HRT offers substantial benefits in this regard. When counseling women about the potential benefits of HRT, one must also consider and discuss the potential side effects and risks.

Risks and Side Effects of Hormone Replacement Therapy

The principal safety concerns with regard to HRT have centered on the risks of breast cancer, endometrial cancer, and thromboembolic disorders. In addition, some women note side effects during treatment with various regimens of hormone replacement. The most commonly reported are breast tenderness, breakthrough bleeding, and mood symptoms.

The relationship between HRT and *breast cancer* has sparked considerable debate in the medical community over the last decade (195). Most of the data on the risk of breast cancer with HRT are derived from observational studies. Numerous studies of this nature have failed to document a significant association between HRT and breast cancer (196–202). Other studies show small increases in the relative risk of breast cancer with HRT use (203–205). However, the Nurses Health Study (206) sparked the most concern with its finding that current users of HRT experienced an increased risk of breast cancer. Experts have advised caution in interpreting this study given that HRT users were at increased risk for breast cancer based on their alcohol consumption and had a higher surveillance rate with mammography.

Meta-analyses of these data have not resolved the issue. Although several meta-analyses have failed to show marked increases in relative risk for breast cancer with HRT use (207–210), the Collaborative Group found a 2.3% annual increase in the risk of breast cancer in a re-analysis of more than 160,000 women (211). These investigators found only localized disease, less aggressive tumors, and better survival in recent or current users of HRT. Other studies have shown that HRT reduces overall mortality rates (212,213) and the risk of fatal breast cancer (214) in a general population. Conclusive data on this issue from large clinical trials are lacking. One small, long-term clinical trial of high-dose estrogen in the presence of cyclic progestin failed to demonstrate an increased risk of breast cancer at the end of a 22-year follow-up period (215). Thus, if estrogen has an effect on breast cancer development, the effect is small. Perhaps, estrogen acts more as a promoter of breast cancer than a carcinogen, as evidenced by the less aggressive tumors with a better prognosis described by the Collaborative Group.

Although the effect of estrogen replacement therapy on breast cancer remains controversial, the risk of *endometrial cancer* with use of unopposed estrogen therapy is well documented (relative risk of 4 to 7) (216–218). Investigators now know that the addition of progestin to an estrogen replacement regimen can prevent the increased incidence of endometrial cancer seen with unopposed estrogen (219–223). Thus, it has become standard to treat women without a uterus with unopposed estrogen and women with a uterus with combined estrogen-progestin replacement therapy.

Because of the well-known association between high-dose oral contraceptives and thromboembolic disease, investigators have examined the effect of low doses of estrogen, as used for HRT, on the risk of *deep venous thrombosis and pulmonary embolism*. Although earlier studies failed to show a significant influence of estrogen replacement therapy on

the risk of venous thrombosis (224–226), more recent studies showed that current users of HRT have an elevated risk of both deep venous thromboembolism (227,228) and pulmonary embolism (229). Therefore, it is prudent to use estrogen replacement therapy with caution in patients who are at increased risk of these events, such as women with cancer, trauma, immobilization, or altered thrombotic profile (protein C or S deficiency, factor V Leiden mutation, antiphospholipid antibody syndrome).

In addition to concern for these safety issues with HRT, many women are reluctant to initiate or continue hormonal therapy because of anticipation of nuisance side effects. The most common of these are breakthrough bleeding, breast tenderness, mood changes, and worry about weight gain. Although transvaginal ultrasound and endometrial biopsy may be necessary to exclude endometrial hyperplasia or neoplasia, the incidence of endometrial disease in women taking combined hormonal regimens is extremely low (230). Mastodynia is common with initiation of HRT but tends to subside with continued treatment. Fears of weight gain with HRT are not well founded in the literature (231). Few women experience adverse mood changes with estrogen therapy, but some depressive symptoms do occur with concomitant progestin use. These can be minimized in an individual patient by manipulating the type, dose, or route of administration of the progestin.

Choices in Hormone Replacement Therapy

Once a woman has chosen to initiate HRT, she and her physician are faced with myriad options in hormonal preparations and routes of delivery, as well as nonhormonal alternatives (Table 13.3). It is beyond the scope of this chapter

TABLE 13.3. CHOICES IN HORMONE REPLACEMENT THERAPY

Estrogen therapy
  Oral preparations
    Conjugated equine estrogens
    Estrone
    Esterified estrogens
    Micronized estradiol
    Triestrogen preparations (estriol, estrone, estradiol)
  Transdermal/transvaginal preparations
    Estradiol
  Parenteral preparations
    Estradiol valerate or cypionate
Concomitant progestin therapy
  Oral preparations
    Medroxyprogesterone acetate
    Micronized progesterone
    Norethindrone and levonorgestrel
  Transdermal/transvaginal preparations
    Progesterone creams and intravaginal gels
    Combined patch (estradiol/norethindrone)
Selective estrogen receptor modulators (SERMs)
  Raloxifene
Phytoestrogens

to review in detail all the relevant literature on the various postmenopausal HRT regimens and alternatives. A brief review of this topic follows. Readers are referred to more extensive reviews on this topic for further information (232–236).

Traditional *estrogen therapy* during menopause has relied on the use of preparations containing ethinyl estradiol or conjugated estrogens. These are available in oral, transdermal, and various preparations. Most women can be successfully treated with these preparations, which are available in a variety of dosages. As reviewed previously, these estrogens are well studied for their efficacy in relieving perimenopausal symptoms and in preventing a variety of chronic diseases of advanced age.

Women with a uterus must be treated with concomitant *progestin therapy.* The most common progestin preparations contain medroxyprogesterone acetate or micronized progesterone. Other progestin alternatives include norethindrone or other C19 nortestosterones, megestrol, and the newer vaginal progesterone preparation (Crinone, Wyeth-Ayerst). Combination estrogen-progestin formulations are now available in both oral and transdermal forms.

Although the benefits of estrogen replacement therapy are well documented, many women have been reluctant to begin or continue estrogen therapy because of concern for breast or endometrial cancer. Efforts to develop compounds that mimic the beneficial effects of estrogen in the bone and the cardiovascular system but act as estrogen antagonists at the level of the breast and uterus have been spurred by the knowledge that estrogen acts through two receptor types, α and β (237). α Receptors predominate in the breast, liver, and uterus, whereas β receptors are found predominately in blood vessels, bone, urogenital tract, and lungs. The ovary and central nervous system express both receptors. This information and other knowledge have helped us to understand the selective effects of a *raloxifene,* a newer therapy for postmenopausal women. This compound was approved by the United States Food and Drug Administration as an alternative to standard HRT for prevention of osteoporosis. Raloxifene belongs to a class of compounds termed selective estrogen receptor modulators (SERMs) (233,238). Other SERMs, such as tamoxifen and clomiphene, have been in clinical use for many years but are used for clinical indications other than postmenopausal replacement therapy. Raloxifene improves bone mineral density and lowers total and low-density lipoprotein cholesterol (239,240). Although studies are ongoing, raloxifene has been shown not to induce endometrial hyperplasia or polyp formation at 1 year of use (241). Hot flushes are not alleviated with raloxifene, and its effects on cardiovascular morbidity and mortality and Alzheimer's disease remain undefined. Further studies are in progress to define the long-term effects of raloxifene on heart disease, hip fracture, breast and endometrial cancer, and overall mortality. In addition, other SERMs are in various stages of development and clinical trials.

Public interest in "natural" and herbal therapies has led to considerable discussion about *phytoestrogens* in the lay and scientific literature. Phytoestrogens are plant-derived compounds with estrogenic activity (234). Phytoestrogens, which fall into three main classes (isoflavones, coumestans, and lignans), are found in a variety of food sources (Table 13.4). The principal estrogenically active compounds within each class are genistein and daidzein (isoflavones), coumestrol (a coumestan), and enterodiol and enterolactone (lignans). These phytoestrogens display weak estrogenic and antiestrogenic actions *in vivo* and *in vitro* (242). Preliminary studies in animals and humans have suggested that phytoestrogens may reduce hot flushes, lead to a more favorable lipid profile, improve bone mineral density, and inhibit breast cancer progression in animal models and human cell lines. However, further study of phytoestrogens in long-term randomized controlled trials is necessary to define the role and safety of phytoestrogens fully as an alternative to standard HRT.

Discovery that circulating levels of *dehydroepiandrosterone* (DHEA) decline with age has led many women to begin or consider DHEA supplementation in the menopause. However, studies demonstrating the safety and efficacy of this therapy in postmenopausal women are lacking. In fact, some preliminary evidence suggests that elevations in DHEA may be associated with an abnormal lipid profile, carbohydrate intolerance, and increased risk of breast cancer (236). Thus, the use of DHEA should not be recommended to postmenopausal women as an alternative to estrogen replacement therapy.

Many *nonhormonal therapies* exist for treating various individual symptoms and diseases that occur in the menopausal period (235). Examples include clonidine for hot

TABLE 13.4. SOURCES OF PHYTOESTROGENS

Isoflavones
  Soybeans and soybean products (soy milk, soy meal, tofu)
  Lentils
  Beans (kidney, lima, broad, haricot)
  Chickpeas
Coumestans
  Alfalfa
  Soybean sprouts
  Clover
Lignans
  Wheat and wheat germ
  Barley and hops
  Rye
  Rice
  Brans and oats
  Various fruits (cherries, apples, pears)
  Various vegetables (carrots, onion, fennel) and vegetable oils
  Garlic
  Sunflower seeds and linseed

From Murkies AL, Wilcox G, Davis SR. Phytoestrogens. *J Clin Endocrinol Metab* 1998;83:297–303, with permission.

flushes, bisphosphonates and calcitonin for osteoporosis, lubricants for vaginal dryness, and lifestyle modifications for reduction of cardiovascular disease. However, the response to many of these agents is either not as effective as estrogen therapy or can be enhanced by concomitant estrogen therapy. In addition to these standard nonhormonal therapies, the use of various herbal medicines for the alleviation of menopausal symptoms has become common. These herbal preparations include evening primrose oil, ginseng, black cohosh, dong quai, and chamomile (236). Clinical studies of these compounds are lacking or limited and fail to reveal true efficacy and safety.

Thus, choices for HRT are vast. For most women, standard estrogen replacement therapy with the appropriate use of concomitant progestin therapy represents the best option for treatment. However, each patient in conjunction with the physician needs to consider specific needs and concerns in deciding whether to initiate HRT and then in selecting the most appropriate treatment regimen.

SUMMARY

The impact of reproductive aging on the health and well-being of women is significant and includes age-related infertility and other childbearing issues, potentially debilitating perimenopausal symptoms, and elevated risks for cardiovascular disease, osteoporosis, Alzheimer's disease, urogenital atrophy and incontinence, and other chronic diseases. As women continue to delay childbearing and the postmenopausal segment of our population grows in the new millennium, these issues will become increasingly important.

Reproductive aging in women appears to result primarily from ovarian factors. Clinically, this is evident in the success that egg donation programs have enjoyed. The underlying physiologic basis for ovarian aging involves attrition in follicular numbers, beginning before birth and culminating in near exhaustion of follicular stores at menopause. This decline in primordial follicle numbers is accompanied by qualitative and quantitative changes in both the somatic (granulosa cells) and germ cell (oocyte) components of the ovary. The underlying mechanisms that lead to ovarian aging have yet to be fully understood; however, this senescent process is likely to involve a complex interaction between genetic and environmental influences. These appear to include familial influences, free-radical and hypoxic damage, and activation of programmed cell death or apoptosis.

The clinical management of issues that arise as a result of reproductive aging is complex. Women in their 30s and 40s can experience not only infertility, but also increased rates of miscarriage and aneuploidy, as their ovaries enter the menopausal transition. It is important to detect diminished ovarian reserve in women undergoing infertility therapy because the presence of this condition is associated with markedly poorer success rates with natural and assisted conceptions. Most clinicians are using basal (day 3) FSH and estradiol levels to screen for diminished ovarian reserve, although the clomiphene citrate challenge test is more sensitive. With further study, other tests such as the day 3 inhibin B level may prove to be useful indicators of diminished ovarian reserve. Efficacious infertility treatment options, other than egg donation, are limited for women with premature ovarian failure or diminished ovarian reserve. Women entering the menopausal transition also need to be counseled about their risk for spontaneous miscarriage and aneuploidy. In women using egg donation, the risk of these latter complications is related to the age of the donor rather than to the age of the recipient.

The impact of reproductive aging also reaches beyond childbearing concerns. Women on average are now spending about 30 years of their life in the menopausal state. The hypoestrogenism that results from senescence of the human ovary has a significant impact on the health and well-being of perimenopausal and postmenopausal women. Symptoms of hot flushes, vaginal dryness, irregular bleeding, and urinary incontinence are common. In addition, the menopausal state is a risk factor for many chronic diseases: cardiovascular disease, osteoporosis, Alzheimer's disease, and others.

Fortunately, HRT has been shown to improve many of the symptoms of the perimenopause and menopause and to reduce the long-term sequelae of hypoestrogenism on the risk of the chronic diseases previously mentioned. For most women, estrogen replacement therapy is beneficial, although compliance with therapy remains low. Concomitant progestin therapy is indicated in women with a uterus to prevent estrogen-induced endometrial hyperplasia and carcinoma. Many different preparations and routes of administration for estrogen and progesterone are now available to suit individual needs and preferences. Alternatives to standard HRT include SERMs, phytoestrogens, and other targeted nonhormonal therapies. These may be useful in women in whom standard HRT regimens are not tolerated, are contraindicated, or are not desired by the patient. Further study is necessary, however, to determine whether they afford the same benefit as estrogen therapy.

10 KEY POINTS

1. Reproductive aging is clinically evident, in the form of impaired fertility and increased spontaneous abortion and aneuploidy rates, long before the menstrual irregularities of the perimenopause.

2. Reproductive aging in women is primarily the result of diminished ovarian function.

3. A decrease in follicular number and a decline in the quality of the ovarian follicle result from a decrease in competence of both granulosa cells and the oocyte.

4. The ovarian theory of reproductive aging asserts that

a deficiency in inhibin B results from both diminished follicular stores and qualitative changes in granulosa cell function and leads to a monotropic rise in early follicular serum FSH.

5. Evidence of diminished granulosa cell function associated with reproductive (follicular) aging includes decreased steroid and growth factor production, altered cell cycle dynamics, decreased numbers of granulosa cells per follicle, and increased granulosa cell apoptosis.

6. Meiotic spindle abnormalities and increased rates of aneuploidy reflect the effects of reproductive aging on the oocyte.

7. HRT is directed toward prevention of short-term (vasomotor symptoms) and long-term estrogen deprivation effects in estrogen-sensitive tissues: bone (osteoporosis), blood vessels (coronary artery disease), urogenital mucosa (vaginal atrophy, urinary incontinence), brain (Alzheimer's disease), eye (macular degeneration), and collagen (loss of skin tugor, peridontal disease, pelvic organ prolapse).

8. Estrogen replacement therapy must be used with caution in women who are at an increased risk of deep venous thrombosis or pulmonary embolism, such as those with a history of cancer, trauma, immobilization, protein C or S deficiency, factor V Leiden mutation, or antiphospholipid antibody syndrome.

9. Alternatives to estrogen replacement therapy include SERMs and phytoestrogens.

10. Concomitant progestin therapy is indicated in women taking estrogen replacement therapy who have not had a prior hysterectomy, to prevent estrogen-induced endometrial hyperplasia or carcinoma.

REFERENCES

1. Federation CECOS, Schwartz D, Mayaux MJ. Female fecundity as a function of age: results of artificial insemination in 2193 nulliparous women with azoospermic husbands. *N Engl J Med* 1982;306:404–406.

2. Menken J, Trussell J, Larsen U. Age and infertility. *Science* 1986;233:1389–1394.

3. Warburton D, Fraser FC. Spontaneous abortion risks in man: data from reproductive histories collected in a medical genetics unit. *Hum Genet* 1964;16:1–25.

4. Smith KE, Buyalos RP. The profound impact of patient age on pregnancy outcome after early detection of fetal cardiac activity. *Fertil Steril* 1996;65:35–40.

5. Hook EB. Rates of chromosome abnormalities at different maternal ages. *Obstet Gynecol* 1981;58:282–285.

6. Fonteyn VJ, Isada NB. Nongenetic implications of childbearing after age thirty-five. *Obstet Gynecol Surv* 1988;43:709–720.

7. Ventura SJ. *Trends and variations in first births to older women, 1970–1986.* Vital Health Statistics 21 (47). Hyattsville, MD: National Center for Health Statistics, United States Department of Health and Human Services, Public Health Service, 1989.

8. Society for Assisted Reproductive Technology and the American Society for Reproductive Medicine. Assisted reproductive technology in the United States and Canada: 1995 results generated from the American Society for Reproductive Medicine/Society for Assisted Reproductive Technology Registry. *Fertil Steril* 1998;69:389–398.

9. Sowers MR, La Pietra MT. Menopause: its epidemiology and potential association with chronic diseases. *Epidemiol Rev* 1995;17:287–302.

10. Hill K. The demography of menopause. *Maturitas* 1996; 23:113–127.

11. Khaw KT. Epidemiology of the menopause. *Br Med Bull* 1992;48:249–261.

12. Dasmahapatra A. Endocrinology of aging. *Clin Consult Obstet Gynecol* 1992;4:8–19.

13. Navot D, Bergh PA, Williams MA, et al. Poor oocyte quality rather than implantation failure as a cause of age-related decline in female fertility. *Lancet* 1991;337:1375–1377.

14. Rabinovici J, Jaffe RB. Development and regulation of growth and differentiated function in human and subhuman primate fetal gonads. *Endocr Rev* 1990;11:532–557.

15. Baker TG. A quantitative and cytological study of germ cells in human ovaries. *Proc R Soc Lond* 1963;158:417–433.

16. Block E. Quantitative morphological investigations of the follicular system in women. *Acta Anat* 1952;14:108–123.

17. Gougeon A, Ecochard R, Thalabard JC. Age-related changes of the population of human ovarian follicles: increase in the disappearance rate of non-growing and early-growing follicles in aging women. *Biol Reprod* 1994;50:653–663.

18. Faddy MJ, Gosden RG, Gougeon A, et al. Accelerated disappearance of ovarian follicles in mid-life: implications for forecasting menopause. *Hum Reprod* 1992;7:1342–1346.

19. Faddy MJ, Gosden RG. A model conforming the decline in follicle numbers to the age of menopause in women. *Hum Reprod* 1996;11:1484–1486.

20. Costoff A, Mahesh VB. Primordial follicles with normal oocytes in the ovaries of postmenopausal women. *J Am Geriatr Soc* 1975;23:193–196.

21. Richardson SJ, Senikas V, Nelson JF. Follicular depletion during the menopausal transition: evidence for accelerated loss and ultimate exhaustion. *J Clin Endocrinol Metab* 1987;65:1231–1237.

22. Gougeon A. Dynamics of follicular growth in the human: a model from preliminary results. *Hum Reprod* 1986;1:81–87.

23. Sherman BM, Korenman SG. Hormonal characteristics of the human menstrual cycle throughout reproductive life. *J Clin Invest* 1975;55:699–706.

24. Sherman BM, West JH, Korenman SG. The menopausal transition: analysis of LH, FSH, estradiol and progesterone concentrations during menstrual cycles of older women. *J Clin Endocrinol Metab* 1976;42:629–636.

25. Reyes FI, Winter JSD, Faiman C. Pituitary-ovarian relationships preceding the menopause. I. A cross-sectional study of serum follicle-stimulating hormone, luteinizing hormone, prolactin, estradiol and progesterone levels. *Am J Obstet Gynecol* 1977;129:557–564.

26. Lee SJ, Lenton EA, Sexton L, et al. The effect of age on the cyclical patterns of plasma LH, FSH, oestradiol and progesterone in women with regular menstrual cycles. *Hum Reprod* 1988;3:851–855.

27. Lenton EA, Sexton L, Lee S, et al. Progressive changes in LH and FSH and LH:FSH ratio in women throughout reproductive life. *Maturitas* 1988;10:35–43.

28. Hee J, MacNaughton J, Bangah M, et al. Perimenopausal patterns of gonadotrophins, immunoreactive inhibin, oestradiol and progesterone. *Maturitas* 1993;18:9–20.

29. Burger HG, Dudley EC, Hopper JL, et al. The endocrinology of the menopausal transition: a cross-sectional study of a popula-

tion-based sample. *J Clin Endocrinol Metab* 1995;80:3537–3545.

30. Buckler HM, Evans CA, Mamtora H, et al. Gonadotropin, steroid, and inhibin levels in women with incipient ovarian failure during anovulatory and ovulatory rebound cycles. *J Clin Endocrinol Metab* 1991;72:116–124.

31. Batista MC, Cartledge TP, Zellmer AW, et al. Effects of aging on menstrual cycle hormones and endometrial maturation. *Fertil Steril* 1995;64:492–499.

32. Klein NA, Battaglia DE, Miller PB, et al. Ovarian follicular development and the follicular fluid hormones and growth factors in normal women of advanced reproductive age. *J Clin Endocrinol Metab* 1996;81:1946–1951.

33. Santoro N, Brown JR, Adel T, et al. Characterization of reproductive hormonal dynamics in the perimenopause. *J Clin Endocrinol Metab* 1996;81:1495–1501.

34. Blake EJ, Adel T, Santoro N. Relationships between insulin-like growth hormone factor-1 and estradiol in reproductive aging. *Fertil Steril* 1997;67:697–701.

35. Soules MR, Battaglia DE, Klein NA. Inhibin and reproductive aging in women. *Maturitas* 1998;30:193–204.

36. Ying S. Inhibins, activins and follistatins: gonadal proteins modulating the secretion of follicle-stimulating hormone. *Endocr Rev* 1988;9:267–293.

37. Groome NP, Illingworth PJ, O'Brien M, et al. Detection of dimeric inhibin throughout the human menstrual cycle by two-site enzyme immunoassay. *Clin Endocrinol* 1994;40:717–723.

38. Groome NP, Illingworth PJ, O'Brien M, et al. Measurement of dimeric inhibin B throughout the human menstrual cycle. *J Clin Endocrinol Metab* 1996;81:1401–1405.

39. Fraser HM, Groome NP, McNeilly AS. Follicle-stimulating hormone-inhibin B interactions during the follicular phase of the primate menstrual cycle revealed by gonadotropin-releasing hormone antagonist and antiestrogen treatment. *J Clin Endocrinol Metab* 1999;84:1365–1369.

40. Lenton EA, De Kretser DM, Woodward AJ, et al. Inhibin concentrations throughout the menstrual cycles of normal, infertile, and older women compared with those during spontaneous conception cycles. *J Clin Endocrinol Metab* 1991;73:1180–1190.

41. Klein NA, Battaglia DE, Fujimoto VY, et al. Reproductive aging: accelerated ovarian follicular development associated with a monotropic follicle-stimulating hormone rise in normal older women. *J Clin Endocrinol Metab* 1996;81:1038–1045.

42. Klein NA, Illingworth PJ, Groome NP, et al. Decreased inhibin B secretion is associated with the monotropic FSH rise in older, ovulatory women: a study of serum and follicular fluid levels of dimeric inhibin A and B in spontaneous menstrual cycles. *J Clin Endocrinol Metab* 1996;81:2742–2745.

43. Hofmann GE, Danforth DR, Seifer DB. Inhibin-B: the physiologic basis of the clomiphene citrate challenge test for ovarian reserve screening. *Fertil Steril* 1998;69:474–477.

44. Burger HG, Cahir N, Robertson DM, et al. Serum inhibins A and B fall differentially as FSH rises in perimenopausal women. *Clin Endocrinol* 1998;48:809–813.

45. Reame NE, Wyman TL, Phillips DJ, et al. Net increase in stimulatory input resulting from a decrease in inhibin B and an increase in activin A may contribute in part to the rise in follicular phase follicle-stimulating hormone of aging cycling women. *J Clin Endocrinol Metab* 1998;83:3302–3307.

46. Danforth DR, Arbogast LK, Mroueh J, et al. Dimeric inhibin: a direct marker of ovarian aging. *Fertil Steril* 1998;70:119–123.

47. Santoro N, Adel T, Skurnick JH. Decreased inhibin tone and increased activin A secretion characterize reproductive aging in women. *Fertil Steril* 1999;71:658–662.

48. Seifer DB, Scott RT, Bergh PA, et al. Women with declining ovarian reserve may demonstrate a decrease in day 3 serum inhibin-B before a rise in day 3 FSH. *Fertil Steril* 1999;72:63–65.

49. Seifer DB, Naftolin F. Moving toward an earlier and better understanding of the perimenopause. *Fertil Steril* 1998;69:387–388.

50. Seifer DB, Gardiner AC, Ferreira KA, et al. Apoptosis as a function of ovarian reserve in women undergoing *in vitro* fertilization. *Fertil Steril* 1996;66:593–598.

51. Chun SY, Billig H, Tilly JL, et al. Gonadotropin suppression of apoptosis in cultured preovulatory follicles: mediatory role of endogenous insulin-like growth factor I. *Endocrinology* 1994;135:1845–1853.

52. Luciano AM, Pappalardo A, Ray C, et al. Epidermal growth factor inhibits large granulosa cell apoptosis by stimulating progesterone synthesis and regulating the distribution of intracellular free calcium. *Biol Reprod* 1994;51:646–654.

53. Pellicer A, Mari M, de los Santos MJ, et al. Effects of aging on the human ovary: the secretion of immunoreactive α-inhibin and progesterone. *Fertil Steril* 1994;61:663–668.

54. Klein NA, Battaglia DE, Miller PB, et al. Circulating levels of growth hormone, insulin-like growth factor-I and growth hormone binding protein in normal women of advanced reproductive age. *Clin Endocrinol* 1996;44:285–292.

55. Seifer DB, Gardiner AC, Lambert-Messerlian G, et al. Differential secretion of dimeric inhibin in cultured luteinized granulosa cells as a function of ovarian reserve. *J Clin Endocrinol Metab* 1996;81:736–739.

56. King KL, Cidlowski JA. Cell cycle and apoptosis: common pathways to life and death. *J Cell Biochem* 1995;58:175–180.

57. Meikrantz W, Schlegel R. Apoptosis and the cell cycle. *J Cell Biochem* 1995;58:160–174.

58. Seifer DB, Honig J, Penzias AS, et al. Flow cytometric analysis of deoxyribonucleic acid in human granulosa cells as a function of chronological age and ovulation induction regimen. *J Clin Endocrinol Metab* 1992;75:636–640.

59. Seifer DB, Charland C, Berlinsky D, et al. Proliferative index of luteinized granulosa cells varies as a function of ovarian reserve. *Am J Obstet Gynecol* 1993;169:1531–1535.

60. Eichenlaub-Ritter U. Genetics of oocyte ageing. *Maturitas* 1998;30:143–169.

61. Sherman SL, Takaesu N, Freeman SB, et al. Trisomy 21: association between reduced recombination and nondisjunction. *Am J Hum Genet* 1991;49:608–620.

62. Angell RR, Xian J, Keith J, et al. First meiotic division abnormalities in human oocytes: mechanism of trisomy formation. *Cytogenet Cell Genet* 1994;65:194–202.

63. Angell R. First-meiotic-division nondisjunction in human oocytes. *Am J Hum Genet* 1977;61:23–32, 1997.

64. McIntosh JR. Spindle structure and the mechanisms of chromosome movement. In: Dellarco VL, Voytek PE, eds. *Aneuploidy: etiology and mechanisms.* New York: Plenum, 1985.

65. Szollosi D. Mammalian eggs aging in the fallopian tubes. In: Blandau, RJ, ed. *Aging gametes: their biology and pathology.* Basel S. Karger, 1975.

66. Egozcue J. Cellular aspects of *in vitro* fertilization: ultrastructural and cytogenetic studies of human gametes and zygotes. *Rev Biol Cell* 1987;13:1–104.

67. Sathananthan AH. Ultrastructure of the human egg. *Hum Cell* 1997;10:21–38.

68. Pickering SJ, Johnson MH, Braude PR, et al. Cytoskeletal organization in fresh, aged and spontaneously activated human oocytes. *Hum Reprod* 1988;3:978–989.

69. Battaglia DE, Goodwin P, Klein NA, et al. Influence of maternal age on meiotic spindle assembly in oocytes from naturally cycling women. *Hum Reprod* 1996;11:2217–2222.

70. Volarcik K, Sheean L, Goldfarb J, et al. The meiotic competence of *in vitro* matured human oocytes is influenced by donor age: evidence that folliculogenesis is compromised in the reproductively aged ovary. *Hum Reprod* 1998;13:154–160.

71. Gras L, McBain J, Trounson A, et al. The incidence of chromosomal aneuploidy in stimulated and unstimulated (natural) uninseminated human oocytes. *Hum Reprod* 1992;7:1396–1401.

72. Eichenlaub-Ritter U, Chandley AC, Gosden RG. The CBA mouse as a model for age-related aneuploidy in man: studies of oocyte maturation, spindle formation and chromosome alignment during meiosis. *Chromosoma* 1988;96:220–226.

73. Brook JD, Gosden RG, Chandley AC. Maternal ageing and aneuploid embryos: evidence from the mouse that biological and not chronological age is the important influence. *Hum Genet* 1984;66:41–45.

74. Eichenlaub-Ritter U, Boll I. Nocodazole sensitivity, age-related aneuploidy, and alterations in the cell cycle during maturation of mouse oocytes. *Cytogenet Cell Genet* 1989;52:170–176.

75. Warburton D. Human female meiosis: new insights into an error-prone process. *Am J Hum Genet* 1997;61:1–4.

76. Messinger SM, Albertini DF. Centrosome and microtubule dynamics during meiotic progression in the mouse oocyte. *J Cell Sci* 1991;100:289–298.

77. Albertini DF. Regulation of meiotic maturation in the mammalian oocyte: interplay between exogenous cues and the microtubule cytoskeleton. *Bioessays* 1992;14:97–103.

78. Wickramasinghe D, Ebert KM, Albertini DF. Meiotic competence acquisition is associated with the appearance of M-phase characteristics in growing mouse oocytes. *Dev Biol* 1991; 143:162–172.

79. Battaglia DE, Klein NA, Soules MR. Changes in centrosomal domains during meiotic maturation in the human oocyte. *Mol Hum Reprod* 1996;2:845–851.

80. Doxsey SJ, Stein P, Evans L, et al. Pericentrin, a highly conserved centrosome protein involved in microtubule organization. *Cell* 1994;76:639–650.

81. George MA, Pickering SJ, Braude PR, et al. The distribution of α- and γ-tubulin in fresh and aged human and mouse oocytes exposed to cryoprotectant. *Mol Hum Reprod* 1996;2:445–456.

82. Guerrier P, Colas P, Neant I. Meiosis reinitiation as a model system for the study of cell division and cell differentiation. *Int J Dev Biol* 1990;34:93–109.

83. Buendia B, Draetta G, Karsenti E. Regulation of the microtubule nucleating activity of centrosomes in *Xenopus* egg extracts: role of cyclin-A–associated protein kinase. *J Cell Biol* 1992; 116:1431–1442.

84. Winston NJ. Stability of cyclin B protein during meiotic maturation and the first mitotic cell division in mouse oocytes. *Biol Cell* 1997;89:211–219.

85. Hunt T. Cell cycle arrest and c-*mos*. *Nature* 1992;355:587–588.

86. Pal SK, Torry D, Serta R, et al. Expression and potential function of the c-*mos* proto-oncogene in human eggs. *Fertil Steril* 1994;61:496–503.

87. Araki K, Naito K, Haraguchi S, et al. Meiotic abnormalities of c-*mos* knockout mouse oocytes: activation after first meiosis or entrance into third meiotic metaphase. *Biol Reprod* 1996; 55:1315–1324.

88. Duesbery NS, Choi T, Brown KD. CENP-E is an essential kinetochore motor in maturing oocytes and is masked during *mos*-dependent, cell cycle arrest at metaphase II. *Proc Natl Acad Sci U S A* 1997;94:9165–9170.

89. Perez GI, Robles R, Knudson CM, et al. Prolongation of ovarian lifespan into advanced chronological age by *Bax*-deficiency. *Nat Genet* 1999;21:200–203.

90. Hunt P, LeMaire R, Embury P, et al. Analysis of chromosome behavior in intact mammalian oocytes: monitoring the segregation of a univalent chromosome during female meiosis. *Hum Mol Genet* 1995;4:2007–2012.

91. Torgerson DJ, Avenell A, Russell IT, et al. Factors associated with onset of menopause in women aged 45–49. *Maturitas* 1994;19:83–92.

92. Cramer DW, Xu H, Harlow BL. Family history as a predictor of early menopause. *Fertil Steril* 1995;64:740–745.

93. Torgerson DJ, Thomas RE, Campbell MK, et al. Alcohol consumption and age of maternal menopause are associated with menopause onset. *Maturitas* 1997;26:21–25.

94. Torgerson DJ, Thomas RE, Reid DM. Mother and daughters menopausal ages: is there a link? *Eur J Obstet Gynecol Reprod Biol* 1997;74:63–66.

95. Snieder H, MacGregor AJ, Spector TD. Genes control the cessation of a woman's reproductive life: a twin study of hysterectomy and age at menopause. *J Clin Endocrinol Metab* 1998;83:1875–1880.

96. Krauss CM, Turksoy RN, Atkins L, et al. Familial premature ovarian failure due to interstitial deletion of the long arm of the X chromosome. *N Engl J Med* 1987;317:125–131.

97. Veneman TF, Beverstock GC, Exalto N, et al. Premature menopause because of inherited deletion in the long arm of the X-chromosome. *Fertil Steril* 1991;55:631–633.

98. Epstein CJ, Martin GM, Schultz AL, et al. Werner's syndrome: a review of its symptomatology, natural history, pathologic features, genetics and relationship to the natural aging process. *Medicine* 1966;45:177–221.

99. Bundey S. Clinical and genetic features of ataxia-telangiectasia. *Int J Radiat Biol* 1994;66:S23–29.

100. Bodnar AG, Ouellette M, Frolkis M, et al. Extension of life-span by introduction of telomerase into normal human cells. *Science* 1998;279:349–352.

101. Linskens MHK, Feng J, Andrews WH, et al. Cataloging altered gene expression in young and senescent cells using enhanced differential display. *Nucleic Acids Res* 1995;23:3244–3251.

102. Swisshelm K, Ryan K, Tsuchiya K, et al. Enhanced expression of an insulin growth factor-like binding protein (mac25) in senescent human mammary epithelial cells and induced expression with retinoic acid. *Proc Natl Acad Sci U S A* 1995;92:4472–4476.

103. Kumazaki T, Robetorye RS, Robetorye SC, et al. Fibronectin expression increases during *in vitro* cellular senescence: correlation with increased cell area. *Exp Cell Res* 1991;195:13–19.

104. Seshadri T, Campisi J. Repression of c-fos transcription and an altered genetic program in senescent human fibroblasts. *Science* 1990;247:205–209.

105. Dimri GP, Hara E, Campisi J. Regulation of two E2F-related genes in presenescent and senescent human fibroblasts. *J Biol Chem* 1994;269:16180–16186.

106. Stein GH, Drullinger LF, Robetorye RS, et al. Senescent cells fail to express cdc2, cycA and cycB in response to mitogen stimulation. *Proc Natl Acad Sci U S A* 1991;88:11012–11016.

107. Tilly JL. Apoptosis and ovarian function. *Rev Reprod* 1996; 1:162–172.

108. Fujino Y, Ozaki K, Yamamasu S, et al. DNA fragmentation of oocytes in aged mice. *Hum Reprod* 1996;11:1480–1483.

109. Tolmasoff JM, Ono T, Cutler RG. Superoxide dismutase: correlation with life span and specific metabolic rate in primate species. *Proc Natl Acad Sci U S A* 1980;77:2777–2781.

110. Martin GM, Austad SN, Johnson TE. Genetic analysis of aging: role of oxidative damage and environmental stresses. *Nat Genet* 1996;13:25–34.

111. Tilly JL, Tilly KI. Inhibitors of oxidative stress mimic the ability of follicle-stimulating hormone to suppress apoptosis in cultured rat ovarian follicles. *Endocrinology* 1995;136:242–252.

112. Okatani Y, Morioka N, Wakatsuki A, et al. Role of the free

radical-scavenger system in aromatase activity of the human ovary. *Horm Res* 1993;39[Suppl 1]:22–27.

113. Van Blerkom J, Davis PW, Lee J. ATP content of human oocytes and developmental potential and outcome after *in vitro* fertilization and embryo transfer. *Hum Reprod* 1995; 10:415–424.

114. Tarin JJ. Aetiology of age-associated aneuploidy: a mechanism based on the "free radical theory of ageing." *Hum Reprod* 1995;10:1563–1565.

115. Gaulden ME. Maternal age effect: the enigma of Down's syndrome and other trisomic conditions. *Mutat Res* 1992; 296:69–88.

116. Van Blerkom J. The influence of intrinsic and extrinsic factors on the developmental potential and chromosomal normality of the human oocyte. *J Soc Gynecol Invest* 1996;3:3–11.

117. Friedman CI, Danforth DR, Herbosa-Encarnacion C, et al. Follicular fluid vascular endothelial growth factor concentrations are elevated in women of advanced reproductive age undergoing ovulation induction. *Fertil Steril* 1997;68:607–612.

118. Van Blerkom J, Antczak M, Schrader R. The developmental potential of the human oocyte is related to the dissolved oxygen content of follicular fluid: association with vascular endothelial growth factor levels and perifollicular blood flow characteristics. *Hum Reprod* 1997;12:1047–1055.

119. Maroulis GB. Effect of aging on fertility and pregnancy. *Semin Reprod Endocrinol* 1991;9:165–175.

120. Hughes EG, King C, Wood EC. A prospective study of prognostic factors in *in vitro* fertilization and embryo transfer. *Fertil Steril* 1989;51:838–844.

121. Toner JP, Philput CB, Jones GS, et al. Basal follicle-stimulating hormone level is a better predictor of *in vitro* fertilization performance than age. *Fertil Steril* 1991;55:784–791.

122. Jacobs SL, Metzger DA, Dodson WC, et al. Effect of age on response to human menopausal gonadotropin stimulation. *J Clin Endocrinol Metab* 1990;71:1525–1530.

123. Roest J, van Heusden AM, Mous H, et al. The ovarian response as a predictor for successful *in vitro* fertilization treatment after the age of 40 years. *Fertil Steril* 1996;66:969–973.

124. Piette C, de Mouzon J, Bachelot A, et al. *In vitro* fertilization: influence of woman's age on pregnancy rates. *Hum Reprod* 1990;5:56–59.

125. Corson SL, Dickey RP, Gocial B, et al. Outcome in 242 *in vitro* fertilization-embryo replacement or gamete intrafallopian transfer-induced pregnancies. *Fertil Steril* 1989;51:644–650.

126. Craft I, Al-Shawaf T, Lewis P, et al. Analysis of 1071 GIFT procedures: the case for a flexible approach to treatment. *Lancet* 1988;1:1094–1098.

127. Padilla SL, Garcia JE. Effect of maternal age and number of *in vitro* fertilization procedures on pregnancy outcome. *Fertil Steril* 1989;52:270–273.

128. Penzias AS, Thompson IE, Alper MM, et al. Successful use of gamete intrafallopian transfer does not reverse the decline in fertility in women over 40 years of age. *Obstet Gynecol* 1991;77:37–39.

129. Navot D, Rosenwaks Z, Margalioth EJ. Prognostic assessment of female fecundity. *Lancet* 1987;2:645–647.

130. Scott RT Jr, Hofmann GE. Prognostic assessment of ovarian reserve. *Fertil Steril* 1995;63:1–11.

131. Pearlstone AC, Fournet N, Gambone JC, et al. Ovulation induction in women age 40 and older: the importance of basal follicle-stimulating hormone level and chronological age. *Fertil Steril* 1992;58:674–679.

132. Scott RT, Toner JP, Muasher SJ, et al. Follicle-stimulating hormone levels on cycle day 3 are predictive of *in vitro* fertilization outcome. *Fertil Steril* 1989;51:651–654.

133. Sharara FI, Scott RT, Seifer DB. The detection of diminished ovarian reserve in infertile women. *Am J Obstet Gynecol* 1998;179:804–812.

134. Muasher SJ, Oehninger S, Simonetti S, et al. The value of basal and/or stimulated serum gonadotropin levels in prediction of stimulation response and *in vitro* fertilization outcome. *Fertil Steril* 1988;50:298–307.

135. Cahill DJ, Prosser CJ, Wardle PG, et al. Relative influence of serum follicle stimulating hormone, age and other factors on ovarian response to gonadotrophin stimulation. *Br J Obstet Gynaecol* 1994;101:999–1002.

136. Hansen LM, Batzer FR, Gutmann JN, et al. Evaluating ovarian reserve: follicle stimulating hormone and oestradiol variability during cycle days 2–5. *Hum Reprod* 1996;3:486–489.

137. Scott RT, Hofmann GE, Oehninger S, et al. Intercycle variability of day 3 follicle-stimulating hormone levels and its effect on stimulation quality in *in vitro* fertilization. *Fertil Steril* 1990;54:297–302.

138. Martin JSB, Nisker JA, Tummon IS, et al. Future *in vitro* fertilization pregnancy potential of women with variably elevated day 3 follicle-stimulating hormone levels. *Fertil Steril* 1996;65:1238–1240.

139. Nasseri A, Mukherjee T, Grifo JA, et al. Elevated day 3 serum follicle stimulating hormone and/or estradiol may predict fetal aneuploidy. *Fertil Steril* 1999;71:715–718.

140. Tanbo T, Dale PO, Abyholm T, et al. Follicle-stimulating hormone as a prognostic indicator in clomiphene citrate/human menopausal gonadotrophin-stimulated cycles for *in-vitro* fertilization. *Hum Reprod* 1989;6:647–650.

141. Loumaye E, Billion JM, Mine JM, et al. Prediction of individual response to controlled ovarian hyperstimulation by means of a clomiphene citrate challenge test. *Fertil Steril* 1990;53: 295–301.

142. Tanbo T, Dale PO, Lunde O, et al. Prediction of response to controlled ovarian hyperstimulation: a comparison of basal and clomiphene citrate-stimulated follicle stimulating hormone levels. *Fertil Steril* 1992;57:819–824.

143. Scott RT, Leonardi MR, Hofmann GE, et al. A prospective evaluation of clomiphene citrate challenge test screening of the general infertility population. *Obstet Gynecol* 1993;82:539–544.

144. Scott RT, Opsahl MS, Leonardi MR, et al. Life table analysis of pregnancy rates in a general infertility population relative to ovarian reserve and patient age. *Hum Reprod* 1995;10:1706–1710.

145. Mukherjee T, Copperman AB, Lapinski R, et al. An elevated day three follicle-stimulating hormone: luteinizing hormone ratio (FSH:LH) in the presence of a normal day 3 FSH predicts a poor response to controlled ovarian hyperstimulation. *Fertil Steril* 1996;65:588–593.

146. Winslow KL, Toner JP, Brzyski RG, et al. The gonadotropin-releasing hormone agonist stimulation test: a sensitive predictor of performance in the flare-up *in vitro* fertilization cycle. *Fertil Steril* 1991;56:711–717.

147. Ranieri DM, Quinn F, Makhlouf A, et al. Simultaneous evaluation of basal follicle-stimulating hormone and 17β-estradiol response to gonadotropin-releasing hormone analogue stimulation: an improved predictor of ovarian reserve. *Fertil Steril* 1998;70:227–233.

148. Fanchin R, de Ziegler D, Olivennes F, et al. Exogenous follicle stimulating hormone ovarian reserve test (EFORT): a simple and reliable screening test for detecting "poor responders" in *in-vitro* fertilization. *Hum Reprod* 1994;9:1607–1611.

149. Smotrich DB, Widra EA, Gindoff PR, et al. Prognostic value of day 3 estradiol on *in vitro* fertilization outcome. *Fertil Steril* 1995;64:1136–1140.

150. Licciardi FL, Liu HC, Rosenwaks Z. Day 3 estradiol serum concentrations as prognosticators of ovarian stimulation re-

sponse and pregnancy outcome in patients undergoing *in vitro* fertilization. *Fertil Steril* 1995;64:991–994.

151. Seifer DB, Lambert-Messerlian G, Hogan JW, et al. Day 3 serum inhibin-B is predictive of assisted reproductive technologies outcome. *Fertil Steril* 1997;67:110–114.

152. Society for Assisted Reproductive Technology and the American Society for Reproductive Medicine. 1996 Assisted reproductive technology success rates: national summary and fertility clinic reports. Available at http://www.cdc.gov/nccdphp/drh/art96/ Accessed April 5, 1999.

153. Cohen J, Scott R, Alikani M, et al. Ooplasmic transfer in mature human oocytes. *Mol Hum Reprod* 1998;4:269–280.

154. McKinlay SM, Brambilla DJ, Posner JG. The normal menopause transition. *Am J Hum Biol* 1992;4:37–46.

155. Treolar AE, Boynton RE, Behn BG, et al. Variation of the human menstrual cycle through reproductive life. *Int J Fertil* 1967;12:77–126.

156. Cramer DW, Barbieri RL, Xu H, et al. Determinants of basal follicle-stimulating hormone levels in premenopausal women. *J Clin Endocrinol Metab* 1994;79:1105–1109.

157. Kaufert PA, Gilbert P, Tate R. Defining menopausal status: the impact of longitudinal data. *Maturitas* 1987;9:217–226.

158. Ditkoff EC, Crary WG, Cristo M, et al. Estrogen improves psychological function in asymptomatic postmenopausal women. *Obstet Gynecol* 1991;78:991–995.

159. Samsioe G, Jansson I, Mellstrom D, et al. Occurrence, nature and treatment of urinary incontinence in a 70-year-old female population. *Maturitas* 1985;7:335–342.

160. Oldenhave A, Jaszmann LJB, Haspels AA, et al. Impact of climacteric on well-being: a survey based on 5213 women 39–60 years old. *Am J Obstet Gynecol* 1993;168:772–780.

161. Kuhn FE, Rackley CE. Coronary artery disease in women: risk factors, evaluation, treatment, and prevention. *Arch Intern Med* 1993;153:2626–2636.

162. National Center for Health Statistics. *Vital statistics of the United States, 1992,* vol II: *Mortality,* Part A. DHHS publication 96–1101. Hyattsville, MD: National Center for Health Statistics, United States Department of Health and Human Services, Public Health Service, 1996.

163. American Heart Association. *Heart and stroke statistical update.* Dallas: American Heart Association, 1997.

164. Lerner DJ, Kannell WB. Patterns of coronary heart disease morbidity and mortality in the sexes: a 26-year follow-up of the Framingham population. *Am Heart J* 1986;111:383–390.

165. Stampfer MJ, Willett WC, Colditz GA, et al. A prospective study of postmenopausal estrogen therapy and coronary heart disease. *N Engl J Med* 1985;313:1044–1049.

166. Bush TL, Barrett-Connor E, Cowan LD, et al. Cardiovascular mortality and noncontraceptive use of estrogen in women: results from the Lipid Research Clinics Program Follow-up Study. *Circulation* 1987;75:1102–1109.

167. Henderson BE, Paginini-Hill A, Ross RK. Estrogen replacement therapy and protection from acute myocardial infarction. *Am J Obstet Gynecol* 1988;159:312–317.

168. Wolf PH, Madans JH, Finucane FF, et al. Reduction of cardiovascular disease-related mortality among postmenopausal women who use hormones: evidence from a national cohort. *Am J Obstet Gynecol* 1991;164:489–494.

169. Falkeborn M, Persson I, Adami HO, et al. The risk of acute myocardial infarction after oestrogen and oestrogen-progestogen replacement. *Br J Obstet Gynecol* 1992;99:821–828.

170. Folsom AR, Mink PJ, Sellers TA, et al. Hormonal replacement therapy and morbidity and mortality in a prospective study of postmenopausal women. *Am J Public Health* 1995;85:1128–1132.

171. Hemminki E, McPherson K. Impact of post-menopausal hormone therapy on cardiovascular events and cancer: pooled data from clinical trials. *BMJ* 1997;315:149–153.

172. Hulley S, Grady D, Bush T, et al. Randomized trial of estrogen plus progestin for secondary prevention of coronary heart disease in postmenopausal women. *JAMA* 1998;280:605–613.

173. The Women's Health Initiative Study Group. Design of the Women's Health Initiative Clinical Trial and Observational Study. *Control Clin Trials* 1998;19:61–109.

174. Writing Group for the PEPI Trial. Effects of estrogen or estrogen/progestin regimens on heart disease risk factors in postmenopausal women: the Postmenopausal Estrogen/Progestin Interventions (PEPI) Trial. *JAMA* 1995;273:199–208.

175. Koh KK, Mincemoyer R, Bui MN, et al. Effects of hormone-replacement therapy on fibrinolysis in postmenopausal women. *N Engl J Med* 1997;336:683–690.

176. White MM, Zamudio S, Stevens T, et al. Estrogen, progesterone, and vascular reactivity: potential cellular mechanisms. *Endocr Rev* 1995;16:739–751.

177. Melton LJ III. How many women have osteoporosis now? *J Bone Miner Res* 1995;10:175–177.

178. Miller CW. Survival and ambulation following hip fractures. *J Bone Joint Surg Am* 1978;60:930–934.

179. Ray NF, Chan JK, Thamer M, Melton LJ. Medical expenditures for the treatment of osteoporotic fractures in the United States in 1995: report from the National Osteoporosis Foundation. *J Bone Miner Res* 1997;12:24–35.

180. Writing group for the PEPI Trial. Effects of hormone therapy on bone mineral density: results from the postmenopausal estrogen/progestin interventions (PEPI) trial. *JAMA* 1996;276:1389–1396.

181. Lindsay R. The menopause: sex steroids and osteoporosis. *Clin Obstet Gynecol* 1987;30:847–859.

182. Johnson RE, Specht EE. The risk of hip fracture in postmenopausal females with and without estrogen exposure. *Am J Public Health* 1981;71:138–144.

183. Paganini-Hill A, Ross RK, Gerkins VR, et al. Menopausal estrogen therapy and hip fractures. *Ann Intern Med* 1981;95:28–31.

184. Cauley JA, Seely DG, Ensrud K, et al. Estrogen replacement therapy and fractures in older women. *Ann Intern Med* 1995;122:9–16.

185. Lindsay R, Bush TL, Grady D, et al. Therapeutic controversy: estrogen replacement in menopause. *J Clin Endocrinol Metab* 1996;81:3829–3838.

186. Paganini-Hill A, Henderson VW. Estrogen replacement therapy and risk of Alzheimer disease. *Arch Intern Med* 1996;156:2213–2217.

187. Tang M-X, Jacobs D, Stern Y, et al. Effect of oestrogen during menopause on risk and age at onset of Alzheimer's disease. *Lancet* 1996;348:429–432.

188. Kawas C, Resnick S, Morrison A, et al. A prospective study of estrogen replacement therapy and the risk of developing Alzheimer's disease: the Baltimore Longitudinal Study of Aging. *Neurology* 1997;48:1517–1521.

189. Yaffe K, Sawaya G, Lieberburg I, et al. Estrogen therapy in postmenopausal women: effects on cognitive function and dementia. *JAMA* 1998;279:688–695.

190. Baldereschi M, Di Carlo A, Lepore V, et al. Estrogen-replacement therapy and Alzheimer's disease in the Italian Longitudinal Study on Aging. *Neurology* 1998;50:996–1002.

191. Furner SE, Davis FG, Nelson RL, et al. A case-control study of large bowel cancer and hormone exposure in women. *Cancer Res* 1989;49:4936–4940.

192. Kampman E, Potter JD, Slattery ML, et al. Hormone replacement therapy, reproductive history, and colon cancer: a

multicenter, case-control study in the United States. *Cancer Causes Control* 1997;8:146–158.

193. Troisi R, Schairer C, Chow W-H, et al. A prospective study of menopausal hormones and risk of colorectal cancer (United States). *Cancer Causes Control* 1997;8:130–138.

194. Eye-Disease Case-Control Study Group. Risk factors for neovascular age-related macular degeneration. *Arch Ophthalmol* 1992;110:1701–1708.

195. Agarwal SK, Judd HL. Estrogen replacement therapy and breast cancer. *Fertil Steril* 1999;71:602–603.

196. Dupont WD, Page DL. Menopausal estrogen replacement therapy and breast cancer. *Arch Intern Med* 1991;151:67–72.

197. Kaufman DW, Palmer JR, de Mouzon J, et al. Estrogen replacement therapy and the risk of breast cancer: results from the case-control surveillance study. *Am J Epidemiol* 1991;134:1375–1385.

198. Palmer JR, Rosenberg L, Clarke EA, et al. Breast cancer risk after estrogen replacement therapy: results from the Toronto Breast Cancer Study. *Am J Epidemiol* 1991;134:1386–1395.

199. La Vecchia C, Negri E, Franceschi S, et al. Hormone replacement therapy and breast cancer risk: a cooperative Italian study. *Br J Cancer* 1995;72:244–248.

200. Schuurman AG, van den Brandt PA, Goldbohm RA. Exogenous hormone use and the risk of postmenopausal breast cancer: results from the Netherlands cohort study. *Cancer Causes Control* 1995;6:416–424.

201. Stanford JL, Weiss NS, Voigt LF, et al. Combined estrogen and progestin hormone replacement therapy in relation to risk of breast cancer in middle-aged women. *JAMA* 1995;274:137–142.

202. Newcomb PA, Longnecker MP, Storer BE, et al. Long-term hormone replacement therapy and risk of breast cancer in postmenopausal women. *Am J Epidemiol* 1995;142:788–795.

203. Risch HA, Howe GR. Menopausal hormone usage and breast cancer in Saskatchewan: a record-linkage cohort study. *Am J Epidemiol* 1994;139:670–683.

204. Schairer C, Byrne C, Keyl PM, et al. Menopausal estrogen and estrogen-progestin replacement therapy and risk of breast cancer (United States). *Cancer Causes Control* 1994;5:491–500.

205. Colditz GA, Hankinson SE, Hunter DJ, et al. The use of estrogens and progestins and the risk of breast cancer in postmenopausal women. *N Engl J Med* 1995;332:1589–1593.

206. Colditz GA, Stampfer MJ, Willett WC, et al. Type of postmenopausal hormone use and risk of breast cancer: 12–year follow-up from the Nurses' Health Study. *Cancer Causes Control* 1992;3:433–439.

207. Armstrong BK. Oestrogen therapy after the menopause: boon or bane? *Med J Aust* 1988;148:213–214.

208. Sillero-Arenas M, Delgado-Rodriguez M, Rodigues-Canteras R, et al. Menopausal hormone replacement therapy and breast cancer: a meta-analysis. *Obstet Gynecol* 1992;79:286–294.

209. Colditz GA, Egan KM, Stampfer MJ. Hormone replacement therapy and risk of breast cancer: results from epidemiologic studies. *Am J Obstet Gynecol* 1993;168:1473–1480.

210. Grady D, Rubin SM, Petitti DB, et al. Hormone therapy to prevent disease and prolong life in postmenopausal women. *Ann Intern Med* 1992;117:1016–1037.

211. Collaborative Group on Hormonal Factors in Breast Cancer. Breast cancer and hormone replacement therapy: collaborative reanalysis of data from 51 epidemiological studies of 52,705 women with breast cancer and 108,411 women without breast cancer. *Lancet* 1997;350:1047–1059.

212. Criqui MH, Suarez L, Barrett-Connor E, et al. Postmenopausal estrogen use and mortality: results from a prospective study in a defined, homogeneous community. *Am J Epidemiol* 1988;128:606–614.

213. Grodstein F, Stampfer MJ, Colditz GA, et al. Postmenopausal hormone therapy and mortality. *N Engl J Med* 1997;336:1769–1775.

214. Willis DB, Calle EE, Miracle-McMahill HL, et al. Estrogen replacement therapy and risk of fatal breast cancer in a prospective cohort of postmenopausal women in the United States. *Cancer Causes Control* 1996;7:449–457.

215. Nachtigall MJ, Smilen SW, Nachtigall RD, et al. Incidence of breast cancer in a 22-year study of women receiving estrogen-progestin replacement therapy. *Obstet Gynecol* 1992;80:827–830.

216. Ziel HK, Finkle WD. Increased risk of endometrial carcinoma among users of conjugated estrogens. *N Engl J Med* 1975;293:1167–1170.

217. Smith DC, Prentice R, Thompson DJ, et al. Association of exogenous estrogen and endometrial carcinoma. *N Engl J Med* 1975;293:1164–1167.

218. Baker DP. Estrogen-replacement therapy in patients with previous endometrial carcinoma. *Compr Ther* 1990;16:28–35.

219. Thom MH, White PJ, Williams RM, et al. Prevention and treatment of endometrial disease in climacteric women receiving estrogen. *Lancet* 1979;2:455–457.

220. Gambrell RD Jr, Babgnell CA, Greenblatt RB. Role of estrogens and progesterone in the etiology and prevention of endometrial cancer: a review. *Am J Obstet Gynecol* 1983;146:696–707.

221. Persson I, Adami H-O, Bergkvist L, et al. Risk of endometrial cancer after treatment with oestrogens alone or in conjunction with progestogens: results of a prospective study. *BMJ* 1989;298:147–151.

222. Voigt LF, Weiss NS, Chu J, et al. Progestagen supplementation of exogenous oestrogens and risk of endometrial cancer. *Lancet* 1991;338:274–277.

223. Persson I, Yuen J, Bergkvist L, et al. Cancer incidence and mortality in women receiving estrogen and estrogen-progestin replacement therapy: long term follow-up of a Swedish cohort. *Int J Cancer* 1996;67:327–332.

224. Boston Collaborative Drug Surveillance Program. Surgically confirmed gallbladder disease, venous thromboembolism and breast tumors in relation to postmenopausal estrogen therapy. *N Engl J Med* 1974;290:15–19.

225. Petitti DB, Wingerd J, Pellegrin F, et al. Risk of vascular disease in women: smoking, oral contraceptives, noncontraceptive estrogens, and other factors. *JAMA* 1979;242:1150–1154.

226. Devor M, Barrett-Connor E, Renvall M, et al. Estrogen replacement therapy and the risk of venous thrombosis. *Am J Med* 1992;92:275–282.

227. Daly E, Vessey MP, Hawkins MM, et al. Risk of venous thromboembolism in users of hormone replacement therapy. *Lancet* 1996;348:977–980.

228. Jick H, Derby LE, Myers MW, et al. Risk of hospital admission for idiopathic venous thromboembolism among users of postmenopausal oestrogens. *Lancet* 1996;348:981–983.

229. Grodstein F, Stampfer MJ, Goldhaber SZ, et al. Prospective study of exogenous hormones and risk of pulmonary embolism in women. *Lancet* 1996;348:983–987.

230. Woodruff JD, Pickar JH, the Menopause Study Group. Incidence of endometrial hyperplasia in postmenopausal women taking conjugated estrogens (Premarin) with medroxyprogesterone acetate or conjugated estrogens alone. *Am J Obstet Gynecol* 1994;170:1213–1223.

231. Reubinoff BE, Wurtman J, Rojansky N, et al. Effects of hormone replacement therapy on weight, body composition, fat distribution, and food intake in early postmenopausal women: a prospective study. *Fertil Steril* 1995;64:963–968.

232. McKinney KA, Thompson W. A practical guide to prescribing hormone replacement therapy. *Drugs* 1998;56:49–57.

233. Goldstein SR. Selective estrogen receptor modulators: a new category of therapeutic agents for extending the health of post-menopausal women. *Am J Obstet Gynecol* 1998;179:1479–1484.

234. Murkies AL, Wilcox G, Davis SR. Phytoestrogens. *J Clin Endocrinol Metab* 1998;83:297–303.

235. Kessel B. Alternatives to estrogen for menopausal women. *Proc Soc Exp Biol Med* 1998;217:38–44.

236. Taffe AM, Cauffield J. "Natural" hormone replacement therapy and dietary supplements used in the treatment of menopausal symptoms. *Lippincotts Prim Care Pract* 1998;2:292–302.

237. Saunders PT. Oestrogen receptor beta (ER beta). *Rev Reprod* 1998;3:164–171.

238. Bryant HU, Dere WH. Selective estrogen receptor modulators: an alternative to hormone replacement therapy. *Proc Soc Exp Biol Med* 1998;217:45–52.

239. Delmas PD, Bjarnason NH, Mitlak BH, et al. The effects of raloxifene on bone mineral density, serum cholesterol concentrations, and uterine endometrium in postmenopausal women. *N Engl J Med* 1997;337:1641–1647.

240. Walsh BW, Kuller LH, Wild RA, et al. Effects of raloxifene on serum lipids and coagulation factors in healthy postmenopausal women. *JAMA* 1998;279:1445–1451.

241. Goldstein SR, Scheele WH, Symanowski SM, et al. Uterine safety considerations for selective estrogen receptor modulators. *Menopause* 1997;4:250.

242. Price KR, Fenwick GR. Naturally occurring oestrogens in foods: a review. *Food Addit Contam* 1985;12:73–106.

243. Soules MR, Bremner WJ. The menopause and climacteric: endocrinologic basis and associated symptomatology. *J Am Soc Geriatr* 1982;30:547–561.

14

BREAST FROM BIRTH THROUGH MENOPAUSE

LISA D. YEE

As organs of the integumentary system, the *mammary glands* are specialized sweat glands that develop under hormonal influences. In women, the breasts differentiate into milk-producing glands during pregnancy. This chapter addresses breast physiology throughout a woman's life, as well as some common disease processes of the breasts.

ANATOMY

Bounded posteriorly by the pectoralis major, serratus anterior, and external oblique muscles, the breast extends transversely from the sternum to the midaxillary line and vertically from the second to the sixth or seventh ribs. The axillary tail of Spence reaches laterally into the axilla. Fibrous bands known as Cooper's suspensory ligaments join the deep pectoral fascia, which covers the pectoralis major and serratus anterior muscles, to the superficial pectoral fascia encasing the breast (Fig. 14.1).

The *breast* is composed of skin, glandular epithelial tissue, and adipose and fibrous connective tissue. The glandular tissue of the breast consists of 15 to 20 lobes radially arranged around the nipple. Each lobe is drained at the nipple by a collecting duct, with convergence of some of these main ducts, so roughly only 5 to 10 are present at the nipple. The collecting duct undergoes sequential branching to the terminal ductal lobular units. No anastomoses exist between ducts. Terminal ductal lobular units are composed of lobules feeding into intralobular terminal ducts, which, in turn, lead into extralobular ducts. Lobules are groupings of tubulosaccular or spheric alveoli emptying into a common duct. Twenty to 40 lobules comprise a lobe. Connective tissue surrounds the alveoli, lobules, and lobes.

Collecting ducts end as papillae on the nipple. The nipple and surrounding areola are covered with pigmented epithelium, with underlying circular and radial muscle fibers. Sebaceous glands of Montgomery are located at the areola, secreting a protective lipidlike substance. Areolar glands are rudimentary milk glands that enlarge during pregnancy. Lymphatic vessels from the breast drain primarily into the ipsilateral axillary lymph nodes, although some lymphatic drainage from the medial breast is to the ipsilateral internal mammary lymph node chain.

The arterial blood supply to the breast enters primarily from the superomedial or superolateral aspects and consists of branches of the internal mammary artery, lateral thoracic artery, and intercostal arteries. Branches from the thoracoacromial artery enter the deep aspect of the breast. The arterial network formed in the subcutaneous fat sends branches into the breast. Superficial and deep venous plexus drain into the internal thoracic, lateral thoracic, upper intercostal, and external jugular veins. Sensory nerves to the breast arise from branches of the lateral and anterior cutaneous branches of intercostal nerves two through six, as well as branches from the supraclavicular nerves.

EMBRYONIC DEVELOPMENT

During the fourth week of fetal development, the mammary ridges appear as bilateral epidermal thickenings between the axillary and inguinal areas. Most of the mammary ridge will ultimately regress, preserved only in the pectoral region. By the sixth week, the mammary glands appear as solid protrusions of epidermis into the underlying mesenchymal tissue. Secondary mammary buds sprout from these primary buds and lead to the formation of lactiferous ducts. From the mesenchyme, fat and fibrous tissues develop around the ducts. At later stages, a mammary pit is formed from depression of the epidermis at the origin of the gland, with nipple formation occurring perinatally as a result of mesenchymal proliferation under the areolar area.

Although absence of the nipple and breast is extremely rare, the presence of an extra breast or nipple occurs in about 1% of females (1). These congenital abnormalities represent errors in the development of the mammary ridge. Supernumerary nipples or breasts typically appear just below the normal gland; however, these extra structures can also be present in the axillary or inguinal areas. Supernumerary nipples are often mistaken for pigmented nevi. Lack of mesenchymal proliferation in the area of the mammary pit leads to an inverted nipple. The size of a woman's breasts

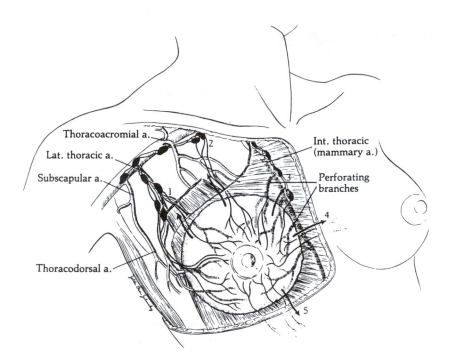

FIGURE 14.1. Arterial supply and lymphatic drainage of breast. *Black arrows* indicate direction of lymph flow: 1, pectoral and axillary nodes; 2, infraclavicular nodes; 3, internal thoracic chain of nodes; 4, flow to contralateral breast; 5, flow to anterior abdominal wall and diaphragm.

may differ slightly, but a large difference can also occur as a congenital abnormality, often in association with poorly developed pectoral muscles.

Highly regulated cell-cell and cell-matrix interactions occur during development of the duct system of the breast. Branching morphogenesis appears to require both stimulatory growth factors and local inhibitory signals to generate a discrete ductal and lobular network (2). Growth factors such as transforming growth factor-β, epidermal growth factor, and basic fibroblast growth factor have been implicated in mammary gland development (3–5). Differential expression of integrins, which are transmembrane glycoprotein receptors for extracellular matrix proteins, as well as adhesion molecules, may also occur during breast morphogenesis (6).

BIRTH THROUGH PUBERTY

At *birth,* the mammary gland is composed of simple branched ducts, with epithelium that is responsive to hormonal stimulation. Enlarged mammary glands and nipple secretions may occur in newborn infants, as a result of maternal hormones received through the placental circulation. Further development of the main lactiferous ducts of the infant breast occurs with the hormonal changes at puberty. Interactions between the mammary epithelium and mesenchymal tissues such as the mammary fat pad are also vital to breast morphogenesis and development (7,8). An increase in the fat and connective tissue of the breasts occurs at *puberty.*

Female sexual development begins with breast budding

(thelarche), followed by pubic hair growth (adrenarche), and then onset of menstruation (menarche). Puberty is induced by the hypothalamic gonadotropin-releasing hormones. Follicle-stimulating hormone released by cells of the anterior pituitary gland leads to maturation of the primordial ovarian follicles into graafian follicles. β-Estradiol and other estrogens secreted by these follicles stimulate growth of the main lactiferous ducts and formation of lobules and alveoli. Increased stromal and adipose tissue also appears. On full maturation of the ovarian follicle 1 to 2 years after menarche, ovulation occurs, and progesterone is released by the corpus luteum. Development of the ductal system, with growth of ducts, lobules, and alveoli, requires both progesterone and estrogen. Elongation and branching of the ducts occurs; lobules form from the continued branching of the ducts (9). Further differentiation of the lobules occurs with pregnancy and lactation, with lobules acquiring greater numbers of alveoli.

Breast development in the absence of hair growth suggests exogenous estrogen exposure, possibly through estrogen-containing creams or medications. Estrogen-producing ovarian tumors can also induce premature thelarche. Idiopathic premature thelarche can also occur.

MENSTRUAL CYCLE CHANGES

Histologic changes in the glandular and stromal tissue of the breast occur in accordance with hormonal changes during the *menstrual cycle* (10,11). The proliferative phase breast is characterized by small lobules with condensed stromal tissue. During the follicular phase of the menstrual cycle,

TABLE 14.1. MENSTRUAL CYCLE CHANGES

Follicular Phase	Luteal Phase
Endocrine changes	Endocrine changes
LH rises and peaks midcycle at ovulation	LH decreases after the midcycle peak
FSH decreases with a small rise midcycle	FSH decreases after the midcycle peak, rises at the end
Estrogen rises and peaks just before ovulation	Estrogen peaks midphase, declines by the end
Progesterone rises at midcycle	Progesterone increases, declines by the end
Histologic changes in the breast	Histologic changes in the breast
Epithelial proliferation	Secretory changes
Ductal epithelial sprouting	Ductal dilatation

FSH, follicle-stimulating hormone; LH, luteinizing hormone.

the ovarian graafian follicles secrete increased amounts of estrogen, leading to the proliferation of breast ductal epithelium. Ovulation occurs at the time of maximal estrogen production, followed by the luteal phase, with a rise in progesterone levels. The midluteal phase is notable for ductal dilatation and secretory differentiation of the epithelial cells in the alveoli. Proliferation appears to peak in the luteal phase, with the simultaneous peak of progesterone and estrogen (12,13). In the secretory phase, the lobules are enlarged, with vacuolization of the myoepithelial cells and apocrine secretion from the alveolar cells. The stroma is loose and edematous. Sex steroid hormone levels drop at the time of menstruation, with resulting regression of the secretory epithelium and stromal edema (Table 14.1).

Mastalgia may occur in the luteal phase, and it typically decreases on completion of the menses. Breast enlargement from proliferative changes and edema occurs at this point in the menstrual cycle, and the pain is likely related to the resulting increased tissue pressure (14, 15).

PREGNANCY

Regulated by luteal and placental estrogen and progesterone, prolactin, placental lactogen, and chorionic gonadotropin, the breast undergoes major proliferative changes during *pregnancy*. New ducts and acini are formed. Proliferation continues throughout the pregnancy, with mitotic activity at its peak in the first trimester (16). During weeks 3 to 4, ductular sprouting and branching and lobular formation occur in response to estrogen stimulation. By weeks 5 to 8, the breasts are markedly enlarged, with prominent superficial veins. Increased progesterone levels during the second trimester induce the formation of lobules. Prolactin steadily increases during pregnancy and stimulates epithelial proliferation. In the second trimester, prolactin stimulates the secretion of colostrum into the alveoli. Human placental lactogen is secreted by the placenta and may have a lactogenic effect in addition to prolactin. At this point, engorgement of the aloveoli with colostrum, myoepithelial cell

hypertrophy, and increased adipose and connective tissue account for progressive breast enlargement. Although the alveoli are usually composed of two cell layers, during the second trimester of pregnancy, the alveoli evolve into monolayer units of colostrum-producing cells. Progesterone exerts an inhibitory effect on complete milk production and prevents stimulation of alveolar cells by prolactin.

LACTATION

The rapid drop in progesterone at parturition leads to lactogenesis. *Lactation* is then maintained through the action of prolactin. Parturition and suckling stimulate the release of oxytocin from the posterior pituitary. Oxytocin then triggers the contraction of myoepithelial cells surrounding the alveoli engorged with milk and leads to the transit of milk through the ductal system to the nipple. Acute increases in prolactin occur with suckling, with resulting increased milk production. Cessation of nursing leads to regression of most of the proliferative changes, with resorption of milk.

Milky discharge can persist into the postlactation period for several years. *Galactorrhea* can occur in premenopausal women who have had children regardless of breast-feeding history. Hypothyroidism in adolescents and hyperthyroidism in women can produce abnormal lactation. Rarely, a pituitary adenoma produces excess prolactin and resulting galactorrhea. Certain medications, such as phenothiazines, metoclopramide, oral contraceptives, reserpine, tricyclic antidepressants, and methyldopa, may also cause hyperprolactinemia. In women with bilateral galactorrhea occurring more than 2 years after lactation, prolactin and thyroid hormone levels should be checked.

FIBROCYSTIC CHANGES

Fibrocystic changes present clinically as breast lumpiness or nodularity, often with tenderness and pain unrelated to the menstrual cycle. Histologically, fibrocystic changes encompass different forms of hyperplasia, with benign proliferation of glandular epithelium and stromal tissue. Formation of microcysts and gross cysts results from ductal hyperplasia and dilatation. Some common findings include ductal epithelial hyperplasia, duct papillomatosis, apocrine metaplasia, and adenosis. The incidence of fibrocystic changes increases with age, and the condition affects 50% of women 40 to 55 years old. Resolution occurs with menopause, however.

Fibrocystic changes are likely related to the hormonal influences of estrogen and progesterone and represent a physiologic response of the breast tissue rather than a true disease entity. An imbalance in the relative levels of estrogen, which stimulates duct epithelial growth, and progesterone, which regulates alveolar growth, may lead to the changes. Alterations in the hormonal responsiveness of the breast to these hormones, as mediated by such hormones as prolactin or other growth factors, may also be involved.

Consumption of caffeine and other methylxanthines may contribute to mastalgia and fibrocystic changes (17–19). A role for altered lipid metabolism is supported by the alleviation of symptoms with evening primrose oil (20). Use of the synthetic androgen danazol leads to decreased estrogen production and improvement in breast pain (21); however, side effects including menstrual irregularity, virilization, and hepatic dysfunction may prove limiting.

Macrocysts result from duct hyperplasia and dilatation and predominantly occur in women aged 40 to 55 years (22). Although these lesions often present as palpable, tender breast masses, gross cysts can also appear as asymptomatic nodules noted on mammography and ultrasound examinations. Fine-needle aspiration of cysts typically yields yellow, green, or brown fluid. Bloody cyst fluid suggests an intracystic or cystic neoplasm and requires excisional biopsy for further evaluation. Surgical excision should be performed for a persistent palpable mass or for a cyst recurring after multiple aspirations (23). Whereas intervention is not needed for asymptomatic simple cysts detected by ultrasound, complex cystic structures merit excision. Cytologic examination of cyst fluid is not generally useful.

Proliferative changes without atypia are associated with only a slightly increased risk of developing breast cancer, with a relative risk of 1.5 to 1. Atypical ductal and lobular hyperplasia confers a moderately increased risk of 5-fold, with a greater 11-fold increased risk noted in women with both atypical hyperplasia and a family history of breast cancer (24). Women with biopsies demonstrating proliferative changes with atypia require close surveillance and may be candidates for chemopreventive measures (25,26).

Lobular neoplasia, also known as lobular carcinoma *in situ,* refers to a proliferation of cells in the terminal ducts of the lobules, such that the ducts become distended and the lumen is effaced (27). Lobular neoplasia is a histologic marker for an increased risk of developing breast cancer, but it is not a malignant lesion, as erroneously implied by the term lobular carcinoma in situ. There is a continuum of changes from lobular hyperplasia to atypical lobular hyperplasia to lobular neoplasia. Lobular neoplasia often exists in a setting of proliferative cystic disease (28). The risk of developing breast cancer ranges from 17.1% to 32%, with involvement of either breast regardless of the site of the lobular neoplasia (29). A clinically silent lesion, lobular neoplasia presents as an incidental finding in biopsies obtained for other reasons. One often notes a long interval between the initial biopsy and the identification of cancer, which can be of any type. The amount of lobular neoplasia present in the breast does not appear to correlate with a more rapid or likely progression to cancer (30). Rather, the presence of lobular neoplasia signifies a malignant predisposition of the breast parenchyma, which likely requires certain hormonal, chemical, cellular, or other cues for progression to carcinoma. Although bilateral prophylactic mastectomies can be considered as a treatment option, close surveillance with regular breast examination and mammography is the recommended course of action (31). Additional treatment options await further advances in chemoprevention.

NIPPLE DISCHARGE

Nipple discharge that is serous, brown, gray, or green may be associated with fibrocystic changes. Whereas discharge after nipple stimulation is of little consequence, spontaneous, unilateral nipple discharge suggests underlying breast disease and necessitates evaluation and treatment. Bloody nipple discharge requires terminal duct excision for a pathologic diagnosis. Intraductal papillomas are the most common cause of bloody nipple discharge, but bloody fluid can also signify underlying breast cancer. Clear, serous drainage is infrequently associated with breast cancer, and excisional biopsy of the affected duct or ducts is also indicated in this instance. Ductograms and cytologic examination of the nipple discharge are not generally employed.

INFECTIONS

Infections of the breast most commonly affect lactating women. The symptoms of mastitis include breast tenderness, redness, induration, swelling, and increased warmth of the affected site, often with involvement of only one area of the breast. *Staphylococcus aureus* is the usual pathogen. Inflammatory breast cancer, which presents with erythema and edema of the breast skin, should also be included in the differential diagnosis.

Mastitis can progress to a *breast abscess,* which presents a painful, tender mass or area of swelling with associated erythema and induration. For deep abscesses, needle aspiration can be performed to confirm the diagnosis, before treatment with incision and drainage. Antistaphylococcal antibiotics are recommended for accompanying cellulitis and soft tissue inflammation. Nonpuerperal mastitis may result from mixed bacterial infections, however. A lactating breast should be mechanically emptied and temporarily withheld from further nursing. Additionally, the possibility of underlying cancer must be excluded with biopsy of the abscess cavity at the time of incision and drainage. Squamous metaplasia of the terminal ducts may result in periareolar abscesses, recurrent abscesses, or periareolar fistulas; these problems often necessitate treatment by terminal duct excision (32).

MENOPAUSE

Menopause results from the gradual and progressive loss of ovarian function. The end of follicular development leads to decreased production of estrogen and progesterone. In response to these hormonal changes, the epithelial and stromal tissues of the breast involute, with regression of the lobules. A gradual process, the atrophy and disappearance of lobules is usually incomplete, because lobular remnants may persist. Additionally, the extent and timing of menopausal involution are highly variable, such that atrophy may not occur or may involve only certain parts of the breast (33). Involution of the glandular tissue is accompanied by an increase in adipose tissue and hyalinization of the intervening connective tissue.

BENIGN TUMORS

Fibroadenomas, the most common benign tumor of the breast, most frequently occur in women less than 30 years of age. On palpation, these tumors are firm and movable, with smooth and well-demarcated borders. Fibroadenomas can be bilateral and multiple. These tumors may spontaneously regress as well as enlarge, and giant fibroadenomas can develop in adolescents. A fibroadenoma consists of a proliferative connective tissue stroma with atypical groupings of ducts. Such a tumor may, in fact, represent massive hypertrophy of a breast lobule, which presumably occurs in response to hormonal signals (33). Thus, normal variations in lobules may include simple hypertrophy, namely, an increase in the number and size of lobules with excessive elaboration of the surrounding connective tissue, as well as the fibroadenoma. Fibroadenomas are hormonally responsive, with lactational changes noted during pregnancy (34). A cellular fibroadenoma may be difficult to distinguish from a benign or malignant phyllodes tumor. Whether malignant transformation of a fibroadenoma can occur is unclear, but it is unlikely (27). Biopsy is required for diagnosis.

Other benign tumors of the breast include tubular adenomas, lactating adenomas, and lipomas. Intramammary lymph nodes can also occur, presenting as a mammographic finding rather than a palpable finding.

MALIGNANT DISEASE

One in 8 women will develop *breast cancer.* The risk increases with age, and about 78% of breast cancers occur in women older than 50 years. Women less than 35 years of age comprise 6% of breast cancer patients, with 0.3% in the age range of 20 to 29 years. Between 1973 and 1991, the incidence of invasive breast cancer rose by 24%, at an estimated annual average increase of 1.7% (35). Mortality rates, however, have remained stable, with increased 5-year survival rates from 72% in 1973 to 80.4% in 1986. Lower breast cancer survival rates are noted in the African-American population in comparison with white women: 65.8% versus 81.6% 5-year relative survival rates for all stages between 1983 to 1990. Moreover, younger women tend to fare worse than older women, with 5-year relative survival rates of 76.3% for ages less than 45 years and 82.7% for ages 65 to 74 years in the period 1986 to 1990.

As with other malignant diseases, breast cancers likely result from the clonal expansion of cells carrying multiple genetic mutations. Genetic susceptibility resulting from mutations in such inherited genes as *BRCA1, BRCA2,* and *p53* is significant, but it involves a minority of patients with breast cancer. Other contributory nongermline mutations represent acquired defects. Risk factors for developing breast cancer appear to relate to increased exposure to estrogen and progesterone, such as through early menarche, late menopause, postmenopausal obesity, alcohol consumption, and hormone replacement therapy (36). Environmental estrogen exposure may also represent an important risk factor (37).

Invasive Breast Cancer

Of invasive breast cancers, invasive ductal carcinoma is the most common histologic type. Invasive lobular carcinoma represents approximately 14% of all invasive breast cancers, with other less frequently noted types including the well-differentiated tubular, mucoid, and papillary carcinomas.

Staging for breast cancer is based on the TNM system, in which T refers to tumor size, N to axillary nodes, and M to metastasis (Table 14.2) (38). Although other tumor features such as estrogen and progesterone receptor status, S-phase fraction, nuclear or histologic grade, and *HER-2/neu* overexpression may have prognostic value, tumor size and lymph node involvement remain the strongest predictors of prognosis (39).

Surgical treatment of invasive breast cancer includes the options of mastectomy with axillary dissection or breast-conserving therapy with lumpectomy, axillary dissection, and breast irradiation. Clinical trials demonstrating the ef-

TABLE 14.2. STAGING OF BREAST CANCER[a]

TNM definitions
Primary tumor

Tx	Primary tumor cannot be assessed
T0	No evidence of primary tumor
Tis	Carcinoma *in situ*: intraductal carcinoma, lobular carcinoma *in situ*, or Paget's disease of the nipple with no tumor
T1	Tumor 2 cm or less in greatest dimension
T1a	0.5 cm or smaller
T1b	More than 0.5 cm, but not more than 1 cm in greatest dimension
T1c	More than 1 cm, but not more than 2 cm in greatest dimension
T2	Tumor more than 2 cm but not more than 5 cm in greatest dimension
T3	Tumor more than 5 cm in greatest dimension
T4	Tumor of any size with direct extension to chest wall or skin
T4a	Extension to chest wall
T4b	Edema (including peau d'orange), ulceration of the skin of the breast, or satellite skin nodules confined to the same breast
T4c	Both (T4a and T4b)
T4d	Inflammatory carcinoma (see definition in text)

Regional lymph node involvement
Clinical

Nx	Regional lymph nodes cannot be assessed (e.g., previously removed)
N0	No regional lymph node metastasis
N1	Metastasis to movable ipsilateral axillary node(s)
N2	Metastasis to ipsilateral axillary lymph node(s) fixed to one another or to other structures
N3	Metastasis to ipsilateral internal mammary lymph node(s)

Pathologic

pNx	Regional lymph node metastasis cannot be assessed
pN0	No regional lymph node metastasis
pN1	Metastasis to movable ipsilateral axillary node(s)
pN1a	Only micrometastasis (none larger than 0.2 cm)
pN1b	Metastasis to lymph node(s), any larger than 0.2 cm
pN1bi	Metastases in one to three lymph nodes, any more than 0.2 cm in greatest dimension
pN1bii	Metastases to four or more lymph nodes, any more than 0.2 cm and all less than 2 cm in greatest dimension
pN1biii	Extension of tumor beyond the capsule of a lymph node metastasis less than 2 cm in greatest dimension
pN1biv	Metastasis to a lymph node 2 cm or more in greatest dimension
pN2	Metastasis to ipsilateral axillary lymph nodes that are fixed to one another or to other structures
pN3	Metastasis to ipsilateral internal mammary lymph node(s)

Distant metastases

Mx	Presence of distant metastases cannot be assessed
M0	No distant metastasis
M1	Distant metastasis (including metastases to ipsilateral supraclavicular node(s)

Stage Grouping

Stage 0	Tis, N0, M0
Stage I	T1, N0, M0
Stage IIA	T0, N1, M0
	T1, N1,[b] M0
	T2, N0, M0
Stage IIB	T2, N1, M0
	T3, N0, M0
Stage IIIA	T0, N2, M0
	T1, N2, M0
	T2, N2, M0
	T3, N1, M0
	T3, N2, M0
Stage IIIB	T4, any N, M0
	Any T, N3, M0
Stage IV	Any T, any N, M1

[a]Definitions for classifying the primary tumor (T) are the same for clinical and pathologic classification. If the measurement is made by physical examination, the examiner should use T1, T2, or T3. If other measurements, such as mammographic or pathologic, are used, the examiner can use the subsets of T1.
[b]The prognosis of patients with N1a is similar to that of patients with pN0.
From Fleming ID, Cooper JS, Henson DE, et al. eds. *AJCC Cancer staging manual,* 5th ed. Philadelphia: Lippincott–Raven, 1997, with permission.

ficacy of less radical surgery led to the replacement of the radical mastectomy, which involves resection of the breast with underlying pectoralis major and minor muscles and an extensive axillary dissection, by the modified radical mastectomy. Modified radical mastectomy involves the removal of the entire breast as a total or simple mastectomy, along with the ipsilateral axillary contents. Breast reconstruction can be performed immediately or as a delayed procedure. Alternatively, removal of the tumor with negative tissue margins, axillary dissection, and whole-breast irradiation offers the same overall survival as a modified radical mastectomy in patients with stage I or II breast cancer, with tumors less than or equal to 4 cm (40). Risk factors for local recurrence include no breast irradiation, positive or close surgical margins, and extensive ductal carcinoma *in situ* (DCIS), which are associated with recurrence rates of 25% to 43%, 20% to 35%, and 20% to 25%, respectively (41).

Contraindications to breast conservation include prior breast irradiation, first- or second-trimester pregnancy, two or more gross tumors in separate breast quadrants, and diffuse indeterminate or suspicious appearing calcifications on mammography (42). A large tumor relative to breast size, tumor situated beneath the nipple, a history of connective tissue disease, and a large breast size are relative contraindications to lumpectomy or radiation.

The role of axillary dissection in the surgical treatment of breast cancer continues to evolve. Axillary dissection yields primarily diagnostic, rather than therapeutic, information. Knowledge of the nodal status guides decisions regarding adjuvant chemotherapy. Clinical examination is an inaccurate measure of axillary involvement, and therefore node dissection has been required for accurate staging. An adequate axillary dissection removes 10 or more lymph nodes in an *en bloc* fashion for histologic evaluation. For axillary adenopathy noted on clinical examination, complete axillary dissection is recommended. However, axillary dissection is not clearly therapeutic for patients without clinical evidence of axillary involvement. Additionally, tumor features such as estrogen receptor expression, lymphovascular invasion, and histologic differentiation influence decisions for adjuvant chemotherapy despite node-negative disease. Given the lack of therapeutic benefit, postoperative morbidity, and possible long-term complications of lymphedema associated with axillary dissection, other means of evaluating nodal status have been investigated. For example, sentinel node biopsy techniques aimed at identifying the first draining axillary lymph node offer a sensitive and accurate means of determining the presence of nodal disease (43–45).

Systemic adjuvant therapy has proven benefit for stage I and II disease. Although women with tumors less than or equal to 0.5 cm greatest diameter (T1a) and without lymph node involvement may derive little additional benefit from systemic therapy, adjuvant treatment can be considered for those with T1b, node-negative disease associated with unfavorable tumor features. For patients with tumors greater than 1 cm in diameter, systemic therapy with cytotoxic agents and/or the antiestrogen tamoxifen for estrogen receptor–positive tumors is warranted. Well-tested regimens include cyclophosphamide, methotrexate, and 5-fluorouracil (CMF), doxorubicin and cyclophosphamide (AC), and cyclophosphamide, doxorubicin, and 5-fluorouracil (CAF). Numerous prospective, randomized clinical studies of adjuvant therapies are in progress to address such issues as the role of taxanes, dose-density, high-dose chemotherapy and stem-cell rescue, and biologic therapies like trastuzumab, the recombinant human monoclonal antibody to Her2/neu protein.

Neoadjuvant chemotherapy is used for patients with locally advanced primary breast cancer, such as T3, T4 or N2, N3 breast cancers, followed by surgical resection, additional systemic therapy, and radiation treatments. *Inflammatory breast cancer* is defined by dermal lymphatic invasion, which leads to the characteristic erythema and edema of the breast skin known as *peau d'orange*. This special clinicopathologic entity is treated as other locally advanced breast cancers, with systemic chemotherapy as the first step in treatment. Preoperative chemotherapy is also under investigation for operable primary breast cancer (46).

Systemic therapy for metastatic breast cancer includes hormonal and cytotoxic agents. Hormonal therapy can be considered for patients with estrogen and progesterone receptor–positive tumors, metastases involving only bone or soft tissue, and limited, asymptomatic visceral disease. Tamoxifen is the hormonal agent of choice for patients previously untreated with this antiestrogen. However, prior tamoxifen therapy necessitates the use of second-line interventions such as progestin, aromatase inhibitors in postmenopausal women, androgens, and oophorectomy in premenopausal women. Patients with tumors negative for estrogen and progesterone receptors, symptomatic visceral metastases, and disease unresponsive to hormonal therapies require chemotherapy. Chemotherapy regimens are based on the history of prior drug treatment, but they generally entail doxorubicin-based combinations, taxines, or CMF.

Ductal Carcinoma *In Situ*

DCIS is a noninvasive breast cancer in which the malignant duct cells have not penetrated the basement membrane of the duct. Histologic types include solid, cribiform, papillary, and comedo-type DCIS, with the last representing a lesion with a greater tendency to invasion. DCIS can also be evaluated for low- to high-grade nuclear features. In certain instances, low-grade DCIS is difficult to distinguish from atypical ductal hyperplasia. Progression from atypical ductal hyperplasia to DCIS to invasive cancer may occur.

DCIS typically presents as an area of abnormal microcalcifications on a mammogram, less frequently first identified as a mass on clinical or radiologic examination. Clusters of granular or linear calcifications, occasionally in a linear, ductal pattern, are suggestive of DCIS. DCIS may diffusely involve the breast as either multifocal disease in a quadrant or multicentric disease distributed throughout the breast.

Treatment options include mastectomy or lumpectomy. Removal of the breast as a simple or total mastectomy is essentially curative. Although lymph nodes may be removed with the axillary tail of the breast, formal axillary dissection or sampling is not indicated for this noninvasive cancer. Breast reconstruction can be performed immediately at the time of the mastectomy or on a delayed basis. Certain patients can also be offered a breast-conserving procedure: wide excision of the cancer as a lumpectomy with negative tumor margins, coupled with postoperative radiation treatments to the entire breast (47–49). Disease amenable to breast conservation is localized and excised with tumor-free margins (50). Indications for consideration of mastectomy include large tumor size relative to the breast, multicentricity of disease, involved excision margins, and comedo-type histologic features (49,51). Although ipsilateral breast recurrence rates are generally less than 10% with wide local excision and breast irradiation, 50% of these lesions are invasive rather than *in situ* cancers. Thus, careful selection of patients with DCIS for breast-conserving therapy is essential, because invasive recurrence has potential for metastases and death.

Phyllodes Tumors

Phyllodes tumors are stromal neoplasms that can be either benign or malignant, with malignant potential judged by tumor size and margin characteristics, cellular atypia, and mitotic activity (52,53). Overgrowth of the stromal component appears to be associated with a poorer prognosis (54). Phyllodes tumors are typically benign in adolescence. Although both benign and malignant phyllodes tumors can recur locally, recurrence of a malignant phyllodes tumor indicates aggressive disease with systemic spread. Treatment options include wide excision with normal tissue margins or simple mastectomy for large tumors that cannot be locally excised (55–57). Because malignant phyllodes tumors disseminate hematogenously and rarely to the axillary lymph nodes, axillary dissections are performed only in instances of clinically apparent nodal involvement.

Other Malignant Breast Diseases

Rarely, lymphomas and sarcomas of the breast occur, each constituting less than 1% of malignant breast neoplasms. Primary lymphoma of the breast carries a poor prognosis. Treatment consists of systemic chemotherapy, with local control achieved by means of limited surgery and radiation therapy (58,59). Total mastectomy is generally the recommended treatment for sarcomas of the breast, with postoperative radiation added for close margins (60).

10 KEY POINTS

1. The breast is a specialized gland of the integumentary system.

2. In the embryo, the mammary gland evolves from the mesenchymal tissue in the mammary ridge.

3. The breast develops in response to hormonal changes throughout life.

4. Pregnancy is associated with hormonally induced proliferative and secretory changes, with lactation induced by hormonal and physical stimuli after parturition.

5. Menopause is associated with involution of the breast glandular tissue.

6. Fibrocystic changes most likely represent the physiologic response of breast tissue to hormones such as estrogen and progesterone.

7. Benign breast tumors such as fibroadenomas occur most commonly in younger women and may represent a localized proliferative response.

8. Risk factors for breast cancer are multifactorial, including genetic susceptibility and estrogen exposure.

9. Lobular neoplasia (or lobular carcinoma *in situ*) and atypical ductal hyperplasia are nonmalignant, histologic findings associated with an increased risk for breast cancer.

10. Breast cancer treatment involves a multimodality approach, often with the administration of radiation therapy and systemic treatment in addition to surgery.

REFERENCES

1. Moore KL. *The developing human,* 3rd ed. Philadelphia: WB Saunders, 1982:438.
2. Moffat DF, Going JJ. Three dimensional anatomy of complete duct systems in human breast: pathological and developmental implications. *J Clin Pathol* 1996;49:48–52.
3. Silberstein GB, Daniel CW. Reversible inhibition of mammary gland growth by transforming growth factor-beta. *Science* 1987;237:291–293.
4. Coleman S, Silberstein GB, Daniel CW. Ductal morphogenesis in the mouse mammary gland: evidence supporting a role for epidermal growth factor. *Dev Biol* 1988;127:304–315.
5. Gomm JJ, Smith J, Ryall GK, et al. Localization of basic fibroblast growth factor and transforming growth factor beta 1 in the human mammary gland. *Cancer Res* 1991;51:4685–4692.
6. Anbazhagan R, Bartek J, Stamp G, et al. Expression of integrin subunits in the human infant breast correlates with morphogenesis and differentiation. *J Pathol* 1995;176:227–232.
7. Anbazhagan R, Bartek J, Monaghan P, et al. Growth and development of the human infant breast. *Am J Anat* 1991;192:407–417.
8. Knight CH, Peaker M. Development of the mammary gland. *J Reprod Fertil* 1982;65:521–536.
9. Monaghan P, Perusinghe NP, Cowen P, et al. Peripubertal human breast development. *Anat Rec* 1990;226:501–508.
10. Longacre TA, Bartow SA. A correlative morphologic study of human breast and endometrium in the menstrual cycle. *Am J Surg Pathol* 1986;10:382–393.
11. Vogel PM, Georgiade NG, Fetter BF, et al. The correlation of

histologic changes in the human breast with the menstrual cycle. *Am J Pathol* 1981;104:23–34.

12. Going JJ, Anderson TJ, Battersby S, et al. Proliferative and secretory activity in human breast during natural and artificial menstrual cycles. *Am J Pathol* 1988;130:193–204.

13. Ferguson DJ, Anderson TJ. Morphological evaluation of cell turnover in relation to the menstrual cycle in the "resting" human breast. *Br J Cancer* 1981;44:177–181.

14. Milligan D, Drife JO, Short RV. Changes in breast volume during normal menstrual cycle and after oral contraceptives. *BMJ* 1975;4:494–496.

15. Fowler PA, Casey CE, Cameron GG, et al. Cyclic changes in composition and volume of the breast during the menstrual cycle, measured by magnetic resonance imaging. *Br J Obstet Gynaecol* 1990;97:595–602.

16. Ferguson DJ, Anderson TJ. A morphological study of the changes which occur during pregnancy in the human breast. *Virchows Arch A Pathol Anat Histopathol* 1983;401:163–175.

17. Minton JP, Abou-Issa H, Reiches N, et al. Clinical and biochemical studies on methylxanthine-related fibrocystic breast disease. *Surgery* 1981;90:299–304.

18. Boyle CA, Berkowitz GS, LiVolsi VA, et al. Caffeine consumption and fibrocystic breast disease: a case control epidemiologic study. *J Natl Cancer Inst* 1984;72:1015–1019.

19. La Vecchia C, Franceschi S, Parazzini F, et al. Benign breast disease and consumption of beverages containing methylxanthines. *J Natl Cancer Inst* 1985;74:995–1000.

20. Gateley CA, Mansel RE. Management of the painful and nodular breast. *Br Med Bull* 1991;47:284–294.

21. Gateley CA, Miers M, Mansel RE, et al. Drug treatments for mastalgia: 17 years experience in the Cadiff Mastalgia Clinic. *J R Soc Med* 1992;85:12–15.

22. Hughes LE, Bundred NJ. Breast macrocysts. *World J Surg* 1989;13:711–714.

23. Leis HP Jr. Gross breast cysts: significance and management. *Contemp Surg* 1991;39:13–20.

24. Dupont WD, Page DL. Risk factors for breast cancer in women with proliferative breast disease. *N Engl J Med* 1985;312:146–151.

25. Noguchi M, Rose DP, Miyazaki I. Breast cancer chemoprevention: clinical trials and research. *Oncology* 1996;53:175–181.

26. Powles TJ. Status of antiestrogen breast cancer prevention trials. *Oncology* 1998;12[Suppl 5]:28–31.

27. Carter D. *Interpretation of breast biopsies.* New York: Raven, 1984:76–94.

28. Rosen PP, Lieberman PH, Braun DW Jr, et al. Lobular carcinoma *in situ* of the breast. *Am J Surg Pathol* 1978;2:225–251.

29. Page DL, Kidd TE Jr, Dupont WD, et al. Lobular neoplasia of the breast: higher risk for subsequent invasive cancer predicted by more extensive disease. *Hum Pathol* 1991;22:1232–1239.

30. Haagensen CD, Lane N, Lattes R, et al. Lobular neoplasia (so-called lobular carcinoma *in situ*) of the breast. *Cancer* 1978;42:737–769.

31. Andersen JA. Lobular carcinoma *in situ* of the breast: an approach to rational treatment. *Cancer* 1977;39:2597–2602.

32. Meguid MM, Oler A, Numann PJ, et al. Pathogenesis-based treatment of recurring subareolar breast abscesses. *Surgery* 1995;118:775–782.

33. Parks AG. The micro-anatomy of the breast. *Ann R Coll Surg Engl* 1959;25:235–251.

34. O'hara MF, Page DL. Adenomas of the breast and ectopic breast under lactational influences. *Hum Pathol* 1985;16:707–712.

35. Ries LAG, Miller BA, Hankey BF, et al. *SEER Cancer Statistics Review, 1973–1991: tables and graphs.* NIH publication No. 94-2789. Bethesda, MD: National Institutes of Health, 1994.

36. King SE, Schottenfeld D. The "epidemic" of breast cancer in the U.S.: determining the factors. *Oncology* 1996;10:453–462.

37. Arnold SF, Klotz DM, Collins BM, et al. Synergistic activation of estrogen receptor with combinations of environmental chemicals. *Science* 1996;272:1489–1492.

38. Fleming ID, Cooper JS, Henson DE, et al., eds. *AJCC cancer staging manual,* 5th ed. Philadelphia: Lippincott–Raven, 1997.

39. Mansour EG, Ravdin PM, Dressler L. Prognostic factors in early breast carcinoma. *Cancer* 1994;74:381–400.

40. Fisher B, Redmond C, Poisson R, et al. Eight-year results of a randomized clinical trial comparing total mastectomy and lumpectomy with or without irradiation in the treatment of breast cancer. *N Engl J Med* 1989;320:822–828.

41. Balch CM, Singletary SE, Bland KI. Clinical decision-making in early breast cancer. *Ann Surg* 1993;93:207–225.

42. Winchester DP, Cox JD. Standards for breast-conservation treatment. *CA Cancer J Clin* 1992;42:134–162.

43. Giuliano AE, Kirgan DM, Guenther JM, et al. Lymphatic mapping and sentinel lymphadenectomy for breast cancer. *Ann Surg* 1994;220:391–401.

44. Krag DN, Weaver DL, Alex JC, et al. Surgical resection and radiolocalization of the sentinel lymph node in breast cancer using a gamma probe. *Surg Oncol* 1993;2:335–340.

45. Turner RR, Ollila DW, Krasne DL, et al. Histopathologic validation of the sentinel lymph node hypothesis for breast carcinoma. *Ann Surg* 1997;226:271–278.

46. Fisher B, Brown A, Mamounas E, et al. Effect of preoperative chemotherapy on local-regional disease in women with operable breast cancer: findings from National Surgical Adjuvant Breast and Bowel Project B-18. *J Clin Oncol* 1997;15:2483–2493.

47. Fisher E, Sass R, Fisher B, et al. Pathologic findings from the National Surgical Adjuvant Breast Project (Protocol 6) I. Intraductal carcinoma (DCIS). *Cancer* 1986;57:197–208.

48. Fisher B, Costantino J, Redmond C, et al. Lumpectomy compared with lumpectomy and radiation therapy for the treatment of intraductal breast cancer. *N Engl J Med* 1993;328:1581–1586.

49. Frykberg ER, Bland KI. Overview of the biology and management of ductal carcinoma *in situ* of the breast. *Cancer* 1994;74:350–361.

50. Faverly DRG, Burgers L, Bult P, et al. Three dimensional imaging of mammary ductal carcinoma *in situ*: clinical implications. *Semin Diagn Pathol* 1994;11:193–198.

51. Silverstein MJ, Waisman JR, Gamagami P, et al. Intraductal carcinoma of the breast (208 cases): clinical factors influencing treatment choice. *Cancer* 1990;66:102–108.

52. Norris HJ, Taylor HB. Relationship of histologic features to behavior of cystosarcoma phyllodes. *Cancer* 1967;2:2090–2099.

53. Pietruszka M, Barnes L. Cystosarcoma phyllodes: a clinicopathologic analysis of 42 cases. *Cancer* 1978;41:1974–1983.

54. Ward RM, Evans HL. Cystosarcoma phyllodes: a clinicopathologic study of 26 cases. *Cancer* 1986;58:2282–2289.

55. Chua CL, Thomas A, Ng BK. Cystosarcoma phyllodes: a review of surgical options. *Surgery* 1989;105:141–147.

56. Salvadori B, Cusumano F, Del Bo R, et al. Surgical treatment of phyllodes tumors of the breast. *Cancer* 1989;63:2532–2536.

57. Palmer ML, De Risi DC, Pelikan A, et al. Treatment options and recurrence potential for cystosarcoma phyllodes. *Surgery* 1990;170:193–196.

58. El-Ghazawy IMH, Singletary SE. Surgical management of primary lymphoma of the breast. *Ann Surg* 1991;214:724–726.

59. Abbondanzo SL, Seidman JD, Lefkowitz M, et al. Primary diffuse large B-cell lymphoma of the breast: a clinicopathologic study of 31 cases. *Pathol Res Pract* 1996;192:37–43.

60. Callery CD, Rosen PP, Kinne DW. Sarcoma of the breast: a study of 32 patients with reappraisal of classification and therapy. *Ann Surg* 1985;201:527–532.

15

UTERUS FROM BIRTH TO MATURITY

WILLIAM A. BENNETT
BRYAN D. COWAN

NORMAL EMBRYONIC DEVELOPMENT

Three important embryologic tissues are responsible for the development of the normal female genital system (1). The ovarian oocytes are derived from yolk sac derivatives, the lower genital tract evolves from the urogenital tissues, and the fallopian tubes, uterus, and upper vagina are derived from the müllerian ductal system. Furthermore, a close relationship exists between the developing urinary and the müllerian systems. In this chapter, we focus on the development of only the müllerian structures.

Development of the urinary and reproductive structures occurs in consecutive waves, commencing high in the abdominal cavity and progressing downward toward the pelvis. Table 15.1 shows the interrelationships and sequence of events in the development of the urinary system, müllerian system, and external genitalia.

The first developing structure of the genitourinary system is the *pronephros,* or primitive kidney. This structure appears bilaterally early in the third or fourth week after conception. It is first seen high in the abdominal cavity and subsequently develops toward the pelvis. During its development, a bulge forms in the mesoderm, and multiple tubules form. The multiple tubules of the pronephric ducts continue to develop, but the pronephros is nonfunctional in the human.

At 4 to 9 weeks of gestation, the *mesonephros* forms as a lateral ductal element in the area of the pronephros and replaces the pronephros completely. It is composed of tubules in the mesodermal core (Fig. 15.1). The mesonephros probably has some rudimentary function, but like the pronephros, it degenerates and is ultimately replaced by the definitive kidney, the *metanephros.* An important mesonephric duct (wolffian) develops in the mesonephros and persists in the adult male as the vas deferens. However, it degenerates in the female at week 10.

The metanephric tubules arise in the same manner as the pronephric and mesonephric tubules. These tubular structures appear in the sixth or seventh week, but they form low in the abdominal cavity. The metanephric ducts are outpouches from the lower end of the mesonephric duct and are called *ureteric buds.* These grow upward (not downward like other formations) and eventually form the definitive *ureters.*

The direct ancestor of the uterus is the *paramesonephric (müllerian) duct.* In the sixth week, a new duct is formed on the lateral mesonephros (Fig. 15.1). At first, this is a blind cord that grows toward the pelvis. Subsequently, it becomes canalized and is recognized as the paramesonephric duct. Both the wolffian and müllerian ducts originate before sexual differentiation is grossly observable and therefore are common to both sexes. In the male, however, the müllerian duct degenerates in the tenth week because of the Sertoli cell product, müllerian-inhibitory substance. In the female, the müllerian duct persists to give rise to the uterus.

The right and left müllerian ducts grow toward each other, cross the wolffian duct, and meet in the midline during the ninth week (Fig. 15.2). The müllerian epithelium throughout the genital tract becomes columnar, thus constituting the characteristic mucosa in the fallopian tubes, the endometrium, the cervix, and the upper portion of the vagina. The cloacal endoderm of the lower portion of the vagina becomes stratified squamous epithelium. The urogenital sinus (junction between columnar and squamous epithelium) represents the separation portion of these two migrating tissue types.

MÜLLERIAN ANOMALIES

Müllerian anomalies occur as a consequence of failed formation (agenesis) or fusion defects of the embryonic müllerian duct (2). Fusion defects are further classified into vertical fusion defects, which affect attachment to the urogenital septum, and lateral fusion defects, which affect lateral exposition of the müllerian ducts. Müllerian anomalies are often classified into six subgroups that are listed in Table 15.2.

The most important clinical presentations of müllerian abnormalities are the obstructive anomalous fusion or canalization events. These include imperforate hymen, transverse vaginal septum, longitudinal vaginal septum, and vaginal atresia.

Imperforate hymen is reported to occur in 1 in 5,000 live female births (3). The diagnosis is usually made before adolescence, but it may present in the peripubertal time with a complaint of amenorrhea and cyclic pelvic pain.

TABLE 15.1. DEVELOPMENT OF THE UTERUS

Age	Glands	Urinary Tract	Ducts	External Genitalia
3–4 wk	Primordial germ cells	Pronephros (nonfunctional) tubules and ducts	Pronephric	
4–9 wk		Mesonephros or wolffian body (temporary function) tubules and ducts	Mesonephric	Cloaca
5th wk	Urogenital ridge			
6th wk	Indifferent gonad: germinal and core epithelium	Mesonephros or kidney (permanent) tubules and ducts	Paramesonephric or müllerian	Cloaca subdivides genital tubercle
7th wk	Male type cords			Anal and urethral membranes rupture
8th wk	Testis and ovary			Urethral and labioscrotal folds, phalus and glans
9th wk			Müllerian ducts fuse at tubercle	Sex distinguishable
10th wk			Müllerian ducts degenerate	
11th wk			Seminal vesicles, epididymis vas deferens	
12th wk	Ovary descent complete		Walls form	
5 mo	Testes at inguinal ring		Sinus epithelium grows in vaginal cleft	
8 mo	Testis descent complete		Rapid uterine growth	

Transverse vaginal septum is uncommon. It is estimated to occur in 1 in 75,000 live female births (3). There is marked variation in the clinical presentation varying from a small annular ring to a completely obstructed vaginal membrane. Clinical symptoms depend on both the width and the location of the anomaly. With complete obstruction, amenorrhea and cyclic pain are the common presenting symptoms. In addition to a transverse orientation, vaginal septa are known to occur in the longitudinal axis.

Longitudinal septa most often occur in association with abnormalities of uterine fusion, but they may develop as a single isolated occurrence. Longitudinal septa are usually asymptomatic, but they may prolong the menses.

Vaginal atresia occurs when the inferior portion of the vagina is replaced by fibrous tissue, and it should be differentiated from müllerian agenesis (4). In vaginal atresia, the inferior portions of the vagina fail to form, but the müllerian structures (cervix and uterus) are intact. The classic presentation is primary amenorrhea and a midline pelvic mass. Müllerian agenesis, often called *Rokitansky-Küstner-Hauser syndrome,* is defined as congenital absence or hypoplasia of the uterine corpus, cervix, and proximal portion of the vagina. The incidence ranges between 1 in 4,000 and 1 in 10,000 female births. Ovaries and fallopian tubes are usually absent. Complete vaginal agenesis occurs in 75% of affected patients, but approximately 25% of patients have a short vaginal pouch.

Other anomalies associated with *incomplete müllerian fusion* include uterus didelphys with unilateral imperforate vaginal septum. This condition represents a syndrome associated with ipsilateral renal agenesis and is the most common fusion defect that presents with symptoms during adolescence. *Nonobstructing fusion defects* include uterus unicornis, bicornuate uterus, and uterus didelphys, and are infrequently diagnosed during the adolescent years because

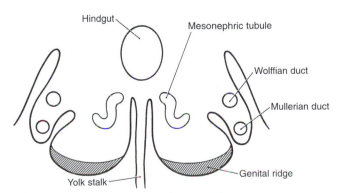

FIGURE 15.1. Transverse section through a 7-week embryo showing thickening of the celomic epithelium, genital ridge, and mesonephric duct.

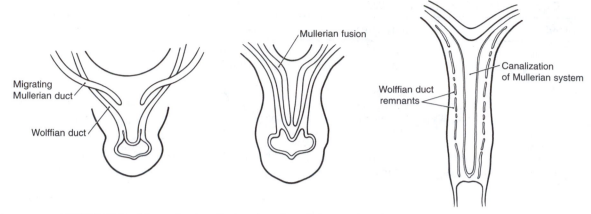

FIGURE 15.2. Schematic of müllerian ductal medial migration, fusion, and canalization during normal female embryonic development.

they are nonobstructive and are not associated with a symptom. These conditions can be associated with obstetric consequences (embryonic loss, preterm labor, or malpresentation), but they are not usually associated with pain or abnormal bleeding.

Obstetric Consequences of Uterovaginal Anomalies

Uterovaginal anomalies may affect fertility and obstetric outcome. Women with müllerian agenesis and complete cervical atresia require hysterectomy and are functionally sterile. In contrast, imperforate hymen should be treated with hymenotomy, because these women do not generally have impaired fertility or obstetric sequelae. Subfertility is documented in patients with transverse vaginal septum, partial cervical atresia, and vaginal atresia.

In contrast to vaginal and cervical abnormalities, the

obstetric sequelae of uterine abnormalities are variable. For example, women with an asymmetric uterus and a rudimentary uterine horn generally have unimpaired fertility. Similarly, women with uterus didelphys or a unilateral uterine horn do not have reduced fertility, but they are affected by preterm labor and malpresentation. In contrast, women with a uterine septum can suffer from repeated early pregnancy loss.

STRUCTURE AND FUNCTION OF UTERINE MUSCLE

Organization of the uterus is similar to other organs that contain smooth muscle (gastrointestinal tract, airways, and blood vessels). The myometrium consists predominantly of muscle cells, but it also contains fibroblast, blood and lymphatic vessels, immune cells, and connective tissue. The uterine wall is composed of at least three distinct layers. The innermost is the *endometrium,* the middle section is the *myometrium,* and the outer layer represents the serosa or *peritoneum.*

The myometrium is composed of two distinct sections. The first is the outer longitudinal muscle layer, and the second is an inner circular structure. The outer longitudinal muscle layer consists of a network of smooth muscles that are generally oriented in the long axis of the uterus. The bundles interconnect and form a network over the surface of the uterus. Each bundle is composed of cells arranged in the long axis of the bundle. In the human, cells of the inner layer are arranged concentrically around the longitudinal axis of the uterus, and bundle formation is diffuse.

The functional unit of myometrium is the smooth muscle cell. These are long spindle-shaped and irregular cells. The size of smooth muscle cells varies considerably among different species, and the human uterus is composed of

TABLE 15.2. CLASSIFICATION OF MÜLLERIAN ANOMALIES

1. Agenesis
   Vagina
   Cervix
   Uterus
   Fallopian tube
   Any combination
2. Unicornuate uterus
   Connected, nonconnected, with or without cavity
3. Uterus didelphys
4. Bicornuate uterus
   Complete
   Partial
   Arcuate
5. Septate uterus
   Partial
   Complete
6. Exposed to diethylstilbestrol

larger cells than most species. The plasma membrane of the smooth muscle cell is the barrier that divides muscle cells from their extracellular environment. The membrane is responsible for the excitable properties of the muscle cells. Uterine smooth muscle cells have an extensive cytoplasmic reticulum system, consisting of a network of tubules within the cytoplasm. The major functions of the cytoplasmic reticulum are those of storage of calcium, and a site for protein synthesis. Calcium is generally stored in the smooth endoplasmic reticulum, whereas protein synthesis occurs in the rough endoplasmic reticulum.

Contraction of smooth muscle cells occurs through the interaction of myosin and actin filaments (as in skeletal muscle). The ability of myometrial cells to contract depends on the distribution of specialized ions that cross the plasma membranes. Sodium and calcium ions are higher outside the cell than inside, whereas potassium ions are higher within the cells. These ionic gradients allow muscle cells to respond when small changes in membrane permeability result in significant movements of ions down their electrochemical gradients. The resting membrane potential of the smooth muscle envelope is about -45 mV. Contraction and relaxation of the myometrium result from the cyclic depolarization and repolarization of the muscle cell (*action potentials.*) As in other excitable tissues, the action potential in smooth muscle results from voltage changes of membrane ionic permeabilities. The *depolarization* phase results from an inward current carried principally by calcium ions. The outward current (*repolarization*) is carried by potassium ions. The contractile event of uterine smooth muscle is initiated by a rise of intracellular free ionized calcium to a concentration of approximately 10^{-5} M. The noncontractile calcium concentration is approximately 10^{-7} M.

Effective myometrial contractility during parturition requires propagation and coordination of myometrial contractility. Propagation and coordination of myometrial contractility are sustained by gap junctions between myometrial cells (6). *Gap junctions* are channels that connect the interiors of two cells. The channels are composed of proteins (*connexins*) that span the plasma membrane to form pores. In all species studied, the onset and progression of labor contractile activity are associated with large numbers of gap junctions between myometrial cells. Gap junctions are present in greater numbers in tissues from women who are undergoing cesarean section and who are in labor, compared with women who are not in labor. Estrogens promote the synthesis of gap junctions in the myometrium, antiestrogen compounds prevent gap junction formation, progesterone inhibits development of gap junction formation at term, antiprogesterone compounds induce preterm development of gap junctions, and prostaglandins have a complex (agonistic-antagonistic) role in gap junction formation (5).

Nitric oxide is a ubiquitous effector of various smooth muscle functions (7). L-Arginine is the immediate substrate for nitrate oxide, and when it is added to strips of myometrium, a substantial relaxation of contractile activity occurs. Inhibitors of nitric oxide syntase (L-NAME) reverse the effect. Curiously, the administration of L-NAME in pregnant rats induced severe hypertension with growth retardation and proteinuria. This finding suggests that inhibition of nitric oxide synthesis is involved in the generation of preeclampsia.

PARTURITION

A new model of *parturition* has evolved that involves two processes. The first is a preparatory process controlled by genomic mechanisms that increase or decrease specific molecules that regulate the force and frequency of phasic contractions of labor. These genomic factors include increases in gap junctions, ion pumps, systems for myofilament interaction, and receptors for oxytocin. Once the preparatory process is complete, successful labor may succeed without any additional assistance. Oxytocin and other agonists (prostaglandins, endothelins) may stimulate contractility to accelerate labor. Thus, these agents may be facilitory rather than essential.

LEIOMYOMAS

Leiomyomas are benign tumors of muscle cell origin. They are commonly referred to as *fibroids* or *fibromyomas.* Leiomyomas are the most frequent pelvic tumor, and their peak incidence occurs in the fifth decade. These tumors are discovered in one of four white women and in one of two black women.

All myomas develop from the myometrium and begin as an intramural structure. As they grow, they remain attached to the myometrium with a pedicel of varying width and thickness. Myomas are classified into subgroups by the relative anatomic relation to the position in the layer of the uterus (Fig. 15.3) (8). The three most common sites of myomas are intramural, subserosa, and submucosal. Special classifications exist for broad ligament myomas and parasitic myomas.

The direction of growth determines whether the myoma is located just below the endometrium (submucosal) or just beneath the serosa (subserosal). Only 5% to 10% of myomas are submucosal, and these lesions are usually the most troublesome clinically.

The origin of uterine leiomyomas is incompletely understood. Each tumor is "monoclonal," resulting from an original single muscle cell. All the cells have an identical electrophoretic expression of glucose-6 phosphate dehydrogenase, a unique mitochondrial marker (9).

The stimulus for growth is unclear. Myomas are rare before menarche, and most diminish in size after menopause

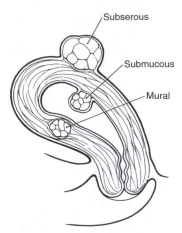

FIGURE 15.3. Anatomic sites of uterine leiomyomas.

or oophorectomy. Estrogen receptor content is higher in myomas than in the surrounding myometrium (10,11), but the dependence of these tumors on estrogen stimulation is unclear. Growth hormone may also regulate leiomyomatous growth.

Symptoms related to uterine fibroids include abnormal uterine bleeding, pelvic pain, pelvic pressure, infertility, and pregnancy complications. The types of symptoms expressed by the patient depend on the size and location of the fibroids. Submucosal fibroids typically generate abnormal bleeding patterns, whereas large mural fibroids can produce pelvic heaviness or pain.

The incidence of malignant degeneration is low and is estimated to be approximately 0.3% to 0.7% (12). Growth of a uterine myoma after menopause is a disturbing symptom, and rapid growth of a uterine fibroid represents the classic symptom of leiomyosarcoma.

Most uterine myomas may be diagnosed by pelvic examination. Transvaginal sonography substantially improves diagnostic accuracy, and sonohysterography has been introduced as a tool that can delineate the proximity of a uterine fibroid to the mucosa (13). Computed tomography and magnetic resonance imaging studies of uterine myomas are rarely indicated. In general, the three treatment options for uterine fibromas are observation, hysterectomy, and myomectomy. Observation should be planned for women who have no symptoms and uterine fibroids smaller than 5.0 cm. Hysterectomy should be recommended for patients who have completed childbearing and who have symptomatic uterine fibroids. Myomectomy should be offered to patients who desire pregnancy and who have symptomatic uterine fibroids or uterine fibroids 6.0 cm or larger. Submucosal fibroids have been successfully treated with hysteroscopic resection without the need for laparotomy (14).

Treatment with a gonadotropin-releasing hormone (GnRH) agonist has been used to shrink fibroids (15). This therapy reduces fibroids to approximately 45% of their pretreatment volume within 12 weeks. This therapy can be an effective adjunct for presurgical size reduction, to control bleeding and symptoms, and as a mechanism to treat patients with complex medical problems. Unfortunately, discontinuation of the therapy usually results in return of the uterine size and symptoms. Thus, GnRH agonist therapy is generally regarded as an adjunct before surgical treatment and not a primary treatment.

Finally, a novel treatment of selective embolization of uterine fibroids has been described (16). This has been accomplished in only a few patients, and longer longitudinal studies will be required to determine its efficacy.

It is difficult to estimate reproductive outcome after myomectomy (17). Estimates range from 10% to 45% of clinical pregnancies. As a confounding complication, approximately 25% of all patients who have had a previous myomectomy will subsequently undergo hysterectomy.

ENDOMETRIAL RESPONSES TO OVARIAN HORMONES

Ovarian Menstrual Cycle and the Endometrium

In primates, the ovarian steroid hormones estrogen (estradiol; E_2) and progesterone prepare the endometrium for implantation and pregnancy (18). This involves changes in endometrial morphology and function that are initiated during the normal menstrual cycle.

The patterns of steroid and gonadotropic hormone levels during the normal menstrual cycle are depicted in Fig. 15.4. At the end of the cycle, circulating levels of E_2 and progesterone are low. This triggers the release of high-amplitude pulses of GnRH from the hypothalamus and results in a premenstrual rise in follicle-stimulating hormone (FSH) from the anterior pituitary. This release of FSH leads to the recruitment of a cohort of ovarian follicles.

Hormonal changes during the follicular phase of the cycle are accompanied by obligatory changes in the morphology of the endometrium (Fig. 15.5A–D). In fact, we argue that a major purpose of ovarian hormone production is to develop and mature the endometrium, the site for subsequent embryonic attachment. During the 24 hours preceding the initiation of menstrual flow, the coiling of the uterine arteries and arterioles leads to ischemia and necrosis of the upper portion of the endometrium. The coiled arteries then relax, and the endometrium detaches from the basal layer, a process leading to the release of endometrial tissue and shedding of the vessels. Endometrial regeneration begins within 48 hours after the initiation of menses. This repair process continues until day 5 to 6 of the cycle and results in the replacement of the epithelium in the spongiosum portion of the endometrium. In response to increasing levels of E_2, there is proliferation of uterine

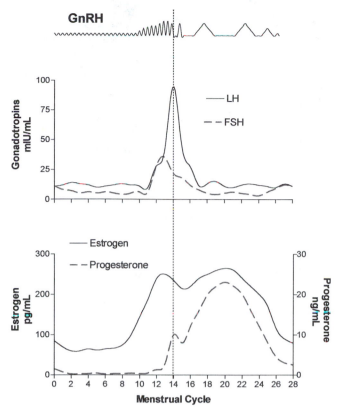

FIGURE 15.4. Changes in ovarian steroid and gonadotropic hormones during the human menstrual cycle.

on about day 10, leading to increased lengthening and coiling of the endometrial glands. During the late proliferative to early luteal stages of the cycle (days 11 through 14), the rapidly growing glands become tortuous.

Around the midpoint of the human menstrual cycle, surges of luteinizing hormone (LH) and FSH are initiated by positive E_2 feedback. This midcycle gonadotropin surge triggers follicle rupture, oocyte release, luteinization of granulosa cells, and the synthesis of progesterone.

The second phase of the menstrual cycle is the luteal phase, which usually lasts for 12 to 14 days in the absence of pregnancy. In the 72 hours after ovulation, LH-transformed (luteinized) granulosa and theca cells form a structure called the corpus luteum. High levels of progesterone production by the corpus luteum are maintained for 11 to 14 days after ovulation. The functional life span of the corpus luteum depends on high-amplitude, low-frequency pulses of LH produced by the anterior pituitary. Unless luteotropic support in the form of embryonic human chorionic gonadotropin (hCG) from the embryo rescues the corpus luteum, regression occurs. A rapid decline in peripheral levels of progesterone and E_2 occurs during the last 4 to 5 days of the human menstrual cycle. This removes the anterior pituitary from negative feedback inhibition and results in increased production and secretion of FSH in response to GnRH from the hypothalamus.

The endometrium is a complex uterine tissue that lies nearest to the lumen and is composed of epithelial, stroma, vascular, and lymphoid tissues. The commonly cited description of endometrial maturity relates the morphology to the proliferative phase, then ascribes secretory changes beginning on day 16 (19). More recently, the histologic features of the endometrium have been correlated with the

epithelial and stromal cells. During the early follicular phase, the endometrial glands are straight, short, and narrow, and the stroma is compact. Later in the follicular phase (days 8 to 10), the glands become elongated and mitotically active. Glycogen production and storage by the glands are initiated

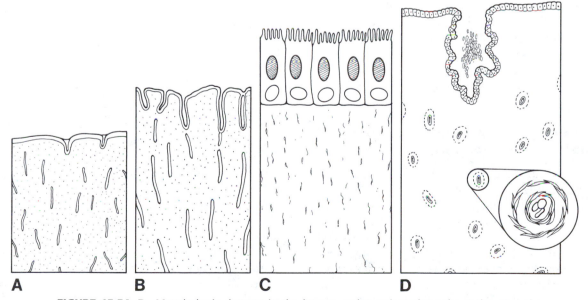

FIGURE 15.5A–D. Morphologic changes in the human endometrium throughout the normal menstrual cycle.

peak of LH secretion (LH + 0), and the secretory changes are then described relative to that reference point (20). The early secretory phase of the endometrium is characterized by tortuous glands and a pseudostratified epithelium. In response to progesterone, glycogen accumulates in the basal portion of the glandular epithelium. By day 17, the nuclei of the glandular epithelial cells appear as an orderly row, with homogenous cytoplasm above and vacuoles underneath. During the midluteal phase, these vacuoles spread, and the nuclei are basally located. The stroma becomes highly edematous, and "predecidual" cells appear as small cells with dense nuclei and filamentous cytoplasm. Stromal cells then surround the spiral arteries (day 23), underlie the surface epithelium (day 25), and, by day 27, the upper endometrial stoma appears as a sheet of well-developed cells resembling decidua. By the end of nonfertile cycles, the endometrial glands are dilated, and the glandular epithelium displays a saw-toothed appearance with shrunken nuclei and rough apical surfaces.

Endometrial Hormone Receptors

The changes in endometrial morphology and function during the human menstrual cycle are related to both the circulating levels of *progesterone* and E_2 and the distribution of specific receptors for these hormones in the endometrium.

Progesterone receptors and *estrogen receptors* are present in the uterine stroma and epithelium (Fig. 15.6) during the proliferative phase of the cycle (21). These receptors increase in concentration during the time-dependent progression of the follicular phase. However, after ovulation (luteal phase), only stromal progesterone receptors persist through the cycle. Therefore, epithelial responses to progesterone in the secretory phase are likely mediated by stromal-derived paracrine factors. These observations underscore the concept that local paracrine communication occurs within the uterus when steroid-dependent changes of the endometrium. Increasingly, evidence emphasizes the role of cytokines and growth factors in these processes.

Cytokine Regulation of Endometrial Morphology and Function

In addition to direct effects through specific receptors on endometrial stromal and epithelial cells, ovarian hormones also act indirectly through induction of *growth factors* and *cytokines*. These substances act both as autocrine intermediaries in the uterine response to steroids and as paracrine regulators of invading trophoblast during pregnancy. Endometrial growth factors most often associated with steroid-induced changes in the endometrium are members of the *insulin-like growth factor* (IGF) and *epidermal growth factor* (EGF) families (Table 15.3).

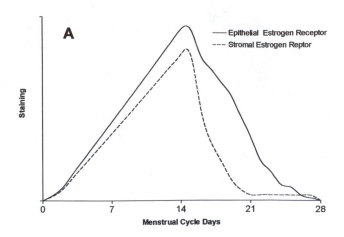

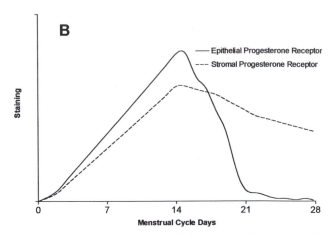

FIGURE 15.6. Levels of endometrial receptors for estrogen **(A)** and progesterone **(B)** during the menstrual cycle.

IGF-I and IGF-II stimulate mitosis in a wide variety of tissues (22). In the rat uterus, E_2 enhances IGF production (23). Endometrial IGF-II transcripts are most abundant during the early follicular phase, whereas IGF-I is expressed later during this period (24). Receptors for IGF-I and IGF-II have been identified in the rat (25) and human (26) endometrium during the proliferative and secretory phases. Expression of IGF-I receptors in the rat uterus is upregulated by E_2 (27). In the human, levels of IGF-I peptide and receptor levels vary with the menstrual cycle, with the highest expression in the late proliferative and early secretory phases (24).

The study of IGF is complicated by the presence of IGF-binding proteins (IGFBP). These binding proteins may function in the transport of IGFs and modulate IGF action within target tissues (28). IGFBP-1 has been isolated to the epithelial and stromal cells of the mouse uterus and may be regulated by E_2 (29). In humans, the uterine glandular epithelium expresses messenger RNA (mRNA) for IGFBPs during the secretory phase. Three different IGF-binding

TABLE 15.3. GROWTH FACTORS AND CYTOKINES EXPRESSED BY THE HUMAN ENDOMETRIUM

Growth Factor	Cellular Source	Proposed Function
Colony-stimulating factor 1 (CSF-1)	Epithelial cells	Macrophage recruitment Trophoblast differentiation Implantation Embryo development
Epidermal growth factor (EGF)	Epithelial cells	Cell proliferation Myometrial contraction Preembryo development
Insulin-like growth factor I and II (IGF-I and IGF-II)	Stromal cells	Cell proliferation
Interleukin-1 (IL-1)	Macrophages Endothelial cells Epithelial cells	Implantation Menstruation
Interleukin-6 (IL-6)	Endothelial cells	Angiogenesis
Leukocyte inhibitory factor (LIF)	Epithelial cells	Implantation
Transforming growth factor-α (TGF-α)	Epithelial cells Decidua	Cell proliferation Preembryo development
Tumor necrosis factor-α (TNF-α)	Epithelium Decidua	Cell proliferation Preembryo development
Granulocyte colony-stimulating factor (G-CSF)	Epithelium Decidua	Trophoblast differentiation Embryo development
Interferon- (IFN-γ)	T cells	Inhibition of cell proliferation

From Bulmer JN. Cellular constituents of human endometrium in the menstrual cycle and early pregnancy. In: Bronson RA, Alexander NJ, Anderson DJ, et al, eds. *Reproductive immunology.* Cambridge, Blackwell Science, Inc., 1996, with permission.

proteins have been identified (IGFBP-1, IGFPB-2, and IGFPB-3).

Estrogens induce EGF mRNA and peptide in the rat uterus (30), and EGF exerts estrogenic effects on uterine growth (31). Expression of EGF is higher in stromal cells than in glandular epithelial cells during the follicular phase, and stromal levels increase during the luteal phase (32).

An increasing body of evidence suggests that other endometrial growth factors are important in endometrial development as well (Table 15.3). Receptors for the ligands are known to exist, and genomic knockout models have demonstrated failed reproduction for many of these factors. Several macrophage-associated cytokines are produced by the uterine epithelium including colony-stimulating factor 1 (CSF-1), granulocyte-macrophage colony-stimulating factor (GM-CSF), and tumor necrosis factor-α (TNF-α) (34–37). The administration of CSF-1 into the rodent uterine lumen results in macrophage recruitment to the luminal-epithelial border (38). After mating in mice, GM-CSF production by the uterine epithelium increases dramatically (39). GM-CSF acts both as a mitogen and chemoattractant for monocytes and macrophages (40). Macrophages are thought to play a role in the phagocytosis of dead sperm and response to foreign antigens at mating and to produce cytokines during implantation that potentiate blastocyst development and uterine receptivity (41).

Immune Cells and the Human Endometrium

In addition to stromal and epithelial cells, the human uterus contains immunocompetent cells that vary in number throughout the menstrual cycle. The main leukocytic populations of the human endometrium include T cells, large granular lymphocytes, and macrophages (Table 15.4). Levels of T cells and macrophages remain relatively constant during the cycle, but large granular lymphocytes populate the stroma in the late secretory phase.

During the menstrual cycle, most *T cells* express the CD8 surface antigen (T-suppressor/T-cytotoxic), and the ratio of these cells to CD4$^+$ T cells (T-helper/T-inducer) is approximately 4:1. During the secretory phase (days 18 to 21), the proportion of T CD8$^+$ cells increases (42). In the preimplantation phase, 22% of stromal leukocytes are CD8$^+$ cells, and only 8% are CD4$^+$.

Large granular lymphocytes are present in pregnant and nonpregnant endometrium. They are present in low levels in the proliferative endometrium, but they increase during the late secretory phase and early pregnancy. After the first trimester of pregnancy, the numbers of large granular lymphocytes decline, and they are virtually absent at term.

Macrophages (CD14$^+$, CD68$^+$ cells) account for 33% of the bone marrow–derived cells in the endometrium

TABLE 15.4. LEUKOCYTIC CELL POPULATIONS OF THE HUMAN ENDOMETRIUM

Cell Type	Proposed functions	
	In vitro	*In vivo*
CD^{3+} cell	—	Immunosuppression
	—	Cytokine production
	—	Intrauterine host defense
CD14$^+$ macrophage	Phagocytosis	Intrauterine immune responses
	Immunosuppression	Immunosuppression
	Cytokine production	Control placental growth
	Antigen presentation	Removal of tissue debris
CD56$^+$ large granular lymphocyte	NK cell activity	Limit trophoblast invasion
	Lysis trophoblast	Immunosuppression
	Immunosuppression	Control placental growth
	Cytokine production	Intrauterine host defense

From Bulmer JN. Cellular constituents of human endometrium in the menstrual cycle and early pregnancy. In: Bronson RA, Alexander NJ, Anderson DJ, et al, eds. *Reproductive immunology*. Cambridge, Massachusetts, Blackwell Science, Inc., 1996, with permission.

during the proliferative phase. They increase slightly during the secretory phase from day 24 to day 27. Endometrial macrophages are localized around endometrial glands, are dispersed throughout the stroma, and occasionally are isolated between surface and glandular epithelial cells.

ENDOMETRIAL RESPONSES TO PREGNANCY

Decidualization of the Human Endometrium

Around the time of implantation, the uterus undergoes complex changes, collectively referred to as *decidualization*. In some species (i.e., rodents), these changes occur only in response to the implanting embryo or other artificial stimuli. In humans, however, they are spontaneously initiated during the nonpregnant menstrual cycle. Decidualization is most pronounced in species in which implantation involves trophoblast penetration of the uterine epithelium and subsequent stromal invasion. During the luteal phase, under the influence of progesterone, uterine epithelium apocrine secretion increases, and stromal cells surrounding the spiral arteries and arterioles differentiate. Both epithelial and stromal events demonstrate cycle-specific changes during decidualization.

In nonfertile cycles, the decidua functionalis (compacta and spongiosa) is shed during menstruation. If pregnancy occurs, these alterations are sustained and extended. The presence of the early embryo distinguishes three regions of the endometrium: (a) decidua basalis, which underlies the embryo; (b) decidua capsularis, which lies over the embryo; and (c) decidua parietalis, which covers the remainder of the uterine surface. The glandular epithelium within the decidua spongiosa exhibits secretory activity during the first trimester.

Functional Aspects of Decidualization

Secretion of the epithelial glands is maximal during the initial 2 to 3 weeks of pregnancy. Secretions of these glands may provide nutrients for the early embryo before the establishment of maternal blood supply to the intervillous space. In species with a superficial implantation (i.e., horses, sheep, pigs), the embryo undergoes extensive modification in the uterine cavity, and uterine secretions probably are critical for the nourishing of the early conceptus. However, in humans, uterine luminal fluid apparently has limited nutritional value.

Nonetheless, large quantities of glycogen, mucins, and glycoproteins are secreted by the epithelium into the luminal glands (Table 15.5). These secretions may influence trophoblast behavior in the first 14 days of gestation. The most abundant glandular protein is PP14, which is a major epithelial protein product (43). PP14 is a member of the β-lactoglobin family and may modulate uterine natural killer (NK) cell activity. MUC-I is another intensively studied epithelial secretory product (44). It displays high polymorphism characterized by unique glycosylation at specific periods of the menstrual cycle. Two specific sialoglycan epitopes are added to the molecule only in the luteal phase. Although the function of MUC-I is unknown, investigators have suggested that the unique cell surface glycans participate in implantation or become involved with vascular endothelial injury.

During decidualization, stromal cells are transformed from small, densely packed cells to large polygonal cells with an open vesicular nucleus. Despite these dramatic morphologic changes, the role that decidual cells play in early pregnancy is only partially understood. Decidualized stromal cells secrete a variety of growth factors including fibroblast growth factor, EGF, and various extracellular matrix proteins including laminin, collagen, and fibronectin. Major soluble proteins produced by stromal cells are

TABLE 15.5. SIGNALING MOLECULES OF THE ENDOMETRIUM

Growth Factors	Epithelial Factors	Stromal Factors
Epidermal growth factor (EGF)	Polymorphic epithelial mucin (MUC-1)	Soluble-IGF binding protein (placental protein 12) + Prolactin
Insulin-like growth factor 1 (IGF-I)	Progestin-associated epithelial protein (placental protein 14)	Extracellular matrix
Colony-stimulating factor 1 (CSF-I)	Heat shock protein 27 (HSP-27)	
Platelet-derived growth factor (PDGF)	Uteroglobin Other species	Laminin
Fibroblast growth factor (FGF)		Collagen Fibronectin
Transforming growth factor α (TGF-α)	Uteroferrin: porcine	
Transforming growth factor β (TGF-β)	Lactotransferrin: mouse Uteroglobin: rabbit	
Interleukin 6 (IL-6)	Protease inhibitors	

IGF, insulin-like growth factor
EGF, epidermal growth factor
CSF, colony stimulating factor
PDGF, platelet-derived growth factor
FGF, fibroblast growth factor
TGF, transforming growth factor
IL, interleukin
MUC, polymorphic epithelial mucin
PAEP, progestin-associated epithelial protein
HSP, heat shock protein
PP, placental protein
IGFBP, IGF, binding protein

prolactin (PRL), IGFBP-1, and renin. IGFBP-1 is secreted in response to progesterone, EGF, and insulin. IGFBP-1 binds to cell surfaces and causes increased cell migration in cells expressing α_5/β_1 integrins, an adhesion molecule found on trophoblast. This interaction may regulate the coordinated migration of trophoblast through the endometrial stroma.

PRL secretion increases in response to steroid hormones, EGF, fibroblast growth factor, IGF-I, and the free α subunit of hCG and is inhibited by interleukin-1 (IL-1), TNF-α, and endothelin (45,46). High levels of PRL are found in the decidua and amniotic cavity during pregnancy. This hormone may mediate amniotic fluid volume and ion content. PRL may also influence the recruitment and retention of decidual NK cells and macrophages. It has been described as an evolutionary precursor of IL-2, and evidence suggests that PRL is required for lymphocyte proliferation in response to IL-2 (47).

Uterine Epithelium and Implantation

Implantation is initiated when the embryonic trophectoderm adheres to the uterine luminal epithelium. Because epithelial surfaces normally do not adhere to other cells, the uterine epithelium is thought to become receptive to the blastocyst under the influence of steroid hormones.

This period of uterine receptivity has been described as the "window of implantation" and is well characterized in laboratory animals. However, human blastocysts readily adhere to adult tissues that do not undergo cyclic changes resulting from steroid hormones. In contrast, the human uterus is normally "hostile" to implantation and only becomes receptive under the correct hormonal stimulus. The specific modifications in the human uterine luminal epithelium that make it receptive to blastocyst adhesion and implantation remain undefined.

The uterine epithelial surface expresses a complex pattern of carbohydrate antigens, some of which may be relevant to implantation (48–51). The Lea antigen is of particular interest because it is localized to the apical surface of luminal epithelium. In addition, the production of lactoaminoglycans, such as keratan sulfate, is increased in glands during the secretory phase (49). MUC-1 is a lactoaminoglucan localized at the apical cell surface of glandular and luminal epithelium (51). The production of MUC-1 increases dramatically during the secretory phase and, as mentioned before, undergoes specific modifications to two sialoglycan epitopes during the luteal phase of the cycle. The functional significance of these hormonally regulated glycans is unknown, although in mice they promote blastocyst attachment and spreading *in vitro* (50).

The implanting human embryo encounters various matrices, substrates, and basement membranes (Table 15.6). These include fibronectin, laminin, heparan, entactin, tenascin, and chondroitin sulfate. These may all assist in guiding and anchoring the embryo as it penetrates the luminal epithelium and moves through the uterine stroma. These matrix substrates also interact with adhesion molecules that are expressed on cell surfaces. Fibronectin is thought to guide and respond to various differentiating and migrating cell types including trophoblast. These migrating cell types attach to fibronectin through integrins. During the late secretory phase, the extracellular matrix is substantially remodeled. In the proliferative and early secretory phase, the extracellular matrix is dense and fibrillar. However, the late secretory stroma extracellular matrix is radically remodeled to contain little fibrillar collagen. Large amounts of laminin are also expressed in the uterus, together with collagen IV, and in blood vessel and gland basement membranes during the midsecretory phase. Laminin may facilitate embryonic adhesion because collagen type III levels decline and type IV collagen levels increase in the decidua. A dense network of collagen IV, fibronectin, and fibrillar proteins declines late in the secretory phases. These changes may facilitate trophoblast invasion and water access (edema).

Integrins function as important mediators of cell-cell interactions (Table 15.6). Their expression by uterine epithelial cells varies with the stage of the menstrual cycle (52). The α_1 and α_4 integrin subunits are expressed by the glandular epithelium during the luteal phase. The β_3 subunit appears on day 19, and its expression then continues into pregnancy. These three subunits are coexpressed from days 20 through 24, concurrent with implantation. In addition, β_1 and α_v integrin subunits are expressed constitutively by uterine epithelial cells. Heterodimers expressed during the time of implantation include α_v/β_3, α_v/β_1, α_4/β_1, and α_1/β_1 (53). The integrin dimer α_v/β_3 engages in cell-cell interactions, and the α_4/β_1 binds the extracellular matrix components

TABLE 15.6. ADHESION MOLECULE EXPRESSION BY THE HUMAN ENDOMETRIUM THAT MAY MEDIATE BLASTOCYST ATTACHMENT AND IMPLANTATION

Adhesion Molecule	Ligand	Integrin Subunits
LFA-1	ICAM −1, −2, −3	α L/B-2
VLA-1	Laminin	α 1/B-1
VLA-2	Collagen	α 2/B-1
VLA-3	Fibronectin, collagen, laminin	α 3/B-1
VLA-4	VCAM-1, fibronectin	α 5/B-1
VLA-6	Laminin	α 6/B-1
Vitronectin receptor	Vitronectin	α v/B-1
LFA-2	LFA-3	

From Bulmer JN. Cellular constituents of human endometrium in the menstrual cycle and early pregnancy. In: Bronson RA, Alexander NJ, Anderson DJ, et al. eds. *Reproductive immunology.* Cambridge, Blackwell Science, Inc., 1996, with permission.

fibronectin and VCAM, a member of the immunoglobulin G superfamily. The roles of α_v/β_1 and α_4/β_1 are less well understood.

Cytokines may also contribute to the receptivity of the endometrium to the implanting blastocyst. In humans, uterine macrophages, epithelial cells, and trophoblasts produce IL-1, and the IL-1 receptor is maximally expressed in the endometrium (54) during the luteal phase. The administration of IL-1 receptor antagonists during the preimplantation period in mice blocks blastocyst implantation.

The uterine growth factor leukemia-inhibitory factor (LIF) may also play a critical role in the implantation process. Peaks of LIF secretion have been noted in the mouse uterus at the time of estrus (55) and just before implantation (56). Blastocysts fail to implant in LIF-deficient females, whereas the transfer of these embryos to normal females results in successful pregnancy (57). This finding suggests that LIF expression by the endometrium is a prerequisite for implantation during murine pregnancy. The human uterus also displays a similar pattern of LIF expression throughout the menstrual cycle and during early pregnancy.

Vascular Development and Implantation

A key event in implantation is the establishment of adequate blood supply to tissues of the maternal-fetal interface. In primates, this is achieved on the maternal side by growth of the spiral arteries, which provide adequate blood supply to the placenta. Although ovarian steroids play key roles in many implantation processes, the principal agents regulating angiogenesis are local peptides that may be modulated by ovarian steroids.

Growth factors such as EGF, transforming growth factor-α, and CSF-1 have wide-ranging effects on ectodermal, mesenchymal, and endothelial cells. These factors may provide generalized support for angiogenesis during implantation. An important growth factor that has been associated with angiogenesis in the human endometrium is vascular endothelial growth factor (VEGF). VEGF is a dimeric peptide with four splice variants encoding proteins of 189, 165, 145, and 121 amino acids (58). In the proliferative phase of the menstrual cycle, VEGF is expressed in epithelial and stromal portions of the endometrium. During the luteal phase, VEGF expression is limited to the epithelial glands with the stroma lacking VEGF mRNA. The intensity of mRNA expression declines as pregnancy continues. VEGF is highly expressed at the placental site, and the cell types involved have been identified as macrophages. This finding raises the possibility that maternal macrophages, attracted to the implanting placenta, may facilitate the development of maternal blood vessels supplying the placenta. In terminal villi, VEGF expression has been localized to Hofbauer's cells, which are fetal macrophages. Therefore, macrophage-derived VEGF may regulate angiogenesis in both compartments of the maternal-fetal interface.

Summary

Endometrial responses to pregnancy are mediated systemically through the production of ovarian steroid hormones and locally by the release of cytokines and growth factors. This communication between mother and fetus regulates such critical processes as decidualization, implantation, and the establishment of adequate blood supply to the fetoplacental unit.

ONCOGENIC ENDOMETRIAL AND MYOMETRIAL RESPONSES OF THE MATURE UTERUS

Epidemiology

Uterine cancer is the fourth leading cancer in women, with an estimated 36,000 cases and 6,000 deaths in the United States during 1996 (59). Most (approximately 97%) of all uterine cancers arise from the glands of the endometrium and thus are termed *endometrial adenocarcinomas.* The average age of diagnosis for endometrial cancer is 63 years, and 75% of women with endometrial carcinoma are postmenopausal (60).

Most risk factors associated with endometrial cancer involve exposure to excessive E_2 (Table 15.7). Prolonged elevations in E_2 result in a continued stimulation of the endometrium and subsequent endometrial hyperplasia. Women with endometrial hyperplasia in the absence of atypical cytologic findings have a low risk of developing endometrial cancer, whereas those with atypical cytologic results display a 23% increased risk of developing uterine cancer over the next 10 years (61).

Obesity is cited as a risk factor for endometrial cancer, thought to be related to increased endogenous estrogen produced by adipose tissue. The increased risk is positively correlated with the degree of obesity; women who are more

TABLE 15.7. ESTIMATED RISK RATIOS (RATIO OF RISK TO WOMEN WITH FACTORS/RISK OF WOMEN WITHOUT FACTORS) FOR FACTORS RELATED TO ENDOMETRIAL CANCER

Risk Factor	Risk Ratio
Sequential oral contraceptives	7.0
Unopposed estrogen therapy	6.0
Overweight	
20–50 lb	3.0
> 50 lb	10.0
No children (versus 1 child)	2.0
No children (versus 5 children)	5.0
Late menopause (> 52 yr versus > 49 yr)	2.4
Diabetes mellitus	2.7
Tamoxifen therapy	2.2
Combination oral contraceptives	0.5

From Rose PG. Endometrial carcinoma. *N Engl J Med* 1996;335:640–648, with permission.

than 50 lb overweight have a 10-fold increased rate of endometrial cancer. Early menarche and late menopause are also risk factors for endometrial carcinoma, because of a longer exposure of the endometrium to estrogen. Ovarian tumors in women often produce estrogen, and 5% to 15% of these patients have concurrent endometrial carcinomas.

One-fourth of women with endometrial cancer are premenopausal, and 5% are less than 40 years old. Most of these women are either obese or have conditions that result in high levels of unopposed E_2 (e.g., polycystic ovarian disease). Pregnancy provides a degree of protection from endometrial cancer by interrupting the continued stimulation of the endometrium by E_2. For this reason, nulliparity is viewed as a risk factor for endometrial carcinoma.

Unopposed E_2 treatments were used for the treatment of menopausal symptoms in the late 1960s and early 1970s. This type of therapy has since been associated with an eightfold increase in the incidence of endometrial cancer. The replacement of continuous E_2 therapy with combined estrogen-progesterone preparations resulted in a decrease in endometrial cancer rates in the United States. However, a worldwide increase in the incidence of endometrial cancer has been reported, even in countries where unopposed E_2 is not prescribed. This worldwide increase has been attributed to increased longevity.

Tamoxifen, a synthetic estrogen antagonist used in the treatment of breast cancer, has also been shown to be a risk factor for endometrial cancer. In contrast to its effects on malignant breast tumors, tamoxifen has estrogenic effects on the endometrium and increases the risk of endometrial carcinoma. Patients who have received tamoxifen therapy are reported to have approximately a 2.2-fold increase in endometrial cancer (62).

Current oral contraceptives are predominantly progesterone, and this hormone has been shown to provide protection from endometrial cancer. Women who take combined oral contraceptives for at least 12 months lower their risk of developing endometrial cancer by about half, and protection persists for at least 10 years after the oral contraceptive is discontinued.

Endometrial Changes

Hyperplasia

Nonmalignant changes in endometrial histology are classified as cystic hyperplasia, adenomatous hyperplasia, and atypical adenomatous hyperplasia. *Hyperplasia* refers to an inactive or nonproliferating endometrium with cystic changes. These changes are prominent in endometrium of some postmenopausal women. A preferred designation of these changes is *inactive endometrium with cystic changes.* No premalignant potential exists in patients with inactive endometrium and only cystic changes. The term adenomatous hyperplasia emphasizes the number of glands and the subsequent crowding that occurs. Endometrial glands in adenomatous hyperplasia proliferate at the expense of the stroma. This results in a crowding of endometrial glands until adjacent glands are only separated by a delicate band of fibrous stroma. In atypical hyperplasia, cytologic atypia is manifested by nuclear enlargement, hyperchromasia, or irregular shape. These changes are associated with an increased risk of progression to adenocarcinoma. Patients who display these changes are often divided into mild, moderate, and severe atypical adenomatous hyperplasia. Severe atypical hyperplasia is characterized by anaplasia or lessened differentiation of the glands. The lining of these glands exhibits pronounced variations in size, shape, cytoplasmic staining, and polarity. The nuclei are irregularly shaped with marked variations in size and staining qualities. This condition has often been referred to as carcinoma *in situ* of the endometrium, or stage 0 cancer of the endometrium.

Endometrial Carcinoma

Early diagnosis of *endometrial carcinoma* often occurs when patients present with postmenopausal vaginal bleeding. The association of postmenopausal bleeding with endometrial cancer increases with age. Evaluation of women with these symptoms includes a pelvic examination, Papanicolaou smear, and endometrial histologic assessment. In addition, the use of endometrial thickness determined by transvaginal ultrasound has become an increasingly popular adjunct in the evaluation of women with postmenopausal bleeding.

Surgery is the initial treatment option for most patients with endometrial carcinoma. The prognosis after surgical treatment depends greatly on the resulting operative and pathologic findings. A surgical staging system has replaced the previous clinical staging scheme (Table 15.8). In a population study of patients with uterine carcinoma, 81% had stage I, 11% stage II, 6% stage III, and 2% stage IV disease. Survival rates for these groups after 5 years were 83%, 73%, 52%, and 27%, respectively (63).

Endometrial curettage samples also can provide important insights into the histologic type and grade of the tumor.

Squamous metaplasia is not an independent prognostic factor when it is correlated with tumor grade. Therefore, in respect to clinical relevance, only three cell types of endometrial carcinomas need to be distinguished: endometrioid adenocarcinoma, papillary serous carcinoma, and clear cell carcinoma. Papillary serous endometrial carcinomas are particularly aggressive, and extrauterine metastasis is found in up to 72% of patients. Five-year survival rates for this type of endometrial carcinoma are between 36% and 40% for stage I and II disease, whereas survival for more than 5 years in patients with stage III or IV disease is rare.

Grading of endometrial tumors is based on the architecture of the tumor and reflects the amount of nonglandforming tumor. Tumors with grades I, II, and III display solid growth patterns in less than 5%, 6% to 50%, and more than 50% of the tumor, respectively. Tumor grade is highly predictive of the extent of disease and the probability of nodal involvement. Tumor grade is also correlated with survival.

Two subgroups of women diagnosed with endometrial carcinomas have been described with different disease courses. Women with type I endometrial cancers typically have estrogen-related risk factors such as obesity, nulliparity, and unopposed E_2 therapy. The prognosis for these women with early endometrial cancers is excellent. Women with type II endometrial cancer have adverse histologic features including poorly differentiated tumors, papillary serous and clear cell tumors, deep myometrial invasion, and extrauterine disease. Risk factors for type II endometrial cancer have not been identified.

Biologic Markers

Both estrogen and progesterone receptors have been used as markers of endometrial carcinoma. High levels of these receptors correlate with enhanced tumor differentiation, myometrial invasion, a lower incidence of nodal metastasis, and better survival rates (64). Chromosomal criteria such as DNA aneuploidy have been associated with poor survival rates in women with endometrial cancer. Overexpression of the human neu gene may also provide an important

TABLE 15.8. SYSTEM FOR THE SURGICAL STAGING OF UTERINE CARCINOMA

Stage	Grade	Features
IA	1, 2, or 3	Tumor limited to endometrium
IB	1, 2, or 3	Invasion of less than half the myometrium
IC	1, 2, or 3	Invasion of more than half the myometrium
IIA	1, 2, or 3	Endocervical glandular involvement only
IIB	1, 2, or 3	Cervical stromal invasion
IIIA	1, 2, or 3	Tumor invading serosa or adnexa or malignant peritonical cytology
IIIB	1, 2, or 3	Vaginal metastosis
IIIC	1, 2, or 3	Metastasis to pelvic or paraaortic lymph nodes
IVA	1, 2, or 3	Tumor invasion of the bladder or bowel mucosa
IVB	1, 2, or 3	Distant metastasis including intraabdominal or inguinal lymph nodes

prognostic factor in uterine cancer. This gene is expressed in a larger percentage of women with metastatic disease compared with patients who disease is restricted to the uterus (65). In addition, mutations of the *p53* tumor-suppressor gene have been identified in some endometrial carcinomas (66). These mutations also are associated with advanced tumor stage, poor tumor differentiation, absence of progesterone receptors, and a poor prognosis.

Treatment

Surgical intervention is the appropriate initial treatment for 92% to 96% of women with endometrial carcinoma. Ultrasonography and magnetic resonance imaging can be performed to provide information concerning the depth of myometrial invasion. At surgery, peritoneal cytologic sampling, abdominal exploration, palpation and biopsy of suspicious lesions and nodes, and abdominal hysterectomy with bilateral oophorectomy are performed. Pelvic and para-aortic lymph node biopsies are performed when pathologic specimens obtained at curettage or hysterectomy have features indicating a poor prognosis such as grade 3, serous or clear cell tumor, middle or deep myometrial invasion, or tumor extension to the cervix or adnexa. On the basis of pathologic features, women may be classified as having a low, intermediate, or high risk of recurrence. After surgery, the extent of disease can be determined and the field for adjuvant radiation therapy can be tailored to treat the pelvis, the pelvis and the paraaortic region, or the whole abdomen. Primary radiation therapy is reserved for women who are poor surgical risks, including the elderly and those with multiple medical problems. In these patients, no differences in survival have been reported in patients receiving primary radiation therapy compared with surgery.

10 KEY POINTS

1. Müllerian anomalies occur as a consequence of formation (agenesis) or fusion defects of the embryonic müllerian duct.

2. Changes in endometrial morphology and function during the menstrual cycle are related to both circulating levels of progesterone and estrogen and the presence of specific receptors for these hormones in the endometrium.

3. Growth factors and cytokines can act as autocrine intermediates in the uterine response to steroids and as paracrine regulators of invading trophoblast during pregnancy.

4. The major endometrial leukocyte populations include T cells, large granular lymphocytes, and macrophages.

5. In species with invasive types of implantation, the endometrium undergoes complex changes referred to as decidualization.

6. The implanting human embryo encounters various extracellular matrix components that may assist in guiding and anchoring the embryo as it penetrates the luminal epithelium and moves through the uterine stroma.

7. Integrins function as important mediators of cell-cell interactions.

8. A key event in implantation is the establishment of adequate blood supply to tissues of the maternal-fetal interface.

9. Uterine cancer is the fourth leading cancer in women in the United States, with an estimated 36,000 cases and 6,000 deaths per year.

10. Prolonged exposure to estrogen results in continual stimulation of the endometrium and subsequent endometrial hyperplasia.

REFERENCES

1. Hampton HL. Mullerian anomalies. In: Cowan BD, Seifer DB, eds. *Clinical reproductive medicine.* Philadelphia: JB Lippincott, 1997.
2. Golan A, Layer R, Bukovsky I, et al. Congenital anomalies of the Müllerian system. *Fertil Steril* 1989;51:747–755.
3. Hampton HL. Role of the gynecologic surgeon in the management of urological anomalies in adolescents. *Curr Opin Obstet Gynecol* 1990;2:812–818.
4. Tolhurst DE, van der Helm TW. The treatment of vaginal atresia. *Surg Gynecol Obstet* 1991;172:407–414.
5. Neulen J, Breckwoldt M. Placental progesterone, prostaglandins and mechanisms leading to initiation of parturition in the human. *Exp Clin Endocrinol* 1994;102:195–202.
6. Garfield RE, Blennerhassett MG, Miller SM. Control of myometrial contractility: role and regulation of gap junctions. *Oxf Rev Reprod Biol* 1988;10:436–490.
7. Norman JE, Cameron IT. Nitric oxide in the human uterus. *Rev Reprod* 1991;1:61–68.
8. Buttram VC, Reiter RC. Uterine leiomyomata: etiology, symptomatology, and management. *Fertil Steril* 1981;36:433–445.
9. Nilbert M, Strombeck B. Independent origin of uterine leiomyomas with karyotypically identical alterations. *Gynecol Obstet Invest* 1992;33:246–248.
10. Sadan O, van Iddekinge B, van Gelderen CJ, et al. Oestrogen and progesterone receptor concentrations in leiomyoma and normal myometrium. *Ann Clin Biochem* 1987;24:263–267.
11. Soules MR, McCarty KS. Leiomyomas: steroid receptor content. *Am J Obstet Gynecol* 1982;143:6–11.
12. Leibsohn S, d'Ablaing G, Mishell DR Jr, et al. Leiomyosarcoma in a series of hysterectomies performed for presumed uterine leiomyomas. *Am J Obstet Gynecol* 1990;162:968–974.
13. Goldberg JM, Falcone T, Attaran M. Sonohysterographic evaluation of uterine abnormalities noted on hysterosalpingography. *Hum Reprod* 1997;12:2151–2153.
14. Verkauf BS. Changing trends in treatment of leiomyomata uteri. *Curr Opin Obstet Gynecol* 1993;5:301–310.
15. Schlaff WD, Zerhouni EA, Huth JAM, et al. A placebo-controlled trial of a depot gonadotropin-releasing hormone analogue (leuprolide) in the treatment of uterine leiomyomata. *Obstet Gynecol* 1989;74:856–862.
16. Goodwin SC, Vedantham S, McLucas B, et al. Preliminary experience with uterine artery embolization for uterine fibroids. *J Vasc Interv Radiol* 1997;8:517–526.
17. Gehlbach DL, Sousa RC, Carpenter SE, et al. Abdominal myomectomy in the treatment of infertility. *Int J Gynaecol Obstet* 1993;40:45–50.

18. Brenner RM, Slayden OD. Cyclic changes in the primate oviduct and endometrium. In: Knobil E, Neill JD, eds. *The physiology of reproduction,* 2nd ed. New York: Raven, 1994.

19. Noyes RW, Hertig AT, Rock J. Dating the endometrial biopsy. *Fertil Steril* 1950;1:3–25.

20. Hansard LJ, Walmer DK. Descriptive histology: the gold standard for clinically evaluating the endometrium. *Infertil Reprod Clin North Am* 1995;6:281–292.

21. McClellan MC, West NB, Tacha DE, et al. Immunohistochemical localization of estrogen receptors in the macaque reproductive tract with monoclonal antiestrophilins. *Endocrinology* 1984; 114:2002–2014.

22. Rechler MM, Nissley SP. Insulin-like growth factors. In: Sporn MB, Roberts AB, eds. *Peptide growth factors and their receptors I.* New York: Springer-Verlag, 1991.

23. Murphy LJ, Friesen HG. Differential effects of estrogen and growth hormone on uterine and hepatic insulin like growth factor I gene expression in the ovariectomized hypophysectomized rat. *Endocrinology* 1988;122:325–332.

24. Zang XM, Rossi MJ, Masterson BJ, et al. Insulin-like growth factor I (IGF-I), IGF-I receptors, and IGF binding proteins 1-4 in human uterine tissue: tissue localization and IGF-I action in endometrial stromal and myometrial smooth muscle cells *in vitro. Biol Reprod* 1994;50:1113–1125.

25. Ghahary A, Murphy LJ. Regulation of uterine insulin-like growth hormone receptors by estrogen and variation throughout the estrous cycle. *Endocrinology* 1989;125:597–604.

26. Talavera F, Reynolds RK, Roberts JA, et al. Insulin-like growth factor I receptors in normal and neoplastic human endometrium. *Cancer Res* 1990;50:3019–3024.

27. Murphy LJ, Ghahary A. Uterine insulin-like growth factor-I: regulation of expression and its role in estrogen-induced uterine proliferation. *Endocr Rev* 1990;11:443–453.

28. Giudice LC, Lamson G, Rosenfeld RG, et al. Insulin-like growth factor-II (IGF-II) and IGF binding proteins in human endometrium. *Ann N Y Acad Sci* 1991;626:295–307.

29. Murphy LJ. Estrogen induction of insulin-like growth factors and myc proto-oncogene expression in the uterus. *J Steroid Biochem Mol Biol* 1991;40:223–230.

30. DiAugustine RP, Petrusy P, Bell GI, et al. Influence of estrogens on mouse uterine epidermal growth factor precursor protein and messenger ribonucleic acid. *Endocrinology* 1988;122:2355–2363.

31. Nelson KG, Tabahashi T, Bossert ML, et al. Epidermal growth factor replaces estrogen in the stimulation of female genital-tract growth and differentiation. *Proc Natl Acad Sci U S A* 1991; 88:21–25.

32. Wang D, Fujii S, Konishi I, et al. Expression of c-erb-2 protein and epidermal growth factor receptor in normal tissues of the female genital tract and in the placenta. *Virchows Arch A Pathol Anat Histopathol* 1992;420:385–393.

33. Bulmer JN, Cellular constituents of human endometrium in the menstrual cycle and early pregnancy. In: Bronson RA, Alexander NJ, Anderson DJ, et al., eds. *Reproductive immunology.* Cambridge, Blackwell Science, Inc., 1996.

34. Pollard JW, Bartocci A, Arceci R, et al. Apparent role of the macrophage growth factor, CSF-I, in placental development. *Nature* 1987;330:484–486.

35. Chen HL, Yang Y, Hu XL, et al. Tumor necrosis factor-alpha mRNA and protein are present in human placental and uterine cells at early and late stages of gestation. *Am J Pathol* 1991;139:327–335.

36. Robertson SA, Seamark RF. Granulocyte macrophage colony stimulating factor (GM-CSF) in the murine reproductive tract: stimulation by seminal factors. *Reprod Fertil Dev* 1990;2: 359–368.

37. Hunt JS, Chen HL, Hu XL, et al. Analysis of tumor necrosis factor-alpha gene expression in virgin and pregnant normal and osteopetrotic (op/op) mice. *Biol Reprod* 1993;49:441–452.

38. Wood GW, De M, Sanford T, et al. Macrophage colony stimulating factor controls macrophage recruitment to the cycling mouse uterus. *Dev Biol* 1992;152:336–343.

39. Robertson SA, Mayrhofer G, Seamark RF. Uterine epithelial cells synthesize granulocyte-macrophage colony-stimulating factor and interleukin-G in pregnant and nonpregnant mice. *Biol Reprod* 1992;46:1069–1079.

40. Robertston SA, Seamark RF. Granulocyte macrophage colony stimulating factor (GM-CSF) in the murine reproductive tract: stimulation by seminal factors. *Reprod Fertil Dev* 1990; 2:359–368.

41. Hunt JS. Cytokine networks in the utero placental unit: macrophages as pivotal regulatory cells. *J Reprod Immunol* 1989; 16:1–17.

42. Warren MA, Li TC, Klentzeris LD. Cell biology of the endometrium: histology, cell types, and menstrual changes. In: Chard T, Grudzinskas JG, eds. *The uterus.* Cambridge: Cambridge University Press, 1994:94–124.

43. Seppala M, Koistinen R, Rutanen EM. Uterine endocrinology and paracrinology: insulin-like growth factor binding protein-I and placenta protein 14 revisited. *Hum Reprod* 1994;9:917–925.

44. Hey NA, Graham RA, Seif MW, et al. The polymorphic epithelial mucin MUC in human endometrium is hormonally regulated with maximal expression in the implantation phase. *J Clin Endocrinol Metab* 1994;78:337–342.

45. Blithe DL, Richards RG, Skarulis MC. Free alpha molecules from pregnancy stimulate secretion of prolactin from human decidual cells: a novel function for free alpha in pregnancy. *Endocrinology* 1991;129:2257–2259.

46. Chao HS, Myers SE, Handiverger S. Endothelin inhibits basal and stimulated release of prolactin by human decidual cells. *Endocrinology* 1993;133:505–510.

47. Clevenger CV, Altman SW, Prystowsky MB. Requirement of nuclear prolactin for interleukin-2–stimulated proliferation and T lymphocytes. *Science* 1991;253:77–79.

48. Mazar MT, Duncan DA, Younger JB. Endometrial biopsy in the cycle of conception: histologic and lectin histochemical evaluation. *Fertil Steril* 1989;51:764–769.

49. Graham RA, Li TC, Cooke ID, et al. Keratan sulfate as a secretory product of human endometrium: cyclic expression in normal women. *Hum Reprod* 1994;9:926–930.

50. Carson DD, Wilson OF, Dutt A. Glycoconjugate expression and interactions at the cell surface of mouse uterine epithelial cells and peri-implantation stage embryos. *Trophoblast Res* 1990;4211–241.

51. Hey NA, Kliman HJ. Trophoblast infiltration. *Reprod Med Rev* 1994;3:137–157.

52. Lessey BA, Castlebaum NJ, Buck CA, et al. Further characterization of endometrial integrins during the menstrual cycle and in pregnancy. *Fertil Steril* 1994;62:497–506.

53. Lessey BA, Domjanovich L, Coutifaris C, et al. Integrin adhesion molecules in the human endometrium. *J Clin Invest* 1992; 90:188–195.

54. Simon C, Frances A, Piquette G, et al. Interleukin-I system in the materno-trophoblast unit in human implantations: immunohistochemical evidence for autocrine/paracrine function. *J Clin Endocrinol Metab* 1994;78:847–854.

55. Shen MM, Leder P. Leukemia inhibitory factor is expressed by the preimplantation uterus and selectively blocks primitive ectoderm formation *in vitro. Proc Natl Acad Sci U S A* 1992;89:8240–8244.

56. Bhatt H, Brunet LJ, Stewart CL. Uterine expression of leukemia

inhibitory factor coincides with the onset of blastocyst implantation. *Proc Natl Acad Sci U S A* 1991;88:11408–11411.

57. Stewart CL, Kaspar P, Brunet LJ, et al. Blastocyst implantation depends on maternal expression of leukemia inhibitory factor. *Nature* 1992;359:76–79.

58. Charnock-Jones DS, Sharkey AM, Rajput-Williams J, et al. Identification and localization of alternatively spliced mRNAs for vascular endothelial growth factor in human uterus and estrogen regulation in endometrial carcinoma cell lines. *Biol Reprod* 1993;48:1120–1128.

59. Rose PG. Endometrial carcinoma. *N Engl J Med* 1996;335: 640–648.

60. Gallup DG, Stock RJ. Adenocarcinoma of the endometrium in women 40 years of age and younger. *Obstet Gynecol* 1984; 64:417–420.

61. Kurman RJ, Kaminski PF, Norris HJ. The behavior of endometrial hyperplasia: a long-term study of "untreated" hyperplasia in 170 patients. *Cancer* 1985;56:403–412.

62. Fisher B, Costantino JP, Redmond CK, et al. Endometrial cancer in tamoxifen-treated breast cancer patients: findings from the National Surgical Adjuvant Breast and Bowel Project (NSABP) B-14. *J Natl Cancer Inst* 1994;86:527–537.

63. Abeler VM, Kjorstad KE. Endometrial adenocarcinoma in Norway: a study of a total population. *Cancer* 1991;67:3093–3103.

64. Creasman WT. Prognostic significance of hormone receptors in endometrial cancer. *Cancer* 1993;71[Suppl]:467–470.

65. Berchuck A, Rodriguez G, Kinney RB, et al. Overexpression of HER-1/neu in endometrial cancer is associated with advanced stage disease. *Am J Obstet Gynecol* 1991;164:15–21.

66. Kohler MF, Berchuck A, Davidoff AM, et al. Overexpression and mutation of p53 in endometrial carcinoma. *Cancer Res* 1992;52:1622–1627.

16

THE FALLOPIAN TUBE IN HEALTH AND DISEASE

BRADLEY T. MILLER
MARK LEONDIRES

In the middle of the 15th century, Fallopius first described the human oviduct. Since that time, years of painstaking research have demonstrated that the human oviduct is a remarkable organ. The oviduct is responsible for sperm and egg transport, fertilization, embryo incubation, and transport of the embryo to the uterine cavity. Before assisted reproductive technology (ART), women without properly functioning oviducts were, for all practical purposes, sterile. Attempts at conservative and corrective surgery have met with some success on mildly diseased oviducts. Today, clinical pregnancy rates per embryo transfer in ART have surpassed the 50% mark (1). In some ART programs, young patients with pure tubal disease have clinical pregnancy rates per embryo transfer as high as 75%. Obviously, our skills of replacing oviductal function have improved immensely over the past 10 years.

A major dilemma for this century will be the selection between ART and corrective tubal surgery. In today's managed-care setting, health care dollars are scarce, and the bottom line will be what is the most cost-effective way to bring home a baby. Many clinicians have experienced a dramatic change in the way tubal disease is approached. Several years ago, ART availability was limited, and aggressive tubal reconstruction was routinely performed. There has been a dramatic change in the way tubal disease is approached. At present, highly successful *in vitro* fertilization (IVF) programs are available throughout the United States, and as a result tubal reconstructive surgery is less commonly performed. Although our understanding of tubal physiology is impressive, there is still no diagnostic test of tubal function. Clinically, one can readily assess tubal patency and gross anatomy, but these factors may have little to do with normal tubal function.

This chapter reviews both the normal and abnormal physiology of the human oviduct. As with many investigations into human physiology, animal models have been used extensively, especially the rat, rabbit, and subhuman primates. Human data for normal physiology come from iatrogenic and naturally occurring tubal dysfunction. The pathophysiology of the following disease processes is reviewed as well: pelvic inflammatory disease (PID), diethyl-stilbestrol (DES) exposure, tuberculosis (TB), endometriosis, and ectopic pregnancy. Finally, other relevant topics such as the utility of salpingectomy for hydrosalpinx before IVF are discussed. Ultimately, the clinician should have a better understanding of the oviduct in both health and disease, and the result should be improved patient care.

ANATOMY AND PHYSIOLOGY OF THE HUMAN OVIDUCT

Embryology

The female internal reproductive structures—oviducts, uterus, and upper two-thirds of the vagina—are formed from the müllerian or paramesonephric ducts. The elaboration of this system occurs in the absence of müllerian-inhibiting substance (MIS), a product of the embryonic testis. Important to remember is that the fetal gonad has the potential to differentiate into either a testis or an ovary. Male differentiation depends on a gene product found on the short arm of the Y chromosome known as sex region Y (SRY). Although SRY is considered to be the main factor leading to gonadal differentiation into a testis, other important regions for male differentiation have been identified on autosomes (2,3). After gonadal sexual determination, testosterone is produced; this is crucial in the elaboration of the primordial male internal structures along the wolffian duct. Concurrently, the embryonic testis secretes MIF, which leads to regression of the primordial female internal structures known as the müllerian ducts. The müllerian ducts persist and develop in the absence of gonads or hormonal influence. Therefore, in the female, because of the lack of testosterone and MIF, the primordia of male sex accessory organs regress, and the müllerian duct begins to develop and differentiate during the eighth week of gestation.

A close association exists among the mesonephros (wolffian duct), paramesonephros (müllerian duct), and the metanephros (differentiates into the ureter and kidney), which, in the early embryo, are arranged closely at their cephalic ends in a medial to lateral fashion, respectively. Near their caudal ends, the müllerian and metanephric ducts cross over the wolffian ducts and come to lie medial to the wolffian ducts. Not only is the development of an abnormal urinary collection system related to normal müllerian differentiation, but abnormal wolffian duct regression in the female is also associated with abnormalities of the renal collecting system.

The *müllerian ducts* in the human embryo become apparent at about the 37th day of gestation. At their cephalic ends, the müllerian ducts maintain a position lateral and parallel to that of the mesonephric ducts or wolffian ducts. At their caudal ends, the two müllerian ducts are juxtaposed. These juxtaposed caudal segments extend down to the urogenital sinus and fuse to become the uterus and the upper two-thirds of the vagina. The fallopian tubes or oviducts are formed from the most cephalic lateralized portions of the müllerian ducts. These cephalic segments of the müllerian ducts continue to differentiate by developing ostia, canalizing, and differentiating into the fully developed fallopian tube. During this time, the wolffian duct system degenerates. Degeneration of this duct is not complete and can manifest itself in the adult female as Gartner's duct cysts in the upper two-thirds of the vagina and as a sessile hydatid cyst just below the tubal ostia. Other vestiges of the embryonic ductal system, which are considered to be müllerian in origin, are appendix vesiculosa or cysts of Morgagni, which are pedunculated cystic structures arising at the tubal ostia. These cysts are found frequently and are considered harmless. Clinically, they are at risk for torsion, which can present as peritonitis or dysmenorrhea and, depending on their anatomic appearance, may need to be removed when encountered during surgery.

Congenital defects of the fallopian tube occur at a frequency of 1 in 500 to 700 and can be classified as complete absence, segmental absence, accessory ostia, and multiple lumina (4). Complete failure of the müllerian system to develop leads to absent tubes, uterus, and upper two-thirds of the vagina. This syndrome is known as müllerian agenesis or Mayer-Rokitansky-Küster-Hauser syndrome. In this syndrome, one often sees a fibromuscular streak of remnant müllerian tissue. The ovaries in these women are usually completely normal. Unilateral failure of the müllerian duct to develop can lead to unicornuate uterus, which often has a normally functioning single oviduct with two normal ovaries. This is an important example of the different embryologic origins of the ovaries and müllerian structures. Complete absence with an otherwise normal uterus or partial absence of the ampullary portion of the tube can be present, but it is rare. This may be secondary to a developmental defect or possibly to torsion with subsequent necrosis and autoamputation (5). In addition, segmental atresias have been reported but are uncommon. Luminal defects, most likely secondary to a failure of proper canalization, exist as well. More frequent than defects secondary to inadequate tubal development are anomalies of excesses, which can present as an accessory tubal ostia, ampullae, or supernumerary oviducts. Supernu-

merary oviducts are rare, but they run along the length of the primary tube. They may or may not be associated with a supernumerary ovary.

With consideration of the embryologic development of the tube, one should realize that any congenital tubal defect may also be associated with defects of the renal system. This is presumably secondary to the reasons explained previously, that is, the close embryologic proximity of the primordia of the female internal reproductive structures and the renal system. The ovarian structures are unique in their embryologic development and are not usually abnormal in patients with müllerian anomalies.

Anatomy

The *oviducts* extend outward from the uterus from the superolateral portion and end by draping around the ovary. They can be divided anatomically into four distinct segments: interstitial, isthmic, ampullary, and infundibular. Fallopian tubes are between 8 and 14 cm in length and consist of three layers: a serosal coat, a muscular layer, and a mucosal lining. The muscular layers make up the myosalpinx, with the outer layer longitudinal in direction, an inner circular layer, and depending on the portion of the oviduct, a third inner longitudinally orientated layer. The inner mucosal layer makes up the endosalpinx, which contains both motile ciliated cells and secretory cells. Cyclic changes in this layer coincide with the female menstrual cycle. In short, during the follicular phase of the cycle, increased ciliation and mitotic activity are observed, and in the luteal phase, decreased ciliation and mitotic activity are noted. This response is mediated at least partially by the dominant steroid hormones of the menstrual cycle—estrogen and progesterone. The myosalpinx and the endosalpinx allow the oviduct to perform its critical role in ovum pickup, gamete transport, and embryo transport.

Caudal to the fallopian tube is the mesosalpinx, which serves as the tubal mesentery containing blood supply and enervation. The main blood supply is from a superior branch of the uterine artery, which extends along the superior aspect of the mesosalpinx to anastomose with the tubal branch of the ovarian artery. This ovarian branch supplies the distal two-thirds of the oviduct. This vascular arrangement is extremely variable, possibly having additional branches and various uterine-ovarian vessel anastomoses. The lymphatic drainage of the oviduct runs to the lymphatic network below the hilus of the ovary. This region receives lymphatic flow from the uterus, tube, and ovary, which drains to either the paraaortic or lumbar lymph nodes.

Oviductal Segments

Interstitial Segment

The *interstitial segment,* also known as the intramural or cornual segment, is the narrowest portion of the tube. It lies within the uterine wall and is approximately 1 cm in length. Anatomically, the course of the interstitial portion of the tube is curved rather than straight as it merges with the endometrial cavity in a funnel-like fashion. The luminal diameter of this segment is the smallest of the entire oviduct at 100 μm. This portion of the tube forms the uterotubal junction. This region, along with ampullary-isthmic junction (AIJ) found more distally, is postulated to play a role in the passage of the embryo into the uterus and sperm into the ampulla.

The myosalpinx has three distinct muscular layers, as does the uterus. Enervation of the interstitial myosalpinx is mainly through adrenergic-noradrenergic fibers, which are organized to facilitate either contractility or relaxation (6,7). The outer longitudinal layer, which runs the length of the entire oviduct, blends with the myometrium at the uterotubal junction and has primarily α-adrenoreceptors. There are two inner muscular layers in this segment and in the isthmic segment. Both these layers primarily have β-adrenoreceptors. The middle layer is circular, and the innermost layer is longitudinal. This inner longitudinal layer is lost at the AIJ. Although it is likely that the muscular aspect of the interstitial segment plays a role in sperm and embryo transport, surgical data suggest that it is not essential for fertility. This is evidenced by a pregnancy rate of up to 50% after bilateral tubal reimplantation of the isthmic portion of the tube into the posterior uterine fundus necessitated by proximal tubal obstruction (PTO) (8).

The endosalpinx in the interstitial region is made up of three to four low, broad mucosal folds, which become more complex in the distal portions of the oviduct. In addition, the epithelial surface of the endosalpinx is endowed with less cilium than the more distal portions of the oviduct. Cilial function is important in gamete transport and is discussed as it relates to the ampullary and infundibular regions of the tube. Pathologic states involving the interstitial portion of the tube can be embryologic, infectious, and mechanical. If severe, these states can lead to PTO, which may account for up to 33% of all cases of tubal occlusion (9). The differential diagnosis of PTO includes obliterative fibrosis, chronic tubal inflammation, endometriosis, chronic ectopic pregnancy, tubal polyps, and congenital disease, and it is discussed later in this chapter.

Isthmic Segment

The *isthmic segment* of the oviduct is the portion closest to the uterus. It is not as narrow as the interstitial aspect of the tube; its luminal diameter enlarges from 100 μm to 1 mm as it makes the transition to the ampullary region of the oviduct. This region of the tube is 1 to 3 cm in length and, like the interstitial region, has a three-layer myosalpinx. In contrast to the larger-caliber ampullary portion of the tube, the myosalpinx is thicker in this region, with a high concentration of connective tissue. This portion of the tube is able to contract and has a high muscular-to-lumen ratio

with dense adrenergic enervation enabling it to respond to both contractile and relaxation agents. The AIJ is the essential mediator of gamete and embryo transport. The endosalpinx has three to five primary folds that become more numerous and complex toward the ampulla. In addition, the isthmic region of the endosalpinx contains more glandular cells than ciliated cells.

The functional aspects of the isthmus are related to the role of the AIJ in regulation of the passage of sperm, ovum, and embryo within the oviduct. Whether this portion of the tube can truly act as a sphincter is debated; most likely, it acts in concert with the interstitial segment, which has a similar muscular arrangement and enervation. As described earlier, there is a differential arrangement of the enervation, with the outer layer mostly α-adrenergic and the two inner layers mostly β-adrenergic (6,7). In general, estrogens stimulate tubal motility, and progesterone inhibits tubal motility (10,11). Estrogen potentiates the activation of α-receptors, and progesterone potentiates the activation of β-receptors. Strom et al. in 1983 found that stimulation of the α-adrenoreceptor in the rabbit led to reduction or cessation of transisthmic flow, whereas stimulation of the β-adrenoreceptors led to an increase in transisthmic flow (12). Therefore, an interpretation of this system would be that the relatively estrogenic environment facilitates cessation of intratubal flow inhibiting embryo passage into the uterus. Conversely, the progestational environment of the luteal phase facilitates tubal relaxation and flow of the early embryo toward the uterus. The direction of propulsive forces of the tube as it changes through the menstrual cycle is shown graphically in Fig. 16.1.

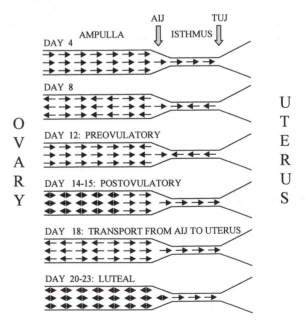

FIGURE 16.1. Direction of propulsive forces in the human oviduct throughout the ovulatory cycle. AIJ, ampulla-isthmic junction; TUJ, tubouterine junction. (From Pulkkinen MO, Talo A. Tubal physiologic consideration in ectopic pregnancy. *Clin Obstet Gynecol* 1987;30:164, with permission.)

It would be simplistic to assume that the adrenergic-noradrenergic enervation is the only system involved in tubal motility and function. Many other factors are apparently involved in tubal muscular function, most notably the prostaglandin family of agents. An added level of complexity relates to the change in effect of prostaglandins, depending on the stage of the menstrual cycle and relative hormonal concentrations. *In vitro* prostaglandin $F_{2\alpha}$ ($PGF_{2\alpha}$) stimulated oviductal contractility in human oviductal tissue, whereas prostaglandin E_1 (PGE_1) and prostaglandin E_2 (PGE_2) inhibited contractility. Contrary to their differential effects on tubal contractility, $PGF_{2\alpha}$, PGE_1, and PGE_2 all stimulate ciliary activity *in vitro* [13]. Numerous other pharmacologic agents have been shown to have an effect on tubal contractility including: ergot derivatives, substance P, neuropeptide Y, oxytocin, copper chloride, and vasoactive intestinal peptide [14–19]. The function of the isthmic segment of the oviduct is mediated by many known and likely, unknown factors.

Although this portion of the tube holds many components likely essential for optimal fertility, it is evident that the entire isthmic segment is not necessary for fertility. Furthermore, the muscular component is not necessary for fertility. Muscular deletion is seen at the sites of fistulization after failed isthmic sterilization. Notably in these regions, there was ciliary function but no muscularis layer in histologic sections of these successfully functioning oviducts [20]. In humans, a subtotal resection of the isthmic portion of the tube does not interfere with fertility [21]. Therefore, this segment of the tube is the most appropriate choice for occlusion in cases of voluntary sterilization because anastomoses of this region result in pregnancy rates approaching 70%.

Ampullary Segment

The *ampullary region* of the oviduct may be the most essential segment for optimum fertility. It represents the longest segment of the oviduct and ranges from 1 to 2 cm in luminal diameter. It is drastically different from the more proximal isthmic portion in many regards. The muscular-to-luminal ratio changes in that there is a thin myosalpinx and the inner longitudinal layer is lost. The endosalpingeal mucosal folds expand to become a complex labyrinth leaving little luminal space. This arrangement forces the recently ovulated cumulus mass and ovum to be in close contact with the endosalpingeal epithelium at all times. Fertilization most likely occurs in the distal ampulla. The epithelium of the endosalpinx is made up of approximately 40% to 50% ciliated cells. The cilia of both the ampulla and the fimbriae beat synchronously and propagate currents toward the uterus at a frequency of approximately seven times per minute [22–24].

Corresponding to the estrogen-predominated and progesterone-predominated portions of the menstrual cycle is a repeating process of ciliation and deciliation. Estrogen not only prevents deciliation, but also it can actually increase the number of ciliated cells. Progesterone acts in an antagonistic fashion decreasing ciliation and the number of ciliated cells [25]. Notably, maximum ciliation occurs during the periovulatory period. As described by Verhage et al., there has been considerable disagreement in the literature on the behavior of the ciliated cells during the menstrual cycle [26]. These investigators confirmed that the epithelial cells of the endosalpinx in both the fimbriae and the ampulla achieved their maximal height during the late follicular phase. In addition, deciliation and atrophy were found to occur in the luteal phase, most notably in the fimbriae. In addition, in the early follicular phase, approximately 10% to 12% of the cells formed new cilia in both the ampulla and the fimbriae. Donnez et al. confirmed these observations and described the effects of estrogen and progesterone on the tubal epithelium [27].

Brenner and Slayden described changes in endosalpingeal cells throughout the menstrual cycle of 27 cynomologus macaques. These investigators examined ciliated cell height, percentage of ciliation, secretory cell height, degree of mitotic activity, content of glycogen and secretory granules, presence of apoptotic bodies, and presence of macrophages containing nuclear and cellular fragments. On the basis of these histologic parameters, they defined a tubal cycle, which consists of eight different stages: preciliogenic, ciliogenic, ciliogenic-ciliated, ciliated-ciliogenic, ciliated-secretory, early regression, late regression, and full regression (Fig. 16.2). These stages are roughly equivalent to the ovarian stages of the menstrual cycle: full regression corresponds to the late luteal phase; preciliogenic and ciliogenic corresponds to menses and early follicular stage; ciliogenic-ciliated corresponds to the midfollicular stage; ciliated-ciliogenic corresponds to the late follicular stage; ciliated-secretory corresponds to the periovulatory stage; early regression corresponds to the early luteal stage; and late regression corresponds to the midluteal stage [28]. These changes are most pronounced in the fimbriae, less so in the ampulla, and least in the isthmus. This finding is in contrast to secretory tip extension, which is least in the fimbriae, larger in the ampulla, and greatest in the isthmus. This may relate to the importance of ciliary function to optimal tubal function in the infundibulum and ampulla and the importance of oviductal secretions to optimal function of the isthmic portion of the fallopian tube.

Although fertilization occurs in the ampulla and this segment is the longest portion of the oviduct, its fundamental role in fertility can be questioned. Ampulloampullary anastomoses are considered one of the least successful tubal repairs, but pregnancies are reported. The lower success rates are thought to be secondary to the complexity of the mucosal folds and microsurgical capacity to reapproximate properly. Improper alignment may lead to impaired transport of the cumulus mass. Halbert concluded that one requires at least 50% of the ampullary regions at anasto-

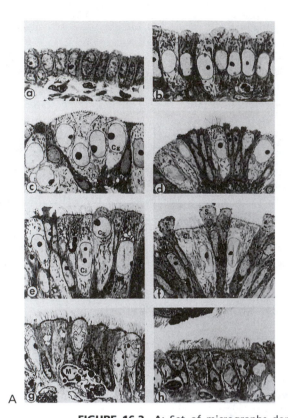

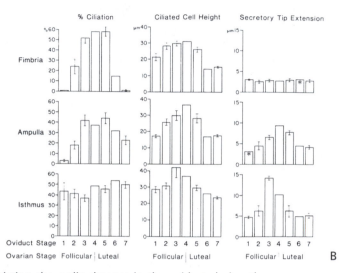

FIGURE 16.2. A: Set of micrographs depicting the cyclic changes in the oviduct during the menstrual cycle in macaques: a, full regression: fimbria; the epithelial cells are maximally atrophied and dedifferentiated, and their nuclei are maximally shriveled, ×1050; b, preciliogenic: ampulla; all the cells are hypertrophied, and their nuclei are swollen; no basal bodies can be seen by light microscopy, ×1050; c, ciliogenic: fimbria; ciliogenic (Cg) cells are light, hypertrophied cells with swollen nuclei and enlarged nucleoli; basal bodies (*arrows*) are present in the apical cytoplasm. The dark cells are future secretory cells, ×1050; d, ciliogenic-ciliated: ampulla; most of the light cells are ciliogenic, but a few have become ciliated; the dark cells are future secretory cells, ×1050; e, ciliated-ciliogenic: ampulla; most of the light cells have become ciliated (Ci), but some are still ciliogenic (Cg); the dark cells are secretory, ×1050; f, ciliated-secretory: ampulla; the light cells are ciliated, and the dark cells are secretory; note the pronounced degree of secretory tip extension, ×1050; g, early regression: fimbria; large numbers of macrophages (M) filled with nuclear and cellular fragments are present in the epithelium, ×1050; h, late regression: ampulla; the epithelium consists of atrophied ciliated and secretory cells with shriveled nuclei; deciliation is more extensive in some regions than others during this phase, ×1050. **B:** Comparison of percentage of ciliation, cell height, and secretory tip extension in the fimbria, ampulla, and isthmic regions of the oviduct of cynomologus macaques at different times during the menstrual cycle. The data are grouped according to the oviductal staging sequence described in the text. For convenience of presentation in graphic form, the oviductal stages are given group numbers as follows: group 1, ampullary epithelial folds preciliogenic-ciliogenic (n = 3); group 2, ciliogenic-ciliated (n = 6); group 3, ciliated-ciliogenic (n = 3); group 4, ciliated-secretory (n = 2); group 5, early regression (n = 4); group 6, late regression (n = 2); and group 7, full regression (n = 7). Data are presented as means with standard error bars where appropriate. The *asterisk* represents the sample of n = 1. (From Adashi E, Rock J, Rosenwaks Z, eds. *Reproductive endocrinology, surgery, and technology.* Philadelphia: Lippincott-Raven, 1995:329–330, with permission.)

moses to result in a successful intrauterine pregnancy (29). In the rabbit, surgical reversal and anastomoses of a 1-cm ampullary segment prevented pregnancy for several months. This finding suggests reestablishment of proper ciliary function or realignment of mucosal folds. Clinically, often the success of neosalpingostomy or fimbrioplasty depends on the amount of damage to the endosalpinx of this portion of the tube. If the ampulla is integral in retaining and

nurturing the cumulus mass, as the site of conception, and releases the embryo to the isthmus at the proper time, one can postulate that its mucosal folds and ciliary action are crucial.

Pathologic states that affect this portion of the tube relate to infection, partial or total tubal occlusion, and hydrosalpinges. Distal tubal obstruction is a significant cause of tubal dysfunction and is discussed later.

Infundibular Segment

The *infundibulum,* the most distal portion of the oviduct, is trumpet shaped and about 1 cm in length. Its muscular layer is thin, but its complement of ciliated cells is about 60% to 80%. Approximately 25 fimbriae are arranged at the most distal portion of the infundibulum, which funnel into a complex folding pattern within the infundibulum. Frequently, a single fimbria is actually attached to the ovary and this is known as the *fimbria ovarica.* The cilia in this region beat continuously and generate a current heading in the uterine direction.

Close proximity of the fimbria to the ovary and cumulus oocyte mass are essential, but even without the presence of an attachment, the anatomic arrangement facilitates this process. The mobility of the infundibulum is perhaps augmented by the normal peristaltic action of the intestinal tract. In fact, many pregnancies have been documented in patients with one oviduct and one ovary on opposite sides of the pelvis (30,31). The process of cumulus pickup by the fimbria and transport into the tubal ostia has been observed directly in rabbits and monkeys (32). This process seems mostly dependent on the complex interaction between the granulosa cells surrounding the ovum and the ciliary activity of the fimbria that provides a fluid current-promoting cumulus mass transport to the ampulla. In addition, surrounding the ovum is the cumulus oophorus, which contains enzymes important for ovum pickup and successful fertilization (33).

The role of cilial action cannot be considered totally essential because women with Kartagener's syndrome, characterized by a congenital lack of cilial function, are fertile (29,34). Other evidence supporting the nonfundamental aspect of the infundibulum is that the ampulla can functionally replace the infundibulum and fimbriae. There are several reports of women who have undergone fimbriectomy for sterilization who achieved pregnancy without reconstruction (35,36). In addition, reversing fimbriectomy by cuff or ampullary salpingostomy has led to pregnancy with a 35% success rate (37,38). Pathologic states that affect the infundibular portion of the tube are related to infection leading to ineffective ovum pickup, restricted tubal motility secondary to pelvic adhesive disease, and partial or total fimbrial obstruction secondary to salpingitis.

In summary, each part of the fallopian tube has a physiologic role in optimizing sperm, ovum, and embryo transport. The absence or alteration of these parts does not preclude fertility. This finding is further supported by successful fertility after various forms of tubal anastomoses. Both the type and site of anastomoses relate to a favorable surgical outcome. When segments of the ampulla or isthmus are missing or shortened significantly, postsurgical fertility is reduced (39). The minimum length after anastomoses necessary to provide a favorable prognosis for pregnancy is considered to be 3 to 5 cm (40,41). There are reports of pregnancies with as little as 1 cm of ampulla if the total tubal length is 3 cm. In fact, a pregnancy rate of 50% has been reported with 3 to 4 cm of postsurgical length, but length greater than 5 cm can yield pregnancy rates as high as 70% (42).

Fallopian Tube Function

The transport of gametes and embryos through the fallopian tube involves an integrated balance of propulsive forces to accomplish: ovum pickup, pro-ovarian sperm transport, prouterine ovum transport, a 2- to 3-day delay at the AIJ, and embryo transport to the uterus.

Ovum Pickup

Ovum pickup is partially dependent on proximity. A combination of tubal musculature, anatomic approximation, and bowel peristaltic activity ensure passage of the fimbria past the ovarian site of ovulation. When ovum pickup is considered from this perspective, the effects of pelvic and paratubal adhesions on fertility are easy to appreciate. Other factors that likely aid in ovum pickup are the prouterine currents generated by the constant beating of the cilia and the rapid absorption of oviductal fluid into the lymphatic system. We know from clinical scenarios of absent tubal musculature and immotile cilia syndromes that these factors are not essential for ovum transport through the fallopian tube. Likely the most important factor is peritoneal fluid, which, when coupled with anatomic approximation to the lumen, facilitates transport of the cumulus mass (43).

Transport of Gametes

Transport of gametes in their uniting directions is influenced by cyclic changes in electrical activity. These changes precede mechanical activity and reflect its force. The human oviduct consists of areas that have pacemaker properties and areas with no intrinsic pacemaker activity to spread. This activity is higher in the ampulla than in the isthmus and is lower in the AIJ. All areas may have pacemaker properties that remain latent because of a lower frequency than that of the dominant pacemaker. Waves spread in both directions, except at the ends of the oviduct (43–46).

These waves are propagated in a coordinated fashion dependent on hormonal, adrenergic, and prostaglandin mediators. This activity has best described by Talo and Pulkinnen. As seen in Fig. 16.2 during menstruation, the electrical activity spreads from the ostium to the uterotubal junction and theoretically prevents menstrual blood from entering into the abdominal cavity. As the menstrual cycle progresses, the activity from the distal end becomes coordinated and prouterine in direction around day 12 to facilitate the transport of the ovum to the AIJ. Concurrently, activity initiating at the uterine end spreads in the opposite direction toward the AIJ and thus facilitates sperm transport. After ovulation, on cycle days 14 to 15, ampullary tubal activity is variable, delaying ovum transport for approximately 72 hours. The size of the cumulus mass and the narrowing diameter of the ampulla (1 mm) may further facilitate this arrest of the ovum at the AIJ. In addition, the smaller percentage of ciliated cells in the isthmus region may diminish prouterine flow.

Sperm transport is through a combination of self-propulsion, retrograde myometrial contractions, pro-ovarian contractions in the interstitial and isthmic segments of the oviducts, and oviductal secretions. Although after ejaculation the largest concentration of sperm are held in the cervix and high concentrations are found in the uterus, the number of sperm reaching the ampullary region is approximately 200. The relatively consistent numbers of sperm reaching the ampulla was shown by Ahlgren to persist during a period of 2 to 34 hours after sexual intercourse. However, in women with hydrosalpinges, many thousands of sperm were seen (47). The mechanisms of constancy in the normal oviduct are not well understood, but additional observations do support tubal factors, which regulate sperm transport.

Although the average ejaculate holds 280 million sperm, it is now understood that sperm after entry into the oviduct are distributed in two ways. First, a few are rapidly transported to the ampullary region, and sperm can be found there as soon as 6 minutes after coitus. The second phase of sperm transport involves retention of most of the spermatozoa in the proximal isthmus until about the time of ovulation with concomitant suppression of capacitation and the acrosome reaction (48,49). Oviductal secretions and binding to isthmic endosalpingeal cells may further play a role in retention of sperm in the isthmus until ovulation (50,51). Capacitation of spermatozoa followed by hyperactivated motility occurs after a period of retention in the oviduct. Only after capacitation can the sperm bind and penetrate the zona pellucida and achieve fertilization.

Oviductal Transport of the Early Embryo

Concurrent with ovulation, sperm are released from the isthmus into the ampulla and fertilize the ova. The human ova/zygote/embryo stays in the ampulla about 72 hours, rapidly crosses the oviductal isthmus, and reaches the uterus at about 80 hours after ovulation. Entry into the uterine cavity occurs at the 7-to 12-cell stage, which corresponds with 2 to 3 days after ovulation based on IVF cleavage rates (52,53). As discussed earlier, a combination of ciliary, hormonal, muscular, and electrical changes coordinate to allow the early embryo to travel through the isthmus into the uterus. As shown in Fig. 16.2, by cycle day 18, the predominant direction of flow from the AIJ is prouterine. In addition, the cumulus mass dissolution allows the early embryo to pass through the narrow isthmus and the interstitial region of the tube at 100 μm. No consensus exists on

how the embryo is rapidly transported to the uterus through the isthmus and interstitial segments of the oviduct after about a 2- to 3-day retention period in the ampulla. A combination of passive and active factors likely integrates to achieve this end: dissipation of the cumulus mass, relaxation of the tubal musculature, localized myoelectrical activity, and changing levels of estrogen, progesterone, prostaglandins, and other tubal and embryonic secretions.

INFECTIOUS CAUSES OF OVIDUCTAL DISEASE

A causal relationship between infectious agents and tubal disease has long been established. The sequelae of tubal infections have included infertility, PID, pelvic pain, and ectopic pregnancy. Tuboperitoneal factors may be responsible for up to 50% of female infertility, and, specifically, tubal disease may represent as much as 30% of female infertility.

Pelvic Inflammatory Disease

Classically, *Chlamydia trachomatis* and *Neisseria gonorrhoeae* lead to a polymicrobial infection resulting in what is called *PID*. Other less common causes have included various anaerobic bacteria, staphylococci, streptococci, coliform bacilli, and, rarely, Herpes simplex virus. Typically, these pathogens infect the oviducts by hematogenous or lymphatic spread and invade from the serosa to the muscularis. Although uncommon, they can be responsible for a case of PID associated with a procedure or a delivery.

In contrast, chlamydial and gonorrheal infections ascend through the endocervix and uterine cavity to the endosalpinx and result in salpingitis. *N. gonorrhoeae* is a major cause of acute and chronic salpingitis and is known to invade and spread along the mucosal surface. However, in the United States, chlamydia may be responsible for the majority of the cases of PID. Marana et al. found that infertility patients having normal-appearing tubes had a high prevalence of chlamydial colonization of the oviductal mucosa (54). Of 34 patients with negative history and a normal pelvis, 6 had isolates of chlamydia in at least one oviduct. Another study found 15% of patients with tubal factor infertility had positive chlamydial cultures (55). Even with a negative culture, there has been well-documented evidence of a prior chlamydial infection. Anestad et al. compared women having tubal disease and negative cultures for chlamydia with pregnant controls. The prevalence of immunoglobulin G (IgG) IgG and IgM antibodies for chlamydia was found to be significantly higher in the infertility group (56).

PID can be classified into three groups: acute, chronic, or a granulomatous inflammatory response. Oviductal damage is a major sequela of PID, resulting in infertility and ectopic pregnancy. As stated previously, ascending infections are the most common cause of PID; however, other causes include postoperative, postprocedural, and puerperal infections, as well as secondary infection from appendicitis or TB. Only 40% of women having tubal factor infertility with evidence of previous intraperitoneal inflammation have a history of PID (57). The effects of recurrent PID can be devastating and underline the need for aggressive treatment in those at risk or with a positive history. In a large retrospective study of 415 women with known PID, the incidence of tubal obstruction after their first, second, and third episode of PID was 13%, 35%, and 75%, respectively (58). After only a single episode of PID, there was a 6-fold increased risk of extrauterine pregnancy with a 20% rate of infertility (58). This increased risk of ectopic pregnancy was confirmed in a prospective cohort of patients with PID (59).

At laparoscopy, acutely infected oviducts grossly appear edematous and inflamed. If the condition is severe, purulent exudate is often found at the fimbrial end. The infection may incorporate the adjacent ovary to become a tuboovarian abscess, which is potentially a life-threatening condition. Microscopically, gonococcal salpingitis is characterized as an infiltrate of polymorphonuclear leukocytes that begins in the epithelial plicae, extends into the lumen, and leads to a purulent exudate. Fibrin and sloughed mucosal epithelium may be found within the lumen. The resulting pyosalpinx reveals a transmural inflammatory reaction with a marked decrease in wall thickness. The cellular components of the exudate eventually include both lymphocytes and plasma cells in the lumen. Nongonococcal salpingitis is similar to the gonococcal variety, except a purulent exudate is absent. As expected by its mode of infection, nongonococcal salpingitis reveals a perivascular infiltrate with a resulting serosal inflammatory response. There is extension into the muscularis in severe cases; however, the mucosa is rarely involved.

The true prevalence of chronic or, more accurately, subclinical salpingitis is difficult to determine. Both the patient and the gross appearance of the oviduct may appear completely normal, as demonstrated in Fig. 16.3. Previously infected oviducts display readily recognized histologic changes such as flattened mucosal plicae, degenerated secretory cells, decreased ciliary beat frequency, and deciliation (Fig. 16.4). These findings are present in patients with overt and silent PID (57). The deciliatory effects of both gonorrhea and chlamydial infection have been well documented, whereas *Mycoplasma hominis* has been shown to have a direct ciliostatic effect (60,61). Clinical studies suggest that both the number and quality of cilia are of critical importance to future fecundity. Vasquez et al. reported no conceptions when the fimbriae contained fewer than than 54% cilia and also noted that marked deciliation occurs after tubal sterilization and ectopic pregnancy (62). Therefore, deciliation is a common pathologic finding in all inflammatory tubal responses. Although, the exact mechanism is still unknown, cytokines are likely to play a role in these adverse effects on the oviductal epithelium.

Tuberculosis

Other infectious causes, such as the tubercle bacillus, can also result in significant tubal damage. *TB* is usually the result of *Mycobacterium tuberculosis* or, occasionally, *M. bovis*. This mycobacterium is an obligate aerobe, replicating in approximately 24 hours, recognized by its acid-fast staining, and typically involving the respiratory system as the primary site of infection. Oviduct involvement occurs by hematogenous spread in more than half the cases, although a descending lymphatic infection is also possible (63). A primary genital infection is rare (64), as is sexual transmission of the disease.

Tuberculous salpingitis only accounts for 1% of tubal factor infertility in the United States, compared with 5% to 10% in developing countries around the world (65). The decrease of TB in the United States has been attributed to both screening and aggressive treatment of the disease (66); however, some investigators believe that the incidence may increase as immigrants arrive from developing countries (67). The chronic granulomatous inflammation that results from TB affects the endosalpinx, myosalpinx, and serosa. Genital TB involves both oviducts more than 90% of the time, with the endometrium involved more than 50% of the time, followed by the ovaries and the cervix (68). TB has a tendency to infect the endometrium and the oviduct by hematogenous spread. A progressive infection starts in the mucosa and proceeds to the muscularis and then to the serosa.

An infected oviduct may look normal or slightly edematous, but in as many as half the cases of genital TB, the oviducts are rigid, thickened, and patent, with everted fimbriae and a distended ampulla (69,70). The intramural and isthmic segments may remain unaffected, or both may resemble salpingitis isthmica nodosa (SIN) with nodules within the wall. However, PTO with intratubal adhesions is not uncommon. The ampulla reveals the earliest signs of infections and has the most severe pathologic changes (71). The fimbria is usually spared with or without peritubal adhesions (67). Because of the extensive and transmural nature of granulomatous salpingitis, tubal repair carries a poor prognosis with a risk of reactivation of the infection (72).

The acute phase of TB salpingitis results from the coalescing of the caseated granulomas to form a pyosalpinx (66). The oviduct is enlarged and mobile, and it contains both caseous material and purulent exudate that results from a secondary infection. The oviduct may resemble a "tobacco pouch" because of the saclike distention of the pyosalpinx. Later in its course, chronic TB salpingitis is characterized by oviducts with multiple nodules on their serosal surface near the mesosalpinx border. The oviductal wall is thick-

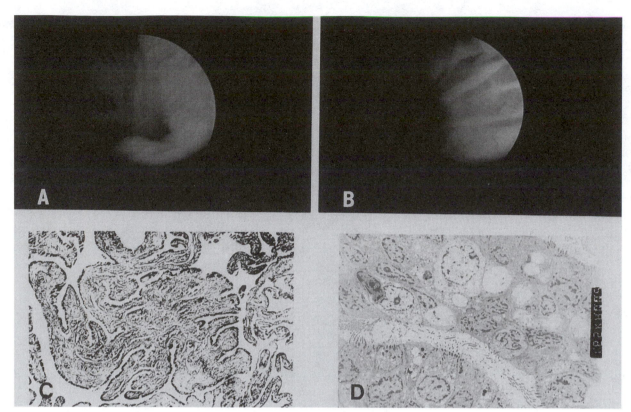

FIGURE 16.3. Normal fallopian tube. Salpingoscopy reveals normal-looking mucosa in the ampullary **(A)** and infundibular **(B)** regions. A thin section of the ampulla **(C)**, embedded in epoxy and stained by hematoxylin and eosin (×8), shows normal ciliated endosalpinx. Electron microscopy **(D)** shows evidence of normal homogeneous cytoplasm, abundant mitochondria, columnar-shaped cells, normal nuclei, and a normal complement of cilia. (From Hershlag A, Seifer D, Carcangiu ML, et al. Salpingoscopy: light microscopic and electron microscopic correlations. *Obstet Gynecol* 1991;77:339–405. Reprinted from the American Society for Reproductive Medicine, with permission.)

ened, nodular, and contains calcified granulomas. In addition, one usually sees dense adhesions involving the oviduct and the adnexa. This chronic form of TB has become more common because of the early recognition and treatment of the disease.

Microscopically, the oviduct reveals classic tuberculous granulomas and a chronic inflammatory infiltrate composed of mainly lymphocytes. Epitheloid cells and multinucleated giant Langhans' cells are commonly seen. Histologic examination demonstrates an extensive, full-thickness involvement of the oviduct. Some of the tubercles may undergo what is called *caseation necrosis*. After developing a caseous center, the tubercles liquefy and coalesce to form a pyosalpinx. The mucosal epithelium overlying these areas is destroyed and develops ulcers composed of granulation tissue surrounded by a pyogenic membrane. The tubal epithelium may also reveal edematous proliferation so complex that it may be confused with adenocarcinoma (69,70). As the oviduct heals, characteristic calcium deposits appear, and there is increased hyalinization and fibrosis. The pathophysiology is unique, and the following findings on hysterosalpingogram (HSG) are strongly predictive of granulomatous salpingitis: midampullary occlusions appearing as a rosette, a pipelike isthmic region with or without diverticulum, a beaded appearance of the lumen with dilation alternating with stenosis, intratubal adhesions, possibly calcified pelvic lymph nodes, and intrauterine synechiae (74).

Nontubercular Granulomatous Disease

Other less common causes of granulomatous disease that involve the oviduct include infections with *Actinomyces israelii, Schistosoma haematobium,* sarcoidosis, inflammatory bowel disease, and *Enterobius vermicularis* infection. A foreign body reaction to mineral oil and, more recently, talc has been implicated as well in granulomatous salpingitis. The pathophysiology of these disorders is similar to that of tuberculous salpingitis.

Actinomyces israelii is an anaerobic organism that typically inhabits the entire gastrointestinal tract to include the oral cavity. Salpingitis from *Actinomyces* infection is rare (74), and it may occur after a procedure such as insertion of an intrauterine device (75). The pelvic infection typically involves the adnexa, with a proclivity for the right side (76). The purulent exudate contains the well-described sulfur granules appearing as small yellow specks composed of colo-

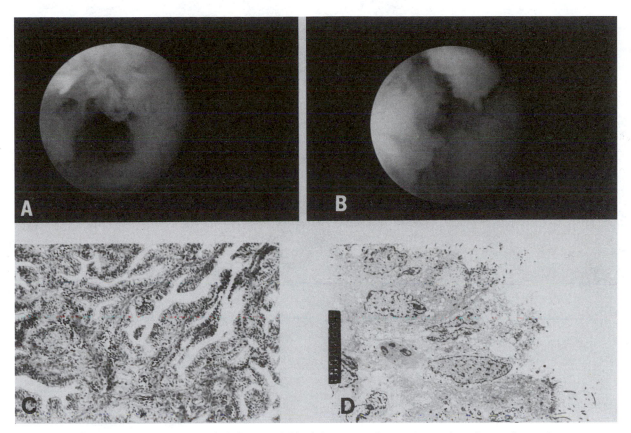

FIGURE 16.4. Moderate tubal disease. Rigid salpingoscopy shows attenuation of ampullary epithelial folds **(A)** with absence of secondary folds and widening of spaces between the primary folds **(B)**. Histologic examination **(C)** of the infundibulum of the same tube shows evidence of conglutination and muscular hypertrophy of the fimbrial stalk (hematoxylin and eosin, ×8). On electron microscopy **(D)**, the epithelial cells are cuboidal, with sparse numbers of cilia per cell. The nuclei are swollen, and large vacuoles are present. (From Hershlag A, Seifer D, Carcangiu ML, et al. Salpingoscopy: light microscopic and electron microscopic correlations. Obstet Gynecol 1991;77:339–405. Reprinted from the American Society for Reproductive Medicine, with permission.)

nies of *Actinomyces.* The granules have a dense woven pattern in their center, and toward the periphery the filaments are radiant. Unlike in TB, caseation necrosis does not occur.

Again, rarely seen in the United States, *schistosomiasis* is common in other parts of the world (77). *Schistosoma haematobium* infection involves the pelvic organs by way of hematogenous spread. In this case, the ova deposited in the veins cause the granulomatous reaction. The oviduct may appear normal or nodular because of a fibrotic reaction that results from an acute infection.

Pinworm or *Enterobius vermicularis* infestation results from an ascending infection of the lower genital tract. Fibrous nodules result from both the ova and the organism itself (78). Both can be identified within the granulomatous nodules usually surrounded by lymphocytes and eosinophils. Foreign body giant cells and Charcot-Leyden crystals can also be identified.

Sarcoidosis is a systemic disease that primarily infects the respiratory system and rarely causes salpingitis. *Inflammatory bowel disease,* specifically Crohn's disease, has also been reported to cause salpingitis (79). Various substances have

been noted to elicit a foreign body granulomatous reaction. *Contrast media (oil-based media), talc, and lubricants* have all been implicated. The appearance of the oviduct in this type of granulomatous salpingitis is much like the others. Microscopically, in addition to the multinucleated giant cells, one may also see foamy histiocytes when oil-based media are used.

COMMON SEQUELAE OF PELVIC INFLAMMATORY DISEASE

Adhesions

In addition to the effects on the cilia, more advanced PID may also result in *tubal obstruction* and *peritubal adhesions* (Fig. 16.5). Obviously, adhesions that restrict tubal mobility or prevent fimbrial-ovarian contact can result in infertility. These adhesions may be filmy and easily resected or dense and vascular, encasing the entire adnexa. A few studies have proposed a prospective scoring system that is based on tubal wall thickness, extent and character of adhesions, and

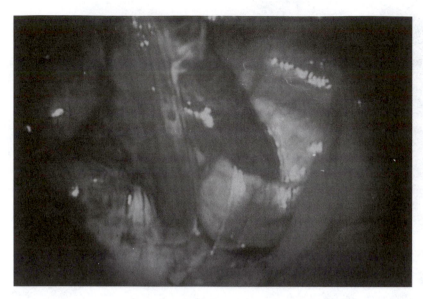

FIGURE 16.5. Peritubal adhesions. Filmy adhesions encase the fimbria and ovary.

percentage of ciliated cells, to determine future fecundity (80,81). However, other than these crude physical and radiographic observations, there remains no diagnostic test of oviductal function.

As stated earlier, the assessment of tubal function has been primarily from direct visualization of the outside of the tube or by imaging the interior tubal architecture by HSG. Beginning in the 1980s, the first attempt was made to visualize the tubal mucosa directly by salpingoscopy at the time of laparotomy or laparoscopy as demonstrated in Fig. 16.3 (82). Later in the decade, Kerin was the first to pioneer the transcervical approach known as *falloposcopy* (83). Falloposcopy provides readily available, atraumatic, minimally invasive, and direct visualization of the entire tubal lumen. With advancing technology, transcervical cannulation of the fallopian tube using a linear everting catheter is now possible in an office setting. This system uses a 0.5-mm falloposcope, with a magnification of 40 that is guided to the tubal lumen by the everting catheter, which does not require hysteroscopy or use of an anesthetic (84). A prospective study comparing the linear everting falloposcope with conventional HSG found that the falloposcope provided more complete information on tubal disorders in 40% of the cases (85). At some point in the near future, this novel falloposcopy system may replace HSG in the evaluation of the fallopian tube.

Hydrosalpinx

As discussed earlier, chronic salpingitis may result in normal-appearing oviducts or in more involved cases, fibrous adhesions that may be both intraluminal and extraluminal. Severe cases cause the oviduct to be grossly abnormal and to appear as a distended, thin-walled, translucent cystic structure. As the pyosalpinx undergoes fibrin deposition, the fimbriae become completely fused, creating a distal

obstruction. Over time, the purulent exudate is replaced with a clear transudate resulting in a *hydrosalpinx* (Fig. 16.6). On a microscopic level, the acute inflammatory response is replaced with lymphocytes and plasma cells, consistent with a chronic inflammation. The plicae of the oviduct become shortened with a fibrous stroma, and the epithelium also becomes shortened, more cuboidal, and deciliated (86–88). A patient may have a simple single cavity hydrosalpinx or a multicystic structure formed by the adhesion of the plicae folds to each other. Microsurgery can restore tubal patency in more than 75% of hydrosalpinges; however, the resulting intrauterine pregnancy rate is only 10% to 35% (89). The establishment of normal ciliary function of the epithelial cells plays an important role in the success of corrective tubal surgery (90,91). Distal tubal disease with decreased ciliary function can result in poor cumulus mass retrieval by the fimbria and poor containment and transport by the ampulla. Additionally, fibrous adhesions that limit tubo-ovarian mobility, reduce ovarian surface area, and compromise ovulatory function can negatively affect normal oviductal function.

Although deciliation and a decreased percentage of ciliated cells have been well documented in hydrosalpinges, other investigators have reported a normal percentage of ciliated cells (92). There may be a certain amount of time required for the epithelial cells to regenerate their cilia, or possibly the cilia present function abnormally. No one has examined the oviducts in women who have had an intrauterine pregnancy after tubal surgery for the presence or function of the ciliated cells. One study documented a lack of cilia in women who did not conceive in more than a year (81). Attempts have been made to create an animal model of a hydrosalpinx. Distal ligation of the rabbit oviduct resulted in flattening of the plicae, but no change in ciliation or ovum transport in the ampullae (93). In oviducts that were ligated both proximally and distally, deciliation oc-

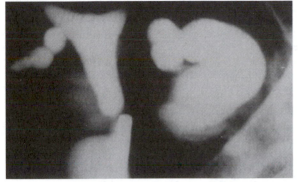
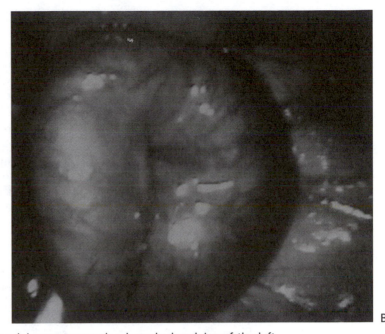

A   B

FIGURE 16.6. Hydrosalpinx. **A:** A hysterosalpingogram reveals a large hydrosalpinx of the left oviduct. Note the absence of mucosal folds and the distal occlusion. **B:** At laparoscopy, the oviduct appears dilated and thin walled, with prominent vascularity.

curred, along with the expected loss of mucosal plicae (94,95). Other investigators have documented more subtle changes in the oviduct such as loss of adrenergic enervation and a decrease in both estrogen and progesterone receptors (96,97). In the animal models, neosalpingostomy resulted in the regeneration of the ciliated cells, and this was enhanced by estrogen treatment. Unfortunately, it would be almost impossible to confirm these results in the human oviduct. We can speculate that neosalpingostomies and the endogenous estrogen levels in women may result in normal oviductal function in some patients with hydrosalpinx. However, many unanswered questions remain. How long should one wait before attempting to conceive after reparative tubal surgery or an ectopic pregnancy? Does the length of time between the formation of a hydrosalpinx and subsequent repair affect the outcome?

Hydrosalpinx and In Vitro *Fertilization*

In the age of ART, a controversy has emerged on the effect of hydrosalpinges on IVF success rates. Some investigators have hypothesized that hydrosalpinx fluid could leak into the uterine cavity and could result in decreased endometrial receptivity or direct embryo toxicity or could simply interfere with embryo endometrial interaction (98). In patients with documented hydrosalpinges, endometrial cavity fluid has been demonstrated before embryo transfer during IVF (99). This fluid is mostly a serous transudate having low protein and bicarbonate concentrations and electrolyte concentrations similar to those of serum (100). Other factors, such as potential embryo or endometrial toxins, have yet to

be identified. Multiple retrospective studies in the literature have compared the effects of hydrosalpinges on IVF implantation and pregnancy rates (101–112). All but one study demonstrated a significant decrease in implantation and pregnancy rates (107). However, until a randomized prospective study with proper controls is performed, the question will remain unanswered. Are the hydrosalpinges that form during controlled ovarian hyperstimulation more significant than those noted at baseline? How can one determine whether a hydrosalpinx is communicating, and must fluid be in the uterine cavity at the time of embryo transfer for it to have an effect? The answers to these questions remain speculative.

In vitro models have included mouse embryo culture systems, examination of markers of implantation, and cytotrophoblast culture systems. Although an embryotoxic effect has been demonstrated in a mouse embryo culture system, this cannot be extrapolated to human embryos at the time of implantation (113). One study examined the effect of hydrosalpinges on markers of endometrial receptivity (114). These investigators prospectively compared the expression of $\alpha_v\beta_3$ integrin in 103 women with hydrosalpinges to 55 infertile and 44 fertile controls. There was significantly less expression of $\alpha_v\beta_3$ integrin in those patients with hydrosalpinges when compared with both control groups. These investigators were also able to demonstrate a 70% increase in expression of $\alpha_v\beta_3$ integrin after corrective tubal surgery. These findings are in agreement with another study reporting that hydrosalpinx fluid actually increased human trophoblast production of β-human chorionic gonadotropin (β-hCG) and trophouteronectin, a protein important in implantation (115). Therefore, decreased endometrial receptivity may play more of a role than embryotoxicity in lowering embryo implantation rates. To make a statement that all patients undergoing IVF with hydrosalpinges require salpingectomies would be premature at this time. A prudent course would be to counsel patients objectively and to make decisions regarding salpingectomy on a case-by-case basis.

Ectopic Pregnancy

The incidence of ectopic pregnancies has increased dramatically over the last 20 years, probably because of an increased prevalence of PID and better diagnostic modalities (116,117). Conversely, mortality has decreased as a result of improved diagnosis and treatment. As many as 95% of ectopic pregnancies occur in the oviducts, and, as indicated earlier, these pregnancies are a common sequela of salpingitis. In one large series of ectopic pregnancies, the most common histologic finding was chronic salpingitis (118). Both medical treatment and conservative surgery have resulted in excellent tubal patency rates; however, recurrence rates remain significant (119,120). A key factor may be the normal function of the ciliated epithelial cells. Studies have revealed that both deciliation and a decrease in cell height occur in oviducts containing ectopic pregnancies (121,122). One important question is this: Is there a certain time frame in which the oviductal epithelium needs to heal from an ectopic pregnancy, or is the resulting damage permanent? Obviously, any oviductal damage resulting in difficulty in retrieving or transporting the oocyte may lead to an ectopic pregnancy.

The damage may be related to tubal surgery, endometriosis, PID, intrauterine devices, DES exposure, SIN, or unexplained infertility. Women with ciliary dysfunction, such as in Kartagener's syndrome, are not infertile and do not have a higher incidence of ectopic pregnancy (123). Other postulated causes of ectopic pregnancies are abnormalities in myoelectric contractility and an imbalance between estrogen and progesterone levels. Advanced reproductive age has been known to be a risk factor for ectopic pregnancies. Myosalpinx contractility was noted to be impaired in postmenopausal women (124). An embryo may become trapped in the ampullae if the isthmic region of the oviduct is unable to transport it to the uterine cavity. One study noted the absence of myoelectric activity in the oviductal region containing the ectopic gestation, whereas the other oviductal contractility occurred toward the ectopic from both directions. One possible explanation is that progesterone secreted locally from the placenta may induce tubal relaxation by activation of the β receptors (125). This effect of progesterone can be reversed by the injection of $PGF_{2\alpha}$, a stimulant of tubal contractility, which resulted in the termination of the ectopic pregnancy (126). The high serum levels of estrogens may be responsible for the myoelectric activation elsewhere in the oviduct by activation on the α receptors

in the myosalpinx. Others have postulated that the myoelectric dysfunction is simply the result of mechanical stretch at the dilated segment (127). Each abnormality may have some role in the overall pathophysiology of ectopic pregnancies.

Oviductal diverticulum, specifically SIN, has been postulated as a predisposing factor for ectopic pregnancy. Several studies have shown that in as many as half the oviducts with ectopic pregnancies, SIN is found in the isthmic regions compared with only 5% in control oviducts (128–130). Ectopic pregnancies are located in the ampullary segment of the oviduct in as many as 80% of the cases, as demonstrated in Fig. 16.7 (131). Many hypotheses have been offered on why this is the case. The embryo is delayed, it may be too large for transport through the isthmic region, the ampullae may be more receptive to implantation than the muscular isthmic region, or myoelectrical transport through the isthmic region is dysfunctional. The last possibility may be the result of SIN and may thereby predispose the ampullae to a large percentage of ectopic pregnancies.

SIN is known to be mainly a disease of the proximal oviduct, affecting the isthmic region 63% of the time and the proximal ampullary region 37% of the time (129). The isthmus becomes fibrotic and hypertrophied by SIN, with a resulting loss of contractility (132,133). Therefore, the embryo is unable to be transported to the uterine cavity, and a functional block results. Once the embryo has reached the blastocyst stage, implantation is likely to occur in the proximal ampullae. However, the isthmic region of the oviduct is the next most common location for an ectopic pregnancy.

This condition may represent an isthmic segment that is only partially damaged, which results in the blastocyst's being trapped there. Rarely, ectopic pregnancies occur in the cornual or interstitial segments of the oviduct and can invade the thick muscularis to become extraluminal. The incidence of underlying disease in patients with these ectopic pregnancies is relatively high, and a follow-up HSG is recommended to rule out SIN.

Linear salpingostomies by operative laparoscopy have now become the operative treatment of choice for almost all tubal ectopic pregnancies. Although recurrent ectopic risks are significant at around 12% to 16%, the intrauterine pregnancy rate is greater than 50% (134–139). This would indicate that the oviduct is capable of regaining normal function. One study revealed that ciliary transport is preserved and ampullary architecture was near normal (140). Some investigators have advocated segmental resection and anastomosis for isthmic ectopic pregnancies as a result from the high probability of SIN, but linear salpingostomies in this region have been reported to be successful. More and more patients with ectopic pregnancies are treated with methotrexate, and resulting patency and pregnancy rates have been good (141–144). However, the effect on oviduc-

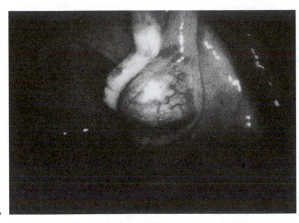
A

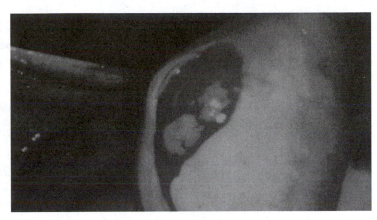
B

FIGURE 16.7. **A:** An ampullary ectopic pregnancy at the time of laparoscopy. **B:** A linear salpingostomy along the antimesenteric border revealing the ectopic gestation within the lumen.

tal physiology after methotrexate treatment remains unknown.

Methotrexate protocols using a single dose (50 mg per meter square of body surface area given intramuscularly) have been more widely adopted than multiple doses by practitioners. Single dose is less expensive, associated with fewer side effects and requires less intensive monitoring than multiple dose. Serum chorionic gonadotropin levels are measured on days 1, 4, and 7. If chorionic gonadotropin levels decline less than 15% between days 4 and 7, the protocol is repeated. When levels decline by 15% or more between days 4 and 7, serum chorionic gonadotropin is measured weekly until levels are less than 15 mlU/ml. Approximately 20% of women require more than one cycle of treatment of methotrexate. Time to resolution (less than 15 mlU/ml) is approximately 35 to 42 days. Approximately 25% of treated women will have self-limiting abdominal pain 4 to 7 days after receiving an initial dose of methotrexate, most likely due to either tubal abortion or stretching of the fallopian tube by hematoma. Although short term success (resolution of the ectopic pregnancy) is comparable to surgery, long-term pregnancy rates have yet to be compared with salpingostomy in a large randomized trial.

Persistent Ectopic Pregnancy

With the advent of conservative surgical and medical treatments for ectopic pregnancies, a relatively new complication of persistent ectopic pregnancy (PEP) has emerged. The reported rate of PEP after conservative surgical treatment has varied from 3% to 20% (145), whereas the reported rate of PEP after salpingectomy or conservative surgery by laparotomy is much lower (146). Several possible explanations have been offered for this observed higher PEP rate in the conservative treatment group. These include the "milking" of a distal ectopic pregnancy from the end of the tube, failure to explore and evacuate the medial segment of the tube, performance of the surgical procedure before

7 weeks' estimated gestational age, a more sensitive quantitative β-hCG assay, use of mechanical removal techniques instead of a pressure irrigator, and failure to irrigate the entire abdominal cavity thoroughly (145).

The most accepted method of diagnosing a PEP is to obtain weekly quantitative β-hCG determinations. If the level plateaus or increases, the diagnosis is made. Whether the patient is symptomatic or not is not important, as long as the patient has a nonsurgical abdomen and is hemodynamically stable. Methotrexate, administered intramuscularly at 50 mg/m^2, has become the mainstay for treatment of a PEP; a cumulative pregnancy rate of 59% at 36 months was reported in one study in which 32 patients attempted to become pregnant after treatment (147). One randomized prospective trial examined the efficacy of prophylactic methotrexate (1 mg/kg) given within the first 24 hours after salpingostomy and found that the incidence of PEP was decreased from 14.5% in the controls to 1.9% in the treatment group (148). The side effects were reported to be mild, occurring in only 5% of those treated and resolving spontaneously. In an attempt to predict patients who would require methotrexate, Spandorfer et al. reported that there were no cases of PEP when the first postoperative β-hCG declined by 77% or more when compared with the initial preoperative value (149), although a decrease of less then 50% on postoperative day 1 carried a 3.51 relative risk of PEP. Regardless of which conservative treatment modality was offered to the patient, the physician is obliged to follow the quantitative β-hCG value to undetectable levels and to encourage patient compliance.

NONINFECTIOUS OVIDUCTAL DISEASE

Endometriosis

The relationship between *endometriosis* and oviductal function remains controversial. In the severe form of the disease, dense fibrous adhesions can result in tubal obstruction or torsion or restriction of tubal motility, or they can completely engulf the ovary. The controversy lies in the effects of minimal or mild cases of endometriosis. The incidence of endometriosis is approximately 10% of women of the reproductive age, and it may be present in as many as one-third of all infertile women. One hypothesis for mild endometriosis as a cause of oviductal dysfunction is that an inflammatory reaction takes place (150). Other investigators have not found an association between an inflammatory reaction and endometriosis (151). However, endometriosis may result in other subtle changes in oviductal ciliation or fluid composition. One study revealed that peritoneal fluid from women with endometriosis contained a protein called ovum capture inhibitor that prevented cumulus-fimbrial interaction (152).

Chronic endometriosis results in a fibrous reaction that leads to scarring and adhesion formation. Active endometriosis on the serosal surface appears much like the classic lesions elsewhere in the pelvis. The lesion may be blue, black, red, or clear and may appear as small, raised spots about 0.5 cm in diameter. Microscopically, the serosal lesion contains the classically described endometrial glands surrounded by endometrial stroma with small blood vessels. The scarred lesions contain fibrin deposition, hemosiderin-laden macrophages, and residual endometrial glands and stroma. The disease process typically spares the muscularis and the fimbria.

Endometriosis may also involve the mucosal surface of the oviduct, especially the isthmic region. PTO results from endometriosis approximately 10% of the time (153–156). Corrective surgery by tubocornual anastomosis resulted in a poor pregnancy rate of 0% to 12% when compared with a pregnancy rate of 40% for other causes of PTO (154,156). At 1 year after surgery, more than 50% of the operated oviducts were reoccluded, perhaps in part because of surgical technique, but recurrence of the endometriosis is probable. Other investigators have shown improved pregnancy rates that correlate with final tubal length by performing a wide excision of the affected segment (157,158). A tubal ligation may protect some women from developing or worsening their endometriosis, but it leaves the proximal stump at risk for disease (159,160). The incidence of proximal tubal disease in these patients increases from the time of sterilization (161).

Salpingitis Isthmica Nodosa

SIN is described as nodular thickening in the isthmic segment of the oviduct, in which diverticula lined by mucosal epithelium penetrate the myosalpinx. SIN was first described in the late 18th century by Chiari (162), and it has been implicated in up to 5% of cases of female infertility. The disease can be bilateral or unilateral, affecting mainly women of reproductive age (129,163). SIN is rarely found in premenopausal girls or postmenopausal women

(164,165). In a retrospective series, the prevalence was increased in African Americans and Jamaicans (128). In advanced SIN, the isthmic nodularity and periglandular hypertrophy of the muscularis result in fibrosis and ultimately proximal obstruction.

As mentioned in the previous section, SIN has been strongly associated with *ectopic pregnancies;* approximately 50% of patients with ectopic pregnancies have documented SIN versus only 1% of fertile controls at the time of tubal sterilization (129,166). In PTO, SIN is reported to occur in 23% to 60% of cases (155,156,167,168). Reports have varied on the location and percentage of bilateral disease; however, most cases appear to be bilateral and occupy the isthmic region of the oviduct (163). Rarely is only the distal segment or entire oviduct involved (129).

Microscopically, one sees multiple randomly spaced nodules containing structures with a glandular appearance throughout the muscularis. Typically, the communication between the diverticula and the oviductal lumen is not seen (Fig. 16.8); however, serial sections reveal the connection in most cases (129). The nodularity results from both hyperplasia and hypertrophy of the muscularis surrounding the glandlike structures. The epithelium is composed of few ciliated cells and low columnar to cuboidal cells, identical to those seen in the oviductal lumen. Similar to endometriosis are the endometrial-like stromal cells that occupy areas near the diverticula; however, endometriosis can be easily excluded by the identification of oviductal epithelium in the glandlike structures. There appears to be no relation between the two disease processes.

Other similar histologic processes that are related to SIN include *endosalpingiosis* and endosalpingoblastosis. In the former, the oviductal epithelium lines a simple cyst and does not have the hyperplastic smooth muscle, as seen in SIN. *Endosalpingoblastosis* has been used to describe diverticula within the myosalpinx after tubal ligation by electrocautery. Although the glandlike structures are lined by oviductal epithelium, again they lack the reactive hypertrophy in the smooth muscle. Still other investigators maintain that these are not distinct processes (154).

The exact cause of SIN is unknown, but the condition is believed to be acquired. Postulated causes include congenital, as in DES exposure (169), hormonal (170,171), mechanical (132), and inflammatory (129,153,155,171). An infectious origin is strongly supported by the literature based on histologic, serologic, and historical data. In a series of women with obstructive SIN, all had histologic evidence of chronic inflammation, and almost half had high antibody titers to chlamydia (172). Other investigators have documented a history of prior pelvic infection and histologic evidence that is characteristic of chronic inflammation in patients with SIN (155). Although the evidence for an infectious origin is strong, hormonal and mechanical factors may still play a role.

On HSG, the finding of multiple diverticula giving a

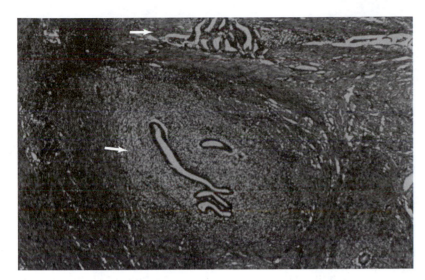

FIGURE 16.8. Salpingitis isthmica nodosa. Cross section through the isthmus demonstrating the relatively few plicae in the lumen (*bottom arrow*). The diverticula are readily visible and are separated by broad bands of smooth muscle (*top arrow*).

honeycombed appearance in the isthmic region of the oviduct is essentially diagnostic for SIN (Fig. 16.9). Other conditions with similar radiographic findings include endosalpingiosis, TB, oviductal endometriosis, and dye extravasation. The incidence of SIN on HSG is approximately 4% (173). At hysteroscopy, SIN has been associated with endosalpingeal hyperplasia of the oviductal ostium (174). Laparoscopically, the diagnosis can be made by observing indurations and nodular thickening of the isthmus. Typically, the serosal surface is smooth and intact, and it reveals the diverticula on chromotubation.

The standard treatment for SIN has been segmental resection with a tubocornual anastomosis. Although this operation is not routinely performed, several studies have recommended performing a tubocornual anastomosis when the diagnosis is made (132,166,175–177). The reasoning

behind this recommendation is the high incidence of both infertility and ectopic pregnancy in patients with documented SIN (132,166). Also of importance is the progressive nature of SIN, which, in some cases, can lead to complete proximal occlusion in as little as 1 year (178). Success rates after microsurgical tubocornual anastomosis are encouraging, with a 57.7% pregnancy rate and a 15% ectopic pregnancy rate in a series with PTO (176). When SIN was identified as the cause of the PTO, similar success rates were reported (175,177). SIN is associated with documented oviductal disease and significant morbidity. The disease process is progressive and is probably hormonally driven; however, the inciting cause is most likely infectious. Those patients with a history of infertility, sexually transmitted disease, or ectopic pregnancy should undergo prompt investigation with HSG.

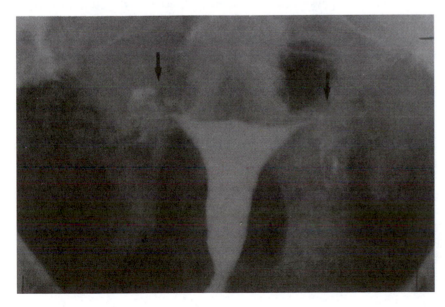

FIGURE 16.9. A hysterosalpingogram that reveals the characteristic radiographic findings of salpingitis isthmica nodosa. The honeycombed appearance (*arrows*) is readily visible in the isthmic region.

Transcervical Tubal Cannulation

The treatment of PTO that does not result from SIN can be achieved by one of several outpatient techniques. The most common are fluoroscopically controlled transcervical tubal cannulation (TCTC) and hysteroscopic TCTC. Other less commonly performed TCTC techniques include ultrasonographic, tactile control, and the newer procedure of operative falloposcopy (179). Patency and cumulative pregnancy rates have been reported to be 75% and 50%, respectively; however, no prospective randomized controlled trials have been conducted. When compared with tubal resection and primary anastomosis, TCTC had similar pregnancy rates but a much lower ectopic pregnancy rate (180). A study by Ransom and Garcia evaluated 43 patients with documented bilateral PTO at laparoscopy but otherwise normal-appearing tubes (181). All patients underwent attempted TCTC, and those not demonstrating patency underwent microsurgical resection and anastomosis. The cumulative pregnancy rate for the 22 patients who had successful TCTC was 68% versus 56% for the 21 patients requiring resection and anastomosis after attempted TCTC. Of those patients who were conceiving, all were successful within the first year after their procedure. TCTC has also been used to recannulate patients with failed patency after a sterilization reversal procedure (182) and as a means of transferring gametes or embryos in ART (183). TCTC does appear to have a role in the treatment of unipolar PTO; however, its usefulness in other tubal conditions remains to be seen.

Endosalpingiosis

In 1930, Sampson described the presence of oviductal-type epithelium outside the tubal lumen as *endosalpingiosis* (184). The original article mainly referred to the outgrowth of mucosal epithelium into the operative side after a tubal ligation or salpingectomy. However, the term now applies to mucosal epithelium found anywhere on a peritoneal surface, and documented cases have included the tube, ovary, uterus, omentum, and bowel. Typically, a lesion appears as a small, clear cyst about 0.5 cm in diameter. Microscopically, the fluid-filled cyst is lined by oviductal mucosal epithelium. Ciliated cells are prominent, but all types are present.

The origin is unknown; however, mucosal epithelial sloughing after salpingitis and metaplasia of the mesothelium have both been postulated (185). As in SIN, endosalpingiosis has been associated with ectopic pregnancy. This disease is distinguished from SIN by the lack of the characteristic myosalpingeal hypertrophy found in SIN. Endosalpingiosis of the oviductal muscularis has been documented in ectopic pregnancies after tubal ligation of the isthmic region through electrocautery (186). Tuboperitoneal fistulas were noted in some of the cases, although it is unlikely that an embryo could pass through one of these defects to become lodged in the ampullae. In contrast, electrocautery of the more distal ampullary segment resulted only in fibrosis and not in endosalpingiosis. This finding supports thr performance of ampullary ligations or the use of nonelectrical modalities.

OVIDUCTAL FLUID

Since the advent of IVF, much time and money have been spent on the creation of *human tubal fluid* (HTF) as a culture medium for human embryos. HTF is basically a balanced salt solution (sodium chloride, potassium chloride), containing buffers (bicarbonate), an energy source (glucose, lactate, pyruvate), a protein source (maternal albumin), and antibiotics. To maintain proper pH and temperature, embryo culture dishes are placed in an incubator having both temperature and carbon dioxide control capabilities. As mentioned in the introduction, embryo implantation rates and IVF pregnancy rates have improved significantly over the last 10 years; however, a large excess of embryos must be grown in culture to select the best ones for transfer. Poor culture conditions can harm healthy embryos, but it is unclear what percentage of oocytes from a cohort of follicles is already destined to become poor-quality embryos. Regardless of this finding, efforts have been made to improve HTF culture media by adding various growth factors (187–189) or by coculturing with bovine oviductal epithelial cells (190), although some investigators have reported success by simply placing the embryos in groups (191,192). Whether oviductal fluid with its numerous proteins plays a crucial role in early embryo development remains unclear. Ectopic pregnancies, although rare, can occur completely outside the oviductal environment. Oviductal fluid may have a more important role in oviductal physiology and endometrial receptivity.

Oviductal fluid is composed of various salts and macromolecules, which vary in concentration along with the pH and the osmolality during the menstrual cycle (193). Many of the glycoproteins and various growth factors secreted by the oviductal epithelium show cycle variation and may depend on steroid hormones.

Examples include calbindin-D9K, a calcium transport protein, and epidermal growth factor (EGF), which are both regulated by changing estrogen levels. Other secreted factors can be regulated by the embryo itself, such as oviductal mitogen factor, which activates transcription, or by a disease process such as endometriosis. Ovum capture inhibitor is expressed by the fimbrial epithelial cells in women with endometriosis, and this may predispose these patients to infertility even in the mildest cases. The ratio of oviductal fluid to peritoneal fluid varies throughout the cycle and has been implicated in potentiating sperm capacitation within the oviducts.

Although these observations are interesting, only a few of these oviductal growth factors have been well characterized by *in vitro* studies. Both EGF and transforming growth factor (TGF), along with their common receptor, are expressed in the human oviduct (194). They are predominantly expressed in the ampullary segment and are present in both ciliated and nonciliated epithelial cells, myosalpinx, and the vascular smooth muscle. Both ligands and the receptor appear to be estrogen dependent, and only EGF is involved in estrogen-induced oviductal cell growth (194). This finding was confirmed by immunohistochemical studies showing EGF and TGF-α expression to be the greatest in the late follicular phase (195). Therefore, this estrogen-induced expression of growth factors may be critical to periovulatory oviductal function.

Another interesting protein is leukemia-inhibitor factor (LIF), a member of the TGF-β family. LIF is required for murine implantation and prevents stem cell differentiation in the bone morrow (196). LIF was found in the human oviduct expressed mainly by the epithelial cells, predominantly in the distal segments, and did not show cycle variation (197). Although estradiol and progesterone did not affect LIF expression, TGF-β increased expression in both stromal and epithelial oviductal cells (197). The highest expression of LIF was found in ectopic pregnancy, a finding suggesting a role for inflammatory cytokines and growth factors in ectopic pregnancies. LIF has not been added to embryo culture media and appears not to be needed for embryo growth, whereas its relation to endometrial receptivity remains unknown.

Oviductal fluid may even be involved with species-specific sperm binding of the zona pellucida. A high-molecular-weight glycoprotein (OGP) is expressed during the late follicular phase and is secreted by the nonciliated epithelial cells throughout the oviduct (198,199). This group also demonstrated that OGP associates with the human zona pellucida *in vitro* and enhances sperm binding to the zona pellucida, but it inhibited sperm binding when baboon OGP was added (200,201). Therefore, human OGP is key to species-specific sperm binding to the zona pellucida and is probably estrogen dependent.

SUMMARY

The oviduct is a remarkable organ that is always in a state of flux and is capable of performing multiple functions simultaneously. Other than complete obstruction or near-complete absence, few conditions exist in which the oviduct is considered nonfunctional. Animal models have provided a valuable insight into basic tubal physiology; however, events peculiar to human oviducts, such as ectopic pregnancy, have yet to be answered. We have become extremely adept at diagnosing and recreating tubal patency, yet to date there remains no test of oviductal function. Many

different myoelectrical, hormonal, epithelial, biochemical, and mechanical actions work in concert to result in normal function of the oviduct. There appears to be redundancy in the system, because any individual component can be absent or severely damaged and pregnancy can still occur. However, it does seem logical to have such an intricate system that is ultimately responsible for continued existence of the species.

10 KEY POINTS

1. The embryologic origin and development of the female internal reproductive structures depends on the absence of MIS.

2. If a müllerian anomaly is present, one should be concerned about and rule out abnormalities in the urologic tract.

3. The functions of the ampullary segment of the oviduct include regulation of sperm and ovum transport, ovum retention and embryo release, being the location of fertilization, and nurture of the early embryo.

4. The oviduct's cycle depends on ovarian steroid production and actively remodels both its ciliary and secretory cells throughout this cycle to achieve optimum function.

5. The cilia, although not essential, play a critical role in oviductal function and may require time to regenerate after an episode of PID, tubal surgery, or ectopic pregnancy.

6. PID continues to be a significant cause of both overt and occult tubal disease and calls for aggressive antibiotic treatment when the condition is diagnosed.

7. Hydrosalpinges are generally associated with a poor pregnancy outcome after surgical repair and may adversely affect endometrial receptivity in IVF embryo transfers.

8. Tuberculous salpingitis is relatively uncommon in developed countries; however, the granulomatous inflammatory response results in extensive oviductal damage and makes reparative surgery unsuccessful.

9. SIN is found only in women of reproductive age, it is associated with infertility and ectopic pregnancy, and it has a cause that is unknown but is suspected to be infectious.

10. The oviduct can be assessed for patency and gross disease by laparoscopy, salpingoscopy, and HSG; however, an instrument for assessment of oviductal function does not exist.

ACKNOWLEDGMENTS

We would like to thank Mr. Kevin Phelps for the preparation of the manuscript and Drs. James Segars and John Frattarelli for their careful review and comments.

REFERENCES

1. Denis AL, Guido M, Adler RD, et al. Antiphospholipid antibodies and pregnancy rates and outcome in *in vitro* fertilization patients. *Fertil Steril* 1997;67:1084–1090.
2. Bruening W, Bardeesy N, Silverman B, et al. Germline intronic and exonic mutations in the Wilm's tumor gene (WT1) affecting urogenital development. *Nat Genet* 1992;1:144–148.
3. Tommerup N, Schempp W, Meinecke P, et al. Assignment of an autosomal sex reversal locus (SRA1) and camptomelic dysplasia (CMPD1) to 17q24.3-q25.1. *Nat Genet* 1993;4:170–174.
4. Paterson P, Chan C. Congenital absence of fallopian tube segments. *Aust N Z J Obstet Gynecol* 1980;25:130–131.
5. Bates GW, Abide JK. Bilateral autoamputation of the fallopian tubes. *Fertil Steril* 1982;25:130.
6. Wilhelmsson L, Lindblom B. Adrenergic responses of the various smooth muscle layers at the human uterotubal junction. *Fertil Steril* 1980;33:280–282.
7. Wilhelmsson L, Lindblom B, Wiqvist N. The human uterotubal junction: contractile patterns of different smooth muscle layers and the influence of prostaglandin E2, prostaglandin F2alpha, and prostaglandin I2 *in vitro*. *Fertil Steril* 1979;32:303–307.
8. Peterson EP, Musich JR, Behrman SJ. Uterotubal implantation and obstetric outcome after previous sterilization. *Am J Obstet Gynecol* 1977;128:662–667.
9. Donnez J, Casanas-Roux F, Nisolle-Pochet M, et al. Surgical management of tubal obstruction at the uterotubal junction. *Acta Eur Fertil* 1987;18:5–9.
10. Lindblom B, Hamberger L, Wiqvist N. Differentiated contractile effects of prostaglandins E and F on the isolated circular and longitudinal smooth muscle of the human oviduct. *Fertil Steril* 1978;30:553–559.
11. Lindblom B, Hamberger L, Ljung B. Contractile patterns of isolated oviductal smooth muscle under different hormonal conditions. *Fertil Steril* 1980;33:283–287.
12. Strom C, Dahlstrom A, Lindblom B, et al. Effects of intraluminal administration of adrenoreceptor agonist on transisthmic flow in the rabbit oviduct. *Biol Reprod* 1983;29:295.
13. Gelety T, Chaudhuri G. Prostaglandins in the ovary and fallopian tube. *Ballieres Clin Obstet Gynecol* 1992;6:707.
14. Lundin S, Forman A, Richberger T, et al. Immunoreactive oxytocin and vasopressin in the non-pregnant human uterus and oviductal isthmus. *Acta Endocrinol* 1989;120:239.
15. Helm G, Ekman R, Owman C. Cyclic fluctuation of vasoactive intestinal polypeptide measured radioimmunologically in various regions of the human fallopian tube. *Int J Fertil* 1987;32:467.
16. Ottesen B, Gram B, Fahrenkrug J. Neuropeptides in the female genital tract: effect on vascular and non-vascular smooth muscle. *Peptides* 1983;4:387.
17. Coutinho EM, Maia H, Nascimento L. The response of the human Fallopian tube to ergonovine and methyl-ergonovine *in vivo*. *Am J Obstet Gynecol* 1976;126:48–54.
18. Heinrich D, Reinecke M, Gauwerky JF, et al. Immunohistochemical and biological evidence for a neuromodulator function of neuropeptide Y in the human oviduct. *Arch Gynecol Obstet* 1987;241:127–132.
19. Larsson B, Ljung B, Hamberger L. The influence of copper on the *in vitro* motility of the human Fallopian tube. *Am J Obstet Gynecol* 1976;125:682–690.
20. McComb P, Fleige-Zahradka B. The fallopian tube: pathophysiology. In: Keye W, et al., eds. *The fallopian tube: pathophysiology.* Philadelphia: WB Saunders, 1995:444.
21. Winston RM. Microsurgical tubocornual anastomosis for reversal of sterilization. *Lancet* 1977;1:284–285.
22. Blandau R. Gamete transport: comparative aspects. In: Hafez E, Blandau R, eds. *The mammalian oviduct.* Chicago: University of Chicago Press, 1969:129.
23. Christoph F, Dennis K. Ciliary activity in the human oviduct. *Br J Obstet Gynecol* 1977;84:216.
24. Gaddum-Rosse P, Blandau R, Thiersch J. Ciliary activity in the human and *Macaca nemestrina* oviduct. *Am J Anat* 1973;138:269–275.
25. Donnez J, Casanas-Roux F, Caprasse J, et al. Cyclic changes in ciliation, cell height, and mitotic activity in human tubal epithelium during reproductive life. *Fertil Steril* 1985;43:554–559.
26. Verhage H, Bareither M, Jaffe R, et al. Cyclic changes in ciliation secretion and cell height of the oviductal epithelium in women. *Am J Anat* 1979;156:505–521.
27. Donnez J, Casanas-Roux F, Ferin J, et al. Changes in ciliation and cell height in human tubal epithelium in the fertile and post-fertile years. *Maturitas* 1983;5:39.
28. Brenner R, Slayden O. The fallopian tube cycle. In: Adashi E, Rock J, Rosewaks Z, eds. *Reproductive endocrinology, surgery and technology.* Philadelphia: Lippincott–Raven, 1995:325.
29. Halbert S. Function and structure of the fallopian tube. In: Gomel V, ed. *Microsurgery in female infertility.* Boston: Little, Brown, 1983:7.
30. Ben-nun I, Fejgin M, Gruber A, et al. Transperitoneal ovum migration in women with unilateral congenital ovarian absence. *Acta Obstet Gynecol Scand* 1988;665:67.
31. First A. Transperitoneal migration of ovum or spermatozoon. *Obstet Gynecol* 1954;3:431.
32. McComb P, Langley L, Villalon M, et al. The oviductal cilia and Kartagener's syndrome. *Fertil Steril* 1986;46:412–416.
33. Suchanek E, Grizelj V, Kozaric Z, et al. Histochemical demonstration of a Δ^5, 3β-hydroxysteroid dehydrogenase activity of cumulus cells related to the maturity and developmental potential of recovered oocytes. *Fertil Steril* 1990;54:873.
34. Bleau G, Richer C, Bousquet D. Absence of dynein arms in cilia of endocervical cells in a fertile women. *Fertil Steril* 1978;362:30.
35. Metz KG. Failures following fimbriectomy: a further report. *Fertil Steril* 1978;30:269–273.
36. Metz KG. Failures following fimbriectomy. *Fertil Steril* 1977;28:66–71.
37. Gomel V. Impact of microsurgery in gynecology. *Clin Obstet Gynecol* 1980;23:301.
38. Novy M. Tuboplasty after fimbriectomy. In: Sciara J, Zatuchni G, Speidel J, eds. *Reversal of sterilization.* Hagerstown, MD: Harper & Row, 1978:143.
39. Winston RM. Microsurgery of the fallopian tube: from fantasy to reality. *Fertil Steril* 1980;34:521–530.
40. Gomel V. Microsurgical reversal of female sterilization: a reappraisal. *Fertil Steril* 1980;33:587–597.
41. Cantor B. Transplantation and replantation of the fallopian tubes and ovaries: a technique for patients undergoing pelvic irradiation. *Fertil Steril* 1983;39:231–234.
42. Silber SJ, Cohen R. Microsurgical reversal of female sterilization: the role of tubal length. *Fertil Steril* 1980;33:598–601.
43. Pulkkinen M. Oviductal function is critical for very early human life. *Ann Med* 1995;27:307.
44. Talo A, Pulkkinen MO. Electrical activity in the human oviduct during the menstrual cycle. *Am J Obstet Gynecol* 1982;142:135–147.
45. Pulkkinen MO, Talo A. Myoelectrical activity in the human oviduct with tubal pregnancy. *Am J Obstet Gynecol* 1984;148:151–154.
46. Pulkkinen MO, Jaakkola UM. Low serum progesterone levels and tubal dysfunction: a possible cause of ectopic pregnancy. *Am J Obstet Gynecol* 1989;161:934–937.

47. Ahlgren M. Sperm transport to and survival in the human fallopian tube. *Gynecol Invest* 1975;6:206.

48. Bielfeld P, Jayendran R, Zanefield L. Human spermatozoa do not undergo the acrosome reaction during storage in the cervix. *Int J Fertil* 1991;36:302.

49. Croxatto H, Faundes A, Medel M, et al. Studies on sperm migration in the human female genital tract. In: Hagez E, Thibault C, eds. *The biology of spermatozoa.* Basel: Karger, 1975:56.

50. Burkman L, Overstreet J, Datz D. A possible role for potassium and pyruvate in the modulation of sperm motility in the rabbit oviductal isthmus. *J Reprod Fertil* 1984;71:367.

51. Khatchadourian C, Menezo Y, Gerard M, et al. Catecholamines within the rabbit oviduct at fertilization time. *Hum Reprod* 1987;2:1.

52. Croxatto H. The duration of egg transport and its regulation in mammals. In: Coutinho E, Fuchs F, eds. *Physiology and genetic of reproduction,* part B. 1974, New York: Plenum, 1974:159.

53. Croxatto HB, Ortiz ME, Diaz S, et al. Studies on the duration of egg transport by the human oviduct. II. Ovum location at various intervals following luteinizing hormone peak. *Am J Obstet Gynecol* 1978;132:629–634.

54. Marana R, Lucisano A, Leone F, et al. High prevalence of silent chlamydia colonization of the tubal mucosa in infertile women. *J Fertil Steril* 1990;88:295–305.

55. Shepard MK, Jones RB. Recovery of *Chlamydia trachomatis* from endometrial and fallopian tube biopsies in women with infertility of tubal origin. *Fertil Steril* 1989;52:232–238.

56. Anestad G, Lundeo O, Moen M, et al. Infertility and chlamydia infection. *Fertil Steril* 1987;46:412–416.

57. Patton DL, Moore DE, Spadoni LR, et al. A comparison of the fallopian tube's response to overt and silent salpingitis. *Obstet Gynecol* 1989;73:622–630.

58. Westrom L, Bengtsson LPH, Mardh P-A. Incidence, trends, and risks of ectopic pregnancy in a population of women. *BMJ* 1981;282:15.

59. Westrom L. Effect of acute pelvic inflammatory disease on fertility *Am J Obstet Gynecol* 1975;121:707–713.

60. Vasquez G, Winston RML, Boeckx W, et al. The epithelium of human hydrosalpinges: a light optical and scanning microscopic study. *Br J Obstet Gynaecol* 1983;90:764–770.

61. Baldetorp B, Mardh P-A, Westrom L. Studies on ciliated epithelia of the human genital tract. *Sex Transm Dis* 1983; 11[Suppl]:363–365.

62. Vasquez G, Boeckx W, Winston RML, et al. Human tubal mucosa in reproductive microsurgery. In: Crosgnain PG, Rubin BL, eds. *Microsurgery in female infertility.* London: Academic Press, 1980;41.

63. Dellepiane G. The pathogenesis of tuberculosis of the female genital organs. In: Rippmann ET, Wenner RS, eds. *Latent female genital tuberculosis.* Basel: Karger, 1966:16–22.

64. Bateman BG, Nunley WC, Kitchin JD III. Surgical management of distal tubal obstruction: are we making progress? *Fertil Steril* 1987;48:523–542.

65. Schaefer G. Tuberculosis of the female genital tract. *Clin Obstet Gynecol* 1970;13:965–998.

66. Woodruff JD, Pauerstein CJ. *The fallopian tube: structure, function, pathology, and management.* Baltimore: Williams & Wilkins, 1969.

67. Bateman BG, Nunley WC Jr, Kitchin JD 3rd, et al. Genital tuberculosis in reproductive-age women: a report of two cases. *J Reprod Med* 1986;31:287–290.

68. Schaefer G. Female genital tuberculosis. *Clin Obstet Gynecol* 1976;19:223.

69. Daly JW, Monif GRG. Mycobacteria. In: Monif GRG, ed.

Infection diseases in obstetrics and gynaecology, 2nd ed. Philadelphia: Harper & Row, 1982:301.

70. Novak ER, Woodruff JD. *Novak's gynecologic and obstetric pathology,* 8th ed. Philadelphia: WB Saunders, 1979:328.

71. Hall JE. *Applied gynecologic pathology.* New York: Appleton-Century-Crofts, 1963.

72. Gomel V, McComb P. Microsurgery in gynecology. In: Silber SJ, ed. *Microsurgery.* Baltimore: Williams & Wilkins, 1979: 143–145.

73. McComb P, Gomel V, Rowe T. Investigation of tuboperitoneal causes of female infertility. In: Insler V, Lunenfeld B, eds. *Infertility.* London: Churchill Livingstone, 1986:213–240.

74. Braby HH, Dougherty CM, Mickal A. Actinomycosis of the female genital tract. *Obstet Gynecol* 1964;23:580–583.

75. Dische FE, Burt IJ, Davidson, NJ, et al. Tubo-ovarian actinomycosis associated with intrauterine contraceptive devices. *J Obstet Gynaecol Br Common* 1974;81:724–729.

76. Paalman RJ, Dockerty MB, Mickal A. Actinomycosis of the female genital tract. *Obstet Gynecol* 1964;23:580–583.

77. Frost O. Bilharzia of the fallopian tube. *S Afr Med J* 1975;49:1201–1203.

78. Majmudar B, Henderson PH III, Semple E. Salpingitis isthmica nodosa: a high-risk factor for tubal pregnancy. *Obstet Gynecol* 1983;62:73–78.

79. Wheeler JE. Pathology of the fallopian tube. In: Kurman RJ, ed. *Blaustein's pathology of the female genital tract,* 3rd ed. New York: Springer-Verlag, 1987.

80. Boer-Meisel ME, te Velde ER, Habbema JDF, et al. Predicting the pregnancy outcome in patients treated for hydrosalpinx: a prospective study. *Fertil Steril* 1986;45:23–29.

81. Donnez J, Casanas-Roux F. Prognostic factors of fimbrial microsurgery. *Fertil Steril* 1986;46:200–204.

82. Henery-Suchet J, Loffredo V, Tequier L, et al. Endoscopy of the tube (tuboscopy): its prognostic value for tuboplasties. *Acta Eur Fertil* 1985;16:139–145.

83. Kerin J, Surrey E, Anderson R, et al. Falloposcopy: microendoscopy of the human fallopian tube from the uterotubal ostium to the fimbria using a transcervico-uterine approach. In: *Proceedings of the fifth World Congress on In Vitro Fertilization and Alternate Assisted Reproduction,* Jerusalem, 1989.

84. Bauer O, Diedrich K, Bacich S, et al. Transcervical access and intra-luminal imaging of the fallopian tube in the non-anesthetized patient: preliminary results using a new technique for fallopian access. *Hum Reprod* 1992;7[Suppl 1]:7–11.

85. Venezia R, Zangara C, Knight C, et al. Initial experience of a new linear everting falloposcopy system in comparison with hysterosalpingography. *Fertil Steril* 1993;60:771–775.

86. David A, Garcia C, Czernobilsky B. Human hydrosalpinx: histologic study and chemical composition of fluid. *Am J Obstet Gynecol* 1969;105:400.

87. Patek E, Nilsson L. Hydrosalpinx simplex as seen by the scanning electron microscope. *Fertil Steril* 1977;28:962.

88. Vasquez G, Winston RML, Boeckx W, et al. The epithelium of human hydrosalpinges: a light optical and scanning electron microscopic study. *Br J Obstet Gynecol* 1983;90:764.

89. McComb PF, Paleologou A. The intussusception technique for the therapy of distal oviductal occlusion at laparoscopy. *Obstet Gynecol* 1991;78:443–447.

90. Bateman BG, Nunley WC, Kitchin JD III. Surgical management of distal tubal obstruction: are we making progress? *Fertil Steril* 1987;48:523–542.

91. Donnez J, Casanas-Roux F. Prognostic factors of fimbrial microsurgery. *Fertil Steril* 1986;46:200–204.

92. Patton DL, Moore DE, Hicks LA, et al. Tubal morphology and physiology in women with silent salpingitis. Presented at the

42nd meeting of the American Fertility Society, Burmingham, Alabama, 1986, and the 18th annual meeting of the Canadian Andrology Society, Toronto, 1986.

93. Halbert SA, Paton DL. Hydrosalpinx: effect of chronic oviductal dilation on egg transport. *Fertil Steril* 1987;35:69.

94. Vemer HM, Boeckx WD, Vasquez G, et al. Experimental hydrosalpinx and salpingostomy in rabbits. *Eur J Obstet Gynecol Reprod Biol* 1984;18:95.

95. Donnez J, Caprasse J, Casanas-Roux F, et al. Morphologic study of mechanically induced hydrosalpinges in rabbits. *Acta Eur Fertil* 1985;16:257.

96. Devoto L, Pino AM, Las Heras JL, et al. Estradiol and progesterone nuclear and cytosol receptors of hydrosalpinx. *Fertil Steril* 1984;42:594.

97. Donnez J, Caprasse J, Casanas-Roux F, et al. Loss of adrenergic innervation in induced rabbit hydrosalpinx. *Gynecol Obstet Invest* 1986;21:213.

98. Andersen AN, Yue Z, Meng FJ, et al. Low implantation rate after *in-vitro* fertilization in patients with hydrosalpinges diagnosed by ultrasonography. *Hum Reprod* 1995;10:576–579.

99. Mansour RT, Aboulghar MA, Serour GI, et al. Fluid accumulation of the uterine cavity before embryo transfer: a possible hindrance for implantation. *J In Vitro Fertil Embryo Transfer* 1991;8:157–159.

100. David A, Garcia CR, Czernobilsky B. Human hydrosalpinx. Histologic study and chemical composition of fluid. *Am J Obstet Gynecol* 1969;105:400–411.

101. Mansour RT, Aboulghar MA, Serour GL, et al. Fluid accumulation of the uterine cavity before embryo transfer: a possible hindrance for implantation. *J In Vitro Fertil Embryo Transfer* 1991;8:157–159.

102. Strandell A, Waldenstrom U, Nilsson L, et al. Hydrosalpinx reduces *in-vitro* fertilization in patients with hydrosalpinges diagnosed by ultrasonography. *Hum Reprod* 1994;9:861–863.

103. Andersen AN, Yue Z, Meng FJ, et al. Low implantation rate after *in-vitro* fertilization in patients with hydrosalpinges diagnosed by ultrasonography. *Hum Reprod* 1994;9:1935–1938.

104. Kassabji M, Sims JA, Butler L, et al. Reduced pregnancy outcome in patients with unilateral or bilateral hydrosalpinx after *in vitro* fertilization. *Eur J Obstet Gynecol Reprod Biol* 1994;56:129–132.

105. Vandromme J, Chasse E, Lejeune B, et al. Hydrosalpinges in *in-vitro* fertilization: an unfavorable prognostic feature. *Hum Reprod* 1995;10:576–579.

106. Shelton KE, Butler L, Toner JP, et al. Salpingectomy improves the pregnancy rate in *in-vitro* fertilization patients with hydrosalpinx. *Hum Reprod* 1996;11:523–525.

107. Sharara FL, Scott Jr RT, Marut EL, et al. *In-vitro* fertilization outcome in women with hydrosalpinx. *Hum Reprod* 1996;11:526–530.

108. Akman MA, Garcia JE, Damewood MD, et al. Hydrosalpinx affects the implantation of previously cryopreserved embryos. *Hum Reprod* 1996;111:1013–1014.

109. Katz E, Akman MA, Damewood MD, et al. Deleterious effect of the presence of hydrosalpinx on implantation and pregnancy rates with *in vitro* fertilization. *Fertil Steril* 1996;66:122–125.

110. Fleming C, Hull MGR. Impaired implantation after *in vitro* fertilization treatment associated with hydrosalpinx. *Br J Obstet Gynecol* 1996;103:268–272.

111. Puttemans PJ, Brosens IA. Salpingectomy improves *in vitro* fertilization outcome in patients with a hydrosalpinx: blind victimization of the fallopian tube? *Hum Reprod* 1996;11:2079–2081.

112. Andersen AN, Lindhard A, Loft A, et al. The infertile patient with hydrosalpinges: IVF with or without salpingectomy? *Hum Reprod* 1996;11:2081–2084.

113. Mukherjee T, Cooperman AB, McCaffrey C, et al. Hydrosalpinx fluid has embryotoxic effects on murine embryogenesis: a case for prophylactic salpingectomy. *Fertil Steril* 1996;66:851–853.

114. Meyer WR, Castelbaum AJ, Somkuti S, et al. Hydrosalpinges adversely affect markers of endometrial receptivity. *Hum Reprod* 1997;12:1393–1398.

115. Sawin SW, Ricardo Lovet de Mola J, Monzon-Bordonaba F, et al. Hydrosalpinx fluid enhances human trophoblast viability and function *in vitro*: implications for embryonic implantation assisted reproduction. *Fertil Steril* 1997;68:65–71.

116. Vessey MP, Hohnson B, Doll R, et al. Outcome of pregnancy in women using intrauterine device. *Lancet* 1974;1:495.

117. Lehfeldt H, Tietze C, Gorstein F. Ovarian pregnancy and the intrauterine device. *Am J Obstet Gynecol* 1970;108:1005–1009.

118. Kliener GJ, Roberts TW. Current factors in the causation of tubal pregnancy. *Am J Obstet Gynecol* 1967;99:21.

119. Langer R, Raziel A, Ron-El R, et al. Reproductive outcome after conservative surgery for unraptured tubal pregnancy—a 15 year experience. *Fertil Steril* 1990;53:227.

120. Mecke H, Semm K, Lehmann-Willenbrock E. Results of operative pelviscopy in 202 cases of ectopic pregnancy. *Int J Fertil* 1989;34:93.

121. Peretz BA, Linenbaum ES, Beach D. Ectopic pregnancy effects on the ispilateral fallopian tube epithelium: an ultrastructural study. *Eur J Obstet Gynecol Reprod Biol* 1984;17:19.

122. Vasquez G, Winston RML, Brosens IA. Tubal mucosa and ectopic pregnancy. *Br J Obstet Gynecol* 1983;90:468–474.

123. Vasquez G, Winston RML, Brosens IA. Tubal mucosa and ectopic pregnancy. *Br J Obstet Gynaecol* 1983;90:468–474.

124. Pulkkinen MO, Talo A. Tubal physiologic consideration in ectopic pregnancy. *Clin Obstet Gynecol* 1987;30:164.

125. Csapo Al. Progesterone "block." *Am J Anat* 1956;98:273.

126. Lindblom B, Hahlin M, Kallfelt B, et al. Local prostaglandin F2a injection for termination of ectopic pregnancy. *Lancet* 1987;1:776.

127. Pulkkinen MO, Talo A. Myoelectrical activity in the human oviduct with tubal pregnancy. *Am J Obstet Gynecol* 1984;148:151.

128. Persaud V. Etiology of tubal ectopic pregnancy: radiologic and pathologic studies. *Obstet Gynecol* 1970;36:257–263.

129. Majmudar B, Henderson PH, Semple E. Salpingitis isthmica nodosa a high-risk factor for tubal pregnancy. *Obstet Gynecol* 1983;62:73–78.

130. Green LK, Kott ML. Histopathologic finding in ectopic tubal pregnancy. *Int J Gynecol Pathol* 1989;8:255–262.

131. Breen JL. A 21 year survey of 654 ectopic pregnancies. *Am J Obstet Gynecol* 1970;106:1004–1019.

132. Honore LH. Salpingitis isthmica nodosa in female infertility and ectopic pregnancy. *Fertil Steril* 1978;29:164–168.

133. Wrork DH, Broders AC. Adenomyosis of the fallopian tube. *Am J Obstet Gynecol* 1942;44:412–432.

134. Bruhat MA, Manhes H, Mage G, et al. Treatment of ectopic pregnancy by means of laparoscopy. *Fertil Steril* 1980;33:411.

135. DeCherney AH, Romero R, Naftolin F. Surgical management of unruptured ectopic pregnancy. *Fertil Steril* 1981;35:21.

136. Cartwright PSW, Herbert CM III, Maxson WS. Operative laparoscopy for the management of tubal pregnancy. *J Reprod Med* 1986;31:589–591.

137. Pouly JL, Mahnes H, Mage G, et al. Conservative laparoscopic treatment of 321 ectopic pregnancies. *Fertil Steril* 1986;46:1093.

138. DeCherney AH, Diamond MP. Laparoscopic salpingostomy for ectopic pregnancy. *Obstet Gynecol* 1987;70:948.

139. Vermesh M, Silva PD, Rosen GF, et al. Management of unruptured ectopic gestation by linear salpingostomy: a prospective

randomized clinical trial of laparoscopy versus laparotomy. *Obstet Gynecol* 1989;73:400.

140. McComb PF. Linear ampullary salpingotomy heals better by secondary versus primary closure. *Acta Eur Fertil* 1985; 16:401–404.

141. Pansky M, Golan A, Bukovsky I, et al. Nonsurgical management of tubal pregnancy: necessity in view of the changing clinical appearance. *Am J Obstet Gynecol* 1991;164:888–895.

142. Stovall TG, Ling FW, Buster JE. Reproductive performance after methotrexate treatment of ectopic pregnancy. *Am J Obstet Gynecol* 1990;1620–1624.

143. Stovall TG, Ling FW, Gray LA, et al. Methotrexate treatment of unruptured ectopic pregnancy: a report of 100 cases. *Obstet Gynecol* 1991;77:749–753.

144. Mitchell DE, McEwain HF, McCarthy JA, et al. Hysterosalpingographic evaluation of tubal patency after ectopic pregnancy. *Am J Obstet Gynecol* 1987;157:618–621.

145. Yao M, Tulandi T. Current status of surgical and nonsurgical management of ectopic pregnancy. *Fertil Steril* 1997;67:421–433.

146. Seifer DB, Gutmann J, Grant WD, et al. Comparison of persistent ectopic pregnancy after laparoscopic salpingostomy versus salpingostomy at laparotomy for ectopic pregnancy. *Obstet Gynecol* 1993;81:387–382.

147. Seifer DB, Silva PD, Grainger DA, et al. Reproductive potential after treatment for persistent ectopic pregnancy. *Fertil Steril* 1994;62:194–196.

148. Graczykowski JW, Mishell DR. Methotrexate prophylaxis for persistent ectopic pregnancy after conservative treatment by salpingostomy. *Obstet Gynecol* 1997;89:118–122.

149. Spandorfer SD, Sawin SW, Benjamin I, et al. Postoperative day 1 serum human chorionic gonadotropin level as predictor of persistent ectopic pregnancy after conservative surgical management. *Fertil Steril* 1997;68:430–434.

150. Surrey ES, Halme J. Endometriosis as a cause of infertility. *Obstet Gynecol Clin North Am* 1989;16:79–91.

151. Forrest J, Buckley CH, Fox H. Pelvic endometriosis and tubal inflammatory disease. *Int J Gynecol Pathol* 1984;3:343.

152. Suginami H, Yano K. An ovum capture inhibitor (OCI) in endometriosis peritoneal fluid: an OCI-related mechanism responsible for fimbrial failure of ovum capture. *Fertil Steril* 1988;50:648.

153. Fortier J, Haney AF. The pathologic spectrum of uterotubal junction obstruction. *Obstet Gynecol* 1985;65:93–98.

154. Donnez J, Casanas-Roux F. Prognostic factors influencing the pregnancy rate after microsurgical cornual anastomosis. *Fertil Steril* 1986;46:1089–1092.

155. Punnonen R, Soederstroem KO, Alanen A. Isthmic tubal occlusion: etiology and histology. *Acta Eur Fertil* 1984;15:39–42.

156. Donnez J, Casanas-Roux F. Histology: a prognostic factor in proximal tubal occlusion. *Eur J Obstet Gynecol Reprod Biol* 1988;29:33–38.

157. Harper MJK. Gamete and zygote transport. In: Knobil E, Neil J, eds. *The physiology of reproduction.* New York: Raven, 1988:103–134.

158. Gamely V. Results of reconstructive infertility surgery. In: Gomel V, ed. *Microsurgery in female infertility.* Boston: Little, Brown, 1983:236.

159. Donnez J, Casanas-Roux F, Ferin J, et al. Tubal polyps, epithelial inclusions, and endometriosis after tubal sterilization. *Fertil Steril* 1984;41:564–568.

160. Rock JA, Parmley TH, King TM, et al. Endometriosis and the development of tuboperitoneal fistulas after tubal ligation. *Fertil Steril* 1981;35:16–20.

161. Vasquez G, Winston RML, Boeckx W, et al. Tubal lesions subsequent to sterilization and their relation to fertility after attempts at reversal. *Am J Obstet Gynecol* 1980;138:86–92.

162. Chiari H. Zur pathologischen Anatomie des Eileitercatarrhs. *Z Heilkd* 1887;8:457–473.

163. Creasy JF, Clark RL, Cuttino JT, et al. Salpingitis isthmica nodosa: radiologic and clinical correlates. *Radiology* 1985; 154:597–600.

164. Chen KTK. Bilateral papillary adenofibromas of the fallopian tubes. *Am J Clin Pathol* 1981;75:229–231.

165. Wrork DH, Brokers AC. Adenomyosis of fallopian tube. *Am J Obstet Gynecol* 1942;44:412–432.

166. Ohm RJ, Hoots G, Garvin AJ. Isthmic ectopic pregnancy and salpingitis isthmica nodosa. *Fertil Steril* 1987;48:756–760.

167. Campbell JS, Nigam S, Hurtig A, et al. Mineral oil granulomas of the uterus and parametrium and granulomatous salpingitis with Schaumann bodies and oxalate deposits. *Fertil Steril* 1964;15:278–287.

168. Jansen RPS. Tubal resection and anastomosis. II. Isthmic salpingitis. *Aust N Z J Obstet Gyneacol* 1986;26:300–304.

169. Shen CC, Bausal M, Purrazzella R, et al. Benign glandular inclusions in lymph nodes, endosalpingiosis, and salpingitis isthmica nodosa in a young girl with clear cell adenocarcinoma of the cervix. *Am J Surg Pathol* 1983;7:293–300.

170. Newbold RR, Bullock BC, McLachlan JA. Diverticulosis and salpingitis isthmica nodosa (SIN) of the fallopian tube. *Am J Pathol* 1984;117:333–335.

171. Benjamin CL, Beaver DC. Pathogenesis of salpingitis isthmica nodosa. *Am J Clin Pathol* 1951;21:212–222.

172. Punnonen R, Soderstrom KO. inflammatory etiology of salpingitis isthmica nodosa: a clinical, histological and ultrastructural study. *Acta Eur Fertil* 1986;17:199–203.

173. Creasy JL, Clark RL, Cuttino JT, et al. Salpingitis isthmica nodosa: radiologic and clinical correlates. *Radiology* 1985; 154:597.

174. Vancaillie T, Schmidt EH. The uterotubal junction. *J Reprod Med* 1988;33:629–634.

175. McComb PF, Moon Y. Prostaglandin E and F concentration in the fimbria of the rabbit fallopian tube increases at the time of ovulation. *Acta Eur Fertil* 1985;16:423–426.

176. McComb PF. Microsurgical tubocornual anastomosis for occlusive cornual disease: reproducible results without the need for tubouterine implantation. *Fertil Steril* 1986;46:571–574.

177. McComb PF, Lee NH, Stephenson MD. Reproductive outcome after microsurgery for proximal and distal occlusions in the same fallopian tube. *Fertil Steril* 1991;56:134–135.

178. McComb PF, Rowe TC. Salpingitis isthmica nodosa: evidence it is a progressive disease. *Fertil Steril* 1989;51:542–525.

179. Lederer KJ. Transcervical tubal cannulation and salpingoscopy in the treatment of tubal infertility. *Curr Opin Obstet Gynecol* 1993;5:240–244.

180. Das K, Nagel TC, Malo JW. Hysteroscopic cannulation for proximal tubal obstruction: a change for the better? *Fertil Steril* 1995;63:1009–1015.

181. Ransom MX, Garcia AJ. Surgical management of cornual-isthmic tubal obstruction. *Fertil Steril* 1997;68:887–891.

182. Lang EK, Dunaway HH. Transcervical recanalization of strictures in the postoperative fallopian tube. *Radiology* 1994; 191:507–512.

183. Bauer O, Diedrich K. Transcervical tubal transfer of gametes and embryos. *Curr Opin Obstet Gynecol* 1994;6:178–183.

184. Sampson JA. Postsalpingectomy endometriosis (endosalpingiosis). *Am J Obstet Gynecol* 1930;20:443–480.

185. Zinsser KR, Wheeler JE. Endosalpingiosis in the omentum: a study of autopsy and surgical material. *Am J Surg Pathol* 1982;6:109–117.

186. McCausland A. Endosalpingiosis ("endosalpingoblastosis")

following laparoscopic tubal coagulation as an etiologic factor in ectopic pregnancy. *Am J Obstet Gynecol* 1982;143: 12–24.

187. Paria BC, Dey SK. Preimplantation embryo development *in vitro*: cooperative interactions among embryos and role of growth factors. *Proc Natl Acad Sci U S A* 1990;87:4756–4760.

188. Pampfer S, Arceci RJ, Pollard JW. Role of colony stimulating factor-1 (CSF-1) and other lympho-hematopoietic growth factors in mouse preimplantation development. *Bioassays* 1991; 13:535–540.

189. Liu LPS, Chan STH, Ho PC, et al. Human oviduct cells produce high molecular weight factors that improve the development of mouse embryo. *Mol Hum Reprod* 1995;10:2781–2786.

190. Wiemer KE, Hoffman DI, Maxson WS, et al. Embryonic morphology and rate of implantation of human embryos following coculture on bovine oviductal epithelial cells. *Hum Reprod* 193;8:97–101.

191. Moessner J, Dodson WC. The quality of human embryo growth is improved when embryos are cultured in group rather than separately. *Fertil Steril* 1995;64:1034–1035.

192. Almagor M, Bejar C, Kafka I, et al. Pregnancy rates after communal growth of preimplantation human embryos *in vitro*. *Fertil Steril* 1996;66:394–397.

193. Sayegh R. Mastroianni L Jr. Recent advances in our understanding of tubal function. *Ann N Y Acad Sci* 1991;626:266–275.

194. Adachi K, Kurachi H, Homme H, et al. Estrogen induces epidermal growth factor (EGF) receptor and its ligands in human fallopian tube: involvement of EGF but not transforming growth factor-alpha in estrogens-induced tubal cell growth *in vitro*. *Endocrinology* 1995;136:2110–2119.

195. Morishige K, Kurachi H, Amemiya K, et al. Menstrual stage specific expression epidermal growth factor and transforming growth factor and the human oviduct and their role in early embryogenesis. *Endocrinology* 1993;133:199–207.

196. Stewart C, Kaspar P, Brunet L, et al. Blastocyst implantation depends on maternal expression of leukemia inhibitory factor. *Nature* 1992;359:76–79.

197. Keltz MD, Altar E, Buradagunta S, et al. Modulation of leukemia inhibitory factor gene expression and protein biosynthesis in the human fallopian tube. *Am J Obstet Gynecol* 1996; 175:1611–1619.

198. Arias EB, Verhage HG, Jaffe RC. Complementary deoxyribonucleic acid cloning and molecular characterization of an estrogen-dependent human oviductal glycoprotein. *Biol Reprod* 1994;51:685–694.

199. O'Day-Bowman MB, Mavrogianis PA, Fazleabas AT, et al. A human oviduct-specific glycoprotein: synthesis, secretion, and localization during the menstrual cycle. *Microsc Res Tech* 1995;32:57–59.

200. O'Day-Bowman MB, Mavrogianis PA, Reuter LM, et al. Association of oviduct-specific glycoproteins with human and baboon (*Papio anubis*) ovarian oocytes and enhancement of human sperm binding to human hemizonae following *in vitro* incubation. *Biol Reprod* 1996;54:60–69.

201. Schmidt A, Mavrogianis PA, O'Day-Bowman MB, et al. Species-specific effect of oviductal glycoproteins on hamster sperm binding to hamster oocytes. *Mol Reprod Dev* 1997; 46:201–207.

202. Hershlag A, Seifer D, Carcangiu ML, et al. Salpingoscopy: light microscopic and electron microscopic correlations. Obstet Gynecol 1997;77:339–405.

17

BASIC INFERTILITY: ETIOLOGY AND THERAPY

ANDREW J. LEVI
ERIC A. WIDRA

Fertility issues have plagued man- and womankind alike for time immemorial. They are referenced in the Bible; the command to "be fruitful and multiply, and replenish the earth" (Genesis 1:28), prompted Sarah to urge her husband Abraham to have relations with her handmaid Hagar, to assess his fertility and extend his family (1). In 1554, Mary Tudor married Phillip II of Spain, and her infertility and inability to produce a son prevented the formation of a Roman Catholic Anglo-Spanish dynasty. In the late 18th century, Charles II's wife, Catherine of Braganza proved infertile allowing the succession of James II, a Roman Catholic, leading to the Glorious Revolution of 1788 and preservation of English Protestantism (2). In the years to come, however, great strides were made in infertility evaluation and treatment, and by the late 19th century, a keener understanding of female reproductive physiology and male factor infertility developed (3). These discoveries subsequently propelled fertility medicine into the 20th century and into the era of assisted reproductive technology (4).

While great advances in fertility have been made in the 20th century, infertility continues to impact as many as 15% of couples trying to conceive. Although innovative testing, data analysis, and reproductive techniques continue to evolve, patients still suffer from infertility. Thus, the inability for a couple to conceive remains a major obstacle encountered by the physician. The purpose of this chapter is to guide the physician through a basic infertility workup and to give insight into the current treatment options available.

Infertility is defined as the inability to attain a pregnancy after 1 year of regular unprotected coitus. It affects approximately 15% of the population in developed countries. Of these couples, about 30% of cases can be attributed to a strictly female factor, about 30% to a male factor, with the remaining roughly 40% attributable to a combined or unexplained etiology (Fig. 17.1). The impact of infertility on the emotional and psychological state of the couple is marked. The financial burden of an infertility workup and subsequent therapy can also be dramatic; the total costs of a single successful *in vitro fertilization* (IVF) delivery in the United States have been estimated to be $50,000 to $100,000 (5,6). Despite significant advances, infertility still remains a devastating medical and financial reality to many.

For the last decade or so, the birth rate has remained steady at 1.8 births per woman after a rapid decrease from the postwar baby boom from 1946 to 1964 (7). This decrease in fertility is most likely the result of the postponement of marriage, the emphasis upon the establishment of a career, and the widespread use of contraception and voluntary sterilization. In addition to a stable birth rate, the fecundity rate, representing the ability to attain a viable birth within a single menstrual cycle, has remained unchanged. From 1982 to 1988, one in 12 women reported impaired fecundity, representing nearly 5,000,000 women (8).

Infertility services appear to be underused. In one study, only 43% of women reporting impaired fecundity actually consulted an infertility service. In terms of the general population, about 2.3% of reproductive age women (1.26 million women in 1988) received some sort of advice or treatment in regard to impaired fertility (9). Thus, although millions of women suffer from decreased fecundity, less than one half of these women seek assistance.

Predicting conception remains difficult. Many women deemed infertile may in fact have had a prior early pregnancy loss that was not clinically detected (10). Many studies have been performed in efforts to predict which couples have the greatest chances at conception, and some have concluded that spontaneous cures for infertile couples are common (11–15). Nonetheless, the fact remains that after 1 and 2 years, 15% and 5% of couples, respectively, will remain infertile.

The workup of the infertile couple can be time-consuming and emotionally exhausting. However, the importance of attention to detail cannot be overemphasized. Etiologies including male factor, anovulation, tubal disease, cervical factor, luteal phase defect, and occult ovarian failure must all be considered and explored. The typical workup involves the identification of risk factors through an in-depth, tailored history and physical, as well as testing to document ovulation, possible postcoital test, hysterosalpingogram, semen analysis, possible laparoscopy, and often, investigation

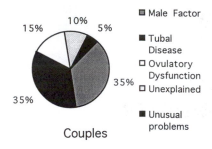

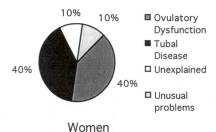

FIGURE 17.1. Causes of Infertility in couples and in women. (From Speroff L, Glass RH, Kase NG. *Clinical gynecologic endocrinology and infertility,* 5th ed. Baltimore: Williams & Wilkins, 1994, with permission.)

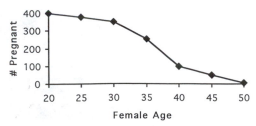

FIGURE 17.2. Historical fertility rates per 1,000 women as a function of age. (From Menken J, Trussell J, Larsen U. Age and infertility. *Science* 1986;233:1389–1394, with permission.)

of menstrual cycle day 3 hormone concentrations. Maternal age plays an important role and must be taken into account during infertility diagnosis and treatment.

AGING AND REPRODUCTION

Time is the enemy of reproduction. While spontaneous pregnancy rates approach 30% per cycle in presumed fertile couples in their 20s, only about 5% of women over the age of 40 will ultimately achieve a term pregnancy (16). This fact alone has great impact in our society, as women delay childbearing due to later marriage, career, and financial concerns. First births among women age 30 to 40 years old continue to increase, and it is estimated that in the year 2000, nearly 10% of all births in the United States will occur in women between the ages of 45 to 49 (17). When a woman with fertility issues seeks evaluation, her age must have impact on the pace of the workup and course of treatment. While the definition of infertility normally encompasses 12 months of reproductive failure, this doctrine may be relaxed in older patients.

Studies clearly show that fertility in women begins to wane at the age of 30, and markedly so by the age of 35 (18). Compared to women age 20 to 24, women in the age groups 25 to 29, 30 to 34, and 35 to 39 have fertility rates reduced by about 6%, 14%, and 37%, respectively; after age 40, rates decrease more dramatically (19) (Fig.

17.2). While diminished coital frequency may contribute to this decrease, ovarian, chromosomal, and uterine factors probably contribute more. Oocyte quality has been shown to decline with age in studies of the effects of age on the response to human menopausal gonadotropin (HMG) stimulation and IVF outcome (20,21). In addition, older patients undergoing IVF with donor oocytes show significantly higher pregnancy rates and lower miscarriage rates compared to matched patients using their own eggs (22). Uterine receptivity may also be decreased in older females, contributing further to declining pregnancy rates; some, however, have found that with donor ova, women in their 50s still have the capacity to sustain a pregnancy (23,24). Lastly, women in their mid- to late 30s have a higher rate of spontaneous abortions due to abnormal fetal karyotypes. Thus, these factors combine to account for the marked decrease in fertility rates in women of advanced reproductive age.

Clearly, one would not instruct a 40-year-old woman with a complaint of infertility for 6 months to return in several months without evaluation. While such a patient would most likely undergo testing and evaluation similar to that of her younger counterpart, there are other markers of fertility that might be explored. As will be discussed, cycle day 3 hormone concentrations, including follicle-stimulating hormone (FSH), luteinizing hormone (LH), and estradiol might be examined. Once adequate ovarian reserve has been documented, the infertility evaluation should proceed in a manner to elicit other etiologies of infertility unrelated to age. It should be made clear to the patient, however, that as time elapses, her chances of achieving a pregnancy continue to decline.

THE INFERTILITY EVALUATION

History and Physical Examination

A detailed history and physical is the cornerstone of a thorough infertility workup. For the female partner, age, duration of infertility, contraceptive history, and obstetric history are all essential. The menstrual history is of paramount importance as well. Ovulatory dysfunction is a leading cause of female infertility. Polycystic ovary syndrome

(PCOS), or chronic anovulation, is the most common cause of anovulatory infertility, and may affect nearly one quarter of reproductive age women (25–27). A diagnosis of chronic anovulation is primarily a clinical one, originally described by Stein and Leventhal in 1935. They reported the triad of hirsutism, obesity, and irregular menses; however, it is now thought that aside from hirsute features, the other clinical features previously described are not always reliable in predicting the disorder (27). About 70% of these women complain of physical changes associated with hyperandrogenism. Other sequelae of anovulation include increased risks of endometrial cancer, cardiovascular disease, and insulin-dependent diabetes mellitus (28). Polycystic ovarian disease itself may also be a risk factor for recurrent early miscarriage (29).

Because of the high prevalence of chronic anovulation, it must be considered in all patients with menstrual irregularities. Patients typically present with complaints of irregular menses and infertility, and bleed following a progesterone challenge. An endometrial biopsy should be done in patients with long-standing oligo-ovulation to rule out endometrial hyperplasia. While weight loss and oral contraceptive pills are first-line therapies for this disorder, other treatments are necessary in the patient desiring pregnancy and will be discussed later in this chapter (28).

A history of pituitary symptoms, such as headache with associated visual changes, or galactorrhea suggests hyperprolactinemia. These patients may also present with polymenorrhea, oligomenorrhea, and decreased libido in conjunction with infertility (30). Hyperprolactinemia, which impedes fertility by interfering with the pulsatile secretion of gonadotropin-releasing hormone (GnRH) or by shortening the luteal phase, may affect upward of 15% of infertile women (31,32). Serum prolactin concentrations should be checked in the morning while fasting in the absence of recent sexual activity. It is also important to rule out underlying hypothyroidism as a cause of hyperprolactinemia; increased levels of thyroid-releasing hormone (TRH) will induce hyperprolactinemia and lead to ovulatory dysfunction and amenorrhea. Hence, in addition to a serum prolactin, a screening for thyroid-stimulating hormone (TSH) is recommended for infertile patients. Those with hyperprolactinemia and galactorrhea should undergo pituitary imaging to rule out a macroadenoma or suprasellar extension.

The gynecologic history should include a thorough sexual history including a history of all sexually transmitted diseases and pelvic inflammatory disease, which might be responsible for tubal pathology. The number of prior sexual partners and prior IUD use should be documented as well. The patient's Pap smear history should be explored, and any therapies for abnormal smears should be investigated; cervical conization or cryocautery for dysplasia may be the etiology for a cervical infertility factor. Recent use of oral contraceptives or long-acting hormonal contraception may result in prolonged but reversible amenorrhea or anovulation. A history of dyspareunia or pain on deep penetration may implicate endometriosis. Adequate coital frequency should also be confirmed (28).

The patient's current medicines should be reviewed. Drugs such as phenothiazines, thioxanthines, and butyrophenes can all cause a drug-induced hyperprolactinemia and infertility. This is also true for certain antihistamines, antidepressants, antihypertensives, and antiemetics (30).

Much can be ascertained from a careful physical examination. Signs of hyperandrogenism should be noted, and PCOS suspected. The breasts should be examined for any evidence of nipple discharge. Cervical cultures for gonorrhea, chlamydia, and, in some cases, mycoplasma and ureaplasma should be obtained. There is still ongoing debate about whether the latter organisms are causes of female infertility (33,34). Treatment with doxycycline for mycoplasma and ureaplasma, however, has not been shown to increase pregnancy rates (35).

The bimanual exam may reveal a fixed uterus or nodularity of the uterosacral ligaments, suggestive of endometriosis or adhesive disease. A pelvic mass may be discovered at the time of exam. Uterine leiomyoma may be found for the first time, and, while an uncommon etiology of infertility, it can distort the endometrial cavity. This can both compromise the vascular and nutrient supply to certain areas and impede sperm transport through the uterus and fallopian tubes (36). Uterine myoma also is associated with recurrent spontaneous abortion and fetal wastage, most likely secondary to increased uterine irritability and contractility with pregnancy (37).

In the assessment of the male partner, a history of proven fertility may help to rule out a male factor. However, secondary causes for male infertility should be explored. All male partners should be queried regarding any history of chronic medical illnesses, in particular, and chronic respiratory illnesses that can be associated with poor sperm motility or obstructive azoospermia. Any trauma to the reproductive system should be elicited, as should any occupational exposures to environmental toxins. The male partner's pubertal development should be discussed. A thorough sexual history should be taken, focusing on issues regarding libido and potency, as well as a history of any sexually transmitted diseases (38). A history of a varicocele may be important and will be discussed later in this chapter.

Documentation of Ovulation

Regular menses usually means regular ovulation. In the case of the infertile patient, however, the documentation of ovulation is a necessary step. Historically, a number of methods have been used to detect ovulation, including basal body temperature (BBT) charting, documentation of the LH surge, serum progesterone levels, ultrasound visualization of mature follicles, as well as other less used methods, including cervical mucus scoring and measurement of oral and vaginal electrical resistance. BBT charting is still used by many physicians as it is a simple, inexpensive, well-studied test for ovulation; it is recommended by some as a good starting point for testing (39). BBT charting relies on the thermogenic properties of progesterone; in the luteal phase, the production of progesterone is responsible for a sharp rise of 0.4° to 0.6°F and is a presumptive indicator of ovulation. The shortcomings of this method include that it is retrospective; a female's fertile days are generally the 6 days prior to ovulation (40). BBT testing may support ovulatory status but is not useful in the timing of sexual intercourse, and the BBT method can predict the actual day of the LH surge in only about one third of cases at best (41). Additionally, some ovulatory women have paradoxically monophasic BBT charts. BBTs can also be affected by stress, medications, illness, changes in diet, and disorders of sleep (42). BBT charting is a relatively easy and economical method to document ovulatory status as long as its limitations are understood.

Urinary LH kits rely on monoclonal antibodies and enzyme-linked immunosorbent assay (ELISA) techniques to predict ovulation by detecting surging LH levels. Studies show that this is a relatively accurate method, and that in about 95% of cases, ovulation could be predicted within 14 to 26 hours after the documented surge (43). Urinary LH kits are often used in conjunction with intrauterine insemination in attempts to increase fecundity (44).

Ultrasound and serum luteal phase progesterone measurements can be used to assess ovulatory status. Although ultrasound can be used to document ovulation, the exact time of ovulation cannot be specifically ascertained in this manner. Ultrasound can be use to monitor pre-, peri-, and postovulatory events, and is most useful in the realm of ovulation induction (45). Perhaps the most accurate method involves luteal phase progesterone measurements. A single value greater than 3 ng/mL has been shown to be representative of a secretory endometrium and consistent with ovulation (46). Some advocate measurements in at least two cycles to ensure adequate documentation, each measured at about day 20 of the menstrual cycle (47).

Evaluation of Luteal Function

The evaluation of luteal function is performed to rule out a luteal phase defect (LPD), a disorder of inappropriate endometrial maturation that may cause infertility and recurrent abortion. LPD is not secondary to a defective endometrium per se; rather, disordered endometrial development occurs secondary to abnormal folliculogenesis and subsequent aberrant corpus luteum function (48,49). This leads to a endometrium incapable of sustaining blastocyst implantation and ongoing pregnancy. The normal luteal phase lasts about 11 to 15 days, with phases of less than 10 days considered abnormal. Inadequate luteal phases may be of normal length but suffer from inadequate levels of progester-

one. Estimates regarding the incidence of LPD vary, but it probably occurs in 3% to 4% of infertile couples (50). LPDs occur more often in infertile women, and may affect women with endometriosis and unexplained infertility more than women with tubal disease (51,52).

The diagnosis of a luteal phase defect is made by histologic examination of an endometrial biopsy. To ensure appropriate dating, the endometrial biopsy is typically performed in the late luteal phase, around day 26 of the menstrual cycle. The criteria of Noyes et al. (53) are used to date the endometrium based on a 28-day cycle, and an out-of-phase biopsy of 3 days or more confirms a diagnosis of LPD.

The use of endometrial biopsy to diagnose LPD is not without debate, as some question its usefulness when performed in the setting of infertility (54,55). Different pathologists have read the same biopsies as being histologically greater than 2 days apart, which has led some to question the consistency of its interpretation. Additionally, many use LH kits to date ovulation, and this has been shown to breed further inconsistencies in the interpretation of the endometrial biopsy (56). Endometrial biopsies are therefore typically performed in two cycles when a luteal phase defect is suspected.

Semen Analysis, Sperm Penetration Assay, and Immunobead Test

Obvious contributions of a male factor to a couple's infertility should be identified in the early stages of the infertility evaluation. Male infertility is most easily evaluated by a semen analysis. Since there is much variability between individual specimens, two or more specimens are generally obtained at a minimum of 2-week intervals. The couple is asked to abstain from coitus for 2 to 3 days prior to the test. The male partner then generates a specimen that should be delivered to the andrology lab within 1 hour, and should be maintained at ambient temperature. The specimen should be collected in a reservoir devoid of any spermicides, which are found in many types of condoms. The specimen should not be obtained from the withdrawal technique during coitus, as sperm may be lost in such a process.

As shown in Table 17.1, the normal values for semen

TABLE 17.1 WORLD HEALTH ORGANIZATION CRITERIA FOR SEMEN ANALYSIS

Criterion	Value
Volume	≥2 mL
Concentration	≥20 million/mL
Motility-total forward	≥50%
Motility-rapid forward	≥75%
Morphology	≥30%
White blood cells	≤1 million/mL

From WHO. *Laboratory manual for the examination of human semen and sperm-cervical mucus interaction,* 3rd ed. Cambridge, England: Cambridge University Press, 1992, with permission.

analysis as determined by the World Health Organization (WHO), are minimum volume of 2.0 mL; minimum sperm concentration of 20 million/mL; at least 50% of sperm with forward progression, or at least 25% with rapid progression within 1 hour of ejaculation; morphology of at least 30% normal forms; 1 million or less white blood cells per milliliter (57). The average sperm count in "normal" males approaches 80 million sperm per milliliter, but such concentrations are not necessary for fertilization to occur; counts as low as one million sperm per milliliter have resulted (rarely) in fertilization (58). Significant declines in pregnancy rates may first occur with counts as low as 5 million sperm per milliliter, although oligospermia is usually defined as < 20 million sperm per milliliter (59). Assisted reproductive techniques require few motile sperm, with most laboratories inseminating oocytes with 100,000 motile sperm (60).

Sperm morphology is important as it is representative of spermatogenic development (61). While the WHO has its own classifications for the determination of what is morphologically "normal," other criteria have been introduced, designed to predict *in vitro* function. Kruger and colleagues (62–64) have proposed a strict criteria for sperm morphology as indicators for IVF prognosis. In sum, it has been shown when using strict criteria and omitting certain sperm morphologies considered "normal" by WHO criteria, higher IVF fertilization rates occur at a threshold of > 14% normal morphology. Patients with < 4% normal morphology had the lowest rates of fertilization *in vitro,* while those with morphologies between 4% and 14% had intermediate oocyte fertilization rates. While these results cannot be directly translated to *in vivo* performance, they strongly suggest that abnormal sperm forms are functionally impaired and most likely have reduced fertilizing capacity (65).

The sperm penetration assay (SPA) is a diagnostic test that measures the ability of sperm ability to undergo capacitation and acrosome reaction, penetrate the ooplasm, and undergo chromatin condensation within ova cytoplasm (61). The SPA utilizes zona pelucida-free golden hamster eggs; with the zona removed, fertilization by foreign mammalian sperm can occur. These zona-free ova are incubated with human sperm in culture media, and the percentage of fertilized eggs is subsequently compared to that of a known fertile sperm specimen. While the SPA is thought to reflect the fertilization ability of a given sperm specimen, its prognostic value has been questioned (66). The SPA is often used as an adjunct prior to IVF, as a poor SPA may predict a poor IVF outcome (28).

The immunobead test is performed to identify sperm antibodies, an uncommon but significant cause of male infertility. Beads labeled with antiimmunoglobulin G (anti-IgG), anti-IgA, and anti-IgM are mixed with sperm and are examined under microscopy. The specific sperm antibody moiety can be identified in this manner, as well as the location of the antibody in relation to sperm head and tail.

Antibody attachment to the head or tail may interfere with sperm fusion and motility, respectively (28). The immunobead test is also commonly used in conjunction with the sperm penetration assay before embarking on IVF.

The Postcoital Test

The postcoital test (PCT), or Sims-Huhner test, was first described by the American gynecologist James Marion Sims in 1866 and again by Max Huhner in 1913. For over 100 years, it has been a part of the infertility evaluation to assess for cervical factor infertility. It is performed at or around the time of ovulation. The PCT analyzes the characteristics of the cervical mucus, including amount, viscosity, cellularity, spinnbarkeit, as well as the concentration and motility of sperm recovered. Patients generally abstain from intercourse for 2 to 3 days prior to testing and present for evaluation 2 to 24 hours after coitus. A specimen is then obtained and examined both grossly and under light microscopy.

The validity of the postcoital test continues to be debated; many feel that it is a poor predictor of pregnancy (67,68). A single abnormal PCT does not necessarily correlate with a poor prognosis for future pregnancy. In one study, over 50% of patients had a negative PCT; after multiple tests and analysis of other variables, the incidence of negative tests dropped to about 30% (69). Reproducibility of the test is invariably poor, with sperm number often the only reproducible factor (70). Moreover, sperm number and motility do not always correlate with fertility, but may simply be associated with good cervical mucus, especially with higher sperm counts (71). It may be that the presence of a single motile sperm in recovered cervical mucus may represent the ability of sperm to survive in cervical mucus and migrate to the fallopian tubes (72).

One European study was performed to assess the uniformity of the postcoital test (73). It was found that while the PCT was used in over 70% of teaching hospitals in Western Europe, there was little consistency in utilization and methodology. Over half the doctors relied on BBT charting or menstrual history to determine ovulation, deemed by many as unreliable in prospectively documenting ovulation. In addition, over 50 time intervals were utilized by physicians in regard to the time interval between coitus and the PCT. Less that half of physicians used a magnification of 400- to assess sperm in cervical mucus, as recommended by WHO guidelines. In addition, cutoff points for a "normal" test varied markedly between physicians. The PCT was also ranked by the doctors responding in the study as the least useful of the routine tests used in an infertility evaluation.

The utility of the postcoital test is limited. Adequate cervical mucus with sperm recovery and motility are not dependable markers of fertility. Inadequate cervical mucus may be secondary to a follicular maturation defect, resulting in poor estradiol production and a consequent cervical mucus abnormality (74). However, the postcoital test continues to be extensively utilized in the evaluation of infertility. It should be interpreted with caution; multiple tests are recommended before initiating therapy based solely on its results.

The Hysterosalpingogram

The hysterosalpingogram (HSG) is a valuable diagnostic tool in the investigation of infertility, with well over 200,000 performed each year in the United States alone (75). Some believe that the HSG can be as accurate as laparoscopy for the diagnosis of tubal disease (76). The purpose of the HSG is to assess tubal patency and pathology, as well as to ascertain defects in the endometrial cavity. The test is typically performed in the early follicular phase with the injection of dye into the cervix, uterus, and tubes utilizing spot films under fluoroscopy with image intensification. Typically, water-soluble dye is used versus oil-soluble dye secondary to faster absorption and decreased risk of infection (28). About 5 cc of dye is injected through the cannulated cervix, with three films taken (without dye, as dye spills from the fallopian tube(s), and as dye spreads through the peritoneal cavity). Some advocate premedicating with an oral nonsteroidal antiinflammatory agent to minimize cramping during the procedure. Dye typically chooses the path of least resistance, and it is not uncommon to see dye spillage from a single tube only; in these cases, the nonfilling tube is typically normal (27,77).

The risk of infection from hysterosalpingogram in the general population is thought to be about 1%, although some studies quote a higher incidence of close to 3% (78). Patients at high risk for pelvic infection are typically cultured and placed on prophylactic antibiotics, such as doxycycline, for at least 2 days prior to the HSG. The highest rates of post-HSG infection are seen in those patients with a history of infertility, a previous episode of pelvic inflammatory disease, or an adnexal mass or tenderness on exam. While patients with a history of sexually transmitted diseases should be cultured and receive prophylactic antibiotics prior to the HSG, those deemed high-risk should probably bypass the HSG and proceed with laparoscopy (78).

While the HSG is considered by most to be an integral part of an infertility evaluation, it is not without controversy. Although an abnormal HSG may be an excellent predictor of severe pelvic disease, a normal HSG does not ensure tubal patency and a normal pelvis. Retrospective studies in patients who underwent an HSG and subsequent laparoscopy support this point (79,80). Additionally, some believe that the HSG itself performed with either water- or oil-soluble dye may be therapeutic and enhance fertility rates; they advocate at least a 3- to 6-month waiting period before initiating any further fertility treatment (81,82). This practice, however, is not adhered to uniformly.

Transvaginal Ultrasound

Transvaginal ultrasound (TVUS) offers the opportunity to rule out possible organic pathology which may contribute to infertilty. Examples of such pathology include endometriomas, hydrosalpinges, leiomyomata and/or polyps. TVUS sensitivity can be markedly enhanced in detecting submucosal leiomyomata and/or endometrial polyps by injection of 8–10 cc of normal saline into the endometrial cavity prior to ultrasound examination. When TVUS is combined with saline infusion it is referred to as a sonohysterogram. HSG however, offers the advantage of important information regarding tubal diameter and patency not readily available during a sonohysterogram.

Cycle Day 3 Hormones and Tests to Assess Ovarian Reserve

Many women seeking fertility therapy have regular menses. After thorough evaluation, the etiology of their infertility cannot be defined, and they are then assigned a diagnosis of unexplained infertility. It has been suggested that these women have impaired ovarian function or oocyte quality. In the last decade or so, much work has been done in the area of defining laboratory parameters that may yield insight into a woman's reproductive potential. Initially, these studies were performed in the realm of controlled ovarian hyperstimulation (COH) and assisted reproductive techniques such as IVF–embryo transfer (ET), but are now being extrapolated and utilized in the general infertility population.

Follicle-stimulating hormone (FSH), measured in the early follicular phase, was the first marker of ovarian reserve to be investigated and defined. The early work of Navot et al. (83), Muasher et al. (84), and Scott et al. (85) demonstrated that increasing basal FSH concentrations measured on cycle day 3 were predictive of poor controlled ovarian hyperstimulation response and IVF outcome. Women with basal FSH measurements > 25 mIU/mL have minimal chances of achieving a pregnancy, while those with levels < 15 mIU/mL have the best prognosis; women with intermediate levels have variable pregnancy rates (85) (Fig. 17.3).

The hypothesis explaining these findings is that those women with higher basal FSH levels have a developing cohort of follicles that are less endocrinologically active than their counterparts with lower basal FSH levels and higher pregnancy rates. Determinants of serum FSH early in the cycle include ovarian estradiol and inhibin, a dimeric peptide hormone that suppresses pituitary FSH secretion. Poor-quality folliculogenesis and diminished ovarian function may result in impaired inhibin production and mildly elevated FSH. Not until complete oocyte depletion at menopause do castrate levels of inhibin and estradiol lead to very high elevations of FSH (28).

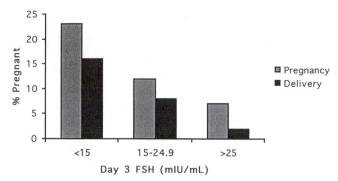

FIGURE 17.3. Cycle day 3 follicle-stimulating hormone (FSH) concentrations and *in vitro* fertilization (IVF) outcome. (From Scott RT, Toner JP, Muasher SJ, et al. Follicle-stimulating hormone levels on cycle day 3 are predictive of in vitro fertilization outcome. *Fertil Steril* 1989;51:651–654, with permission.)

Although the age-related decline in fertility is well substantiated, it has been postulated that basal FSH levels are a more reliable predictor of IVF outcome than age (86). Some stress the relative importance of both, as in the setting of a 42-year-old woman with a low basal FSH. Such a patient would not be assured that her chances of achieving a pregnancy were good based on a favorable FSH with no regard to her advanced reproductive age. It has also been shown that women with one ovary have significantly higher basal FSH levels than matched counterparts with both ovaries; those having previous unilateral oophorectomy and undergoing COH and IVF had more canceled cycles and lower overall pregnancy rates (87,88).

The clomiphene citrate challenge test (CCCT) and stimulatory response to leuprolide acetate are well-studied techniques to assess prognosis for COH and IVF, and when appropriate, may be useful adjuncts in the general infertile population. The CCCT, as described by Loumaye et al. (89), involves the administration of 100 mg of clomiphene citrate to the patient on days 5 to 9 of her cycle, and measuring FSH levels on day 3 (prestimulatory) and day 10 (poststimulatory). Patients with elevated day 10 FSH concentrations are less likely to respond to COH and conceive with IVF. It may be that clomiphene citrate-stimulated FSH levels are more predictive of IVF outcome than basal FSH levels by themselves (90). It has also been shown that the serum estradiol response during the CCCT does not correlate with pregnancy rates (91).

In the leuprolide acetate stimulation test, the quantity and pattern of estradiol production is defined. Patients are given leuprolide acetate doses subcutaneously on cycle days 1 to 5, and a serum estradiol is obtained each day. Results fall into one of four response patterns, each correlating with varying pregnancy outcomes. Such data are useful in determining a patient's prognosis for COH and IVF, as well as for the adjustment of stimulation protocols (92).

Other markers of reproductive potential have been studied in relation to IVF outcome, including cycle day 3 levels of estradiol, inhibin, and the cycle day 3 FSH/LH ratio (93–96). Smotrich et al. (93) showed that patients with elevated day 3 estradiol levels (> 80 pg/mL) have a poor pregnancy prognosis and should be counseled accordingly. Such elevated estradiol levels are hypothesized to be secondary to decreased late luteal inhibin levels, resulting in transiently elevated FSH levels and consequent elevated estradiol levels. Day 3 FSH levels, however, in such a scenario might be normal secondary to negative feedback from the elevated estrogen. The work of Seifer et al. (94,95) showed that higher cycle day 3 levels of inhibin-B are associated with higher pregnancy rates and may be a better marker of reproductive outcome than FSH or estradiol, thus confirming the current explanatory hypothesis for these findings. Lastly, Mukherjee et al. (97) determined that the basal cycle day 3 FSH/LH ratio may be a useful indicator of ovarian reserve prior to embarking on a COH protocol, especially in those patients with normal basal FSH levels who have previously stimulated poorly.

While these studies deal almost exclusively with COH and IVF, ovarian reserve screening has been examined in the general infertile population as well. While basal levels of FSH, estradiol, and inhibin have not been evaluated, the CCCT is a valuable test for such patients as long as its limitations are understood. Scott et al. (98) determined that about 10% of infertile patients have abnormal CCCTs, with increasing incidence in patients over the age of 30 who would have otherwise been categorized as suffering from unexplained infertility (98). Patients with normal ovarian reserve (normal CCCTs) were noted to have significantly higher pregnancy rates, but did experience a decline in rates with increasing maternal age (99). Abnormal tests were infrequent in women less than 30 years old (3%), and increased in incidence with advancing age.

Therefore, these laboratory tests can be used to distinguish patients with diminished ovarian reserve from those with unexplained infertility with normal oocytes. Based on this work, it may be advisable to screen patients older than 30 years of age who have a diagnosis of unexplained infertility with a CCCT or leuprolide acetate stimulation test, as well as to measure cycle day 3 serum concentrations of estradiol and inhibin. It is important to recognize, although it is uncommon, that some women will achieve a pregnancy despite normal testing, the corollary being that normal test results do not in any way ensure a patient of reproductive success.

Laparoscopy

A diagnostic laparoscopy is typically performed at the end of the infertility evaluation. It allows for direct visualization of the pelvis and may detect pathology not apparent on hysterosalpingogram. Approximately 50% of patients undergoing laparoscopy have adhesive disease, endometriosis, or other pelvic pathology. The results at laparoscopy concur with a prior HSG in about two thirds of cases (28). In many cases, operative laparoscopy can be performed in patients with pelvic adhesions and gross endometriosis. In addition, chromopertubation can be performed to assess tubal patency. If a patient has had a previous laparoscopy, a repeat laparoscopy may be indicated, especially in cases where abnormalities were identified but not treated, or in conditions such as endometriosis, where a high likelihood of progression can be expected (100).

TREATMENT

The treatment of infertility has undergone a revolution in recent years. The last 5 to 10 years have seen dramatic increases in pregnancy rates with assisted reproductive technologies (ARTs) such as IVF and gamete intrafallopian transfer (GIFT). Pregnancy rates in selected groups of patients often exceed 40% per attempt in the best centers. New medications utilizing recombinant DNA technology are on the horizon and hold the promise of more efficient and better tolerated therapies.

The most dramatic changes have occurred in the treatment of severe sperm abnormalities. The introduction of intracytoplasmic sperm injection (ICSI) has given us a tool to treat men with few or no sperm in the ejaculate (101). Couples in which the man was previously considered sterile, and those with azoospermia or severe oligospermia can now conceive and deliver their own genetic offspring with surprising degrees of success (101–104).

However, the news is not all good. Despite these advances, serious barriers to success still exist. While we can better understand the effects of aging on reproduction, little progress has been made in overcoming these effects and achieving viable pregnancies, without resorting to donated oocytes (16–23). Premature ovarian failure and recurrent pregnancy loss affect many couples and are notoriously resistant to treatment.

Recent studies have also questioned the long-term safety of some fertility drugs. While far from conclusive, these studies suggest a link between clomiphene citrate and ovarian cancer. These potential risks raise the threshold for instituting treatment, counseling patients, and ensuring efficacy (105–107).

Changes in the financing of health care have had their impact, too. The costs of much infertility treatment are not covered by managed care organizations, leaving patients to decide between treatment, continuing infertility, or going into debt to pay for these sometimes expensive therapies. As a society we have still not decided whether we value this area of medicine and its impact enough to insist on its coverage under insurance plans (5,6).

Deciding when and how to administer treatment is increasingly difficult. While numerous articles have been written about the efficacy of various treatments, many suffer from methodologic handicaps. All too often, these studies are poorly controlled or report per cycle pregnancy rates rather than cumulative success determined by life-table analysis or other appropriate methods. Because infertility patients present with heterogeneous diagnoses, the literature often fails to draw clear distinctions based on specific diagnoses. Whenever possible, recommendations will be based on studies presenting cumulative data.

We will therefore attempt to define treatment by diagnosis. However, since many studies treat milder degrees of endometriosis, unexplained infertility, and mild sperm disorders similarly, we will do the same. It is hoped that this results in a functional stratification of patients and treatments into ovulation disorders, tubal disease, endometriosis, infertility with minimal abnormalities (unexplained, mild endometriosis, mild sperm disorders), and severe sperm abnormalities. Excellent reviews have been prepared on this topic; except for their lack of coverage of the revolution caused by ICSI, they remain rather accurate (108).

A final caution must be sounded in regard to interpreting success rates for patients. Studies presented in the literature use a wide variety of end points. While clinical pregnancy rates are very useful measures by which to compare techniques, they do not reflect the patient's goal—delivery of a healthy baby. Clinicians must remember that spontaneous abortions and other complications of pregnancy are a function of maternal age, number of gestations, and other, often inapparent, clinical factors. These issues must be acknowledged and clearly presented prior to treatment. Doctors and patients, therefore, must be careful consumers of fertility treatments, selecting high-quality centers and protocols with straightforward and reliable statistical information.

The Physiology of Ovulation

A thorough appreciation of ovarian physiology is fundamental in the practice of ovulation induction and assisted reproductive techniques. The ovaries contain a maximum of 6 million follicles by the seventh month of fetal life, only a third of which survive through the neonatal period. At the time of menarche, only about 400,000 follicles remain, and throughout a woman's reproductive life perhaps 500 of these follicles will achieve dominance and be ovulated. To comprehend ovarian stimulation protocols in the treatment of infertility, an understanding of folliculogenesis, development, and ovarian dynamics is necessary.

By the fifth week of fetal life, germ cells migrate from the yolk sac to the gonadal ridge and form the indifferent gonad. Once stroma arises between the oocytes, primordial follicles have developed. These follicles remain quiescent until recruited and subsequently develop into preantral follicles. This period is also known as the gonadotropin-independent period of folliculogenesis, and it is not known exactly what causes such follicles to commence development. It is known that these first stages of development occur in the absence of circulating gonadotropins and are a part of folliculogenesis that cannot be manipulated by assisted reproductive techniques. Once the preantral follicles begin to accumulate follicular fluid and enlarge, they become antral or graafian follicles. This period of folliculogenesis is referred to as the FSH-dependent or gonadotropin-dependent portion of follicular development and is rapid in comparison to the preantral period (109). Stimulation protocols take advantage of this gonadotropin-dependent portion of folliculogenesis, the mechanisms of which are better understood.

At the end of the luteal phase of the menstrual cycle, a cohort of four to eight follicles are selectively stimulated by FSH, initiating the process of recruitment. As the corpus luteum regresses, estradiol, progesterone, and inhibin levels wane, and the hypothalamic-pituitary-ovarian axis is no longer suppressed. The cohort of follicles are physiologically equivalent, and remain so throughout the period of recruitment, which ends with menses of the prior menstrual cycle. Ovarian stimulation protocols take advantage of this physiologic equivalence to drive multiple follicles to maturity. By day 5 to 7 of the current menstrual cycle, selection of the dominant follicle proceeds. Increased mitotic activity within the granulosa cells of the selected follicle subsequently occurs, the mechanism of which, however, is not well understood (110). As the selected follicle achieves dominance, it grows rapidly. Granulosa cell estradiol serves to increase FSH receptors within the growing follicle, and, by negatively feeding back upon the hypothalamus and pituitary, effectively withdraws the gonadotropins needed by the remaining cohort of follicles. Apoptosis of the granulosa cells of the unselected follicles ensues, and follicular atresia inevitably occurs (111). FSH levels remain high in the microenvironment of the dominant follicle and are necessary for granulosa cell development and differentiation (112). Local autocrine and paracrine peptides also contribute to the development and survival of the dominant follicle.

As the dominant follicle matures, estradiol and FSH act to upregulate LH and FSH in anticipation of the LH/FSH surge preceding ovulation (109). Follicular estradiol production occurs via the actions of both LH-induced theca cells and FSH-induced granulosa cells, referred to classically as the two-cell/two gonadotropin hypothesis (113). While the decreasing plasma estradiol in the late luteal phase acts to stimulate FSH production and follicular recruitment, the increasing estradiol production in the follicular phase reflects the differentiation and maturation of the dominant follicle (114). Hence, estradiol levels can be monitored during ovulation induction protocols as a marker of follicular development.

The importance of FSH to the dominant follicle cannot be overemphasized. FSH binding to its receptor (a G-protein transmembrane receptor) in the dominant follicle directly increases estradiol output and also potentiates progesterone production by granulosa cells (115). In addition to

stimulating granulosa cell mitosis, FSH induces the expression of LH receptors in the dominant follicle, which are necessary for ovulation. LH is critical not only in the triggering of ovulation and subsequent corpus luteum support but also in the synthesis of androgenic precursors to estradiol during development of the Graffian follicle (116). Ovarian steroidogenesis is always LH-dependent, but only FSH is required for folliculogenesis (28).

Follicular development is a complex process dependent on both paracrine and autocrine regulators. In addition to FSH, LH, progesterone, estradiol, and inhibin, intraovarian peptides including insulin-like growth factor-I, epidermal growth factor, transforming growth factor-α, basic fibroblast growth factor, transforming growth factor-β, interleukin-1, and tumor necrosis factor-α, luteinization inhibitor, and oocyte maturation inhibitor may play roles in granulosa cell maturation and ovarian folliculogenesis (112,117,118). As mentioned previously, inhibin, a nonsteroidal granulosa cell product, is closely associated with the inhibition of FSH secretion and may be one of the critical mediators of folliculogenesis (119–121). Inhibin directly suppresses pituitary FSH release and magnifies FSH withdrawal from the follicular cohort destined for atresia. This helps to assure dominance of the selected follicle (28). Inhibin may also play a more direct role in follicular atresia and may directly modulate theca and granulosa cell steroidogenesis (112).

In sum, assisted reproductive technologies seek to enhance these signaling pathways, particularly in the recruitment of follicles and in the attempts to bring a larger cohort to dominance (122).

Ovulation Disorders

Anovulation and oligo-ovulation are pleiomorphic disorders with a variety of causes. Careful attention to the diagnostic evaluation will result in treatment appropriately directed at the underlying cause.

Although the evaluation of hyperprolactinemia is beyond the scope of this chapter, when it is identified as the cause of oligo- or amenorrhea, with or without galactorrhea, a dopamine agonist is the treatment of choice. Bromocriptine is a lysergic acid derivative originally developed for the treatment of Parkinson's disease. Given at relatively low doses (2.5 to 10 mg daily), it very effectively lowers serum prolactin levels and restores normal ovulation. Approximately 80% of hyperprolactinemic patients with microademas will ovulate within 6 weeks of treatment (123,124). Orthostatic hypotension, with manifestations including faintness, nausea, and headache, is the most common adverse effect. Starting at low doses or using a vaginal preparation may limit these symptoms (28,124). Patients who cannot tolerate or do not respond to these medications may benefit from treatment with other agents such as pergolide or cabergoline (125,126).

Hypothyroidism is often cited as a cause of absent or

abnormal ovulation. There are scant data, however, on the magnitude of this problem. For the few women in whom this is the sole cause of their infertility, thyroid replacement should have dramatic results. Patients with significant hyperthyroidism will usually have more serious symptoms requiring treatment (28). Needless to say, for the infertility patient with known thyroid disease, careful surveillance is necessary.

The luteal phase defect may rightly be considered a consequence of abnormal ovulation. Treatment with luteal progesterone supplementation or clomiphene in the follicular phase has been advocated (48,127). A comparative study by Murray et al. (128) using life-table analysis and pregnancy as an end point found these treatments to be equally effective.

These conditions constitute only a small proportion of the disorders of ovulation. Hypogonadotropic hypogonadism (WHO group I), the polycystic ovary syndrome (hypothalamic-pituitary dysfunction, WHO group II), and premature ovarian failure (POF, hypergonadotropic hypogonadism, WHO group III) represent the majority of cases. We will consider therapy for each in turn.

Hypogonadotropic Hypogonadism

While rare causes of hypothalamic anovulation such as Kallmann's syndrome do occur, the typical patient exhibits changes secondary to stress, exercise, weight loss, or anorexia nervosa. The metabolic consequences of these conditions is suppression of hypothalamic GnRH pulsatile secretion (28,129). There is evidence that this is brought about through increased levels of cortisol or dopamine (130,131).

Regardless of the cause, treatment should be directed at restoring GnRH pulsatility or exogenously supplying GnRH or gonadotropins. While weight gain and decreased exercise or stress will often restore normal function, they can be difficult to achieve (132). Thus, ovulation induction may be necessary. Since these patients are already hypoestrogenic, clomiphene citrate is an inappropriate agent; injectable gonadotropins are the treatment of choice for these patients. Gonadotropins may be derived from the urine of menopausal women and are prepared as either FSH alone or combinations of FSH and LH. Most recently through the application of recombinant DNA technology it is now possible to produce human gonadotropins without having to derive them from human fluids. Thus, recombinant production can be virtually 100% pure, devoid of contamination and offer greater batch to batch consistency. Recombinant products are produced in vitro by genetically engineered mammalian cells [Chinese hamster ovary (CHO) cells]. Clinical studies have demonstrated similar pharmacokinetic characteristics between recombinant FSH and urinary FSH preparations. Recombinant products offer the advantage of less painful subcutaneous administration

in contrast to the less purified, older urinary preparations which require intramuscular administration.

The mechanism of action is direct stimulation of follicular receptors, thereby activating follicular recruitment and growth. Ovulation is usually triggered by a large dose of human chorionic gonadotropin (hCG), mimicking the LH effect on the preovulatory follicle. These medications are expensive and require careful monitoring of estrogen levels and follicular growth with ultrasound to help prevent multiple gestation and the hyperstimulation syndrome. When managed by an experienced practitioner, this therapy has a cumulative pregnancy rate of 90% over 6 months in this patient population (28,133). GnRH can also be administered by a pulsatile subcutaneous pump. This is physiologically appealing treatment and it has a high success rate. However, given the expense and inconvenience of this treatment and the high success rates with gonadotropins alone, its utility is questionable (134,135).

Polycystic Ovary Syndrome

The woman with PCOS is the prototypic oligoanovulatory patient. Speroff et al. (28) present a very complete description of this fascinating condition. Briefly, the patient with PCOS has infrequent or absent menses, and normal estrogen and gonadotropin levels, although the LH concentration may significantly exceed FSH, the well-known inverted LH:FSH ratio. These women may be obese, hirsute, and hyperandrogenic, but these findings, like the polycystic ovaries themselves, are neither constant nor necessary for the diagnosis. While weight loss in obese PCOS patients may be very beneficial, medical ovulation induction is usually necessary (28).

Clomiphene citrate is the drug of first choice for these patients. Clomiphene is a weakly estrogenic, nonsteroidal chemical related to diethylstilbestrol. It is a racemic mixture of enclomiphene and the biologically active zuclomiphene (136,137). The polycystic ovary contains multiple follicles at an intermediate stage of development, producing physiologically static amounts of estrogen without normal feedback communication to the pituitary. Clomiphene inhibits hypothalamic estrogen receptor replenishment, thus mimicking a hypoestrogenic environment. GnRH pulsatility increases as does FSH and LH secretion (137,138). Provided with additional FSH stimulation, follicles can escape from their suppressed, often hyperandrogenic, state and resume development. Normal estrogen feedback is restored and ovulation occurs (139).

Approximately 80% of properly selected women will ovulate, and as many as half will become pregnant. Patients in whom no other factor exists can expect a cumulative pregnancy rate in excess of 60% over 6 months (28,139,140) (Fig. 17.4). Clomiphene is typically given on days 5 to 9 of a normal or pharmacologically induced menstrual cycle. The starting dose is 50 mg and is increased by 50 mg in

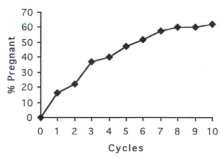

FIGURE 17.4. Cumulative pregnancy rates in clomiphene-treated polycystic ovary syndrome (PCOS) patients. (From Kettel LM, Hummel WP. Ovulation induction in the estrogenized anovulatory patient. *Semin Reprod Endocrinol* 1996;14:309–315, with permission.)

subsequent cycles until ovulation is achieved as evidenced by serum progesterone levels or biphasic temperature charts. Ovulation can be timed with urinary LH detector kits (139,140). Most women who conceive do so at or below the 150-mg dose; much lower rates of ovulation and pregnancy occur at 200 to 250 mg (28,139,140). Once regular ovulation is achieved, treatment is continued for up to 6 months in the absence of pregnancy; success beyond this time period is unlikely. Further, two recent studies have implicated clomiphene in the pathogenesis of ovarian cancer. While this is far from an established risk, it may be duration dependent (105,106). Thus, continuing clomiphene beyond the likely window of effectiveness should be done with caution and ample informed consent.

Multiple gestations occur in approximately 5% of pregnancies and are uniformly composed of twins. Miscarriage rates are not increased. Severe hyperstimulation syndrome is rare (28).

Clomiphene is not without its pitfalls. The antiestrogenic effect of clomiphene may manifest itself in poor cervical mucus production. A postcoital test is recommended, and while exogenous estrogen has been suggested to correct a mucus problem, no data validate this practice (140,141). If the postcoital test is poor, intrauterine insemination may be valuable, however, data supporting this practice are also scant. Suggested adjuncts to clomiphene therapy for patients resistant to traditional regimens have included hCG triggering of ovulation, extended clomiphene treatment, and the addition of dexamethasone or bromocriptine. Studies utilizing these treatments are small; given the potential consequences and low yield of long-term clomiphene exposure, resistant patients may fare better with gonadotropin administration. The interested reader is referred to Speroff et al. (28) for a review of these adjuncts.

Most recently, a novel approach to inducing ovulation in women with PCOS has been the oral administration of Metformin, an insulin sensitizing agent. As insulin resistance with compensatory hyperinsulinemia may contribute to the hyperandrogenism and chronic annovulation associated with PCOS, Metformin, a biguanide, has been demon-

strated to be effective alone and in combination with Clomiphene in inducing ovulation. Metformin interferes with hepatic gluconeogensis by an unknown mechanism. Thus, Metformin reduces insulin secretion which results in less insulin binding to thecal IGF-1 receptors in the ovary and thus less androgen production in response to LH. The most commonly reported side effects are nausea and diarrhea. Metformin's beneficial effect of decreasing serum androgens and inducing ovulation should be demonstrated within 3 months of its use. Renal function (serum BUN, Cr) should be normal prior to and during treatment in order to minimize the infrequent complication of lactic acidosis.

Despite the trappings of gonadotropin therapy mentioned earlier, it is very effective for patients resistant to clomiphene. Patients who have not had a complete anatomic evaluation prior to clomiphene induction should consider a laparoscopy prior to initiating gonadotropin treatment (28). With careful monitoring, pregnancy rates in these patients utilizing gonadotropins and hCG can reach 40% per cycle (28,142–144). The utility of intrauterine insemination in these patients is unclear. Current published data do not resolve the issue satisfactorily.

The mechanism of action of gonadotropins is the same as in hypothalamic amenorrhea; however, women with PCOS have higher estrogen levels and large numbers of intermediate follicles. Multifollicular recruitment therefore occurs at lower doses. Consequently, multiple gestation rates range from 10% to 30%, and PCOS patients are at highest risk for severe hyperstimulation syndrome. While careful serum and ultrasound monitoring can assess and limit these risks, they cannot be eliminated (28,143).

Even with the use of these potent agents, some patients fail to conceive. Some cannot be safely stimulated due to multiple gestation and hyperstimulation risks, others do not conceive for unknown reasons. IVF is a viable alternative for these patients. In fact, many overstimulated PCOS patients can be converted to this procedure directly. Cumulative pregnancy and delivery rates at 6 months have been reported as 82% and 69%, respectively (145).

Finally, surgical treatment of the polycystic ovary has been used to induce ovulation. A variation on the traditional wedge resection, laparoscopic cautery of the ovarian cysts results in reduction of circulating androgens and estrogens. This may allow reinstitution of normal pituitary control or easier induction with clomiphene. Concerns over surgical risks and the development of postoperative adhesions has limited the use of this technique (28,146,147).

Premature Ovarian Failure (POF) in Hypergonadotropic Hypogonadism

This condition, also called premature menopause, is characterized by anovulation, very high FSH and LH levels, and symptoms of hypoestrogenism. Once rare causes of elevated gonadotropins and medical conditions associated with this

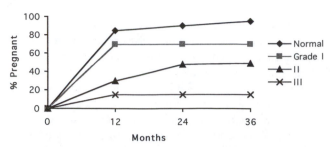

FIGURE 17.5. Cumulative pregnancy rates after surgical treatment of tubal disease, stratified by severity of disease. (From Hull MGR. Infertility treatment: relative effectiveness of conventional and assisted conception methods. *Hum Reprod* 1992;7:785–796, with permission.)

disease have been ruled out, referral for donor oocytes is the appropriate course of treatment in this most frustrating of conditions. Protocols utilizing high-dose gonadotropins or corticosteroids rarely result in pregnancy. While spontaneous remissions and pregnancies do occasionally occur, they can be neither predicted nor effected. Hormone replacement and psychological support offer far more benefit to these young women (28,148).

Tubal and Pelvic Infectious Disease

Prior to the development of the assisted reproductive technologies, surgical correction was the only option for women with pelvic or tubal disease. Despite great effort at refining surgical techniques with operative laparoscopy and microsurgical techniques, cumulative pregnancy rates in most series are under 30% (108). In fact, the most dramatic results have been in anastomoses of proximally obstructed or previously ligated normal tubes, illustrating the importance of normal distal and internal tubal anatomy for function (108,149).

There is a clear hierarchy of tubal disease in regard to its response to surgical intervention. Laparoscopic lysis of peritubal adhesions with otherwise normal anatomy may have 3-year cumulative pregnancy rates in excess of 50% (108,150). By contrast, fimbrial disease, distal occlusion, and occlusion with hydrosalpinx demonstrate rapidly declining response to surgery with cumulative rates of 45% down to 16% after 3 years (150–152). In studies where careful attention was paid to grade the severity of tubal disease, pregnancy rates pre- and postoperatively correlated with the degree of damage. Treatment of severe disease in this study brought the 3-year pregnancy rate from approximately 5% up to only 15%. In fact, surgical treatment of even the mildest disease failed to bring success rates up to those of controls, illustrating once again the sensitivity of the fallopian tube to damage (108,150,153) (Fig. 17.5).

A methodologically sound trial of surgery for distal tubal disease demonstrated cumulative pregnancy rates above 15% only in patients with unilateral disease, calling into question the value of treatment for bilateral distal disease.

Moreover, the risk of subsequent ectopic pregnancy after salpingitis or surgery is significant and must be considered when evaluating the propriety of surgical intervention (150–153).

In vitro fertilization, by contrast, offers couples with tubal disease per cycle pregnancy rates exceeding the multiyear cumulative rates after surgery. Cumulative IVF rates in leading centers routinely exceed 60% after three to six cycles (28,108,154,155). These procedures, while costly, are minimally invasive and have lower risks of complications and ectopic pregnancy than tubal surgery (108,154,155). Patients with even minimal disease treated surgically who fail to conceive within a year should consider IVF (108,156).

Ironically, recent data have suggested that surgery may be a valuable adjunct to IVF in patients with unilateral or bilateral hydrosalpinx. While final resolution of this issue awaits the results of a randomized trial now in progress, several publications have suggested that surgical removal, drainage, or proximal ligation of hydrosalpinges may dramatically improve IVF success rates. The current hypothesis is that reflux of tubal fluid is embryotoxic (157–160).

Endometriosis

The treatment outcomes for moderate and severe endometriosis [American Society for Reproductive Medicine (ASRM) stage III and IV] have been reported to be similar to that of severe tubal disease (108,161). However, a life-table analysis and meta-analysis of surgery for moderate and severe endometriosis by Adamson and Pasta (162) reported 3-year pregnancy rates of 50% to 60%, a much greater improvement than that seen in other tubal disease. In fact, this group also reported high pregnancy rates after laparoscopic treatment of endometriosis only if fimbrial disease was absent (163), confirming the work by Olive and Martin (164). These studies may be detecting differential effects on the tubal mucosa due to the different pathogenesis of these diseases.

Patients with severe anatomic destruction by this disease should consider IVF. Although one longitudinal study found a large numerical difference in 3-year pregnancy rates between IVF and expectant management postoperatively (52% vs. 27%), this was not statistically significant ($p = .09$), probably due to the small sample size. Some have demonstrated per cycle and cumulative pregnancy rates similar to those in tubal factor patients, while others have shown IVF success to decrease with stage of disease (28,108,165,166).

The surgical treatment of lesser degrees of endometriosis has been more controversial as studies have suffered from poor controls, inadequate numbers, and postoperative use of adjunctive therapy (discussed below) (108,167). However, a Canadian group has reported a relatively large series of infertile patients randomized to operative or diagnostic laparoscopy for minimal and mild endometriosis. The cumula-

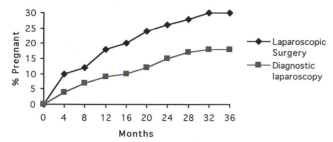

FIGURE 17.6. Cumulative pregnancy rates after laparoscopic surgical treatment of minimal or mild endometriosis vs. expectant management. (From Marcoux S, Maheux R, Bérubé S, Canadian Collaborative Group on Endometriosis. Laparoscopic surgery in infertile women with minimal or mild endometriosis. *N Engl J Med* 1997;337:217–222, with permission.)

tive pregnancy rates (30.7% vs. 17.7%) were significantly higher ($p = .006$) in the laparoscopic treatment group (168) (Fig. 17.6).

Finally, although hormonal treatment of endometriosis with progestational agents, danazol, or GnRH agonists may be very beneficial for painful symptoms, a similar positive effect has not been demonstrated for fertility (28,169,170).

Infertility with Minimal Abnormalities

This heterogeneous group of patients consists of couples with unexplained infertility, those with minimal or mild endometriosis (ASRM stages I and II), and those with lesser degrees of sperm dysfunction. While it can be argued that lumping them together in this fashion is artificial, much of the available literature is likewise constituted. When possible, we will present treatment data specific to a particular diagnosis.

When selecting treatment for these disorders, the duration of infertility and the age of the female partner must be of primary concern. Infertility of greater than 3 years' duration is associated with declining success as is increasing age (108,171). Women over 39 years of age should consider more aggressive forms of treatment, e.g., ART. The treatment strategies applied to these patients include expectant management; intrauterine insemination (IUI); COH, i.e., the deliberate recruitment of multiple follicles using clomiphene or gonadotropins with or without IUI; and ART.

Intrauterine Insemination and Clomiphene

Few studies have systematically addressed the use of IUI alone for the treatment of unexplained infertility. One early study by Kerin suggested that IUI alone offered per cycle pregnancy rates of up to 21% for the first three to four cycles but others have failed to duplicate this finding (108,172–175). A more recent study of patients with cervical, male factor, and idiopathic infertility found cumulative and per cycle pregnancy rates of 38% and 6% to 12%,

respectively; however, there was no control group for comparison (176).

The use of clomiphene alone or in combination with IUI may be of modest benefit. Many investigators have failed to find a significant improvement in pregnancy rates with clomiphene. However, one well-designed trial of clomiphene and IUI by Deaton et al. (177) did detect a statistically significant but modest improvement in cycle fecundity (108). While enthusiasm for clomiphene needs to be balanced against potential long-term risks, these therapies may be appropriate for young women with shorter durations of infertility.

Controlled Ovarian Hyperstimulation

Gonadotropins administered to ovulatory women will reliably induce the development of multiple ovarian follicles that will release multiple eggs after the administration of hCG. The data evaluating this treatment for patients with minimal or no apparent abnormalities are difficult to interpret. Studies vary dramatically in regard to study design, inclusion criteria, use of controls, variables tested, end points, and statistical methods. Some trials limit inclusion to rigorously defined unexplained infertility or endometriosis, while others consider these groups as well as those with male factor or cervical factor infertility together. Studies have evaluated COH vs. clomiphene or expectant management, the use of IUI or timed intercourse, or various combinations of these measures (178–184).

The largest and best controlled trials indicate that there is probably an improvement in cycle fecundity and cumulative pregnancy rates in women with unexplained infertility or ASRM stage I and II endometriosis (178–182). Treatment cycle fecundity of 13% to 19% vs. 5% to 9% for controls has been reported with differences in cumulative pregnancy rates after four to six cycles of 34% to 60% vs. 15% to 24% (178–182). In many of these studies, "control" patients continued to receive therapy such as clomiphene or IUI alone, confounding the results and possibly underestimating the effectiveness of COH.

The impact of IUI in combination with COH is even less clear. The literature is conflicting on this subject but, overall, suggests that IUI is beneficial (185–189). In fact, a small but well-designed trial by Olive's group (190) demonstrated a significant benefit of two IUIs per treatment cycle.

It is important to keep in mind that these treatment successes, while often compelling, come at significant costs. Increased utilization of medical technology and the higher incidence of multiple gestation are two prominent examples of the consequences of infertility treatment. Unfortunately, the understandable reluctance of investigators and patients to accept randomization to prolonged periods of expectant management has hampered our ability to develop a clear picture of effective treatment for these types of infertility.

Assisted Reproductive Technologies

As with all the treatments mentioned above, a subgroup of patients will fail to conceive. For these couples, as well as those with advanced reproductive age or long-standing infertility (greater than 3 years), ART is the appropriate therapy. IVF, GIFT, and zygote intrafallopian transfer (ZIFT) have all been used to treat patients with unexplained infertility. Success rates in this group are similar to those seen with tubal infertility (28,191,192). While GIFT was initially thought to hold an advantage over IVF for patients with patent tubes, this difference has not held up (28,108). Cumulative pregnancy rates after six cycles often exceed 60% (108,192). Moreover, ART has given us insight into possible mechanisms for unexplained infertility. Some women with this diagnosis produce oocytes with absent or significantly lower fertilization rates, presumably responsible for their infertility (193). These women may be treated with donated oocytes or offered adoption.

Male Factor Infertility—Sperm Disorders

We will confine our discussion to treatments of varicocele, seminal antisperm antibodies, and severe oligo- or azoospermia. Milder degrees of abnormality are considered in the previous section.

Varicocele

Varicocele is a relatively common finding in men. Its incidence in infertile couples has been reported to be as high as 35% to 45%; one study reported an 81% incidence in secondary infertility (194–196). While it is clear that a varicocele may cause abnormalities in the semen analyisis, this is not always the case (196,197). Furthermore, surgical treatment may not be universally beneficial. Studies of varicocele repair are poorly controlled and often report changes in sperm parameters rather than pregnancy rates (196).

One well controlled study showed a minimal improvement in motility after surgery without a significant improvement in pregnancy rates (197). Men with severely depressed sperm parameters or who are symptomatic may benefit more from surgery, and we recommend urologic evaluation in these cases.

Antisperm Antibodies

Seminal antibodies directed at sperm can occur after vasectomy, torsion, testicular trauma, or infection (28). Their presence is suggested by agglutination on the semen analysis and confirmed with the immunobead test. Glucocorticoid treatment of men with these antibodies, while appealing in concept, has not met with great success. Extended therapy has resulted in 9-month cumulative pregnancy rates of only 27% at the cost of the established risks of steroid treatment (108).

The popularity of treating this disorder with IUI has not been affected by the lack of data supporting its use. Poor recovery of motile sperm after immunobead separation or swim-up indicates the use of IVF techniques (28).

ART for Sperm Disorders

As recently as 1992, the carefully prepared review by Hull (frequently cited in this chapter) reported modest results using IVF and micromanipulation techniques for nonimmune sperm disorders, and no effective treatment for azoospermia. High concentrations of sperm per oocyte and varying degrees of zona pellucida dissection resulted in fertilization rates of 11% to 56% and maximal per cycle pregnancy rates of less than 20%, confirming the correlation between sperm number and function (108).

While some groups improved on these numbers, it is the introduction of ICSI that has revolutionized the treatment of male factor infertility. In 1992, van Steirteghem's group (101) reported that mechanical injection of a single sperm into an oocyte can result in fertilization, cleavage, clinical pregnancy, and delivery. Since that time, multiple groups have reported pregnancy rates equal to or in excess of those for tubal factor after ICSI. Sperm have been utilized from the ejaculate, from frozen specimens, and after epididymal aspiration. Recently, immature sperm from testicular tissue have resulted in pregnancy and delivery, giving men with both obstructive and nonobstructive azoospermia the ability to reproduce (102–104). Prior to ICSI, donor insemination was the only choice for these couples. In fact, the only limitations on the success of these treatments are the same as for other disorders: age of the female and, possibly, duration of infertility (198,199).

Follow-up of children born after ICSI has to date been uniformly reassuring (200). However, new data reported by Pryor et al. (201) suggest that many sperm disorders could be due to microdeletions of the Y chromosome and that ICSI may permit genetically transmissible male infertility. Evaluation of this hypothesis will take years, but given the progress made in treating male infertility to date, this may not be an issue in the future. Another similar and important consideration exists for obstructive azoospermia due to congenital bilateral absence of the vas deferens. The genetic defect responsible for this condition is often the same as that for cystic fibrosis (CF). The female partner should be screened for the known CF mutations before pursuing ICSI.

SUMMARY

This is a time of rapid and exciting changes in the evaluation and treatment of infertility. An efficient and careful evaluation, with constant regard to the woman's age at presentation, will result in an appropriate diagnosis for most couples. The prognostic value of early follicular testing, be it day 3 FSH, estradiol or inhibin-B, and the clomiphene challenge test, can be invaluable in selecting the appropriate treatment.

Ovulation disorders and severe tubal disease are relatively straightforward to treat. Unexplained infertility and minor degrees of endometriosis are more of a therapeutic challenge. Inconsistency in the literature has left the decision to move on to more aggressive and expensive treatment a difficult one. Some conclusions, however, can be drawn. Women over 35, and certainly those over 39, and those with long-standing infertility are more likely to require ART for conception, and early referral is appropriate.

Once complex, the treatment options for severe male infertility have been made much clearer with the astonishing success of ICSI. It is hoped that emerging ideas in implantation and genetics will find other forms of infertility yielding as easily to treatment in the next edition of this book.

10 KEY POINTS

1. As many as 15% of couples will be affected by impaired fertility, resulting in substantial physical, emotional, and financial costs.

2. Constant attention must be paid to the age of the female partner and the duration of the infertility; the chance of successful conception declines steadily with age, most dramatically after 39.

3. Ovulation can be most easily documented by serum progesterone concentrations in the luteal phase.

4. Semen analysis should be one of the first tests in the evaluation of infertility, and multiple examinations may be necessary.

5. Cycle day 3 FSH and estradiol concentrations can be used to evaluate ovarian function and offer valuable prognostic information.

6. Approximately 80% of women with PCOS will ovulate on clomiphene citrate, and a majority will conceive within 6 months.

7. Gonadotropins for ovulation induction or hyperstimulation must be administered with caution to limit the risks of multiple gestation and hyperstimulation syndrome.

8. Severe tubal disease and endometriosis are probably best treated with *in vitro* fertilization.

9. Treatment of unexplained infertility is age- and duration-dependent; ovarian stimulation, IUI, and ART have all been used with success.

10. Intracytoplasmic sperm injection (ICSI) has revolutionized the treatment of male infertility and is the treatment of choice for severe oligospermia or azoospermia.

REFERENCES

1. Ober WB. Reuben's Mandrakes: infertility in the Bible. *Int J Gynecol Pathol* 1984;3:299–317.
2. Ober WB. Obstetrical events that shaped Western history. *Yale J Biol Med* 1992;65:201–210.
3. McLane CM, McLane M. A half century of sterility 1840–1890. *Fertil Steril* 1969;20(6):853–870.
4. Chen SH, Wallach EE. Five decades of progress in management of the infertile couple. *Fertil Steril* 1994;62(4):665–685.
5. Shushan A, Eisenberg VH, Schenker JG. Subfertility in the era of assisted reproduction: changes and consequences. *Fertil Steril* 1995;64(3):459–469.
6. Neumann PJ, Gharib SD, Weinstein MC. The cost of a successful delivery with in vitro fertilization. *N Engl J Med* 1994; 331:239–243.
7. Westhoff CF. Fertility in the United States. *Science* 1986; 234(4776):554–559.
8. Mosher WD, Pratt WF. Fecundity and infertility in the United States: incidence and trends. *Fertil Steril* 1991;56:192–193.
9. Wilcox LS, Mosher WD. Use of infertility services in the United States. *Obstet Gynecol* 1993;82:122–127.
10. Wilcox AJ, Weinberg CR, O'Connor JF, et al. Incidence of early loss of pregnancy. *N Engl J Med* 1988;319:189–194.
11. Guzick DS, Grefenstette I, Baffone K, et al. Infertility evaluation in fertile women: a model for assessing the efficacy of infertility testing. *Hum Reprod* 1994;9(12):2306–2310.
12. Bostofte E, Bagger P, Michael A, et al. Fertility prognosis for infertile couples. *Fertil Steril* 1993;59:102–107.
13. Eimers JM, te Velde ER, Gerritse R, et al. The prediction of the chance to conceive in subfertile couples. *Fertil Steril* 1994;61:44–52.
14. Wichmann L, Isola J, Tuohimaa P. Prognostic variables in predicting pregnancy: a prospective follow up study of 907 couples with an infertility problem. *Hum Reprod* 1994; 9(6):1102–1108.
15. Collins JA, Wrixon W, Jancs LB, et al. Treatment-independent pregnancy among infertile couples. *N Engl J Med* 1983; 309:1201–1206.
16. Toner JP, Flood JT. Fertility after the age of 40. *Obstet Gynecol Clin North Am* 1993;20:261–272.
17. Newcomb WW, Rodriguez M, Johnson JWC. Reproduction in the older gravida: a literature review. *J Reprod Med* 1991; 36:839–845.
18. Fédération CECOS, Schwartz D, Mayaux MJ. Female fecundity as a function of age. *N Engl J Med* 1982;306:404–406.
19. Menken J, Trussell J, Larsen U. Age and infertility. *Science* 1986;233:1389–1394.
20. Jacobs SL, Metzger DA, Dodson WC, et al. Effect of age on response to human menopausal gonadotropin stimulation. *J Clin Endocrinol Metab* 1990;71:1525–1530.
21. Van Kooij RJ, Looman CWN, Habbema JDF, et al. Age-dependent decrease in embryo implantation rate after in vitro fertilization. *Fertil Steril* 1996;66:769–775.
22. Sauer MV, Paulson RJ, Lobo RA. Reversing the natural decline in human fertility. *JAMA* 1992;268:1275–1279.
23. Meldrum DR. Female reproductive aging—ovarian and uterine factors. *Fertil Steril* 1993;59:1–5.
24. Navot D, Drews MR, Bergh PA, et al. Age-related decline in female fertility is not due to diminished capacity of the uterus to sustain embryo implantation. *Fertil Steril* 1994;61: 97–101.
25. Hull MGR. Epidemiology of infertility and polycystic ovarian disease: endocrinological and demographic studies. *Gynecol Endocrinol* 1987;1:235–245.
26. Polson DW, Wadsworth J, Adams J, et al. Polycystic ovaries—a common finding in normal women. *Lancet* 1988;1:870–872.
27. Clayton RN, Ogden V, Hodgkinson J, et al. How common are polycystic ovaries in normal women and what is their significance for the fertility of the population? *Clin Endocrinol* 1992;37:127–134.

28. Speroff L, Glass RH, Kase NG. *Clinical gynecologic endocrinology and infertility.* 6th ed. Lippincott Williams & Wilkins, 1999.

29. Sagle M, Bishop K, Ridley N, et al. Recurrent early miscarriage and polycystic ovaries. *Br Med J* 1988;297:1027–1028.

30. Jones EE. Hyperprolactinemia and female infertility. *J Reprod Med* 1989;34:117–126.

31. Bahamondes L, Saboya W, Tambascia M, et al. Galactorrhea, infertility, and short luteal phases in hyperprolactinemic women: early stage of amenorrhea-galactorrhea? *Fertil Steril* 1979;32:476–477.

32. Asukai K, Uemura T, Minaguchi H. Occult hyperprolactinemia in infertile women. *Fertil Steril* 1993;60:423–427.

33. Gnarpe H, Friberg J. T-Mycoplasmas as a possible cause for reproductive failure. *Nature* 1973;242:120–121.

34. De Louvois J, Harrison RF, Blades M, et al. Frequency of mycoplasma in fertile and infertile couples. *Lancet* 1974;1:1073–1075.

35. Harrison RF, Blades M, de Louvois J, et al. Doxycycline treatment and human infertility. *Lancet* 1975;1:605–607.

36. Wallach EE, Vu KK. Myomata uteri and infertility. *Obstet Gynecol Clin North Am* 1995;22:791–799.

37. Buttram VC, Reiter RC. Uterine leiomyomata: etiology, symptomatology, and management. *Fertil Steril* 1981;36:433–445.

38. Swerdloff RS, Wang C, Kandeel FR. Evaluation of the infertile couple. *Endocrinol Metab Clin North Am* 1988;17:301–337.

39. Akin A, Elstein M. The value of the basal temperature chart in the management of infertility. *Int J Fertil* 1975;20:122–124.

40. Wilcox AJ, Weinberg CR, Baird DD. Timing of sexual intercourse in relation to ovulation. *N Engl J Med* 1995;23:1517–1521.

41. Quagliarello J, Arny M. Inaccuracy of basal body temperature charts in predicting urinary luteinizing hormone surges. *Fertil Steril* 1986;45:334–337.

42. McCarthy JJ, Rockette HE. Prediction of ovulation with basal body temperature. *J Reprod Med* 1986;31:742–747.

43. Miller PB, Soules MR. The usefulness of a urinary LH kit for ovulation prediction during menstrual cycles of normal women. *Obstet Gynecol* 1996;87:13–17.

44. Kenigsberg D. New tests for the prediction of ovulation. *Clin Obstet Gynecol* 1989;32:533–540.

45. Baltzer FR. Ultrasonic indices of ovulation. *J Reprod Med* 1996;31:764–769.

46. Israel R, Mishell DR, Stone SC, et al. Single luteal phase serum progesterone assay as an indicator of ovulation. *Am J Obstet Gynecol* 1972;112:1043–1046.

47. Collins JA. Diagnostic assessment of the infertile female partner. In: Barbieri RL, ed. *Current problems in obstetrics, gynecology and fertility.* Chicago: Year Book Medical, 1988:11–42.

48. Ginsburg KA. Luteal phase defect: etiology, diagnosis, management. *Endocrinol Metab Clin North Am* 1992;21:85–104.

49. Soules MR, McLachlan RI, Ek M, et al. Luteal phase deficiency: characterization of reproductive hormones over the menstrual cycle. *J Clin Endocrinol Metab* 1989;69:804–811.

50. Bopp B, Shoupe D. Luteal phase defects. *J Reprod Med* 1993;38:348–356.

51. Batista MC, Cartledge TP, Zellmer AW, et al. A prospective controlled study of luteal and endometrial abnormalities in an infertile population. *Fertil Steril* 1996;65:495–502.

52. Li TC, Dockery P, Cooke ID. Endometrial development in the luteal phase of women with various types of infertility: comparison with women of normal fertility. *Hum Reprod* 1991;6:325–330.

53. Noyes RW, Hertig AT, Rock J. Dating the endometrial biopsy. *Fertil Steril* 1950;1:3–25.

54. Davidson BJ, Thrasher TV, Seraj IM. An analysis of endometrial biopsies performed for infertility. *Fertil Steril* 1987;48:770–774.

55. Peters AJ, Lloyd RP, Coulam CB. Prevalence of out-of-phase endometrial biopsy specimens. *Am J Obstet Gynecol* 1992;166:1738–1746.

56. Smith S. Determining the time of the urinary luteinizing hormone surge: does it facilitate the interpretation of endometrial biopsy results? *J Reprod Med* 1992;37:785–788.

57. WHO. *Laboratory manual for the examination of human semen and sperm-cervical mucus interaction,* 3rd ed. Cambridge, England: Cambridge University Press, 1992.

58. Sokol RZ, Sparkes R. Demonstrated paternity in spite of severe idiopathic oligospermia. *Fertil Steril* 1987;47:356–358.

59. Jouannet P, Feneaux D. Sperm analysis. *Ann Biol Clin* 1987;45:335–339.

60. Wolf DP, Sokoloski JE, Quigley MM. Correlation of human in vitro fertilization with a hamster egg bioassay. *Fertil Steril* 1983;40:53–59.

61. Bar-Chama N, Lamb DJ. Evaluation of sperm function: what is available in the modern andrology laboratory? *Urol Clin North Am* 1994;21:443–446.

62. Kruger TF, Acosta AA, Simmons KF, et al. New method of evaluating sperm morphology with predictive value for human in vitro fertilization. *Urology* 1987;30:248–251.

63. Kruger TF, Acosta AA, Simmons KF, et al. Predictive value of abnormal sperm morphology in in vitro fertilization. *Fertil Steril* 1988;49:112–117.

64. Kruger TF, Menkveld R, Stander FSH, et al. Sperm morphologic features as a prognostic factor in in vitro fertilization. *Fertil Steril* 1986;46:1118–1123.

65. Eggert-Kruse W, Reimann-Andersen J, Rohr G, et al. Clinical relevance of sperm morphology assessment using strict criteria and relationship with sperm-mucus interaction in vivo and in vitro. *Fertil Steril* 1995;63:612–624.

66. O'Shea DL, Odem RR, Cholewa C, et al. Long-term follow-up of couples after hamster egg penetration testing. *Fertil Steril* 1993;60:1040–1045.

67. Griffith CS, Grimes DA. The validity of the postcoital test. *Am J Obstet Gynecol* 1990;162:615–620.

68. Gibor Y, Garcia CJ, Cohen MR, et al. The cyclical changes in the physical properties of the cervical mucus and the results of the postcoital test. *Fertil Steril* 1970;21:20–27.

69. Harrison RF. The diagnostic and therapeutic potential of the postcoital test. *Fertil Steril* 1981;36:71–75.

70. Glatstein IZ, Best CL, Palumbo A, et al. The reproducibility of the postcoital test: a prospective study. *Obstet Gynecol* 1995;85:396–400.

71. Collins JA, So Y, Wilson EH, et al. The postcoital test as a predictor of pregnancy among 355 infertile couples. *Fertil Steril* 1984;41:703–708.

72. Jette NT, Glass RH. Prognostic value of the postcoital test. *Fertil Steril* 1972;23:29–32.

73. Oei SG, Keirse MJNC, Bloemenkamp KWM, et al. European postcoital tests: opinions and practice. *Br J Obstet Gynaecol* 1995;102:621–624.

74. Check JH, Dietterich C, Lauer C, et al. Ovulation-inducing drugs versus specific mucus therapy for cervical factor. *Int J Fertil* 1991;36:108–112.

75. Karande VC, Pratt DE, Rabin DS, et al. The limited value of hysterosalpingography in assessing tubal status and fertility potential. *Fertil Steril* 1995;63:1167–1171.

76. Henig I, Prough SG, Cheatwood M, et al. Hysterosalpingography, laparoscopy and hysteroscopy in infertility: a comparative study. *J Reprod Med* 1991;36:573–575.

77. Mol BWJ, Swart P, Bossuyt PMM, et al. Is hysterosalpingography an important tool in predicting fertility outcome? *Fertil Steril* 1997;67:663–669.

78. Stumpf PG, March CM. Febrile morbidity following hystero-

salpingraphy: identification of risk factors and recommendations for prophylaxis. *Fertil Steril* 1980;33:487–492.

79. Opsahl MS, Miller B, Klein TA. The predictive value of hysterosalpingraphy for tubal and peritoneal infertility factors. *Fertil Steril* 1993;60:444–448.

80. Swart P, Mol BWJ, van der Veen F, et al. The accuracy of hysterosalpingraphy in the diagnosis of tubal pathology: a meta-analysis. *Fertil Steril* 1995;64:486–491.

81. Cundiff G, Carr BR, Marshburn PB. Infertile couples with a normal hysterosalpingogram. *J Reprod Med* 1995;40:19–24.

82. Mackey RA, Glass RH, Olson LE, et al. Pregnancy following hysterosalpingraphy with oil and water soluble dye. *Fertil Steril* 1971;22:504–507.

83. Navot D, Rosenwaks Z, Margalioth EJ. Prognostic assessment of female fecundity. *Lancet* 1987;2:645–647.

84. Muasher SJ, Oehninger S, Simonetti S, et al. The value of basal and/or stimulated serum gonadotropin levels in prediction of stimulation response and in vitro fertilization outcome. *Fertil Steril* 1988;50:298–307.

85. Scott RT, Toner JP, Muasher SJ, et al. Follicle-stimulating hormone levels on cycle day 3 are predictive of in vitro fertilization outcome. *Fertil Steril* 1989;51:651–654.

86. Toner JP, Philput CB, Jones GS, et al. Basal follicle-stimulating hormone level is a better predictor of in vitro fertilization performance than age. *Fertil Steril* 1991;55:784–791.

87. Pearlstone AC, Fournet N, Gambone JC, et al. Ovulation induction in women age 40 and older: the importance of basal follicle-stimulating hormone level and chronological age. *Fertil Steril* 1992;58:674–679.

88. Khalifia E, Toner JP, Muasher SJ, et al. Significance of basal follicle-stimulating hormone levels in women with one ovary in a program of in vitro fertilization. *Fertil Steril* 1992;57:835–839.

89. Loumaye E, Billion J-M, Mire J-M, et al. Prediction of individual response to controlled ovarian hyperstimulation by means of a clomiphene citrate challenge test. *Fertil Steril* 1990;53:295–301.

90. Tanbo T, Dale PO, Lunde O, et al. Prediction of response to controlled ovarian hyperstimulation: a comparison of basal and clomiphene citrate-stimulated follicle-stimulating hormone levels. *Fertil Steril* 1992;57:819–824.

91. Scott RT, Illions EH, Kost ER, et al. Evaluation of the significance of the estradiol response during the clomiphene citrate challenge test. *Fertil Steril* 1993;60:242–246.

92. Padilla SL, Bayati J, Garcia JE. Prognostic value of the early serum estradiol response to leuprolide acetate in in vitro fertilization. *Fertil Steril* 1990;53:288–294.

93. Smotrich DB, Widra EA, Gindoff PR, et al. Prognostic value of day 3 estradiol on in vitro fertilization outcome. *Fertil Steril* 1995;64:1136–1140.

94. Seifer DB, Lambert-Messerlian G, Hogan JW, et al. Day 3 serum inhibin-B is predictive of assisted reproductive technologies outcome. *Fertil Steril* 1997;67:110–114.

95. Seifer DB, Gardiner AC, Lambert-Messerlian G, et al. Differential secretion of dimeric inhibin in cultured luteinized granulosa cells as a function of ovarian reserve. *J Clin Endocrinol Metab* 1996;81:736–739.

96. McLachlan RI, Robertson DM, Healy DL, et al. Circulating immunoreactive inhibin levels during the normal human menstrual cycle. *J Clin Endocrinol Metab* 1987;65:954–961.

97. Mukherjee T, Copperman AB, Lapinski R, et al. An elevated day three follicle-stimulating hormone: luteinizing hormone ration (FSH:LH) in the presence of a normal day 3 FSH predicts a poor response to controlled ovarian hyperstimulation. *Fertil Steril* 1996;65:588–593.

98. Scott RT, Leonardi MR, Hofmann GE, et al. A prospective

99. evaluation of clumiphene citrate challenge test screening of the general infertility population. *Obstet Gynecol* 1993;82:539–544.

99. Scott RT, Opsahl MS, Leonardi MR, et al. Life table analysis of pregnancy rates in a general infertility population relative to ovarian reserve and patient age. *Hum Reprod* 1995;10:1706–1710.

100. Wallach EE. Unexplained infertility. In: Wallach EE, Zasur HA, eds. *Reproductive medicine and surgery.* St. Louis: Mosby-Year Book, 1995, 459–467.

101. Palermo G, Joris H, Devroey P, et al. Pregnancies after intracytoplasmic injection of single spermatozoon into an oocyte. *Lancet* 1992;340:17–18.

102. Nagy Z, Liu J, Cecile J, et al. Using ejaculated, fresh, and frozen-thawed epididymal and testicular spermatozoa gives rise to comparable results after intracytoplasmic sperm injection. *Fertil Steril* 1995;63:808–815.

103. Silber SJ, Van Steirteghem A, Nagy Z, et al. Normal pregnancies resulting from testicular sperm extractin and intracytoplasmic sperm injection for azoospermia due to maturation arrest. *Fertil Steril* 1996;66:110–117.

104. Devroey P, Nagy P, Tournaye H, et al. Outcome of intracytoplasmic sperm injection with testicular spermatozoa in obstructive and non-obstructive azoospermia. *Hum Reprod* 1995;10:1015–1018.

105. Whittemore AS. The risk of ovarian cancer after treatment for infertility. *N Engl J Med* 1994;331:805–806.

106. Rossing MA, Daling JR, Weiss NS, et al. Ovarian tumors in a cohort of infertile women. *N Engl J Med* 1994:331:771–778.

107. Bristow RE, Karlan BY. Ovulation induction, infertility, and ovarian cancer risk. *Fertil Steril* 1996;66:499–507.

108. Hull MGR. Infertility treatment: relative effectiveness of conventional and assisted conception methods. *Hum Reprod* 1992;7:785–796.

109. Irianni F, Hodgen G. Mechanism of ovulation. *Endocrinol Metab Clin North Am* 1992;21:19–38.

110. Hillier S, Reichert L, Van Hall E. Control of preovulatory follicular estrogen biosynthesis in the human ovary. *J Endocrinol Metab* 1981;52:847–856.

111. Spencer S, Cataldo N, Jaffe R. Apoptosis in the human female reproductive tract. *Obstet Gynecol Surv* 1996;51:314–323.

112. Erickson G, Danforth D. Ovarian control of follicle development. *Am J Obstet Gynecol* 1995;172:736–747.

113. Ryan KJ, Petro Z. Steroid biosynthesis by human ovarian granulosa and theca cells. *J Clin Endocrinol Metab* 1966;26:46–52.

114. Le Nestour E, Marraoui J, Lahlou N, et al. Role of estradiol in the rise in follicle-stimulating hormone levels during the luteal-follicular phase transition. *J Clin Endocrinol Metab* 1993;77:439–442.

115. Erickson G. Physiologic basis of ovulation induction. *Semin Reprod Endocrinol* 1996;14:287–297.

116. McNatty KP, Makris A, Osathamondh R. Effects of luteinizing hormone on steroidogenesis by thecal tissue from human ovarian follicles in vitro. *Steroids* 1980;36:53–63.

117. Adashi E. Intraovarian peptides: stimulators and inhibitors of follicular growth and differentiation. *Endocrinol Metab Clin North Am* 1992;21:1–17.

118. Danforth D. Endocrine and paracrine control of oocyte development. *Am J Obstet Gynecol* 1995;172:747–752.

119. Roseff S, Bangah L, Kettel M, et al. Dynamic changes in circulating inhibin levels during the luteal-follicular transition of the human menstrual cycle. *J Clin Endocrinol Metab* 1989;69:1033–1039.

120. McLachlin R, Robertson D, Healy D, et al. Circulating immu-

noreactive inhibin levels during the normal human menstrual cycle. *J Clin Endocrinol Metab* 1987;65:954–961.

121. Strauss J, Steinkampf MP. Pituitary-ovarian interactions during follicular maturation and ovulation. *Am J Obstet Gynecol* 1995;172:726–735.

122. Strickler R, Radwanska E, Williams D. Controlled ovarian hyperstimulation regimens in assisted reproductive technologies. *Am J Obstet Gynecol* 1995;172:766–773.

123. Cuellar FG. Bromocriptine mesylate (parlodel) in the management of amenorrhea/galactorrhea associated with hyperprolactinemia. *Obstet Gynecol* 1980;55:278–284.

124. Brue T, Lancranjan I, Louvet J-P, et al. A long-acting repeatable form of bromocriptine as long-term treatment of prolactin-secreting macroadenomas: a multicenter study. *Fertil Steril* 1992;57:74–80.

125. Lamberts SWJ, Quik RFP. A comparison of the efficacy and safety of pergolide and bromocriptine in the treatment of hyper-prolactinemia. *J Clin Endocrinol Metab* 1991;72:635–641.

126. Brue T, Pellegrini I, Gunz G, et al. Effects of the dopamine agonist CV 205–502 in human prolactinomas resistant to bromocriptine. *J Clin Endocrinol Metab* 1992;74:577–584.

127. Downs KA, Gibson M. Clomiphene citrate therapy for luteal phase defect. *Fertil Steril* 1983;39:34–38.

128. Murray DL, Reich L, Adashi EY. Oral clomiphene citrate and vaginal progesterone suppositories in the treatment of luteal phase dysfunction: a comparative study. *Fertil Steril* 1989;51:35–41.

129. Berga SL, Mortola JF, Suh B, et al. Neuroendocrine aberrations in women with functional hypothalamic amenorrhea. *J Clin Endocrinol Metab* 1989;68:301–308.

130. Olster DH, Ferin M. Corticotropin-releasing hormone inhibits gonadotropin secretion in the ovariectomized rhesus monkey. *J Clin Endocrinol Metab* 1987;65:262–267.

131. Berga SL, Loucks AB, Rossmanith WG, et al. Acceleration of luteinizing hormone pulse frequency in functional hypothalamic amennorrhea by dopamine blockade. *J Clin Endocrinol Metab* 1991;72:151–156.

132. Bullen BA, Skrinar GS, Beitins IZ, et al. Induction of menstrual disorders by strenuous exercise in untrained women. *N Engl J Med* 1985;312:1349–1353.

133. Yuen BH, Pride S. Induction of ovulation with exogenous gonadotropins in anovulatory infertile women. *Semin Reprod Endocrinol* 1990;8:186–197.

134. Carr JS, Reid RL. Ovulation induction with gonadotropin-releasing hormone (GnRH). *Semin Reprod Endocrinol* 1990; 8:174–185.

135. Braat DDM, Schoemaker R, Schoemaker J. Life table analysis of fecundity in intravenously gonadotropin-releasing hormone-treated patients with normogonadotropic and hypogonado-tropic amenorrhea. *Fertil Steril* 1991;55:266–271.

136. Ernst S, Hite G, Cantrell JS, et al. Stereochemistry of geometric isomers of clomiphene: a correction of the literature and a reexamination of structure-activity relationships. *J Pharm Sci* 1976;65:148–150.

137. Clark JH, Markaverich BM. The agonistic-antagonistic properties of clomiphene: a review. *Pharmacol Ther* 1982;15:467–519.

138. Kerin JF, Liu JH, Phillipou G, et al. Evidence for a hypothalamic site of action of clomiphene citrate in women. *J Clin Endocrinol Metab* 1985;61:265–268.

139. Kettel LM, Hummel WP. Ovulation induction in the estro-genized anovulatory patient. *Semin Reprod Endocrinol* 1996; 14:309–315.

140. Gysler M, March CM, Mishell DR, et al. A decade's experience with an individualized clomiphene treatment regimen including its effect on the postcoital test. *Fertil Steril* 1982;37:161–167.

141. Bateman BG, Nunley WC, Kolp LA. Exogenous estrogen ther-apy for treatment of clomiphene citrate-induced cervical mucus abnormalities: is it effective? *Fertil Steril* 1990;54:577–579.

142. Flamingni C, Venturoli S, Paradisi R, et al. Use of human urinary follicle-stimulating hormone in infertile women with polycystic ovaries. *J Reprod Med* 1985;30:184–188.

143. Garcea N, Campo S, Panetta V, et al. Induction of ovulation with purified urinary follicle-stimulating hormone in patients with polycystic ovarian syndrome. *Am J Obstet Gynecol* 1985;151:635–640.

144. Buvat J, Buvat-Herbaut M, Marcolin G, et al. Purified follicle-stimulating hormone in polycystic ovary syndrome: slow administration is safer and more effective. *Fertil Steril* 1989; 52:553–559.

145. Homburg R, Berkowitz D, Levy T, et al. In vitro fertilization and embryo transfer for the treatment of infertility associated with polycystic ovary syndrome. *Fertil Steril* 1993;60:858–863.

146. Kovacs G, Buckler H, Bangah M, et al. Treatment of anovulation due to polycystic ovarian syndrome by laparoscopic ovarian electrocautery. *Br J Obstet Gynecol* 1991;98:30–35.

147. Daniell JF, Miller W. Polycystic ovaries treated by laparoscopic laser vaporization. *Fertil Steril* 1989;51:232–236.

148. Rebar RW, Connolly HV. Clinical features of young women with hypergonadotropic amenorrhea. *Fertil Steril* 1990;53: 804–810.

149. McComb P. Microsurgical tubocornual anastomosis for occlusive cornual disease: reproducible results without the need for tubouterine implantation. *Fertil Steril* 1986;46:571–577.

150. Audibert F. Therapeutic strategy in tubal infertility. *Ann NY Acad Sci* 1993:460–468.

151. Dlugi AM, Reddy S, Saleh WA, et al. Pregnancy rates after operative endoscopic treatment of total (neosalpingostomy) or near total (salpingostomy) distal tubal occlusion. *Fertil Steril* 1994;62:913–920.

152. Schlaff WD, Hassiakos DK, Damewood MD, et al. Neosalpin-gostomy for distal tubal obstruction: prognostic factors and impact of surgical technique. *Fertil Steril* 1990;54:984–990.

153. Mage G, Pouly J-L, de Joliniere JB, et al. A preoperative classification to predict the intrauterine and ectopic pregnancy rates after distal tubal microsurgery. *Fertil Steril* 1986;46:807–810.

154. Society for Assisted Reproductive Technology and the American Society for Reproductive Medicine. Assisted reproductive technology in the United States and Canada: 1994 results generated from the American Society for Reproductive Medicine/Society for Assisted Reproductive Technology Registry. *Fertil Steril* 1996;66:697–705.

155. Alsalili M, Yuzpe A, Tummon I, et al. Cumulative pregnancy rates and pregnancy outcome after in-vitro fertilization: > 5000 cycles at one centre. *Hum Reprod* 1995;10:470–474.

156. Penzias AS, DeCherney AH. Is there ever a role for tubal surgery? *Am J Obstet Gynecol* 1996;174:1218–1223.

157. Kassabji M, Sims JA, Butler L, et al. Reduced pregnancy outcome in patients with unilateral or bilateral hydrosalpinx after in vitro fertilization. *Eur J Obstet Gynecol Reprod Biol* 1994; 56:129–132.

158. Mansour RT, Aboulghar MA, Serour GI, et al. Fluid accumulation of the uterine cavity before embryo transfer: a possible hindrance for implantation. *J In Vitro Fertil Embryo Transfer* 1991;8:157–159.

159. Strandell A, Waldenstrom U, Nilsson L, et al. Hydrosalpinx reduces in-vitro fertilization/embryo transfer rates. *Hum Reprod* 1994;9:861–863.

160. Vandromme J, Chasse E, Lejeune B, et al. Hydrosalpinges in in-vitro fertilization: an unfavourable prognostic feature. *Hum Reprod* 1995;10:576–579.

161. Am Soc for Reprod Med. Revised American Society for Repro-

ductive Medicine classification fo endometriosis: 1996. *Fertil Steril* 1997;67:817–821.

162. Adamson GD, Pasta DJ. Surgical treatment of endometriosis-associated infertility: meta-analysis compared with survival analysis. *Am J Obstet Gynecol* 1994;171:1488–1505.

163. Adamson GD, Hurd SJ, Pasta DJ, et al. Laparoscopic endometriosis treatment: is it better? *Fertil Steril* 1993;59:35–44.

164. Olive DL, Martin DC. Treatment of endometriosis-associated infertility with CO_2 laser laparoscopy: the use of one- and two-parameter exponential models. *Fertil Steril* 1987;48:18–23.

165. Kodama H, Fukuda J, Karube H, et al. Benefit of in vitro fertilization treatment for endometriosis-associated infertility. *Fertil Steril* 1996;66:974–979.

166. Matson PL, Yovich JL. The treatment of infertility associated with endometriosis by in vitro fertilization. *Fertil Steril* 1986;46:432–434.

167. Nezhat C, Crowgey S, Nezhat F. Videolaseroscopy for the treatment of endometriosis associated with infertility. *Fertil Steril* 1989;51:237–240.

168. Marcoux S, Maheux R, Bérubé S, Canadian Collaborative Group on Endometriosis. Laparoscopic surgery in infertile women with minimal or mild endometriosis. *N Engl J Med* 1997;337:217–222.

169. Hughes EG, Fedorkow DM, Collins JA. A quantitative overview of controlled trials in endometriosis-associated infertility. *Fertil Steril* 1993;59:963–970.

170. Telimaa S. Danazol and medroxyprogesterone acetate inefficacious in the treatment of infertility in endometriosis. *Fertil Steril* 1988;50:872–875.

171. Collins JA, Rowe TC. Age of the female partner is a prognostic factor in prolonged unexplained infertility: a multicenter study. *Fertil Steril* 1989;52:15–20.

172. Martinez AR, Bernardus RE, Vermeiden JPW, et al. Basic questions on intrauterine insemination: an update. *Obstet Gynecol Surv* 1993;48:811–828.

173. Kerin JF, Peek J, Kirby C, et al. Improved conception rate after intrauterine insemination of washed spermatozoa from men with poor semen quality. *Lancet* 1984;1:533–534.

174. Kirby CA, Flaherty SP, Godfrey BM, et al. A prospective trial of intrauterine insemination of motile spermatozoa versus timed intercourse. *Fertil Steril* 1991;56:102–107.

175. Campana A, Sakkas D, Stalberg A, et al. Intrauterine insemination: evaluation of the results according to the woman's age, sperm quality, total sperm count per insemination and life table analysis. *Hum Reprod* 1996;11:732–736.

176. Friedman AJ, Juneau-Norcross M, Sedenmsky B, et al. Life table analysis of intrauterine insemination pregnancy rates for couples with cervical factor, male factor, and idiopathic infertility. *Fertil Steril* 1991;55:1005–1007.

177. Deaton JL, Gibson M, Blackmer KM, et al. A randomized, controlled trial of clomiphene citrate and intrauterine insemination in couples with unexplained infertility or surgically corrected endometriosis. *Fertil Steril* 1990;54:1083–1088.

178. Dodson WC, Haney AF. Controlled ovarian hyperstimulation and intrauterine insemination for treatment of infertility. *Fertil Steril* 1991;55:457–467.

179. DiMarzo SJ, Kennedy JF, Young PE, et al. Effect of controlled ovarian hyperstimulation on pregnancy rates after intrauterine insemination. *Am J Obstet Gynecol* 1992;166:1607–1613.

180. Fedele L, Bianchi S, Marchini M, et al. Superovulation with human menopausal gonadotropins in the treatment of infertility associated with minimal or mild endometriosis: a controlled randomized study. *Fertil Steril* 1992;58:28–31.

181. Aboulghar MA, Mansour RT, Serour GI, et al. Ovarian super-stimulation and intrauterine insemination for the treatment of unexplained infertility. *Fertil Steril* 1993;60:303–306.

182. Nulsen JC, Walsh S, Dumez S, et al. A randomized and longitudinal study of human menopausal gonadotropin with intrauterine insemination in the treatment of infertility. *Obstet Gynecol* 1993;82:780–786.

183. Vollenhoven B, Selub M, Davidson O, et al. Controlled ovarian hyperstimulation using human menopausal gonadotropin in combination with intrauterine insemination. *J Reprod Med* 1996;41:658–664.

184. Lu PY, Chen ALJ, Atkinson EJ, et al. Minimal stimulation achieves pregnancy rates comparable to human menopausal gonadotropins in the treatment of infertility. *Fertil Steril* 1996;65:583–587.

185. Karlström P-O, Torbjörn B, Lundkvist Ö. A prospective randomized trial of artificial insemination versus intercourse in cycles stimulated with human menopausal gonadotropin or clomiphene citrate. *Fertil Steril* 1993;59:554–559.

186. Melis GB, Paoletti AM, Ajossa S, et al. Ovulation induction with gonadotropins as sole treatment in infertile couples with open tubes: a randomized prospective comparison between intrauterine insemination and timed vaginal intercourse. *Fertil Steril* 1995;64:1088–1093.

187. Hurst BS, Tjaden BL, Kimball A, et al. Superovulation with or without intrauterine insemination for the treatment of infertility. *J Reprod Med* 1992:237–241.

188. Arcaini L, Bianchi S, Baglioni A, et al. Superovulation and intrauterine insemination vs. superovulation alone in the treatment of unexplained infertility. *J Reprod Med* 1994:614–618.

189. Serhal PF, Katz M, Little V, et al. Unexplained infertility—the value of Pergonal superovulation combined with intrauterine insemination. *Fertil Steril* 1988;49:602–606.

190. Silverberg KM, Johnson JV, Olive DL, et al. A prospective, randomized trial comparing two different intrauterine insemination regimens in controlled ovarian hyperstimulation cycles. *Fertil Steril* 1992;57:357–361.

191. Devroey P, Staessen C, Camus M, et al. Zygote intrafallopian transfer as a successful treatment for unexplained infertility. *Fertil Steril* 1989;52:246–249.

192. Gürgan T, Urman B, Yarali H, et al. The results of in vitro fertilization–embryo transfer in couples with unexplained infertility failing to conceive with superovulation and intrauterine insemination. *Fertil Steril* 1995;64:93–97.

193. Ezra Y, Simon A, Laufer N. Defective oocytes: a new subgroup of unexplained infertility. *Fertil Steril* 1992;58:24–27.

194. Jarow JP, Coburn M, Sigman M. Incidence of varicoceles in men with primary and secondary infertility. *Urology* 1996;47:73–76.

195. Takihara H, Sakatoku J, Cockett ATK. The pathophysiology of varicocele in male infertility. *Fertil Steril* 1991;55:861–868.

196. Schlesinger MH, Wilets IF, Nagler HM. Treatment outcome after varicocelectomy. *Urol Clin North Am* 1994;21:517–529.

197. Gorelick JI, Goldstein M. Loss of fertility in men with varicocele. *Fertil Steril* 1993;59:613–616.

198. Nagy ZP, Liu J, Joris H, et al. The result of intracytoplasmic sperm injection is not related to any of the three basic sperm parameters. *Hum Reprod* 1995;10:1123–1129.

199. Devroey P, Godoy H, Smitz J, et al. Female age predicts embryonic implantation after ICSI: a case-controlled study. *Hum Reprod* 1996;11:1324–1327.

200. Bonduelle M, Legein J, Buysse A, et al. Prospective follow-up study of 423 children born after intracytoplasmic sperm injection. *Hum Reprod* 1996;11:1558–1564.

201. Pryor JL, Kent-First M, Muallem A, et al. Microdeletions in the Y chromosome of infertile men. *N Engl J Med* 1997;336:534–539

ENVIRONMENTAL INFLUENCES AND REPRODUCTION

JODI ANNE FLAWS
FADY I. SHARARA

Female reproduction requires the appropriate function and interaction of many organs, including the hypothalamus, pituitary, breast, ovaries, uterus, and external genitalia. Several factors (including socioeconomic status, behavior, physical structure, biologic processes, and exposure to toxicants) can alter normal function of the reproductive organs and thus lead to adverse reproductive outcomes. This chapter reviews the environmental factors that have been associated with adverse female reproduction in humans, wildlife, and laboratory animals—mainly the reproductive effects of environmental chemicals and toxicants including endocrine disrupters, phytoestrogens, diethylstilbestrol, heavy metals, phthalates, solvents, industrial pollutants, pesticides, herbicides, fungicides, and cigarette smoke (Table 18.1).

ENVIRONMENTAL CHEMICALS

Endocrine Disrupters

Endocrine disrupters are exogenous substances that cause adverse health outcomes in an intact organism or its progeny via changes in endocrine function (1–6). Endocrine-disrupting chemicals often mimic hormones, block hormone action, or trigger inappropriate hormone activity (1–3). Women are exposed to endocrine disrupters in the workplace, home, community, or during medical care, and wildlife are exposed during food and water consumption (1,2).

Phthalates, phytoestrogens, pesticides, herbicides, and some industrial waste products are known endocrine disrupters (1,2,7–9). These chemicals exert a wide variety of effects on the reproductive system of a vast number of species (1,2,8,10). In marine mollusks, endocrine disrupters can induce morphologic changes in the female reproductive organs (2). In fish, they often cause hermaphroditism and reduced fertility (8,11,12). In birds, endocrine disrupters produce abnormal clutch size, female-female pairing, wasting, and embryonic deformity (2,10,13,14). In reptiles, endocrine disrupters are thought to induce abnormalities in sexual development (1,5,15). In mammals, they may be responsible for reproductive failure in Great Lakes minks and reproductive impairment in the Florida panther (2,16).

In humans, the effects of endocrine disrupters on reproductive function are not well characterized. Some studies suggest that environmental exposures to endocrine disrupters are associated with an increase in the incidence of breast cancer, precocious puberty, and early menopause (2,17). Other studies, however, have been unable to document such associations (18).

Natural Estrogens

Many reproductive toxicants are naturally present in plants and food sources such as soy products, legumes, and grains. Plant-derived estrogens and xenoestrogens (e.g., phytoestrogens) adversely affect the reproductive system of many species (1,3,19–22). In rats, phytoestrogen exposure results in persistent estrus, altered pituitary hormone levels, and precocious puberty (19–21,23). Phytoestrogens also alter uterine growth, block implantation of fertilized eggs, inhibit ovulation, and induce oocyte degeneration (21,24). In sheep, clover-derived phytoestrogens have been linked to abnormalities in cyclicity as well as infertility (25,26). In women, the effects of phytoestrogens on reproduction are equivocal. Some studies suggest that phytoestrogens are beneficial because they reduce the risk of uterine cancer, breast cancer, and menopausal hot flashes (22,27,28). Other studies indicate that phytoestrogens are harmful because they alter the length of the menstrual cycle and possibly cause premature breast growth in children (28,29).

Diethylstilbestrol (DES)

From 1950 to 1971, a synthetic estrogen known as diethylstilbestrol (DES) was used in an attempt to prevent miscarriages and pregnancy complications in women (30,31). During that time, approximately 5 to 10 million Americans were exposed to DES either during pregnancy (DES mothers) or gestation (DES daughters and sons) (30–33). In 1971, DES use was banned when it was noted that DES daughters were at risk for developing a rare form of vaginal cancer known as clear-cell adenocarcinoma (31,33–35). Studies on DES daughters suggest that DES exposure increases the risk for development of non–clear-cell mucinous

TABLE 18.1 CHEMICALS THAT ALTER FEMALE REPRODUCTION

Chemical	Species	Documented Reproductive Effects
Endocrine disruptors	Mollusks	Morphologic changes
	Fish	Hermaphroditism, reduced fertility
	Birds	Abnormal clutch size, female-female pairing, deformity
	Reptiles	Abnormal sexual development
	Mammals	Reproductive failure, impairment, possible cancers
Natural estrogens	Rats	Persistent estrus, precocious puberty, inhibition of ovulation
	Sheep	Infertility, abnormal cyclicity
	Women	Reduced cancer and hot flashes, premature breast growth
Diethylstilbestrol	Women	Cancer, menstrual irregularities, infertility, premature birth
Heavy metals	Rats	Altered hormone levels, birth defects, follicular depletion
	Mice	Altered hormone levels, birth defects
	Women	Spontaneous abortion, birth defects
Phthlates	Rodents	Spontaneous abortion, birth defects, abnormal cyclicity
Solvents	Rodents	Decreased pup survival, increased fetal resorption, birth defects
	Women	Spontaneous abortion, infertility, abnormal cyclicity
Industrial chemicals	Mice	Birth defects, follicular depletion, abnormal cyclicity
	Rats	Follicular depletion, ovarian neoplasms, birth defects
	Monkeys	Infertility, endometriosis
	Women	Spontaneous abortion, infertility, subfecundity
Pesticides	Wildlife	Reproductive failure
	Rodents	Abnormal cyclicity, decreased fertility, precocious puberty
	Women	Spontaneous abortion, preterm birth, infertility, cancer
Herbicides/fungicides	Rodents	Abnormal cyclicity, anovulation, fetotoxicity
Cigarette smoke	Rodents	Infertility, follicular depletion, premature ovarian failure
	Women	Subfecundity, infertility, follicular depletion, early menopause

adenocarcinomas consisting of atypical, irregular glands lined by endocervical, intestinal, and endometrial epithelium (36). In addition, several studies associate DES exposure with menstrual irregularities, infertility, breast cancer, ectopic pregnancies, miscarriages, and premature births (30,31,37).

Heavy Metals

Lead, mercury, cadmium, and manganese are known reproductive toxicants. Humans and wildlife are exposed to lead in paint, water, food, soil, and air. In the United States, it is estimated that more than 42 million people are exposed to lead through drinking water and that 52% of residential homes contain unacceptable levels of lead (38). These exposures are known to exert a variety of adverse effects. In rodents, lead suppresses follicle-stimulating hormone (FSH), affects gonadotropin-receptor binding in the ovary, and alters steroid metabolism (39,40). In women, lead increases the risk of complications during pregnancy and may cause spontaneous abortion, miscarriage, intrauterine death of the fetus, or preterm delivery (41–45). It also results in low birth weight, fetal growth retardation, and delays in behavioral and mental development (41,43–47).

Mercury permeates the environment and workplace in three different forms: organic mercury, elemental mercury, and inorganic mercury. Organic mercury is used as a fungicide in paints and during some industrial processes. Elemen-

tal mercury is used in dental amalgam fillings, thermometers, batteries, gold mining, and the production of some chlorine-containing chemicals. Inorganic mercury is used in electrical equipment, fungicides, antiseptics, and several brands of skin-lightening cream. These creams often contain mercury levels well above the Food and Drug Administration limit of 1 part per million (48). All three forms of mercury are thought to adversely affect female reproductive health (40,48–53). Organic mercury increases the risk of spontaneous abortion and birth defects such as microencephaly, cerebral palsy, and mental retardation (40,54–56). Elemental mercury is thought to increase the risk of spontaneous abortion, menstrual irregularities (e.g., hypermenorrhea or dysmenorrhea), and severe menstrual cramps (40,56,57). Inorganic mercury has been reported to cause menstrual irregularities (57).

Cadmium exposure occurs during welding, soldering, painting, mining, ceramics, fish consumption, and cigarette smoking (see Cigarette Smoke, below), and has been linked to a variety of adverse reproductive outcomes in laboratory animals and women (58–63). In rodents, cadmium causes structural birth defects (e.g., cleft palate, exencephaly, anophthalmia, and microphthalmia), delays lung development, induces respiratory distress syndrome, and adversely affects the nervous system (59,60,64). It also decreases production of human chorionic gonadotropin and inhibits placental transfer of oxygen and nutrients to the fetus, placing the fetus at risk for damage or death (61,65).

Manganese is naturally abundant in grains, cloves, and tea. Although low levels of manganese are required for normal growth and development, high levels interfere with some reproductive processes (63,66–68). In pregnant mice, manganese exposure leads to the birth of growth-retarded fetuses and/or fetuses with encephaly (68). In rats, manganese reduces the number of ovarian follicles and causes persistent corpora lutea (66,67). It also induces developmental abnormalities, including angulated or irregularly shaped clavicles, femurs, fibulas, humerus, scapulas, tibias, and/or ulnas (69). In humans, the effect of manganese on reproduction is equivocal. In one Australian population, manganese exposure was associated with a higher than expected number of stillbirths and clubfoot (63). There also have been reports of severe weakness, muscle atrophy, scoliosis of the spine, mild joint abnormalities, clumsiness, and tremor in children exposed to high levels of manganese during development (63).

Phthalates

Phthalates are commonly used in the manufacturing of automotive, medical, and household products (e.g., plastic wraps, beverage containers, and linings of metal cans). It is not clear whether phthalates alter reproduction in women; however, several studies indicate that they adversely affect reproductive function in laboratory animals (70–73). In mice and rats, phthalates cause spontaneous abortions and birth defects (71). In rats, phthalates prolong the estrous cycle, suppress or delay ovulation, and reduce the size of the preovulatory follicles (70,71).

Solvents

Solvents are widely used in electronics, health care products, dry-cleaning, auto repair, laboratories, varnish strippers, glues, and paints. They also are present as contaminants in drinking water (74,75). Solvents such as perchloroethylene (PCE), toluene, xylene, and styrene are known to affect reproductive function in a variety of species (76–81).

PCE is used in dry cleaning and vapor degreasing. It is extremely volatile, and thus rapidly enters the body via inhalation or dermal absorption (82,83). Once PCE enters the body, it can adversely affect reproductive function (84–86). In rats and mice, gestational exposure to PCE decreases pup survival, reduces fetal body weight, and increases the number of resorbed fetuses (76,87). In women, PCE exposure is associated with an increased risk of infertility and spontaneous abortion (42,77,84–88).

Toluene is present in glues, coatings, inks, paints, cleaning agents, and gasoline additives. In laboratory animals, gestational exposure to toluene reduces fetal weight and delays skeletal development (89). In women, toluene exposure increases the risk of spontaneous abortion by two- to fivefold and lengthens the menstrual cycle (76,89,90).

Xylene is commonly used in paints, lacquers, varnishes, gasoline, insecticides, rubber products, plastics, and leather production. In rodents, xylene increases the number of fetal resorptions, delays fetal development, and reduces birth weight (91). It also lowers the blood levels of progesterone and estrogen, blocks cyclicity, and prevents ovulation (91). In humans, xylene has been reported to increase the risk of spontaneous abortion and induce a rare birth defect known as caudal regression (76,91,92).

Styrene is used to make reinforced plastics, rubber products, and polyester resins. In rats, styrene lengthens the estrous cycle and induces embryonic death (76,81,92,93). In women, the reproductive effects of styrene exposure are unclear. Some studies demonstrate that it interferes with menstrual cyclicity, whereas others show no effect of sytrene on menses (94,95).

Industrial Chemicals

Thousands of industrial chemicals are released into the workplace or environment where they pose a human health hazard. For the most part, these chemicals have not been well studied, and thus their effects on the reproductive system are poorly understood. To date, there are several reports on four industrial chemicals: ethylene oxide, 4-vinylcyclohexene (VCH), 2,3,7,8-tetrachlorodibenzo-*p*-dioxin (TCDD), and polychlorinated biphenyls (PCBs). Ethylene oxide is a sterilizing chemical that is routinely used in dental offices. In laboratory animals, it causes malformations, fetal loss, and abnormal gestation lengths (96,97). In humans, ethylene oxide increases the risk of spontaneous abortion (98,99). In one study, the age-adjusted relative risks for spontaneous abortion, preterm birth, and postterm abnormalities among exposed women were 2.5, 2.7, and 2.1, respectively (98).

VCH and a metabolite of VCH, 4-vinylcyclohexene diepoxide (VCD), are produced during the manufacturing of synthetic rubber, insecticides, and flame retardants. Both VCH and VCD are released into the environment as gases and thus, there is potential for wildlife and human exposure. In mice, VCH causes destruction of oocytes in primordial follicles and induces ovarian neoplasms (100,101). In rats, VCD has several effects on the ovary (101–108). For example, it depletes the pool of primordial ovarian follicles, alters protein synthesis, and increases expression of genes involved in programmed cell death (Fig. 18.1) (105,107,108). In women, the effects of VCH or VCD on reproductive function are virtually unknown. This is largely because few women work or live near industries that produce VCH and VCD, thus making epidemiologic studies difficult.

TCDD is released into the environment during the bleaching of paper pulp, production of some pesticides, and incineration of chlorine-containing waste. It poses a health hazard because it persists in the environment and food chain, accumulates in adipose tissue, and is found in human

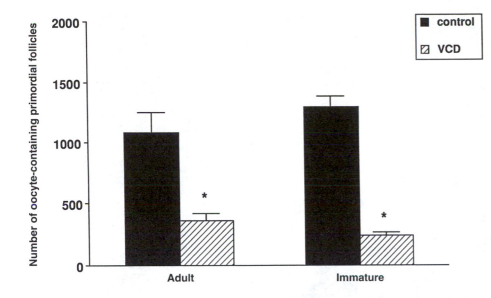

FIGURE 18.1. Effect of 4-vinylcyclohexene diepoxide (VCD) on rat primordial follicles. Adult (58 days) and immature (28 days) rats were given intraperitoneal injections of vehicle or VCD (80 mg/kg, 0.57 mmol/kg) for 30 days. On day 31, ovaries were removed, histologically processed, and used to count the number of oocytes contained in primordial follicles. Bars with * are significantly different from control ($n = 20$; $p < .05$). (From Flaws JA, Doerr JK, Sipes IG, et al. Destruction of preantral follicles in adult rats by 4-vinylcyclohexene diepoxide. *Reprod Toxicol* 1994;8:509–514, with permission.)

breast milk (109). In rats, *in utero* and lactational exposure to TCDD alters estrous cyclicity, decreases fertility, and induces abnormal development of the vaginal canal (Fig. 18.2) (9,102,110,111). It also causes partial to complete clefting of the phallus, decreases ovarian weight by 25%, and induces cystic endometrial hyperplasia (110). In adult rats, TCDD inhibits ovulation, decreases serum levels of luteinizing hormone and FSH, and increases estradiol levels (112–114). In monkeys, TCDD has been shown to alter hormone levels, decrease fertility, and cause endometriosis (115–117). In women, the effects of TCDD on the reproductive system are not well defined. A few studies, however, have evaluated the effect of TCDD on women (9,118). In 1976, women living near Seveso, Italy, were exposed to TCDD when the Icmesa factory exploded and released high levels of TCDD, as well as other toxicants, into the environment (118). Studies on these women suggest that TCDD does not alter the rates of spontaneous abortion, cytogenetic abnormalities, and birth defects compared to those for the entire Italian population (118). However, TCDD did appear to increase the number of females born 9 months after the explosion (48 females vs. 26 males) (119). The reason for the excess female births is unknown, but Mocarelli et al. (119) suggest that TCDD may modify the hormonal balance present during gestation, selectively cause spontaneous miscarriage of male fetuses, or directly affect genes responsible for sex determination.

PCBs were once used in the production of electrical transformers, capacitators, hydraulic fluids, plasiticizers, and adhesives. These chemicals were banned in the United States in 1977, but still persist in the environment and food chain today (120–123). In laboratory animals, PCBs reduce progesterone levels, stimulate uterine growth, prolong the estrous cycle, cause subfecundity, and induce spontaneous abortions (124–127). They also prolong

gestation periods, decrease birth weight, and reduce litter size (125,126). In women, PCB exposure is associated with prenatal death, infertility, fetal growth retardation, and abnormally low levels of thyroid hormone in nursing infants (79,121,128–133).

Pesticides

Pesticides are routinely used in the home, workplace, and agriculture as pest control agents and lawn care products. They also are present in many paints, glues, metal-working fluids, household disinfectants, food packaging materials, and cosmetics. In addition, many banned pesticides persist in the environment and food chain, posing a human health hazard (134–144).

Dichlorodiphenyltrichloroethane (DDT) was banned in 1972 when it was noted to adversely affect wildlife. However, sufficient levels persist in the environment today and are linked to recent reproductive failures (2,7). For example, DDT exposure partially accounts for the decline in the alligator population observed in Lake Apopka, Florida (1,5). It also contributes to a decline in the bald eagle population; bald eagles have difficulty producing viable offspring after eating Great Lakes fish contaminated with DDT (2). In pregnant women, DDT exposure is associated with low birth weight, small skull circumference, and cognitive, motor, and behavioral deficits in the fetus (145).

Organochlorine pesticides such as methoxychlor and chlordecone (kepone) have several effects on the female reproductive system (146–152). In rodents, methoxychlor accelerates vaginal opening, induces abnormal estrous cyclicity, inhibits luteal function, blocks implantation, reduces fertility, decreases litter size, and stimulates the number of epidermal growth factor receptors in the uterus (152,154,155). Kepone causes persistent vaginal estrus,

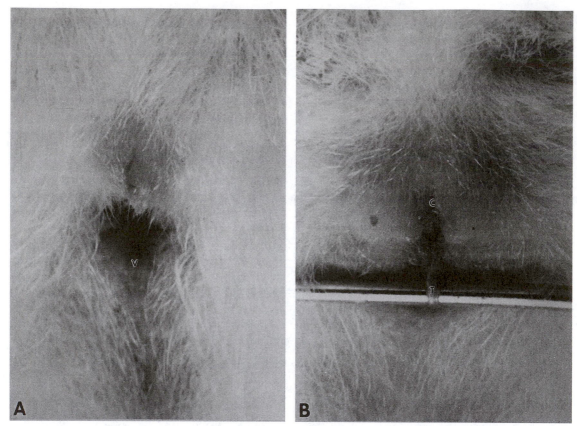

FIGURE 18.2. Morphologic appearance of vaginas in control and 2,3,7,8-tetrachlorodibenzo-*p*-dioxin (TCDD)-treated rats. Pregnant dams were treated with a single dose of TCDD (1 µg/kg) or vehicle on gestation day 15. Female offspring were monitored for abnormal external genitalia and vaginas on postnatal days 2 to 200. **A:** A representative micrograph of the external genitalia and vagina of a control rat on postnatal day 45. **B:** A micrograph of the cleft clitoris and vaginal thread present in a TCDD-exposed pup on postnatal day 45. The thread is lifted from the vaginal opening by a paper clip. V, vagina; C, cleft clitoris; T, vaginal thread. (From Flaws JA, Sommers RJ, Silbergeld EK, et al. *Toxicol Appl Pharmacol* 1997;147:351–362, with permission.)

anovulation, and tonic levels of serum estradiol (146, 148,150,151). In humans, organochlorine pesticides are found in breast milk and adipose tissue, and are thought to be associated with an increased risk of breast cancer, spontaneous abortion, and preterm delivery (134,135, 153,156–158).

Organophosphate pesticides (e.g., parathion, malathion, and diazanon) have not been well studied in laboratory animals or humans. A few animal studies indicate that organophosphate pesticides inhibit the growth of ovarian follicles, induce premature ovulation, and cause poor oocyte development (150,159). In addition, studies show that organophosphate pesticides decrease the levels of luteinizing hormone and progesterone in the blood (159).

Herbicides and Fungicides

Herbicides and fungicides are widely used for turf management of lawns, golf courses, parks, recreation areas, and highways. Additionally, herbicides are used by the federal government for elimination of marijuana crops. The effects of herbicides and fungicides on human health have not been elucidated. Several animal studies, however, indicate that these chemicals cause fetotoxicity, pseudopregnancy, anestrus, ovarian regression, and anovulation (160,161).

Cigarette Smoke

Cigarette smoke is known to contain more than 4,000 chemical compounds, including 43 known carcinogens/poisons and over 300 polycyclic aromatic hydrocarbons. Among these compounds are the addictive chemical nicotine and its metabolites. These chemicals are known to cause vasoconstriction, reduce tissue oxygenation, and concentrate in many tissues (162). In one study, investigators monitored the levels of the nicotine metabolite cotinine in human tissues (162,163). This metabolite was detected in blood, urine, saliva, semen, and follicular fluid in both active and passive smokers (164–167). Cotinine immunostaining has been visualized in the nucleus and cytoplasm of granulosa-lutein cells from active and passive smokers, with mean scores higher in active smokers than those in passive smokers or nonsmokers (Fig.18.3) (168).

Cadmium also is found in cigarette smoke. In humans, cadmium accumulates in the ovaries of smokers and in follicular fluid of smokers undergoing *in vitro* fertilization (169,170). In laboratory animals, cadmium exposure produces an increased proportion of oocytes and embryos with chromosomal anomalies. It also results in a lower number of oocytes reaching metaphase II (171,172).

One of the best studied components of cigarette smoke is the carcinogen known as benzo(a)pyrene (BP) (173). In mice, BP exposure leads to a significant increase in abnormal oocytes and somatic mutations (174,175). In women smokers, Shamsuddin and Gan (176) have shown that BP leads to DNA adduct formation. BP-DNA adducts were found in luteal cells, oocytes of primordial follicles, tunica media of arteries, and corpora albicans. In nonsmokers, BP-DNA adducts were absent in the vascular media and stroma (176).

Cigarette smoke also contains methyl isocyanate, a poison responsible for killing 2,000 people when accidentally

released into the air in Bhopal, India, in 1984. Additionally, it contains benzene, a known toxicant that, in trace amounts (10 μg), forced the 1990 recall of Perrier water. A one-pack-a-day smoker inhales 100 times that amount each day. Lastly, cigarette smoke is composed of acetone, ammonia, arsenic, butane, carbon monoxide, cyanide, DDT, formaldehyde, lead, methanol, polonium 210 (a cancerous radioactive element), and naphthalene—all of which are known carcinogens or reproductive toxicants. In a year, the average smoker takes in the equivalent of 250 chest x-rays from the polonium exposure.

Humans are exposed to the chemicals in cigarette smoke though both active and passive smoking. In the United States, it is estimated that 23.1% of women (about 23 million) and 28.2% of men actively smoke cigarettes, and that approximately 3,000 adolescents become regular smokers each day (177–180). It also is estimated that 60% of nonsmokers (including children) are exposed to tobacco smoke daily. These active and passive exposures are associated with many adverse health outcomes. Cigarette smoke is estimated to kill more people than AIDS, car accidents, alcohol, homicides, illegal drugs, suicides, and fires combined (181–183). In the United States, 400,000 smokers die each year of smoking-related complications such as heart disease, lung cancer, oral cancer, gum disease, chronic bronchitis, and emphysema. In addition, passive smoking results in approximately 3,000 lung cancer deaths each year (184–186).

The effects of cigarette smoking on female reproduction are less clear than the nonreproductive effects. However, several epidemiologic studies have revealed a consistent and highly significant incidence of infertility or subfecundity among smokers compared to nonsmokers (187,188). Of 13 studies evaluating natural conception, all but one demonstrated a negative association between smoking and fertility, with an odds ratio for conception or live births ranging from 0.33 to 1.0 (180,187–190). In another study, smoking was associated with a small increased risk of pregnancy loss (odds ratio of 0.83–1.8) (187). Weinberg and co-workers (189) have shown that prenatal exposure to cigarette smoke is associated with reduced fecundity. In their study of 221 couples, prenatal exposure resulted in a 50% reduction in fecundity [95% confidence interval (CI): 0.4–0.8], even after adjusting for multiple covariates. Kandel and co-workers (190) have found that maternal smoking during pregnancy increases the odds of smoking in their adolescent daughters by a factor of 4, even after controlling for postnatal smoking, implying a possible prenatal effect of nicotine or other substances found in cigarette smoke on the developing fetal brain. This effect was not observed in boys of smoking mothers; the reason for this difference between boys and girls is not clear, but could relate to the sexual dimorphism of the brain (190).

Several studies also indicate that smoking may alter the success rate of assisted reproductive technologies (ARTs).

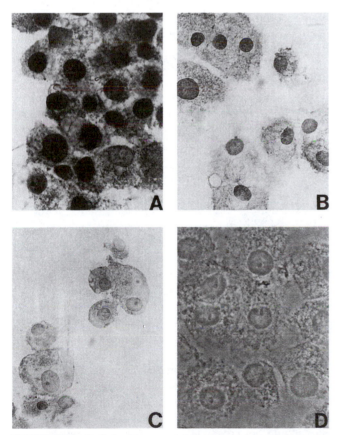

FIGURE 18.3. Cotinine immunostaining in granulosa-lutein cells. **A:** Active smoker. Note strong to moderate immunostaining intensity. **B:** Passive smoker. Note weak staining. **C:** Nonsmoker. Note weak to no immunoreactivity. **D:** Negative control. ×787. (From Zenzes MT, Puy LA, Bielecki R. Immunodetection of cotinine protein in granulosa-lutein cells of women exposed to cigarette smoke. *Fertil Steril* 1997;68:76–82, with permission.)

Eight studies evaluating the effect of smoking on ART yielded a common odds ratio for conception of 0.62 (95% CI: 0.47–0.83). One study found that active smokers had a 50% reduction in implantation rate and ongoing pregnancy rate compared to nonsmokers, and that women who quit smoking before their treatment cycle had the same pregnancy rate as nonsmokers (191). Another study found a significantly lower live birth rate in smokers compared to nonsmokers (10.5% vs. 33.3%) in women undergoing gamete intrafallopian transfer (GIFT) (192). Lastly, one study indicates that ovarian reserve is diminished in smokers aged 35 to 39 (odds ratio: 2.8; 95% CI: 1.2–7.99) compared to nonsmokers aged 35 to 39 (Fig. 18.4) (193).

Although several studies indicate that smoking alters reproductive health, only limited data are available regarding potential mechanisms by which smoking results in infertility, subfecundity, and ART failure in women. In laboratory animals, chemicals in cigarette smoke increase the rate of follicular destruction and accelerate the loss of reproductive function (194–196). They also affect meiotic maturation in oocytes, resulting in oocytes with diploid complements (197,198). In the human, several studies suggest that the mechanism also involves follicular depletion (199–204). Women who smoke become menopausal 1 to 4 years earlier than age-matched nonsmokers, indicating that cigarette smoke accelerates follicular loss and results in entry into the climacteric at an early age (204–206). In addition, women who smoke have high FSH levels, an indicator of diminished ovarian reserve. In one study, Cooper and co-workers (207) evaluated 290 women aged 38 to 49, of whom 31 (11%) were active smokers (207). Basal FSH (drawn on cycle days 2 to 4) was 66% higher in active smokers, and 39% higher in passive smokers compared to nonsmokers (207). Further, Sharara et al. (193) have demonstrated that basal or stimulated FSH levels are higher in smokers compared to nonsmokers.

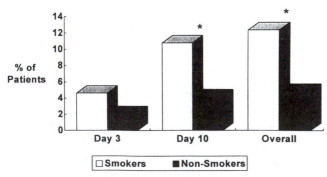

FIGURE 18.4. The incidence of diminished ovarian reserve as evidenced by abnormal clomiphene citrate challenge tests is significantly increased in women ages 35 to 39 who smoke cigarettes compared to age-matched nonsmoking controls. (From Sharara FI, Beatse SN, Leonardi MR, et al. Cigarette smoking accelerates the development of diminished ovarian reserve as evidenced by the clomiphene citrate challenge test. *Fertil Steril* 1994;62:257–262, with permission.)

SUMMARY

Many studies have assessed the effects of endocrine disrupters, phytoestrogens, diethylstilbestrol, heavy metals, phthalates, solvents, industrial pollutants, pesticides, herbicides, fungicides, and cigarette smoke on female reproduction. When viewed as a whole, these studies provide evidence that chemical exposures can lead to adverse reproductive outcomes (e.g., infertility, subfecundity). Individual studies, however, often contain bias, confounders, design problems, or inadequate methodology. Thus, continued research in this area is needed to fully understand the potential effects of chemicals on female reproduction. Continued research also is needed to evaluate the effects of thousands of untested chemicals or chemical mixtures on the reproductive system. Lastly, future efforts need to focus on methods that reduce or eliminate known reproductive toxicants. Such efforts may help to reduce or eliminate chemical-induced infertility, subfecundity, pregnancy loss, and developmental defects.

10 KEY POINTS

1. Many environmental chemicals affect reproduction in animals and humans.

2. Environmental toxicants include phytoestrogens, DES, heavy metals, phthalates, chemical solvents, industrial pollutants, pesticides, herbicides, and fungicides, among others.

3. Adverse effects include subfertility, infertility, birth defects, abnormal genitalia, ovulatory defects, oocyte anomalies, abnormal folliculogenesis, and cancers of the ovary, uterus, breast, and external genitalia.

4. Chemical and environmental toxicants may result in similar reproductive adverse effects in laboratory animals and humans.

5. Cigarette smoke contains more than 4,000 chemicals, including 43 known carcinogens/toxicants and over 300 polycyclic aromatic hydrocarbons.

6. About 23 million women currently smoke, and 3,000 adolescents become regular smokers each day.

7. Women who smoke cigarettes enter menopause 1 to 4 years earlier than nonsmokers. This also applies to passive smokers.

8. Prenatal exposure to cigarette smoke reduces fecundity by 50%.

9. Active smoking results in delayed fecundity and infertility, in both natural and assisted reproduction.

10. More research is needed to clarify further the adverse effects of environmental toxicants on reproduction, and steps should be actively taken to minimize exposure.

REFERENCES

1. Chapin RE, Stevens JT, Hughes CL, et al. Endocrine modulation of reproduction. *Fundam Appl Toxicol* 1996;29:1–17.

2. Colborn T, vom Saal FS, Soto AM. Developmental effects of endocrine-disrupting chemicals in wildlife and humans. *Environ Health Perspect* 1993;101:378–384.

3. McLachlan JA, Arnold SF. Environmental estrogens: found internally, certain compounds are important biological signals; found in the environment, they can become just so much noise. *Am Sci* 1996;84:452–461.

4. Kelce WR, Wilson EM. Environmental antiandrogens—developmental effects, molecular mechanisms, and clinical implications. *J Mol Med* 1997;75:198–207.

5. Guillette LJ, Gross TS, Masson GR. Developmental abnormalities of the gonad and abnormal sex hormone concentrations in juvenile alligators from contaminated and control lakes in Fla. *Environ Health Perspect* 1994;102:680–688.

6. McLachlan JA, Korach KS. Estrogens in the environment III. Global health implications. *Environ Health Perspect* 1995;103:3–4.

7. Fry DM. Reproductive effects in birds exposed to pesticides and industrial chemicals. *Environ Health Perspect* 1995;103:165–171.

8. Gilbertson M. Effects on fish and wildlife populations. In: Kimbrough RD, Jensen AA, eds. *Halogenated biphenyls, terphenyls, naphthalenes, dibenzodioxins, and related products.* Amsterdam: Elsevier Science, 1989, 1–518.

9. Couture LA, Abbott BD, Birnbaum LS. A critical review of the developmental toxicity and teratogenicity of 2,3,7,8-tetrachlorodibenzo-p-dioxin: recent advances toward understanding the mechanism. *Teratology* 1990;42:619–627.

10. Tillet DE, Ankley GT, Giespy JP, et al. Polychlorinated biphenyl residues and egg mortality in double-breasted cormorants from the Great Lakes. *Environ Toxicol Chem* 1992;11:1281–1288.

11. Walker MK, Peterson RE. Potencies of polychlorinated dibenzo-p-dioxins, dibenzofurans, and biphenyl congeners for producing early life stage mortality in rainbow trout (Oncorhyncus mykiss). *Aquatic Toxicol* 1991;21:219–238.

12. Leatherland J. Endocrine and reproductive function in Great Lakes salmon. In: Colborn T, Clement C, eds. *Chemically induced alterations in sexual and functional development: the wildlife/human connection.* Princeton, NJ: Princeton Scientific, 1992:129–145.

13. Shugart G. Frequency and distribution of polygony in Great lakes herring gulls in 1978. *Condor* 1980;82:426–429.

14. Kubiak TJ, Harris HJ, Smith LM, et al. Microcontaminants and reproductive impairment of the Forster's tern on Green Bay, Lake Michigan—1983. *Arch Environ Contam Toxicol* 1989;18:706–727.

15. Bishop CA, Brooks RJ, Carey JH, et al. The case for a cause-effect linkage between environmental contamination and development in eggs of the common snapping turtle (Chelydra s. serpentina) from Ontario, Canada. *J Toxicol Environ Health* 1991;33:521–547.

16. Aulerich RJ, Ringer RK, Iwamoto S. Reproductive failure and mortality in mink fed on Great Lakes fish. *J Reprod Fertil* 1973;suppl 19:365–376.

17. Davis DL, Axelrod D, Osborne MP, et al. Environmental influences on breast cancer risk. *Sci Med* 1997;May-June:56–63.

18. Safe SH. Environmental and dietary estrogens and human health: is there a problem? *Environ Health Perspect* 1995;103:346–351.

19. Whitten PL, Lewis C, Russel E, et al. Phytoestrogen influences on the development of behavior and gonadotropin function. *Proc Soc Exp Biol Med* 1995;208:82–86.

20. Levy JR, Faber KA, Ayyash L, et al. The effect of prenatal exposure to the phytoestrogen genistein on sexual differentiation in rats. *Proc Soc Exp Biol Med* 1995;208:60–66.

21. Whitten PL, Lewis C, Naftolin F. A phytoestrogen diet induces the premature anovulatory syndrome in lactationally exposed female rats. *Biol Reprod* 1993;49:1117–1121.

22. Baird DD, Umbach DM, Lansdell L, et al. Dietary intervention study to assess estrogenicity of dietary soy among postmenopausal women. *J Clin Endocrinol Metab* 1995;80:1685–1690.

23. Faber KA, Hughes CL Jr. Dose-response characteristics of neonatal exposure to genestein on pituitary responsiveness to gonadotropin releasing hormone and volume of the sexually dimorphic nucleus of the preoptic area (SDN-POA) in postpubertal castrated female rats. *Reprod Toxicol* 1993;7:35–39.

24. Whitten PL, Russel E, Naftolin F. Influence of phytoestrogen diets on estradiol action in the rat uterus. *Steroids* 1994;59:443–449.

25. Seawright AA. Directly toxic effects of plant chemicals which may occur in human and animal foods. *Nat Toxins* 1995;3:227–232.

26. Adams NR. Detection of the effects of phytoestrogens on sheep and cattle. *J Anim Sci* 1995;73:1509–1515.

27. Adlercreutz H. Phytoestrogens. Epidemiology and a possible role in cancer protection. *Environ Health Perspect* 1995;103:103–112.

28. Herman C, Adlercreutz T, Goldin BR, et al. Soybean phytoestrogen intake and cancer risk. *J Nutr* 1995;125:757S–770S.

29. Whitten PL, Lewis C, Russell E, et al. Potential adverse effects of phytoestrogens. *J Nutr* 1995,125:771S–776S.

30. Berger MJ, Goldstein DP. Impaired reproductive performance in DES-exposed women. *Obstet Gynecol* 1980;55:25–27.

31. Giusti RM, Iwamoto K, Hatch EE. Diethylstilbestrol revisited: a review of the long-term health effects. *Ann Intern Med* 1995;122:778–788.

32. Salle B, Sergeant P, Awada A, et al. Transvaginal ultrasound studies of vascular and morphological changes in utero exposed to diethylstilbestrol in utero. *Hum Reprod* 1996;11:2531–2536.

33. Herbst AL, Scully RE. Adenocarcinoma of the vagina in adolescence. A report of 7 cases including 6 clear-cell carcinomas (so-called mesonephromas). *Cancer* 1970;25:745–757.

34. Hanselaar A, van Loosbroek M, Schuurbiers O, et al. Clear cell adenocarcinoma of the vagina and cervix—an update of the Central Netherlands Registry showing twin age incidence peaks. *Cancer* 1997;79:2229–2236.

35. Giusti RM, Iwamoto K, Hatch EE. Diethylstilbestrol revisited. a review of the long-term health effects. *Ann Intern Med* 1995;122:778–788.

36. DeMars LR, Van Le L, Huang I, et al. Primary non-clear-cell adenocarcinomas of the vagina in older DES-exposed women. *Gynecol Oncol* 1995;58:389–392.

37. Colton T, Greenberg ER, Noller K, et al. Breast cancer in mothers prescribed diethylstilbestrol in pregnancy. Further follow-up. *JAMA* 1993;269:2096–2100.

38. Agency for Toxic Substances and Disease Registry. *Toxicological profile for lead.* Georgia: U.S. Department of Health and Human Services. Public Health Service, 1993.

39. Hamilton A. *Industrial poisons in the United States.* New York: Macmillan, 1925:1.

40. Goyer RA. Toxic effects of metals. In: Amdur MO, Doull J, Klaassen CD, eds. *Casarett and Doull's toxicology: the basic science of poisons.* New York: McGraw-Hill, 1993, 582–635.

41. Saric M. Reproduction and exposure to lead. *Ann Acad Med Singapore* 1984;13:383–388.

42. Lindbohm ML, Taskinen H, Kyyronen P. Effects of parental occupational exposure to solvents and lead on spontaneous abortion. *Scand J Work Environ Health* 1992;18:37–39.

43. Murphy MJ, Graziano JH, Popovac D. Past pregnancy outcomes among women living in the vicinity of a lead smelter in Kosovo, Yugoslavia. *Am J Public Health* 1990;80:33–35.

44. Hu H. Knowledge of diagnosis and reproductive history among survivors of childhood plumbism. *Am J Public Health* 1991; 81:1070–1072.

45. Goyer RA. Transplacental transport of lead. *Environ Health Perspect* 1990;89:101–105.

46. McMichael AJ, Vimpani GV, Robertson EF. The Port Pirie Cohort Study: maternal blood lead and pregnancy outcome. *J Epidemiol Community Health* 1986;40:18–25.

47. Needleman HL, Rabinowitz M, Leviton A. The relationship between prenatal exposure to lead and congenital anomalies. *JAMA* 1984;251:2956–2959.

48. Alsaleh I, Aldoush I. Mercury content in skin-lightening creams and potential hazards to the health of Saudi Women. *J Toxicol Environ Health* 1997;51:123–130.

49. Gold EB, Tomich E. Occupational hazards to fertility and pregnancy outcome. *Occup Med* 1994;9:435–469.

50. Hanf V, Forstmann A, Costea JE, et al. Mercury in urine and ejaculate in husbands of barren couples. *Toxicol Lett* 1996; 88:227–231.

51. Oskarsson A, Schultz A, Skerfving S, et al. Total and inorganic mercury in breast milk in relation to fish consumption and amalgam in lactating women. *Arch Environ Health* 1996;51: 234–241.

52. Vimy MJ, Hooper DE, King WW, et al. Mercury from maternal silver tooth fillings in sheep and human breast milk—a source of neonatal exposure. *Biol Trace Element Res* 1997; 56:143–152.

53. Burbacher T, Rodier R, Weiss B. Methylmercury developmental neurotoxicity. a comparison of effects in humans and animals. *Neurotoxicol Teratol* 1990;12:191–202.

54. Myers GJ, Davidson PW, Cox C, et al. Summary of the Seychelles Child Development Study on the relationship of fetal methylmercury exposure to neurodevelopment. *Neurotoxicology* 1995;16:711–716.

55. Myers GJ, Marsh DO, Davidson PW, et al. Main neurodevelopmental study of Seychelles children following in utero exposure to methylmercury from a maternal fish diet: outcome at six months. *Neurotoxicology* 1995,16:653–664.

56. Cordier S, Deplan F, Handereau L, et al. Paternal exposure to mercury and spontaneous abortions. *Br J Ind Med* 1989, 15:517–529.

57. Ericson A, Kallen B. Pregnancy outcome in women working as dentists, dental assistants, or dental technicians. *Int Arch Occup Environ Health* 1989,61:329–333.

58. Paksy K, Varga B, Lazar P. Zinc protection against cadmium-induced infertility in female rats. Effect of zinc and cadmium on the progesterone production of cultured granulosa cells. *Biometals* 1997,10:27–35.

59. Whelton BD, Bhattacharyya MH, Carnes BA, et al. Female reproduction and pup survival and growth for mice fed a cadmium-containing purified diet through six consecutive rounds of gestation and lactation. *J Toxicol Environ Health* 1988; 24:321–343.

60. Levin A, Miller RK. Fetal toxicity of cadmium in the rat: decreased utero-placental blood flow. *Toxicol Appl Pharmacol* 1981;58:297–306.

61. Levin AA, Plautz JR, di Sant' Agnes PA, et al. Cadmium: placental mechanisms of fetal toxicity. *Placenta* 1981; 3:303–318.

62. Sikorsky R, Juzkiewicz T, Paszkowski T, et al. Women in dental surgeries: reproductive hazards in occupational exposure to metallic mercury. *Int Arch Occup Environ Health* 1987; 59:551–557.

63. Tsuchiya H, Shima S, Kurita H, et al. Effects of maternal exposure to six heavy metals on fetal development. *Environ Contam Toxicol* 1987;38:580–587.

64. Daston GP. Toxic effects of cadmium on the developing rat lung. II. Glycogen and phospholipid metabolism. *J Toxicol Environ Health* 1982;9:51–61.

65. Weir PJ, Miller RK, et al. Cadmium toxicity in the perfuse human placenta. *Toxicol Appl Pharmacol* 1990;105:156–171.

66. Corella Vargas R. High levels of manganese in the diet of rats (Rattus norvegicus albinicus). I. Effect on reproduction. *Arch Latinoam Nutr* 1984;34:457–465.

67. Laskey JW, Rehnberg GL, Hein JF, et al. Effects of chronic manganese (Mn304) exposure on selected reproductive parameters in rats. *J Toxicol Environ Health* 1982;8:677–687.

68. Sanchez DJ, Domingo JL, Liobet JM, et al. Maternal and developmental toxicity of manganese in the mouse. *Toxicol Lett* 1993;69:45–52.

69. Treinen KA, Gray TJ, Blazak WF. Developmental toxicity of mangafodipir trisodium and manganese chloride in Sprague-Dawley rats. *Teratology* 1995;52:109–115.

70. Davis BJ, Maronpot RR, Heindel JJ. Di-(2-ethylhexyl) phthalate suppresses estradiol and ovulation in cycling rats. *Toxicol Appl Pharmacol* 1994;128:216–223.

71. Heindel JJ, Gulati DK, Mounce RC, et al. Reproductive toxicity of three phthalic acid esters in a continuous breeding protocol. *Fundam Appl Toxicol* 1989;12:508–518.

72. Jobling S, Reynolds T, White R, et al. A variety of environmentally persistent chemicals, including some phthalate plasticizers, are weakly estrogenic. *Environ Health Perspect* 1995;103: 582–587.

73. Narotsky MG, Weller EA, Chinchilli VM, et al. Nonadditive developmental toxicity in mixtures of trichloroethylene, di(2-ethylexyl)phthalate, and heptachlor in a 5 × 5 × 5 design. *Fundam Appl Toxicol* 1995;27:203–216.

74. Wrensch M, Swan S, Lipscomb J, et al. Pregnancy outcomes in women potentially exposed to solvent-contaminated drinking water in San Jose, California. *Am J Epidemiol* 1990;131: 283–300.

75. Aschengrau A, Ozonoff K, Paulu C, et al. Cancer risk and tetrachloroethene-contaminated drinking water in Massachusetts. *Arch Environ Health* 1993;48:284–292.

76. MacFarland HN. Toxicology of solvents. *Am Ind Hyg Assoc J* 1986;47:704–707.

77. Lindbohm ML, Taskinen H, Sallmen M, et al. Spontaneous abortions among women exposed to organic solvents. *Am J Ind Med* 1990;17:449–463.

78. Lindbohm ML, Taskinen H, et al. Effects of parental occupational exposure to solvents and lead on spontaneous abortion. *Scand J Work Environ Health* 1992;18:37–39.

79. Lipscomb JA, Fenster L, Wrensch M, et al. Pregnancy outcomes in women potentially exposed to occupational solvents and women working in the electronics industry. *J Occup Med* 1991;33:597–604.

80. Eskenazi B, Bracken MB, Halford TR. Exposure to organic solvents and hypertensive disorders of pregnancy. *Am J Ind Med* 1988;14:177–188.

81. Baker EL. A review of recent research on health effects of human occupational exposure to organic solvents. *J Occup Med* 1994;36:1079–1092.

82. Wallace D, Groth E, et al. Upstairs, downstairs: perchlorethylene in the air in apartments above New York City dry cleaners. *Consumers Union* 1995, 1—57.

83. Popp W, Muller G, Baltes-Schmitz B, et al. Concentrations of tetrachloroethene in blood and trichloroacetic acid in urine in workers and neighbors of dry-cleaning shops. *Int Arch Occup Env Health* 1992;63:393–395.

84. Sallmen M, Lindbohm ML, Kyyronen P, et al. Reduced fertility among women exposed to organic solvents. *Am J Ind Med* 1995;27:699–713.

85. Bosco MG, Figa-Talamanca I, Salerno S. Health and reproductive status of female workers in dry cleaning shops. *Int Arch Occup Env Health* 1987;59:295–301.

86. Ahlborg G. Pregnancy outcome among women working in laundries and dry-cleaning shops using tetrachlorethylene. *Am J Ind Med* 1990;17:567–575.

87. Windham GC, Shusterman D, Swan SH, et al. Exposure to organic solvents and adverse pregnancy outcome. *Am J Ind Med* 1991;20:241–259.

88. Eskenazi B, Fenster L, Hudes M, et al. A study of the effect of perchlorethylene exposure on the reproductive outcomes of wives of dry-cleaning workers. *Am J Ind Med* 1991;20:593–600.

89. Donald JM, Hooper K, Hopenhayn-Rich C. Reproductive and developmental toxicity of toluene: a review. *Environ Health Perspect* 1991;94:237–244.

90. Taskinen H, Kyyronen P, Hemminki K, et al. Laboratory work and pregnancy outcome. *J Occup Med* 1994;36:311–319.

91. Ungvary G, Tatrai E, Hudak A. Studies on the embryotoxic effects of ortho-, meta-, and para-xylene. *Toxicology* 1980; 18:61–74.

92. Ungvary G. The possible contribution of industrial chemicals (organic solvents) to the incidence of congenital defects caused by teratogenic drugs and consumer goods—an experimental study. *Prog Clin Biol Res* 1985;163B:295–300.

93. Taskinen H. Effects of parental occupational exposure on spontaneous abortion and congenital malformation [review]. *Scand J Work Environ Health* 1990;16:297–314.

94. Harkonen H, Holmberg PC. Obstetrics histories of women occupationally exposed to styrene. *Scand J Work Environ Health* 1982;8:74–77.

95. Harkonen H, Tola S, Korkala ML, et al. Congenital malformations and styrene exposure. *Ann Acad Med* 1984;13:404–407.

96. Generoso WM, Cain KT, Krishna M, et al. Heritable translocation and dominant lethal mutation induction with ethylene oxide in mice. *Mutat Res* 1980,129:89–102.

97. LaBorde JB, Kimmel CA. The teratogenicity of ethylene oxide administered intravenously to mice. *Toxicol Appl Pharmacol* 1980;56:16–22.

98. Rowland AS, Baird DD, Shore DL, et al. Ethylene oxide exposure may increase the risk of spontaneous abortion, preterm birth, and postterm birth. *Epidemiology* 1996;7:363–368.

99. Hemminki R, Mutanen P, Saloniemi I, et al. Spontaneous abortions in hospital staff engaged in sterilizing instruments with chemical agents. *Br Med J* 1982;285:1461–1463.

100. Grizzle TB, George JD, Fail PA, et al. Reproductive effects of 4-vinylcyclohexene in Swiss mice assessed by a continuous breeding protocol. *Fundam Appl Toxicol* 1994;22:122–129.

101. Smith BJ, Mattison DR, Sipes IG. The role of epoxidation in 4-vinylcyclohexene-induced ovarian toxicity. *Toxicol Appl Pharmacol* 1990;105:372–381.

102. Murray FJ, Smith FA, Nitschke KD, et al. Three-generation reproduction study of rats given 2,3,7,8-tetrachlorodibenzo-p-dioxin (TCDD) in the diet. *Toxicol Appl Pharmacol* 1979; 50:241–252.

103. Bevan C, Stadler JC, Elliott GS, et al. Subchronic toxicity of 4-vinylcyclohexene in rats and mice by inhalation exposure. *Fundam Appl Toxicol* 1996;32:1–10.

104. Springer LN, Tilly JL, Sipes IG, et al. Enhanced expression of bax in small preantral follicles during 4-vinylcyclohexene diepoxide-induced ovotoxicity in the rat. *Fundam Appl Toxicol* 1996;139:402–410.

105. Flaws JA, Doerr JK, Sipes IG, et al. Destruction of preantral follicles in adult rats by 4-vinylcyclohexene diepoxide. *Reprod Toxicol* 1994;8:509–514.

106. Flaws JA, Salyers KL, Sipes IG, et al. Reduced ability of rat preantral ovarian follicles to metabolize 4-vinyl-1-cyclohexene

107. Springer LN, Flaws JA, Sipes IG, et al. Follicular mechanisms associated with 4-vinylcyclohexene diepoxide-induced ovotoxicity in rats. *Reprod Toxicol* 1996;10:137–143.

108. Springer LN, McAsey ME, Flaws JA, et al. Involvement of apoptosis in 4-vinylcyclohexene diepoxide-induced ovotoxicity in rats. *Toxicol Appl Pharmacol* 1996;139:394–401.

109. Smith AH. Infant exposure assessment for breast milk dioxins and furans derived from waste incineration emissions. *Risk Anal* 1987;7:347–353.

110. Gray LE Jr, Ostby JS. In utero 2,3,7,8-tetrachlorodibenzo-p-dioxin (TCDD) alters reproductive morphology and function in female rat offspring. *Toxicol Appl Pharmacol* 1995;133: 285–294.

111. Mably TA, Moore RW, Goy RW, et al. In utero and lactational exposure of male rats to 2,3,7,8-tetrachlorodibenzo-p-dioxin. 2. Effects on sexual behavior and the regulation of LH secretion in adulthood. *Toxicol Appl Pharmacol* 1992;114:108–117.

112. Li X, Johnson DC, Rozman KK. Reproductive effects of 2,3,7,8-tetrachlorodibenzo-p-dioxin (TCDD) in female rats: ovulation, hormonal regulation, and possible mechanism(s). *Toxicol Appl Pharmacol* 1995;133:321–327.

113. Kociba RJ, Keeler PA, Park GN, et al. 2,3,7,8-tetrachlorodibenzo-p-dioxin. Results of a 13 week oral toxicity study in rats. *Toxicol Appl Pharmacol* 1976;35:553–574.

114. McConnell EE, Moore JA, Haseman JK, et al. The comparative toxicity of chlorinated dibenzo-p-dioxins in mice and guinea pigs. *Toxicol Appl Pharmacol* 1978;44:335–356.

115. Allen JR, Barsotti DA, Lambrecht LK, et al. Reproductive effects of halogenated aromatic hydrocarbons on nonhuman primates. *Ann NY Acad Sci* 1979;320:419–425.

116. Barsotti DA, Abrahamson LJ, Allen JR. Hormonal alterations in female rhesus monkeys fed a diet containing 2,3,7,8-TCDD. *Bull Environ Contam Toxicol* 1979;21:463–469.

117. Rier SE, Martin DC, Bowman RE, et al. Endometriosis in rhesus monkeys (Macaca mulatta) following chronic exposure to 2,3,7,8-tetrachlorodibenzo-p-dioxin. *Fundam Appl Toxicol* 1993;21:433–441.

118. Mocarelli P, Marocchi A, Brambilla P, et al. Effects of dioxin exposure in humans at Seveso, Italy. Banbury report 35. In: Gallo MA, Schenplein RJ, van der Heijden KA, eds, *Biological basis for risk assessment of dioxins and related compounds.* 1991: 95–110.

119. Mocarelli P, Brambilla P, Gerthoux PM, et al. Change in sex ratio with exposure to dioxin. *Lancet* 1996;348:409.

120. Johansen HR, Alexander J, Rossland OJ, et al. PCDDs, PCDFs, and PCBs in human blood in relation to consumption of crabs from a contaminated Fjord area in Norway. *Environ Health Perspect* 1996;104:756–764.

121. Kimbrough RD. Polychlorinated biphenyls (PCBs) and human health: *an update. Crit Rev Toxicol* 1995;25:133–163.

122. Bright DA, Dushenko WT, Grundy SL, et al. Effects of local and distant contaminant sources: polychlorinated biphenyls and other organochlorines in bottom-dwelling animals from an Arctic estuary. *Sci Total Environ* 1995;160–61:265–283.

123. Dewailly E, Ayotte P, Bruneau S, et al. Innuit exposure to organochlorines through the aquatic food chain in Arctic Quebec. *Environ Health Perspect* 1993;101:618–620.

124. Gellert RJ, Wilson C. Reproductive function in rats exposed prenatally to pesticides and polychlorinated biphenyls (PCB). *Environ Res* 1979;18:437–443.

125. Li MH, Hansen LG. Enzyme induction and acute endocrine effects in prepubertal female rats receiving environmental PCB/PCDF/PCDD mixtures. *Environ Health Perspect* 1996;104: 712–722.

diepoxide in vitro. *Toxicol Appl Pharmacol* 1994;126:286–294.

126. Lindenau A, Fischer B, Speiler P, et al. Effects of persistent chlorinated hydrocarbons on reproductive tissues in female rabbits. *Hum Reprod* 1994;9:772–780.

127. Tilson HA, Davis GJ, McLachlan JA, et al. The effects of polychlorinated biphenyls given prenatally on the neurobehavioral development of mice. *Environ Res* 1979;18:466–474.

128. Leoni V, Fabiani L, Marinelli G, et al. PCB and other organochlorine compounds in blood of women with or without miscarriage: a hypothesis of correlation. *Ecotoxicol Environ Saf* 1989;17:1–11.

129. Pastides H, Calabrese EJ, Hosmer DW, Jr et al. Spontaneous abortion and general illness symptoms among semiconductor manufacturers. *J Occup Med* 1988;30:543–551.

130. Taylor PR, Stelma JM, Lawrence CE. The relation of polychlorinated biphenyls to birth weight and gestational age in the offspring of occupationally exposed mothers. *Am J Epidemiol* 1989;129:395–406.

131. Rogan WJ, Gladen BC, Hung KL, et al. Congenital poisoning by polychlorinated biphenyls and their contaminants in Taiwan. *Science* 1988;241:334–336.

132. Jacobson JL, Jacobson SW, Humphrey HE. Effects of in utero exposure to polychlorinated biphenyls and related contaminants on cognitive functioning in young children. *J Pediatr* 1990;116:38–45.

133. Fein GG, Jacobson JL, Jacobson SW, et al. Prenatal exposure to polychlorinated biphenyls: effects on birth size and gestational age. *J Pediatr* 1984;105:315–320.

134. Mobed K, Gold EB, Schenker MB. Occupational health problems among migrant and seasonal farmworkers. *West J Med* 1992;157:367–373.

135. Nurminen T. Maternal pesticide exposure and pregnancy outcome. *J Occup Environ Med* 1995;37:935–940.

136. Hemminki K, Niemi ML, Saloniemi I, et al. Spontaneous abortions by occupation and social class in Finland. *Int J Epidemiol* 1980;9:149–153.

137. Lindbohm ML, Hemminki K, Kyyronen P. Parental occupational exposure and spontaneous abortions in Finland. *Am J Epidemiol* 1984;120:370–378.

138. McDonald AD, McDonald JC, Armstrong B, et al. Occupation and pregnancy outcome. *Br J Ind Med* 1987;44:521–526.

139. McDonald AD, McDonald JC, Armstrong B, et al. Congenital defects and work in pregnancy. *Br J Ind Med* 1988;45:581–588.

140. Schwartz DA, Newsum LA, Heifetz RM, et al. Parental occupation and birth outcome in an agricultural community. *Scand J Work Environ Health* 1986;12:51–54.

141. Schwartz DA, Lo Gerfo JP. Congenital limb reduction defects in the agricultural setting. *Am J Public Health* 1988;78:654–658.

142. Fenster L, Coye MJ. Birthweight of infants born to Hispanic women employed in agriculture. *Arch Environ Health* 1990;45:46–52.

143. Restrepo M, Munoz N, Day NE, et al. Prevalence of adverse reproductive outcomes in a population occupationally exposed to pesticides in Colombia. *Scand J Work Environ Health* 1990;16:232–238.

144. Rupa DS, Reddy PP, Reddi OS. Reproductive performance in population exposed to pesticides in cotton fields in India. *Environ Res* 1991;55:123–128.

145. Dar E, Kanarek MS, Anderson HA, et al. Fish consumption and reproductive outcomes in Green Bay, Wisconsin. *Environ Res* 1992;59:189–201.

146. Eroschenko VP. Estrogenic activity of the insecticide chlordecone in the reproductive tract of birds and mammals. *J Toxicol Environ Health* 1981;8:731–742.

147. Metcalf JL, Laws SC, Cummings AM. Methoxychlor mimics the action of 17 beta-estradiol on induction of uterine epidermal growth factor receptors in immature female rats. *Reprod Toxicol* 1996;10:393–399.

148. Uphouse L. Effects of chlordecone on neuroendocrine function of female rats. *Neurotoxicology* 1985;6:191–210.

149. Lemonica IP, Garrido Dos Santos AM, Bernardi MM. Effect of administration of organochlorine pesticide (dicofol) during gestation on neurobehavioral development of rats. *Teratology* 1992;46:25A.

150. Ecobichon DJ. Toxic effects of pesticides. In: Amdur MO, Doull J, Klaassen CD, eds. *Casarett and Doull's toxicology.* New York: McGraw-Hill, 1995, 643–690.

151. Guzelian PS. Comparative toxicology of chlordecone (kepone) in humans and experimental animals. *Annu Rev Pharmacol Toxicol* 1982;22:89–113.

152. Eroschenko VP, Cooke PS. Morphological and biochemical alterations in reproductive tracts of neonatal female mice treated with the pesticide methoxychlor. *Biol Reprod* 1990;42:573–583.

153. Falck F Jr, Ricci A Jr, Wolff MS, et al. Pesticides and polychlorinated biphenyl residues in human breast lipids and their relation to breast cancer. *Arch Environ Health* 1992;47:143–146.

154. Gray LE, Jr, Ostby JS, Ferrell JM, et al. Methoxychlor induces estrogen-like alterations of behavior and the reproductive tract in the female rat and hamster. Effects on sex behavior, running wheel activity, and uterine morphology. *Toxicol Appl Pharmacol* 1988;96:525–540.

155. Gray LE Jr, Ostby JS, Ferrell JM, et al. A dose-response analysis of methoxychlor-induced alterations of reproductive development and function in the rat. *Fundam Appl Toxicol* 1989; 12:92–108.

156. Saxena MC, Siddiqui MK, Seth TD, et al. Organochlorine pesticides in specimens from women undergoing spontaneous abortion, premature or full-term delivery. *J Anal Toxicol* 1981; 5:6–9.

157. Bercovici B, Wassermann M, Cucos S, et al. Serum levels of polychlorinated biphenyls and some organochlorine insecticides in women with recent and former missed abortions. *Environ Res* 1983;30:169–174.

158. Zhang J, Cai W, Lee DJ. Occupational hazards and pregnancy outcomes. *Am J Ind Med* 1992,21:397–408.

159. Rattner BA, Michael SD. Organophosphorous insecticide induced decrease in plasma luteinizing hormone concentration in white-footed mice. *Toxicol Lett* 1985;24:65–69.

160. Cooper RL, Stoker TE, Goldman JM, et al. Effect of atrazine on ovarian function in the rat. *Reprod Toxicol* 1996;10:257–264.

161. Goldman JM, Parrish MB, Cooper RL, et al. Blockade of ovulation in the rat by systemic and ovarian intrabursal administration of the fungicide sodium dimethyl-dithiocarbamate. *Reprod Toxicol* 1997;11:185–190.

162. Jensen JA, Goodson WH, Hopf HW, et al. Cigarette smoking decreases tissue oxygen. *Arch Surg* 1991;126:1131–1134.

163. Rosenberg J, Benowitz NL, Jacob P, et al. Disposition kinetics and effects of nicotine. *Clin Pharmacol Ther* 1980;28:517–522.

164. Wall MA, Johnson J, Jacob P, et al. Cotinine in the serum, saliva, and urine of non-smokers, passive smokers, and active smokers. *Am J Public Health* 1988;78:699–701.

165. Vine MF, Hulka BS, Margolin BH, et al. Cotinine concentrations in semen, urine, and blood of smokers and non-smokers. *Am J Public Health* 1993;83:1335–1338.

166. Zenzes MT, Reed TE, Wang P, et al. Cotinine, a major metabolite of nicotine, is detectable in follicular fluids of passive smokers in in vitro fertilization therapy. *Fertil Steril* 1996;66:614–619.

167. Weiss T, Eckert A. Cotinine levels in follicular fluid and serum of IVF patients: effect of granulosa-luteal function in vitro. *Hum Reprod* 1989;4:482–485.

168. Zenzes MT, Puy LA, Bielecki R. Immunodetection of cotinine protein in granulosa-lutein cells of women exposed to cigarette smoke. *Fertil Steril* 1997;68:76–82.

169. Varga B, Zsolnai B, Paksy K, et al. Age dependent accumulation of cadmium in the human ovary. *Reprod Toxicol* 1993;7:225–228.

170. Zenzes MT, Krishnan S, Krishnan B, et al. Cadmium accumulation in follicular fluid of women in in vitro fertilization-embryo transfer is higher in smokers. *Fertil Steril* 1995;64:599–603.

171. Watanabe T, Shimada T, Endo A. Mutagenic effects of cadmium on mammalian oocyte chromosomes. *Mutat Res* 1979;67:349–356.

172. Pisa J, Cibulka J, Ptacek M. Effect of subcutaneous application of a single cadmium dose on oocyte maturation in vitro. *Physiol Bohemoslov* 1990;39:185–190.

173. Phillips DH. Fifty years of benzo(a)pyrene. *Nature* 1983;303:468–472.

174. Davidson GE, Dawson GW. The induction of somatic mutations in mouse embryos by benzo(a)pyrene. *Arch Toxicol* 1977;38:99–103.

175. Basler A, Rohrborn G. Chromosome aberrations in oocytes of NMRI mice and bone marrow cells of Chinese hamsters induced with 3,4-benzpyrene. *Mutat Res* 1976;38:327–332.

176. Shamsuddin AK, Gan R. Immunocytochemical localization of benzo(a)pyrene-DNA adducts in human tissues. *Hum Pathol* 1988;19:309–315.

177. Kessler DA. Nicotine addiction in young people. *N Engl J Med* 1995;333:186–189.

178. Lynch BS, Bonnie RJ, eds. *Growing up tobacco free: preventing nicotine addiction in children and youths.* Washington, DC: National Academy Press, 1994:3.

179. Department of Health and Human Services. *Preventing tobacco use among young people: a report of the surgeon general.* Washington, DC: Government Printing Office, 1994;5:58.

180. Kendrick JS, Merritt RK. Women and smoking: an update for the 1990s. *Am J Obstet Gynecol* 1996;175:528–535.

181. Centers for Disease Control and Prevention. Cigarette smoking among adults—United States, 1993. *MMWR* 1994;43:925–930.

182. Cigarette smoking—attributable mortality and years of potential life lost—United States. *MMWR* 1993;42:645–649.

183. Bartecchi CE, MacKenzie TD, Schrier RW. The human costs of tobacco use. *N Engl J Med* 1994;330:907–912.

184. Steenland K. Passive smoking and the risk of heart disease. *JAMA* 1992;267:94–99.

185. Fielding JE. Smoking: health effects and control. *N Engl J Med* 1985;313:491–498.

186. Fielding JE, Phenow KJ. Health effects of involuntary smoking. *N Engl J Med* 1988;319:1452–1460.

187. Hughes EG, Brennan BG. Does cigarette smoking impair natural or assisted fecundity? *Fertil Steril* 1996;66:679–689.

188. Zenzes MT. Cigarette smoking as a cause of delay in conception. *Reprod Med Rev* 1995;4:189–205.

189. Weinberg CR, Wilcox AJ, Baird DD. Reduced fecundability in women with prenatal exposure to cigarette smoking. *Am J Epidemiol* 1989;129:1072–1078.

190. Kandel DB, Wu P, Davies M. Maternal smoking during pregnancy and smoking by adolescent daughter. *Am J Public Health* 1994;84:1407–1413.

191. Van Voorhis BJ, Dawson JD, Stovall DW, et al. The effects of smoking on ovarian function and fertility during assisted reproduction cycles. *Obstet Gynecol* 1996;88:785–791.

192. Chung PH, Yeko TR, Mayer JC, et al. Gamete intrafallopian transfer. Does smoking play a role? *J Reprod Med* 1997;42:65–70.

193. Sharara FI, Beatse SN, Leonardi MR, et al. Cigarette smoking accelerates the development of diminished ovarian reserve as evidenced by the clomiphene citrate challenge test. *Fertil Steril* 1994;62:257–262.

194. Mattison DR. The effects of smoking on fertility from gametogenesis to implantation. *Environ Res* 1982;28:410–433.

195. Mattison DR, Plowchalk DR, Meadows MJ, et al. The effect of smoking on oogenesis, fertilization, and implantation. *Semin Reprod Endocrinol* 1989;7:291–304.

196. Blackburn CW, Peterson A, Hales HA, et al. Nicotine, but not cotinine, has a direct toxic effect on ovarian function in the immature gonadotropin-stimulated rat. *Reprod Toxicol* 1994;8:325–331.

197. Racowsky C, Hendricks RC, Baldwin KV. Direct effects of nicotine on the meiotic maturation of hamster oocytes. *Reprod Toxicol* 1989;3:13–21.

198. Zenzes MT, Wang P, Casper RF. Cigarette smoking may affect meiotic maturation of human oocytes. *Hum Reprod* 1995;10:3213–3217.

199. Gindoff PR, Tidey GF. Effects of smoking on female fecundity and early pregnancy outcome. *Semin Reprod Endocrinol* 1989;7:305–313.

200. Michnovicz JS, Hershcopf RJ, Naganuma H, et al. Increased 2-hydroxylation of estradiol as a possible mechanism for the anti-estrogenic effect of cigarette smoking. *N Engl J Med* 1986;315:1305.

201. Yeh J, Barbieri RL. Effects of smoking on steroid production, metabolism, and estrogen-related disease. *Semin Reprod Endocrinol* 1989;7:326–334.

202. Barbieri RL, McShane PM, Ryan KJ. Constituents of cigarette smoke inhibit human granulosa cell aromatase. *Fertil Steril* 1986;46:232–236.

203. Adena MA, Gallagher HG. Cigarette smoking and the age of menopause. *Ann Hum Biol* 1982;9:121–130.

204. Jick H, Porter J. Relationship between smoking and age of natural menopause. *Lancet* 1977;1:1354–1355.

205. Everson RB, Sandler DP, Wilcox AJ, et al. Effect of passive exposure to smoking on age at natural menopause. *Br Med J* 1986;293:792.

206. Midgette AS, Baron JA. Cigarette smoking and the risk of natural menopause. *Epidemiology* 1990;1:474–480.

207. Cooper GS, Baird DD, Hulka BS, et al. Follicle-stimulating hormone concentrations in relation to active and passive smoking. *Obstet Gynecol* 1995;85:407–411.

19

CONTRACEPTION

LISA M. KEDER

The ability to prevent or delay conception is an important and modern development. A substantial portion of women's lives will be spent in the reproductive years. For sexually active women, selection of a contraceptive agent depends on many factors: the woman's perception of her likelihood of conceiving, the strength of her motivation to prevent pregnancy, her understanding of the risks and benefits of particular contraceptives, and her partner's understanding of the method. Additionally, the availability and affordability of contraceptives can affect their use.

As clinicians, we are a trusted source of information for our patients. We must understand the physiologic basis for the mechanism of action, risks, benefits, and side effects of contraceptives in order to accurately counsel patients. This chapter reviews this information.

COMBINED ORAL CONTRACEPTIVES

Over 10 million women in the United State use oral contraceptive pills (OCPs). Twenty-seven percent of contraceptive users rely on oral contraceptives, making them the most frequently used, reversible method. Since their introduction in 1960, combined oral contraceptives have undergone a progressive reduction in dosage. Most pills contain ethinyl estradiol, although there are two available that contain mestranol. Mestranol is the 3-methyl ether of ethinyl estradiol and is converted to ethinyl estradiol in the body. The majority of prescriptions are now written for pills containing 35 μg or less of ethinyl estradiol. Several pills with 20 μg are currently available, and ongoing research is investigating the use of even lower doses. Combined oral contraceptives also contain one of eight progestins: norethindrone, norethindrone acetate, ethynodiol diacetate, norgestrel, levonorgestrel, desogestrel, gestodene, or norgestimate. Most combined pill packs contain 21 days of active pills and 1 week of nonhormonal placebo pills. Monophasic pills contain a constant dose of estrogen and progestin, while triphasic pills vary the dose of progestin, estrogen, or both.

Mechanism of Action

Combined oral contraceptives prevent ovulation. Both the estrogen and progestin components inhibit follicle-stimulating hormone (FSH) and luteinizing hormone (LH) by decreasing the production of gonadotropin-releasing hormone (GnRH). The progestin component is particularly effective at inhibiting the midcycle LH surge (1). Addition of ethinyl estradiol potentiates the effect of the progestin, probably by increasing the intracellular content of progesterone receptors. Ethinyl estradiol also prevents shedding of the endometrium (2).

Suppression of follicular development requires at least 7 days of uninterrupted use of oral contraceptives, although gonadotropin levels begin to fall after the first day of use (3). Resumption of gonadotropin release occurs rapidly after discontinuation of pills, and the development of new follicles may occur during the pill-free interval (4). Hence, delay in starting a new cycle may lead to contraceptive failure.

Combined oral contraceptives are also known to affect cervical mucus, causing it to thicken. Sperm penetration is inhibited by this mechanism (5). Progestins cause changes in the endometrium that make it unreceptive for implantation. However, there is no direct evidence that this contributes to the effectiveness of oral contraceptives.

Efficacy

Currently available, low-dose, oral contraceptives (even those containing 20 μg of ethinyl estradiol) have equivalent failure rates to higher dose pills. In carefully monitored efficacy trials, annual failure rates are approximately 0.1% (6). However, it is widely recognized that the in-use failure rate is much higher. Recent data from the National Survey of Family Growth corrected for abortion underreporting suggest that, in the United States, the first year failure rate for oral contraceptives is 7% to 8% (7).

Combined oral contraceptives have no long-term effect on fertility. In women attempting conception after discontinuation of oral contraceptives, the pregnancy rate as well as the incidence of infertility are similar to the general population (8). Additionally, the incidence of postpill amenorrhea is similar to the incidence of secondary amenorrhea, suggesting that there is no significant delay in the resumption of ovulation for most women (9).

Side Effects

Early studies indicated that oral contraceptive use was associated with myocardial infarction (MI). However, reanalysis of that data suggests the observed relationship may have been due to smoking. Compelling evidence now exists that oral contraceptives containing less than 50 μg of ethinyl estradiol do not increase the risk of MI in women who do not smoke (10). However, it does appear that oral contraceptives amplify the risk of MI in smokers. One case-control study found that the risk of MI was not increased in nonsmoking OCP users, but that the relative risk of MI was 30 for OCP users who smoked more than 30 cigarettes per day, and 8.7 in smokers who did not use OCPs (11). Another study found the relative risk of MI in heavy smokers using oral contraceptives was 20.8, while the risk of oral contraceptive use alone was not increased (12). The physiologic basis for this relationship has not been completely elucidated; however, it is felt to be due to increased vascular reactivity in combination with increased thrombotic tendency. Oral contraceptive use is contraindicated in women older than 35 who smoke. Table 19.1 reviews the absolute contraindications to OCP use.

A great deal of attention in the past has focused on the effect of oral contraceptives on serum lipids. Combined oral contraceptives containing high doses of progestins are associated with an unfavorable lipid profile. Of currently available pills, only those with fixed dose combinations of levonorgestrel increase low-density lipoproteins. The other formulations available—triphasic levonorgestrel, all norethindrone, and third-generation pills (those containing gestodene, norgestimate, or desogestrel)—are either lipid neutral or increase high-density lipoproteins. Initially, there was concern that the adverse lipid profile induced by some OCPs might lead to atherosclerosis and thereby increase women's risk of cardiovascular disease. However, epidemiologic data and animal studies do not support a relationship between previous oral contraceptive use and cardiovascular risk (11,13).

TABLE 19.1. CONTRAINDICATIONS TO COMBINED ORAL CONTRACEPTIVE USE

History of thrombosis or thromboembolism, cerebral vascular accident, coronary artery disease, myocardial infarction
Significantly impaired liver function
Hypertriglyceridemia
Breast cancer
Pregnancy
Smoking in woman older than 35
Undiagnosed vaginal bleeding

Several recent studies have examined the relationship between stroke and low-dose oral contraceptive use. A recent pooled analysis of two U.S. studies found no increased risk of ischemic or hemorrhagic stroke in women using low-dose oral contraceptives. However, women with a history of migraine headaches had a higher risk of both types of stroke (14). World Health Organization (WHO) data show no increased risk of stroke among healthy, nonsmoking women in Europe, but did find an increase for women in developing countries. This was felt to be because cardiovascular risk factors were not detected, and therefore prescribing practices differed (15,16). Smoking and hypertension in and of themselves both increase the risk of stroke.

Venous thromboembolism (VTE) is related to oral contraceptive use, but not to smoking. The risk of VTE is related to the estrogen dose of pills. The precise mechanism of this effect is unknown. Estrogen does increase the production of clotting factors. However, studies have shown that both monophasic and multiphasic low-dose oral contraceptives have no significant clinical impact on the coagulation system because increased thrombin formation is offset by increased fibrinolytic activity. However, there is evidence that an increase in clotting factors associated with an increase in platelet activity occurs in women using 30- to 35-μg pills (17). Several studies have demonstrated a higher risk for pills containing gmore than 50 μg of ethinyl estradiol. Others have shown a higher risk for 50-μg pills in comparison to 30- or 35-μg pills. It is unknown if sub–30-μg pills will convey an even lower risk. In comparison to nonusers, the risk of VTE is three- to fourfold higher in users of 30- to 35-μg pills.

The relationship between progestational agent and VTE was recently raised by the publication of several studies that reported an increased risk among women using pills containing gestodene and desogestrel. The first of these was a hospital case-control study performed by the WHO. It found that women using desogestrel- or gestodene-containing pills had a relative risk of VTE 2.6 times that of women using levonorgestrel pills (18). A second case-control study, known as the transnational study, found a similarly increased risk of 1–5 fold (19). The third study evaluated cohort data from the General Practice Research Database in the United Kingdom, and found the risk of VTE to be about twice that of levonorgestrel users (20). Data from a previous study of Leiden factor V thrombophilia were also analyzed and revealed an elevated risk of 2.3 (21). Despite the similar findings of all these studies, their publication spurred a significant debate among experts in the field. Many felt the results were not biologically plausible since desogestrel and gestodene have no significant impact in and of themselves on clotting parameters (17). Others suggested that the results were affected by pervasive bias among all the studies.

The most convincing arguments came on the basis of preferential prescribing and the healthy user effect. The newer products containing desogestrel and gestodene were marketed as being less androgenic and having less impact on lipids. Thus, clinicians may have provided oral contraceptives containing these agents to women who were considered at higher risk (preferentially prescribed). Women who are satisfied with an oral contraceptive tend to stay with that product, while those who have problems are more likely to switch. Therefore, those using an older product tend to be healthy and free of side effects. This is known as the healthy user effect or attrition of susceptibles. In an attempt to evaluate the effect of these biases, the transnational study group reanalyzed its data to look at duration of use, and found that among first-time users there was no difference in VTE risk between second- and third-generation oral contraceptive users. Two additional studies were then published supporting the contention that bias contributed to the initial results. A case-control study in the United Kingdom found that the risk was similar among all formulations when subjects were matched by year of birth (22). Another study found no increased risk for the new progestins when the data were adjusted for duration of use (23). The relationship between progestagen and thrombosis was also criticized on the basis that it was not biologically plausible. Thrombosis risk is felt to be related to estrogen dose, and there is no mechanism known by which progestagens would induce thrombophilia. One group attempted to evaluate the mechanism and reported that women using second- and third-generation oral contraceptives have different sensitivities to activated protein C, which is important in preventing thrombosis (24). However, this research was criticized as having a great deal of overlap in results among test groups and, to date, has not been corroborated by another laboratory (17).

Thus, there is good evidence that substantial bias created the perception that progestagen type is related to thrombosis risk. However, there is undoubtedly still a risk of thrombosis associated with pill use. The relative risk of low-dose pill use is 3 to 4 with an incidence of about 15 per 100,000 women-years of use. Women who have a personal history of idiopathic thrombosis should not be prescribed oral contraceptives. Women with a family history of idiopathic thrombosis should undergo evaluation for an underlying abnormality of the coagulation system, including testing for Leiden factor V mutation before initiating oral contraceptive use (25).

Clinically significant hypertension does not occur with current low-dose OCPs; however, small increases in blood pressure may occur (26). Occasionally, patients may experience an idiosyncratic reaction and have clinically important blood pressure changes. This is felt to be due to an effect on the renin-angiotensin system and may take as long as 6 months to resolve. Because of the added risk of oral contraceptive use in women with hypertension, blood pressure screening should be performed at intake and on an annual basis thereafter. Women with hypertension who are adequately treated may use oral contraception under close supervision with frequent blood pressure monitoring (25).

Carbohydrate metabolism is affected by the progestin component of the pill, which increases insulin resistance. Although older, high-dose pills significantly impaired glucose tolerance, changes with low-dose pills are minimal and not felt to be clinically significant. However, hyperinsulinemia is a risk factor for cardiovascular disease. It is unclear whether the small effect that low-dose OCPs exert on insulin secretion will have any long-term effect on risk. Population-based studies have not detected any increase in the incidence of diabetes related to oral contraceptive use. The Royal College of General Practitioners Oral Contraception Study and the Oxford Family Planning Association Study found no difference in the incidence of diabetes mellitus among current, past, or non-users of the pill (27). Likewise, the Nurses' Health Study found no increase in risk of type II diabetes mellitus in either current or former users. Moreover, women with a history of gestational diabetes also do not appear to be at increased risk because of OCP use (28).

The use of oral contraceptives in overtly diabetic women has been controversial. However, the risk of use is important to clarify because of complications associated with pregnancy and diabetes as well as the need for planning pregnancies at a time of optimal glycemic control. Klein et al. (29) examined data from the Wisconsin Epidemiologic Study of Diabetic Retinopathy. They found that former or current use of oral contraceptives was not associated with severity of retinopathy or hypertension. However, this was not a controlled trial and preferential prescribing may have significantly influenced the results. Another historical cohort study of college-aged women did not find any difference in renal or retinal complications in diabetic OCP users (30).

Early studies of oral contraceptives indicated that their use might be associated with an increased incidence of benign gallbladder disease in the first year of use (31). This was thought to be because cholesterol saturation rises in bile of oral contraceptive users (32). Subsequently, a number of studies have been published that put this relationship in question. A 1993 meta-analysis summarized the findings of the nine best-designed studies done up to that point. This analysis found that there was an overall odds ratio of 1.4 for the development of gallstones (33). However, the authors also found that there was an apparent dose-response relationship with the estrogen content of the pill. A follow-up study published in 1994, using data from the Royal College of General Practitioners, found no significant risk in gallbladder disease (34). Thus, it seems likely that with today's low-dose pills, oral contraceptives do not contribute significantly to the incidence of gallbladder disease.

The relationship of oral contraceptive use to cancer is one of the most widely misunderstood effects of oral contraceptives, despite a great deal of research in this area.

Breast cancer is of primary concern to American women because of its prevalence. Many early large cohort studies found no relationship between oral contraceptive users and nonusers in breast cancer incidence (35–37). However, these studies were done with higher-dose oral contraceptives than are currently in use. Additionally, they involved women spacing pregnancies rather than women delaying their first pregnancy. Later studies examined the use of oral contraceptives in young women and nulliparous women. The Cancer and Steroid Hormone Study conducted by the Centers for Disease Control examined these issues. Overall no increased risk of breast cancer was found in women using oral contraceptives, even with long-term use, use by women younger than 20, and use before first pregnancy. Moreover, birth control pills did not amplify the risk associated with family history of breast cancer (38). Despite this reassuring information, not all research has been consistent. A number of studies have indicated that oral contraceptives may be associated with an increased risk of premenopausal breast cancer in women who have used birth control pills over an extended time (39–42). Other work has had contradictory results. Most recently, the Collaborative Group on Hormonal Factors in Breast Cancer pooled data from 54 epidemiologic studies. This analysis found a small increased risk for current users of oral contraceptives that dropped to zero by 10 years after discontinuation (43). Additionally, cancers in current and recent OCP users were less advanced clinically than in women who never used OCPs. Some authors have hypothesized that the observed risk in young women and current users is related to detection bias, since women on oral contraceptives are more likely to receive frequent health care, or to a promotional effect resulting in growth of a preexistent tumor.

Thus, the long-term use of oral contraceptives does not appear to increase the overall risk of breast cancer even in women with a family history. However, there may be a slight increased risk with current use or an increase in detection. Because breast cancer is rare in young women, the public health impact of this risk is small in comparison to the benefits of oral contraceptive use.

Several studies have found an increase in the incidence of cervical dysplasia and carcinoma-in-situ in women using oral contraceptives for more than 1 year (44–47). However, the risk factors for dysplasia follow those of a sexually transmitted disease. It is widely recognized that exposure to human papillomavirus (HPV) is a major risk factor for dysplasia. Additionally, women using oral contraceptives are more likely to undergo Pap smear screening and therefore more likely to have dysplasia diagnosed. Women using barrier methods of contraception may have lower risk due to prevention of HPV transmission. These facts confound the study of cervical intraepithelial neoplasia and oral contraceptives. Early research examining this relationship failed to control adequately for sexual behavior. One subsequent study that controlled for sexual activity and frequency of screening did not show an increased risk of invasive cervical cancer among oral contraceptive users (48). However, the WHO studied the issue and found an increased risk even controlling for screening bias (46). Many authorities feel that there is minimal risk of invasive squamous cell carcinoma associated with oral contraceptive use and that the apparent risk identified represents detection bias. Additionally, OCP use does not seem to affect the natural history of HPV infection (49). However, most also agree that recent studies identifying an increased risk of cervical adenocarcinoma are convincing (50–52). The relative risk is approximately 2. From a physiologic basis this increased risk is difficult to understand given the decreased risk of endometrial adenocarcinoma associated with pill use. However, it has been hypothesized that the increase in cervical ectropion that occurs in OCP users results in increased exposure of the endocervical glandular tissue. Therefore, women using oral contraceptives should undergo regular cytologic screening.

The health benefits of oral contraceptives have not received as much attention as the risks (Table 19.2). However, there is good epidemiologic evidence to suggest that oral contraceptives provide substantial protection against endometrial carcinoma. Overall, the risk of endometrial cancer is reduced by half in ever users of the pill in comparison to never users (47). The reduction of risk increases with increasing duration of use and persists for at least 15 years after discontinuation (53). Moreover, the protective effect is greatest in nulliparas and women of low parity who are at greatest risk. The physiologic basis for this protection is an effect of the progestin component of the pill. The predominant influence of all combined OCPs on the endometrium is an atrophic pattern.

Although endometrial cancer is more common, epithelial ovarian cancer has a high mortality rate. Therefore, the protective effect of oral contraceptives against ovarian cancer is an important finding and one of the few preventive strategies we can offer to women for this cancer. A reduction in risk is found in women who have used OCPs for a short time, 3 to 6 months. However, there appears to be an increasing reduction in risk with increasing duration of use. Ovarian epithelial cancer risk is decreased as much as 80% in women who have used oral contraceptives for 10 years

TABLE 19.2. HEALTH BENEFITS OF ORAL CONTRACEPTIVES

Decreased risk of ovarian cancer
Decreased risk of endometrial cancer
Less dysmenorrhea and mittelschmerz
Decreased menstrual flow and lower incidence of anemia
Improved cycle control
Decreased risk of pelvic inflammatory disease

(54–56). This reduction in risk extends to women with a family history of ovarian cancer who carry either the *BRCA1* or *BRCA2* mutation. Their risk is reduced by 60% when OCPs are used for 6 years or longer (57). The mechanism by which OCPs create this protection is unclear. However, since the risk of ovarian carcinoma is felt to be related to the total number of ovulations in a woman's life, prevention of ovulation may be the explanation.

Health risks are of utmost concern to women considering oral contraceptive use. However, once OCPs are initiated, side effects are frequent reasons for discontinuation or inconsistent use. Breakthrough bleeding is common in the first few months of OCP use. As many as 30% of women will experience this side effect within the first month. The progestin component of oral contraceptives results in a relatively thin endometrium, while the estrogen content provides some stability to it. Breakthrough bleeding is felt to be a result of decidualization in which the endometrium is prone to break down, resulting in irregular bleeding. During early oral contraceptive use, irregular bleeding will often resolve with time. Bleeding that develops later during use may require supplemental estrogen or a change in oral contraceptive formulation. Breakthrough bleeding is more common in women using lower dose oral contraceptives and is often precipitated by missed pills or pills taken off of an established schedule (58,59). Cycle control is also affected by cigarette smoking. In one study smokers were 47% more likely to have breakthrough bleeding than nonsmokers (60). This is felt to occur because smokers metabolize the estrogenic component of pills more quickly, resulting in lower serum levels.

Amenorrhea can also occur in OCP users. This, again, is a result of a relative paucity of endometrial growth. Although it is not known to lead to any long-term health effects, it can be anxiety provoking. The incidence of amenorrhea appears to increase with duration of pill use. Occasionally, it can be overcome with a change in pill formulation. Alternatively, oral estrogen supplements can be used to increase endometrial proliferation (25).

Another concern that affects compliance with oral contraceptives is weight gain. Adolescents, in particular, commonly believe that OCPs cause weight gain. Research has failed to demonstrate a consistent relationship between increased body weight and oral contraceptive use (61–63).

One birth control pill has been approved by the U.S. Food and Drug Administration (FDA) for the treatment of acne. This pill is a tricyclic containing ethinyl estradiol and norgestimate. In a randomized, double-blind, placebo-controlled trial, this OCP formulation decreased total acne lesion count by 53%, which was significantly greater than the placebo (64). Research has also demonstrated that acne improves in users of other oral contraceptive formulations (65,66). Other health benefits of OCPs include a reduction in the incidence of endometriosis, dysmenorrhea, and menorrhagia (25).

PROGESTERONE-ONLY PILLS

Progesterone-only birth control pills (POPs) contain a lower amount of progestin than do combined oral contraceptives. In the United States there are three available pills in two formulations, 350 μg of norethindrone or 75 μg of levonorgestrel. In contrast to combined pills, which are taken for 21 days out of a 28-day cycle, progesterone-only pills are taken daily. Desogestrel-only pills are available in Europe.

Mechanism of Action

Progesterone only pills do not inhibit ovulation as reliably as do combined pills. Ovulation is inhibited in approximately half of POP users. The remainder of the contraceptive effect is due to thickening of cervical mucus, slowing of ovum transport, and atrophy of the endometrium. The relative importance of these factors has not been elucidated (67).

Efficacy

Like combined oral contraceptives, the efficacy of POPs is highly user dependent. Failure rates of 1.1 to 9.6 per 100 women have been reported for the first year of use (68). However, failure rates of less than 1 per 100 women-years of use have been found among compliant users (67). Younger women and women with body weight greater than 155 pounds have higher failure rates (67). It is recommended that POP be taken at the same time every day and that a backup method be used for 48 hours if a pill is taken more that 3 hours late (25). This advice is based on the fact that sperm penetration is unimpaired 24 hours after administration of POPs. A recent comparative trial suggests that desogestrel-only pills have a lower failure rate in comparison to levonorgestrel-only pills (69).

Side Effects

Progestin-only pills are more likely than combined pills to create menstrual disturbances. Approximately 40% of users will continue to have regular menstrual cycles. As many as 30% of users will have intermenstrual bleeding in the first 4 months of use. Irregular bleeding is the most common reason for POP discontinuation (70). Breast tenderness also occurs more frequently than with combined oral contraceptives. Additionally, women using POPs have more functional ovarian cysts (71).

POPs are frequently used in lactating women. POPs do not adversely affect the quality or quantity of breast milk. In combination with the effect of lactation on ovulation, they often result in prolonged amenorrhea, which is well tolerated in the postpartum period (72,73). Moreover, POPs may attenuate the bone loss associated with breastfeeding (74). There appears to be no relationship between

POP use and myocardial infarction, thromboembolism, or cerebrovascular accident (75,76). POPs do not appear to increase the risk of breast cancer, and they decrease the risk of endometrial cancer by even a larger degree than do combined oral contraceptives (77,78). No studies have directly assessed mood disorders in women using POPs, but one study evaluating sexuality and well-being found they have no adverse impact on the former and an improvement in the latter (79).

SUBDERMAL IMPLANTS

Norplant is a series of six Silastic capsules containing levonorgestrel. The capsules are implanted beneath the skin in a fan-like pattern. They release an average of 30 μg of levonorgestrel per day and continue this release for at least 5 years. When placed within 7 days from the onset of normal menses, the system is effective within 24 hours of insertion.

Mechanism of Action

Immediately after insertion the level of circulating levonorgestrel is sufficient to inhibit ovulation. The rate of release declines over the first year of use to a level lower than that in users of oral progesterone only pills. Norplant is felt to have three major mechanisms of action. Levonorgestrel inhibits the LH surge at the level of the pituitary and hypothalamus. This mechanism is probably most active within the first 2 years of use. With increasing duration of use there is increasing evidence of ovulation based on progesterone levels (80). Norplant is also felt to work by its effect on cervical mucus. Normal sperm penetration is dependent on the quantity and quality of mucus. Norplant thickens and decreases cervical mucus (81). The third postulated mechanism of action is at the level of the endometrium. Constant exposure to levonorgestrel prevents maturation of the endometrium. This could prevent implantation. However, fertilization has not been observed in Norplant users (82).

Efficacy

Norplant is one of the most effective contraceptives ever developed. Once implanted, its effectiveness is not user dependent, thus its theoretical effectiveness mirrors its in-use effectiveness. In a multicountry international trial involving over 2,000 women, the first-year pregnancy rate was 0.2. However, all but one of the pregnancies in this trial were present at the time of Norplant insertion. Removing those from the analysis decreases the first-year failure rate to 0.09 (83). Table 19.3 describes pregnancy rates over the 5-year life span. Medications that speed hepatic microsomal metabolism may impair Norplant's effective-

TABLE 19.3. PREGNANCY RATE BY YEAR OF NORPLANT USE

Year	Rate (%)
1	0.2
2	0.2
3	0.9
4	0.5
5	1.1

From Sivin I. International experience with Norplant and Norplant-2 contraceptives. *Stud Fam Plann* 1988;19:81–94, with permission.

ness by lowering serum levonorgestrel levels. In initial studies with Norplant, there was a higher failure rate among women weighing more than 70 kg. Since those initial data were compiled, the Silastic capsule has been reformulated and is less dense. Thus, serum levels are higher. However, heavier women may have a higher failure rate in the fourth or fifth years of use. This rate is not higher than the failure rate of other contraceptives, such as combined pills (25).

There are no long-term effects of Norplant on future fertility. After removal, the level of levonorgestrel becomes too low to measure within 48 hours. Ovulation generally resumes within the first month, and pregnancy rates in the first year after removal are similar to those in women who have not been using contraception (84).

Side Effects

Menstrual irregularity occurs in 80% of women during the first year of use. Bleeding patterns may include irregular episodes of bleeding and prolonged spotting. Oligomenorrhea or amenorrhea occurs in approximately 10% of women. Menstrual cycle disturbances are less frequent after the first year of use. Approximately 60% to 70% of women will experience regular cycles by the third year of use (85). Although the total number of bleeding days may increase in Norplant recipients, the overall blood loss appears to be less than in normally menstruating women (86).

Headache is a common side effect of hormonal contraceptives. Approximately 20% of Norplant removals are performed because of headaches. There is no evidence that such headaches are a significant health problem. Weight gain is also a concern for hormonal contraceptive users. Initial research showed marked differences in weight gain or loss, depending on the population studied. One follow-up study of 75 Norplant users found no increase in body weight over 5 years of use (87). Other side effects of Norplant include acne, galactorrhea, mastalgia, and hyperpigmentation over the area of insertion. Additionally, the incidence of simple ovarian cysts is increased. There are no significant effects of Norplant on carbohydrate metabolism, liver function, blood coagulation, blood chemistries, or cortisol levels (25). Hormonal agents are also known to affect mood. There are case reports of mood disorders developing

TABLE 19.4. CONTRAINDICATIONS TO NORPLANT USE

Active thrombosis or thromboembolism
Acute liver disease
Breast cancer
Undiagnosed vaginal bleeding
Concomitant use of medications that induce hepatic micro-
   somal enzymes
Lower incidence of ovarian cysts
Lower incidence of benign breast disease
Improvement in acne

in women using Norplant (88). However, one study that evaluated depressive symptoms found no increase in Norplant users (89). Table 19.4 reviews the contraindications to Norplant use.

DEPO-PROVERA

Depot medroxyprogesterone acetate (DMPA), 150 mg, is administered as an intramuscular injection every 3 months.

Mechanism of Action

DMPA inhibits ovulation by blocking the LH surge. In order for it to be effective within a cycle, it must be administered within 5 days of the onset of menses. Although its primary mechanism of action is felt to be prevention of ovulation, DMPA also thickens cervical mucus and disturbs normal endometrial maturation.

Efficacy

A number of studies have evaluated the efficacy of DMPA and its dosing. The WHO evaluated 100 versus 150 mg given every 3 months and found the higher dose to be more effective (90). The largest multicenter study examining efficacy found a failure rate of 0.32 per 100 women-years of use (91). An interesting finding was that massaging the area of injection might decrease efficacy. Compliance with injection schedule is an important contribution to user effectiveness. However, as with Norplant, the lack of daily compliance makes the in-use failure rate similar to its theoretical failure.

Side Effects

As with the other progestin-only methods of contraception, irregular bleeding is a common side effect of DMPA. As with Norplant, this bleeding rarely leads to a decrease in hemoglobin. However, it is a common reason for discontinuation. Seventy percent of DMPA users have irregular bleeding in the first year of use. Over time, many progress

to amenorrhea. After 1 year of use 50% of women will be amenorrheic, and after 5 years 80%. Other side effects include mood changes, decreased libido, hair loss, and weight gain. Weight gain is of particular concern, as it may be a deterrent to use. Although the package insert for DMPA suggests that women can expect to gain 5 pounds within 1 year of use, other studies do not support a significant increase in weight (92).

The initial attempt at approval of DMPA as a contraceptive in the United States was delayed due to concern that it might increase the risk of breast cancer, since it was found to cause breast tumors in beagles. This was subsequently found to be an effect specific to dogs. WHO data suggest there may be a slight increase in risk of breast cancer in the first 4 years of DMPA use (93). However, this study and others have not found any increase in risk with duration of use or overall increase. Thus, DMPA may accelerate the growth of existing tumors, or women using DMPA may be more likely to have cancer detected. Moreover, a study that pooled the results of this research suggested no elevation in risk for women who had ever used DMPA (94). Likewise, WHO data have not found any increased risk of invasive cervical cancer. Depo-Provera decreases the risk of endometrial cancer and may decrease the risk of ovarian cancer (25).

Another issue that has raised concern with long-term DMPA use is its effect on bone density. Estrogen levels in DMPA users are similar to those found in the follicular phase of normally cycling women. A cross-sectional study that compared DMPA users, postmenopausal women, and premenopausal women found that DMPA use was associated with a lower average bone density than in premenopausal women, but not as low as in postmenopausal women (95). However, this study was limited by its cross-sectional design. Additionally, smoking was not controlled for as a risk factor for osteoporosis. The same researcher found that, following discontinuation of DMPA, bone density increased. Another cross-sectional study found that women exposed to DMPA had lower bone mineral density, especially among women ages 18 to 21 (96). This study did control for smoking and other risk factors. A prospective study compared adolescents using oral contraceptives, Norplant, and DMPA, and found that DMPA users experienced bone loss in comparison to the others who gained bone density (97). Further research examining this issue is ongoing. In deciding whether to prescribe DMPA to adolescents, it is important to weigh the risks of pregnancy (which is also associated with bone loss) against this side effect.

DMPA does not affect long-term fertility. However, in comparison to women using other contraceptive methods, DMPA users have a delay in return to full fertility of 9 months after their last injection. However, by 18 months after the last injection 90% of women desiring fertility will have conceived (98). Therefore, women planning pregnancy within the next 12 months are not good candidates for this contraceptive.

Hormonal contraceptives have been associated with mood changes. However, no increase in depressive symptoms was found in one prospective study of DMPA users (99).

INTRAUTERINE DEVICE

The intrauterine device (IUD) has been manufactured in many shapes over the last century. IUDs currently available in the United States include the Paraguard copper-containing IUD (internationally known as the TCu-380A) and the Progestasert progesterone-containing IUD. The TCu-380A is currently FDA approved for 10 years of continuous use. The progesterone-containing IUD releases 65 μg of progesterone per day and must be replaced yearly. The progesterone has a local effect on the endometrium and decreases menstrual cramping and blood loss. An extended use, levonorgestrel-containing IUD is currently available in Europe, but has not yet been approved for use in the U.S. Although widely used internationally, the IUD has declined in popularity in the U.S. over the last decade. Currently, less than 1% of contraceptive users rely on the IUD. This drop in use is felt to be in relation to publications that implicated the IUD in tubal infertility and to recognition that the Dalkon Shield was associated with pelvic inflammatory disease (PID). More recent data reaffirm the safety of currently available IUDs.

Mechanism of Action

The mechanism of action of the IUD is important to some women and clinicians who are ethically opposed to a postfertilization, preimplantation effect. It is commonly believed that the major mechanism of action is to cause an intrauterine inflammatory reaction that prevents implantation. This hypothesis has been examined in multiple animal models. Unfortunately, the IUD's effect is highly species dependent, ranging from ovulation suppression to inhibition of implantation; therefore, animal studies cannot be generalized to humans (100).

Detection of a postfertilization, preimplantation effect requires that an embryo-specific substance be detectable to measure the rate of conception in IUD users and nonusers. Human chorionic gonadotropin (hCG) has been used for this purpose. It is first produced by the blastocyst about 5 days after fertilization. Implantation occurs 2 to 3 days later. A number of studies have evaluated increases in hCG as a marker of postfertilization pregnancy loss. The majority of these have found a much lower rate of hCG positivity in women using IUDs than in women attempting conception, indicating that IUD users form embryos less frequently than nonusers (100).

Sperm function and migration are also altered by IUD use. Copper affects sperm motility. Additionally, a number

of studies have reported decreased sperm recovery from tubes in IUD users. These studies have examined excised tubes after artificial insemination or coitus. In general they report a lower recovery rate for IUD users and specifically for those using a copper-containing IUD (100). Recovery of eggs has also been attempted. Transcervical flushing of the endometrial cavity yielded eight eggs in 36 control women and one in 65 IUD users. Another study found that ova were less commonly found in the tubes or endometrial cavities of women using copper-containing IUDs than in controls. Women wearing inert or progesterone-containing IUDs had similar recovery rates to controls (101).

The precise mechanism of IUD action is still undetermined. To date, data indicate that embryos are formed at lower rates in IUD users and refute the commonly held belief that embryos are destroyed within the uterine cavity. Copper-containing IUDs likely inhibit sperm migration into the upper genital tract and may directly affect ova.

Efficacy

The efficacy of individual IUDs varies by the device. Inert IUDs such as the Lippes Loop have higher failure rates than active IUDs containing copper or progesterone. Moreover, an increase in copper surface area is associated with greater efficacy (102). The TCu-380A has a failure rate of less than one per 100 women per year. Its cumulative pregnancy rate after 7 years of use is 1.5 per 100 woman-years of use (Table 19.5). Failure rates are higher among women 25 years of age or younger. The progesterone-containing IUD is only indicated for 1 year of use and has a reported life-table failure rate between 1.3 and 2.0. The levonorgestrel IUD releases 20 μg per day and has now been used for up to 10 years continuously. It has a failure rate equivalent to or lower than that of the copper-containing IUD. Additionally, it is associated with less menstrual bleeding (100).

Side Effects

A common misperception of both clinicians and patients is that the IUD is a risky contraceptive choice. Most of the adverse events associated with IUD use are related to devices

TABLE 19.5. INTRAUTERINE DEVICE (IUD) EXPERIENCE IN THE FIRST YEAR OF USE

Device	Pregnancy Rate	Expulsion Rate	Removal Rate
TCu-380A	0.5–0.8	5	14
Progesterone IUD	1.3–1.6	2.7	9.3
Levonorgestrel IUD	0.2	6	17

From Sivin I, Schmidt F. Effectiveness of IUDs: a review. *Contraception* 1987;36:55–84, with permission.

that are not currently in use. Therefore, clarifying the rate of adverse side effects is important.

Insertion of an IUD can be complicated by perforation of the uterus. WHO data indicated that perforation occurs between 0.4 and 1.1 times per 1,000 insertions. The rate is similar among different types of IUDs and higher among inexperienced clinicians. When perforation is recognized, the IUD should be removed as soon as possible.

The most common reason for dissatisfaction with the IUD is related to menstrual cycle changes. Multiple studies have shown an increase in menstrual blood loss with use of plastic- and copper-containing IUDs. In one study, the Copper-T-200 increased blood loss by 50% over baseline menstruation (103). In contrast, the progesterone- and levo-norgestrel-containing IUDs are associated with a decrease in menstrual blood loss. The reason for increased menstrual flow is not completely understood. However, it has been shown that there is an increase in fibrinolytic activity in the tissue (104). Additionally, it is felt that alterations in the balance of prostaglandin may contribute since nonsteroidal antiinflammatory drugs reduce blood loss in IUD users (105). Progesterone-releasing IUDs decrease blood loss through a local effect on the endometrium. The stroma becomes thin with few glands, and cyclic changes are suppressed. Intermenstrual bleeding is also common in the first few months of IUD use. This decreases with duration of use and most likely occurs because of superficial erosion of the endometrium with microvascular bleeding into the uterine cavity. IUD-associated bleeding and pain are the most common causes for requested removal. In the first year of use, 7% to 12% of women request removal for these reasons. Overall, bleeding side effects account for 40% to 50% of all reasons for discontinuation.

Infectious complications of IUD use were examined in the Women's Health Study (106). This case-control study evaluated IUD use and the risk of hospitalization for PID. IUD use was found to have an odds ratio of 1.6. However, this study included women who used the Dalkon Shield, an IUD that was associated with a high rate of infectious complications. When a reanalysis of data was performed excluding Dalkon Shield users, an increased risk of PID was found only in women who had been wearing the device for 4 months or less. Moreover, the risk of PID did not increase in the 5 years thereafter (107). IUD insertion is known to cause transient contamination of the endometrial cavity (108). However, the most significant risk factor for PID in IUD users is sexual behavior. Studies have shown that unmarried, noncohabitating women and women with multiple partners are at increased risk. The Dalkon Shield had a multifilament string. This string has been hypothesized to lead to ascending contamination of the endometrial cavity. Investigators have also examined the relationship between the presence or absence of an IUD monofilament string and infection. A recent meta-analysis of this data concluded that a tail string did not increase the risk of PID

in IUD users (109). A number of studies have examined the effect of prophylactic antibiotics at the time of IUD insertion. One study conducted in Kenya showed a lower rate of unplanned clinic visits postinsertion, and showed a 31% lower rate of infection in doxycycline users; however, this decrease was not statistically significant (110). Other studies using doxycycline have failed to show any benefit. Likewise, in a recent United States trial, azithromycin did not affect the frequency with which women sought postinsertion medical attention. The authors of this study concluded that the risk of salpingitis related to IUD insertion is negligible in women who are appropriately screened (111).

The effect of the IUD on future fertility is also of concern to women selecting this method. Skjeldestad (112) reviewed the literature regarding this topic and concluded that the IUD has no harmful effect on subsequent fertility in women after their first childbirth. However, nulliparous women may be at increased risk of tubal infertility.

Other researchers have found that there is no increased risk of infertility among IUD users who have one sex partner (113).

BARRIER CONTRACEPTIVES AND SPERMICIDES

Barrier contraceptives include male and female condoms, the diaphragm, and the cervical cap. These devices are used in conjunction with spermicide.

Mechanism of Action

The spermicide most widely used is nonoxynol-9, which is a surface agent that damages the sperm cell membrane. Barrier contraceptives may act both as physical barriers to progression of the sperm into the female upper genital tract and as a mechanism to hold spermicide in a location at which it is maximally effective.

Efficacy

Spermicides have a highly variable rate of efficacy as reported in clinical trials. Their in-use failure rate is approximately 20% (114). Although there are an array of differing vehicles for spermicide administration, there are no comparative data among them. Spermicides require application 10 to 30 minutes prior to sexual intercourse and some may last as long as 8 hours (25).

Male condoms are reported to break in 1% to 12% of incidents of vaginal intercourse (25). Their first year failure rate is approximately 9% (114). Application of vaginal spermicide is recommended as a routine practice with condoms. Although some condoms come lubricated with nonoxynol-9, it is not known if this adds to their efficacy. Condoms are made of latex, polyurethane, or sheep intestine. Latex and polyurethane condoms are impermeable to sexually transmitted diseases. Most condoms marketed in the United States are manufactured of latex. However, recently two polyurethane condoms have been developed. Polyurethane is felt to hold an advantage in that it is not associated with contact allergy as is latex, it is odorless, and is resistant to oil-based lubricants. However, a randomized, controlled trial of latex and polyurethane condoms found significantly higher breakage and slippage rates for the polyurethane condom as well as a higher failure rate (115).

The female condom is also made of polyurethane. It is prelubricated with silicon. Based on data submitted to the FDA for its approval process, the first-year failure rate of the female condom was 21% in typical use (116).

The diaphragm and cervical cap are both made of latex and are routinely used with spermicide. The failure rate of the diaphragm itself, without the use of spermicide, has never been studied. The first-year failure rate for the diaphragm and cervical cap reported by the National Survey of Family Growth, and corrected for abortion under reporting, was 14% (7). Previously, data have suggested that the cap has a greater failure rate for parous women than for nulliparous.

Side Effects

Spermicides have no known effect on long-term fertility. Although concern was raised in the past regarding a relationship with congenital anomalies, epidemiologic studies have failed to find any association (117). Spermicides, however, do provide some protection against sexually transmitted disease and therefore may have a beneficial effect in reducing upper genital tract infection that might adversely effect fertility (118,119).

The diaphragm is associated with an increased incidence of urinary tract infections in comparison with oral contraceptives (120). No relationship has been identified between diaphragm or cervical cap usage and toxic shock syndrome. Additionally, there appears to be no increased risk of dysplasia in cap users (121). Latex sensitivity is an increasing public health concern (122). Most male condoms, the diaphragm, and cervical cap are made of latex. The estimated incidence of latex allergy in the general population is approximately 1%. However, it is substantially higher in health

care workers. Latex allergy or sensitivity has been reported in male condom users (123).

EMERGENCY CONTRACEPTION

Emergency contraception or postcoital contraception is the use of a drug or device to prevent pregnancy after intercourse. It has been suggested that the widespread use of emergency contraception could have a substantial impact of the rate of unplanned pregnancy in the United States (124). Currently, there are two products marketed in the U.S. for postcoital contraception: levonorgestrel alone (75 μg), and a combined pill of ethinyl estradiol (100 μg) and levonorgestrel (50μg). These doses are repeated 12 hours after the initial administration. The insertion of a copper-containing IUD and oral administration of a single dose of 600 mg of mifepristone (RU-486) are also effective postcoital contraceptive approaches (Table 19.6).

Mechanism of Action

The most commonly recognized agent for postcoital contraception is a combination of ethinyl estradiol and levonorgestrel, also known as the Yuzpe regimen. These medications work by inhibiting or delaying ovulation. They appear to have a minimal effect on the endometrium when given postovulation, and are therefore unlikely to inhibit implantation. Although less research has been done with levonorgestrel alone, it is felt to have a similar mechanism of action. Mifepristone, when given prior to ovulation, significantly delays the onset of menstruation and thus appears to inhibit ovulation. In the luteal phase, mifepristone delays endometrial maturation and therefore may interfere with implantation. The IUD is known to adversely affect sperm. Additionally, when inserted after ovulation, it causes endometrial changes that are felt to impair implantation (125).

Efficacy

The efficacy of postcoital contraceptives is difficult to assess. Currently most studies report an effectiveness rate as the percentage of expected pregnancies that were prevented by the use of emergency contraception. The calculation of

TABLE 19.6. POSTCOITAL CONTRACEPTIVE OPTIONS

Method	Timing	Dose	Efficacy
Levonorgestrel (Plan B)	Within 72 hours	75 μg, two doses spaced by 12 hours	85%
Ethinyl estradiol and norgestrel (Preven, Ovral)	Within 72 hours	100 μg ethinyl estradiol and 50 μg levonorgestrel, two doses spaced by 12 hours	60%–75%
Copper IUD	Up to 5 days	Single insertion	99%
Mifepristone (RU-486)	Within 72 hours	Single dose	100%

expected pregnancies is based on the cycle day on which intercourse occurred and the probability of pregnancy on that cycle day. This is obviously prone to some error: the day of ovulation is generally determined based on the day of expected next menses, and for a particular woman ovulation may vary by several days from cycle to cycle. A recent randomized trial found that levonorgestrel alone was 85% effective in comparison to the Yuzpe regimen, which was 57% effective (126). This study also demonstrated that the sooner either regimen was initiated, the more effective it was. A previous meta-analysis had estimated a 74% efficacy for the Yuzpe regimen (127). Mifepristone has been used in two randomized trials without a reported failure (125). Copper-containing IUDs are 99% effective (128).

Side Effects

The biggest drawback of the Yuzpe regimen is the incidence of nausea and vomiting associated with the estrogen content. Nausea occurs in approximately 50% and vomiting in 20%. Levonorgestrel alone has a lower incidence of nausea (23%) and vomiting (6%). For both methods, disturbances in the menstrual cycle occur in as many as 40% of women, with 28% experiencing a delay in onset of menses of 3 days or longer (126). Other reported side effects include dizziness, fatigue, breast tenderness, and headache. Levonorgestrel causes less dizziness and fatigue (126). Although there have been reported cases of venous thromboembolism in users of emergency contraception, it is not clear if there is a causal relationship. The risk of thromboembolism associated with pregnancy is significantly higher than that associated with oral contraceptive use. Currently, the WHO and the International Planned Parenthood Federation have stated there are no absolute contraindications to the combined estrogen and progestin regimen, except existing pregnancy. However, this regimen should not affect an established pregnancy nor is there any reason to believe it is teratogenic (129).

The insertion of an IUD is contraindicated in women at risk of sexually transmitted infections. Therefore, the use IUDs as postcoital contraceptives is limited. Side effects of of IUD insertion include pain, heavier menstruation, a small risk of infection, and spotting. Mifepristone also causes nausea in approximately 40%, but vomiting occurs in only 3% of users. However, because mifepristone may delay ovulation, it is associated with a delay in menstruation of 3 days or more in 50% of women (130). This provokes anxiety in women who are awaiting menstruation to assure that they are not pregnant.

SUMMARY

A woman's reproductive years generally encompass many more years of contraceptive need than years of childbearing. During early sexual activity, when she is choosing to delay childbirth, she may be very concerned about the efficacy and reversibility of her chosen contraceptive. Later, during years of spacing births, efficacy may not play as prominent a role. At the conclusion of childbearing, minimizing side effects and maximizing efficacy become paramount. No one contraceptive method is right for every woman, nor is one contraceptive method right for an individual woman at all points in her reproductive years. Accurate knowledge of the risk, benefits, use, and efficacy of the available contraceptive methods will assist clinicians in counseling women appropriately about their choices.

10 KEY POINTS

1. Combined oral contraceptives are the most frequently used method of reversible contraception in the United States. They inhibit ovulation and have a low failure rate when used correctly.

2. The health benefits of oral contraceptives include reduction in the risk of ovarian and endometrial carcinoma. A small risk of venous thromboembolism is associated with combined oral contraceptive use. No increased risk of myocardial infarction exists in normotensive, nonsmoking women. The risk of breast cancer detection is higher in women currently using oral contraceptives. An increased risk of adenocarcinoma of the cervix is associated with combined oral contraceptive use.

3. Progesterone-only birth control pills thicken cervical mucus. They must be taken on a strict schedule to ensure efficacy. They are particularly appropriate for lactating women and women who cannot take estrogen.

4. Norplant, a subdermal levonorgestrel implant system, inhibits ovulation and thickens cervical mucus. It is a highly effective contraceptive that minimizes user error. Irregular bleeding is a frequent side effect.

5. Depot medroxyprogesterone acetate inhibits ovulation for 12 weeks after a single 150-mg intramuscular injection. Amenorrhea is a common side effect and becomes more common with extended use.

6. Two intrauterine devices are currently marketed in the United States. Paraguard is a copper-containing IUD that can remain in place for 10 years. Progestasert contains progesterone and must be replaced after 1 year of use. Currently available data regarding the mechanism of action of copper-containing IUDs suggest that they prevent conception.

7. Condoms have regained popularity as a contraceptive method and are effective in preventing transmission of sexually transmitted infections. Polyurethane condoms are now available for individuals with latex sensitivity. However, they may be associated with a higher rate of slippage. Female condoms made of polyurethane have a higher failure rate than male condoms.

8. The diaphragm and cervical cap are used in conjunction with spermicide. These devices have an intrinsically higher failure rate than the hormonal contraceptive methods, but minimize side effects.

9. Two hormonal emergency contraceptives are now available in the United States. New data suggest that levonorgestrel alone is superior to the combination of levonorgestrel and ethinyl estradiol in both effectiveness and reduction in side effects.

10. Insertion of a copper IUD or oral administration of mifepristone (RU-486) is also an effective emergency contraceptive approach.

REFERENCES

1. Mishell DR Jr, Kletzky OA, Brenner PF, et al. The effect of contraceptive steroids on hypothalamic-pituitary function. *Am J Obstet Gynecol* 1977:128:60–74.

2. Lobo RA, Stanczyk FZ. New knowledge in the physiology of hormonal contraceptives. *Am J Obstet Gynecol* 1994;170:499–507.

3. Molloy BG, Coulson KA, Lee JM, et al. "Missed pill" conception: fact or fiction? *Br Med J* 1985;290:1474–1475.

4. Killick S, Eyong E, Elstein M. Ovarian follicular development in oral contraceptive cycles. *Fertil Steril* 1987;48:409–413.

5. Elstein M, Morris SE, Groom GV, et al. Studies on low-dose oral contraceptives: cervical mucus and plasma hormone changes in relation to circulating D-norgestrel and 17-ethynyl-estradiol concentrations. *Fertil Steril* 1976;27:892–899.

6. Elstein M. Consensus paper. Low dose contraceptive formulations: is further reduction in steroid dosage justified? *Adv Contracept* 1994;10:1–4.

7. Fu H, Darroch JE, Haas T, et al. Contraceptive failure rates: new estimates from the 1995 National Survey of Family Growth. *Fam Plann Perspect* 1999;31:56–63.

8. Royal College of General Practitioners. The outcome of pregnancy in former oral contraceptive users. *Br J Obstet Gynaecol* 1976;83:608–616.

9. Furuhjelm M, Carlstrom K. Amenorrhea following use of combined oral contraceptives. *Acta Obstet Gynecol Scand* 1973;52:373–379.

10. Carr BR, Ory H. Estrogen and progestin components of oral contraceptives: relationship to vascular disease. *Contraception* 1997;55:267–272.

11. Rosenberg L, Palmer JR, Lesko SM, et al. Oral contraceptive use and the risk of myocardial infarction. *Am J Epidemiol* 1990;131:1009–1016.

12. Croft P, Hannaford PC. Risk factors for acute myocardial infarction in women: evidence from the Royal College of General Practitioners' oral contraceptive study. *Br Med J* 1989;298:165–168.

13. Colditz GA, and the Nurses' Health Study Research Group. Oral contraceptive use and mortality during 12 years of follow-up: the Nurses' Health Study. *Ann Intern Med* 1994;120:821–826.

14. Schwartz SM, Petitti DB, Siscovick DS, et al. Stroke and use of low-dose oral contraceptives in young women: a pooled analysis of two US studies. *Stroke* 1998;29:2277–2284.

15. WHO Collaborative Study of Cardiovascular Disease and Steroid Hormone Contraception. Haemorrhagic stroke, overall stroke risk and combined oral contraceptives: results of an international multicentre case-control study. *Lancet* 1996;348:505–510.

16. WHO Collaborative Study of Cardiovascular Disease and Steroid Hormone Contraception. Ishaemic stroke and combined oral contraceptives: results of an international multicentre case-control study. *Lancet* 1996;348:498–505.

17. Speroff L. Oral contraceptives and arterial and venous thrombosis: a clinician's formulation. *Am J Obstet Gynecol* 1998;178:S25–S36.

18. WHO Collaborative Study of Cardiovascular Disease and Steroid Hormone Contraception. Venous thromboembolic disease and combined oral contraceptives results of international multicentre case-control study. *Lancet* 1995;348:1575–1582.

19. Spitzer WO, Lewis MA, Heinemann LA, et al. Third generation oral contraceptives and risk of venous thromboembolic disorders: an international case-control study. *Br Med J* 1996;312:83–88.

20. Jick H, Jick SS, Gurewich V, et al. Risk of idiopathic cardiovascular death and nonfatal venous thromboembolism in women using oral contraceptives with differing progestagen components. *Lancet* 1995;346:1589–1593.

21. Bloemenkamp KW, Rosendaal FR, Helmerhorst FM, et al. Enhancement by factor V Leiden mutation of risk of deep-vein thrombosis associated with oral contraceptives containing a third-generation progestagen. *Lancet* 1995;346:1593–1596.

22. Farmer RD, Lawrenson RA, Thompson CR et al. Population-based study of risk of venous thromboembolism associated with various oral contraceptives. *Lancet* 1997;349:83–88.

23. Lidegaard O, Edstrom B, Kreiner S. Oral contraceptives and venous thromboembolism: a case-control study. *Contraception* 1998;57:291–301.

24. Rosing J, Tans G, Nicolaes GA, et al. Oral contraceptives and venous thrombosis: different sensitivities to activated protein C in women using second and third generation oral contraceptives. *Br J Haematol* 1997;97:233–238.

25. Speroff L, Darney PD. *A clinical guide for contraception,* 2nd ed. Baltimore: Williams & Wilkins, 1996.

26. Kovacs L, Bartfai G, Apro G, et al. The effect of the contraceptive pill on blood pressure: a randomized controlled trial of three progestogen-oestrogen combinations in Szeged, Hungary. *Contraception* 1986;33:69–77.

27. Hannaford PC, Kay CR. Oral contraceptives and diabetes mellitus. *Br Med J* 1989;299:1315–1316.

28. Grimes DA, Wallach M, eds. *Modern contraception.* Totowa, NJ: Emron, 1997.

29. Klein BE, Moss SE, Klein R. Oral contraceptives in women with diabetes. *Diabetes Care* 1990;13:895–898.

30. Garg SK, Chase HP, Marshall G, et al. Oral contraceptives and renal and retinal complications in young women with insulin-dependent diabetes mellitus. *JAMA* 1994;271:1099–1102.

31. Royal College of General Practitioners. *Oral contraceptives and health.* London: Pitman Medical, 1974:57–59.

32. Bennion LJ, Ginsberg RL, Gernick MB, et al. Effects of oral contraceptives on the gallbladder bile of normal women. *N Engl J Med* 1976;294:189–192.

33. Thijs C, Knipschild P. Oral contraceptives and the risk of gallbladder disease: a meta analysis. *Am J Public Health* 1993;83:1113–1120.

34. Vessey M, Paainer R. Oral contraceptive use and benign gallbladder disease revisited. *Contraception* 1994;50:167–173.

35. Romieu I, Willett WC, Colditz GA, et al. Prospective study of oral contraceptive use and risk of breast cancer in women. *J Natl Cancer Inst* 1989;81:1313–1321.

36. Royal College of General Practitioners Oral Contraceptive Study. Further analyses of mortality in oral contraceptive users. *Lancet* 1981;1:541–546.

37. Cancer and Steroid Hormone Study, CDC and NICHD. Oral contraceptive use and the risk of breast cancer. *N Engl J Med* 1986;315:405–411.

38. UK National Case-Control Study Group. Oral contraceptive use and breast cancer risk in young women. *Lancet* 1989;1:973–982.

39. McPherson K, Vessey MP, Neil A, et al. Early oral contraceptive use and breast cancer: results of another case-control study. *Br J Cancer* 1987;56:653–660.

40. Stadel BV, Rubin GL, Webster LA, et al. Oral contraceptives and breast cancer in young women. *Lancet* 1985;2:970–973.

41. Brinton LA, Daling JR, Liff JM, et al. Oral contraceptives and breast cancer risk among younger women. *J Natl Cancer Inst* 1995;87:827–835.

42. La Vecchia C, Negri E, Franceschi S, et al. Oral contraceptives and breast cancer: a cooperative Italian study. *Int J Cancer* 1995;60:163–167.

43. Collaborative Group on Hormonal Factors in Breast Cancer: Breast cancer and hormonal contraceptives: collaborative reanalysis of individual data on 52,705 women with breast cancer and 108,411 women without breast cancer. *Lancet* 1997;350:1047–1059.

44. Brinton LA. Oral contraceptives and cervical neoplasia. *Contraception* 1991;43:581–595.

45. Delgado-Rodriquez M, Sillero-Arenas M, Martin-Moreno JM, et al. Oral contraceptives and cancer of the cervix uteri: a meta-analysis. *Acta Obstet Gynecol Scand* 1992;71:368–372.

46. Ye Z, Thomas DB, Ray RM, and the WHO Collaborative Study of Neoplasia and Steroid Contraceptives. Combined oral contraceptives and risk of cervical carcinoma in situ. *Int J Epidemiol* 1995;24:19–26.

47. Prentice FL, Thomas DB. On the epidemiology of oral contraceptives and disease. *Adv Cancer Res* 1987;49:285–401.

48. Irwin KL, Roser-Bixby L, Oberle MW, et al. Oral contraceptives and cervical cancer risk in Costa Rica: detection bias or causal association? *JAMA* 1988;259:59–64.

49. Ley C, Bauer HM, Reingold A, et al. Determinants of genital human papilloma virus infection in young women. *J Natl Cancer Inst* 1991;83:997–1003.

50. Brinton LA, Reeves WC, Brenes MM, et al. Oral contraceptive use and risk of invasive cervical cancer. *Int J Epidemiol* 1990;19:4–11.

51. Ursin G, Peters RK, Henderson BE, et al. Oral contraceptive use and adenocarcinoma of the cervix. *Lancet* 1994;344:1390–1394.

52. Thomas DB, Ray RM, and the World Health Organization Collaborative Study of Neoplasia and Steroid Contraceptives. Oral contraceptives and invasive adenocarcinomas and adenosquamous carcinomas of the uterine cervix. *Am J Epidemiol* 1996;144:281–289.

53. The Cancer and Steroid Hormone Study of the Centers for Disease Control and National Institute of Child Health and Human Development. Combination oral contraceptive use and the risk of endometrial cancer. *JAMA* 1987;49:285–401.

54. The Cancer and Steroid Hormone Study of the Centers for Disease Control and National Institute of Child Health and Human Development. The reduction in risk of ovarian cancer associated with oral contraceptive use. *N Engl J Med* 1987;316:650–655.

55. Whittemore AS, Harris R, Itnyre J, and the Collaborative Ovarian Cancer Group. Characteristics relating to ovarian cancer risk: collaborative analysis of 12 US case-control studies. II. Invasive epithelial ovarian cancers in white women. *Am J Epidemiol* 1992;136:1184–1203.

56. Rosenberg L, Palmer JR, Zauber AG, et al. A case-control study of oral contraceptive use and invasive epithelial ovarian cancer. *Am J Epidemiol* 1994;139:654–661.

57. Narod SA, Risch H, Moslehi R, et al. Oral contraceptives and the risk of hereditary ovarian cancer. *N Engl J Med* 1998;339:424–428.

58. Akerlund M, Rode A, Westergaard J. Comparative profiles of reliability, cycle control and side effects of two oral contraceptive formulations containing 150 μg desogestrel and either 30 μg or 20 μg ethinyl oestradiol. *Br J Obstet Gynaecol* 1993;100:832–838.

59. Saleh WA, Burkman RT, Zacur HA, et al. A randomized trial of three oral contraceptives: comparison of bleeding patterns by contraceptive types and steroid levels. *Am J Obstet Gynecol* 1993;168:1740–1745.

60. Rosenberg MJ, Waugh MS, Steven CM. Smoking and cycle control among oral contraceptive users. *Am J Obstet Gynecol* 1996;174:628–632.

61. Rosenberg M. Weight change with oral contraceptive use and during the menstrual cycle: results of daily measurements. *Contraception* 1998;58:345–349.

62. Carpenter S, Neinstein LS. Weight gain in adolescent and young adult oral contraceptive users. *J Adolesc Health Care* 1986:7:342–344.

63. Moore LL, Valuck R, McDougall C, et al. A comparative study of one-year weight gain among users of medroxyprogesterone acetate, levonorgestrel implants, and oral contraceptives. *Contraception* 1995;52:215–219.

64. Lucky AW, Henderson TA, Olson WH, et al. Effectiveness of norgestimate and ethinyl estradiol in treating moderate acne vulgaris. *J Am Acad Dermatol* 1997;37:746–754.

65. Lemay A, Dewailly SD, Grenier R, et al. Attenuation of mild hyperandrogenic activity in postpubertal acne by a triphasic oral contraceptive containing low doses of ethynyl estradiol and d,l-norgestrel. *J Clin Endocrinol Metab* 1990;71:8–14.

66. Wishart JM. An open study of Triphasil and Diane 50 in the treatment of acne. *Australas J Dermatol* 1991;32:51–54.

67. Chi I. The safety and efficacy issues of progestin-only contraceptives: an epidemiologic perspective. *Contraception* 1993;47:1–21.

68. Trussell J, Kost K. Contraceptive failure in the United States: a critical review of the literature. *Stud Fam Plann* 1987;18:237.

69. Collaborative Study Group on the Desogestrel-Containing Progestogen-Only Pill. A double-blind study comparing the contraceptive efficacy, acceptability and safety of two progestogen-only pills containing desogestrel 75 micrograms/day or levonorgestrel 30 micrograms/day. *Eur J Contracept Reprod Health Care* 1998;3:169–178.

70. Broome M, Fotherby K. Clinical experience with the progestogen-only pill. *Contraception* 1990;42:489.

71. Tayob Y, Adams J. Jacobs HS, et al. Ultrasound demonstration of increased frequency of functional ovarian cyst in women using progestogen-only oral contraception. *Br J Obstet Gynaecol* 1985;92:1003–1009.

72. McCann MF, Moggia AV, Higgins JE, et al. The effects of progestin-only oral contraceptive (levonorgestrel 0.03 mg) on breast-feeding. *Contraception* 1989;40:635–648.

73. Dunson TR, McLaurin VL, Grubb GS, et al. A multicenter clinical trial of a progestin-only oral contraceptive in lactating women. *Contraception* 1993;47:23–35.

74. Caird LE, Reid-Thomas V, Hannan WJ, et al. Oral progestogen-only contraception may protect against loss of bone mass in breast-feeding women. *Clin Endocrinol* 1994;41:739–745.

75. Heinemann LA, Assmann A, DoMinh T, et al. Oral progestogen-only contraceptives and cardiovascular risk: results from the Transnational Study on Oral Contraceptives and the Health of

Young Women. *Eur J Contracept Reprod Health Care* 1999;4:67–73.

76. World Health Organization Collaborative Study of Cardiovascular Disease and Steroid Hormone Contraception. Cardiovascular disease and use of oral and injectable progestogen-only contraceptives and combined injectable contraceptives: results of an international, multicenter, case-control study. *Contraception* 1998;57:315–324.

77. Skegg DC, Paul C, Spear GF, et al. Progestogen-only oral contraceptives and risk of breast cancer in New Zealand. *Cancer Causes Control* 1996;7:513–519.

78. Weiderpass E, Adami HO, Baron JA, et al. Use of oral contraceptive and endometrial cancer risk. *Cancer Causes Control* 1999;10:277–284.

79. Graham CA, Ramos R, Bancroft J, et al. The effects of steroidal contraceptives on the well-being and sexuality of women: a double-blind, placebo-controlled, two-centre study of combined and progestogen-only methods. *Contraception* 1995;52:363–369.

80. Brache V, Alvarez-Sanchez F, Faundes A, et al. Ovarian endocrine function through five years of continuous treatment with NORPLANT subdermal contraceptive implants. *Contraception* 1990;41:169–177.

81. Croxatto HB, Diaz S, Salvatierra AM, et al. Treatment with Norplant subdermal implants inhibits sperm penetration through cervical mucus in vitro. *Contraception* 1987;36:193–201.

82. Segal SJ, Alvarez-Sanchez F, Brache V, et al. Norplant implants: the mechanism of contraceptive action. *Fertil Steril* 1991;56:273–277.

83. Sivin I. International experience with Norplant and Norplant-2 contraceptives. *Stud Fam Plann* 1988;19:81–94.

84. Sivin I, Stern J, Diaz S, et al. Rates and outcomes of planned pregnancy after use of Norplant capsules, Norplant II rods, or levonorgestrel-releasing or copper TCu 380Ag intrauterine contraceptive devices. *Am J Obstet Gynecol* 1992;166:1208–1213.

85. Shoupe D, Mishell DR Jr, Bopp BL, et al. The significance of bleeding patterns in Norplant implant users. *Obstet Gynecol* 1991;77:256–260.

86. Shoupe D, Mishell DR. NORPLANT: subdermal implant system for long-term contraception. *Am J Obstet Gynecol* 1989;160:1286–1292.

87. Pasquale SA, Knuppel RA, Owens AG, et al. Irregular bleeding, body mass index, and coital frequency in Norplant contraceptive users. *Contraception* 1994;50:109–116.

88. Wagner KD. Major depression and anxiety disorders associated with Norplant. *J Clin Psychiatry* 1996;57:152–157.

89. Westhoff C, Truman C, Kalmuss D, et al. Depressive symptoms and Norplant contraceptive implants. *Contraception* 1998;57:241–245.

90. WHO. A multicentered phase II comparative clinical trial of depot-medroxyprogesterone acetate given three-monthly at doses of 100 mg or 150 mg: I. Contraceptive efficacy and side effects. *Contraception* 1986;34:223–235.

91. Schwallie PC and Assenzo JR. Contraceptive use-efficacy study utilizing medroxyprogesterone acetate administered as an intramuscular injection once every 90 days. *Fertil Steril* 1973;24:331–339.

92. Mainwaring R, Hales HA, Stevenson K, et al. Metabolic parameter, bleeding and weight changes in U.S. women using progestin only contraceptives. *Contraception* 1995;51:149–153.

93. WHO Collaborative Study of Neoplasia and Steroid Contraceptives. Breast cancer and depot-medroxyprogesterone acetate: a multinational study. *Lancet* 1991;338:833–838.

94. Skegg DC, Noonan EA, Paul C, et al. Depot medroxyprogesterone acetate and breast cancer: a pooled analysis of the World Health Organization and New Zealand studies. *JAMA* 1995;273:799–804.

95. Cundy T, Evans M, Roberts H, et al. Bone density in women receiving depot medroxyprogesterone acetate for contraception. *Br Med J* 1991;303:13–16.

96. Scholes D, Lacroiz AZ, Ott SM et al. Bone mineral density in women using depot medroxyprogesterone acetate for contraception. *Obstet Gynecol* 1999;93:233–238.

97. Cromer BA, Blair JM, Mahan JD, et al. A prospective comparison of bone density in adolescent girls receiving depot medroxyprogesterone acetate (Depo-Provera), levonorgestrel (Norplant), or oral contraceptives. *J Pediatr* 1996;129:671–676.

98. Schwallie PC, Assenzo JR. The effect of depot-medroxyprogesterone acetate on pituitary and ovarian function and the return of fertility following its discontinuation: a review. *Contraception* 1974;10:181–202.

99. Westhoff C, Truman C, Kalmuss D, et al. Depressive symptoms and Depo-Provera. *Contraception* 1998;57:237–240.

100. Croxatto HB, Ortiz ME, Valdez E. IUD mechanisms of action. In: Bardin CW, Mishell DR, eds. *Fourth International Conference on IUDs*. Newton, MA: Butterworth-Heinemann, 1994:44–62.

101. Alvarez F, Brache V, Fernandez E, et al. New insights on the mode of action of the intrauterine contraceptive device in women. *Fertil Steril* 1988;49:768–773.

102. Tatum HJ. Intrauterine contraception. *Am J Obstet Gynecol* 1972;112:1000–1023.

103. Rybo G. The IUD and endometrial bleeding. *J Reprod Med* 1978;20:175–182.

104. Larsson B, Liedholm P, Astedt B. Increased fibrinolytic activity in the endometrium of patients using copper IUD. *Int J Fertil* 1975;20:77–80.

105. Anderson AB, Haynes PJ, Guillebaud J, et al. Reduction of menstrual blood loss by prostaglandin-synthetase inhibitors. *Lancet* 1976;1:774–776.

106. Burkman RT, and the Women's Health Study. Association between intrauterine device and pelvic inflammatory disease. *Obstet Gynecol* 1981:57:269–276.

107. Lee NC, Rubin GL, Ory HW, et al. Type of intrauterine device and the risk of pelvic inflammatory disease. *Obstet Gynecol* 1983;62:1–6.

108. Mishell DR, Bell JH, Good RG, et al. The intrauterine device: a bacteriologic study of the endometrial cavity. *Am J Obstet Gynecol* 1966;96:119–126.

109. Ebi KL, Piziali RL, Rosenberg M, et al. Evidence against tailstrings increasing the rate of pelvic inflammatory disease among IUD users. *Contraception* 1996;53:25–32.

110. Sinei SK, Schultz KF, Lamptey PR, et al. Preventing IUCD-related pelvic infection: the efficacy of prophylactic doxycycline at insertion. *Br J Obstet Gynaecol* 1990;97:412–419.

111. Walsh TL, Grimes D, Frezieres R, et al. Randomized controlled trial of prophylactic antibiotics before insertion of intrauterine devices. IUD Study Group. *Lancet* 1998;351:1005–1008.

112. Skjeldestad FE. Conception rates post IUD removal. In: Bardin CW, Mishell DR, eds. *Fourth International Conference on IUDs*. Newton, MA: Butterworth-Heinemann, 1994:63–74.

113. Cramer DW, Schiff I, Schoenbaum SC, et al. Tubal infertility and the intrauterine device. *N Engl J Med* 1985;312:941–947.

114. Trussell J, Vaughan B. Contraceptive failure, method-related discontinuation and resumption of use: results from the 1995 National Survey of Family Growth. *Fam Plann Perspect* 1999;31:64–72, 93.

115. Frezieres RG, Walsh TL, Nelson AL, et al. Evaluation of the efficacy of a polyurethane condom: results from a randomized, controlled clinical trial. *Fam Plann Perspect* 1999;31:81–87.

116. Trussell J, Sturgen K, Strickler J, et al. Comparative contraceptive efficacy of the female condom and other barrier methods. *Fam Plann Perspect* 1994;26:66–72.

117. Einarson TR, Koren G, Mattice D, et al. Maternal spermicide use and adverse reproductive outcome: a meta-analysis. *Am J Obstet Gynecol* 1990;162:655–660.

118. Niruthisard S, Roddy RE, Chutivongse S. Use of nonoxynol-9 and reduction in rate of gonococcal and chlamydial cervical infections. *Lancet* 1992;339:1371–1375.

119. Kelaghan J, Rubin GL, Ory HW, et al. Barrier-method contraceptives and pelvic inflammatory disease. *JAMA* 1982;248:184–187.

120. Fihn SD, Latham FH, Roberts P, et al. Association between diaphragm use and urinary tract infection. *JAMA* 1985;254:240–245.

121. Gollub EL, Sivin I. The Prentif cervical cap and Pap smear results: a critical appraisal. *Contraception* 1989;40:343.

122. Liss GM, Sussman GL. Latex sensitization: occupational versus general population prevalence rates. *Am J Ind Med* 1999;35:196–200.

123. Levy DA, Khouader S, Leynadier F. Allergy to latex condoms. *Allergy* 1998;53:1107–1108.

124. Trussell J, Ellertson C, Stewart F. The effectiveness of the Yuzpe regimen of emergency contraception. *Fam Plann Perspect* 1996;28:58–64.

125. Glasier A. Emergency postcoital contraception. *N Engl J Med* 1997;337:1058–1064.

126. World Health Organization Task Force on Postovulatory Methods of Fertility Regulation. Randomised controlled trial of levonorgestrel versus the Yuzpe regimen of combined oral contraceptives for emergency contraception. *Lancet* 1998;352:428–433.

127. Trussell J, Stewart F. The effectiveness of postcoital contraception. *Fam Plann Perspect* 1992;24:262–264.

128. Trussell J, Ellertson C. Efficacy of emergency contraception. *Fertil Control Rev* 1995;4:8–11.

129. Glasier A. Safety of emergency contraception. *JAMWA* 1998;53:219–221.

130. Von Hertzen H. Research on Mifepristone and levonorgestrel in comparison with the Yuzpe regimen. *JAMWA* 1998;53:222–224.

SEXUALLY TRANSMITTED DISEASES

PARUL KRISHNAMURTHY
A. GEORGE NEUBERT
PETER A. SCHWARTZ

An understanding of the microbiology, diagnosis, and treatment of sexually transmitted diseases (STDs) is of vital importance in the provision of health care to women. This chapter provides an overview of the common STDs encountered in practice in the United States today. A review of STDs causing vaginal discharge, genital ulceration, and genital skin lesions is provided. The risk factors for STDs include adolescence, multiple sexual partners, nonwhite race, low socioeconomic status, nonbarrier contraception, previous history of STDs, and use of intravenous drugs and/or crack cocaine. Treatment of STDs includes alleviation of symptoms, microbiologic cure, and prevention of transmission. Prevention and control of STDs involves screening, education, and counseling of those at risk on ways to reduce or eliminate their risk of STDs. HIV infection can modify the clinical presentation and features of other STDs, and major genital ulcer diseases have been associated with an increased risk of acquiring and transmitting HIV.

SEXUALLY TRANSMITTED DISEASES CAUSING VAGINAL DISCHARGE

Chlamydia Trachomatis

Chlamydia trachomatis is the most common STD. An estimated 4 million chlamydial infections were reported to the Centers for Disease Control (CDC) in 1993 (1). Chlamydiaceae are obligate intracellular bacteria that were once regarded as viruses. *C. trachomatis* is a mucosal pathogen that exclusively infects humans. Chlamydial infections often elude detection because they produce few or no symptoms, or the symptoms and signs they do produce are nonspecific.

Epidemiology and Transmission

Chlamydial infection is the major cause of pelvic inflammatory disease (PID) in the United States (1). The prevalence of *C. trachomatis* is as low as 3% in asymptomatic women to as high as 20% in patients attending a STD clinic (2). However, a prevalence rate close to 10% is detected in asymptomatic young women using ligase chain reaction

(LCR)-based tests (3). Chlamydia is detected in 30% to 60% of women with gonorrhea or those with prior exposure to gonorrhea (4). It has been estimated that eradication of genital chlamydial infections could eliminate 80% of tubal factor infertility and 50% of tubal pregnancies (5). Oral contraceptives users, though at increased risk of cervical infection with *C. trachomatis*, have a decreased risk of chlamydial PID (6).

Other diseases caused by chlamydia are ocular trachoma and lymphogranuloma venereum (LGV). Ocular trachoma affects 500 million people worldwide, primarily young children. It is associated with conditions of poor hygiene and is prevalent in the Middle East and sub-Saharan Africa (7). LGV, unusual in Europe and United States, is characterized by a primary ulcerative genital lesion that may progress to genital hyperplasia, rectal fistulae, and sinus tract formation. Chlamydial infections such as inclusion conjunctivitis and neonatal pneumonia are transmitted from mother to infant during birth. In contrast to trachoma, inclusion conjunctivitis does not lead to blindness (8).

Microorganism and Pathogenesis

C. trachomatis resembles bacteria in that it has a cell envelope, but resembles viruses in that it is an obligatory intracellular organism. Chlamydiae have a unique life cycle, with an intracellular replicative form, the reticulate body (RB), and an extracellular infective form, the elementary body (EB) (9). The extracellular, metabolically inert EB attaches to the columnar epithelium and enters the host cell through a process of endocytosis. When inside the phagosome, the EB is transformed to become the RB. RB is the metabolically active form that parasitically uses the host's adenosine triphosphate (ATP) supplies to replicate by binary fission. The infected cell is now characterized by a microscopically visible, iodine-stainable inclusion that contains the maturing RBs. The process of maturation involves the conversion of the progeny from reticulate to elementary bodies, which are released from the host cell by exocytosis. The released EBs may then infect other cells.

C. trachomatis behaves similarly to other Gram-negative

bacteria, insomuch as antibiotics inhibit it. As a Gram-negative bacterium, the organism has an outer membrane that contains lipopolysaccharide and other antigens; however, it lacks a peptidoglycan layer. The lipopolysaccharide may contribute to the virulence of the organism and is a major antigenic component of the organism. Within the genus trachomatis, there are three LGV types, LGV1 to LGV3, 12 trachoma types, and types D through K, which cause genital and occasionally eye infections (8).

Clinical Manifestations

The organism produces an inflammatory response that involves the superficial epithelium as well as the submucosa. The primary site of chlamydial infection in women is the endocervix, the signs of which include mucopurulent discharge, and an edematous, friable cervix. Similar to gonococci, *C. trachomatis* is also a cause of urethritis, bartholinitis, proctitis, and salpingitis. Approximately 20% of cases of acute PID are associated with *C. trachomatis* infections, and about one-third of women with untreated chlamydial infection of the genital tract will develop acute PID. As many as 70% to 80% of women identified as having chlamydial genital tract infections are asymptomatic. These silently infected individuals serve as a large reservoir to sustain transmission within a community (8). Both acute and chronic forms of chlamydial infections can lead to sequelae of infertility, ectopic pregnancy, or chronic pelvic pain syndrome. Reiter's syndrome, characterized by polyarticular arthritis, conjunctivitis, and stomatitis, occurs in <1% of women with chlamydial infections. Reiter's syndrome is strongly associated with the human leukocyte antigen (HLA)-B27 haplotype, where an exaggerated immune response to chlamydial antigens is thought to underlie the inflammation at involved target organs (10).

Diagnosis and Differential

C. trachomatis can be diagnosed by cytology, culture, direct detection of antigen or nucleic acids, and serologic testing. Sites of infection with recovery of the organism include infected cells of the urethra, cervix, rectum, conjunctiva, nasopharynx, and material aspirated from the fallopian tubes. The finding of mucopurulent discharge from the endocervix that appears yellow on a white cotton-tipped swab yields a presumptive diagnosis of mucopurulent cervicitis (MPC). The differential diagnosis includes gonococcal cervicitis, chlamydial cervicitis, herpetic cervicitis, chronic dysplastic changes due to human papillomavirus (HPV) disease, and cervical inflammation due to chronic vaginitis. For collecting specimens from the cervix, it is first necessary to remove all secretions from the cervix with a large swab, which is then discarded. A Dacron-tip swab or endocervical brush is inserted 1 to 2 cm into the endocervical canal, rotated for 10 to 30 seconds, and withdrawn without touch-

ing any vaginal surfaces. The swab is then placed in the appropriate transport medium or swabbed onto a slide prepared for direct fluorescent antibody (DFA) testing (8). Wood-shafted and calcium alginate swabs depress the recovery of this organism. Transport to the laboratory is time and temperature sensitive. Ideally the swab should be transported in chlamydial transport medium on a cold pack at 2°C to 8°C and arrive at the laboratory within 4 hours. Chlamydia are obligate intracellular bacteria; hence, living host cells are required to support their growth. The usual medium is cycloheximide-treated or irradiated McCoy cells. Iodine-positive inclusion bodies may be visualized 48 to 72 hours after the cell culture is infected with material from the patient. Alternatively, specific fluorescent antibody stain may be used to verify the presence of the organism. When performed in experienced laboratories, the sensitivity and specificity of culture is 70% to 90% and 100%, respectively (11). Despite the limitations, culture is the diagnostic method of choice in situations with legal implications, when the possibility of a false-positive test is unacceptable (8).

Although culture remains the gold standard for diagnosis of chlamydia infection, it is expensive, takes up to 72 hours, and few laboratories have the expertise to provide reliable results. Antigen detection and nucleic acid hybridization techniques offer the advantages of automated tests with rapid and accurate diagnosis. Studies indicate that nucleic acid amplification methods are more sensitive than culture and as specific (12). Both polymerase chain reaction (PCR) and LCR are *in vitro* nucleic acid amplification techniques that exponentially amplify specific targeted DNA sequences to enhance sensitivity. An additional advantage is the possibility of detecting the presence of both *C. trachomatis* and *Neisseria gonorrhoeae* in the same sample. Hence, an expanded gold standard has been defined as a positive culture or at least one specimen (from the cervix or urine) confirmed to be positive by LCR testing (3). The LCR is becoming the nonculture method of choice.

Diagnosis of genital chlamydial infection can also be successfully performed using first voided urine (FVU) specimens. The FVU specimen allows rapid and reliable testing for both chlamydia and gonorrhea without pelvic examination, as is required with culture and immunoassay methods. The sensitivity is over 95%, with few, if any, false positives (12). However, for women with symptoms, it is advisable also to perform a pelvic examination. Universal *C. trachomatis* screening programs with PCR or LCR through the FVU testing may contribute to the early detection of chlamydial infections because most infections are asymptomatic or minimally symptomatic. Early detection of asymptomatic chlamydial infections could lead to secondary prevention of PID and adverse pregnancy outcomes. The cost-effectiveness of universal testing requires further study (13,14). Serologic testing has limited value for diagnosis of urogenital infection in adults, because it does not provide timely and accurate information for the diagnosis of acute infections. However, serologic tests are useful in studies of PID and infertility, where the active infection is no longer present (15,16). Detection of *C. trachomatis*–specific immunoglobulin M (IgM) is useful in diagnosis of neonatal infections. Negative serology in the neonate can reliably exclude chlamydial infection (8).

Treatment (Table 20.1)

For several years, the standard therapy for uncomplicated genital tract infection has been doxycycline 100 mg orally twice a day for 7 days, with erythromycin as a first alternative. Although more expensive than doxycycline, single-dose azithromycin is currently the appropriate first choice for the treatment of chlamydial infection. Administration of the single-dose agent can be directly observed, thereby ensuring compliance, which is especially important in treating asymptomatic patients (17). With azithromycin, high tissue bioavailability and a tissue half-life of 67 hours allow for a short dosing period with high antimicrobial activity at sites of infection (17). It has been documented that there are effective levels of azithromycin in the cervical mucus more than a week after administration of a single 1-g dose (18). Alternative regimens include erythromycin base (less effective than doxycycline and azithromycin) 500 mg orally four times a day for 7 days, or ofloxacin (as effective as doxycycline and azithromycin) 300 mg orally twice a day for 7 days. Doxycycline and azithromycin are highly efficacious for chlamydia; hence, routine test of cure is not necessary. A test of cure may be considered 3 weeks after completion of treatment with erythromycin. Continued excretion of dead organisms may result in false-positive results with PCR testing for up to 3 weeks following completion of treatment. Rescreening women several months after treatment might be effective for detecting reinfection.

Patients should be instructed to abstain from sexual intercourse for 7 days after single-dose therapy, or until completion of a 7-day regimen. Sex partners should be evaluated, tested, and treated if they had sexual contact with the patient during the 60 days preceding onset of symptoms in the patient or diagnosis of chlamydia. The most recent sex partner should be treated even if the time of the last sexual contact was >60 days before onset or diagnosis. Patients should be instructed to avoid sexual intercourse until therapy is completed and their sex partners and themselves no longer have symptoms.

Interactions with Pregnancy

Genital chlamydial infection during pregnancy is associated with complications such as premature birth and postpartum endometritis (19). The prevalence of *C. trachomatis* infection among pregnant women usually is >5%, regardless of race/ethnicity or socioeconomic status (1). Neonatal conjunctivitis, which develops 5 to 12 days postpartum, occurs in approximately 30% of infants born to infected women. Marked conjunctival erythema, edema, and a watery ocular discharge characterize neonatal inclusion conjunctivitis. The neonate may also develop otitis, mucopurulent rhinitis, or pneumonia. A chlamydial etiology should be considered for all infants aged ≤30 days who have conjunctivitis. Approximately 10% to 20% of infants delivered vaginally to infected mothers develop chlamydial pneumonia, with onset from 1 to 3 months of age. In 1987, total direct and indirect costs of chlamydial infection in infants, including treatment of conjunctivitis and hospitalization for pneumonia, were estimated to be $54 million (20). Infants born to mothers who have untreated chlamydia are at high risk for infection; however, the efficacy of prophylactic antibiotic treatment is unknown. Infants born to women with untreated chlamydial infections should be monitored closely but not treated emphirically. *C. trachomatis* infection of the nasopharynx, urogenital tract, and rectum may persist for more than a year. However, sexual abuse must be considered a possible cause in preadolescent children.

The CDC recommends screening all pregnant women for *C. trachomatis*. Urine samples from pregnant women contain inhibitors of the LCR assay. Therefore, screening for *C. trachomatis* by LCR on urine samples from pregnant women is not recommended (21). Recommended treatments of infected women include 500 mg oral erythromycin base four times a day for 7 days, or oral amoxicillin 500 mg three times a day for 7 days (Table 20.2). Side effects such as nausea, vomiting, diarrhea, and abdominal pain are not uncommon with erythromycin. In a study of pregnant women with chlamydial infection, azithromycin was significantly more effective and better tolerated than erythromycin (22). Erythromycin base 250 mg orally four times a day for 14 days is another alternative. Erythromycin estolate is contraindicated during pregnancy because of drug-related hepatotoxicity.

TABLE 20.1. TREATMENT OF CHLAMYDIAL INFECTION (NOT PREGNANT)

Drug	Dose (PO)	Duration of Therapy
Azithromycin[a] *or*	1 g	Single dose
Doxycycline[a] *or*	100 mg b.i.d.	7 days
Erythromycin base *or*	500 mg q.i.d.	7 days
Erthromycin ethylsuccinate *or*	800 mg q.i.d.	7 days
Ofloxacin	300 mg b.i.d.	7 days

[a]Recommended regimen.
From Centers for Disease Control and Prevention. 1998 Guidelines for treatment of sexually transmitted diseases. *MMWR* 1998;47(RR-1):54, with permission.

TABLE 20.2. TREATMENT OF CHLAMYDIAL INFECTION IN PREGNANCY

Drug	Dose (PO)	Duration of Therapy
Erythromycin base[a] *or*	500 mg q.i.d.	7 days
Amoxicillin[a] *or*	500 mg t.i.d.	7 days
Erythromycin base *or*	250 mg q.i.d.	14 days
Erythromycin ethylsuccinate *or*	800 mg q.i.d.	7 days
Erythromycin ethylsuccinate *or*	400 mg q.i.d.	14 days
Azithromycin[a]	1 g	Single dose

[a]Recommended regimen.
From Centers for Disease Control and Prevention. 1998 Guidelines for treatment of sexually transmitted diseases. *MMWR* 1998;47 (RR-1):56, with permission.

Gonorrhea

Albert Neisser, first described *N. gonorrhoeae* in 1879 in patients with symptoms of gonococcal urethritis, cervicitis, and conjunctivitis. *N. gonorrhoeae* is an aerobic, nonmotile, non–spore-forming, Gram-negative intracellular diplococcus with a distinctive kidney bean shape. Although most of the *Neisseria* species can colonize in humans, *N. gonorrhoeae*, when present, is always considered a clinically significant pathogen. *N. gonorrhoeae* is the most fastidious member of the genus. Complex growth requirements including vitamins, amino acids, and iron are supplied by enriched media such as the modified Thayer Martin and the New York City media (23).

Microorganism and Pathogenesis

The cell wall of *N. gonorrhoeae* is a trilaminar structure that consists of an outer membrane, peptidoglycan, and an inner cytoplasmic membrane. The pathogenesis of gonococcal infections is due to mediators of adhesion, inflammation, and mucosal invasiveness produced by the organism (24). The outer cell membrane consists of a lipo-oligosaccharide (LOS) capsule, and various proteins. Traversing the entire membrane are antigenically variable pili. These pili are filamentous projections responsible for mucosal adhesion. Outer membrane opa and porin proteins play a role in adherence of the cells to the epithelium and host cell endocytosis, respectively. The outer membrane proteins have significant phase and antigenic variability, which permit repeated gonococcal infections. The capsule of *N. gonorrhoeae* is composed of lipid A and a core oligosaccharide that lacks the O-antigenic side chains present in other Gram-negative bacteria. LOS induces an intense inflammatory response and local production of tumor necrosis factor-α (TNF-α), which is believed to be responsible for most of the tissue damage of salpingitis. The LOS also induces phagocytosis, and aids bacterial adherence to cells and lysis of host cells (25). Peptidoglycan forms the major cell wall constituent. Inhibition of peptidoglycan synthesis provides the mechanism of action for the penicillins and cephalosporins. The inner cytoplasmic membrane contains penicillin-binding proteins. Emergence of resistant strains may be due to plasmid-mediated penicillinase production or chromosomally mediated alterations in penicillin-binding proteins.

Epidemiology and Transmission

N. gonorrhoeae is a leading cause of STD. In the United States, an estimated 600,000 new infections with this mucosal pathogen occur each year (1). Because gonococcal infections in women may be asymptomatic, an important component of gonorrhea control in the United States continues to be the screening of women at high risk for STDs. Infections caused by this organism are usually localized to the mucosal surfaces at primary sites of inoculation. Sites such as the urogenital tract, the anorectal canal, and the pharynx provide the susceptible mucosal surfaces necessary for infection. In menarchal women, the cervical epithelium provides the primary site of infection, whereas in premenarchal women the gonococcus may infect the nonestrogenized vaginal epithelium. Contact during parturition can infect the ocular conjunctiva. Localized infections may produce a pronounced purulent response, or they may be entirely asymptomatic. Spread from the initial infection site can lead to severe disseminated disease.

Clinical Manifestations

In women, the endocervical canal is the primary site of gonorrheal infection. Gonococcal infection may be asymptomatic in up to 50% of women (26). In 70% to 90% of

TABLE 20.3. CRITERIA FOR DIAGNOSIS OF PID

Minimal Criteria[a]
Lower abdominal tenderness
Adnexal tenderness
Cervical motion tenderness

Additional Criteria
Oral temperature >38.3°C
Abnormal cervical or vaginal discharge
Elevated erythrocyte sedimentation rate
Elevated C-reactive protein level
Laboratory documentation of cervical infection with *Neisseria gonorrhoae* or *Chlamydia trachomatis*

Definitive Criteria
Histopathologic evidence of endometritis on endometrial biopsy
Transvaginal sonography or imaging techniques showing thickened fluid-filled tubes with or without free pelvic fluid or tubo-ovarian complex
Laparoscopic abnormalities consistent with PID

[a]Empiric treatment is indicated in sexually active women considered at risk for PID if all three findings are present.
From Centers for Disease Control and Prevention. 1998 Guidelines for treatment of sexually transmitted diseases. *MMWR* 1998;47 (RR-1): 80, with permission.

TABLE 20.4. INDICATIONS FOR IN-HOSPITAL TREATMENT OF PELVIC INFLAMMATORY DISEASE

Pregnancy	WBC >11,000 mm³
Poor compliance	Failure to improve with outpatient therapy
Suspected peritonitis	Inability to take PO medications
Suspected tuboovarian abcess	Immunosuppressive illness
Temperature >38°C	Presence of an intrauterine device (IUD)

Adapted from Centers for Disease Control and Prevention. 1998 Guidelines for treatment of sexually transmitted diseases. *MMWR* 1998;47(RR-1):81–82, with permission.

infected women, the urethra is also infected. The incubation period for gonococcal cervicitis is around 10 days. When symptoms do occur, they are usually more pronounced during menses. Women may experience cervical discharge, urinary symptoms such as frequency and dysuria, dyspareunia, intermenstrual bleeding, increased menstrual flow, and occasionally tenesmus. The typical appearance of the cervix includes friability with edema and erythema. Fever, lower abdominal pain, and adnexal and cervical tenderness may indicate PID that requires differentiation from other surgical diagnoses; 10% to 40% of infected women may develop PID leading to infertility, chronic pelvic pain, and ectopic pregnancy. PID is seen more commonly during menses, in women who douche, and in women who have had a previous episode of PID. The criteria for the diagnosis of PID are discussed in Table 20.3. However, the clinical features of PID are often enigmatic, and single historical, clincal or laboratory finding or combination thereof lacks high sensitivity and specificity for the diagnosis of PID. The decision regarding inpatient versus outpatient therapy of PID is based on the clinical presentation (Table 20.4). Approaches to the treatment of PID are varied and include both primarily parenteral-based (Table 20.5) and enteral-based (Table 20.6) options. Patients may develop sudden onset of pain in the right upper abdominal quadrant due to perihepatitis. Disseminated gonococcal infection (DGI) occurs in approximately 0.5% to 3% of persons with *N. gonorrhoeae* infections. DGI is more common in women, occurring usually 7 to 10 days after menstruation (26). DGI may manifest as arthritis-dermatitis, endocarditis, or meningitis. In perinatally infected infants, gonorrhea may lead to blindness, destructive septic arthritis, and neonatal sepsis (1).

Diagnosis

Diagnosis of cervical gonococcal infection may be based on an endocervical culture, Gram stain, or identification of gonococcal enzymes, antigens, or nucleic acids in genital secretions. The Gram stain revealing Gram-negative intracellular diplococci is highly sensitive and specific in men. However, in women, while the specificity of the endocervical Gram-stained smear is 95% to 100%, the sensitivity is only about 50%. The normal vaginal and rectal flora is composed of Gram-negative coccobacilli, which can resemble *N. gonorrhoeae;* hence, diagnosis must be confirmed by culture. The use of cultures also allows performance of antimicrobial testing. *N. gonorrhoeae* is a fastidious and fragile organism. The best method for culture and transport

TABLE 20.5. INPATIENT TREATMENT OF PELVIC INFLAMMATORY DISEASE

Regimen	Drug	Dose	Duration of Therapy
A	Cefotetan[a]	2 g IV every 12 hours	24 hours after clinical improvement
	or		
	Cefoxitin[a]	2 g IV every 6 hours	24 hours after clinical improvement
	and		
	Doxycycline	100 mg IV or PO every 12 hours (PO preferred route)	14 days
B	Clindamycin	900 mg IV every 8 hours	24 hours after clinical improvement[b]
	and		
	Gentamicin	2 mg/kg IV load followed by 1.5 mg/kg every 8 hours	24 hours after clinical improvement[b]

[a]Either drug should be combined with doxycycline.
[b]Parenteral therapy is followed by clindamycin 450 mg PO q.i.d. and doxycycline 100 mg PO b.i.d. for a total of 14 days.
Adapted from Centers for Disease Control and Prevention. 1998 Guidelines for treatment of sexually transmitted diseases. *MMWR* 1998;47(RR-1):82–83.

TABLE 20.6. AMBULATORY TREATMENT OF PELVIC INFLAMMATORY DISEASE

Regimen	Drug	Dose	Duration of Therapy
A	Ofloxacin *and*	400 mg b.i.d.	14 days
	Metronidazole	500 mg b.i.d.	14 days
B	Ceftriaxone[a]	250 mg IM	Single dose
	Cefoxitin[a] *and*	2 g IM	Single dose
	Probenecid	1 g PO	Single dose

[a]Either choice is combined with doxycycline 100 mg PO b.i.d. for a total of 14 days. For regimens of drugs such as ceftriaxone and doxycycline that are associated with limitations in anaerobic coverage but excellent clinical performance data, the addition of a 7- to 14-day course of metronidazole is suggested.
From Centers for Disease Control and Prevention. 1998 Guidelines for treatment of sexually transmitted diseases. *MMWR* 1998;47 (RR-1):84, with permission.

is to inoculate onto a suitable enriched selective (i.e., antibiotic containing) agar immediately after specimen collection and placing the medium in an atmosphere of increased CO_2 (3% to 7%). In women, both the endocervix and rectum should be cultured to detect gonococcal infection. Cervical specimens are obtained with the aid of a speculum lubricated with warm water. Excessive cervical mucus should be removed, followed by introducing a noncotton swab into the cervical canal (26). The swab should be moved from side to side and left in place for 10 to 30 seconds and then rolled on a culture plate. Rectal swabs should be inserted about 3 to 4 cm, attempting to avoid fecal contamination. Urethral and oropharyngeal sampling may be helpful in selected patients. After 48 to 72 hours of incubation at 35° to 37°C in a CO_2-enriched, humid atmosphere, up to five different colony types may be seen. These colonies are round, grayish white, and shiny. A presumptive diagnosis of *N. gonorrhoeae* is made after isolation of characteristic colonies followed by a positive oxidase reaction. In potential medicolegal situations such as rape, or diagnosis of gonorrhea infection in a child, only standard culture procedures should be used. Specimens from the vagina, urethra, rectum, or pharynx should be streaked onto selective media for isolation of *N. gonorrhoeae*. All presumptive isolates of *N. gonorrhoeae* should be identified definitively by at least two tests that involve different principles (e.g., biochemical, enzyme substrate, or serologic). Isolates should be preserved to enable additional testing (1).

Culture on selective medium is the current diagnostic gold standard. However, because of time constraints and the urgency to administer treatment, there is growing interest in rapid detection methods. In addition, screening for gonorrhea with single cervical swab cultures is not 100% sensitive because of multiple factors, such as sampling errors, inhibition of growth by components of selective culture media, and loss of viability during specimen transport (27). Rapid detection methods involve detection of outer membrane proteins, gonococcal DNA, or gonococcal ribosomal RNA (rRNA) by

various techniques. The combo probe 2C combines probes against *N. gonorrhoeae* and *C. trachomatis*, and when used with endocervical specimens yields a sensitivity and specificity of 96% and 98.8%, respectively (28). A nucleic acid amplification method and LCR assay with swabs or FVU outperformed culture and other methods for the diagnosis of genital and extragenital gonorrhea (29). LCR has a detection limit of 10 to 100 colony forming units (CFUs)/mL compared to Pace2, which requires 1,000 to 10,000 CFUs/mL (30). In one study, the sensitivities of the *N. gonorrhoeae* LCR assays for the female and male specimens were 97.3% and 98.5%, respectively, with specificities of 99.6% and 99.8%, respectively (30). In settings such as school-based clinics and detention centers, FVU sampling circumvents the technique-dependent nature of swab sampling and the logistic problems associated with transport of specimens for culture. More over, urine LCR testing has the added advantage of testing for two major STD pathogens by using a single urine specimen. LCR is also well suited for distinguishing between very closely related sequences such as those found in *N. gonorrhoeae* and *N. meningitidis* (31). An expanded gold standard has been defined to include all culture-positive as well as culture-negative, confirmed LCR-positive specimens (30). In addition, if LCR-based assays on vaginal and vulvar specimens collected by the patients themselves prove as reliable as endocervical swabs collected by physicians, the convenience and simplicity of the assay procedure will be further improved.

Treatment (Table 20.7)

All patients and their known sexual contacts who receive treatment for gonoccocal disease should also be treated for chlamydia, as coinfection rates range from 30% to 60% (1). Since the introduction of dual therapy, the prevalence

TABLE 20.7. TREATMENT OF UNCOMPLICATED GONOCOCCAL INFECTIONS OF THE CERVIX, URETHRA, RECTUM

Drug	Dose	Duration of Therapy
Cefixime *or*	400 mg PO	Single dose
Ceftriaxone *or*	125 mg IM	Single dose
Ciprofloxacin[a] *or*	500 mg PO	Single dose
Ofloxacin[a] *or* plus Azithromycin	400 mg PO	Single dose
or	1 g PO	Single dose
Doxycycline	100 mg PO b.i.d.	7 days

[a]Not recommended in pregnancy. If patients or their sex partners are likely to have acquired gonococcal infections in Hawaii, the Pacific Islands, or Asia; ceftrixone or cefixime should be used. CDC does not recommend routine treatment of gonorrhea infections with azithromycin because of cost issues and gastrointestinal intolerance to this dose. *MMWR* 2000;49:833–837.
From Centers for Disease Control and Prevention. 1998 Guidelines for treatment of sexually transmitted diseases. *MMWR* 1998;47 (RR-1):61, with permission.

of chlamydial infection has decreased in some populations. Cephalosporins and quinolones have been widely effective, and can be used in a single dose. Directly observed therapy with the administration of medication by health care providers is recommended by the CDC to ensure compliance, minimize transmission, and reduce consequences of untreated infection. Extensive clinical experience indicates that ceftriaxone is safe and effective for the treatment of uncomplicated gonorrhea, curing 99.1% of uncomplicated urogenital and anorectal infections (1). Patients may be treated with either 125 or 250 mg IM in a single dose. Ciprofloxacin is safe, relatively inexpensive, can be administered orally, and in published clinical trials has cured 99.8% of uncomplicated urogenital and anorectal infections. Patients treated for uncomplicated gonorrhea, and who have symptomatic relief, need not return for test-of-cure (1). Reexamination with culture 2 to 3 months after treatment to detect both treatment failures and reinfections may be considered.

Patients with persistent symptoms should be screened for a resistant *N. gonorrhoeae* isolate, reinfection, or persistent infection with another organism. A 2-g dose of azithromycin is active against *N. gonorrhoeae* and *C. trachomatis* in a single-dose regimen. In published susceptibility guidelines, no azithromycin resistance was found (32). However, a 2-g dose of azithromycin causes gastrointestinal upset too often to be recommended. Azithromycin at a dose of 1 g is insufficiently effective, curing only 93% of patients. Spectinomycin, 2 g IM, an aminoglycoside, is an alternative when patients cannot tolerate a cephalosporin or quinolone. A single 2-g IM dose of spectinomycin has been effective in curing over 98% of uncomplicated urogenital and anorectal gonococcal infections (1). However, spectinomycin is only 52% effective against pharyngeal infections.

Sex partners should be evaluated and treated as per the recommendations for chlamydial infections. All patients with gonorrhea should be offered testing for syphilis and human immunodeficiency virus (HIV) infection. Most patients with incubating syphilis are successfully treated with the regimens containing β-lactams but not quinolones or spectinomycin. Hence, patients treated with the latter drugs should have a serologic test for syphilis repeated in 3 months, if the initial test was negative.

Interactions with Pregnancy

The prevalence of gonorrhea in pregnant women in industrialized nations, though generally considered to be about 1%, may be underestimated. Gonorrhea in pregnancy is associated with septic spontaneous abortion, infection after therapeutic termination, premature rupture of membranes, chorioamnionitis, preterm delivery, disseminated gonococcal disease, and postpartum endometritis. Pregnant women should be treated with either a cephalosporin or spectinomycin, but not with quinolones or tetracyclines. Azithromycin, erythromycin, or amoxicillin is recommended for

treatment of presumptive or diagnosed *C. trachomatis* infection during pregnancy.

Ophthalmia neonatorum, a purulent bilateral conjunctivitis, occurs by inoculation of gonococci during delivery through an infected birth canal. The incubation period is approximately 3 days but may be prolonged if an ineffective conjunctival prophylaxis has been used. The condition is largely preventable with the use of antimicrobial preparations instilled into the eyes of every neonate as soon as possible after delivery. The recommended regimens for ophthalmia neonatorum prophylaxis include single applications of aqueous solution of silver nitrate 1%, or erythromycin 0.5% ophthalmic ointment, or tetracycline 1% ophthalmic ointment. In the United States, *C. trachomatis* is probably the most common cause of neonatal infectious conjunctivitis. Though *N. gonorrhoeae* is an uncommon cause of ophthalmia neonatorum, it is especially important, because it may result in blindness. Other manifestations of neonatal gonococcal infection include localized gonococcal infection of the scalp through scalp electrodes, sepsis, meningitis, and arthritis.

Trichomoniasis

M. A. Donne in 1836 first described the flagellated protozoan parasite *Trichomonas vaginalis* after microscopically examining a patient's vaginal discharge (33). In fresh preparations, the organism is pear-shaped with average dimensions of 10 × 7 μm. It has four free anterior flagellae, which appear to arise from a single stalk, and a fifth flagellum embedded in an undulating membrane. An axostyle, which traverses the cell and projects from the posterior end, maintains its rigidity. *T. vaginalis* is one of the three species of trichomonads found in humans and is the only one for which a pathogenic role has been established. *T. vaginalis* is found in the trophozoite form and produces genitourinary tract infections in both males and females. Nonvenereal transmission of infection is rare.

Epidemiology and Transmission

T. vaginalis infects approximately 3 million American women annually (34). However, the accuracy of any estimate is questionable, as *T. vaginalis* is not a reportable STD in the Unites States. Infections are often subclinical, and the sensitivity of the currently employed wet prep for diagnosis is low. Depending on the patient groups studied, Third World countries have reported rates of trichomoniasis that vary from 19% to 47% (35). The organism is commonly found in women with other STDs. Coinfection with trichomoniasis has been reported in 60% of patients with gonorrhea (36). Infection with *T. vaginalis* may play a role in the transmission of herpes simplex virus and increase the host's susceptibility to HIV (37,38).

Clinical Features

Trichomoniasis is asymptomatic in approximately 50% of infected females, while the majority of males present a self-limiting or subclinical infection (39). Trichomoniasis is transmissible between lesbian partners. Deficiency of glycogen in premenarchal and postmenopausal females is not conducive to the growth of *T. vaginalis*. The incubation period ranges from 5 to 28 days, and symptoms often begin or are exacerbated following menses. Trichomonads invade the vagina, endocervix, and the urethra, resulting in vaginitis, pruritus, dysuria, and dyspareunia. Other symptoms include backache, pelvic pressure, and occasionally lower abdominal discomfort. Vaginal discharge is greenish-gray, frothy, and often malodorous. Both symptoms and physical findings in patients with trichomoniasis are highly variable. Only a minority manifest the complete classic picture of a yellowish, frothy, foul-smelling discharge accompanied by inflammatory changes of the vulva, vaginal walls, and cervix (34). The vulva may appear red and erythematous. Intense vaginal inflammation may lead to vaginal edema, hypertrophy, and desquamation. Florid granular vaginitis occurs in severe infection, where the vaginal walls are characterized by dilation of blood vessels and capillary proliferation. The strawberry cervix, the most specific clinical finding for the diagnosis of trichomoniasis, is caused by a high parasite burden. Examination with colposcopy reveals a strawberry cervix in 45% of infected women; however, by visual inspection it is observed in only 2% of infected women (40).

Diagnosis and Differential

Although more commonly associated with bacterial vaginosis, a vaginal pH >4.5 and a positive whiff test (an amine-like fishy odor generated by the addition of potassium hydroxide to vaginal discharge) are positive in approximately 75% of cases with trichomoniasis. A vaginal saline wet mount shows numerous polymorphonuclear neutrophils and trichomonads, recognized by their flagella and characteristic twitching motility. The Papanicolaou stain is frequently inaccurate; hence the Pap smear should not be used as a diagnostic tool. Culture is considered the gold standard for diagnosis of trichomoniasis. Routine culture is not readily performed in the United States due to cost concerns and delays in diagnosis (41). The InPouch TV test (BioMed Diagnostics, Santa Clara, CA) is a disposable culture system that offers superior efficacy and logistic advantages (42). Until further study of the cost-effectiveness, sensitivity, and specificity of the newer technologies such as direct immunofluorescence assay, direct enzyme immunoassay, etc., are established, the wet prep will remain the mainstay for the diagnosis of trichomoniasis because it is an inexpensive, rapid, and a reasonably accurate procedure. Bacterial vaginosis and candidiasis are two other conditions

TABLE 20.8. TREATMENT OF TRICHOMONIASIS

Drug	Dose (PO)	Duration of Therapy
Metronidazole[a] *or*	2 g	Single dose
Metronidazole	500 mg b.i.d.	7 days

[a]Recommended regimen.
From Centers for Disease Control and Prevention. 1998 Guidelines for treatment of sexually transmitted diseases. *MMWR* 1998;47 (RR-1):74, with permission.

associated with vulvovaginal irritation with vaginal discharge.

Treatment (Table 20.8)

Treatment of trichomoniasis is optimized by the use of systemic therapy with one of the 5'-nitroimidazoles. Metronidazole is the only nitroimidazole available for treatment of trichomoniasis in the United States. Cure rates of approximately 90% to 95% have been reported with the recommended regimen of metronidazole 2 g orally in a single dose (1). Advantages of single-dose regimens include lower cost and better compliance. The alternative regimen is oral metronidazole 500 mg twice a day for 7 days (1). Sexual partners should be treated and sexual intercourse should be postponed until both partners are asymptomatic. In the absence of reinfection, treatment failures are usually due to resistance of *T. vaginalis* to metronidazole (1). Most cases of metronidazole resistance are cured with retreatment with metronidazole 500 mg twice a day for 7 days, or metronidazole 2 g once a day for 3 to 5 days. Side effects seen more commonly with larger doses of metronidazole include gastointestinal upset, metallic taste, leukopenia, seizures, and peripheral neuropathy. Patients taking metronidazole should be cautioned to abstain from the use of alcohol, which can cause a disulfuram-like reaction, consisting of severe nausea and vomiting. Patients allergic to metronidazole can be managed by desensitization (1).

Interactions with Pregnancy

A possible relationship has been noted between vaginal trichomoniasis and preterm delivery and premature rupture of membranes. An infected mother can transmit the infection to her newborn female by direct vulvovaginal contamination during a vaginal delivery, or contamination of the urethra and vagina can occur following the infant's ingestion of the trichomonads. Though systemic use of metronidazole is not recommended during the first trimester of pregnancy, there is no evidence that it is teratogenic in humans. Pregnant patients can be treated with 2 g of metronidazole in a single dose (1).

SEXUALLY TRANSMITTED DISEASES CAUSING GENITAL ULCERS

Herpes Simplex Virus Infections

Genital herpes, a recurrent, incurable viral disease, is the commonest cause of sexually transmitted genital ulcer disease (1). Herpes simplex virus (HSV) types 1 and 2 belong to a family of viruses called Herpesviridae. There are eight known human herpesviruses, which include varicella-zoster virus (VZV), Epstein-Barr virus (EBV), and cytomegalovirus (CMV). Human herpesviruses 6 and 7 have been associated with roseola. Herpesviruses are large, enveloped, double-stranded DNA viruses. Both HSV-1 and HSV-2 have relatively short replication cycles, and spread rapidly with high cytopathogenicity in cell culture (43). HSV, like HPV and HIV, can exist in chronic and latent forms (44). HSV-1 infections usually involve the oral cavity and HSV-2 infections cause genital lesions; however, either virus type can infect the oral or genital mucosa. Occasionally, disseminated infection may occur, especially in immuno-compromised individuals and neonates. Infection with HSV is an important cofactor in the development of cervical neoplasm (44).

Epidemiology and Transmission

An epidemic of HSV-2 infections has occurred in the United States in the past two decades (1). It is estimated that approximately 300,000 to 500,000 new cases of genital herpes occur each year in the United States. In some populations, up to 75% of persons are HSV-2 infected (45). Risk factors for the acquisition of genital HSV infection include young age, female gender, black race, and multiple sexual partners. Transmission occurs by direct contact with infected secretions, with either overt infection or asymptomatic excretion of the virus. Many cases of genital herpes are transmitted by persons who are unaware that they have the infection or are asymptomatic when transmission at the rate of 10% to 12% annually (male to female transmission more efficient) occurs. Genital infections with HSV-1 are associated with less asymptomatic shedding. lower rates of recurrence, and lower rates of transmission (43).

Viral Agent and Pathogenesis

Herpesviruses are enveloped viruses with icosapentahedral nucleocapsids, and the viral genome consists of double-stranded DNA (44). HSVs are capable of infecting both the epithelial cells and cells of the nervous system. The replication cycle involves the attachment, penetration, and uncoating of the virus in the host cell nucleoplasm, followed by viral DNA synthesis. This replication cycle occurs over a period of 36 hours. The viral particles become enveloped during the process of egress through the nuclear membrane, are transported through the cytoplasm, and are released by passage through the Golgi bodies or by exocytosis through the cytoplasmic membrane (44). Though herpesviruses can induce cytolysis of the infected cells, the ability to remain latent in the host organism is a remarkable characteristic of herpesviruses. During acute HSV infection, the virus penetrates the skin either on a mucosal surface or through a break. Replication of the virus in the epithelial cells may occur, but within hours the virus enters axons of peripheral nerves and ascends into the dorsal nerve root ganglia, where replication occurs. The virus then spreads back to the mucosal and epithelial skin area, is released from nerve endings and causes the characteristic multiple, bilateral lesions seen with primary infections (46). Commonly, the virus assumes latency in the neuron and subsequent reactivation may occur with either physical or emotional stress.

Clinical Features

HSV-2 is the most common etiology of genital ulcers in the United States followed by syphilis and chancroid (1). Acute primary genital HSV infection is the most severe form of the infection. It occurs following an incubation period of 2 to 7 days and is caused by HSV-2 in 70% to 95% of cases. The disease may be mild to life-threatening. Mild symptoms may go unrecognized. Fever, chills, headache, and malaise are seen in up to 70% of cases. A burning sensation precedes the eruption of vesicles, which can appear on the vulva, perineum, buttocks, cervix, and vagina. These lesions ulcerate and coalesce within 3 to 5 days, and are very painful. The majority of the women (80%) experience dysuria, vaginal discharge, and have prolonged painful bilateral inguinal adenopathy during a primary genital HSV infection (43). Severity of the infection peaks between 8 to 10 days after onset of the infection. Shedding of the virus from genital lesions persists for about 10 to 12 days after the onset of the lesions. Complete healing of the lesions occurs in 3 to 4 weeks. Following primary genital HSV infection, extragenital spread, including the central nervous system, occurs more commonly in women than men. Clinical features include a stiff neck, headache, and photophobia. Fortunately, however, long-term neurologic sequelae are rare.

After the primary infection, latency is established in the trigeminal and autonomic nerve root ganglia for orally acquired lesions and sacral nerve root ganglia for genitally acquired infections (46). Subclinical primary infections may be manifest clinically with subsequent reactivation. Infected individuals remain carriers and it is possible for them to shed virus even while asymptomatic. Some of the factors known to trigger reactivation of a latent herpetic infection are stress, fever, menstruation, sunlight, and injury to the area of reactivation. Recurrent genital HSV infection occurs in 75% and 50% of cases following infection with

HSV-2 and HSV-1, respectively (43). Most patients with primary genital HSV-1 infection have at least one recurrence by 12 months and 20% to 30% will have very frequent recurrences (>10/year) (47). The median number of recurrences per year is five for the first 3 to 4 years after infection. Recurrent genital lesions are characterized by a lack of systemic symptoms and the genital lesions are generally less severe than primary infection. In women, recurrent lesions are usually unilaterally grouped vesicles with mild pain and irritation. During recurrent episodes fewer localized lesions develop, and these heal within 7 to 10 days in immunocompetent persons. Viral shedding from the genital lesions during recurrent infection occurs for 2 to 5 days and in lower quantity than during primary disease. During recurrent disease, viral shedding from the cervix is much less likely compared to the primary episode (43). One third to one half of all HSV reactivations in the genital area are subclinical, and unnoticed lesions especially in the cervical area are the predominant means by which HSV transmission occurs (47). In HIV-infected individuals, reactivation can be a frequent occurrence and lesions may become large, secondarily infected, and resistant to acyclovir.

Diagnosis

Although herpetic lesions are fairly typical in terms of appearance, laboratory confirmation must be obtained. Culture is the best confirmation of an HSV lesion, and because the virus replicates rapidly, culture results may be available within 24 to 48 hours. Cultures should be examined daily and finalized if negative after 5 days of incubation (48). For culture of a newly formed vesicular lesion, unroof the lesion, sample the fluid, and place in viral transport medium. If there is to be any delay in culturing, the specimen should be refrigerated. Other specimens that may yield HSV include cerebrospinal fluid (CSF), urethral swabs, specimens from the cervix, vagina, throat, and conjunctivae (43). Cytologic methods are quicker and more widely available, though only 60% as sensitive as viral isolation. Scrapings or swabs obtained from the base of skin or mucous lesions are stained according to the methods of Wright, Giemsa (Tzanck preparation), or Papanicolaou. The presence of multinucleated giant cells is indicative of either HSV or VZV infection. Immunofluorescent staining of HSV antigens has improved the specificity and sensitivity of cytology. PCR assays that detect HSV DNA are now acknowledged to be the most sensitive assay for detecting HSV in secretions, lesions, tissue, or body fluids. Further standardization is necessary prior to their routine clinical use.

Serologic diagnosis of HSV infection can be useful in diagnosing a primary HSV-1 or HSV-2 infection by demonstrating a fourfold rise in antibody titer in acute and convalescent sera. Serology may also be useful in the diagnosis of nonprimary first episode herpes, which is the acquisition of a new serotype in a person with prior HSV infection.

Serology is unable to predict a recurrent infection due to the lack of correlation between a rising antibody titer and the presence of genital lesions (43).

Treatment (Table 20.9)

Management of patients with first clinical episode of genital herpes includes antiviral therapy and counseling. As clinical recurrences are much less frequent with HSV-1 than with HSV-2 genital infection, HSV typing has prognostic importance and may be useful for counseling purposes. Individuals who present early in the course of the infection or those with severe disease are more likely to benefit from acyclovir therapy (1). Systemic antiviral drugs partially control the symptoms and lesions of herpes episodes. These drugs neither eradicate latent virus nor affect the risk, frequency, or severity of recurrences after the drug is discontinued. Counseling includes information on the potential for recurrences, asymptomatic viral shedding, and sexual and perinatal transmission. Use of condoms during all sexual exposures with uninfected sex partners should be encouraged, and patients should be advised to abstain from sexual activity when prodromal symptoms or lesions are present. Asymptomatic viral shedding within the first 12 months occurs more frequently following genital HSV-2 infection. The risk of neonatal infection should be explained to reproductive-age women.

Acyclovir, valacyclovir, and famciclovir are three antiviral medications that provide clinical benefit for treatment of genital herpes. Acyclovir, similar in structure to the natural nucleoside guanosine, is a highly potent and selective inhibitor of HSV replication (49). HSV-1, HSV-2, and VZV have viral thymidine kinase, which phosphorylates acyclovir to its active triphosphate form. This active triphosphate form inhibits HSV DNA polymerase. Cells not infected with HSV have little thymidine kinase, leading to the selective concentration of acyclovir in HSV-infected cells. Topical therapy with acyclovir is substantially less effective than the systemic drug. Both valacyclovir, and famciclovir have high oral bioavailability. Recommended regimens (Table 20.9) include acyclovir 400 mg orally three times a day for

TABLE 20.9. TREATMENT OF FIRST CLINICAL EPISODE OF GENITAL HERPES

Drug	Dose (PO)	Duration of Therapy
Acyclovir *or*	400 mg t.i.d.	7–10 days
Acyclovir *or*	200 mg 5 times/day	7–10 days
Famciclovir *or*	250 mg t.i.d.	7–10 days
Valacyclovir	1 g b.i.d.	7–10 days

From Centers for Disease Control and Prevention. 1998 Guidelines for treatment of sexually transmitted diseases. *MMWR* 1998; 47(RR-1):21, with permission.

TABLE 20.10. TREATMENT OF EPISODIC RECURRENT GENITAL HERPES

Drug	Dose (PO)	Duration of Therapy
Acyclovir *or*	400 mg t.i.d.	5 days
Acyclovir *or*	200 mg 5 times/day	5 days
Acyclovir *or*	800 mg b.i.d.	5 days
Famciclovir *or*	125 mg b.i.d.	5 days
Valacyclovir	500 mg b.i.d.	5 days

From Centers for Disease Control and Prevention. 1998 Guidelines for treatment of sexually transmitted diseases. *MMWR* 1998; 47(RR-1):23, with permission.

7 to 10 days, or acyclovir 200 mg orally five times a day for 7 to 10 days, or famciclovir 250 mg orally three times a day for 7 to 10 days, or valacyclovir 1 g orally twice a day for 7 to 10 days. Treatment may be extended if healing is incomplete after 10 days of therapy (1). Intravenous acyclovir brings about the quickest resolution of lesions, but is indicated only for severe, disseminated, or neurologic involvement. Intravenous acyclovir is given at a dose of 5 to 10 mg/kg every 8 hours for a period of 7 to 21 days depending on the clinical situation.

Antiviral therapy during recurrent episodes may shorten the duration of lesions (Table 20.10). Symptomatic recurrences are treated with acyclovir 400 mg three times a day for 5 days, or 200 mg five times a day for 5 days, or famciclovir 125 mg twice a day for 5 days, or valacyclovir 500 mg orally twice a day for 5 days. Treatment must be initiated at the first sign of prodrome or genital lesions. Acyclovir prophylaxis can reduce the frequency and severity of HSV recurrences by over 75% and is currently recommended for individuals who experience more than six episodes per year (43). For suppression of recurrences, acyclovir 400 mg twice a day, or famciclovir 250 mg orally twice a day, or valacyclovir 500 mg orally once a day is effective (Table 20.11). The need for ongoing prophylaxis should be evaluated on a yearly basis. Long-term use of acyclovir is associated with nausea, diarrhea, and headache in less than 5% of patients (43). Acyclovir has been used for up to 6 years as daily therapy; however, insufficient experience

TABLE 20.11. DAILY SUPPRESSIVE THERAPY OF GENITAL HERPES

Drug	Dose (PO)
Acyclovir *or*	400 mg b.i.d.
Famciclovir *or*	250 mg b.i.d.
Valacyclovir (<10 recurrences/yr)	500 mg q.i.d.
Valacyclovir (>10 recurrences/yr)	1000 mg q.i.d.

From Centers for Disease Control and Prevention. 1998 Guidelines for treatment of sexually transmitted diseases. *MMWR* 1998; 47(RR-1):23, with permission.

with famciclovir and valacyclovir prevents recommendation of these drugs for >1 year. The extent to which suppressive therapy may prevent HSV transmission is unknown. Acyclovir-resistant herpes is frequently seen in immunocompromised patients. If higher doses of acyclovir fail, intravenous foscarnet may be useful in such patients.

Interactions with Pregnancy

Neonatal herpes, the most severe complication of HSV infection, involves HSV-2 in the majority of cases. The incidence of neonatal herpes is estimated to range from 10 to 50 per 100,000 live births (49). Perinatal infection may occur transplacentally. The usual source of infection, however, is the infected genital tract. The infant may be affected during passage through the birth canal or through ascension of the virus after membrane rupture. Neonatal infection may rarely result from postnatal contact with infected family or hospital staff. The disease manifests in three forms: mucocutaneous lesions, central nervous system disease, and disseminated infection. Perinatal infection may produce symptoms from birth to approximately 4 weeks. Mucocutaneous disease occurs in about 70% of infected infants (44). Signs of serious infection include irritability, jaundice, hepatosplenomegaly, seizures, and coagulopathy. Mortality is about 60% in disseminated disease, and the majority of the survivors of encephalitis will have permanent impairment. Some reduction in mortality is possible with antiviral therapy.

Primary HSV infection during pregnancy may result in congenital infection, abortion, premature labor, or growth retardation. In mothers acquiring primary and nonprimary HSV-2 near term, transmission rates to the neonates are as high as 50% and 25%, respectively. The risk of neonatal infection is tenfold less with reactivated HSV infections. However, cesarean delivery continues to be recommended in those cases with active lesions at the time of labor regardless of primary or nonprimary status (49). Usually, cesarean section is recommended within 4 to 6 hours of membrane rupture; however, even when the membranes have been ruptured longer than 4 to 6 hours, the benefit of abdominal delivery outweighs the risks. The risk of neonatal exposure in asymptomatic women with a history of recurrent genital herpes is 0.1%. Hence, it may be concluded that unless lesions develop near the time of expected delivery, women with a history of recurrent infection may plan to deliver vaginally (44).

Recent studies suggest that acyclovir treatment near term might reduce the rate of cesarean section among women who have frequently recurring or newly acquired genital herpes by decreasing the incidence of active lesions. Pending further study, routine administration of acyclovir to pregnant women who have a history of recurrent genital herpes is not recommended at this time (1).

Syphilis

Venereal syphilis is a systemic disease caused by *Treponema pallidum*. It is claimed that syphilis existed in China 2,000 years ago; however, its introduction to America began with the return of Columbus in 1493 (50). The overall incidence of syphilis, including congenital syphilis, has risen dramatically in recent years. Syphilis may be silent, undetected, or characterized by prolonged asymptomatic periods. Syphilitic genital ulcers may enhance the acquisition and transmission of HIV, and asymptomatic syphilis may be a potent cofactor in the progression of HIV-related immune deficiency (1). *T. pallidum* is a microaerophilic Gram-negative bacterium that stains poorly with Gram's or Giemsa's methods. *T. pallidum* does not grow on standard laboratory media. Diagnosis is based on detection with the use of darkfield or phase-contrast microscopy, and serologic testing.

Epidemiology and Transmission

The annual incidence of syphilis has periodically increased and decreased. In the United States, the rate of primary and secondary cases per 100,000 population was 20.3 in 1990. By 1993 the rate declined to approximately 12 cases per 100,000 population (51). Since surveillance began in 1941, the lowest rate of 3.2 cases per 100,000 people was reported by the Centers for Disease Control and Prevention (CDC) in 1998. Among industrialized nations, the United States has the highest rate of syphilis. It has been estimated that, presently, there may be more than 500,000 cases of unreported and untreated syphilis in the United States (1). Risk factors for infection include poverty, chronic unemployment, prostitution, illicit drug use, and poor education (1). The number of infants born with congenital syphilis increased to 107.2 per 100,000 live births in 1991, followed by a decline in 1992 and 1993. Crack cocaine use and failure to obtain prenatal care are the most important risk factors associated with congenital syphilis (50). Syphilis, therefore, is a major public health problem.

The ratio of male-to-female infection is nearly 1, which suggests that the venereal transmission of syphilis is primarily heterosexual. The site of initial invasion may involve extragenital epithelial tissues, including oropharynx, rectum, and conjunctiva. Contaminated blood may occasionally produce primary infection through accidental needle sticks or blood transfusion. An infant may be infected *in utero* through transplacental passage of spirochetes or from contact with an infectious lesion during passage through the birth canal. *T. pallidum* is extremely susceptible to heat, drying, and disinfectant agents, and does not survive well outside the human host. Transmission by fomites is rare (50).

Microorganism and Pathogenesis

Treponema are members of the order Spirochetales and family Spirochetaceae. The three pathogenic subspecies of *T. pallidum*—pallidum (syphilis), pertenue (yaws), and endemicum (nonvenereal syphilis)—infect only humans (50). Spirochetes are long, slender, helically curved, Gram-negative bacilli with axial filaments and an outer sheath (52). The spirochetes replicate by binary fission in a longitudinal plane of division. *T. pallidum* is morphologically distinct from the other human spirochetal pathogens such as *Borrelia* and *Leptospira* species. Treponema are slender with tight coils, while Borrelia are somewhat thicker with fewer and looser coils. Leptospira resemble Borrelia with minimal morphologic differences, primarily marked curvature at the end of this organism. The axial filaments are flagella-like organelles that facilitate motility of the organisms. Although the axial filaments resemble flagella, they are not external appendages, but wrap around the bacteria's cell wall and are enclosed within the outer sheath (52). *T. pallidum* is a highly motile spiral bacterium, with rigid, uniform, deep spirals. It has a length of 10 to 13 μm and a diameter of 0.13 to 0.15 μm (50). Because of its small size, the organism is below the resolution of the conventional light microscope. Darkfield microscopy reveals both the treponemal cell morphology and its distinctive corkscrew-like motility. *T. pallidum* has not been successfully cultured on artificial culture media, but has been maintained in animal hosts by inoculation. The organism is exquisitely sensitive to penicillin; however, because replication is slow, the bactericidal action of penicillin is also slower than that for conventional rapid-growing organisms (44).

The vast majority of *T. pallidum*'s membrane proteins are lipoproteins. These lipoproteins, including cardiolipin, are immunogenic and are anchored in the cytoplasmic membrane. A notable feature of the organism is a paucity of surface-exposed transmembrane proteins. Limited exposure of antigens on the surface of the treponemes may contribute to its ability to evade the immune system, and explains in part the natural history and chronicity of the infection.

T. pallidum enters the host by either penetrating intact mucous membranes or entering through breaks in the skin. Replication at the site of invasion results in the formation of a local ulcer that constitutes primary syphilis. The hematogenous spread of the spirochetes produces a wide array of symptoms associated with secondary syphilis. In untreated infections, long latent periods may occur followed by tertiary disease. *T. pallidum* has a strong predilection for endothelium (52). Infection elicits a strong, perivascular inflammatory reaction involving lymphocytes, macrophages, and plasma cells, which ultimately leads to endarteritis and progressive tissue destruction. Late manifestations occur due to hypersensitivity reactions to the organisms that are present in relatively low numbers. Tertiary syphilis is characterized by granuloma-like lesions, which are called gumma, and can occur at any site. Immunocompromised patients may present with unusual manifestations and aggressive disease (50).

Clinical Features

Syphilis has been called the "great imitator," because its varied and complex clinical manifestations often mimic many other diseases. Syphilis infection is divided into several stages: incubating, primary, secondary, early latent, late latent, and tertiary (53). Primary syphilis is characterized by the appearance of a chancre and regional lymphadenopathy. The chancre is typically a single, painless ulcer with raised, sharply demarcated margins and a clean, indurated base. The chancre occurs at the site of inoculation, approximately 3 weeks (range 10 to 90 days) after contact with the organism. Incidental antibiotic use can delay or modify the appearance of the chancre (54). In the female patient, primary genital lesions usually occur on the labia. However, chancres can also be located on the cervix and proximal third of the vagina and consequently may go unnoticed. Lymph node enlargement may accompany the chancre, and is usually bilateral, discrete, and nontender. The external genitalia and distal two thirds of the vagina drain to the inguinofemoral nodes, while the cervix and proximal third of the vagina drain to the deep iliac nodes. Thus, chancres at these latter locations may not be accompanied by palpable lymphadenopathy (54). Primary infection may occur at extragenital sites such as the anus, mouth, throat, breasts, fingers, and conjunctiva. Syphilitic genital ulcers need to be differentiated from ulcers due to herpes, chancroid, donovanosis, and LGV. Untreated, the chancre heals within 3 to 6 weeks, possibly due to the establishment of local immunity.

The secondary stage of syphilis occurs from 6 weeks to 6 months following the appearance of the primary lesion. This stage occurs due to the spirochetemia that arises during the incubation or pretreatment stage of syphilis. The characteristic lesion is a maculopapular skin rash involving the entire body, including the palms, soles, and mucous membranes. Nonspecific constitutional symptoms such as fever, weight loss, and malaise are present in up to 50% of patients. Condyloma lata, flat wartlike lesions, which occur at moist intertriginous areas such as anogenital sites, under the breasts, and axillae, also characterize secondary syphilis. These lesions must be differentiated from condyloma acuminata, caused by HPV, which are generally more wartlike and exuberant. Generalized lymphadenopathy often accompanies the skin rash in secondary syphilis. In untreated cases, the secondary stage resolves within 3 to 8 weeks. Although disseminated infection occurs in virtually all infected individuals, multiple secondary lesions arise in only 25% (55).

The secondary phase of syphilis is followed by the latent phase, characterized by a lack of clinically apparent lesions and a positive serologic test for syphilis. In some cases, a latent phase may precede the secondary stage. The disease may be communicable during the first 4 years of latency, after which time the disease is unlikely to be transmitted, except for transplacental infection to the fetus (44). Tertiary or late syphilis is the tissue destructive phase that appears 10 to 25 years after the initial infection in up to 35% of untreated patients (53). Granulomatous lesions called gummas can occur in any organ, with damage occurring secondary to the local immune response, rather than direct injury by the organism. More serious manifestations of tertiary syphilis may include cardiovascular and neurologic effects such as aortic insufficiency, coronary ostial stenosis, tabes dorsalis, dementia, and death. Previous longitudinal observations of patients with untreated syphilis indicate that approximately one third of infected individuals remain latently infected for life, one third undergo spontaneous cure, and the remaining one third develop late manifestations (56).

Diagnosis

The current tests for syphilis include serologic tests and the direct detection of the organism on microscopic examination of material taken from skin lesions or other tissues. Serologic tests for syphilis include nontreponemal and treponemal specific tests. The two commonly used nontreponemal tests, the Venereal Disease Research Laboratory (VDRL) test, and the rapid plasma reagin (RPR) test become positive 1 to 3 weeks after the chancre appears. These tests assay the IgG and IgM anticardiolipin antibody response seen in patients with syphilis and are not specific for *T. pallidum*. Both assays are examples of a flocculation test, in which soluble antigen particles are coalesced to form larger particles, visible as clumps when aggregated by antibody. False-positive reactions occur in about 1% of the general population. A positive test must be confirmed by more specific methods. Conditions that give rise to false-positive reactions include viral infections, malaria, autoimmune diseases, immunization, intravenous drug use, malignancies, cirrhosis, and pregnancy. False-negative tests can occur, with the VDRL being reactive in approximately 75%, 100%, and 96% of patients with primary, secondary, and late syphilis, respectively. It is important to realize that the serologic test may be negative due to the prozone phenomenon, where the concentration of the antibody in a given specimen is so high that flocculation does not occur. Samples suitable for testing include human serum and CSF. The RPR and VDRL tests are advantageous for screening programs, as they are sensitive and inexpensive. The quantitative VDRL test can also be used to measure the effectiveness of therapy. While titers may not decline in all patients, a fourfold decrease in titer after treatment indicates a successful response to treatment. A fourfold increase in titer usually indicates relapse or reinfection. The nontreponemal tests usually decline in titer over 6 to 8 months following adequate treatment. The VDRL and RPR are equally valid, but quantitative results from the two tests cannot be directly compared because RPR titers are often slightly higher than VDRL titers (1). The routine testing scheme does not need to be altered for HIV-positive individuals; however, the antibody response may be delayed in immunosuppressed individuals (57).

Treponemal antibody tests—fluorescent treponemal antibody tests (FTA-ABS) and microhemagglutination assay for antibody to *T. pallidum* (MHA-TP)—are specific and are used to confirm positive VDRL and RPR results. The treponemal tests are comparatively more expensive and complicated to perform. Reactivity in these tests rarely disappears following treatment. If lesions are present, direct microscopic examination, either by darkfield microscopy or direct fluorescent antibody staining for *T. pallidum* (DFA-TP) can be performed. The area surrounding the lesion is cleansed with saline-moistened sterile gauze. The surface of the ulcer is abraded and blotted until serous fluid is expressed. The surface of a clean glass slide is touched to the exudate, allowed to air-dry, and transported in a dust-free container for fluorescent antibody screening (52). The slide containing material for darkfield examination is obtained in a similar manner and must be examined immediately under high-dry magnification (400×). The presence of motile spirochetes confirms the diagnosis. Use of PCR for direct detection of *T. pallidum* in clinical material is currently under study. Preliminary results suggest that this may be an important diagnostic tool in the future.

Treatment (Table 20.12)

Penicillin remains the drug of choice for all stages of syphilis. For purposes of therapy, early syphilis is defined as primary, secondary, or early latent (present for less than 1 year). While the CDC recommends a single IM dose of 2.4 million units of benzathine penicillin G (1.2 million units in each buttock) for early syphilis, some experts recommend two doses of benzathine penicillin G, 2.4 million units, administered 1 week apart (54). Patients with penicillin allergy may be desensitized, or treated with tetracycline (500 mg orally four times a day) or doxycycline (100 mg orally two times a day) for 2 weeks. Treatment with penicillin frequently precipitates the Jarisch-Herxheimer reaction, the exact mechanism of which remains unclear. This is an acute febrile reaction accompanied by headache, myalgia, hypo-

tension, and intensification of skin rash; it usually begins 1 to 2 hours of initiating treatment, and resolves within 24 to 48 hours.

Failure of test titers to decline fourfold within 6 months after therapy for primary or secondary syphilis may be due to treatment failure or reinfection. These patients should be evaluated for HIV infection, and CSF examination should be performed to exclude neurosyphilis. Experts recommend retreatment with three weekly injections of IM 2.4 million units of benzathine penicillin G. After 2 doses of benzathine pencillin as described earlier, the RPR will be seronegative after 1 abd 2 years in primary and secondary syphilis respectively.

A patient with HIV infection, late latent and tertiary stages with normal CSF examination, is treated with three doses of 2.4 million units of benzathine penicillin, administered a week apart. Patients with neurosyphilis need a more prolonged, 10- to 14-day course of IV penicillin. Alternatively, in penicillin-allergic patients, a 4-week course of doxycycline or tetracycline can be used. Penicillin in recommended doses is nearly always effective in eliminating syphilis at any stage except in late tertiary syphilis and HIV infection.

Persons who were exposed within 90 days preceding the diagnosis of primary, secondary, or early latent syphilis in a sex partner might be infected even if seronegative; therefore, such persons should be treated presumptively. Sex partners should be treated presumptively if serologic tests are not available or the opportunity of follow-up is uncertain. Long-term sex partners of patients who have late syphilis should be evaluated clinically and serologically for syphilis and treated accordingly (1).

Congenital Syphilis

The rates of congenital syphilis have increased sharply since 1988. Approximately one case of congenital syphilis occurs for every 80 cases of primary or secondary syphilis in women of reproductive age. Although some proportion of the increase is due to broadening of the case definition for congenital syphilis, most of the increase is due to increased exposure to the disease. Risk factors for maternal syphilis include

TABLE 20.12. TREATMENT OF SYPHILIS

Stage/Drug	Dose	Duration of Therapy
Early latent/benzathine penicillin G	2.4 million units IM	Single dose
Late latent or latent of unknown duration/benzathine penicillin G	2.4 million units IM	Weekly times 3
Tertiary/benzathine penicillin G	2.4 million units IM	Weekly times 3
Neurosyphilis/aqueous crystalline penicillin G	3–4 million units IV q 4 hours	10–14 days

From Centers for Disease Control and Prevention. 1998 Guidelines for treatment of sexually transmitted diseases. *MMWR* 1998;47(RR-1):34–37, with permission.

young age, multigravid, black or Hispanic, prostitution, crack cocaine use, inadequate prenatal care, and HIV infection. Prenatal screening with serologic tests is the most important tool in the identification of infants at risk for development of congenital syphilis. In high-risk populations serologic testing for syphilis should be performed during both early and late gestation. In the high-risk mother, testing should also be performed at the time of delivery. It should also be realized that infection or reinfection could occur between tests. Infection acquired late in pregnancy can be missed, as it may take weeks for antibody titers to become elevated. The likelihood of neurologic involvement in pregnant women appears to be higher than that in nonpregnant individuals. Evaluation for neurosyphilis should be considered in any pregnant woman who is diagnosed as having syphilis (44). Treatment during pregnancy should be the penicillin regimen appropriate for the stage of syphilis. Follow-up serologic assays are indicated at 1-month intervals throughout the pregnancy in women at high risk for reinfection. Pregnant patients allergic to penicillin should be desensitized, because use of erythromycin in this setting is associated with treatment failures. The Jarisch-Herxheimer reaction may induce premature labor or cause fetal distress.

Transplacental infection of the fetus can occur during any stage of maternal syphilis and at any time during the pregnancy. The probability that the organism will be transmitted to the fetus may be as high as 95%. Much of the damage associated with congenital syphilis appears to have an immunologic component. Transmission of infection later in pregnancy is associated with significant damage, secondary to the improved fetal immune competence seen at this time. Ultrasound findings such as hepatosplenomegaly and hydrops are suggestive of fetal syphilis. No infant should be discharged without the serologic status of the mother having been documented at least once during pregnancy (44). Without treatment, one fourth of infected fetuses die before birth, and another one fourth die shortly after birth. The remainder of the affected infants are said to have early congenital syphilis if symptoms appear within the first 2 years of life and late congenital syphilis if symptoms develop after the age of 2 years. Hepatosplenomegaly and rash are the most common manifestations of early congenital syphilis, which usually presents at delivery or within 3 to 7 weeks after delivery.

LOW-PREVALANCE SEXUALLY TRANSMISSIBLE INFECTIONS

Table 20.13. provides a comparison of the various diseases causing genital ulceration. Chancroid, granuloma inguinale (GI), and LGV are the so-called minor venereal diseases. This does not imply that these diseases are unimportant, but that the prevalence of these conditions in North America is low. International travel and immigration are frequently responsible for transporting the so-called tropical diseases into the United States. Although genital ulcer disease in the United States is most frequently caused by herpes, syphlis, or chancroid, GI and LGV should be considered in the differential diagnosis. Genital ulcer disease is an important cofactor for HIV transmission. Evaluation of all patients with genital ulcers should include a serologic test for syphilis and diagnostic evaluation for herpes. Specific tests such as darkfield examination for *T. pallidum*, culture or antigen test for HSV, and culture for *Haemophilus ducreyi* may be performed depending on test availability and clinical suspicion. However, even after complete diagnostic evaluation, at least 25% of patients who have genital ulcers have no laboratory-confirmed diagnosis (1).

Chancroid

H. ducreyi, a Gram-negative intracellular rod, is the causative agent of chancroid. Although only a few thousand cases of chancroid occur in the United States each year, chancroid has become endemic in the United States, and underreporting has been widespread. Prostitution and crack cocaine use are significant risk factors for infection (58). An estimated 10% of patients with chancroid may be coinfected with *T. pallidum* or HSV (1). Chancroid typically presents as one or more painful ulcers on the vulva, vagina, cervix, or anus appearing 4 to 7 days after exposure. The ulcer has soft, ragged edges. The base is composed of gray or yellow granulation tissue that bleeds easily. Painful, unilateral, inguinal lymphadenopathy is seen in 50% of the patients, which may progress to suppurative lymphadenitis (59). Lesions in women may be mildly symptomatic and may go undiagnosed. The Gram stain of chancroidal ulcer secretions may show Gram-negative coccobacilli in chains or clusters with a "school of fish" appearance. Gram stain, however, lacks adequate sensitivity and specificity for definitive diagnosis. *H. ducreyi* may be cultured with difficulty from clinical material on chocolate agar made selective with vancomycin and supplemented with vitamins and fetal calf serum. Colonies are yellow-gray, granular, and very cohesive (59). PCR testing for bacterial DNA may soon be available. If the initial tests were negative, patients should be retested for syphilis and HIV 3 months after the diagnosis of chancroid (1).

The recommended treatment regimens include single doses of azithromycin 1 g orally or ceftriaxone 250 mg IM, or ciprofloxacin 500 mg orally twice a day for 3 days, or erythromycin base 500 mg orally four times a day for 7 days. The healing time for large ulcers may be over 2 weeks. Inguinal buboes may require aspiration or incision and drainage. Sex contacts during the 10 days preceding the onset of symptoms should be examined and treated, regardless of whether symptoms of the disease are present (1). When compared with single-dose treatments, a 7-day regimen of erythromycin may be a better option for treating

TABLE 20.13. CLINICAL AND LABORATORY FEATURES OF GENITAL ULCERS

Characteristics	Primary Herpes	Syphilis	Chancroid	LGV
Incubation period	2–10 days	1–2 weeks	4–7 days	3–12 days
Primary lesion	Vesicle	Papule	Papule or pustule; erodes after 24–48 hours	Papule, pustule, vesicle
Number of lesions	Multiple	Single	Usually 1–3; 33% of cases multiple	Single
Size	1–3 mm	5–15 mm	2–20 mm	2–10 mm
Appearance	Superficial, erythematous, nonindurated	Raised border; smooth, necrotic base; firm induration	Deep, ragged, purulent base	Elevated, round, variable depth
Pain	Common	Unusual	Very tender	Unusual
Lymphadenopathy	Bilateral, tender	Bilateral, nontender	Unilateral, tender, suppurative	Unilateral, tender, suppurative
Diagnostic test	Viral culture	Darkfield	Gram stain of lesion shows "school of fish" pattern	Complement fixation

LGV, lymphogranuloma venereum.
From Prolog. *Gynecology*, 3rd ed. Washington: American College of Obstetrics and Gynecology, 1997:159, with permission.

HIV-infected patients. No adverse effects of chancroid on pregnancy outcome have been reported. Ciprofloxacin use is contraindicated during pregnancy.

Granuloma Inguinale (Donovanosis)

GI caused by the encapsulated, Gram-negative, nonmotile *Calymmatobacterium granulomatis* bacterium is rarely seen in the United States (44). The sexually transmitted nature of GI is controversial, due to the frequent occurrence of extragenital manifestations. Donovanosis, in most cases, begins as subcutaneous nodules at the site of initial infection, 1 to 12 weeks after exposure (60). These lesions enlarge, necrose, and erode, revealing beefy red granulation tissue. Spread then occurs by autoinoculation of adjacent skin; secondary bacterial contamination is common. The disease is typically painless, and the occurrence of general symptoms or adenopathies is rare (61). In women, the most common sites of infection are the labia minora, fourchette, and labia majora. The causative organism cannot be cultured on standard microbiologic media; hence, diagnosis requires visualization of dark-staining Donovan bodies on tissue crush preparation or biopsy (1).

The recommended treatment regimens include double-strength trimethoprim-sulfamethoxazole one tablet orally twice a day, or doxycycline 100 mg orally twice a day for a minimum of 3 weeks. Alternative regimens include ciprofloxacin 750 mg orally twice a day, or erythromycin base 500 mg orally four times a day for a minimum of 3 weeks. Treatment should be continued until all lesions have healed completely. Sexual contacts within the 60 days preceding the onset of symptoms in the patient should be examined and treated. Pregnant and lactating patients should be treated with erythromycin. Addition of a parenteral aminoglycoside should be strongly considered in pregnant and HIV-infected patients (1).

Lymphogranuloma Venereum

LGV, a rare disease in the United States, is caused by L1, L2, or L3 types of *C. trachomatis* (1). LGV is characterized by three stages (59). The primary, often unnoticed, genital ulcerative stage occurs 3 to 12 days after inoculation. Ulcers typically occur on the vaginal wall. Painful, suppurative, inguinal and/or femoral lymphadenopathy, divided by the inguinal ligament, yields the classic "groove" sign, and is the hallmark of the secondary stage of LGV, which arises 2 to 6 weeks after initial exposure. Perirectal lymphatic drainage of the vagina leads to the symptoms of proctitis in women (44). The tertiary stage is characterized by chronic ulceration, with fistula and stricture formation. The rectum and the vagina are the usual sites of involvement. Elephantiasis of the genitalia may occur secondary to lymphatic stasis. The diagnosis is usually made serologically by complement fixation, and by exclusion of other causes of inguinal lymphadenopathy or genital ulcers (1).

Doxycycline 100 mg orally twice a day for 21 days is the preferred treatment. Pregnant women should be treated with erythromycin 500 mg orally four times a day for 21 days. Sexual contacts should be treated if they had exposure to the patient during the 30 days preceding the onset of symptoms. HIV-infected patients may require prolonged therapy. Buboes may require aspiration or incision and drainage to prevent the formation of inguinal/femoral ulcerations (1).

SEXUALLY TRANSMITTED DISEASES CAUSING GENITAL SKIN LESIONS

Human Papillomavirus

Genital infections caused by HPV are one of the most prevalent STDs in the United States (62). Genital warts have been observed for centuries and described in outbreaks of syphilis in Europe in the late 15th century (63). HPV is a double-stranded DNA virus that cannot be cultured. On the basis of DNA homology, some 80 types of papillomavirus are known, and more than 20 types can infect the female genital tract (44). The most common clinical expression of genital HPV infection is condyloma acuminatum. HPVs are highly associated with the development of genital epithelial malignancies in both sexes.

Epidemiology and Transmission

HPVs are associated with three clinical groups of infections: common warts on nongenital skin of healthy individuals, disseminated cutaneous warts in immunosuppressed individuals, and anogenital infections. Genital HPV infections are recognized as the most common viral STD in the United States. An estimated half million people each year acquire symptomatic genital warts, with a prevalence of 20% to 40% in sexually active groups (64). Genital HPV infections arise after direct contact with an infected sexual partner, transmission occurring in approximately two thirds of such contacts (63). Patients with genital HPV frequently have other STDs. Behavioral risk factors such as multiple sexual partners, sexual experience at an early age, and having a male partner previously married to a woman with cervical cancer have been noted as risk factors for the development of HPV infection (44). Genital HPV types have been associated with conjunctival, nasal, oral, and laryngeal warts. Infants born to mothers who have genital HPV infection may develop laryngeal papilloma, typically caused by HPV 6 or 11.

Microorganism and Pathogenesis

Each HPV virion is a 55-nm, icosahedral particle composed of a circular, double-stranded, covalently closed DNA molecule, surrounded by a protein capsid (65). The absence of an outer membrane may account for the low antigenicity of papillomavirus infections. Typing is based on DNA homology. Most HPV infections are asymptomatic, subclinical, or unrecognized. HPVs are mucosotropic or cutaneotropic and commonly involve the skin, lower uroanogenital tract, oral cavity, and larynx. HPV types 6 and 11 have been shown to be the predominant viral types in classic condylomata acuminata warts, and HPV types 16, 18, 31, 33, 35, 39, 45, 51, and 52 have been recognized for their oncogenic potential (62).

Typically, HPV infections involve only the superficial terminally differentiated epithelial layers (44). In most instances, inoculation of cells with HPV at sites of microtrauma produces colonization with no disease expression. Virus exposure is detected by molecular hybridization of exfoliated cells. In perhaps one in ten exposed individuals, focal transcription and translation leads to disease expression (65). Genital condyloma occurs 6 weeks to 3 months after exposure. This is followed by a period of active lesion growth, which typically lasts 3 to 6 months. After a lag time of several months, there is a host-containment phase, during which lesion growth is slowed. In up to 20% of cases, spontaneous regression may occur. Regression may even be seen in cases of extensive disease. About 9 months from the onset of the first lesion, an equilibrium between lesion growth and host containment is established. At this point, patients diverge into two groups: those who remain in sustained clinical remission, and those who relapse into continued active disease expression (66). Body warmth, moist mucosal areas, and pregnancy hasten growth of genital warts (63). Immunosuppressed individuals are more susceptible to clinical infections and continued active disease.

Clinical Manifestations

Genital HPV infections are classified as latent (asymptomatic), subclinical, or clinical (67). Latent infections have no visible lesions and are detected only by DNA hybridization tests for HPV. Subclinical lesions are identified as a white irregular mosaic surface after application of 5% acetic acid and inspection under magnification. Clinical lesions are identified without the aid of magnification and are typically called condylomata acuminata. Infection in the genital tract may involve the vulva, vagina, cervix, urethra, perianal skin, and rectum. Classic condylomata present in three forms: hyperplastic, flat, and verrucous (63). The hyperplastic condyloma is a large, moist, filiform lesion that frequently presents on the labia. The flat condyloma appears as a small flesh-colored papule on the labia or surrounding tissues. The verrucous condyloma appears as verruca vulgaris on the keratinized skin of the perineum. Perianal involvement occurs in 80% of women with vulvar condylomata and does not necessarily imply anoreceptive sexual exposure. Vulvar itching, vulvar pain and burning, vaginal discharge, bleeding, and dyspareunia can be associated with HPV infections in women.

Association with Gynecologic Neoplasia

Vulvar, vaginal, and anal cancers have been shown to harbor HPV DNA. HPV DNA has been found in as many as 90% of cervical cancers (68). HPV detection is associated with a tenfold or greater risk of cervical neoplasm when compared with controls (69). HPV 16 is the most common type found in squamous carcinoma, while HPV 18 is most common in adenocarcinoma and neuroendocrine-positive, small cell cervical carcinomas (70). Despite these striking associations, type 16 DNA may be found in cells from women without precancerous changes (44). Patients with cervical cancer who are HPV negative have been found to have a significantly increased risk of dying from cervical carcinoma as compared with those who are HPV positive (71). Vulvar intraepithelial neoplasia and vulvar squamous carcinoma in younger women are associated with HPV in most patients, with HPV 16 being the most common (72).

Diagnosis

Visible genital warts constitute a minority of HPV infections. Condylomas are recognized as cauliflower-like projections or flat papular lesions. Molluscum contagiosum may be confused with anogenital warts. The anus, urethra, and oral mucosa should be evaluated. Genital HPV infection is often detected on Pap tests, where the presence of koilocytes is pathognomonic. Koilocytosis is the cytopathic effect induced by HPV infection in the epithelium, and correlates better with results of DNA hybridization than any other single cytologic feature. The koilocyte is a large cell with a hyperchromatic nucleus and a perinuclear halo. In the Bethesda system of cytologic classification, cytologic features of HPV infection are classified as low-grade squamous intraepithelial lesions (LGSIL).

Colposcopy of the vulva, vagina, and cervix is valuable for the diagnosis of subclinical HPV infection. This procedure involves application of 3% to 5% acetic acid for 3 to 5 minutes, followed by examination under magnification. The acetowhite lesions of intraepithelial neoplasia are usually multicentric and/or often extensive. The degree of acetowhite change and sharpness of margins correlates with the severity of the neoplastic process. Routine use of colposcopy as a screening test to detect subclinical or acetowhite genital warts is not recommended. Diagnosis of genital warts can by confirmed by biopsy, although biopsy is rarely necessary. Microscopic examination reveals acanthosis, parakeratosis, and hyperkeratosis, with or without dysplastic changes. Biopsy is indicated if the diagnosis is uncertain, if lesions do not respond to standard therapy, if the disease worsens during therapy, if the patient is immunocompromised, or if warts are pigmented, indurated, fixed, or ulcerated (1).

HPV DNA may be detected by nucleic acid probes. DNA hybridization assays including Southern blot and dot blot for fixed tissue samples, and *in situ* hybridization of gene probes with frozen tissue samples, have mainly been used in research settings. Presently, the most sensitive and relatively inexpensive test is the PCR technique. PCR has been reported to detect as little as one viral genome in 105 cells (73). No data support the use of type specific nucleic acid tests in the routine diagnosis and management of visible genital warts (1). The role of HPV testing in the manage-

ment of women with atypical squamous cells of undetermined significance (ASCUS) is still under study (74).

Treatment

The primary goal of treating visible genital warts is the removal of symptomatic warts, and ablation is the mainstay of therapy. Currently available treatments do not alter the natural history of HPV infection, and removal of warts may or may not decrease infectivity (1). If left untreated, visible genital warts may resolve on their own, remain unchanged, or increase in size or number. Factors that may influence selection of treatment include wart size, wart number, anatomic sites, patient preference, cost, convenience, and physician experience (1). The treatment modality should be changed if substantial improvement has not occurred within three to six treatments. Patients should be warned that ablative therapies may result in scarring in the form of persistent hypo- or hyperpigmentation, and may rarely result in chronic pain syndromes. Table 20.14 lists the various modalities currently available for treatment of HPV infections. Combining modalities does not increase efficacy and may increase complications.

Therapeutic alternatives for patient-administered treatment of extragenital warts includes podofilox 0.5% in a solution or gel form. This agent functions as an antimitotic drug and is relatively inexpensive and safe in its use. Patients occasionally report mild to moderate pain after treatment. The medication is administered with a cotton swab or finger and is applied twice a day for 3 days followed by 4 days of no therapy. A total of four cycles may be repeated. The total area of wart that is treated should not exceed 10 cm², and the total volume of podofilox applied should not exceed 0.5 mL per day. The safety of podofilox during pregnancy has not been established. An alternative for patient-applied therapy includes imiquimod 5% cream. This agent functions as a topically active immune enhancer. Localized mild to moderate irritation is sometimes seen after treatment. Imiquimod 5% cream is applied to warts at bedtime three

TABLE 20.14. TREATMENT OF EXTERNAL GENITAL WARTS

Patient Administered	Provider Administered	Alternative Therapies
Podofilox 0.5% solution or gel		
	Cryotherapy	Intralesional interferon
	Podophyllin resin	
Imiquimod 5% cream	TCA or BCA	
	Surgical removal	Laser ablation

BCA, bilchloroacetic acid; TCA, trichloroacetic acid.
From Centers for Disease Control and Prevention. 1998 Guidelines for treatment of sexually transmitted diseases. *MMWR* 1998; 47(RR-1):89–90, with permission.

times a week up to 16 weeks. It is recommended that the treatment area be washed with mild soap and water 6 to 10 hours after the application. Imiquimod is listed as an FDA class B drug, though no studies in pregnancy have been reported. Imiquimod acts locally with no reported systematic side effects, hence its use during pregancy may be considered safe.

Provider-administered therapy includes alternatives such as cryotherapy, which results in a thermal-induced cytolysis. Pain at the site during the healing process is commonly reported. Repeat applications may be undertaken every 1 to 2 weeks. Podophyllin resin, similar to podofilox, functions as an antimitotic agent. It is commonly compounded with a 10% to 25% tincture of benzoin. The shelf life and stability of these agents can be variable. A small amount of resin is applied to each wart, and then allowed to air dry. Limitation to <0.5 mL of podophyllin or <10 cm² of warts per session is recommended. The resin should be washed off 1 to 4 hours following its application in order to reduce local irritation. Applications may be repeated weekly if necessary. Safe use during pregnancy has not been established.

Trichloro- and bichloroacetic acid destroy warts by causing chemical coagulation of protein. These agents are caustic and should be sparingly applied with a swab and allowed to dry completely. The use of baking soda is helpful in removing any excess acid and preventing surrounding tissue damage. Applications may be repeated weekly. Surgical removal using electrosurgical or sharp dissection techniques may render the patient wart-free, often with a single session of therapy. This approach can also be useful for extensive or intraurethral warts. Alternative therapy such as intralesional interferon and laser surgery should only be used in refractory cases secondary to the high frequency of systemic adverse effects and additional cost associated with these therapies.

Prior to treatment of exophytic cervical and anal warts, high-grade squamous intraepithelial lesions must be excluded. Vaginal warts may be treated with trichloroacetic acid (TCA), bichloroacetic acid (BCA), or podophyllin as described above, restricting treatment to ≤2 cm² per session. The use of a cryoprobe in the vagina is not recommended because of the risk of vaginal perforation and fistula formation. Urethral meatus and oral warts may be treated by cryotherapy with liquid nitrogen or surgical removal.

After visible genital warts have cleared, a follow-up evaluation is not necessary. Recurrences occur most frequently during the first 3 months. Though the presence of genital warts is not an indication for cervical colposcopy, women should be counseled regarding the need for regular cytologic screening. Sex partners may benefit from examination to assess the presence of genital warts or other STDs. Patients and sex partners should be warned that the patient may remain infectious even though warts are not visible. The use of condoms may reduce, but not eliminate, the risk of transmission to uninfected partners. In the absence of coexistent dysplasia, treatment for subclinical infection is not recommended. No therapy has been identified to permanently eradicate infection (1).

Interactions with Pregnancy

Genital warts may first appear or may grow markedly during pregnancy (67). Podophyllin and interferon are contraindicated during pregnancy (1). Large symptomatic lesions may be treated with TCA acid or BCA acid. Because genital warts can proliferate and become friable during pregnancy, many experts advocate their removal after the first trimester by simple excision or electrosurgery under anesthesia (1). Laryngeal papillomatosis, a potentially life-threatening condition that usually appears within the first 5 years of life, is typically caused by HPV types 6 and 11. The route of transmission is not completely understood. It is estimated that 2% to 5% of all births are at risk for neonatal HPV exposure, and vaginal delivery carries a risk of 0.04% of laryngeal infection in the neonate (67). Reports exist of children having developed laryngeal papillomas after being born to women not known to have HPV. Hence, cesarean delivery is not routinely indicated to prevent laryngeal papillomatosis in the neonate. Cesarean section may be indicated if genital warts threaten to obstruct the pelvic outlet or if vaginal delivery would cause excessive bleeding.

Human Immunodeficiency Virus

Infection with HIV produces a spectrum of disease that progresses from a clinically latent or asymptomatic state to the development of acquired immunodeficiency syndrome (AIDS). Though AIDS was first identified and defined by the CDC in 1981, studies suggest that the virus has been present in Africa since the 1950s, and that it first appeared in North America in the mid-1970s. HIV has been isolated from human populations in two serotypes: HIV-1 and HIV-2. HIV-1 was isolated in 1984, and is the most common and virulent in the United States. HIV-2 appears to be less pathogenic than HIV-1 and is prevalent mainly in West Africa (75). Obstetrician-gynecologists are increasingly involved in caring for women with HIV, as 85% of cases in females are among those 15 to 44 years old (76).

Epidemiology and Transmission

The World Health Organization (WHO) estimated that there would be 40 million people infected with HIV by the year 2000. Of these, 10 to 15 million are expected to be women and children. In the United States, an estimated 3 million individuals are infected with HIV, 98% of whom are adults. In 1994, HIV infection was the third leading cause of death among women 25 to 44 years old, and the fifth leading cause of death in girls 1 to 4 years old (77).

Viral cultures have demonstrated the presence of HIV

in many body fluids such as blood, saliva, semen, vaginal secretions, tears, CSF, amniotic fluid, and breast milk. HIV infection appears to be transmitted mainly through sexual intercourse or through blood contamination and less commonly by breast milk (78). Heterosexual transmission has become the most rapidly increasing mode of HIV acquisition, whereas the incidence of HIV transmission in homosexual men and intravenous drug abusers has diminished. Male to female transmission of HIV is three times more efficient than female to male transmission. Anal intercourse, ulcerative STDs, menstruation, and tampon use increase the risk of transmission. Though transmission is more likely to occur in the latter stages of the disease, HIV-infected persons are capable of transmitting the virus at all stages of their disease. There is no evidence to suggest that transmission occurs through exposure to food, fomites, tears, saliva, urine, insects, or casual contact. It is generally accepted that intact skin is an effective barrier to transmission (74). Transmission of HIV through deep kissing and biting is exceedingly rare.

In the United States, the AIDS epidemic has had its greatest impact in women of minority populations. By mid-1995, more than half a million people in the United States had been reported as having AIDS, of whom approximately 14% were women (79). In 1997, women accounted for 21% of AIDS cases in adults, and the proportion of all cases that are young females continues to grow. Moreover, African-American and Hispanic women accounted for 60% and 20%, respectively, of AIDS cases in women (CDC 1997). Over 90% of pediatric AIDS cases are attributed to perinatal transmission from infected mothers. The overall HIV seroprevalence of 0.17% (1% to 2% in some inner city populations) corresponds to nearly 7,000 births to HIV-infected mothers annually in the United States. Assuming a perinatal transmission rate of 20% to 30%, this would result in 1,400 to 2,100 newborns infected with HIV annually. However, more recent estimates of the transmission rates, reflecting implementation of gestational chemoprophylaxis, range from 3% to 10%. Worldwide, the current epidemic results in an estimated 200,000 congenitally infected infants per year. The risk of infection following needlestick injury with infected blood is 1:250, and following transfusion with screened blood bank blood [enzyme-linked immunosorbent assay (ELISA)] is 1:225,000 per unit transfused.

Viral Agent and Pathophysiology

HIV, a member of the Lentivirus family, is an enveloped single-stranded RNA retrovirus. HIV is described as a retrovirus because it encodes the information required to synthesize DNA for integration into the host DNA from an RNA template by means of the reverse transcriptase (RT) enzyme. Both RNA and the RT enzyme are located within the core of the virus, along with core proteins p24 (gag protein) and

p18. The viral envelope contains glycoprotein structures, transmembrane glycoprotein-gp41, and gp120, which resides outside the viral envelope in association with gp41 (79).

The gp120 component binds to the CD4 receptor that is found on T-helper lymphocytes and some macrophages and monocytes. The infected macrophages may have a particularly important role in the development of AIDS-related dementia because the macrophage-monocyte is the major cell type infected in the brain. Also, infection of alveolar macrophages may contribute to pneumonia by a mechanism unrelated to the loss of T-helper cell function. The terms *M-tropic HIV-1* and *T-tropic HIV-1* describe viral forms that are adapted to macrophages and monocytes and T cells, respectively (79). HIV may also infect the placenta (80). In addition to the gp120 and gp41 viral envelope proteins that allow attachment and fusion of viral and host cell membranes, a chemokine receptor named fusin, unique to human cells, is thought to be essential for this interaction (79).

After the viral genome enters a suitable host cell, the viral RT produces a DNA copy of the RNA genome, which becomes integrated into the host genome (79). Once incorporated into the host genome, new viral copies are made, which "bud" through the host cell to infect new cells. The host cell is killed with HIV replication. Approximately 10 billion HIV particles are produced each day, many of which are genetic variants that are more virulent and resistant to drug therapy and less susceptible to immune attack. Plasma virus half-life is about 6 hours, and in untreated patients, each milliliter of blood may contain 60,000 copies of HIV. Increasing viral load and declining CD4 counts renders a patient susceptible to opportunistic infections and neoplasms that rarely affect immunocompetent patients.

Clinical Manifestations

The incubation period after initial infection is 1 to 3 weeks. The modified WHO staging system for HIV infection describes four clinical groups of infection: asymptomatic (group I), mildly symptomatic (group II), moderately symptomatic (group III), and severely symptomatic (group IV).

Group I (CDC Category A)
At the time of initial infection the patient may be asymptomatic, may present with an acute syndrome similar to mononucleosis with accompanying aseptic meningitis, or may present with persistent generalized lymphadenopathy. Fever and sweats; myalgias and arthralgias; pharyngitis and lymphadenopathy; nausea, vomiting, and diarrhea; pruritic maculopapular erythematous rash on trunk and legs; and headaches characterize the acute primary infection. Many of these symptoms seem flulike and if not severe may be ignored. Viremia lasts for 2 to 3 months; humoral antibody and cytotoxic CD8 lymphocytes mount an immune re-

sponse, but do not clear the virus, which persists in lymphoid tissue (77). Antibodies may be detected in most adults 6 to 12 weeks after exposure, but in rare cases the "window phase" before antibodies are detectable is longer (81).

Group II

Patients in this group are classified as being in the latent or mildly symptomatic phase. A rise in viral load leads to slow depletion of CD4 cells. Minor weight loss (<10%), minor mucocutaneous symptoms or signs, and/or recurrent upper respiratory tract infections may occur during this stage of infection.

Group III (CDC Category B)

This group is characterized by progressive weight loss of >10%, fever, and/or unexplained diarrhea of >1 month; pulmonary TB; idiopathic thrombocytopenic purpura; oropharyngeal and persistent vulvovaginal candidiasis; severe cervical dysplasia; and pelvic inflammatory disease.

Group IV (CDC Category C)

This group is defined by the presence of conditions such as *Pneumocystis carinii* pneumonia (PCP), cerebral toxoplasmosis, invasive cervical cancer, and other opportunistic infections that are strongly associated with severe immunodeficiency. In the past, the mean latency period from seroconversion to AIDS was 10 years, and survival after diagnosis of AIDS was 50% at 1 year. However, newer antiretroviral therapy has improved these numbers considerably.

Diagnosis

The early diagnosis of HIV infection is important for several reasons. Treatment is available to slow the decline of immune system function, which in turn prolongs the patient's life as well as the asymptomatic phase of the infection. HIV-infected persons with altered immune function are at increased risk for infections such as PCP, toxoplasmic encephalitis, and others for which preventive measures are now available. HIV affects the efficacy of antimicrobial therapy for some STDs. Finally, the early diagnosis of HIV enables the health care provider to counsel such patients and to assist in preventing HIV transmission to others. Testing for HIV should be offered to all patients since it is often difficult to identify those whose behavior puts them at risk of infection.

Counseling followed by informed consent must be obtained before an HIV test is performed. Some states require written documentation of informed consent. HIV infection usually is diagnosed by using HIV-1 antibody tests. ELISA is usually the first test used for screening, with Western blot (WB), or an immunofluorescence assay (IFA) used as a follow-up test. ELISA, which tests for antibodies to p24

or gp41, has a sensitivity of 99%, but poor specificity. WB measures presence of antibodies to both structural and nonstructural viral proteins, and the result is read as positive, indeterminate, or negative. Detection of antibodies to any two of the following antigens is read as positive: p24, gp41, gp120, and gp160. The achievable false-positive rate of sequentially performed ELISA and WB tests can be less than 0.001%. The average time between infection and development of detectable antibodies is 25 days. HIV antibody is detectable in at least 95% of patients within 6 months after infection. Antibody tests cannot exclude infection that occurred <6 months before the test. Since the prevalence of HIV-2 in the United States is extremely low, testing for HIV-2 is conducted only when indicated by demographic or behavioral information, or when there is clinical suspicion of HIV disease in the absence of a positive test for antibodies to HIV-1. Because HIV antibody crosses the placenta, its presence in a child aged <18 months is not diagnostic of HIV infection. The PCR can detect HIV proviral DNA within the peripheral blood of patients with HIV two to six months or more before seroconversion occurs.

A rapid screening test for detecting HIV antibody—Single Use Diagnostic System for HIV-1 (SUDS) (Murex, Norcross, GA)—is now available. The sensitivity and specificity of the rapid HIV test are comparable to those of ELISA, it is easier to use, and results are available in 5 to 30 minutes. The rapid HIV test eliminates patients' need for a second visit to learn their results. Also, an accurate rapid test would have the utility among pregnant women in labor who do not know their HIV status. It would help identify HIV-infected pregnant patients whose infants might still benefit from the intrapartum and postpartum components of the AIDS Clinical Trials Group (ACTG) 076 regimen. Patients with positive HIV test results must receive behavioral, psychosocial, and medical evaluation and monitoring services.

Laboratory Markers of Disease Progression

The CD4 count and the plasma viral load are comparable to a "train-cliff" scenario: the plasma viral load is indicative of the speed of the train, i.e., disease activity and the immunologic damage that is about to occur, whereas the CD4 count represents the distance to the cliff, i.e., the level of immunosuppression, or the immunologic damage that has already occurred. RT-PCR (Roche Molecular Systems, Branchburg, New Jersey) and bDNA (Chiron, Emeryville, California), are some of the currently available assays to measure plasma HIV-1 viral load. The lower threshold of detection is in the 500 copies/mL range, when a qualitative PCR may become useful. Infections and vaccinations can transiently but substantially increase the plasma viral load (75). Data have conclusively demonstrated that a treatment reduction in plasma HIV-1 RNA viral load is associated with a decrease in the rate of disease progression (82). CD4 count range of 400 to 1,400 cells/mm³ is considered normal, and a count <200 cells/mm³ is associated with increased risk of opportunistic infection and rapid disease progression. Diurnal variation, infections, vaccinations, and corticosteroids may affect CD4 counts; hence, fluctuations of up to 30% may occur that are not attributable to a change in the disease status. Therefore, monitoring trends in CD4 is more important than an isolated value. Some conditions such as tuberculosis, Kaposi's sarcoma, and lymphomas can occur despite normal CD4 counts. Plasma viral load and CD4 counts are to be measured at least quarterly in stable HIV-infected adults as part of their routine evaluation (75).

Management

A single health care source that is able to provide comprehensive care for all stages of HIV infection is preferred. The initial evaluation of the HIV-positive patient begins with a detailed history including sexual history; substance abuse; immunizations; travel; medical conditions such as liver, lung, and kidney disease; and prior history of drug intolerance, which may compromise future drug therapy. Constitutional symptoms such as fever, night sweats, unexplained weight loss, and anorexia are indicative of disease progression, but may also represent the presence of opportunistic infections. Physical exam for women should include a gynecologic exam including tests for *N. gonorrhoeae, C. trachomatis*, a Pap smear, and wet mount examination of vaginal secretions. The genital and perianal areas should be closely examined for evidence of STDs. Unless the CD4 count is < 100 cells/mm³, syphilis serology is usually accurate; however, a lumbar puncture is recommended to exclude neurosyphilis. HSV recurrences are more common and severe in patients with HIV. PID, vaginal candidiasis, and cervical HPV infection with the oncogenic subtypes 16 and 18 are extremely common in women with HIV. Table 20.15 lists Pap smear recommendations in HIV-infected women.

TABLE 20.15. CDC 1998 RECOMMENDATIONS FOR PAP SMEAR SCREENING OF HIV-INFECTED WOMEN

Comprehensive gynecological examination, including Pap smear, genital cultures, wet mount of vaginal secretions, and anal inspection.

If initial Pap smear is normal, then at least one additional Pap smear shoiuld be obtained in 6 months to exclude the possibility of false-negative results on the initial Pap smear

If repeat Pap smear is normal, then obtain annual Pap smears

If any Pap smear shows reactive squamous cellular changes, obtain another Pap smear in 3 months.

If any Pap smear shows squamous intraepithelial lesion or atypical squamous cells of undetermined significance, colposcopic examination with biopsies if necessary of the lower genital tract should be performed.

From the Centers for Disease Control and Prevention. 1998 Guidelines for treatment of sexually transmitted diseases. *MMWR* 1998;47(No. RR-1), with permission.

Baseline investigations in an HIV-positive patient should include plasma HIV RNA viral load, CD4 lymphocyte count, complete blood count, liver and renal profiles, and a chest x-ray. Absolute lymphopenia should raise suspicion of advanced disease. Baseline laboratory investigations also include serology testing for hepatitis B, hepatitis C, syphilis, CMV, and toxoplasmosis. Sputum cultures and smears for mycobacteria should be performed as indicated by the patient's history and physical exam. A tuberculin skin test should be performed annually. The usefulness of anergy testing is controversial. An induration of ≥5 mm should be regarded as a positive response in an HIV-infected patient and prophylaxis with isoniazid 300 mg/day for 12 months should be initiated, along with pyridoxine (50 mg/day) to reduce the risk of isoniazid toxicity. When antigen recognition is still intact, pneumococcal vaccine every 6 years, influenza vaccine annually, tetanus toxoid updates, inactivated polio vaccine if traveling, and hepatitis B vaccine if seronegative should be encouraged. Prophylaxis against opportunistic diseases should be offered on the basis of a low CD4 count and continued indefinitely. At a CD4 count of <200 cells/mm³, PCP prophylaxis with one double-strength tablet of trimethoprim-sulfamethoxazole daily, or dapsone 100 mg daily, or aerosol pentamidine 300 mg once a month is recommended. Prophylaxis for toxoplasmosis is indicated for patients with a CD4 count <100 cells/mm³ and positive serum serology for toxoplasmosis IgG. However, trimethoprim-sulfamethoxazole daily, as indicated for PCP prophylaxis, is also effective for toxoplasma. At a CD4 count <75 cells/mm³, consideration of prophylaxis for *Mycobacterium avium* complex (MAC) with azithromycin 600 mg PO every week should be given. At a CD4 count of <50 cells/mm³ a dilated ophthalmoscopic exam every 3 to 6 months to identify CMV retinitis and fungal prophylaxis with fluconazole 100 to 200 mg daily are encouraged.

Principles of Antiretroviral Therapy

The goal of antiretroviral therapy is aggressive and complete suppression of HIV, because suppression of viral load correlates well with a reduction is disease progression. Monotherapy consistently leads to the selection of resistant strains of HIV and eventually treatment failure. Triple-drug therapy, usually with two nucleoside analogue reverse transcriptase inhibitors (NRTIs) and a nonnucleoside analogue reverse transcriptase inhibitor (NNRTI) or a protease inhibitor, should be offered if plasma RNA viral load is ≥5,000 copies/mL or if the CD4 count is <500 cells/mm³ (83). However, a number of experts recommend levels <500 copies/mL (detection level of current assays) as the target of antiretroviral therapy (75). Drug toxicity, interactions, and intolerance or failure of an expected fall in plasma viral load measurements within 4 to 8 weeks of therapy are indications to modify antiretroviral therapy. The side effects with nucleoside analogue inhibitors such as zidovudine

(AZT) include severe anemia, leukopenia, rash, and myositis. Didanosine and zalcitabine are associated with peripheral neuropathy and pancreatitis. Protease inhibitors such as ritonavir and saquinavir are associated with nausea, diarrhea, fatigue, and liver enzyme abnormalities. Nephrolithiasis may occur in up to 10% of patients taking indinavir. Skin rash is the most common adverse event with nevirapine, which is the first compound within the NNRTI group.

Perinatal Transmission: Reducing the Odds

Between 600,000 and 800,000 infants are born with HIV infection each year, virtually all in the developing world. Health care providers should ensure that all pregnant women are counseled and encouraged to be tested for HIV infection both for their own health and to reduce the risk for perinatal HIV transmission. HIV testing should be performed as early in pregnancy as possible so that informed and timely therapeutic and reproductive decisions can be made. The prevalence of HIV infection may be higher in women who have not received prenatal care, and intrapartum testing with rapid screening tests may be useful. Medical management of HIV infection is essentially the same for pregnant and nonpregnant women. In addition, they should receive appropriate referral for psychological, social, and legal services. CD4 lymphocyte counts and HIV viral load should be measured at least every trimester. Pregnancy among HIV-infected women does not appear to increase maternal morbidity or mortality. Also, asymptomatic HIV infection does not increase the risk of obstetric complications.

Management of HIV infection during pregnancy is directed toward stabilization of HIV disease, prevention of opportunistic infections, and prevention of perinatal transmission. HIV transmission from mother to infant can occur *in utero* (25% to 30%), during labor and delivery (70% to 75%), or through breast-feeding. The mechanisms of intrapartum transmission might include transplacental infection or through mucocutaneous exposure to maternal blood or cervical secretions. HIV-seropositive women in industrialized countries are advised not to breast-feed their babies. In July 1998, the WHO recommended that HIV-infected women in developing countries be given information about the benefits and risks of breast-feeding. Maternal immune depletion and high maternal viral loads have been associated with increased risk of HIV perinatal transmission. However, transmission may be observed across the full range of viral levels. Other STDs, increased duration of membrane rupture, hemorrhage during labor, chorioamnionitis, and invasive procedures during pregnancy and delivery have all been associated with an increased risk of perinatal HIV transmission (84).

Strategies to prevent vertical HIV transmission include maternal nutritional intervention, vaccinations, management of maternal coinfections, bypassing the route of expo-

sure, and most importantly perinatal antiretroviral therapy (84). Connor et al. (85), in a randomized, double-blind, placebo-controlled trial protocol (ACTG 076), demonstrated profound reduction in vertical HIV transmission in mother-infant pairs treated with zidovudine (AZT). The proportion of infants infected at 18 months in the AZT group was 8.3% compared to 25.5% for those who received placebo. HIV-infected pregnant women (14 to 34 weeks' gestation) with CD4 cell count >200/mm^3 who had not received antiretroviral therapy during the current pregnancy were enrolled. The AZT regimen included antepartum AZT (100 mg orally five times daily), intrapartum AZT (2 mg/kg body weight given IV over 1 hour, then 1 mg/kg per hour until delivery), and AZT for the newborn (2 mg/kg orally every 6 hours for 6 weeks). The only observed short-term toxicity in AZT-treated infants was anemia, which was not clinically significant. In ACTG 185, the ACTG 076 regimen was administered to women with advanced HIV infection, and the perinatal HIV transmission rate was reported to be 4.8% (86). Several trials evaluating the efficacy of shorter and less intensive antiretroviral regimens are in progress. An ACTG phase II/III trial evaluating the efficacy of nevirapine (a NNRTI) in preventing HIV transmission is also under way. Preliminary results in Uganda demonstrated that a single nevirapine pill during labor ($3/pill), with the newborn also getting a single dose, cuts the transmission rate in half. These results hold great potential for use in the world's poorer nations. Combination drug regimens with incorporation of AZT to maximally suppress the virus are now recommended during pregnancy (87). Decisions regarding initiation of therapy should be the same for women who are not currently receiving antiretroviral therapy and for women who are not pregnant, with the additional consideration of the potential impact of such therapy on the fetus and infant. Antiretroviral therapy may be withheld during the first trimester. Experience to date with the administration of antiretrovirals other than AZT during pregnancy is quite limited. Several pharmaceutical companies (Glaxo Wellcome, Hoffman-LaRoche, etc.), in cooperation with the CDC, maintain a registry to assess the safety of AZT and other antiretroviral agents.

Cesarean section has been proposed as a means of reducing the risk of exposure, particularly if performed prior to the rupture of membranes. In a French perinatal cohort study, cesarean section appeared to reduce the risk of vertical HIV-1 transmission (88). However, the benefit of cesarean section was only apparent when performed prior to the onset of labor and in mother-infant pairs who received AZT. The International Perinatal HIV Group recently reported a meta-analysis of 15 prospective cohort studies from European and North American centers on the mode of delivery and the risk of vertical transmission (89). The International Perinatal HIV Group included data on 8,533 mother-child pairs, and concluded that elective cesarean section reduces the risk of transmission of HIV-1 from mother to child by

50%, independently of the effects of treatment with AZT. Among mother-child pairs receiving antiretroviral therapy during the prenatal, intrapartum, and neonatal periods, rates of vertical transmission were 2.0% among the 196 mothers who underwent elective cesarean section and 7.3% among the 1,255 mothers with other modes of delivery. The results of the interim analysis of a randomized clinical trial of elective cesarean section in 436 HIV-1 women who were given AZT according to the ACTG 076 protocol and who did not breast-feed provide evidence that elective cesarean section delivery significantly lowers the risk of mother-to-child transmission of HIV-1 without a significantly increased risk of complications for the mother (90). The role of cesarean section in reducing vertical transmission in patients who receive combination antiretroviral therapy and have a low viral load remains to be completely evaluated. Furthermore, cesarean section may carry long-term risks to the mother, especially in areas of economic deprivation. Despite these considerations and others, the American College of Obstetrics and Gynecology Committee on Obstetric Practice has recommended that scheduled cesarean delivery be offered to all HIV-infected women (91).

In summary, to minimize vertical transmission of HIV, women must be identified as HIV-infected as early as possible during pregnancy and offered antiretroviral therapy. Postnatal evaluation of the HIV at-risk infant, beginning immediately after birth, is crucial for early diagnosis and optimal medical management.

10 KEY POINTS

1. *C. trachomatis* is the most common bacterial cause of sexually transmitted disease in the United States, and is the major cause of PID.

2. *N. gonorrhoeae*, like *C. trachomatis*, causes mucopurulent cervicitis, and patients testing positive for *N. gonorrhoeae* should also be treated for chlamydia, as coinfection rates range from 30% to 60%.

3. *T. vaginalis* infection is commonly found in women with other STDs, and may play a role in the transmission of HSV and HIV infections.

4. HSV-2 is the most common cause of genital ulcer disease in the United States.

5. Syphilis infection may be silent, undetected, or characterized by prolonged asymptomatic periods. Tests such as the VDRL and RPR are used to screen for infection, with specific tests such as the FTA-ABS and MHA-TP being used to confirm the diagnosis.

6. Genital ulcer disease is an important cofactor for HIV transmission. Herpes, syphilis, chancroid, GI, and LGV should be considered in the differential diagnosis.

7. Granuloma inguinale (donovanosis), uncommonly seen in the United States, results in genital ulcers that are typically painless, and occurrence of general symptoms or lymphadenopathy is rare.

8. Lymphogranuloma venereum is caused by L1, L2, or L3 types of *C. trachomatis*.

9. Genital HPV infection is the most common viral STD in the United States. HPV types 6 and 11 are the predominant viral types seen in association with condyloma acuminata, while types 16 and 18 are associated with the development of genital epithelial malignancies.

10. The standards of care for HIV-infected women are rapidly evolving. A single health care source that is able to provide comprehensive care for all stages of HIV infection is important for successful treatment.

REFERENCES

1. Centers for Disease Control and Prevention. 1998 guidelines for treatment of sexually transmitted diseases. *MMWR* 1998; 47(RR-1):1–116.
2. Stamm WE, Holmes KK. Chlamydia trachomatis infections of the adult. In: Holmes KK, Mardh P-A, Sparling PF, et al., eds. *Sexually transmitted diseases,* 2nd ed. New York: McGraw-Hill, 1990:181–193.
3. Buimer M, Van Doornum GJJ, Ching S, et al. Detection of *Chlamydia trachomatis* and *Neisseria gonorrhoeae* by ligase chain reaction-based assays with clinical specimens from various sites: implications for diagnostic testing and screening. *J Clin Microbiol* 1996;34(10):2395–2400.
4. Majeroni BA. Chlamydial cervicitis: complications and new treatment options. *Am Fam Physician* 1994;49(8):1825–1832.
5. Paavonen J. Genital *Chlamydia trachomatis* infection in the female. *J Infect* 1992;25(suppl 1):39–45.
6. Grimes DA, Cates W Jr. Family planning and sexually transmitted diseases. In: Holmes KK, Mardh P-A, Sparling PF, et al., eds. *Sexually transmitted diseases,* 2nd ed. New York: McGraw-Hill, 1990:1087–1095.
7. Thylefors B. Development of trachoma control programs and the involvement of natural resources. *Rev Infect* Dis 1985; 7(6):774–776.
8. Forbes BA, Sahm DF, Weissfeld AS. In: *Bailey and Scott's diagnostic microbiology,* 10th ed, New York: Mosby, 1998:751–765.
9. Jones R. *Chlamydia trachomatis.* In: Mandell GR, Bennett JE, Dolin R, eds. *Principles and practice of infectious diseases,* 4th ed. New York: Churchill Livingstone, 1995:1680.
10. Hansfield HH, Pollock PS. Arthritis associated with sexually transmitted diseases. In: Holmes KK, Cates W, Jr., Stamm WE, Lemon SM, eds. *Sexually transmitted diseases,* 2nd ed. New York: McGraw-Hill, 1990:737–751.
11. Relman DA. The identification of uncultured microbial pathogens. *J Infect Dis* 1993;168(1):1–8.
12. Pastemack R, Vuorinen P, Kuukankorpi A, et al. Detection of *Chlamydia trachomatis* infections in women by Amplicor PCR: comparison of diagnostic performance with urine and cervical specimens. *J Clin Microbiol* 1996;34(4):995–998.
13. Chernesky MA, Jang D, Lee H, et al. Diagnosis of *Chlamydia trachomatis* infections in men and women by testing first-void urine by ligase chain reaction. *J Clin Microbiol* 1994;32(11):2682–2685.
14. Paavonen J, Puolakkainen M, Paukku M, et al. Cost-benefit analysis of first-void urine *Chlamydia trachomatis* screening program. *Obstet Gynecol* 1998;92:292–298.

15. Mattila A, Miettinen A, Heinomen PK, et al. Detection of serum antibodies to *Chlamydia trachomatis* in patients with chlamydial and nonchlamydial pelvic inflammatory disease by the IPAzyme *Chlamydia* and enzyme immunoassay. *J Clin Microbiol* 1993; 31(4),998–1000.

16. Sarov I, Kleinman D, Holcberg G, et al. Specific IgG and IgA antibodies to *Chlamydia trachomatis* in infertile women. *Int J Fertil* 1986;31(3):193–197.

17. Martin DH, Mroczkowsli TF, Dalu ZA, et al. A controlled trial of a single dose of azithromycin for the treatment of chlamydial urethritis and cervicitis. *N Engl J Med* 1992;327(13):921–925.

18. Worm AM, Osterlind A. Azithromycin levels in cervical mucus and plasma after a single 1-g oral dose for chlamydial cervicitis. *Genitourin Med* 1995;71(4):244–246.

19. Gencay M, Koskiniemi M, Saikku P, et al. *Chlamydia trachomatis* seropositivity during pregnancy is associated with perinatal complications. *Clin Infect Dis* 1995;21(2):424–426.

20. Washington AE, Johnson RE, Sanders LL Jr. *Chlamydia trachomatis* infections in the United States. What are they costing us? *JAMA* 1987;257(15):2070–2072.

21. Jensen IP, Thorsen P, Moller BR. Sensitivity of ligase chain reaction assay of urine from pregnant women for *Chlamydia trachomatis*. *Lancet* 1997;349:329–330.

22. Bush MR, Rosa C. Azithromycin and erythromycin in the treatment of cervical chlamydial infection during pregnancy. *Obstet Gynecol* 1994;84(1):61–63.

23. Knapp JS, Koumans EH. *Neisseria* and *Branhamella*. In: Murray PR, ed. *Manual of clinical microbiology*, 7th ed. Washington, DC: American Society for Microbiology, 1999:506–603.

24. Gutman LT. Gonococcal infection. In: Remington JS, Klein JO, eds. *Infectious diseases of the fetus and newborn infant.* Philadelphia: WB Saunders, 1995.

25. Salyers AA, Whitt DD. *Bacterial pathogenesis: a molecular approach.* Washington, DC: ASM Press, 1994.

26. Handsfield HH, Sparling PF. *Neisseria gonorrhea*. In: Mandell, GL, Bennett JE, Dolin R, eds. *Principles and practice of infectious diseases.* Vol. 2. Philadelphia: Churchill Livingstone 2000: 2242–2256.

27. Sng EH, Rajan VS, Yeo KL, et al. The recovery of *Neisseria gonorrhea* from clinical specimens: effects of different temperatures, transport times, and media. *Sex Transm Dis* 1982;9:74–78.

28. Iwen PC, Walker RA, Warren KL, et al. Evaluation of the nucleic acid-based test (PACE 2C) for simultaneous detection of *Chlamydia trachomatis* and *Neisseria gonorrhoeae* in endocervical specimens. *J Clin Microbiol* 1995;33(10):2587–2591.

29. Stary A, Ching S, Teodorowicz L, et al. Comparison of ligase chain reaction and culture for detection of *Neisseria gonorrhoeae* in genital and extragenital specimens. *J Clin Microbiol* 1997; 35(1):239–242.

30. Ching S, Lee H, Hook EW III, et al. Ligase chain reaction for detection of Neisseria gonorrhea in urogenital swabs. *J Clin Microbiol* 1995;33(12):3111–3114.

31. Birkenmeyer L, Armstrong AS. Preliminary evaluation of the ligase chain reaction for specific detection of *Neisseria gonorrhoeae.* *J Clin Microbiol* 1992;30(12):3089–3094.

32. Mehaffey PC, Putnam SD, Barret MS, et al. Evaluation of in vitro spectra of activity of azithromycin, clarithromycin, and erythromycin tested against strains of *Neisseria gonorrhoeae* by reference agar dilution disk diffusion and E-test methods. *J Clin Microbiol* 1996;34(2):479–481.

33. Kampmeier RH. Description of *Trichomonas vaginalis* by M. A. Donne. *Sex Transm Dis* 1978;5(3):119–122.

34. Rein MF. *Trichomonas vaginalis*. In: Mandell GL, Douglas RG Jr, Bennett JE, et al., eds. *Principles and practice of infectious diseases,* 4th ed. New York: Churchill Livingstone, 1995:2497.

35. Wawer MJ, McNairn D, Wabwire-Mergen F, et al. Self-adminis-

tered vaginal swabs for population-based assessment of *Trichomonas vaginalis* prevalence. *Lancet* 1995;345(8942):131–132.

36. Judson FN. The importance of coexisting syphilitic, chlamydial, mycoplasmal, and trichomonal infections in the treatment of gonorrhea. *Sex Transm Dis* 1979;6(suppl 2):112–119.

37. Wasserheit JN, Homes KK. Reproductive tract infections: challenges for international health policy, programs, and research. In: Germain A, Holmes KK, Piot P, et al., eds. *Reproductive tract infections: global impact and priorities for women's reproductive health.* New York: Plenum Press, 1992:27–33.

38. Pindak FF, dePindak MM, Hyde BM, et al. Acquisition and retention of viruses by *Trichomonas vaginalis*. *Genitourin Med* 1989;65(6):366–371.

39. Laga M, Manoka A, Kivuvu M, et al. Non ulcerative sexually transmitted diseases as risk factors for HIV-1 transmission in women: results from a cohort study. *AIDS* 1993;7(1):95–102.

40. Krieger JN, Wolner-Hanssen P, Stevens C, et al. Characteristics of *Trichomonas vaginalis* isolates from women with and without colpitis macularis. *J Infect Dis* 1990;161(2):307–311.

41. Lossick JG, Kent HL. Trichomoniasis: trends in diagnosis and management. *Am J Obstet Gynecol* 1991;165(4 part 2):1217–1222.

42. Borchardt KA, Zhang MZ, Shing H. A comparison on the sensitivity of the InPouch, Diamonds, and Trichosel media for detection of Trichomonas vaginalis. American Society for Microbiology, New Orleans, LA, abst. 721, 1996.

43. Sokol DM, Garry RF. In: Borchardt KA, Noble MA, eds. *Sexually transmitted diseases—epidemiology, pathology, diagnosis, and treatment.* New York: CRC Press, 1997:217–294.

44. Larsen B. *Basic science monograph in obstetrics and gynecology,* 2nd ed. 1998:264–265.

45. Johnson RE, Nahmias AJ, Magder LS, et al. A seroepidemiologic survey of the prevalence of herpes simplex virus type 2 infection in the United States. *N Engl J Med* 1989;32:7.

46. Corey L, Spear P. Infections with herpes simplex viruses. *N Engl J Med* 1986;314:686.

47. Benedetti J, Corey L, Ashley R, Recurrence rates of genital herpes after acquisition of symptomatic first-episode infection. *Ann Intern Med* 1994;121:847–854.

48. Forbes BA, Sahm DF, Weissfeld AS, eds, in: *Bailey and Scott's diagnostic microbiology,* 10th ed, New York: Mosby, 1998:963–1028.

49. Corey L. In: Rein MF, ed. *Atlas of Infectious Diseases,* vol 5. Philadelphia: Churchill Livingstone, 1996, Chapter 15.

50. Domingue GD. In: Borchardt KA, Noble MA, eds. *Sexually transmitted diseases—epidemiology, pathology, diagnosis, and treatment.* New York: CRC Press, 1997:131–146.

51. Hook EW III, Marra CM. Acquired syphilis in adults. *N Engl J Med* 1992;326(16):1060–1069.

52. Forbes BA, Sahm DF, Weissfeld AS. In: *Bailey and Scott's diagnostic microbiology,* 10th ed, New York: Mosby, 1998:775–782. Tramont EC. Syphilis in adults: from Christopher Columbus to Sir Alexander Fleming to AIDS. *Clin Infect Dis* 1995; 21(6):1361–1369.

54. Fiumara NJ. In: Rein MF, ed. *Atlas of infectious diseases,* vol 5. Philadelphia: Churchill Livingstone, 1996:9–16.

55. Larsen SA. In: Rein MF, ed. *Atlas of infectious diseases,* vol 5. Philadelphia: Churchill Livingstone, 1996:9–16.

56. Gjestland T. The Oslo study of untreated syphilis. *Acta Derm Venereol (Stockh)* 1955;35(suppl 34):1–368.

57. Larsen SA, Steiner BM, Rudolph AH. Laboratory diagnosis and interpretation of tests for syphilis. *Clin Microbiol Rev* 1995; 8(1):1–21.

58. Schulte JM, Martich F, Schmid GP. Chancroid in the United States 1981–90: a case for underreporting. *MMWR* 1992; 41(SS-3):57–61.

59. Schmid GP. Approach to the patient with genital ulcer disease. *Med Clin North Am* 1990;74:1559–1572.

60. Joseph AK, Rosen T. Laboratory techniques used in the diagnosis of chancroid, granuloma inguinale, and lymphogranuloma venereum. *Dermatol Clin* 1994;12(1):1–8.

61. Passos MRL, Filho JT, Barreto NA. In: Borchardt KA, Noble MA eds. *Sexually transmitted diseases—epidemiology, pathology, diagnosis, and treatment.* New York: CRC Press, 1997:103–116.

62. Krowchuk DP, Anglin TM. Genital human papillomavirus infections in adolescents: implications for evaluation and management. *Semin Dermatol* 1992;11:24–30.

63. Zhang MZ, Borchardt KA, Li Z. In: Borchardt KA, Noble MA. eds. *Sexually transmitted diseases—epidemiology, pathology, diagnosis, and treatment.* New York: CRC Press, 1997: 271–282.

64. Division of STD/HIV Prevention. *Sexually transmitted disease surveillance,* 1992. Atlanta: Centers for Disease Control and Prevention, 1993:28.

65. Reid R. In: Rein MF. ed. *Atlas of infectious diseases,* vol 5. Philadelphia: Churchill Livingstone, 1996:Chapter 12.

66. Reid R, Dorsey JH. Physical and surgical principles of carbon dioxide laser surgery in the lower genital tract. In: Coppleson M, ed. *Gynecologic oncology,* 2nd ed. Edinburgh: Churchill Livingstone, 1992:1087–1131.

67. ACOG Technical Bulletin. *Genital human papillomavirus infections.* 1994;193.

68. Munoz N, Bosch FX, Shah KV, et al. *The epidemiology of human papillomavirus and cervical cancer.* IARC science publication 119. Lyons, France: International Agency for Research on Cancer 1992:3–23.

69. Schiffman MH. Recent progress in defining the epidemiology of human papillomavirus infection and cervical neoplasia. *J Natl Cancer Inst* 1992;84:394–398.

70. Johnson TL, Kim W, Plieth DA, et al. Detection of HPV 16/18 DNA in cervical adenocarcinoma using polymerase chain reaction (PCR) methodology. *Mod Pathol* 1992;5:35–40.

71. DeBritton RC, Hildesheim A, De Lao SL, et al. Human papillomaviruses and other influences on survival from cervical cancer in Panama. *Obstet Gynecol* 1993;81:19–24.

72. Crum CP. Carcinoma of the vulva: epidemiology and pathogenesis. *Obstet Gynecol* 1992;79:448–454.

73. Brown DR, Fife KH. Human papillomavirus infection of the genital tract. *Med Clin North Am* 1990;74(6):1455.

74. Koutsky LA. Human papillomavirus testing for triage of women with cytologic evidence of low-grade squamous intraepithelial lesions: baseline date from a randomized trial. *J Natl cancer Inst* 2000;92:397–402.

75. Montaner JSG, O'Shaughnessy MV, Schechter MT. Infection with the human immunodeficiency virus and the acquired immunodeficiency syndrome. In: Borchardt KA, Noble MA eds. *Sexually transmitted diseases—epidemiology, pathology, diagnosis, and treatment.* New York: CRC Press, 1997:245–269.

76. Center for Disease Control. AIDS in women—United States. *MMWR* 1990:39:845–846.

77. National Center for Health Statistics. *Annual summary of births, marriages, divorces, and deaths: United States, 1994.* Monthly vital statistics report, vol 43, no 13. Hyattsville, MD: Department of Health and Human Services, Public Health Service, 1994.

78. Larsen B. *Viral infection in obstetrics and gynecology. Basic science monograph in obstetrics and gynecology,* 2nd ed. The American College of Obstetricians & Gynecologists, Washington, D.C., 1998:229–236.

79. Centers for Disease Control and Prevention. First 500,000 AIDS cases—United States, 1995. *MMWR* 1995;44:849–853.

80. Maury W, Pott NJ, Rabson AB. HIV infection of first-trimester and term human placental tissue: a possible mode of maternal-fetal transmission. *J Infect Dis* 1989;160:583–588.

81. Center for Disease Control. Public Health Service guidelines for counseling and antibody testing to prevent HIV infection and AIDS. *MMWR* 1987;36:509–515.

82. O'Brien WA, Hartigan PM, Martin D, et al. Changes in plasma HIV-1 RNA and CD4+ lymphocyte count relative to treatment and progression to AIDS. *N Engl J Med* 1996;334:426–431.

83. Carpenter CCJ, Fischl MA, Hammer SM, et al. Antiretroviral therapy for HIV infection in 1996. Recommendations of an international panel. *JAMA* 1996;276(2):146–154.

84. Stoto MA, Almario DA, McCormick MC, eds. *Reducing the odds preventing perinatal transmission of HIV in the United States.* Washington, DC: National Academy Press, 1999:45–53.

85. Connor EM, Sperling RS, Gelber R, et al. Reduction of maternal-infant transmission of human immunodeficiency virus type 1 with zidovudine treatment. Pediatric AIDS Clinical Trials Group Protocol 076 Study Group. *N Engl J Med* 1994;331(18):1173–1180.

86. Mofenson L. Advances in HIV prevention: prevention of perinatal HIV transmission. Presented at the Fifth Conference on Retroviruses and Opportunistic Infection, Chicago, February 1–5, 1998.

87. Center for Disease Control. Public Health Service recommendations for the use of antiretroviral drugs in pregnant women infected with HIV-1 for maternal health and for reducing perinatal HIV-1 transmission in the United States. *MMWR* 1998; 47:31.

88. Mandelbrot L, Le Cheandec J, Berrebi A, et al. Perinatal HIV-1 transmission: interaction between zidovudine prophylaxis and mode of delivery in the French Perinatal Cohort. *JAMA* 1998; 280:55–60.

89. Read JS. The mode of delivery and the risk of vertical transmission of human immunodeficiency virus type I. A meta-analysis of 15 prospective cohort studies. *N Engl J Med* 1999;340:977–987.

90. Parazzini F. Elective caesarean-section versus vaginal delivery in prevention of vertical HIV-1 transmission: a randomised clinical trial. The European Mode of Delivery Collaboration. *Lancet* 1999;353:1035–1039.

91. ACOG Committee on Obstetric Practice. Schedule cesarean delivery and the prevention of vertical transmission of HIV infection. The Amercian College of Obstetricians & Gynecologists, Washington, D.C., 2000: committee opinion, no. 234.

UROGYNECOLOGY

NEERAJ KOHLI

Urogynecology is the study of the female urogenital tract with emphasis on anatomy and pathophysiology. The evaluation and management of urinary incontinence are emphasized. *Urinary incontinence,* defined as the involuntary loss of urine that is objectively demonstrable and a social or hygienic problem, is a condition that affects approximately 13 million persons in the United States in community and institutional settings. Despite the prevalence of this condition and an estimated annual direct cost of more than $15 billion, most affected persons do not seek help for incontinence primarily because of embarrassment or because they are not aware that help is available (1). Urinary incontinence has a profound psychosocial impact on persons, their families, and caregivers. It can result in loss of self-esteem, social isolation, sexual dysfunction, and a decrease in ability to maintain an independent lifestyle. When patients do seek help, many clinicians are hesitant or inexperienced to discuss, diagnose, or treat the problem. Urinary incontinence is expected to continue to be a significant health care problem in the elderly and institutionalized populations and to increase as the population continues to age. Fortunately, awareness of this health care issue is growing, as more media attention is given to the condition. The following chapter reviews the pathophysiology, diagnosis, and office management of urinary incontinence.

EPIDEMIOLOGY OF INCONTINENCE

Although demographic surveys report that urinary incontinence affects 10% to 35% of adults and at least half of the 1.5 million nursing home residents in the United States, this number is most likely underweighted, because many patients who suffer from this condition are reluctant to report the problem to their health care provider as a result of embarrassment and social stigma. Although the prevalence of urinary incontinence increases with age, the condition should not be considered a normal part of the aging process. Among the population between 15 and 64 years of age, the prevalence of urinary incontinence ranges between 1.5% and 5% in men and from 10% to 30% in women (2). Incontinence is two to three times more common among women than men, primarily because of gender-specific risk factors such as childbirth

and menopause, which adversely affect pelvic support structures and result in stress urinary incontinence. Although urinary incontinence is commonly regarded as a condition affecting older, multiparous women, it is also common in young, nulliparous women, and is particularly associated with strenuous physical exercise.

In the elderly population, urinary incontinence can affect 15% to 30% of women older than 60 years of age and more than 50% of nursing home residents (3). It is one of the major causes of institutionalization of the elderly in the United States even though one-third of all cases may result from transient factors that may be readily treatable or may undergo spontaneous remission. Appropriate diagnosis and management of urinary incontinence in the elderly by the primary care provider can have a profound impact on quality of life and may prevent the need for subsequent nursing home admission. The economic impact of urinary incontinence has been scarcely reported because of the inability to obtain reliable prevalence, risk factor, and cost data, and because of wide diversification of treatment modalities. Recent data, estimated at more than $15 billion annually, do not consider indirect costs such as loss of productivity from morbidity or mortality and time costs of unpaid caregivers who treat and care for incontinent patients. As public awareness of this condition continues to increase, it is expected that the financial costs of treating this disorder will also rise proportionately. Unfortunately, most of these expenditures have been directed toward control measures rather than cure options, and the result has been minimal improvement. Of the reported $15 billion spent annually on this disorder, only 1% of this amount is spent on the diagnosis and permanent treatment of this disorder, whereas 60% is spent on palliative measures (4). Since that study, greater emphasis has been placed on prevention and appropriate diagnosis, to lead to more effective treatment modalities and better overall outcomes.

Because of the increased incidence of incontinence, studies have shown that an effective prevention program would result in a reduction of approximately 50,000 cases annually (5). Reversible conditions or risk factors associated with incontinence are presented in Table 21.1. Although no controlled clinical trial data exist to support that risk factor interventions would result in a significant reduction of the

TABLE 21.1. REVERSIBLE CAUSES AND RISK FACTORS FOR URINARY INCONTINENCE

Immobility or chronic degenerative disease
Impaired cognition
Medications
Morbid obesity
Diuretics
Smoking
Fecal impaction
Delirium
Low fluid intake
Environmental barriers
High-impact physical activities
Diabetes mellitus
Stroke
Estrogen deprivation
Pelvic muscle weakness
Childhood nocturnal enuresis
Race
Pregnancy, vaginal delivery, or episiotomy

incidence, severity, or prevalence of incontinence, these programs are easy to institute and may result in other medically related benefits. These include weight loss and smoking cessation programs, control of hypertension and diabetes, maintenance on estrogen replacement therapy and pelvic muscle exercise programs, and alteration or adjustment of current medications. Patient education and routine follow-up are the cornerstones of an effective risk reduction program with regard to urinary incontinence.

ANATOMY AND PHYSIOLOGY OF THE NORMAL CONTINENCE MECHANISM

The exact mechanism of continence in the healthy adult is incompletely understood. Current concepts emphasize a complex interaction between the bladder and urethra dependent on intact enervation and anatomic support of the bladder neck, especially in women. The bladder is a muscular organ with two primary functions, bladder storage at rest and bladder emptying during contraction. Both phases are regulated by the autonomic nervous system with sympathetic enervation from T-10 to L-2 coming through the hypogastric nerve and parasympathetic enervation coming from S-2 to S-3 through the pelvic plexus. This system can be modulated by somatic nerves that innervate the pelvic floor and external urethral sphincter.

Disorders that affect bladder storage (filling phase) cause urinary incontinence, whereas disorders of emptying (voiding phase) cause voiding dysfunction and urinary retention. In some patients, especially women, abnormalities during filling and voiding may coexist. Because urinary incontinence is primarily related to the storage phase, a detailed description of the physiology of normal micturition (voiding phase) is beyond the scope of this chapter.

The mechanism of *continence* is complex. At rest, the bladder is a muscular reservoir that holds increasing volumes of urine while maintaining a low, resting pressure (accommodation) because of compliance of the bladder wall. Simultaneous sympathetic stimulation of β-adrenergic receptors within the bladder wall and inhibition of parasympathetic activity cause detrusor relaxation. Continence is maintained by a high resting pressure in the urethra at the urethrovesical junction (bladder neck) as a result of the musculature of the internal and external urethral sphincter, mucosal coaptation of the urethral lumen, and sympathetic stimulation of α-adrenergic receptors in the urethra (Fig. 21.1).

During increases in intraabdominal pressure, the pressure gradient between the bladder and the urethra is maintained by equal transmission of pressure to the bladder and proximal urethra to ensure continence. In women, the external urethral sphincter and levator ani muscle complex serve as a secondary continence mechanism by a reflex contraction with resulting bladder neck closure during increased abdominal pressure. In addition, the vagina, slung like a hammock below the urethra by its lateral fascial attachments, functions as a backboard against which the bladder neck is compressed during Valsalva maneuvers. During micturition, a coordinated change in the pressure relationship between the bladder (detrusor muscle) and urethra occurs. Voiding is initiated by voluntary relaxation of the pelvic musculature and urethral sphincter followed by a detrusor contraction mediated by parasympathetic cholinergic receptors in the bladder. With an increase in bladder pressure and a decrease in urethral pressure, the pressure gradient favors micturition, and bladder emptying occurs.

Urinary incontinence may result from abnormal increases in bladder pressure or decreases in urethral pressure that alter the low bladder pressure–high urethral pressure relationship that maintains continence at rest. Abnormal increases in bladder pressure are primarily caused by spontaneous detrusor contractions (detrusor instability) with a reflex relaxation of the urethral sphincter that results in urinary leakage. Increased bladder pressure may also be caused by overfilling of the bladder beyond its capacity and compliance resulting in overflow incontinence. Abnormal

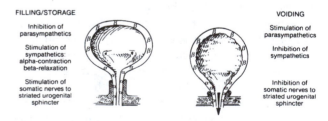

FIGURE 21.1. Physiologic basis of storage and voiding based on characteristic distribution of sympathetic and parasympathetic receptors. (From Walten MD, Karran MM. *Clinical urogynecology.* St. Louis: Mosby–Year Book, 1993:1–19, with permission.)

decreases in urethral pressure may be static or dynamic. A decrease in resting urethral tone can be caused by injury to the sphincter enervation or musculature (intrinsic sphincter deficiency). Abnormal bladder neck function in dynamic states of increased abdominal pressure or Valsalva maneuver is seen in female patients with genuine stress incontinence. With relaxation of the pelvic floor musculature and fascial supports, the proximal urethra exhibits rotational descent outside the zone of abdominal pressure transmission and no longer has a fixed backboard for mechanical compression. As a result, increases in intraabdominal pressure cause only elevated intravesical pressure, which overcomes the resting intraurethral pressure and results in loss of urine.

An adequate understanding of the normal continence mechanism and of specific abnormalities resulting in urinary incontinence is critical in determining the underlying origin and in formulating an effective treatment plan. Diagnostic evaluation is based on understanding normal bladder function at rest and on assessing the lower urinary tract within these parameters.

CLASSIFICATION OF URINARY INCONTINENCE

Urinary incontinence is a symptom, a sign, and a condition. The International Continence Society created a classification of urinary incontinence (6). Accurate diagnosis of the type of incontinence determines the appropriate treatment plan.

Genuine stress incontinence is the involuntary loss of urine that occurs when, in the absence of a detrusor contraction, the intravesical pressure exceeds the maximum urethral pressure. It is most common in women who typically complain of urinary leakage with cough, exercise, laughing, Valsalva maneuver, and other activities that increase intraabdominal pressure. Patients with severe stress incontinence may report constant leakage with minimal exertion. Genuine stress incontinence results from urethral hypermobility or intrinsic sphincter deficiency. Urethral hypermobility, the most common cause of genuine stress incontinence, occurs when the anatomic support of the bladder neck is lost and allows the proximal urethra to be displaced outside the abdominal pressure zone during straining. McGuire et al. classified subtypes I, IIA, and IIB, depending on the amount of descent of the bladder base at rest and with straining (7). This damage to the bladder neck supports may be the result of pregnancy and vaginal delivery, tissue atrophy that results from advancing age and estrogen withdrawal, or continuous stressors such as obesity and chronic coughing. With intrinsic sphincter deficiency, the urethra exhibits decreased resting tone and no longer functions as a sphincter. Even at rest, it loses the ability to maintain a normal continence mechanism. More common in women, this condition is often associated with a history of pelvic radiation, previous antiincontinence surgery, advancing age, and denervation injuries resulting in overt disruption of the sphincteric musculature. These patients most commonly demonstrate a fixed, rigid urethral tube with a nonfunctioning sphincter (lead pipe urethra or type III incontinence). In men, this condition is most often associated with urethral damage that occurs after transurethral resection of the prostate.

Potential stress incontinence can occur in women with advanced pelvic prolapse. These patients initially have loss of bladder neck support and resulting incontinence. Continued prolapse of the anterior vaginal wall results in kinking of the urethra with improvement of incontinent episodes but incomplete bladder emptying. Subsequent reduction of the prolapse with a pessary or surgery without concurrent bladder neck support results in reestablishment of the incontinence symptoms.

Urge incontinence is defined as the involuntary loss of urine associated with a sudden and strong desire to void (urgency). Normal micturition is under voluntary control. Spontaneous uninhibited detrusor overactivity can result in detrusor contractions with reflex urethral relaxation and urinary incontinence. Overactive detrusor function in the absence of a known neurologic abnormality is called *detrusor instability;* overactivity caused by its disturbance of the nervous control mechanisms is termed *detrusor hyperreflexia.* Patients with this condition complain of an inability to control voiding and experience sudden urgency to void that is sometimes insuppressible. These patients commonly report coexisting urinary frequency (more than seven times per day), nocturia (more than once per night) enuresis, and, occasionally, pelvic pain. Although detrusor instability is most often iatrogenic, secondary causes include urinary tract infection, antiincontinence surgery, bladder stones or foreign bodies, and bladder cancer. Suburethral diverticulum, an outpouching of the urethral mucosa, can also occasionally present with irritative bladder symptoms such as urgency and frequency.

Detrusor hyperreflexia with impaired contractility is a rare disorder that may occur in some patients, especially the elderly or patients with neurologic lesions. This paradoxic condition is characterized by detrusor overactivity in combination with decreased detrusor contractility. These patients present with urge incontinence in combination with urinary retention. Diagnosis is difficult because this disorder can mimic other types of incontinence and usually requires complex multichannel urodynamic testing.

Mixed incontinence, a condition characterized by coexisting stress incontinence and urge incontinence, is one of the most common types of incontinence in patients presenting to their primary care physicians. It typically results from compensatory responses that the stress-incontinent patient self-initiates. Once the initial symptom of stress incontinence is noted, the patient begins to urinate frequently to maintain a low residual of urine in the bladder and to minimize the risk of further episodes of stress-related incontinence. As the condition worsens, the degree of urinary frequency increases, and the bladder accommodates to a lower capacity. When the bladder distends beyond its now reduced capacity, the patient experiences sensory urgency or detrusor instability with or without associated urinary leakage and irritative symptoms such as frequency, urgency, and nocturia. Often, however, one symptom, stress, or urge is more bothersome to the patient than the other, and therapeutic intervention is based on the predominant symptom.

Overflow incontinence is the uncontrollable loss of urine associated with overdistention of the bladder. This is usually caused by an underactive or acontractile detrusor or bladder outlet or urethral obstruction leading to overdistention and overflow. Failure of the bladder to empty adequately with large postvoid residuals may by idiopathic, but it is usually found in conjunction with drugs, diabetic neuropathy, spinal cord injury, or radical pelvic surgery that causes denervation of the detrusor muscle. In men, overflow incontinence is associated with obstruction from prostatic hypertrophy or urethral stricture. In women, it can be associated with advanced pelvic prolapse that causes bladder outlet obstruction from kinking of the bladder neck. Increased bladder capacities with a large postvoid residual urine volume clarify the diagnosis.

Other types of incontinence are less common but should be considered in the appropriate clinical context. *Functional incontinence* refers to urine loss that results from factors outside the urinary tract such as chronic impairment of physical or cognitive functioning. This type of incontinence is typically found in the elderly immobile nursing home resident. *Reflex incontinence* is the loss of urine from detrusor hyperreflexia, involuntary urethral relaxation, or both in the absence of the sensation usually associated with the desire to void. This condition is most commonly seen in patients with neuropathic bladder or urethral dysfunction resulting from neurologic injury. *Transient and reversible causes* of incontinence are often identified, particularly in elderly patients. A useful mnemonic for common reversible causes of incontinence is *D I A P P E R S*—delirium, infection, atrophic urethritis, pharmaceuticals, psychologic factors, endocrine disorders, restricted mobility, and stool impaction. Often, treatment of the inciting factor results in immediate cure of urinary leakage. Extraurethral causes of incontinence should be included in the differential diagnosis. This is particularly relevant for women with a history of pelvic surgery, radiation, or obstetric delivery. Causes include urinary fistulas (ureterovaginal, vesicovaginal, or urethrovaginal), ectopic ureter, and urethral diverticulum. A detailed pelvic examination is required for diagnosis.

EVALUATION OF URINARY INCONTINENCE

The evaluation of patients with urinary incontinence is directed toward (a) clarifying a patient's symptoms, (b)

objectively documenting loss of urine, (c) determining the cause of the incontinence, and (d) identifying patients who require further consultation and complex testing. Most patients can be appropriately diagnosed and managed in the primary care setting, and few require outside referrals unless they have a complex condition or desire surgical correction. A step-by-step diagnostic algorithm that includes a history, physical examination, and appropriate office testing is useful in the evaluation of the incontinent patient (Fig. 21.2).

Accurate diagnosis of urinary incontinence begins with a careful review of the patient's history. The history should focus on the duration, characteristics, and severity of the incontinence, with particular attention to precipitating factors and reversible causes. Cystitis, foreign body, or tumor should be suspected in patients with acute onset of symptoms, whereas chronic causes such as urethral hypermobility, intrinsic sphincter deficiency, and idiopathic detrusor instability should be considered for long-standing complaints. Concurrent lower urinary tract symptoms (i.e., dysuria, urgency, pelvic pain, dyspareunia) as well as symptoms related to the gastrointestinal tract (i.e., constipation, fecal incontinence) and genital tract (i.e., pelvic prolapse, abnormal vaginal discharge) should also be discussed. Objective assessment of the patient's incontinence using a bladder diary is recommended. We routinely ask patients to keep a 2-day record of fluid intake, voids, and incontinent episodes with precipitating events before their first visit. This record

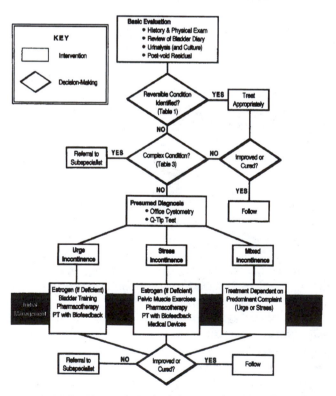

FIGURE 21.2. Diagnosis and treatment algorithm for urinary incontinence for the primary care provider in the office setting.

is subsequently reviewed with the patient to assess whether the patient will benefit from behavioral or dietary modification such as increased fluid intake, change in voiding pattern, or dietary restriction. A detailed medical and surgical history should be obtained to rule out conditions such as diabetes, thyroid disease, spinal cord injury, cerebral vascular accidents, urethral sphincter damage, or fistula. Because incontinence increases with advanced age, a detailed drug history is particularly important given that many of these elderly patients are taking multiple medications. Various medications can induce urinary incontinence directly by acting on the bladder or urethra or indirectly by mechanisms such as inducing cough or pelvic muscle relaxation. Pharmacotherapy may induce any of the subtypes of urinary incontinence previously discussed (Table 21.2). In women, estrogen status should be determined because hypoestrogenism can contribute to recurrent cystitis, detrusor instability, and stress incontinence. Patients should also be questioned about a history of recurrent urinary tract infection, kidney stones, bladder pain, or hematuria (8).

After a general physical examination and mental status assessment, clinical evaluation of the lower urinary tract should begin with a detailed neurologic examination of the perineum and lower extremities. Normal sensation in the perineal dermatomes and the back of the leg confirms intact sensory enervation of the lower urinary tract. Sacral reflex activity is tested by two reflexes. In the anal reflex, stroking the skin adjacent to the anus causes reflex contraction of the external anal sphincter, whereas the sacral (bulbocavernosus) reflex involves contraction of the bulbocavernosus and ischiocavernosus muscles in response to tapping or squeezing of the clitoris. Pelvic floor muscle tone can be assessed by voluntary contraction of the anal sphincter and vagina during a bimanual examination.

In women, a pelvic examination should be performed to assess the external genitalia, perineal sensation, presence of pelvic organ prolapse (cystocele, rectocele, uterine prolapse), estrogen status, and pelvic muscle strength. During inspection, particular attention should be given to the assessment and grading of pelvic organ prolapse to rule out urethral hypermobility and potential stress incontinence. A bimanual examination including a rectovaginal examination should be done to rule out pelvic masses compressing the bladder. In men, a rectal examination should be performed to test for perineal sensation or a rectal mass and to evaluate the consistency and size of the prostate.

The patient should be examined with a full bladder so observation of urine loss can be performed by having the patient cough vigorously, either in the standing or supine position. If instantaneous leakage occurs with cough, stress urinary incontinence is likely, whereas urge incontinence (detrusor instability) should be considered with delayed or sustained leakage. In women, urethral hypermobility resulting from the loss of bladder neck support can most easily be assessed using a simple cotton swab test. A sterile, lubricated cotton swab is inserted transurethrally into the bladder and then is withdrawn slowly until definite resistance is felt, indicating that the cotton swab is at the bladder neck. The resting angle of the cotton swab in relation to the horizontal is measured, the patient is then asked to cough or to perform a Valsalva maneuver, and the maximum straining angle from the horizontal is measured. Although no standardized data are available to differentiate abnormal from normal measurements, most clinicians have adopted a 30-degree deflection as a cutoff for urethral hypermobility.

Initial diagnostic testing should include a postvoid residual to rule out overflow incontinence and incomplete bladder emptying and a urinalysis or urine culture to rule out urinary tract infection. After a normal void, a postvoid residual urine volume is determined using catheterization or bladder scan. Although values for normal bladder emptying may vary with age, a postvoid residual should be less than 25% of the total bladder volume and less than 100 mL. Patients with high postvoid residual measurement may experience overflow incontinence. A catheterized sample of urine should be obtained for urinalysis or urine culture. Clean catch urine specimens are routinely contaminated and do not provide accurate data with regard to urinary tract infection. Cystitis is the leading cause of acute urinary incontinence in younger women. Based on initial evaluation and testing, a preliminary diagnosis can be made. Further office testing such as simple cystometry can be performed at the time of the initial examination, or it may be reserved for subsequent visits. It is an inexpensive test that is easy to perform and provides important initial data; it should be done at the initial evaluation. In addition, it allows simultaneous measurement of a postvoid residual and collection of a catheterized urine specimen.

Cystometry is used to measure the pressure volume relationship of the bladder as it distends and contracts and to determine abnormalities of the bladder with respect to

TABLE 21.2. MEDICATIONS CAUSING INCONTINENCE

Angiotensin-converting enzyme inhibitors	Anticholinergics
Enalapril	Hyoscyamine
Antiparkinsonism agents	Oxybutynin
Benztropine	Antihypertensives
Trihexyphenidyl	Prazosin
Benzodiazepines	Terazosin
Valium	α-Methyldopa
Bethanecol	Reserpine
Cisapride	Beta-blockers
Diuretics	Pindolol
Furosemide	Neuroleptics
Hydrochlorothiazide	Thioridazine
Disopyramide	Chlorpromazine
Alcohol	Haloperidol
Calcium-channel blockers	Clozapine
Verapamil	Over-the-counter cough preparations

detrusor activity, sensation, capacity, and compliance. Complex cystometry (multichannel urodynamics) uses specialized equipment with pressure catheters to record abdominal, bladder, and urethral pressures and to determine specific detrusor activity through subtracted calculations (Fig. 21.3). In contrast, simple cystometry can readily be performed in the office and requires a stopwatch, red rubber catheter, 50-mL syringe, and sterile water or saline. The patient should be initially evaluated with a full bladder. The patient is allowed to void normally in a private setting, and the time to void and amount of urine void are recorded. The patient then returns to the examination room, where a transurethral catheter is inserted into the bladder lumen to check a postvoid residual and to obtain a sterile urine specimen for urinalysis or culture. With the transurethral catheter in place, a 50-mL catheter tip syringe with its bulb removed is attached to the catheter and is held approximately 15 cm above the pubic symphysis. With the patient in the sitting or standing position, the bladder is filled by pouring sterile water or saline into the syringe at a medium fill rate while attempting to keep the water level in the syringe constant (Fig. 21.4). During bladder filling, the patient is asked to report first bladder sensation, initial urge to void, and maximum bladder capacity. Normal values are 100 to 200 mL, 200 to 400 mL, and 400 to 600 mL, respectively. Decreased bladder capacity suggests urgency-frequency syndromes and urge incontinence.

The water level is closely monitored during filling because a rise with or without associated urgency or urinary leakage may indicate an uninhibited bladder contraction suggesting detrusor instability. Unfortunately, rises in intravesical pressure may result from a detrusor contraction or Valsalva maneuver and therefore are not diagnostic of detrusor overactivity. It may be helpful to ask the patient to inspire during a noted rise in intravesical pressure, because women can rarely increase their intraabdominal pressure during

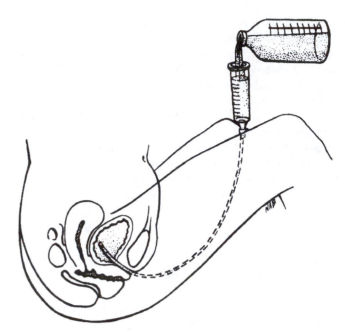

FIGURE 21.4. Simple office cystometry is performed with a catheter, syringe, and fluid.

inspiration. Once the bladder is filled to maximum capacity, the transurethral catheter is removed, and the patient is examined in the supine and standing positions. The patient is asked to perform provocative maneuvers such as coughing, heel jumping, and Valsalva maneuver. Urethral hypermobility and urinary leakage are evaluated. Loss of small amounts of urine simultaneous with cough suggests a diagnosis of stress incontinence. Prolonged loss of urine leaking 5 to 10 seconds after cough or no urine loss with provocation indicates that other causes of incontinence, especially detrusor instability, may be present (9). Patients with reduced bladder capacity with coexisting urge-related complaints most likely have underlying detrusor instability and should be treated accordingly.

Additional evaluation including blood testing, cystometry, and radiographic studies should be considered on an individualized basis. Blood testing including blood urea nitrogen, creatinine, glucose, and calcium determinations is recommended if compromised renal function is suspected or if polyuria is present. Urine cytology and cystoscopy are not necessary in the routine initial evaluation of the incontinent patient, but they may be helpful for patients with persistent symptoms or coexisting hematuria.

After a presumptive diagnosis has been made, the patient should be treated appropriately and reevaluated in 6 to 8 weeks. Referral to a subspecialist depends on various factors such as the clinician's experience and comfort level with the diagnosis and management of urinary incontinence, access to urodynamic testing equipment, and health care referral patterns. However, patients with significant pelvic prolapse and concurrent urinary tract symptoms, recurrent

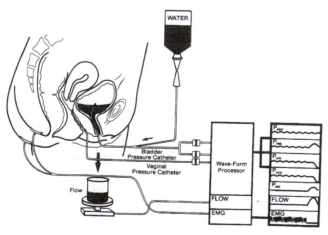

FIGURE 21.3. Complex multichannel urodynamics with pressure catheters allows precise determination of intraabdominal, intraurethral, and detrusor-urethral pressures.

TABLE 21.3. COMPLEX CONDITIONS REQUIRING FURTHER CONSULTATION OR TESTING

Complicated history
Office cystometry inconclusive
Frequency, urgency, and pain syndromes unresponsive to conservative therapy
Stress incontinence before surgical correction
Recurrent urinary loss after previous surgery for stress incontinence
Urge-related symptoms with gross or microscopic hematuria
Nocturnal enuresis unresponsive to previous therapy
Complaints of stress incontinence with absence of urethral hypermobility
Advanced pelvic prolapse before surgical correction
Coexisting neurologic disorders or diabetes mellitus
Urge incontinence unresponsive to previous therapy
Age over 65 yr
Continuous urinary leakage
Lower urinary tract dysfunction after pelvic radiation or radical pelvic surgery

incontinence, anatomic abnormalities, voiding dysfunction, and coexisting neurologic disorders may benefit from a urogynecologic or urologic consultation (Table 21.3). The role of the subspecialist should include comprehensive urodynamic testing, interpretation of these findings, and further management including surgery as appropriate.

TREATMENT OF URINARY INCONTINENCE

The appropriate treatment of urinary incontinence primarily depends on accurate diagnosis of the underlying cause. Patients with isolated urge incontinence (detrusor instability) are best treated with conservative treatment options including bladder retraining and pharmacologic therapy, with the primary goal of expanding bladder capacity to a functional level with resulting inhibition of spontaneous bladder spasms. Patients with detrusor instability refractory to first-line therapy may be candidates for polypharmacotherapy, biofeedback, psychotherapy, or functional electrical stimulation. Surgical treatment of refractory detrusor instability includes bladder distention, sacral neurectomy, and augmentation cystoplasty, but these procedures are associated with significant complications and have produced mixed results. Patients with isolated genuine stress incontinence, resulting from urethral hypermobility or intrinsic sphincter deficiency, may be candidates for conservative therapy including Kegel exercises, pharmacotherapy, physical therapy with biofeedback, electrical stimulation, or medical devices. We recommend an initial course of conservative therapy for all patients with follow-up assessment in 2 to 3 months. Surgery using traditional antiincontinence procedures should be considered for those patients who experience significantly persistent urinary leakage or those who desire surgical correction. Patients with mixed incontinence

should be initially offered a trial of conservative treatment consisting of Kegel exercises, bladder training, and pharmacotherapy, because improvement in the urge component of their incontinence may be sufficient to provide the patient with symptomatic relief and to alleviate the need for further intervention including surgery. Patients with a predominant stress component or persistence of their symptoms after a course of conservative therapy may warrant surgical correction. However, it should be clearly explained to these patients that the course of their detrusor instability is unpredictable after surgery, and it may worsen postoperatively (10). Patients with secondary causes of incontinence (reflex, overflow, functional, anatomic) should be treated on an individual basis. Patients with significant voiding dysfunction, anatomic abnormalities, and recurrent incontinence pose a challenging problem to the primary care provider. These patients often require additional testing or complex procedures, and urogynecologic or urologic consultation is recommended.

Behavioral Modification

Behavioral modification is useful in the treatment of many types of urinary incontinence and may include dietary restriction, toileting assistance, bladder retraining, and pelvic muscle rehabilitation. Patients with urge incontinence may benefit from dietary restriction of caffeine, alcohol, chocolate, and spicy food because these can all cause bladder irritation. Routine or scheduled toileting should be offered to incontinent patients on a consistent schedule and is recommended in the treatment of functional incontinence. The mainstay of treatment for urge and mixed incontinence is bladder training with pharmacotherapy. However, several reports demonstrate that bladder training is effective in reducing episodes of stress incontinence, although the exact origin of this effect is unclear (11). Bladder training (timed voiding) helps to distend the bladder progressively and allows the patient to be regain critical control over voiding patterns. The patient is instructed to void at preassigned times during the waking hours. The initial voiding interval is set at less than the patient's current voiding interval, and this is gradually increased on a weekly basis over an 8-week period. Patients are encouraged to try to suppress the sudden urge to void at times other than these designated intervals. Regular monitoring and positive reinforcement by review of the bladder diary provide continued feedback to the patient.

Pelvic muscle rehabilitation, or Kegel exercises, can reduce the severity of incontinent episodes by strengthening the pelvic muscles and reestablishing support to the bladder neck continence mechanism (12). Although pelvic muscle exercises are used predominantly in the treatment of stress urinary incontinence in women with poor pelvic supports and in men after prostatectomy, evidence indicates that this approach is also useful in patients with urge or mixed incontinence. Unfortunately, only 30% of women can perform pelvic floor exercises correctly after verbal instruction. We recommend simple biofeedback or referral to a physical therapist (13). Simple biofeedback can be performed in the office at the time of the bimanual examination with the clinician's asking the patient to squeeze her levator muscles while two fingers are placed in the vagina. Care must be given to discourage the patient from performing a Valsalva maneuver or tightening her gluteus muscles. Pelvic floor exercises can be enhanced using biofeedback with intravaginal pressure probes or mechanical devices such as graduated vaginal cone weights. A typical regimen of pelvic floor exercises is based on sets of short and long contractions performed two to four times daily. Under this regimen, patients with mild to moderate incontinence can expect 60% to 70% improvement in their symptoms (14).

Electrical stimulation has been shown to be effective in the treatment of stress, urge, and mixed incontinence. This treatment modality involves the use of nonimplantable vaginal or anal sensors or surface electrodes to stimulate a reflex arc in the sacral micturition center and to produce a contraction of the pelvic musculature and urethral sphincter with an accompanying reflex inhibition of the detrusor muscle. This treatment modality is especially useful in the patient who is unable to perform pelvic muscle exercises properly or in patients with an acontractile levator muscle. Electrical stimulation is usually given twice daily for 15 minutes and can be performed in the office or at home using a portable generator. Treatment should be continued for 8 to 12 weeks, depending on the underlying cause and on symptomatic improvement. Several studies addressing long-term follow-up after pelvic floor electrical stimulation have reported cure rates ranging from 54% to 77% (15).

Pharmacotherapy

Pharmacotherapy is the mainstay of the treatment of urge incontinence, but it can also be used for stress urinary incontinence as an adjunct to other nonsurgical modalities or in patients who do not desire surgical correction. Medica-

tions used in the treatment of urinary incontinence function by either relaxing the overactive detrusor muscle in women with urge incontinence or increasing urethral sphincter tone in patients with stress incontinence. Anticholinergic and antispasmodic agents are recommended as first-line pharmacologic therapy for patients with detrusor instability. These medications mediate the parasympathetic control of the bladder and treat detrusor instability by producing bladder relaxation. Commonly used medications are listed in Table 21.4. Oxybutynin has long been considered the primary anticholinergic agent of choice. It also has smooth muscle relaxant and local anesthetic properties. The recommended dose is 2.5 to 5 mg orally three to four times daily, but we find that many elderly patients experience significant side effects at this dosage. We routinely start patients on 2.5 mg orally twice daily and then titrate up based on improvement of symptoms and occurrence of side effects. The primary side effects of anticholinergic medications include dry mouth, constipation, blurred vision, change in mental status, and nausea. These medications are contraindicated in patients with narrow-angle glaucoma. Other anticholinergic agents, including propantheline, dicyclomine hydrochloride, and flavoxate, may be used as second-line agents in patients with a poor response to oxybutinin. Tolterodine has been introduced as a bladder-selective anticholinergic agent that is associated with improved symptoms and reduced side effects. Initial results with its use are encouraging because the drug is well tolerated in most patients.

Imipramine, a tricyclic antidepressant, has been shown to be effective in the treatment of both stress incontinence and urge incontinence. Although the exact mechanism of action is incompletely understood, the drug seems to work by increasing urethral contractility and suppressing involuntary bladder contractions through its anticholinergic properties. The recommended dosage is 25 to 100 mg daily. Side effects include orthostatic hypertension, dry mouth, nausea, and hepatic dysfunction. It is contraindicated in patients taking monoamine oxidase inhibitors.

Calcium channel blockers such as nifedipine, verapamil,

TABLE 21.4. PHARMACOLOGIC AGENTS FOR THE TREATMENT OF URINARY INCONTINENCE

Medication (Trade name)	Dosage	Mechanism of Action	Indication
Oxybutynin (Ditropan)	2.5 mg b.i.d.–5 mg t.i.d.	Anticholinergic/spasmolytic	Urge incontinence
Hyoscyamine (Levsin, Cystospaz)	0.15 mg t.i.d. to q.i.d. 0.375 mg b.i.d. to t.i.d. (extended release)	Anticholinergic	Urge incontinence
Flavoxate (Urispas)	100–200 mg t.i.d. to q.i.d.	Anticholinergic/spasmolytic	Urge incontinence
Tolterodine (Detrol)	2 mg b.i.d.	Anticholinergic	Urge incontinence
Propantheline bromide (Pro-Banthine)	7.5 mg t.i.d.	Anticholinergic	Urge incontinence
Phenylpropanolamine (Entex)	5 mg b.i.d.	α-adrenergic stimulation	Stress incontinence
Pseudoephedrine (Sudafed)	60 mg q.i.d.	α-adrenergic stimulation	Stress incontinence
Imipramine (Tofranil)	25–75 mg daily	Anticholinergic and α-adrenergic stimulation	Urge incontinence Stress incontinence
Estrogen (Premarin)	0.625 mg orally or vaginally, daily	Beneficial effects on urethral mucosa and sphincter	Urge incontinence Stress incontinence

and terodiline work by blocking the influx of extracellular calcium that is important for detrusor muscle contraction. They have been used extensively in the treatment of detrusor instability in Europe but are still currently under investigation for use in the United States. Side effects include dry mouth, blurred vision, headache, and cardiac arrhythmia. At the present time, these agents are not recommended for general use in the treatment of urinary incontinence.

α-Adrenergic agonists, phenylpropanolamine and pseudoephedrine, have little effect on the detrusor muscle but can significantly increase urethral pressure by inducing contraction of the urethral sphincter. These agents are useful in the treatment of genuine stress incontinence, particularly that caused by intrinsic sphincter deficiency. Recommended dosage for phenylpropanolamine is 25 to 100 mg orally in a sustained release form twice daily, and for pseudoephedrine it is 15 to 30 mg orally three times daily. Patients often report improvement in their symptoms within 1 week. Side effects include drowsiness, dry mouth, and hypertension.

Estrogen replacement, either oral or vaginal, should be used as an adjunctive pharmacologic agent for postmenopausal women with stress urinary incontinence or mixed incontinence. Although the exact mechanism by which estrogen therapy improves incontinence symptoms is unknown, various theories have been proposed. Estrogen has been shown to alter the vaginal pH and to decrease the frequency of urinary tract infections. In addition, estrogen-induced cytologic changes in the urethral mucosa may lead to improved coaptation and re-creation of the mucosal seal. Estrogen may also augment periurethral vascularity with improved function of the smooth and striated periurethral muscles (16). Finally, the combination of α-agonists and estrogen may have synergistic effects. Conjugated estrogen can be administered either orally or vaginally, and progestin should be added in patients who have an intact uterus. Side effects include irregular vaginal bleeding, breast tenderness, weight gain, and nausea. Estrogen is contraindicated in patients with a history of breast or gynecologic cancer (17).

Medical Devices

Medical devices for the management of urinary incontinence include absorbent products, vaginal support devices, and urethral products (18). The widespread use of absorbent pads for the symptomatic control of urinary incontinence has prolonged research and technologic advances in the treatment of this socially debilitating condition. Often marketed as "adult diapers" or "absorbent undergarments," these products provide palliative control and often dissuade the patient from seeking medical attention for incontinence that is usually readily treatable. Given the variety of surgical and nonsurgical management options today, the use of absorbent products should be reserved for long-term care of patients with chronic, intractable urinary incontinence.

Medical devices, classified as obstructive or supportive, are designed primarily for the treatment of stress urinary incontinence or mild mixed incontinence resulting from urethral hypermobility or intrinsic sphincter deficiency (Fig. 21.5). Urethral plugs and patches are placed in or over the urethra to occlude the lumen and to prevent urinary leakage with increases in abdominal pressure. Complications include urinary tract infection, hematuria, migration of the device into the bladder, and persistent incontinence. Vaginal devices include diaphragms, pessaries, and tampons. These devices function by providing intravaginal support to the bladder neck during episodes of increased abdominal pressure. Complications related to intravaginal devices are less common and include vaginal discharge and pelvic discomfort. Success rates for medical devices have been found to vary depending on the severity of incontinence. Vierhout and Lose reported subjective success rates ranging from 40% to 60%, depending on the type of device (19).

Surgical Correction

Although a comprehensive discussion of the various *surgical procedures* used in the treatment of your incontinence is beyond the scope of this chapter, it may be helpful to review the major classes of surgery briefly, to provide preliminary information regarding surgical options. Surgery is used primarily in the treatment of genuine stress urinary incontinence resulting from urethral hypermobility or intrinsic sphincter deficiency.

In female patients with urethral hypermobility, the goal of the surgical procedure is to restore normal anatomic bladder neck support and to prevent descent during increased abdominal pressure. This can be done by a retropubic urethropexy, a transvaginal needle suspension procedure, or a suburethral sling. The retropubic urethropexy is per-

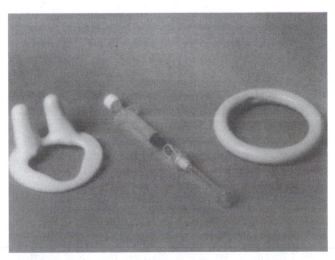

FIGURE 21.5. Medical devices for incontinence include pessary devices with and without support (*left and right*) and urethral plugs (*center*).

formed through a small suprapubic laparotomy incision that provides access to the retropubic space. Vaginal tissue underneath the urethra is then suspended to the pubic symphysis (Marshall-Marchetti-Krantz urethropexy) or Cooper's ligament (Burch colposuspension). Retropubic procedures have been performed laparoscopically with equivalent cure rates on short-term follow-up. The transvaginal needle suspension procedure is mainly performed through the vaginal route with a small abdominal incision. The retropubic space is entered vaginally, and support tissue on either side of the urethra is grasped and sutured in a helical stitch. These sutures are then transferred above the anterior rectus fascia to the suprapubic incision through a long needle carrier. Tiedown over the rectus fascia results in elevation and stabilization of the bladder neck. The suburethral sling is performed in a similar manner, but it uses a synthetic or natural graft underneath the urethra rather than incorporating the periurethral tissue in a helical stitch. Risks of these procedures include bleeding, infection, damage to the lower urinary tract, recurrent incontinence, and postoperative urinary retention. In a metaanalysis performed by Jarvis, the long-term success rates for the retropubic urethropexy, transvaginal needle suspension, and suburethral sling were reported to be 80%, 70%, and 85%, respectively (20).

In patients with intrinsic sphincter deficiency, the goal of the surgical procedure is to restore the normal continence mechanism by compressing the urethra at the bladder neck. This can be done by a suburethral sling, an artificial urinary sphincter, or periurethral collagen injections. The suburethral sling has been previously described. The artificial urinary sphincter involves placement of a mechanical prosthesis around the bladder neck that can inflate and deflate depending on the need for continence or voiding. Periurethral collagen injections involve injection of bulk-enhancing agents, most commonly cross-linked bovine dermal collagen, around the urethra until closure of the internal urethral meatus occurs. This procedure is commonly performed using local anesthesia in the office setting. Risks of these procedures include infection, recurrent incontinence, and postoperative urinary retention.

Newer Techniques

Medical and surgical advances have been made in the treatment of urinary incontinence. Various new medications for the treatment of stress and urge incontinence are expected to be released over the next several years. These include long-acting delivery systems as well as pharmacologic agents that should improve treatment outcomes and reduce the incidence of side effects.

Although pharmacotherapy and behavioral modification are still the mainstay of treatment for detrusor instability, patients with persistent urge incontinence may be candidates for newly introduced implantable nerve root stimula-

tors. The implantable electrode is designed to stimulate the dorsal nerve root of S-2, S-3, and S-4, to reestablish a neurologic equilibrium with relief of persistent urge incontinence. Patients initially undergo placement of a subcutaneous test stimulator on an outpatient basis. Those patients who experience at least a 50% reduction in symptoms are candidates for subsequent placement of a permanent implantable device. Initial results have been encouraging, especially because surgical alternatives for refractory urge incontinence are associated with poor outcomes.

For patients with stress incontinence, new laparoscopic procedures are providing good surgical outcomes with fewer complications and reduced hospital stay. New substances for periurethral injection in the treatment of intrinsic sphincter deficiency are being developed to provide long-lasting results with minimal risk. With increased understanding of this condition and greater media attention, it is expected that more treatment options will be available in the future.

SUMMARY

Urinary incontinence is a condition that affects more than 13 million persons in the United States. This number is expected to continue to grow as the population continues to age. A basic understanding of the pathophysiology of the lower urinary tract is vital in diagnosing and treating this condition. Initial diagnosis can usually be made on the first visit after history and physical examination. Many patients may require basic additional testing that can easily be performed in the office setting. Preliminary treatment modalities either cure or significantly improve the majority of patients. The small subset of patients with a complex presentation or who require surgery will need further consultation and complex urodynamic testing.

A step-by-step algorithm with an understanding of the available treatment options allows the clinician to provide care for this condition and to identify those patients who require subspecialist referral. In either case, this care will probably make a long-lasting impact in the medical, social, and psychologic well-being of patients suffering from this debilitating condition.

10 KEY POINTS

1. Urinary incontinence affects more than 13 million persons in the United States and is two to three times more common in women compared with men.

2. Incontinence and voiding dysfunction result from alterations in the normal anatomy or physiology of the filling phase or emptying phase.

3. Urinary incontinence can be classified based on origin: urge, genuine stress, mixed, overflow, functional, and anatomic.

4. Urinary incontinence in women is related to vaginal childbirth, hypoestrogenism, chronic straining disorders, infection, and aging.

5. The initial evaluation of urinary incontinence includes a detailed medical history, general and focused physical examination, urinalysis, measurement of postvoid residual urine, and simple cystometry with cough stress test.

6. Complex urodynamic and additional testing is indicated in patients with a complicated history, persistent or recurrent incontinence, and complicated medical history, as well as preoperatively.

7. Most patients with urinary incontinence can be treated with conservative regimens consisting of behavioral and dietary modification, exercises, medical devices, and pharmacotherapy.

8. Surgical correction should be reserved for those patients who are unresponsive to conservative therapies, have severe stress incontinence or advanced prolapse, or desire surgical intervention.

9. Optimal patient management requires accurate assessment of the underlying problem, management of patient expectations, and follow-up of compliance and progress.

10. Urinary incontinence is a problem of epidemic proportion but can be easily treated in the office with a logical step-by-step algorithm.

REFERENCES

1. Fantl JA, Newman DK, Collins J, et al. *Urinary incontinence in adults: acute and chronic management.* Clinical practice guideline No. 2, 1996 update. Rockville, MD: United States Department of Health and Human Services, Public Health Service, Agency for Health Care Policy and Research, 1996;2:5–7.
2. Burgio KL, Matthews KA, Engel BT. Prevalence, incidence, and correlates of urinary incontinence in healthy, middle-aged women. *J Urol* 1991;146:1255–1259.
3. Ouslander J, Kane R, Abrass I. Urinary incontinence in elderly nursing-home patients. *JAMA* 1982;248:1194–1198.
4. Baker KR, Bice TW. The influence of urinary incontinence on publicly financed home care services to low income elderly people. *Gerontologist* 1995;35:360–369.
5. Siu AL, Beers MH, Morgenstern H. The geriatric "medical and public health" imperative revisited. *J Am Geriatr Soc* 1995;43: 286–294.
6. International Continence Society Committee on Standardisation of Terminology. The standardisation of terminology of lower urinary tract function. *Scand J Urol Nephrol* 1988;114[Suppl]: 5–19.
7. Mcguire EJ, Fitzpatrick CC, Wan J, et al. Clinical assessment or urethral sphincter function. *J Urol* 1993;50:1452–1454.
8. Jensen JK, Nielsen FR, Ostergard DR. The role of patient history in the diagnosis of urinary incontinence. *Obstet Gynecol* 1994; 83:904–910.
9. Scotti R, Myers D. A simplified urogynecologic workup. *AUGS Q Rep* 1990;8:1–3.
10. Cardozo LD, Stanton SL. Genuine stress incontinence and detrusor instability: a review of 200 patients. *Br J Obstet Gynaecol* 1980;87:184–190.
11. Fantl JA, Wyman JF, Mclish DK, et al. Efficacy of bladder training in older women with urinary incontinence. *JAMA* 1991; 265:609–613.
12. Tchou DCH, Adams C, Varner RE, et al. Pelvic floor musculature exercises in treatment of anatomical urinary stress incontinence. *Phys Ther* 1988;68:652–655.
13. Bump RC, Hurt WG, Fantl JA, et al. Assessment of Kegel pelvic muscle exercise performance after brief verbal instruction. *Am J Obstet Gynecol* 1991;165:322–329.
14. Dougherty M, Bishop K, Mooney R, et al. Graded pelvic muscle exercise: effect on stress urinary incontinence. *J Reprod Med* 1993;39:684–691.
15. Fantl JA, Newman DK, Collins J, et al. *Urinary incontinence in adults: acute and chronic management.* Clinical practice guideline No. 2, 1996 update. Rockville, MD: United States Department of Health and Human Services, Public Health Service, Agency for Health Care Policy and Research, 1996;2:42–43.
16. Bhatia NN, Bergman A, Karram MM. Effects of estrogen on urethral function in women with urinary incontinence. *Am J Obstet Gynecol* 1989;160:176–181.
17. Griebling TL, Kreder KJ. Female urinary incontinence: new management techniques and technologies. *Mediguide Urol* 1998; 11:1–6.
18. Nygaard I. Prevention of exercise incontinence with mechanical devices. *J Reprod Med* 1995;40:89–94.
19. Vierhout ME, Lose G. Preventive vaginal and intra-urethral devices in the treatment of female urinary stress incontinence. *Curr Opin Obstet Gynecol* 1997;9:325–328.
20. Jarvis GJ. Surgery for genuine stress incontinence. *Br J Obstet Gynaecol* 1994;101:371–374.

22

SELECTED GYNECOLOGIC TECHNOLOGIES: MAGNETIC RESONANCE IMAGING, FLOW CYTOMETRY, ASSISTED REPRODUCTIVE TECHNOLOGIES, PREIMPLANTATION GENETIC DIAGNOSIS, AND FIBEROPTICS

LISA DABNEY
ALAN S. PENZIAS

If time travel were possible, the average 19th-century obstetrician or gynecologist would be astounded by the clinical practice of his or her 21st-century colleague. Amid the plethora of new medications and safer and more effective treatment algorithms lies a host of technologic breakthroughs that are used on a daily basis. In fact, many of the technologies are so routine that the modern practitioner rarely ponders their development; rather, he or she simply looks to the answers provided by the tests with hardly a passing thought. This chapter examines the basis of five selected technologies that have changed the face of medicine.

MAGNETIC RESONANCE IMAGING

Magnetic resonance imaging (MRI) works on the principle of nuclear magnetic resonance that involves the absorption of radiofrequencies (RFs) by protons in an external magnetic field. In this section, we discuss the fundamental principles behind the operation of MRI as well as the clinical application of MRI in imaging the female pelvis for both normal and abnormal anatomy.

MRI works on the principle of magnetic fields and the absorption of energy by protons that are placed within the magnetic fields. Within the nucleus of each atom, protons and neutrons spin on their own nuclear axis and thus act as small magnets. In atoms with equal numbers of protons and neutrons, the "spins" cancel each other so the net magnetization in that atom is zero. In atoms with odd numbers of protons, however, there will be a net magnetic force. MRI then can use any atom or element that has an odd number of protons. The favored element, however, is hydrogen. This is because it is abundant in all tissues and because of its properties: it

gives off a high signal. Within a tissue, the individual spins of each atom are usually random and thus cancel each other. However, when an external magnetic force is applied to the atoms, nuclei line up parallel or antiparallel to the magnetic field. This difference results in a net magnetization of the tissue.

The application of the magnetic field is the first step in creating images in MRI. The net magnetization is then intentionally disrupted by introducing a second, much smaller magnetic field that disrupts the alignment magnetized atoms. These are known as *RF pulses*. With time, the nuclei realign through relaxation and give off radio signals that vary in force and time of relaxation. The MRI machine reads the radio signals emitted by the atoms as they return to their baseline state after the RF pulse. Gradient magnetic fields are applied to determine spatial localization of the atoms within the tissues.

After the RF pulse is applied, the nuclei realign with the vector of net magnetization (M), and signal decay is measured. Two mechanisms by which this relaxation occurs can be measured by time: *T1 relaxation* (longitudinal or spin-lattice relaxation) and *T2 relaxation* (spin-spin relaxation). T1 is a measure of how quickly the axis of M realigns with the axis of the applied magnetic field (B). In other words, T1 relaxation is a measure of how quickly the net magnetization returns from the transverse to the longitudinal plane. T1 is an exponential time constant and is equal to the time it takes for 63% of complete recovery of alignment. One excitation does not produce enough signal for an image, so multiple repetitive RF pulses are applied to the tissue. The time between repetitions of RF pulses is known as the *repetition time* (TR). The nuclei must be realigned completely before they can absorb the next RF pulse. For this reason, equilibrium for longitudinal magnetization is eventually reached by using repetitive pulses. This equilibrium depends on T1 and TR. For long TR, more nuclei have realigned with the external magnetic field between pulses, and therefore more nuclei can absorb the next RF pulse to produce a strong signal. For short TR, fewer nuclei absorb successive RF pulses, and the signal is weak.

Changing TR highlights the varying T1 relaxation times of different tissues. For example, fat has a short T1, and therefore most of its nuclei are realigned before successive pulses. For this reason, it appears brighter than tissues with long T1 whose nuclei are not realigned between pulses and therefore cannot absorbs all the pulses. These differences enable the MRI to distinguish between tissues based on T1 relaxation times by manipulating TR, a process known as T1 weighting.

T2 relaxation times refer to the dephasing of nuclei as they precess about the external magnetic field, B. Immediately after the application of the RF pulse, the nuclei "wobble" or precess in phase with each other. However, with time, some precess faster than others, and thus the nuclei are no longer in phase with each other. T2 is an exponential time constant equal to the amount of time it takes for dephasing to reduce transverse magnetization by 63%. The signal produced is measured at some time interval after RF excitation known as echo time (TE). As TE is increased, more dephasing occurs between the RF pulse and signal readout resulting in a larger decrease in signal intensity. Again, tissues can be distinguished by their different T2 by manipulating TE. For example, water has a T2 of greater that 2 seconds, so signal decay will be minimal if TE is 30 milliseconds. It can thus be easily distinguished from muscle with a T2 of 50 milliseconds because its decay will be substantial if TE is set at 30 milliseconds. Manipulating TE to enhance T2 differences is known as T2 weighting.

MRIs use T1 and T2 relaxation times to distinguish among different tissues. An increase in free water content of tissues tends to increase both T1 and T2. Because pathologic changes are often associated with an increase in free water, the MRI can distinguish between normal and pathologic tissues. However, as T1 increases, signal intensity decreases, and as T2 increases, signal intensity increases. If a pulse sequence produced equal T1 and T2 weighting, the effects would cancel each other, and no change would be seen. For this reason, pulse sequences are chosen that cause either T1 or T2 weighting. In general, on T2-weighted images, pathologic tissues appear brighter, and on T1-weighted images, pathologic tissues appear less bright.

Specific pulse sequences have been developed that maximize these effects. The simplest of these is known as the *partial saturation*. This technique exploits differences in T1 among different tissues. Successive pulses with a set TR are applied to tissues. Protons in tissues with short T1, such as fat, return completely to the relaxed state between pulses and are able to absorb more energy from each successive pulse and thus appear bright on the image. Tissues with longer T1 times, such as fluid, appear darker. This method is the simplest and provides the least contrast between normal and pathologic tissues and is used mostly for viewing normal anatomy.

Inversion recovery, another type of pulse sequence, is much more sensitive. This method involves a pulse with a flip angle of 180 degrees to rotate M opposite the magnetic field, followed by a 90-degree pulse that causes the vector M to point in the transverse plane. TR is the time between successive 180-degree pulses. Like the partial saturation sequence, inversion recovery also depends on T1 effects. Because of pulses with varying flip angles, however, T1 effects are maximized.

The third type of pulse sequencing is the most sensitive and is based on mostly T2 effects, which usually vary more among tissues. In this sequence, a 90-degree pulse is used to rotate the vector M into a transverse plane. After some time to allow T2 dephasing to occur, a second 180-degree pulse is applied. This pulse causes the protons to come back in to phase with one another and restores the signal in the transverse plane. In tissues with a long T2, little dephasing occurs, and so these tissues appear brighter than tissues with a shorter T2. The TE in this sequence is the time between the 90-degree pulse and signal measurement. TR is the time between one pulse sequence and the next. This sequence is mostly T2 weighted, and long TRs are used to enhance signal amplitude. TR along with TE can also be shortened in the sequence to bring out differences in T1 resulting in T1 weighting.

Once contrast between tissues is achieved, the MRI signal from various regions of tissues must be localized. This is done by using gradient magnetic fields in which the field strength varies with position. The external magnetic field (B) experienced by each individual proton depends on its location within the gradient. Because of the gradient, the RF pulse needed to excite an individual proton depends on its spatial location. Gradients are applied in different planes to gather information about the spatial relationships of different tissues. This information is gathered by the computer that uses an equation known as the *Fourier transform* to create a gray scale image that corresponds to the tissues. This gives us MRI images (1–3).

MRI is particularly well suited for imaging the female reproductive tract for several reasons. It does not involve ionizing radiation, soft tissue contrast is superb, and multiplanar images can be obtained. T2-weighted scans depict uterine zonal anatomy well including changes under hormonal stimulation. Uterine neoplasms are also well seen. T1-weighted images provide excellent contrast among pelvic smooth muscle, fat, and blood and are good for specific pathology involving hemorrhage or fat-containing lesions. In the next section, we begin with a discussion of normal anatomy and then discuss pathologic conditions of different organ systems.

Uterus

The *uterus* is well demonstrated on T2 images. (It is fairly homogenous on T1 images). The myometrium and endometrium are recognized by high-signal areas and are separated by a low-signal junctional zone. Hormonal changes are easily seen because the endometrium thickness changes in width throughout the cycle. The myometrium can also be seen expanding in the secretory phase on MRI images.

Fibroids are easily seen on MRI. On T2-weighted scans, they have a lower signal intensity than the surrounding uterus, and tumors as small as 0.5 cm can be seen. If cystic degeneration is present, it will be seen as an area of increased signal intensity. MRI is superior to ultrasound because the exact location (subserosal, intramural or submucosal) of the fibroids can be identified. T1-weighted images can be used to distinguish subserosal fibroids from fat.

MRI is helpful in the diagnosis of *adenomyosis.* T2-weighted scans show diffuse thickening of the junctional zone. Low-signal foci, representing ectopic endometrium, can also be seen scattered throughout the myometrium. These lesions can be distinguished from fibroids by their less distinct margins. Occasional bright spots, representing hemorrhage, are seen as well.

MRI can aid in the staging of *endometrial cancer.* Diagnosis with MRI alone is not possible because endometrial cancer, blood clots, and adenomatous hyperplasia all have similar appearances on MRI. They all demonstrate high signal on T2 images. For this reason, histologic diagnosis is mandatory. Once this diagnosis has been made, however, MRI is helpful in determining myometrial invasion. Preservation of the junctional zone is a sensitive indicator for lack of invasion. The overall accuracy in staging was found to be 92% in one study (4). Evaluation of nodes is similar to that with computed tomography. MRI may be better suited to determine spread into adjacent organs because of its excellent soft tissue resolution. Further studies must be done to evaluate this possibility.

Uterine anomalies are also well visualized. MRI is less invasive than a hysterosalpingogram and is usually more informative than ultrasound. Uterine anatomy is best seen on T2-weighted images. *Bicornuate uteri* are easily seen with MRI. A high-signal-intensity endometrium is seen in each horn surrounded by a low-signal junctional zone. The low-signal junctional zone of each horn is separated by an intermediate-signal band of myometrium. These findings are best appreciated on transverse images.

Septate uteri are also best seen on T2-weighted scans. The uterine septum appears as a low-intensity zone separating the endometrial cavity. No junctional zone or myometrium is seen. It can also be distinguished from bicornuate uteri by the wider separation of endometrial cavities usually seen in the latter condition.

A *unicornuate uterus* can usually be appreciated as a smaller deviated uterine cavity. *Arcuate and hypoplastic uteri* can also be seen. *T-shaped uteri* are not as well appreciated and are better seen with a hysterosalpingogram.

Cervix

The *cervix* is best seen on T2-weighted images as well. Two zones can be distinguished, a central zone of high signal intensity corresponding to the cervical epithelium and mucus surrounded by a low-signal zone corresponding to stroma. The parametrium can also be seen as an area of medium high signal intensity surrounding the cervix. The support structures and ligaments of the uterus are generally not well seen.

Early *cervical cancer* is staged clinically, so MRI is not as helpful as in later stages, when it can be used to detect tumor spread to parametrial tissues. On T2 images, cervical cancer appears as a high-intensity mass or a disruption of the architecture of the normally dark cervix. T1 images are useful for detecting extension of the cancer into surrounding fat.

Ovary

The *ovary* is not as well visualized, but it can be found by imaging in the coronal or transverse plane and looking for vascular landmarks. Imaging is particularly difficult in prepubertal girls and postmenopausal women. On T1-weighted images, the ovary has a low to medium signal intensity. On T2-weighted images, ovarian stroma is isointense with fat, and the follicles are hyperintense to fat.

Some *adnexal pathologic processes* can be seen on MRI. This method is most helpful in determining whether masses are ovarian or uterine in origin. Simple follicles and cysts behave like free water and have long T2, so they are seen as low-intensity structures on T1 images with increased intensity on T2 images. Hemorrhagic cysts vary according to time course. Acute hemorrhages are seen as intermediate signals on T1 images and as high signals on T2 images. Chronic hemorrhage is seen as a high-intensity signal on T1 images. The appearance of dermoids on MRI varies according to their composition, but they are usually similar overall to fat and so are seen as a high-intensity signal on T1 and an intermediate signal on T2.

Vagina

The *vagina* can also be seen on MRI. On T1-weighted images, the vagina is uniformly hypointense. On T2-weighted images, the canal and walls can be delineated because the former is hyperintense and the latter appears hypointense.

Vaginal anomalies are also evident on MRI. Complete agenesis is best seen on T2-weighted images. Nothing is seen between the urethra and the rectum. In partial vaginal agenesis, hematometrocolpos may be appreciated by the presence of high-density material, representing menstrual blood, seen filling the vagina and uterus on both T1-weighted and T2-weighted scans. MRI can also be used to measure the distance between the upper vagina and the introitus to determine whether vaginoplasty is feasible. Because many of these anomalies are associated with renal and skeletal anomalies, MRI is also helpful as a noninvasive technique to visualize associated anomalies.

In summary, MRI is a noninvasive and highly accurate method for scanning the pelvis and female genital tract. MRI can distinguish between septate and bicornuate uteri by the presence of intervening myometrium. It can confirm the diagnosis of conditions such as bicornuate uterus, adenomyosis, and vaginal agenesis, diagnoses previously only confirmed by surgery. It is still costly but has a definitive role that will continue to expand as more research and analysis are done (1,4–8).

FLOW CYTOMETRY

Flow cytometry is an evolving field of medicine that uses rapid quantification and qualification of cells and other material to gather information about tissues, cells, and organs. Many of its uses are still under investigation, but it already has many clinical applications and will continue to do so. In this section, we describe the basic concepts of flow cytometry and then discuss specific clinical applications in the field of gynecology.

Flow cytometry evolved from experiments performed over the last 50 years. In the 1940s and 1950s, scientists began to use fluorescence microscopes in conjunction with fluorescent stains for nucleic acids to detect malignant cells. Microscopes were fitted with photodetectors to measure and quantify DNA. Cells were examined slowly, however. In the 1960s, scientists began to develop microscopes that could count and quantify numerous cells at once. This technology was similar to Coulter counters developed around the same time. The latter worked by counting cells as they flowed by the microscope apparatus. The cells were lined up in single file, and analysis was based on increases in electrical resistance caused by each cell as it displaced isotonic saline. Differences were based mostly on cell size, and the early machines were used primarily for sorting red and white blood cells.

These early machines were modified so many other types of cells could be analyzed as well. The basic concept of flow cytometry is the measurement of particle characteristics as the particle flows through a beam of light. Any particle suspended in a fluid can be measured. Not only cells but also chromosomes, DNA, and even latex beads can be measured. Fluorescein dyes are used to gain additional information about the particles under study, so many flow cytometers are referred to as *fluorescein-activated cell sorters.*

The common elements of all flow cytometers are a light source, a fluid stream containing particles for measurement, photodetectors to measure the intensity of light as particles flow through the system, and a computer to analyze changes in the light intensity. In this apparatus, light emerges from a laser source and is focused into a beam as small as 50 μm in diameter. At its focal point, it intersects with the liquid stream of particles so the stream is uniformly illuminated by the light. This is known as the *analysis or observation point.* Surrounding the observation point are lenses to collect the scatter of light, or signal, produced by the particles. Some of the lenses have filters to detect only certain wavelengths of light. The information from the various lenses, or *photodetectors* as they are called, surrounding the analysis point is converted into electrical impulses to be analyzed by a computer into data about the particles under study.

Usually, there are three to four photodetectors at right angles to the light beam. In this way, a certain amount of deflection or scatter of the light must occur for the photodetectors to pick up any signal. Particles that have an irregular surface scatter more light. One lens, or photodetector, is set at 90 degrees to the source beam. Light picked up by this particular photodetector is known as *side scatter light.* The amount of light detected by this photodetector reflects how much scatter is caused by the particle and is called the *granularity signal.*

In addition to side scatter, *forward scatter* caused by the particle is measured as well. This is called the *volume signal* and is determined as follows. A forward-angle photodetector is placed in direct line of the laser beam with an obstruction bar in front of it to prevent much of the illuminating beam from reaching the photodetector. The only light that actually reaches the forward-angle photodetector is light that is bent by the particle so it can go around the obstruction bar. The bending of light depends on the refractive index of the particle under study as well as its size. This signal is known as the *volume signal,* a term that is misleading because size is not the only indicator of forward light scatter.

The wavelength of laser light used by many flow cytometers is usually 488 nm, which corresponds to a blue light. Both forward-angle and side-angle photodetector have blue filters in this case that detect only light with the same wavelength as the source beam. Additional photodetectors within the system have filters to detect other wavelengths of light. This is where the fluorescein dyes are needed.

An unstained particle does not generate its own light, so scattered light would only be registered by the forward and side scatter photodetectors. Fluorescein stains, or *fluorochromes,* emit light when they are excited by lasers, and they enable the particles to scatter the blue light and to emit light of other wavelengths and colors. This light is picked up as signals by photodetectors with filters specific to various wavelengths. The signals from these photodetectors provide information on the staining characteristics of the particle in question.

In summary, light leaves the laser and is reflected, refracted, and changed into various wavelengths. The forward light scatter and side light scatter photodetectors provide information on the physical characteristics of the particle by measuring refraction of light in the same wavelength as the original beam. Other photodetectors are equipped with colored filters to measure fluorescein emissions and thus provide information on the staining characteristics. Each photodetector measures a parameter of the particle, so instruments are named as such by the number of photodetectors they contain. A three-parameter system has three photodetectors, and a six-parameter system has six photodetectors.

Flow cytometers are made up of specific components that can be modified or adjusted: the fluid system, electronics, and data processing. The *fluid system* begins as a reservoir of liquid known as *sheath fluid.* Pressure regulators are used to control the rate of flow through the system. Ideally, the rate should by about 1,000 particles per second. If the rate is too fast, two particles may come through the observation point at the same time, and their signal will become mixed. If the rate is too slow, it markedly increases the analysis time of the sample. Another way to control rate is by adjusting the concentration of particles in the original sample. It is usually about 105 particles/mL. The size of the particles also affects the system. If they are too large, they will clog the system. If they are too small, they will not be distinguished from background noise. The maximum particle size is determined by the nozzle or flow chamber and the size of the focused beam of illuminated light; both must be larger than the particles for study.

The *electronics* of the system can be manipulated by voltage and amplitude changes in the photodetectors. Light signals are changed into electrical impulses by the photodetectors. As the voltage of each photodetector tube is increased, its sensitivity is increased so it can pick up weaker signals. The sensitivity of the photodetectors can also be modified by amplification of the signal once it is detected. Amplification can be on a logarithmic or linear scale, and it can operate at various gains. With *linear amplifiers,* the signal intensity begins at zero. Increasing the gain spreads out the signals so overlapping signals can be better delineated. With *log amplifiers,* the same is true; however, signals that are double in intensity relative to one another will remain the same distance apart regardless of gain or voltage. Linear amplifiers are usually used for analyzing DNA because the DNA content of cells usually does not vary by much more than a factor of 2. Most gynecologic applications involve measurement of DNA and thus use linear amplifiers.

As the photodetectors register signals from the thousands of particles, the intensities are *analyzed,* and the values recorded by means of an *analog-to-digital converter.* The role of this converter is to organize the signals into discreet ranges in the form of a bar graph or histogram. These discrete ranges are divided up into channels that are either 256 or 1,024 in number. Each channel represents a certain light intensity, and the signal of each particle is grouped into a channel that corresponds to the intensity of its signal. The intensity range represented by each channel depends on voltage, gain, and some other parameters that can be adjusted for a given experiment. These parameters are important to understand the relationships among these channels. For example, in a linear system, a signal in channel 200 would correspond to a particle 2.78 times as bright as a signal in channel 72 (200/72 = 2.78). In a log system with a gain that covers 2 decades full scale, the signal in channel 200 would correspond to a particle 10 times as bright as the particle, giving a signal in channel 72. In this system, every 128 channels represent a 10-fold increase in intensity.

Another parameter that can be controlled with flow cytometry is *threshold.* It is a way of filtering out noise in the system. The easiest way to control threshold is to adjust the parameters of the forward scatter photodetector. A channel number for this photodetector can be set so only particles with intensity brighter than the defined channel number are counted by the flow cytometer. Wavelength thresholds can also be used to detect only particles emitting a certain wavelength or color of light.

To review, a particle is illuminated by light that gives off signals detected by the photodetectors. The photodectors transform the signal into electrical impulses that vary in intensity and thus can be classified into channels on a scale from 0 to 255. Each photodetector does this separately, so for one particle, we have several numbers, one for each photodetector. A five-parameter system produces five numbers for each particle. This information can then be used by the computer for data analysis that will be explained in the next section.

Data from a flow cytometer are stored in *flow cytometer standard* and are usually stored in list mode. This means that in a five-parameter system, five bytes of information are stored on each particle. This information then can be analyzed and correlated in many different ways. To organize this information, "gates" are used. A gate is way of defining characteristics of the particles to be used for analysis. Usually, parameters can be set so the computer will only save information on particles whose signals meet certain criteria for analysis. Information on all other particles is lost. This is analogous to a microscopist's disregarding all other white blood cells when counting lymphocyte concentration in the blood.

Once the gate has been defined, the information can be organized in several ways. A histogram can be plotted from the information obtained from one photodetector analyzing a population of particles. The signal intensity produced by each particle is assigned a channel by the system so groups of particles are placed into channels corresponding to the intensity of light they produce. Once the histograms are created, information about the population of cells can be obtained, for example, the median, mean, mode, and range of intensity of the population.

In addition to looking at only one parameter or photodetector, *bit maps* can be made that correlate the information of one parameter with another. Each particle is plotted according to the intensity channels of two chosen parameters, and *dot plots* are created. These dot plots are limited by "black out." If there is a high concentration of dots in one area, the area can only become so dark. Because of this, gradations of highly concentrated areas may be difficult to appreciate. For this reason, *contour plots* are also created. Contour plots are plotted in the same way, except they use three dimensions to represent increasing concentrations, much like a topographic map. Concentrations among various regions of the graph are much more easily seen. Most of the examples that follow use only one-dimensional histograms, but one must understand that two-dimensional histograms can be created as well.

DNA

Analysis of DNA is most directly applicable to analyzing cancer cells to detect major abnormalities in DNA content and proliferation. Flow cytometry can be used to measure nuclei from either frozen, formalin-fixed, or paraffin-embedded tissue. The cells are isolated, and the remaining tissue is digested with pepsin, trypsin, and ribonucleases to remove unwanted protein and RNA and to isolate the nuclei. Stains are then used to stain the DNA. The most common stain used is propidium iodide, which stains double-stranded DNA, absorbs 488-nm light, and fluoresces at wavelengths higher than 600 nm. It is ideal for argon beams. Some other stains are Hoechst 33258, which stains AT pairs on DNA, and Chromomycin A3, which stains GC pairs.

Once the DNA is stained, it is sent through the flow cytometer and is exposed to a laser, usually an argon beam. The cells then fluoresce red in proportion to the amount of DNA present. This red fluorescence is detected by a photodetector with a red filter, and a channel number is assigned to the fluorescent intensity of the cell. As the flow cytometer measures thousands of cells, 1,000 per second and 20,0000 to 100,000 overall, a histogram of the results is created.

DNA content or ploidy can easily be determined by this technique and is used to detect the major DNA abnormalities found in cancerous cells. The amount of DNA in a cell is specific to each organism and is denoted as a 2N, or diploid, concentration of cells. All normal cells have the same amount of DNA, except during meiosis, when they can contain 1N concentration of DNA, and mitosis, when for a brief time during DNA replication they may contain 4N concentration of DNA. Cancer cells, however, may contain large amounts of unusual concentrations of DNA, and these cells are termed *aneuploid.*

Researchers have developed a term known as the *DNA index* to compare the degree of aneuploidy of different tumors to correlate this with outcome for the patient. To calculate the DNA index, cells are first separated into various phases of the cell cycle, G_0, G_1, S, G_2, and M. Cells in G_0 are not cycling and contain 2N amount of DNA. Cells in G_1 are preparing for the initiation of a new cycle and also contain 2N DNA. Cells in S phase are making new DNA, and so the concentration of their DNA varies between 2N and 4N. Cells in G_2 and M are finished with synthesis and are in the process of mitosis, respectively, and both contain 4N amounts of DNA. The DNA index is calculated by measuring the ratio of DNA content of cells in the G_0-G_1 phase in the abnormal population over the DNA content of cells in the G_0-G_1 phase in the normal population. By definition, the DNA index of normal DNA diploid cells is 1.0.

DNA index measurements and ploidy analysis have several shortcomings. Some major chromosomal alterations, such as translocations, do not lead to changes in DNA content. In addition, small deletions or insertions may lead to changes that are too small to be detected by flow cytometry. Changes in DNA content less than about 5%, or two chromosomes, cannot be detected. This problem is created by inherent staining and measurement inconsistencies that lead to nonuniform fluorescence among normal nuclei. This results in wider peaks and what is known as the *coefficient of variation*. A wide peak may represent two populations with DNA indexes that are close to one another, or it may represent one population and a large coefficient of variation. In general, a coefficient of variation greater than 5% becomes uninterpretable.

Another limitation of ploidy analysis involves *tetraploidy,* or abnormal cell lines with a DNA content that is close to double the amount found in normal cells. This arises for two reasons. Normal cells during the M and G_2 phases of the cycle contain 4N amount of DNA. In addition, the flow cytometer cannot always distinguish large particles from clumped particles and thus cannot always distinguish nuclei with double the amount of DNA from two normal nuclei clumped together. *Clumping* can sometimes be detected by looking for peaks at the 6N position.

In addition to DNA content, cell-cycle analysis can also be performed. In this method, the proportion of cells in each phase—G_0, G_1, S, G_2, and M—is determined for a given population. The distribution of the peaks is as follows: the G_1-G_0 cells usually represent the largest peak, the G_2-M cells are usually represented by a smaller peak, and the S-phase cells contain an intermediate amount of DNA between the first two groups and are represented by a peak that spans the first two. Because there is no clear distinction in the peaks between the G_1-G_0 cells and the G_2-M cells, it is frequently difficult to measure these peaks, and different mathematic models have been devised to attempt to estimate the area corresponding to the different peaks. Another difficulty arises when studying two cell populations. The

S-phase region of one population could overlap with the G_2-M compartment of another cell population. Mathematic models and statistics are continually advancing, however, making S-phase calculations more accurate.

Aneuploidy and high proportion of S-phase cells are found in many types of cancers. The ability to perform flow cytometry on paraffin-embedded samples, and thus in pathology archives, has allowed long-term follow-up of cytometry results. With this technology, correlations can be made between abnormal DNA detected by flow cytometry and long-term outcome of cancer patients. The areas discussed next are the specific applications of flow cytometry to the field of gynecology (9–11).

Flow cytometry has been most helpful in cancer research. Its significance is probably most evident in *ovarian cancer.* Survival in ovarian cancer frequently depends more on individual tumor characteristics than on the type of treatment administered. The traditionally used prognostic factors are subjective, and so more objective ways of evaluating tumor characteristics have been sought. Flow cytometry is an objective measure of DNA abnormalities of tumors. Combined with information from CA-125 assays, cell-cycle information, and other tumor markers, it has proven helpful in outcome prediction.

Tumor ploidy seems to be a major prognostic indicator in ovarian cancer. Several researchers studied aneuploidy in tumors and found a rate of about 50% to 80%. Braly et al., in a review of the literature, found that 8 of the 10 studies showed that aneuploidy corresponded to significantly shorter survival times. Prolonged survival of patients with diploid tumors seems to be most significant in those patients with stage III carcinoma (12,13). Some investigators have suggested recommending that these patients have flow cytometry studies done so more aggressive treatment can be offered to patients with aneuploid tumors (14). Patients with stage IV ovarian cancer seem to have uniformly short survival times regardless of ploidy (12).

Tumor ploidy and residual disease after debulking have also been studied. Diploid tumors were found to have less residual disease after debulking. Again in their review of the literature, Braly et al. found that aneuploid tumors generally had more residual disease (12–17).

One of the most promising areas for flow cytometry is in evaluating ovarian tumors of borderline malignancy. In general, patients with these tumors tend to do well, even with advanced disease. However, in a subset of patients, the tumors are more aggressive, and these patients could benefit from adjuvant therapy. Flow cytometry may be helpful in determining which patients fall into this subset. One study analyzed 44 patients. Two had aneuploid tumors, and 1 of the 2 patients died within 7 months after diagnosis (18). In another study, flow cytometry was performed on 64 patients with borderline tumors; 42 were found to be diploid and 22 aneuploid. The 15-year survival rates were 80% and 20%, respectively (19). Flow cytometry seems to

be a promising new tool to determine which patients have more aggressive tumors and need adjuvant therapy.

In addition to ovarian cancer, *cervical cancer* has been studied. Results are not as definitive as in ovarian cancer, but some trends have been observed. Higher proportions of aneuploid cells are seen in late-stage as compared with early-stage carcinoma (20). This is seen in premalignant lesions as well. One study demonstrated higher rates of aneuploidy in cervical intraepithelial neoplasia type III as compared with type I lesions. Higher rates still were demonstrated in the invasive carcinomas evaluated in that study (21).

Aneuploidy has also been compared with histopathologic findings. Distinct correlations are not seen in all studies, but when information on S-phase rates are included as well, tumors with aneuploidy and high S-phase rates have worse histologic grades (22). Studies are conflicting on whether ploidy is a prognostic indicator of survival. Aneuploidy is associated with more vascular invasion and worse histologic grade, but these same tumors tend to be more radiosensitive. This is an important confounder in studies measuring survival of patients with advanced-stage disease. Overall, S-phase rates may be a better overall predictor of poor prognosis, but more studies will be needed (23–26).

Flow cytometry has also been used to analyze tumors in *endometrial carcinoma.* Several studies have shown that aneuploidy confers shorter survival times, higher death rates, and shorter disease-free intervals (26,27). In a study of 52 cases, 14 patients had aneuploid tumors, and 38 had diploid tumors. The mortality rate of those in the former group was 50%, with a median survival time of 17 months. The latter group had a mortality rate of 16% and a median survival time of 27.5 months (28). Aneuploidy has also been correlated with tumor stage. One group of researchers studied 222 endometrial carcinoma specimens (29). Aneuploidy and DNA index increased with worsening stage.

Other reports have examined the use of flow cytometry on *endometrial biopsy specimens.* Rosenberg et al. analyzed 111 curettage specimens. Aneuploidy was detected in 29% of tumors and was correlated with the grade of tumor: 11% in grade 1 tumors versus 42% in grade 3 tumors. S-phase fraction was also studied and was correlated with mortality. When the S-phase fraction was less than 5%, mortality rates were 7%. When the S-phase fraction was greater than 10%, mortality jumped to 49% (30). Another study sampled endometrial curettage specimens and made comparisons with 5-year survival rates. Relapse and mortality correlated with nondiploid status. Twenty-nine percent of 140 specimens were nondiploid but accounted for 50% of recurrences and 54% of deaths in the population studied (31). These data suggest that flow cytometry could be helpful in identifying high-risk patients after endometrial sampling and thus better direct treatment and referrals (32).

In addition to gynecologic cancer, flow cytometry is used in other areas. Researchers are studying the following:

endometrial biopsy dating, karyotype analysis, molar pregnancies as well as sex sorting of sperm. This research is all preliminary but promising.

Sperm

An interesting application of flow cytometry is the *segregation of sperm*. By using a fluorescent probe, sperm can be labeled. The Y-chromosome–containing sperm can be stained with a fluorescent probe that responds at one wavelength, whereas the X-chromosome–containing sperm can be labeled with a probe that responds at another wavelength. By using these fluorescent antibodies, the sperm can be run through the flow cytometer, and the X or Y sperm can be sorted. One report of this technology showed that 29 pregnancies were achieved by this method. Children were of the female gender in 92.9% of the pregnancies (33). Although this ratio is much better than anything reported previously in terms of the actual ability to discriminate between X and Y sperm, the long-term effects of this pretreatment are not fully known. However, as the authors pointed out, the specific dye and laser used in animals resulted in a negative Ames mutagenicity test. Flow cytometry will most likely continue to have a great impact on the field of obstetrics and gynecology in the future.

ASSISTED REPRODUCTIVE TECHNOLOGY

In vitro fertilization (IVF) of a human embryo was first reported in 1978 by a team of British scientists, Steptoe and Edwards. Since that time, thousands of babies have been born with this technology as well as with newer modifications of this technique. This section discusses the principles of IVF as well as other related technologies of gamete intrafallopian transfer (GIFT), zygote intrafallopian transfer, intracytoplasmic sperm injection, and oocyte donation.

IVF was initially designed to help women with severe tubal disease who had difficulty conceiving. Over the last 20 years, modifications have enabled clinicians to offer this technology to couples with unexplained infertility, endometriosis, male factor infertility, and immunologic causes of infertility. Until recently, a woman's age was the limiting factor for treatment, but this is changing as well with the use of donor eggs. IVF and related technologies are now used to treat infertility resulting from a variety of causes.

The first successful attempt at IVF was achieved in a nonstimulated cycle in which oocyte retrieval was timed by monitoring luteinizing hormone. Nonstimulated cycles are still used, but the success rates are low, around 6%. These low rates led to the use of stimulation protocols to improve the chances of successful oocyte retrieval and fertilization. Gonadotropin-releasing hormone agonists and human menopausal gonadotropins are now used to stimulate the development of multiple follicles. Injection of human chori-

onic gonadotropin is then used to trigger ovulation so retrieval can be timed precisely.

During one human menstrual cycle, a single oocyte is ovulated. This oocyte emerges as the dominant one of 15 to 20 immature oocytes that may have begun the process of maturation at the beginning of the cycle. The nondominant follicles undergo a process of atresia, and because they are not selected, they are effectively wasted. The goal of stimulation and superovulation in IVF is to allow full development of multiple follicles instead of the usual single dominant follicle that develops in an unstimulated cycle. *Superovulation protocols* essentially rescue some of the ovarian follicles that would otherwise undergo atresia.

All protocols involve the stimulation of follicles early in development before natural selection of the dominant follicle can occur. Human menopausal gonadotropins have been the standard drug. They are obtained through distillation of the urine of menopausal women, who produce high levels of follicle-stimulating hormone and luteinizing hormone. Newer preparations have included purified and highly purified follicle-stimulating hormone. The highly purified hormone has the advantage of subcutaneous administration, whereas the others must be administered intramuscularly because of impurities. Recombinant technology has allowed the production of human gonadotropins. These medications are currently available and have several advantages over the original product. The first advantage is that they can be produced indefinitely from the cultured cells. This obviates the need to collect urine from postmenopausal women. Moreover, by changing from a human-derived purified product to a recombinant one, theoretically there will be less chance of batch-to-batch variability. Ultimately, recombinant products are expected entirely to replace products currently retrieved and purified from human sources.

In stimulated cycles in assisted reproductive technology, transvaginal ultrasound and estradiol measurements are made frequently. At the appropriate time, ovulation is triggered with human chorionic gonadotropin. This is usually done when several follicles have reached a mature size, 16 to 20 mm, and the estradiol level is approximately 200 pg/mL per mature follicle. The oocytes are retrieved approximately 36 hours after human chorionic gonadotropin injection, most commonly by transvaginal aspiration of follicles. Timing is critical. It must occur before the release of the eggs at ovulation but late enough so the oocytes have time to complete meiosis I and enter meiosis II.

Once the follicles are aspirated, oocytes are identified under a dissecting microscope. They usually can be easily seen because of the cumulus-corona cell complex. The oocytes are not fertilized right away but only after a period of 4 to 6 hours has passed. Fertilization rates are higher if the first polar body is present.

Semen is obtained by masturbation on the day of oocyte retrieval after a 24- to 48-hour period of sexual abstinence. The sperm must be washed and separated from the seminal fluid. This is done using media and centrifugation techniques.

Fertilization is accomplished by adding 50,000 to 100,000 sperm to a culture well containing each egg. Fertilization requires a sequence of carefully orchestrated steps to occur. The sperm binds to recognition sites on the zona pellucida. Once the fertilizing sperm penetrates, a zona reaction occurs that makes it impenetrable to other sperm. This process is accomplished by the release of hydrolytic enzymes that cause hardening of the extracellular layer by cross linking of proteins and the inactivation of sperm receptors. The sperm then penetrates the perivitelline space, and, eventually, fusion of the egg and sperm membrane occurs. This triggers another reaction that results in the completion of meiosis II and release of the second polar body by the egg. At this point, two pronuclei are visible, and this is noted as evidence of successful fertilization and usually occurs after 16 to 20 hours of incubation.

After fertilization, the embryos are incubated for another 72 hours until they reach the four- to eight-cell stage. At this time, the embryos are transferred to the uterine cavity by the transcervical route. The number of embryos transferred depends on the patient's age and clinical history. Typically, a woman less than 35 years of age would receive three embryos, whereas a woman older than 40 years could receive four or more. This approach increases the chances of pregnancy. Viable embryos not otherwise transferred can be cryopreserved for use in subsequent cycles. Transferring more embryos markedly increases the risk of multiple births. The overall incidence with usual practice is 16% to 25% for twins and 1% to 3% for triplets (34). If higher-order multiple births occur, selective reduction has improved the overall success of these pregnancies. An emerging technology that maintains the high pregnancy rate but essentially caps the risk of multiples to twins is the transfer of blastocysts. By allowing embryos to grow for 48 additional hours on top of the traditional 72 hours of culture, some embryos reach the final stage of development before implantation, the blastocyst stage. At that point, two embryos can be returned to the woman's uterus instead of three or more. Progesterone supplements in the form of vaginal suppositories, oral micronized tablets, or intramuscular injection are also given to supplement the corpus luteum in the early weeks of pregnancy (34–40).

Once IVF was applied successfully to patients with infertility from causes other than tubal disease, modifications were made to benefit couples with other causes of infertility. One of these modifications is *GIFT*. GIFT is significantly different from IVF in that fertilization takes place within the body. The process of GIFT is identical to that of IVF for ovarian stimulation. Instead of transvaginal retrieval through ultrasound, however, the follicles are aspirated laparoscopically. Oocytes and spermatozoa are then placed directly into the fimbriated end of the fallopian tube, the number again depending on the patient's age and other relevant clinical factors. The markedly shortened time that the oocytes are kept outside the body, usually less than 15 minutes instead of 72 hours, is another difference. GIFT is suitable for any couple with prolonged infertility, provided the women has at least one normal fallopian tube. Some centers report greater success of GIFT in appropriate couples when compared with IVF (39). The tubal environment may facilitate fertilization and early embryonic development that cannot be duplicated in the *in vitro* environment. Although some reports have supported this claim of superior pregnancy rates, the data are controversial (41), and at present, with improvements in the ability to handle eggs and embryos extracorporeally, the gap in pregnancy rates has narrowed considerably.

A hybrid technique related to both GIFT and IVF is *zygote intrafallopian transfer*. When fertilization is in doubt, eggs are aspirated transvaginally and are inseminated as in routine IVF. The resultant pronuclear embryos are then transferred laparoscopically to the fallopian tube. Allegedly, this allows the embryos to be transported to the uterus through the fallopian tube, where they can develop in a nonartificial environment.

Another modification of IVF has attempted to enhance fertilization through *micromanipulation techniques*. This treatment is most useful for male infertility. A normal ejaculate has a volume of 1.5 to 5 mL and contains more than 20×10^6 sperm/mL with a motility of greater than 60% and greater than 30% normal morphology (42). Oligozoospermia and pregnancy rates are closely correlated. The 1-year pregnancy rate for couples with normal sperm count is 82%, whereas the pregnancy rate drops to 8.7% if the sperm count is less than 1×10^6 (42).

Assisted fertilization refers to techniques that involve mechanical penetration of the egg. Three techniques have been tried. The first one was *zona drilling*, in which a small opening is created in the zona pellucida to provide better access to the sperm. The second type is *subzonal insemination*, in which approximately five sperm are injected just below the zona pellucida. This technique ensures sperm penetration of the zona but increases the risk of polyspermy. These techniques, unfortunately, have low fertilization rates.

In 1992, a breakthrough was made with the introduction of *intracytoplasmic sperm injection* (43). In this technique, a single sperm is selected and is injected into the cytoplasm of the egg. Because only one sperm is used, the risk of polyspermy is eliminated. Pregnancy rates have been promising, around 25% (44), and this technique is possible with epididymal and testicular sperm. Because intracytoplasmic sperm injection bypasses natural selection for sperm, concern has been expressed about an increase in chromosomal or genetic abnormalities in the children. To date, however, spontaneous abortion rates have not been excessively high, and there has not been an increase in chromosomal abnormalities in children born with this technique (37,44). Overall, the obstetric outcome in pregnancies from intracytoplasmic sperm injection is similar to that of conventional IVF. However, the rates of preterm deliveries, low and very low birth weight, and perinatal mortality appear slightly higher than for spontaneous pregnancies when only singletons are considered (45). Further case-controlled studies are needed to determine the causes of these differences.

In addition to treating men with abnormal or reduced sperm counts, the technology of IVF has also enabled women with abnormal or deficient ovaries to achieve pregnancy through *donor oocytes*. Research that led to successful human oocyte donation began in animals. *In vivo* fertilized embryos have been transferred from donor to recipients in many species of mammals. In nonhuman mammals, superovulated donors are inseminated, and then embryos are obtained just before implantation through uterine lavage. The embryos are then transferred to a recipient whose cycle has been synchronized with that of the donor. In the early 1980s, similar techniques were applied to humans. These techniques were first applied to women with ovarian failure. Follicular aspiration with IVF instead of *in vivo* fertilization was attempted with success in 1984 (46). With the addition of sex steroids to stimulate preparation and support of the endometrium, this latter technique was applied to women with dysfunctional ovaries. At that time, donors had to undergo surgical follicular aspiration through laparoscopy or minilaparotomy, which limited the widespread acceptance of this procedure. With the improvement of ultrasound techniques, transvaginal egg retrieval became the standard route of egg retrieval; therefore, the risk to the donors was decreased, thus allowing many more infertile women access to this technique. In 1988, 130 patients underwent 158 preembryo transfers, and 32% of these patients produced a clinical pregnancy, with a 23% live delivery rate. This rate was better than the live delivery rate of standard IVF in the same year (47). This technique has enabled older women reasonable success in the age-related battle against infertility.

Oocyte donation requires that the donor's and recipient's cycles be synchronized. The donor undergoes superovulation and follicular aspiration under ultrasound guidance. Recipients receive hormones to prepare the endometrium for the transfer and hopeful implantation of donor embryos. This is usually done with oral estradiol and intramuscular progesterone given before transfer and continued through the 12th week of pregnancy. If there is difficulty in coordinating cycles, embryos can be cryopreserved and used later.

Oocyte donation is appropriate for women with various causes of infertility. Women with premature ovarian failure from gonadal dysgenesis, radiation, chemotherapy, and immunologic mechanisms can all benefit. It also benefits those with abnormal chromosomes and those who are at high risk of passing on a genetically inherited disease. Its greatest success has been in those women who have age-related infertility, and this is the largest population benefiting from this technique. Oocyte donors are typically women between

the ages of 21 and 34 years. A fertility history in the donors is desirable but not a requirement. Many recipients prefer to recruit their own donor, and in many cases the latter is a sister, other relative, or close friend.

The high success rates of oocyte donation, sometimes greater than 60%, are generally better than those of conventional IVF and reflect the importance of oocyte age in fertility. The finding that recipients do not undergo superovulation also ensures a more natural environment for implantation of the embryo. Achieving pregnancy for a women in her 50s is now possible. The challenge now lies in the prenatal management of these women, who frequently have multiple gestations and high rates of gestational diabetes, hypertension, and preeclampsia. With many women now delaying childbearing until their 40s, this technology will continue to be popular and will play an increasing role in assisted reproductive technology (47–49).

PREIMPLANTATION GENETIC DIAGNOSIS

IVF has afforded medical science access to the earliest stages of human development. Researchers have begun to use this opportunity for the diagnosis of some genetic diseases before implantation has taken place. A single cell, or sometimes two, may be removed from an embryo in the earlier stages of development. The chromosomes can be checked for aneuploidy, or specific genetic defects can be identified by direct DNA testing. Embryos that have been examined by biopsy and have proved normal are returned to the uterus for implantation. This process involves a combination of the latest technologies in molecular biology, genetics, embryology, and assisted reproductive technology. To date, an estimated 50 children, who underwent this sampling as embryos, have been born.

As with any experimental technology, it is first important to identify the population for which it is most useful. *Preimplantation genetic diagnosis* is most helpful for specific groups of patients. The first group comprises those couples who are at risk of having a child with a lethal X-linked disorder for which the biochemical or molecular defect is not yet known. These couples can have sex typing done and have only female embryos returned to the uterine cavity. At worst, the child would be a carrier of the disease, but she would be unaffected. In the second group, one member of a couple carries a translocation, and such couples are at greater risk of chromosomal aneuploidy. The third group comprises those at risk of having a child with a single gene disorder. Preimplantation genetic diagnosis allows screening of the embryos before implantation, with the hope of avoiding a second trimester abortion of an affected fetus.

To perform preimplantation genetic diagnosis, several criteria must first be met. The genetic disease for which the couple is at risk must be one whose DNA defect has been sequenced and for which reliable testing is available. The

DNA of the biopsied cell must be amplified by polymerase chain reaction (PCR). The micromanipulation biopsy technique must provide a high rate of continued growth and development of the preembryo. The diagnosis of disease must be accurate, reproducible, and consistent. The IVF team must have a high "take home baby" rate because the number of embryos available for transfer is reduced by 25% in autosomal disorders and by 50% in X-linked and autosomal dominant disorders. The specifics of these technologies are discussed here, beginning with micromanipulation and biopsy techniques.

Micromanipulation involves the biopsy and handling of one or two blastomeres (the cells of an embryo are called blastomeres) obtained from a developing embryo. Specialized microscopes and biopsy instruments are used for these procedures. These techniques have already been used widely in animal husbandry and agriculture. Preembryos have been cleaved to form twins, with varying results among different animals. *Biopsy of embryos* has also been performed for sex determination. Several studies have documented the success rates of biopsy techniques on preembryos. Four- and eight-cell embryos have undergone biopsy without any adverse effects on *in vivo* or *in vitro* development (50–52). Karyotyping of oocytes and early embryos has also been successfully performed (53).

In humans, biopsy for genetic material can be performed on polar bodies, or blastomeres. The first polar body is formed after the first meiotic division and is found under the zona pellucida. In a heterozygous individual, the polar body has either the normal or mutant allele, with the oocyte having the other allele, provided crossing over has not taken place. Therefore, if a woman is a carrier of a specific genetic condition, she has two alleles in her genome. One allele is the affected or abnormal allele, and the other is the wild-type or normal allele. When the oocyte undergoes meiosis I and the chromosome complement is reduced from diploid (paired chromosomes) to haploid (single chromosomes), one strand of chromosomes remains in the oocyte, and the other is shed in the first polar body. If the polar body is examined by biopsy and contains the affected allele, one can reason that the normal allele must have remained behind in the oocyte. That oocyte can then be used in IVF. If the normal allele is detected in the polar body, one can deduce that the abnormal allele remained inside the nucleus of the egg, and this egg would not be used. *Polar body biopsy* has the advantage of avoiding sampling of the actual embryo and so circumvents any ethical questions raised about this procedure.

Polar body biopsy has several limitations, however. The number of potential healthy preembryos is reduced by half because only those with unaffected oocytes are used. Another problem with polar biopsy concerns crossing over of genes. If crossing over occurs, the oocyte and polar body could be heterozygous for the mutation. The further the gene in question is from the centromere, the more likely that crossing over will occur. For this reason, with genes that are a considerable distance from the centromere, the polar body must be examined with probes for both the normal and affected alleles to make sure that one copy of the gene is present. If one were to only test for the normal gene and to assume that no signal meant the abnormal gene was present, one could be mistaken because of the crossing over effect. A third limitation is that the carrier status of the preembryos is not known because the genes of the sperm are not tested.

An alternative to polar body biopsy is *sampling extraembryonic tissue* at the blastocyst stage. Sampling is done from the trophoectoderm, and limited studies *in vitro* have shown that biopsies have been performed on blastocysts without impeding development (54). Advantages of this technique are several. More cells can be sampled, allowing for more material for genetic diagnosis. In addition, it precludes biopsy of the embryo proper, so persons with moral or ethical objections may find this technique more acceptable. Finally, if cryopreservation is necessary, some evidence suggests that blastocysts may survive thawing better than preembryos (55,56). This approach has several disadvantages as well. Many preembryos do not develop to the blastocyst stage *in vitro* (57). Finally, some concern exists about genetic mosaicism because there have been cases of chorionic villi sampling in which chromosomal abnormalities have been found in the chorionic villi that did not exist in the fetus (52).

The third and most widely adopted biopsy technique involves removing one or two cells (*blastomeres*) from the embryo at the eight-cell stage. By day 3 after fertilization, a human IVF embryo has reached the six- to eight-cell stage, and all cells are still totipotent. Researchers have shown that biopsy of one to two cells does not affect development to the blastocyst stage or pregnancy rates *in vivo* (58,59). Biopsy of day 3 embryos is the technique used by most centers today because it has had the greatest success rates (60).

Once access to the cells is obtained, genetic testing can begin. Three types of testing can be performed: gender identification for X-linked disease, testing for single gene defects, and testing for gene products or biochemical assays. One molecular technique that has revolutionized molecular genetics and made preimplantation genetic diagnosis possible is *PCR*. This technique enables researchers to multiply copies of DNA for analysis by 10^5 or 10^6 within several hours. PCR is based on repetitive cycling of reactions at varying temperatures. The DNA to be amplified is mixed with two single-stranded oligonucleotides or primers that are complementary to target sequences comprising the normal and mutant DNA of the gene in question. An excess amount of the four deoxyribonucleiotide triphosphates and heat-stable TAQ DNA polymerase are added as well.

The PCR reaction then consists of three main steps: denaturing of the DNA, annealing or lining up of the primers to complementary DNA, and extension from the primers to form new strands of DNA. By constantly changing the temperature of the mixture, repeated cycles of these three steps occur, so multiple copies of the target DNA are made. Once the desired DNA has been amplified, detection of gene defects is possible. Sex selection for couples at risk for sex-linked disease has been performed using primers specific for a sequence derived from the Y chromosome. The first successful attempts at preimplantation genetic diagnosis were achieved using this technique. In 1990, several healthy baby girls were born after biopsy and sexing by PCR (59).

Diagnosis of single gene defects has also been possible through PCR. Analysis of DNA is performed through the use of linked markers or, if the gene has been cloned, through the use of specific primers. PCR techniques are now available to detect single copy gene defects in sickle cell disease, thalassemias, hemophilia, cystic fibrosis, Lesch-Nyhan disease, α_1-antitrypsin deficiency, and Duchenne's muscular dystrophy (61). The first report of the use of preimplantation genetic diagnosis for single gene defects was in a couple at risk for cystic fibrosis. This experiment illustrates how PCR is used for detection of these defects. Researchers tested three couples, all carriers for cystic fibrosis. Cells were biopsied on day 3 after fertilization, and PCR was used to amplify the DNA. Probes containing the Δ508 cystic fibrosis mutation as well as normal DNA were used, and DNA fragments were produced that were either 154 bp (normal DNA) or 151 bp (mutant DNA). Unaffected cells produced only 154-bp fragments. Cells that were carriers produced a mixture of 151- and 154-bp fragments. Cells that had only mutant alleles produced only 151-bp fragments. The DNA fragments from each of the cells were mixed first with 154-bp fragments of normal DNA and then with 151-bp fragments of DNA containing the Δ508 mutation in such a way that heteroduplexes were allowed to form. The heteroduplexes were then easily detected by gel electrophoresis because they migrate more slowly.

Carrier and affected individuals were then identified as follows. When the cells in question were mixed with normal DNA and no heteroduplexes formed, then only normal DNA was present, and the cells were unaffected. When the cells in question were mixed with affected DNA and no heteroduplexes formed, then the cells were homozygous recessive for the Δ508 mutation and embryo had cystic fibrosis. Finally, when heteroduplexes formed when the DNA from the cells was mixed with either normal or affected DNA, then the corresponding embryo was a carrier for the disease. One normal and one carrier embryo were used for transfer in two of the couples, respectively. One woman became pregnant and gave birth to a girl free of the deletion in both chromosomes. Unaffected children have also been born to couples at risk for Tay-Sachs disease and Lesch-Nyhan syndrome (60).

Despite its success, PCR also has several drawbacks. Because of its powerful amplification ability from small amounts of DNA, nonspecific copying can occur, either from other sections of the specimen's DNA or from DNA of contaminants. The most worrisome situation is contamination from DNA of the sperm or of maternal cells. Contamination in routine PCR is reduced because many more copies of the target DNA exist than of contaminant DNA, thus increasing the odds that the specimen DNA will be the one that is amplified. With single cells containing only a single copy of the target gene, the risk of misinterpretation from contaminants becomes much more acute. In addition, the number of replication cycles used in conventional DNA is usually around 20 to 40. Forty to 60 cycles are usually needed when a single copy of the target DNA is used. In addition to contamination, PCR presents a second problem with sex typing. With PCR, the presence of an amplified band only indicates that an X or Y chromosome is present and gives no information about copy number. Aneuploidy could easily be missed.

In a second series using PCR for sex typing, one of seven fetuses labeled female by PCR was later found to be male, and the pregnancy was terminated (60). The reason for misdiagnosis was presumed to be amplification failure. Researchers have thus tried a second method for sex typing known as *fluorescent in situ hybridization*. In this technique, fluorescent DNA probes to the target DNA are used to detect the presence of a Y chromosome. To ensure reliability, a dual technique using simultaneous hybridization of one X and two Y probes has been developed. The first series produced five live births after IVF, all of the predicted sex (62). In addition to sex typing and testing for specific genetic mutations, some researchers have also studied biochemical assays. Testing for the gene product has the advantage of diagnosing an inherited disease regardless of the mutation. One group of researchers developed a mouse model for hypoxanthine phosphoribosyl transferase deficiency, which causes Lesch-Nyhan syndrome in humans (61). Preimplantation genetic diagnosis was performed easily with a biochemical microassay. When the same test was tried with humans, however, it was not successful. No hypoxanthine phosphoribosyl transferase activity was observed in any of the embryos tested. This is because, in human embryos, expression of genes begins later in development. No reliable biochemical assays have been developed yet.

Data collected from 14 centers revealed that 34 healthy babies have undergone preimplantation genetic diagnosis. Diseases for which testing is available include cystic fibrosis, Duchenne's muscular dystrophy, fragile X syndrome, Tay-Sachs disease, RhD blood typing, and hemophilia A (63). Among these pregnancies were 3 misdiagnoses. The first was one of sex typing mentioned earlier. The other 2 were misdiagnoses of cystic fibrosis. In both cases, only a single parent carried the Δ508 mutation; the mutation in the other was a rarer type. In these cases, carrier detection in the embryo is essential because these children could be affected if their other copy of the cystic fibrosis gene is a mutation other than Δ508. The exact reason for misdiagnosis was unclear. One possibility could be amplification failure of one allele of the sampled cell's DNA. Another is contamination of sperm DNA. A third is chromosomal mosaicism (60).

Chromosomal mosaicism has been detected in several preimplantation embryos. In one study, 69 embryos were studied (60). Half were analyzed for the sex chromosomes and the other half for the autosomal chromosomes. Fifteen percent of the former were found to be mosaic, and 30% of the latter were found to be mosaic. This finding has implications especially for the diagnosis of dominant disorders and chromosomal abnormalities. For this reason, most centers advocate testing two separate cells in these cases.

Preimplantation genetic diagnosis will likely prove to be a powerful tool for couples at risk of having a child with a genetic disease. As more genes are cloned and more tests are developed, additional couples will be able to take advantage of this technology. Work still needs to be done, but this new technology promises to have a large impact on reproductive medicine in the future.

FIBEROPTICS

This chapter concludes with a discussion of *fiberoptics,* a technology that has been around since the 1970s and one that has probably had the greatest impact on the field of gynecology by making laparoscopic surgery efficient and safe. Fiberoptics enabled light transmission and thus visualization of organs and tissues within the human body. Before 1960, endoscopy used small, hot tungsten bulbs. Visualization was poor, and complications were common because the hot endoscope could easily coagulate and damage bowel and other structures in the abdomen. Fiberoptic cables revolutionized this field. Flexible fibers allowed better visualization through ease of manipulation. In addition, the light reflected through the fibers was a marked improvement over the hot tungsten bulbs and made endoscopy much safer.

Optical fibers are constructed of glass fibers with a relatively high index of refraction surrounded by a sheath with a lower index of refraction. A source at one end of the cable gives off light that is propagated down the optical fiber with little loss by a process known as *total internal reflection.* This is possible because the fibers are made with a length much greater than their diameter (usually 10 to 25 μm). Numerous fibers are packed together in bundles to create the bright light viewed at the other end.

To explain total internal reflection, it is first necessary to review the concepts of reflection and refraction of light. At the interface between two transparent media, rays can be transmitted or reflected. If they are transmitted, they will be bent or refracted. The amount of refraction is determined by Snell's law, $n_1 \sin \alpha_1 = n_2 \sin \alpha_2$, where n is the angle of refraction of each respective interface and α_1 is the angle of the incident ray and α_2 is the angle of the refracted ray. Angle measurements are in relation to the normal, a line perpendicular to the interface. Another principle is that light rays moving from a denser medium will be bent away from the normal, whereas those traveling to a denser medium will be bent toward the normal. Any reflection that occurs will be at an angle equal to the incident in angle.

When light travels from denser to less dense material, the angle of the incident ray can be increased to the point at which the refracted ray forms an angle that is 90 degrees to the normal. In this case, refraction no longer occurs. If the angle of incidence is greater than this angle, known as the *critical angle,* the light rays will only be reflected, a situation known as *total internal reflection.* This property of light holds true even if the fiber is bent, as long as the radius of the bend is much larger than the diameter of the fiber. This process allows the propagation of light along a fiberoptic cable.

Fiberoptic cables are made of multiple thin fibers that enable total internal reflection. Because total internal reflection occurs only when light travels from a dense to a rarer medium, the rods are all encased in a material of lower optical density called *cladding* that ensures maximum capture of light rays. Multiple thin fibers composed of core and cladding are arranged within one light cord to enable transmission of high-intensity light for the length of the bundle. This simple principle is used to make laparoscopy safe and effective (64,65).

SUMMARY

Numerous technologies touch the lives of the practicing obstetrician or gynecologist every day. New technologies seep into practice almost insidiously. Treated with great skepticism initially, they must pass the test of time, but when validated, they become indispensable links in the chain of progress.

10 KEY POINTS

1. MRI can differentiate between healthy and diseased tissue with the use of magnetic fields and RF pulses.

2. MRI has application in evaluating pelvic anatomy including uterine anomalies, fibroids, and endometrial disease.

3. Flow cytometry is a technique that can identify or sort cells on the basis of their DNA content.

4. The DNA content of cells and their stage in the cell cycle can be useful diagnostic tools in evaluating pelvic neoplasms.

5. Flow cytometry has been adapted to sort sperm into

populations of X- and Y-bearing gametes that can then be used for insemination and pregnancy. This technique is in the earliest phases of development and will require further investigation before it becomes more widespread.

6. Assisted reproductive technologies have been in clinical use for 20 years now. The success rates continue to climb with incremental improvements in our ability to handle gametes and embryos.

7. Intracytoplasmic sperm injection is a technique that provides hope to millions of couples with severe male factor infertility. By injecting sperm directly into the eggs of affected couples, fertilization and pregnancies can occur that would not have been possible with conventional treatment.

8. Blastocyst culture is a technique in IVF in which embryos are grown for 5 days instead of 3 after egg retrieval. Most embryos in culture do not survive to the blastocyst stage. However, those that do survive have a high implantation rate, thus limiting the number of embryos needed to be transferred.

9. Preimplantation genetic testing is a way to check on the health of an embryo before it is returned to a woman's body. This technique makes it possible to distinguish between healthy embryos and those that contain potentially lethal disorders.

10. Fiberoptics are routinely used in medicine. The physical principles that make this possible have been readily adapted to numerous areas of medicine. Perhaps the greatest impact is the use of fiberoptic cables that convey light in operative endoscopy.

REFERENCES

1. Young SW. *Magnetic resonance imaging: basic principles,* 2nd ed. New York: Raven, 1988.
2. Johnston DL, Liu P, Wismer GL, et al. Magnetic resonance imaging: present and future applications. *Can Med Assoc J* 1985; 132:765–777.
3. Council on Scientific Affairs. Fundamentals of magnetic resonance imaging. *JAMA* 1987;258:3417–3423.
4. Hricak H, Stern JL, Fisher MR, et al. Endometrial carcinoma staging by MR imaging. *Radiology* 1987;162:297–305.
5. McCarthy S. Gynecologic applications of MRI. *Crit Rev Diagn Imaging* 1990;31:263–281.
6. Hricak H, Alpers C, Crooks LE, et al. Magnetic resonance imaging of the female pelvis: initial experience. *AJR Am J Roentgenol* 1983;141:1119–1128.
7. Hricak H. MRI of the female pelvis: a review. *AJR Am J Roentgenol* 1986;146:1115–1122.
8. McCarthy S. Magnetic resonance imaging of the normal female pelvis. *Radiol Clin North Am* 1992;30:769–775.
9. Givan AL. *Flow cytometry: first principles.* New York: John Wiley & Sons, 1992.
10. Merkel DE, Dressler LG, McGuire WL. Flow cytometry, cellular DNA content, and prognosis in human malignancy. *J Clin Oncol* 1987;5:1690–1703.
11. Orfao A, Ciudad J, Gonzalez M, et al. Flow cytometry in the diagnosis of cancer. *Scand J Clin Lab Invest Suppl* 1995;221: 145–152.
12. Friedlander ML, Hedley DW, Swanson C, et al. Prediction of long-term survival by flow cytometric analysis of cellular DNA content in patients with advanced ovarian cancer. *J Clin Oncol* 1988;6:282–290.
13. Rodenburg CJ, Cornelisse CJ, Heintz PA, et al. Tumor ploidy as a major prognostic factor in advanced ovarian cancer. *Cancer* 1987;59:317–323.
14. Seckinger D, Sugarbaker E, Frankfurt O. DNA content in human cancer: application in pathology and clinical medicine. *Arch Pathol Lab Med* 1989;113:619–626.
15. Braly PS, Klevecz RR. Flow cytometric evaluation of ovarian cancer. *Cancer* 1993;71[Suppl 4]:1621–1628.
16. Trope C, Makar A, Kaern J. DNA flow cytometry as a new prognostic factor in ovarian malignancies: a review. *Acta Obstet Gynecol Scand Suppl* 1992;155:95–97.
17. Friedlander ML, Hedley DW, Taylor IW, et al. Influence of cellular DNA content on survival in advanced ovarian cancer. *Cancer Res* 1984;44:397–400.
18. Friedlander ML, Russell P, Taylor IW, et al. Flow cytometric analysis of cellular DNA content as an adjunct to the diagnosis of ovarian tumours of borderline malignancy. *Pathology* 1984; 16:301–306.
19. Kaern J, Trope C, Kjorstad KE, et al. Cellular DNA content as a new prognostic tool in patients with borderline tumors of the ovary. *Gynecol Oncol* 1990;38:452–457.
20. Strang P. Cytogenetic and cytometric analyses in squamous cell carcinoma of the uterine cervix. *Int J Gynecol Pathol* 1989;8: 54–63.
21. Dudzinski MR, Haskill SJ, Fowler WC, et al. DNA content in cervical neoplasia and its relationship to prognosis. *Obstet Gynecol* 1987;69:373–377.
22. Johnson TS, Adelson MD, Sneige N, et al. Cervical carcinoma DNA content, S-fraction, and malignancy grading. I. Interrelationships. *Gynecol Oncol* 1987;26:41–56.
23. Tribukait B. Clinical DNA flow cytometry. *Med Oncol Tumor Pharmacother* 1984;1:211–218.
24. Jakobsen A. Ploidy level and short-time prognosis of early cervix cancer. *Radiother Oncol* 1984;1:271–275.
25. Rutgers DH, van der Linden PM, van Peperzeel HA. DNA-flow cytometry of squamous cell carcinomas from the human uterine cervix: the identification of prognostically different subgroups. *Radiother Oncol* 1986;7:249–258.
26. Strang P, Eklund G, Stendahl U, et al. S-phase rate as a predictor of early recurrences in carcinoma of the uterine cervix. *Anticancer Res* 1987;7:807–810.
27. Britton LC, Wilson TO, Gaffey TA, et al. Flow cytometric DNA analysis of stage I endometrial carcinoma. *Gynecol Oncol* 1989;34:317–322.
28. Iversen OE. Flow cytometric deoxyribonucleic acid index: a prognostic factor in endometrial carcinoma. *Am J Obstet Gynecol* 1986;155:770–776.
29. Lindahl B, Alm P, Killander D, et al. Flow cytometric DNA analysis of normal and cancerous human endometrium and cytological-histopathological correlations. *Anticancer Res* 1987;7: 781–789.
30. Rosenberg P, Wingren S, Simonsen E, et al. Flow cytometric measurements of DNA index and S-phase on paraffin-embedded early stage endometrial cancer: an important prognostic indicator. *Gynecol Oncol* 1989;35:50–54.
31. Podratz KC, Wilson TO, Gaffey TA, et al. Deoxyribonucleic acid analysis facilitates the pretreatment identification of high-risk endometrial cancer patients. *Am J Obstet Gynecol* 1993; 168:1206–1213.
32. Evans MP, Podratz KC. Endometrial neoplasia: prognostic significance of ploidy status. *Clin Obstet Gynecol* 1996;39:696–706.
33. Fugger EF, Black SH, Keyvanfar K, et al. Births of normal

daughters after MicroSort sperm separation and intrauterine insemination, *in-vitro* fertilization, or intracytoplasmic sperm injection. *Hum Reprod* 1998;13:2367–2370.

34. New reproductive technologies. *Int J Gynaecol Obstet* 1991; 35:274–278.

35. Paulson RJ. *In vitro* fertilization and other assisted reproductive techniques. *J Reprod Med* 1993;38:261–268.

36. Jennings JC, Moreland K, Peterson CM. *In vitro* fertilisation: a review of drug therapy and clinical management. *Drugs* 1996; 52:313–343.

37. Zilberstein M, Seibel MM. Fertilization and implantation. *Curr Opin Obstet Gynecol* 1994;6:184–189.

38. Penzias AS, DeCherney AH. Clinical review 55: advances in clinical *in vitro* fertilization. *J Clin Endocrinol Metab* 1994;78: 503–508.

39. Trounson AO, Wood C. IVF and related technology: the present and the future. *Med J Aust* 1993;158:853–857.

40. Edwards RG, Handyside AH. Future developments in IVF. *Br Med Bull* 1990;46:823–841.

41. Abyholm T, Tanbo T. GIFT, ZIFT, and related techniques. *Curr Opin Obstet Gynecol* 1993;5:615–622.

42. Diedrich K, Felberbaum R, Kupker W, et al. New approaches to male infertility: IVF and microinjection. *Int J Androl* 1995; 18[Suppl 2]:78–80.

43. Palermo G, Joris H, Devroey P, et al. Pregnancies after intracytoplasmic injection of single spermatozoon into an oocyte. *Lancet* 1992;340:17–18.

44. Gordts S, Vercruyssen M, Roziers P, et al. Recent developments in assisted fertilization. *Hum Reprod* 1995;10[Suppl 1]:107–114.

45. Aytoz A, Camus M, Tournaye H, et al. Outcome of pregnancies after intracytoplasmic sperm injection and the effect of sperm origin and quality on this outcome. *Fertil Steril* 1998;70: 500–505.

46. Lutjen P, Trounson A, Leeton J, et al. The establishment and maintenance of pregnancy using *in vitro* fertilization and embryo donation in a patient with primary ovarian failure. *Nature* 1984; 307:174–175.

47. Sauer MV, Paulson RJ. Human oocyte and preembryo donation: an evolving method for the treatment of infertility. *Am J Obstet Gynecol* 1990;163:1421–1424.

48. Sauer MV, Paulson RJ. Oocyte and embryo donation. *Curr Opin Obstet Gynecol* 1995;7:193–198.

49. Morris RS, Sauer MV. New advances in the treatment of infertility in women with ovarian failure. *Curr Opin Obstet Gynecol* 1993;5:368–377.

50. Wilton LJ, Shaw JM, Trounson AO. Successful single-cell biopsy and cryopreservation of preimplantation mouse embryos. *Fertil Steril* 1989;51:513–517.

51. Wilton LJ, Trounson AO. Biopsy of preimplantation mouse embryos: development of micromanipulated embryos and proliferation of single blastomeres *in vitro*. *Biol Reprod* 1989;40: 145–152.

52. Kaufmann RA, Morsy M, Takeuchi K, et al. Preimplantation genetic analysis. *J Reprod Med* 1992;37:428–436.

53. McGowan KD. Preimplantation prenatal diagnosis. *Obstet Gynecol Clin North Am* 1993;20:599–610.

54. Dokras A, Sargent IL, Ross C, et al. Trophectoderm biopsy in human blastocysts. *Hum Reprod* 1990;5:821–825.

55. Fehilly CB, Cohen J, Simons RF, et al. Cryopreservation of cleaving embryos and expanded blastocysts in the human: a comparative study. *Fertil Steril* 1985;44:638–644.

56. Li R, Cameron AW, Batt PA, et al. Maximum survival of frozen goat embryos is attained at the expanded, hatching and hatched blastocyst stages of development. *Reprod Fertil Dev* 1990;2: 345–350.

57. Sauer MV, Bustillo M, Rodi IA, et al. *In-vivo* blastocyst production and ovum yield among fertile women. *Hum Reprod* 1987;2: 701–703.

58. Hardy K, Martin KL, Leese HJ, et al. Human preimplantation development *in vitro* is not adversely affected by biopsy at the 8-cell stage. *Hum Reprod* 1990;5:708–714.

59. Handyside AH, Kontogianni EH, Hardy K, et al. Pregnancies from biopsied human preimplantation embryos sexed by Y-specific DNA amplification. *Nature* 1990;344:768–770.

60. Delhanty JD. Preimplantation diagnosis. *Prenat Diagn* 1994; 14:1217–1227.

61. Monk M. Preimplantation diagnosis of genetic disease. *Ann Med* 1993;25:463–466.

62. Griffin DK, Handyside AH, Harper JC, et al. Clinical experience with preimplantation diagnosis of sex by dual fluorescent *in situ* hybridization. *J Assist Reprod Genet* 1994;11:132–143.

63. Harper JC. Preimplantation diagnosis of inherited disease by embryo biopsy: an update of the world figures. *J Assist Reprod Genet* 1996;13:90–95.

64. Epstein M. Fiber optics in medicine. *Crit Rev Biomed Eng* 1982; 7:79–120.

65. Hulka JF, Reich H. *Textbook of laparoscopy*, 2nd ed. Philadelphia: WB Saunders, 1993.

BASICS OF GYNECOLOGIC ONCOLOGY

W. MICHAEL LIN
CAROLYN Y. MULLER
DAVID SCOTT MILLER

The field of *gynecologic oncology* has matured tremendously over the last several decades. Great strides have been made in clinical research evaluating the many aspects of conventional single or combined therapy. Conventional cancer treatment strategies include single or combination chemotherapy, surgical treatment, or radiation therapy. However, as our knowledge of cancer biology, cancer genetics, and immunology continues to increase rapidly, it has become essential to integrate the basic science of carcinogenesis with present clinical practice, in other words, to translate the "bench to the bedside." The purpose of this chapter is to provide a brief overview of the field of clinical gynecologic oncology, with particular emphasis on a biochemical, genetic, and cellular understanding as it pertains to today's clinical challenges. These principles are the basis of the biologic therapeutic paradigms in clinical research today that may be the successful practices of tomorrow.

EPIDEMIOLOGY

Ovarian Cancer

Ovarian cancer is the second most common genital cancer that affects women in the United States, but it remains the most deadly. Approximately 1 in 70 women in the United States will develop ovarian cancer during their lifetime, a rate that accounts for about 4% of all cancer cases in women. In 1998, investigators estimated that 25,400 new cases of ovarian cancer would be diagnosed in the United States, and an estimated 14,500 women would die of it (1). Ovarian cancer may arise from the germ cells, the stroma, or the epithelial lining covering the ovary or peritoneum. This discussion is limited to epithelial ovarian cancer because this is the most deadly and the best studied on a molecular basis.

Epithelial ovarian cancer is thought to arise from cells sharing a common embryologic origin to the cells covering the peritoneum. During the early part of cancer growth, most tumors remain confined as a cystic growth within these epithelial inclusion cysts within the substrate of the ovary. The tumor eventually penetrates the surface of the ovarian capsule and allows the malignant cells to seed the peritoneal cavity, thereby causing the classic diffuse perito-

neal tumor involvement referred to as *peritoneal carcinomatosis*. The omentum especially is a frequent site of involvement, because its job is to scavenge abnormal cells in the abdomen and pelvis. As a result of the highly vascular fatty tissue, these metastatic lesions tend to grow large and represent the classic *omental cake.*

Epidemiologic studies have identified several risk factors for ovarian cancer. Ovulation appears to be a key factor in ovarian cancer risk. Conditions associated with reduced ovulation are associated with reduced risks. Case-control studies have consistently demonstrated that women who have used oral contraceptives have a 30% to 60% less chance of developing ovarian cancer than women without history of oral contraceptive use (2). Women who have ever been pregnant also have about a 30% to 60% decreased risk of ovarian cancer compared with nulliparous women (3). The protective effects of parity, multiple birth, history of breast feeding, and oral contraceptive use support the *incessant ovulation hypothesis* in which ovarian cancer is thought to be related to the lifetime number of ovulations. Based on this theory, the epithelial covering of the ovary is disrupted at the time of ovulation and undergoes involution and a high metabolic turnover during the repair process. Cellular changes can occur during this repair process, and dysregulation of cellular control genes can lead to an uncontrolled growth advantage and a subsequent early tumor cell. One provocative study by Berchuck et al. linked the number of ovulatory cycles with proliferation-associated DNA damage and an increased risk of developing *p53* mutations within the tumor (4). An association with an increased risk of ovarian cancer in patients receiving ovulation induction has been raised by several investigators but has yet to be well documented (5).

One of the most recently recognized important risk factors for ovarian cancer is family history. Previous estimates of a 5% risk were given to women with an affected first-degree relative and 7% with 2 affected relatives (6). However, much more is known today about causative genes associated with family cancer syndromes. The best studied is the *hereditary breast-ovarian cancer (HBOC) syndrome,* which describes families with an autosomal dominant expression of breast or ovarian cancer through the generations that can manifest through either the maternal or paternal lineage. The germline mutations often involve either the *BRCA1* or *BRCA2* genes, but occasionally other genes may be causative. Unaffected patients who have this germline mutation may be at a 16% to 62% lifetime risk of developing ovarian cancer (7), but it is possible that these patients have a more favorable prognosis (8). Another family cancer syndrome demonstrating an increased risk of ovarian cancer is the *Lynch II syndrome of hereditary nonpolyposis colon cancer.* This syndrome involves a germline mutation in one of several genes (*MSH-2, MLH-1, PMS-1,* and *PMS-2*) involved in the DNA mismatch repair pathway. A careful family history reveals family members affected with colon, endometrial, ovarian, or other gastointestinal primary cancers. The role of the primary caretaker is to identify these patients at risk by taking a thorough family history. Options for genetic counseling, cancer risk assessment, and genetic testing are available with referral. Research is ongoing regarding adequate screening techniques, behavior modification, and prophylactic surgery. Patients at a significant hereditary risk for ovarian cancer may benefit from prophylactic oophrectomy because screening modalities even for high-risk patients have been disappointing.

Most ovarian cancers are diagnosed at an advanced stage at which the 5-year survival rate approaches 30% or less. Newer drugs such as paclitaxel have increased the initial response rate but have not made a substantial impact on survival (9). The significant clinical prognostic factors include stage and grade of the tumor and, most important, the degree of residual tumor left after primary cytoreduction. Other molecular prognostic features, including flow cytometric evaluation (10), *p53* mutational analysis (11), loss of heterozygosity (LOH) studies (11) (loss of tumor-suppressor genes [TSG]), and overexpression of oncogenes such as *HER-2/neu* (11), have been equivocal in independently predicting survival and are not currently clinically useful. We discuss the role of oncogenes and TSGs later in this chapter.

Uterine Carcinoma

Endometrial cancer is the most common genital cancer in the United States. In 1998, investigators estimated that 36,100 new cases would be diagnosed, and that 6,300 women would die of this disease (1).

From epidemiologic studies, it is apparent that reproductive and menstrual risk factors play an important role in most endometrial cancers. Most studies demonstrate a threefold or greater excessive risk for nulliparous women, in particular, for women with a history of infertility and anovulatory cycles (12). Type I endometrial cancer (13), or estrogen-dependent endometrial cancer, is more frequent in situations of unopposed estrogen stimulation such as in obesity, in which there is peripheral conversion of androstenedione to estrone, in Stein-Leventhal syndrome (14),

in the case of estrogen replacement without the use of a progestational agent (15), and in the case of an estrogen-producing tumor (16).

Epidemiologic studies have shown that a woman who is the first-degree relative of a patient affected with endometrial cancer has a personal increased cancer risk. The Lynch II syndrome of hereditary nonpolyposis colon cancer has been well documented, with endometrial carcinoma as the most common extracolonic cancer. Lynch et al. in 1994 described a family with an aggregation of endometrial carcinoma along with other malignant diseases that lacked any classic hereditary cancer syndrome (17). It is now known that loss of function of one of the DNA mismatch repair genes *MSH-2, MSH-3, MLH-1, PMS-2,* and *PMS-1* is found in many of these families predisposed to cancer.

Further evidence for the role of exogenous hormones in the pathogenesis of type I endometrial cancer is derived from studies that have shown that estrogen-progestin combination hormone replacement significantly lowers the risk of endometrial cancer (18). Tamoxifen, an "antiestrogen" with stimulatory effects on the endometrium, has also been implicated in an increased risk of endometrial cancer because of its weak estrogenic effect on the uterine target organ. Fisher et al. from the National Surgical Adjuvant Breast and Bowel Project trial reported an average annual hazard rate of endometrial cancer as 1.2 per 1,000, with a cumulative hazard rate of 6.3 per 1,000 within the first 5 years (19). Because the benefit of tamoxifen in preventing a second breast malignancy or recurrence outweighs this low-level increased risk of endometrial cancer, women who take tamoxifen should report any worrisome signs such as bleeding or abdominal pain promptly to their physician.

Unlike ovarian cancer, women with endometrial cancer are frequently diagnosed at an early stage as a result of recognizing the early warning signs of postmenopausal or irregular bleeding. However, the disease recurs in a small subset of patients with stage I disease. In 1991, Lurain et al. studied 264 patients with clinical stage I endometrial adenocarcinoma and found that, using multivariate analysis, grade 3 tumor, advancing age, lymph node metastasis, and presence of extrauterine spread were the only variables significantly associated with disease recurrence or death (20). Tumor size also appears to be an important prognostic factor because it is observed that the greater the tumor size, the higher the likelihood of lymph node metastasis and the poorer the 5-year survival (21). Flow cytometry provides a rapid, reproducible, and precise method of quantifying cellular DNA contents and determining proliferative activity in tumors. Coleman et al. performed flow cytometry on 21 clinical stage I endometrial carcinomas with nodal metastasis and found aneuploidy in 65%. The ploidy status of the primary tumor correlates with survival; however, little additional information was gained by knowledge of the lymph node ploidy status (22). In addition, other molecular markers, such as *p53* status (23), the mutator phenotype (from defective DNA mismatch repair pathway) (24), and oncogene status such as *HER-2/neu* (25), are being evaluated as prognosticators.

Cervical Cancer

Cervical cancer is the leading cancer among women in developing countries, and is the third most common female genital malignant disease in the United States. In 1998, investigators estimated that 13,700 new cases of cervical cancer would be diagnosed, and an estimated 4,900 women would die of cervical cancer (1).

The incidence of cervical carcinoma is substantially higher among women in lower socioeconomic groups. Case-control studies have shown that sexual behavior is a major risk factor. Risk has been directly related to lifetime number of sexual partners, and it has been inversely related to age at first sexual intercourse (26). Several epidemiologic studies also have demonstrated excess risk of both preinvasive and invasive cervical abnormalities among smokers (27).

While evidence has been mounting in recent years establishing human papillomavirus (HPV) as the etiologic agent in the carcinogenesis of cervical cancer, it is clear that other factors are involved, as the majority of patients with HPV infections do not develop invasive lesions. It is well known that the natural history of cervical dysplasia is characterized by regression in the majority of mild and moderate dysplasia and progression only in a minority of mild, moderate, and even severe dysplasias. To date, there is no clinically useful tool to predict those patients at risk for recurrent dysplasia or progression to invasive cancer.

It is widely accepted that there are multi-step molecular changes leading to malignant transformation from preneoplastic lesions to invasive tumors. However, the sequence of molecular events responsible for cervical carcinogenesis has not been elucidated. To date, there are no reliable biomarkers to predict an individual's cervical dysplasia progression risk. The current management strategies are based on outcomes statistics and issues of patient compliance. This current system often leads to expensive and uncomfortable evaluations and overtreatment.

HPV is a double-stranded DNA virus of approximately 8,000 bp. HPV has more than 70 known subtypes. Types 6 and 11 are the common agents associated with condylomata acuminata, whereas types 16 and to a lesser extent 18 and 31 are oncogenic and play a key role in the oncogenesis of cervical cancer (28). The interaction of the HPV oncoproteins E6 and E7 irreversibly binds the TSGs *p53* and *Rb,* respectively, and elicits their degradation through the ubiquitin pathway. This degradation causes loss of function of critical proteins that regulate the cell cycle and allows uncontrolled cell growth and the loss of apoptosis, or programmed cell death. Present research is under way to evaluate a vaccine against the oncogenic HPV subtypes in cervical

cancer (29). However, millions of women harbor HPV in the lower genital tract, and only a few develop dysplasia or, less commonly, invasive cancer. Data suggest that other critical gene regions are required in cervical carcinogenesis. Critical TSG regions involved in cervical cancer include chromosomes 3p, 5p, 6p, and 11q. Regions of 3p LOH have been found in preneoplasias as well (30). The *FHIT* gene on 3p14.2 has been implicated in cervical carcinogenesis, but its role as a classic TSG has not yet been substantiated (31). Data have linked this gene as a target of smoking in lung cancer (32), and it may prove to be significant to the effects of cigarette carcinogens in cervical cancer as well. HPV subtypes have been studied as a predictor for cervical dysplasia progression, but again these have not proved to be clinically useful.

In 1993, flow cytometry was used to determine the ploidy status of cervical carcinoma and its use as a prognostic indicator. Forty-seven percent of cancers were found to have DNA aneuploidy; however, neither DNA index nor S-phase fraction correlated significantly with recurrence or survival (33).

Vaginal Cancer

Vaginal cancer is a rare genital malignant disease in the United States. In 1998, investigators estimated that 2,000 new cases would be diagnosed, and an estimated 600 women would die of it (1). Most (80% to 90%) carcinomas involving the vagina are metastatic from some other primary site by direct tumor extension, recurrence after complete surgical removal of a primary pelvic tumor, or direct lymphatic or hematogenous routes (34).

Vaginal cancer is primarily a disease of older women, with 60% of tumors occurring among women 60 years old or older. However, in the late 1960s, cases of clear cell adenocarcinoma of the vagina were observed among women between 15 and 22 years of age, and most of these tumors were linked to *in utero* exposure to diethylstilbestrol (35). Many other etiologic factors have been suggested such as trauma to the vagina, the use of pessaries, the presence of leukoplakia, or chronic vaginitis. These risk factors again support the common notion that cancers are more common in tissues that are metabolically active or that must undergo turnover and repair. Higher cellular turnover allows cells to enter the cell cycle in which DNA is susceptible to greater cumulative damage. One case-control study found an association of risks with low socioeconomic status, history of genital warts, or genital irradiation (36).

Vulvar Carcinoma

Vulvar cancer is the fourth most common genital cancer among women in the United States. Investigators estimated that approximately 3,200 new cases would be diagnosed in 1998, and 800 women would die of this disease (1). Approximately 15% to 20% of women with vulvar cancer have a second primary cancer occurring synchronously or metachronously in the cervix, vagina, or anogenital area (37).

Many risk factors common to cervical cancer have been observed for vulvar cancer, such as the number of sexual partners, a history of genital warts, cigarette smoking, and the presence of HPV. It appears that smokers with a history of HPV are at the highest risk, a finding possibly supporting the notion that the oncogenic effect of HPV depends on the presence of other cofactors such as immune alteration or molecular genetic alteration from cigarette smoking, diabetes, or loss of other critical TSG (36,38). Little work has been done on molecular prognosticators; however, it is apparent that a greater percentage of LOH occurs in tumors that are HPV negative (38).

The major prognostic factors in vulvar cancer are tumor size, depth of tumor invasion, nodal spread, and distant metastasis (39,40). Several authors have attempted to define a subpopulation of microinvasive tumors in which the risk of inguinal metastasis is negligible. The current consensus is that only tumors with less than 1 mm stromal invasion fulfill this requirement (41). Lymph node metastasis is the single most important prognostic factor. The presence of inguinal node metastasis routinely results in a 50% reduction of long-term survival (42).

ONCOGENES

A large and diverse body of research conducted over the last 20 years has uncovered much information regarding the molecular origin of cancer. By now, we have a clear view of how two sets of genes, oncogenes and TSGs, participate in carcinogenesis. There are predominantly three classes of genes involved in tumorigenesis: *oncogenes, TSGs,* and *DNA repair genes.* In this section, we focus on oncogenes.

The discovery of oncogenes came about during the research of tumor-causing retroviruses. One of these viruses, the Rous sarcoma virus, was found to carry a specific gene the protein product of which can cause cellular transformation. Such a transforming gene was termed a *viral oncogene,* and its protein product was termed an *oncoprotein.* A single oncogene carried into a chicken cell by the Rous sarcoma virus was able to derail and redirect the entire metabolism of the cell and to force it to grow in a malignant fashion. In 1976, Varmus and Bishop discovered that the oncogene in the Rous sarcoma virus was not a genuinely viral gene at all; instead, it arose directly from a preexisting cellular gene (*proto-oncogene*) that had been captured by an ancestor of the Rous sarcoma virus. Once captured, this gene was used by the virus to transform cells (43). Investigators now know that other nonviral agents such as mutagenic chemicals and x-rays can also activate this proto-oncogene and can convert it into a powerful oncogene.

By the early 1980s, many activated mutant proto-oncogenes were found in human tumors. Oncogenes are mostly responsible for the "liquid" tumors such as leukemias and lymphomas in which normal recombinational events bring these proto-oncogenes erroneously under the promotor of a light- or heavy-chain antibody component. In each case, a change in the sequence structure of these genes or overexpression by an active promotor was determined to be responsible for converting a proto-oncogene into an active oncogene. For example, a *ras* oncogene in human bladder carcinoma was found to have arisen through a single base change that altered the DNA sequence of a precursor proto-oncogene. An *abl* oncogene was created by a chromosomal translocation in myelogenic leukemia. The *myc* oncogene arose through gene amplification in a variety of malignancies, the prototype first described in Burkitt's lymphoma (43).

The growth cycle of a normal cell residing within a tissue is controlled largely by its surroundings. A normal cell rarely, if ever, spontaneously signals itself to proliferate; rather, it receives messages that originate from its environment. These messages are conveyed by growth factors, hormones, or other molecules that target their signal at either the cell surface or within the nucleus. Each cell possesses complex machinery that enables it to receive these signals, to process them, and to launch a growth program. The machinery consists of an array of proteins such as cell surface receptors that function to acquire growth-activating signals and to transmit them throughout the cell. The cytoplasmic signal transducers that become activated by these receptors can then pass signals further into cells and nuclear transcription factors that activate whole cascades of cellular genes. These activated pathways together orchestrate the cell's growth program (44).

Proto-oncogenes encode many of the proteins in this complex signaling circuitry that enable a normal cell to respond to exogenous growth factors. Oncogenic proteins succeed in activating these signaling circuits even in the absence of stimulation by extracellular growth factors. In doing so, they force a cell to grow, even when its surroundings contain none of the cues that are normally required to provoke growth. The proteins encoded by the *ras* proto-oncogene and the *ras* oncogene provide a good example of this mechanism. The protein encoded by the *ras* proto-oncogene usually sits quietly in the cytoplasm of the cell and awaits stimulation by a growth factor receptor at the cell surface. When such a receptor binds its growth factor, it sends a stimulatory signal to the ras protein through receptor tyrosine kinase, which responds by releasing a burst of secondary signals deeper into the cell through the *ras* signaling pathway. The aberrant ras protein specified by a *ras* oncogene acts much more differently. It releases signals into the cell continually, independent of prior stimulation by a growth factor receptor. In effect, the cell is tricked into thinking that it has encountered growth factors in its surrounding when, in fact, none may be present. As an

TABLE 23.1. SOME EXAMPLES OF ONCOGENES IN HUMAN TUMORS

Oncogenes	Tumor Associations	Mechanism of Action	Properties of Gene Products
ERBB2	Mammary, ovarian, and stomach carcinomas	Amplification	Cell surface growth factor receptor
ERBB	Mammary carcinoma, glioblastoma	Amplification	Growth factor receptor
RAF	Stomach carcinoma	Rearrangement	Cytoplasmic serine/threonine kinase
HARAS	Bladder carcinoma	Point mutation	GDP/GTP binding
KIRAS	Lung and colon carcinomas	Point mutation	GDP/GTP binding
NRAS	Leukemia	Point mutation	GDP/GTP binding
MYC	Lymphomas, carcinomas	Amplification, chromosomal translocation	Nuclear transcription factor
NMYC	Neuroblastoma	Amplification	Nuclear transcription factor
LMYC	Small cell lung carcinoma	Amplification	Nuclear transcription factor
BLC2	Follicular and undifferentiated lymphomas	Chromosomal translocation	Cytoplasmic, perhaps mitochondrial
GSP	Pituitary tumor	Point mutation	Cytoplasmic GDP/GTP signal transducer
HST	Stomach carcinoma	Rearrangement	Growth factor
RET	Thyroid carcinoma	Rearrangement	Growth factor receptor
TRK	Thyroid carcinoma	Rearrangement	Growth factor receptor

GDP, guanosine diphosphate; GTP, guanosine triphosphate.

immediate result, proliferation of a *ras*-activated cell now becomes autonomous and no longer responsive to the needs of the tissue around it. The end result is the outgrowth of a large cohort of descendant cells that we see as a tumor.

Many activated or overexpressed oncogenes can be found in human tumor cells. Those currently known have all been proven to be tumorigeneic and cause uncontrolled cellular growth *in vitro* (45). To date, about 50 oncogenes have been identified; however, only about 20 have actually been found in mutant form in human tumors (Table 23.1). The most interesting in gynecologic malignant diseases include *HER-2/neu* in ovarian and endometrial cancer, members of the *ras* family (k-*ras*, h-*ras*), and c-*myc*, and *PRAD1* in cervical cancer. Understanding these mechanisms and pathways may lead to rational therapeutic strategies designed to block the overexpression of these oncogenes. Active clinical studies by the Gynecologic Oncology Group include the treatment of ovarian cancer with a *HER-2/neu* antibody in patients with ovarian cancers that overexpress *HER-2/neu*, because it is estimated that 5% to 32% of ovarian cancers overexpress this oncogene (46). Other oncogenes such as *fos, jun, mad, max, bcl-2,* and others are all important in alternative pathways for apoptosis, and their particular role in gynecologic malignancies, when determined, may provide alternate mechanisms to target for cancer therapeutics.

HER-2/neu

The *HER-2/neu* (c-*erb B2*) proto-oncogene was first identified in studies of NIH 3T3 cells. The studies suggested a direct role for overexpression of *HER-2/neu* in neoplastic transformation. The *HER-2/neu* gene, located on chromosome 17q, encodes a membrane-spanning cell surface glycoprotein of 185 kd. Although the function of the HER-2/neu protein is unknown, it has homology to the receptor for epidermal growth factor, has tyrosine kinase activity, and may function as a receptor for other growth-regulating molecules (47).

In ovarian cancer, various studies have looked at the frequency of overexpression of the *HER-2/neu* oncogene and its prognostic value in survival. Slamon et al. in 1989 reported that 26% of 120 ovarian cancers showed overexpression, with statistically significant correlation between gene amplification and median survival (48). Rubin et al. reported that 24% of their ovarian cancer cases also showed *HER-2/neu* overexpression (49); however, only a marginal prognostic significance ($p = .09$) was observed in advanced stages.

In endometrial cancer, Berchuck et al. studied 95 patients with various stages of endometrial cancer (25). Of 95 cases studied, only 9 (9%) showed overexpression of *HER-2/neu* gene. However, high expression was found in 27% of patients with metastatic disease as compared with 4% of patients with disease confined to the uterus ($p < .005$), a finding suggesting that advanced-stage endometrial cancers are associated with overexpression of the *HER-2/neu* oncogene. In 1992, Hetzel et al. examined 247 cases of endometrial cancer, 37 of which (15%) showed *HER-2/neu* overexpression (50). In 203 patients with stage I disease, the 5-year progression-free survival was 62% for the overexpressed group versus 97% for the group with no appreciable oncogene expression, a finding thereby suggesting that *HER-2/neu* gene expression may be considered a major prognostic factor in endometrial cancer.

HER-2/neu has only been found to be significantly overexpressed in the adenocarcinomas, as described earlier. Studies of squamous carcinomas suggest that alternative oncogenes may be more important. In 1990, Berchuck et al. evaluated 34 cases of squamous cell carcinoma of the cervix, vulva, and vagina for the overexpression of *HER-2/neu* (51). Only 1 of 34 cases showed overexpression, and that patient had distant metastasis. These data suggest that overexpression of *HER-2/neu* gene in squamous cancer of lower genital tract is a rare event.

ras

The *ras* gene family consists of three closely related genes: H-*ras,* K-*ras,* and N-*ras.* These genes encode for 21,000-kd proteins (p21) located in the inner plasma membrane and demonstrate guanosine triphosphatase activity. Mutant p21 produced by specific amino acid substitutions at codon 12, 13, or 61 results in the loss of guanosine triphosphatase activity and activation of gene product (52).

In ovarian cancer, Yaginuma et al. examined 110 ovarian samples ranging from normal, benign, and borderline malignant to malignant tumors (53). They were evaluated for overexpression of *ras* by immunohistochemistry. The frequency and intensity of *ras* p21 expression were observed to increase with the degree of malignancy (81% for malignant serous tumors and 50% for malignant mucinous tumors). This study, however, failed to show a statistically significant relationship between overexpression and clinical prognosis. K-*ras* mutations have been detected in premalignant colon epithelium and may represent an early genetic event in the development of colon carcinoma. Mok et al. investigated 44 cases of borderline ovarian epithelial tumors and 18 cases of invasive ovarian carcinomas to determine the possible involvement of K-*ras* mutation in borderline epithelial ovarian tumors (54). In borderline tumors, 21 of 44 (44%) were found to have K-*ras* mutation at codon 12. Invasive epithelial ovarian cancers had K-*ras* mutations at codon 12 in 7 of 18 (39%), and most were early-stage mucinous tumors. These findings support the notion that borderline ovarian tumors may represent a pathologic continuum between benign and fully invasive disease. Cuatrecasas et al. set out to assess the role of K-*ras* mutations in the pathogenesis of mucinous ovarian tumors (55). A total of 95 cases of benign, borderline, and malignant mucinous ovarian tumors were evaluated. The overall frequency of codons 12 and 13 *ras* mutation was 68% (56% of mucinous cystadenomas, 73% of borderline tumors, and 85% of carcinomas). The result of this study confirmed that K-*ras* mutations do occur in benign and particularly in malignant mucinous ovarian tumors. These findings further support the hypothesis that K-*ras* mutational activation is an early event in mucinous ovarian tumorigenesis.

Mutations in K-*ras* are less frequent in other gynecologic cancers. In 1994, Duggan et al. screened 60 endometrial cancer specimens for point mutations at codons 12 and 13 of the K-*ras* gene (56). In 9 of 60 (15%) cases, K-*ras* overexpression was found. Microdissection was done on 9 specimens in which topographic distribution of the mutant K-*ras* alleles was determined. K-*ras* mutations were detected in the areas of simple and complex hyperplasia with atypia and in adenocarcinoma. K-*ras* mutations were consistently absent in benign epithelium and in simple and complex hyperplasia without atypia. A direct genetic relationship appears to exist between premalignant and malignant endometrial epithelium and the activation of the K-*ras* locus, which is likely to have occurred before clonal expansion of the atypical hyperplasia. Sasaki et al. evaluated 89 samples of endometrial hyperplasia and found the overall incidence of K-*ras* mutation to be 16%, similar to the 18% found in invasive carcinoma. These findings suggest that *ras* mutations may represent an early event in a subset of endometrial carcinomas (57).

Few data are available for *ras* activation in lower genital tract cancers. Lee et al. examined 27 cases of cervical cancer for the expression and the mutation of H-*ras* oncogene (58). In 10 of 27 (37%) cases, strong immunoreaction on p21 protein was observed, whereas 6 of 27 (22%) cases showed point mutation at codon 12 of H-*ras* oncogene. In this small series, no correlation was found between H-*ras* gene alteration and patient survival.

MYC

The signals emitted by growth factor receptors on binding by their ligand are transmitted through an elaborate cascade of molecules that must ultimately reach the cell's nucleus to activate and regulate gene transcription. *MYC* families encode proteins that are predominantly localized in the cell nucleus and are often mediators of the final steps of signal transduction. Many studies have reported the frequency of *myc* gene amplification in ovarian cancer to be in the range of 15% to 35%. Most studies are of small sample size; however, if all the studies are combined, an average of 25% of malignant ovarian tumors will show amplification of *MYC* gene (59).

TUMOR-SUPPRESSOR GENES

The transformation of a normal cell into a cancer cell requires multiple events. First, each normal cell must undergo multiple "hits" to its genome, not just a single change that may activate an oncogene. Loss of function of other cellular regulatory genes is also required. These other genes have been called *antioncogenes;* however, the term *TSG* is now more widely used. Oncogenes are a hyperactivated version of normal cellular growth-promoting genes. By releasing strong, unrelenting growth-stimulating signals into a cell, oncogenes can drive cell growth endlessly. A normal cell also contains genes that encode proteins that turn off these growth signals at appropriate intervals or trigger timed programmed cell death. Indeed, normal cell growth may be regulated by a finely tuned balance achieved between its growth-promoting proto-oncogenes and its growth-regulating TSGs. When the latter lose their function, their negative

TABLE 23.2. EXAMPLES OF TUMOR-SUPPRESSOR GENES

Symptoms (or Tumor)	Name of Gene	Types of Tumor	Cellular Location	Chromosome Localization
Colon carcinoma	DCC	Colon carcinoma	Cytoplasm	18q
Familial adenomatous polyposis	APC	Colon carcinoma	Cytoplasm	5q
Li-Fraumeni syndrome	p53	Carcinomas, leukemia	Nucleus	17p
Neurofibromatosis type 1	NF1	Neurofibromas	Cytoplasm	17q
Neurofibromatosis type 2	NF2	Schwannomas, meningiomas	Cytoplasm	22q
Retinoblastoma	RB	Retinoblastomas, small cell lung carcinomas, osteosarcomas	Nucleus	13q
Wilms' tumor	WT1	Renal cell carcinoma	Nucleus	11p
Hereditary breast-ovarian cancer	BRCA1	Breast and ovarian tumors	Nucleus	17q

effects on cell growth are no longer felt, and cell proliferation may progress uncontrollably (60).

The number of confirmed TSGs discovered to date is relatively small—less than a dozen (Table 23.2). The retinoblastoma (*Rb*) gene, named after the rare childhood eye tumor in which it was discovered, provides a model for many of these genes. Because loss of function of the protein is required for the phenotype (cancer), both copies of the gene must be disturbed. This often results in a mutation of one gene copy with subsequent deletion of the normal or wild-type copy. Many TSGs are responsible for the hereditary cancer syndromes. In these syndromes, a germline mutation occurs in the TSG and is inherited in an autosomal dominant fashion. In these patients, all cells within the body then have one altered copy of the gene. Over time, somatic "hits" occur in target tissues such as the breast, ovary, and retina that allow for deletion or mutation of the second gene copy. Cancers therefore occur at an earlier age in these patients. For example, a father with a germline mutation in the *Rb* gene will have a 50% risk to his children. His child inherits one intact (maternal) and one defective (paternal) *Rb* gene copy. The child will have a 90% probability of sustaining a retinal tumor before the age of 6 or 7 years (61).

TSG function can also be lost through a variety of different mechanisms. Cellular proteins can bind and inactivate normal TSGs and thus may cause the same end result. The HPV oncoproteins E6 and E7 bind wild-type *p53* and *Rb* and cause increased degradation. The end result is inactivation of these regulatory proteins and subsequent uncontrolled cell growth. In addition, particular mutations or deletions within the TSGs themselves can increase production of an abnormal protein that itself may bind to the normal protein generated from the other normal gene copy, thus causing a "dominant negative" mode of action (62). We now know that mutant versions of the *p53* gene have been found in DNA samples prepared from more than half of solid human tumors examined to date, so it is the most common gene associated with human cancer causation. TSGs are critical in embryogenesis, and newer discoveries

in this reproductive field may lead to a greater understanding of the role new TSGs in carcinogenesis.

Retinoblastoma

The *Rb* gene, located on chromosome 13 at the q14 band in humans, spans a region of at least 200,000 bp of genomic DNA and encodes a 105- to 110-kd nuclear phosphoprotein. Structural analysis of the *Rb* locus has revealed a large and complex gene composed of at least 27 exons that codes for 4,700-base mRNA transcript that is expressed not only in retinoblasts but also in most other tissues. *Rb* is believed to restrain cell growth in normal cells by maintaining strict regulation of the G_1 cell-cycle check point, but in tumor cells, when both copies of the *Rb* gene are inactivated, no normal protein is produced, the cells proliferate, and cancer can develop (63). In 1978, Knudson et al. postulated that retinoblastoma and possibly other heritable cancers were a result of the deletion of inactivation of both copies of recessive gene in a single cell (64). In the so-called *two-hit hypothesis*, Knudson suggested that retinoblastoma was initiated by two genetic lesions. His hypothesis recognized that a germline mutation can come from a parent, followed by somatic mutation that occurs "accidentally" or randomly in tissue during one's lifetime.

Various investigations have examined the status of the retinoblastoma gene in ovarian cancer as a result of the numerous LOH studies implicating this gene's locus. LOH on chromosome 13q has been observed in malignant cells from 30% to 61% of the patients with ovarian cancer who were examined (65). Alleles are often lost in serous adenocarcinomas, whereas in nonserous tumors the incidence of LOH is low. Furthermore, LOH at the *Rb* locus was significantly more common in high-grade malignant diseases as compared with invasive low-grade, borderline, and benign tumors. These studies suggested that *Rb* gene was involved in ovarian carcinogenesis; however, direct mutational analysis failed to show any significant protein-altering mutations.

HPV has been implicated in the pathogenesis of cervical cancer. The viral genome is organized into three major regions: two protein-coding regions (early and late gene region) and a noncoding upstream regulating region. The early region has six open-reading frames coding for E1, E2, E4, E5, E6, and E7 proteins. In normal cells not infected with oncogenic HPV, the hypophosphorylated form of RB protein forms complexes with transcription factor E2F. These complex negatively regulate cell growth by repressing transcription of the E2F-dependent gene. The E7 protein of HPV 16 alters this precisely regulated cellular growth control mechanism by binding to *RB* and its related protein and dissociating the E2F-RB complex. This causes the release of transcriptionally active E2F, which can stimulate the transcription of the E2F-dependent gene and causes cell-cycle stimulation (66).

p53

The *p53* gene product has been a constant source of fascination since its discovery over a decade ago. The gene encoding this 53-kd nuclear phosphoprotein was initially considered to be a cellular oncogene because introduction of expression vectors containing mutant *p53* cDNA clones by transfection could transform recipient cells in concert with an activated *RAS* gene. Subsequently, several convergent lines of research indicated, however, that normal (wild-type) *p53* actually functioned as a TSG. To date, *p53* is the most commonly altered gene yet identified in human tumors. The loss of *p53* function can occur through point mutation, allelic loss, rearrangement, and intragenic deletion. The sites of the point mutations are nonrandom; more than 90% of these mutations occur in highly conserved regions within the middle third of the gene (67).

The *p53* gene encodes a nuclear phosphoprotein that exists at low levels in virtually all normal cells. Wild-type *p53* acts as a negative regulator of cell growth and is induced after DNA damage and mediates cell-cycle arrest in the late G_1 phase. In some contexts, wild-type *p53* can induce apoptosis, and in the absence of the wild-type protein leads to resistance to radiation and chemotherapeutic agents. It appears that *p53* mediates growth suppression in part through its specific DNA-binding and transcriptional regulatory abilities (68).

Various studies have looked at the overexpression of *p53* with immunohistochemistry and mutation analysis of *p53* using a combination of polymerase chain reaction and single-strand conformation polymorphism in epithelial ovarian cancer. The frequency of overexpression and mutation varies from 36% to 79% depending on techniques (69–71). Most mutations were base-pair substitutions and most occurred within exons 5 to 8 (72). Kohler et al. investigated *p53* mutations in early-stage ovarian cancer (73). The incidence of *p53* overexpression was lower in cancer confined to the ovaries (stage IA/IB) (15%) than in cancer that had spread outside the ovaries (stage IC/II) (44%). These results suggest that mutation and overexpression of *p53* are less frequent in early-stage ovarian cancer than in advanced cases, and these findings could be interpreted as consistent with the hypothesis that aberrant *p53* expression is a relatively late event in ovarian carcinogenesis that occurs during tumor progression and metastasis.

Zeng et al. set out to clarify whether cystadenomas were precursors for ovarian cancer (74). They sought to find whether mutations in the *p53* TSG could be a marker of malignancy in ovarian tumors. Mutations in the *p53* gene were present in 24 of 46 (52%) of ovarian carcinomas, but they were absent in 21 tumors of low malignant potential and 16 solitary cystadenomas. All of six cystadenocarcinomas with *p53* mutations showed the presence of the same mutation in the adjacent histologic benign cyst. This finding suggests that such cysts are not typical benign cysts, and they may carry a genetic predisposition to carcinogenesis.

In 1995, Liu et al. pointed out that such a progression model of *p53* can be applied clinically (75). For example, a patient with a benign cyst with a *p53* mutation may need to have more vigorous postoperative surveillance. To prove this point, however, many patients with benign cysts will need to be screened for *p53* so the prevalence may be established. Regardless of the prevalence of *p53* in benign cysts, the observation that greater than 50% of ovarian adenocarcinomas have discernible mutations in *p53* immediately suggests that these mutations can be used as a target for the detection of residual disease or for molecular staging. The clinical application suggested is provocative, but it needs further confirmation and a rapid, inexpensive means of testing before generalized acceptance in actual clinical practice.

The role of *p53* status and treatment response has also been well studied. Platinum-based combination chemotherapy has become standard treatment, with responses rate in excess of 70% (76). However, treatment success has been limited by the development of tumor resistance to platinum compounds. Mutation of the *p53* gene is one of the most frequent genetic alterations found in a variety of human cancers, including ovarian carcinoma. Thus, loss of wild-type *p53* function could lead to a relative resistance as a consequence of abrogation of *p53*-dependent apoptosis. In 1996, Righetti el al. examined 33 advanced-stage ovarian carcinomas (77). After initial debulking surgery, patients received high-dose cisplatin therapy. Tumor samples were analyzed for *p53* gene mutations and for *p53* protein accumulation. *p53* mutations were found in 20 cases. Most (12 of 14) of the tumors containing missense mutations associated with p53 protein stabilization were refractory to therapy. A significant correlation has also been found between p53 accumulation and pathologic response to cisplatin-based therapy. These investigators concluded that their results are consistent with a role of *p53* as a direct determinant of the chemosensitivity of ovarian cancer (77).

HPV is critically involved in the pathogenesis of cervical cancer. As discussed previously, the HPV 16 E6 open-reading frame encodes a zinc-binding protein of approximately 150 amino acids that appears to alter cell growth through its effect on *p53*. Binding of HPV 16 or 18 E6 protein to *p53* stimulates degradation of cellular *p53* through a selective ubiquitin-dependent proteolytic pathway. Therefore, the cellular levels of *p53* are low in cells expressing HPV 16 or 18 E6 (66). Benjamin et al. studied 132 patients with stage IB and IIA cervical cancer to investigate the correlation between overexpression of the p53 protein, as detected by immunohistochemistry, and somatic point mutation of the *p53* gene detected by single-strand conformation polymorphism analysis (78). Fifty-eight of 132 (44%) showed overexpression of the p53 protein; however, only 1 of 58 (1.7%) exhibited a point mutation. These results showed that *p53* gene mutation was rarely seen in early-stage cervical cancer, and detection by immunohistochemistry does not predict a somatic mutation in the *p53* gene in cervical cancer.

In endometrial carcinoma, overexpression and mutation of *p53* gene have been observed in 86% of serous carcinomas compared with 20% of endometroid carcinomas (23). This finding suggests a different molecular pathway between type I and type II uterine cancers. In sarcoma, *p53* overexpression and mutation were observed in 59% (79).

We have given a few examples of the role of TSGs in gynecologic cancers. Other known and still many unknown genes will be pivotal to our understanding of carcinogenesis. Clinical correlation remains important, as we strive to improve the results of our conventional therapy and begin to explore novel therapeutics.

BRCA1

Some families suffer from an extraordinarily high incidence of breast and ovarian cancer. Investigators have estimated that 10% of the total observed cases of breast and ovarian cancer may result from an inherited predisposition (80), but the exact number and distribution of predisposing genes are unknown. Building on the results of many genetic linkage studies of hundreds of families with breast cancer and breast-ovarian cancer, multipoint linkage analysis provided evidence that a predisposing gene exists between markers D17S588 and D17S250 on chromosome 17q. Also by examining the fit of the linkage data to different penetration function, the cumulative risks of developing ovarian cancer for the breast-ovarian families were 59% by the age of 50 years and 82% by age 70 years (81).

In 1994, Miki et al. finally mapped the predisposition gene to the region of 17q21, located in the center of a 600-kb region spanning the D17S855 locus (82). The *BRCA1* gene is composed of 22 coding exons distributed over roughly 100 kb of genomic DNA. The transcript is detected in numerous tissues, including breast and ovary, and encodes a predicted protein of 1,862 amino acids. Much of the BRCA1 protein shows no homology to other known proteins, with the exception of a 126-nucleotide sequence at the amino terminus, which encodes a "zinc-finger" motif, a motif that suggests that *BRCA1* functions as a transcription factor. Mutational inactivation of *BRCA1* would thus be expected to affect the expression of other genes involved presumably in the regulation of growth or differentiation in breast and ovarian epithelium.

BRCA1 is responsible for approximately 45% of early-onset hereditary breast cancer and more than 80% cases of hereditary ovarian cancer occurring within the context of HBOC (7). Stratton et al. determined the contribution of *BRCA1* mutations to the incidence of breast and ovarian cancer in the general population (83). Three hundred seventy-four women in a consecutive series of ovarian cancer cases in a single center were evaluated for *BRCA1* gene mutation. In this cohort, 13 of 374 (3%) were identified to have a germline *BRCA1* mutation. Assuming a sensitivity of 70% for their mutational analysis, the actual contribution of mutation in *BRCA1* to ovarian cancer in the general population is about 5%.

In 1995, Shattuck-Eidens et al. conducted a collaborative study of 1,086 women with either breast or ovarian cancer from 9 laboratories in North America and the United Kingdom for *BRCA1* mutations (84). *BRCA1* mutations were identified in a total of 80 patient samples. A total of 38 distinct mutations were found. However, most of the mutations identified were frameshift, accounting for 58% of the 36 different mutations. Three specific mutations appeared relatively common. Mutations predicted to result in a truncated protein accounted for 86% of the mutations. This finding suggests that the high frequency of the protein-terminating mutation and the observation of many recurrent mutation could lead to a relatively simple diagnostic test for *BRCA1* mutations.

In 1996, Rubin et al. tested the hypothesis that ovarian cancers associated with germline mutations of *BRCA1* have distinct clinical and pathologic features as compared with sporadic ovarian cancer (85). Fifty-three patients with germline mutations of *BRCA1* were compared with matched control patients. The median survival for patients with advanced disease and *BRCA1* mutation was 77 months as compared with 29 months for the matched controls ($p <$ .001). These data suggest that cancers associated with a *BRCA1* mutation appear to have a significantly more favorable clinical course. The relatively indolent course of *BRCA1*-related ovarian cancer, however, is not immediately obvious from the data, and the results should be confirmed prospectively.

GROWTH FACTOR RECEPTORS AND SIGNAL TRANSDUCTION

Our understanding of the biologic behavior of malignant cells has been derived from *in vitro* comparison of normal and transformed cells and the study of cell lines established by culturing human cancer cells. Normal human cells display a finite ability to proliferate in cell culture and stop after about 50 cell divisions. Agents such as ultraviolet light, X-rays, certain viruses and chemicals, and tumor cell DNA can be used to establish immortalized fibroblasts and epithelial cell lines to produce cell lines capable of forming tumors in an immunocompromised animal. Transformed cells usually require less serum and supplement to grow and exhibit greater cell population density because of a loss of contact inhibition (86).

During the process of replication, a cell passes through a series of phases culminating in mitosis (M phase), the process in which the cell actively divides. DNA synthesis occurs during the S phase. These two periods are separated by the presynthesis and premitotic phases G_1 and G_2. Cells that are not actively proliferating are in the G_0 phase. Entering into and cycling through the cell cycle appears to be controlled by different regulatory proteins in several pathways (Fig. 23.1).

In certain respects, neoplasia may be viewed as a disorder of cell proliferation in both space and time. *Growth factors,* originally defined as peptides or proteins extractable from living tissues that promoted cell proliferation, have come to be viewed as the means by which these signals are conveyed. In this way, neoplasia can also be viewed as a disorder of cellular communication. *Signal transduction* refers to the biochemical mechanism by which small molecules alter the activities of the intracellular milieu (87).

Two broad mechanisms for signal transduction have emerged. The first involves the growth receptor–associated protein kinases such as tyrosine kinase and serine-threonine kinase. These protein kinases phosphorylate the signals by transferring the γ-phosphate of adenosine triphosphate to the substrate molecules. The second mechanism is found in the generation of secondary messenger molecules such as calcium ion, cyclic adenosine monophosphate, and phospholipid metabolites (87).

In the signal transduction system (Fig. 23.2), the input from the tyrosine kinase results in increased generation of activated *ras* bound to guanosine triphosphate, which, in turn, associates with *raf; raf* then propagates the signal to the microtubule-associated protein kinase (MAPKk), which activates *MAPK; MAPK* phosphorylates a host of substrates, including cytosolic phospholipase A_2, transcription factors, cytoskeletal components, and protein synthesis machinery (87).

The generation of secondary messengers that act on intracellular receptor sites is exemplified by G-protein–coupled receptors. G-proteins interact with adenylate cyclase and certain phospholipases. Consequent hydrolysis of membrane phosphatidylinositol-4,5-bis-phosphate yields inositol-1,4,5-trisphosphate, which releases calcium from internal stores, and diacylglycerol, which activates protein kinase C. The ultimate effect of growth factors is to trigger the enzymatic cascade involving cyclin-dependent kinases that play a critical role in stimulating cells to enter and transit through the cell cycle (87).

The identification of certain cytokines and growth factors has become pivotal in cancer chemotherapy. Stem cell modulators such as erythropoeitin, granulosa-granulocyte colony-stimulating factor and granulocyte-macrophage colony-stimulating factor have revolutionized bone marrow or stem cell transplantion and have allowed a safer method of dose escalation. Despite the relative safety of these treatments, neither dose escalation nor stem cell transplantation has proven significant benefit in the treatment of gynecologic cancers.

TUMOR INVASION, METASTASIS, AND ANGIOGENESIS

Metastasis, the spread of malignant cells from primary lesions to anatomically distant sites, is present in more than 70% of cancer cases at the time of diagnosis. Moreover, occult metastatic disease may remain dormant for many years after removal of the primary tumor and accounts for many unexpected recurrences (88). These dormant malignant cells can reactivate and grow rapidly, to form new metastatic foci that are generally more resistant to conventional therapy. Frequently, metastatic disease is multifocal, making localized surgery, radiation, or chemotherapy ineffective. Thus, recognizing that metastatic disease may be an early event and changing the direction of therapy to affect both local and metastatic disease may lead to improved disease-free survival and cure rates.

Understanding the biologic basis of the metastatic process is one of the major challenges of cancer research today. In gynecologic tumors, distant metastases follow several

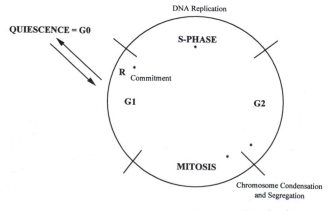

FIGURE 23.1. Schematic representation of cell-cycle phases.

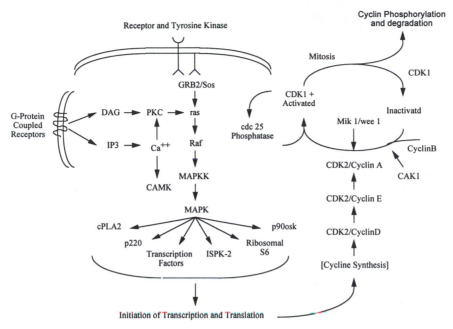

FIGURE 23.2. Signal transduction and regulation of the cell cycle by growth factors.

potential patterns of dissemination, including spread to adjacent and distant serosal surfaces as well as through the capillary and lymphatic networks. Many metastatic sites cannot be predicted on the basis of anatomic considerations alone and may be considered examples of selective organ tropism. Breast cancers often metastasize to the ovary, retinal cancer to the liver, and endometrial cancer to the lung (89).

There are several theoretic mechanisms for the organ tropism of metastases. First, tumor cells circulate equally in all organs, but they preferentially grow only in selected sites. For example, insulin-like growth factors are present in liver and lung and have been shown to be important growth factors for cancers of the breast, ovary (90), endometrium (91), and lung (92). Second, circulating tumor cells may preferentially recognize endothelial cells only in the target organ. This requires that signals on the endothelial cells determine organ specificity (93).

Cancer metastasis consists of a repetitive process of linked, sequential steps involving numerous tumor cell-host interactions. These steps include proliferation of tumor cells, angiogenesis, and three components of invasion: adhesion, proteolysis, and migration.

The initial transforming events that induce malignant cell *proliferation* are followed by local invasion of adjacent tissue by tumor cells. Many of the steps in the metastatic process involve distinct cell–cell and cell–matrix interactions. These include detachment of cancer cells from the primary tumor, adhesion to surrounding extracellular matrix components, and specific contacts between malignant cells and endothelial cells at the site of entrance or exit from the vasculature. These different types of interactions are mediated by distinct classes of receptors present on the tumor cells or endothelial cell surface. The *adhesion* processes are facilitated by different classes of adhesion molecules such as integrins (94), which are transmembrane glycoproteins, or cadherins (95), which are extracellular calcium-dependent cell adhesion molecules. These adhesion molecules and a family of cell surface receptors for the matrix glycoprotein laminin may mediate attachment of cancer cells to the basement membrane and may facilitate invasion of host stroma (96).

In *proteolysis,* extracellular matrix degradation is an important component of the invasive process and occurs in both benign and pathologic conditions. Connective tissues are composed of a mesh of different macromolecules, including collagens, fibronectin, elastin, and proteoglycans. Several experimental studies have demonstrated that in the process of invasion, almost all cells of the tumor-host microenvironment inappropriately overexpress one or more proteolytic enzymes. Plasminogen activator, itself a serine protease, converts plasminogen into plasmin, which, in turn, degrades several extracellular matrix components (97). Two genetically distinct plasminogen activator subtypes are known, urokinase and tissue-type plasminogen activator. High levels of expression of urokinase in human tumors and cancer cell lines have been demonstrated. The other class of protease is matrix metalloproteinase (MMP), which is a family of neutral zinc metalloenzymes secreted as latent proenzymes that require activation through the proteolytic cleavage of an amino-terminal domain. At least 11 different MMPs have been identified to date and are divided into 3 general subclasses according to the substrate specificity: interstitial collagenase, gelatinases, and stromolysins (98).

The ability to *migrate* is another property that characterizes both normal and malignant cells. Locomotion of cancer cells is an active process involving chemokinetic or random movement and chemotactic or directional motility. Several migration factors, or attractants, have been characterized by their ability to target tumor cells to specific secondary sites. Three classes of chemoattractants have been identified: (a) intact and degraded matrix molecules, (b) growth factors, and (c) autocrine or paracrine motility factors. Examples of growth factors that stimulate tumor cell motility include the insulin-like growth factors, hepatocyte growth factor, also known as scatter factor, fibroblast growth factors, and tumor necrosis factor-α (89).

Angiogenesis is a necessary step in the metastatic process both for tumor survival and for tumor progression. *Neovascularization* is a prerequisite for the local expansion of tumor colonies beyond the size restricted by oxygen and nutrient diffusion. Angiogenesis starts with the degradation of the endothelial cell basement membrane by protease secreted by the endothelial cells. MMP1, MMP2, and urokinase have been shown to be secreted by endothelial cells *in vitro* and are necessary for vessel formation *in vivo* (99). After the dissolution of the basement membrane, endothelial cells migrate out of the preexisting vessels toward the source of the angiogenic stimulus. Proliferation of the endothelial cells occurs behind the migrating front and ceases when the cells begin to differentiate to form vascular tubes (100).

Several laboratories have demonstrated that tumors produce a variety of angiogenic factors, including members of the fibroblast growth factor family, vascular endothelial growth factor, epidermal growth factor, and transforming growth factors-α and β (101). Histologic and ultrastructural analyses of tumor vessels have revealed pronounced differences in tumor vessels compared with normal vessels found in mature tissues. The distinction includes differences in the cellular composition of tumor vessels, the basement membrane composition and integrity, and permeability (100). Because of a discontinuous basement membrane, tumor vessels are leaky and are easily penetrated by cancer cells entering the circulation at a high rate (millions of cells daily).

The clinical application of angiogenesis is best seen in cervical preneoplasia and invasive cancer. Colposcopic changes of punctations, mosaic patterns, and atypical vessels represent the progression of neovascularization or angiogenesis. Increased production of angiogenic factors such as vascular endothelial growth factor has been studied in these invasive and preinvasive lesions. These data have been targeted as prognosticators in cervical cancer. In addition, recent advances show promise in future application of antiangiogenic therapy.

Thorpe et al. developed a novel strategy for cancer therapy by the use of immunoconjugate that selectively occludes the vasculature of solid tumors. These investigators demonstrated the feasibility of treating solid tumors by targeting human tissue factor to tumor vascular endothelium in a mouse model. The intravenous administration of the antibody–tissue factor complex to mice with large neuroblastomas resulted in complete tumor regression in 38% of the mice (102). Surely, antiangiogenic therapeutic strategies will be the subject of exciting future clinical research.

TUMOR IMMUNOLOGY

Specific *immune responses* are mediated by two major groups of lymphocytes that arise from a common stem cell: *T (thymus-derived) lymphocytes and B (bone marrow—derived) lymphocytes.* In addition to T cells and B cells, large granular lymphocytes, monocytes, and macrophages also contribute to the function and regulation of immunologic reactions. Cytokines are soluble proteins produced by cells of the immune system that regulate the proliferation and differentiation of leukocytes and other cell types. Several lymphocyte- and macrophage-derived cytokines have been designated *interleukins* and others are *colony stimulating factors.* Antibodies and the complement system are integral parts of the immune system because the interaction of bacterial polysaccharides with complement components or the binding of antibodies with specific antigens can trigger the interaction of molecules within the complement cascade and can attract inflammatory cells while preparing cellular and molecular targets of phagocytosis or lysis (103). Figure 23.3 depicts the interaction of the cellular and humoral immune systems.

Fundamental to understanding the immunology of gynecologic cancers is the concept that tumors have chemically defined antigens on their cell surfaces that differ both quantitatively and qualitatively from those found on normal cells in the host. Proteins, lipids, and various carbohydrates can also serve as tumor-associated antigens. Kutteh et al. in 1996 demonstrated that autologous ovarian tumor-associated antigen was detected in all eight ovarian cancer cell lines (104). Some, but not all, tumor-associated antigens can be recognized by the host and can mediate tumor-specific transplantation resistance to tumor growth. Unfortunately, spontaneous tumors have a weak ability to elicit an immune response as compared with those tumors induced by chemicals or viruses. Differentiation antigens and embryonic or fetal antigens are tumor associated, but they are not necessarily recognized by the host and may not induce resistance to tumor growth. These tumor-associated antigens can, however, prove useful in detecting tumors preoperatively or in monitoring the response of a tumor to systemic chemotherapy. Human tumor-associated antigens have been recognized by human antibodies. Over the last 2 decades, monoclonal antibodies from mice or rats have been used to define new tumor-associated antigens. Nonviable tumor cells and purified antigens can be administered as vaccines to evoke delayed hypersensitivity *in vivo* as well

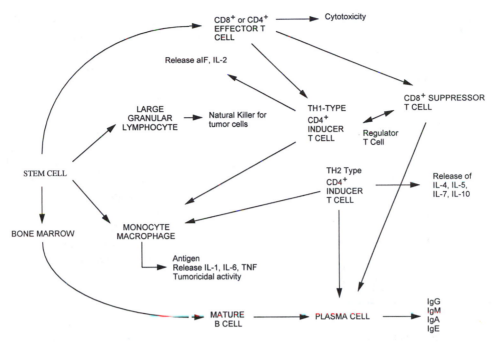

FIGURE 23.3. Diagram of cellular and humoral interaction modulating T-cell and B-cell functions.

as antibodies and T-cell reactivity that can be measured *in vitro*. However, appropriate ethical constraints and the genetic heterogeneity of our human population have precluded challenge with viable tumor cells to demonstrate the relevance of these correlates (103).

PRINCIPLES OF TREATMENT

The management of gynecologic malignant diseases, like that of most cancers, involves multimodal therapy. Because of different pathologic behavior and spread patterns, the treatment of gynecologic cancers differs depending on the site, histology, grade, and stage. However, for many gynecologic cancers, surgery must be combined with chemotherapy or irradiation to provide optimal treatment. The specifics of treatment for each organ site is beyond the scope of this chapter. We discuss the general approach to treatment, the pitfalls, the role of biologic therapeutics, and the novel strategies proposed for future studies based on the enhanced knowledge of molecular gynecologic oncology.

Surgery

The principle of *primary surgical treatment* for cancer is based on the ability to remove the primary tumor completely. Therefore, in general, tumors with large metastatic potential or large multifocal involvement may not be optimal candidates for primary curative surgical therapy. The second role of surgical therapy is in *cancer staging*. This information defines the anatomic location of the tumor, removes the primary site, allows for prognostic information

for the patient and family, and can define the need for additional treatment modalities. The success of primary curative therapy relies on the histopathologic determination of tumor-free or "negative" margins. The limitation here is based on the pathologist's ability to assess residual tumor cells. In general, 10^6 cells are required before they are histologically apparent. The role of molecular pathologic markers is intriguing, because it may be possible to use molecular abnormalities seen in the primary tumor (oncogene overexpression or specific TSG mutations) to determine involvement of apparent negative lymph nodes or surgical margins.

Chemotherapy

Cancer chemotherapy began in the mid 1940s with the accidental demonstration that nitrogen mustard had reproducible activity against lymphomas. Since then, various important chemotherapeutic agents were developed that demonstrated antitumor activity in gynecologic cancers. These agents were discovered basically by trial and error, without the understanding of their biologic mechanism of action. Many of the principles of modern chemotherapy and its toxicities are now derived from knowledge of the growth characteristics of normal and tumor tissues (105). With this knowledge, attempts are being made to combine particular agents, to use agents as radiosensitizers, and to combine these with recombinant growth factor support rationally to optimize tumor kill.

Cell-cycle events have important implications for the cancer chemotherapist. Most chemotherapeutic agents act

TABLE 23.3. MECHANISM OF VARIOUS CHEMOTHERAPEUTIC AGENTS

Agents	Mechanisms
Alkylating agents	Cross-linking DNA
Melphalan	
Cyclophosphamide	
Ifosfamide	
Platinum compounds	Formation of platinum-DNA adduct
Cisplatin	that causes DNA kinking
Carboplatin	
Antimetabolites	
Methotrexate	Inhibition of dihydrofolate reductase
Hydroxyurea	Inhibition of ribonucleotide reductase
Topoisomerase agents	
Topotecan	Inhibition of topoisomerase I
Etoposide	Inhibition of topoisomerase II
Doxorubicin	Inhibition of topoisomerase II
Antimicrotubule agents	
Vincristine	Disruption of microtubules
Paclitaxel	Promotion of microtubule assembly and prevention of depolymerization

primarily by disrupting some aspect of critical DNA, RNA, or protein synthesis that is likely to be more destructive to rapidly proliferating cells. Different sensitivities to chemotherapy are associated with different proliferative states. Rapidly proliferating cells are most sensitive to chemotherapy, whereas cells that slowly proliferate are generally less sensitive (106).

Chemotherapeutic agents have complex mechanisms of action and generally affect tumor cells through several pathways. Nevertheless, certain anticancers drugs are known to depend on proliferation and to be specific to the cell cycle, such as the alkylating agents. Cell-cycle–specific agents depend on the proliferative fraction of the tumor and on the cell cycle. Hydroxyurea, which inhibits ribonucleotide reductase and is used as a radiosensitizer in cervical cancer, is a typical example. Cell-cycle–specific drugs tend to be more effective against tumors with high proliferative rates and high growth fractions, but they are often ineffective against the more slowly growing solid tumors. Table 23.3 shows various chemotherapeutic agents and their respective mechanisms of action.

Drug resistance often compromises the efficacy of chemotherapy. The two broad classes of resistant tumors are those intrinsically resistant to chemotherapy and those that acquire resistance to chemotherapy. Several mechanisms have been identified, and they include defective transport, altered drug activation, altered hormone receptor concentration or affinity, altered DNA repair, gene amplification, defective drug metabolism, altered target protein, and altered intracellular nucleotide pools (105).

Radiation Therapy

Radiation oncology is the clinical and scientific endeavor devoted to the management of patients with cancer by ionizing radiation, alone or combined with other modalities. Radiation effects, whether direct or indirect, are random. The biologically important effects are those concerned with reproductive integrity. It is usually assumed that DNA is the critical target for this radiation effect, although it has not been proved with certainty. Other biologically important effects of radiation such as edema are far more likely to be caused by its action on membranes. At least four possible consequences of radiation interaction with cells can affect long-term reproductive viability of the cell or its progeny: necrosis, apoptosis, accelerated senescence, and terminal differentiation. The most important modifier of the biologic effect of ionizing irradiation is molecular oxygen. For equivalent cell killing, greater doses are required under hypoxic conditions compared with normoxia. Study of the phenomenon reveals that oxygen must be present during irradiation; however, the exact mechanism of the oxygen effects has not been determined definitely. It is believed that oxygen-derived free radicals affect the initial chemical products of interaction of radiation with biologic material.

Several investigators have demonstrated experimentally that the sensitivity of cells to radiation and to most chemotherapeutic agents varies depending on the cell's phase of the proliferative cycle at the time it is exposed to the physical or chemical event. After a single dose of irradiation, the cell-age distribution of surviving cells changes as a result of two factors: (a) preferential killing of cells in the more sensitive phase of the proliferative cycle, leading to an increase in percentage of viable cells in the more resistant phase; and (b) a temporary premitotic cell-cycle block that prevents the progression of proliferating cells through the cell cycle. At least four concepts have been considered that explain the differences in radiosensitivity of tumors:

1. Hypoxia. It is generally accepted that the less responsive tumors either have a high hypoxic fraction or fail to reoxygenate during fractionated irradiation.
2. Proportion of clonogenic cells. Proliferating cells are more radiosensitive.
3. Inherent radiosensitivity of tumor cells.
4. Repair of radiation damage. Repair of sublethal damage is found in almost all tumor cell lines.

Immunotherapy

Research efforts over the past decade have focused on the identification of tumor-associated or tumor-specific *antigens*. The neoplastic state, resulting from the expression of mutated or unregulated oncogenes or TSGs, leads to complex changes in cancer cells with a concomitant expression of certain cellular proteins that are repressed or expressed at much lower levels in normal cells. These proteins include tumor antigens that are recognized as foreign by the host resulting in a specific immune response to tumor cells (107).

Many different *monoclonal antibodies* directed against ovarian cancer-associated antigens have been developed. These antibodies recognize unique or shared markers of epithelial differentiation, blood group substance, mucins, native or oncogene-associated growth factor receptors, or intracellular proteins (108). Specific examples include targeting ERBB2 and the epidermal growth factor receptor.

Emerging technologies have provided an array of *engineered proteins* for preclinical and clinical evaluation. Recombinant approaches include the construction of low molecular weight, single-chain antibody binding domains (sFv) that target ERBB2, TAG-72, and a multitude of other antigens (109). Application of polymerase chain reaction technology to the cloning of antibody-variable segment genes facilitated the rapid development of new sFv (110). In general, these low-molecular-weight compounds show rapid tumor localization and rapid systemic clearance with high ratios of tumor to normal tissue binding.

One of the major limitations of antibody-based therapy has been poor retention in tumors with low ratios of tumor to normal tissue. Tumors usually have reduced vascularity compared with normal tissues and abnormal vessels with minimal smooth muscle content that are unable to regulate blood flow effectively in response to the usual vasoactive agents. Regional therapy offers the possibility for sustained contact between high levels of antibody and tumor, particularly in patients with malignant ascites. However, exposure is not equivalent with penetration, and the ability of antibodies to permeate parenchymal or bulk tumor masses sequestered by adhesion and fibrosis is limited (103).

Antibodies have been conjugated to potent polypeptide toxins of plant and bacterial origin to create immunotoxins. After antibody-directed binding to cell surface antigens, immunotoxins are internalized by endocytosis. The two most widely studied toxins have been *Pseudomonas* exotoxin A (PE) and *Ricin* with A chain (RA). Recombinant forms of PE and RA permit systematic modifications to reduce normal tissue binding and enhance internalization (111). Several phase I clinical trials of immunotoxin were carried out; however, most were terminated largely because of severe neural toxicities (112,113).

Large granular lymphocytes, natural killer cells, and lymphokine-activated killer cells belong to a family of non–major histocompatibility complex–restricted effectors that recognize and lyse a variety of tumors after activation. Regional therapy with lymphokine-activated killer cells and interleukin-2 was considered a strategy for focusing the antitumor response and reducing systemic toxicity. Results after intraperitoneal lymphokine-activated killer cells and interleukin-2 were reported in 20 patients with refractory ovarian cancer (114). Alternatively, there has been considerable interest in using autologous antispecific T lymphocytes, rather than nonspecific lymphokine-activated killer cells, to improve tumor targeting and to reduce host toxicity.

Genetic Counseling, Testing, and Surveillance

Now that genetic testing is commercially available for high-risk patients with a genetic predisposition to cancer, the crucial problem facing the clinician is how to use this information appropriately. The obvious goal of genetic testing is to identify the carrier of the *BRCA1* or other cancer-predisposition gene who is at the greatest risk of developing breast, ovarian, or other cancers. There are many unresolved issues regarding cancer predisposition testing. Most involve the lack of information regarding proven intervention strategies to lessen the risk of cancer development. Optimal surveillance and surgical or behavioral recommendations are yet to be defined.

Genetic testing generates many psychologic and social consequences. Before embarking on *BRCA1* or other genetic testing, one must understand the limitations and the ramifications of the test. The psychologic consequences often involve survival guilt, anger, and a sense of hopelessness. These social consequences can lead to lifestyle changes characterized by destructive behaviors. Issues regarding marriage or childbearing may also be altered. Lynch et al. conducted a familial linkage analysis and gene mutation studies for *BRCA1* genes on 181 members of 14 HBOC families (80). Education and detailed genetic counseling were given to each person before testing and after receiving results. Seventy-eight were positive and 100 were negative for *BRCA1*. The most common reasons given for seeking DNA testing were concerns about risk to children and concern about surveillance and prevention. Prophylactic mastectomy was considered by 35% of women who tested positive, whereas prophylactic oophorectomy was considered an important option by 75% of women who tested positive. Eighty percent of those who tested negative reported emotional relief, whereas more than one-third of those tested positive reported sadness, anger, or guilt. The authors of this study concluded that DNA testing of patients with HBOC syndrome must be performed in the context of genetic counseling, and many complex clinical and nonclinical issues are important in this process (80).

With genetic testing available to the general public, it is essential that a consensus is reached regarding the clinical interpretation of mutation carriers. In 1997, a task force organized by the National Human Genome Research Institute developed recommendations for cancer surveillance and risk reduction for persons carrying mutations in the *BRCA1* or *BRCA2* genes (115). Based on expert opinion concerning presumptive benefit, early breast cancer and ovarian cancer screening is recommended for persons with *BRCA1* mutations, and early breast cancer screening is advised for those with *BRCA2* mutations. The *BRCA1* or *BRCA2* carrier's surveillance includes monthly breast self-examination beginning at age 18 to 21 years, an annual or semiannual breast examination by a clinician beginning at age 25 to 35 years, and annual mammography beginning at age 25 to 35 years. The task force also recommended that *BRCA1* carriers have ovarian cancer surveillance to include annual or semiannual screening using transvaginal ultrasound and CA-125 level determinations beginning at age 25 to 35 years.

Schrag et al. at Brigham and Women's Hospital in Boston performed a decision analysis in comparing prophylactic mastectomy and prophylactic oophorectomy with no prophylactic surgery among women who carried mutations in the *BRCA1* or *BRCA2* gene (116). They calculated that, on average, 30-year old women who carry *BRCA1* or *BRCA2* mutations gain 2.9 to 5.3 years of life expectancy from prophylactic mastectomy and 0.3 to 1.7 years of life expectancy from prophylactic oophorectomy, depending on their cumulative risk of cancer. Surprisingly, among 30-year old women, oophorectomy may be delayed 10 years with little loss of life expectancy. This model suggests that prophylactic mastectomy provides substantial gains in life expectancy and prophylactic oophorectomy has more limited gains for young women with *BRCA1* and *BRCA2* mutations.

The field of cancer predisposition testing is young, and new information will rapidly change recommendations for surveillance and prophylaxis. Numerous familial predisposition syndromes encompass many types of cancer; however, the most recently and thoroughly studied is HBOC. Limitations of the technology for testing and limitations in the understanding of complex molecular interactions that may lessen the predictive risk still limit global clinical application.

Gene Therapy

Little progress has been made in improving survival in patients with gynecologic cancers over the past several decades. Much research has involved altering conventional therapeutics such as dose-intense chemotherapy, radiosensitizing chemotherapy, and high-dose chemotherapy with stem cell rescue (modified bone marrow transplantation). However, nothing has demonstrated a significant impact on survival. Novel therapeutics based on the biologic mechanisms of cancer, that is, actually applying the "bench to the bedside," will be the emphasis of future oncologic research. One such modality is the use of gene therapy to treat cancer on a genetic level.

The principles of *gene therapy* are based on the ability to deliver DNA or related nucleic acid derivatives into a cell as an anticancer agent. The DNA can be delivered to tumor cells or normal cells by infectious or noninfectious vectors. This manipulation may alter a variety of normal or abnormal cellular processes, or it may even introduce new biochemical pathways that did not exist previously. These changes can reverse the tumorigenic phenotype, or they may cause the cell to undergo apoptosis and die. Alternatively, these changes may cause the cell to be more susceptible to death by conventional treatment, may produce a

protein that will stimulate host immunity, or may simply mark tumor cells to follow the progress of conventional cancer treatment (107).

Many different genes and many different delivery systems are used in gene therapy therapeutics, all which are beyond the scope of this chapter. Most are still in animal (preclinical) trials in gynecologic cancers. An example of a target gene is *p53*, a 53-kd nuclear phosphoprotein that binds to DNA and functions as a transcriptional regulator, which plays an important role in cell-cycle control and in the initiation of the apoptosis. Mutation of *p53* gene has been identified in more than 50% of epithelial ovarian cancers. The restoration of *p53* function in tumor cells often induces growth arrest or growth inhibition *in vitro* and loss or reduction of tumorigenicity *in vivo*. Santoso et al. was able to show that the growth of 2,774 cell line cells infected with Ad-CMV-*p53* was inhibited by more than 90% compared with noninfected cells (117). The ability of the adenoviral vector to mediate high-level expression of infected genes and the inhibitory effect of Ad-CMV-*p53* on the 2774 cell line suggest that the Ad-CMV-*p53* could be further developed into a therapeutic agent for ovarian cancer. In a follow-up study, von Gruenigen et al. performed animal studies using a nu/nu mouse xenograft model mimicking microscopic or minimal residual ovarian cancer. Intraperitoneal injection of human OVCAR-3 epithelial ovarian cancer cells resulted in microscopic implants throughout the peritoneal surface of most intraperitoneal organs. These mice then received series of intraperitoneal injection of Ad5-*p53*. The mice tolerated Ad5-*p53* without adverse effects and showed a survival time significantly greater for the adenoviral treated animals versus the control animals (118).

In 1996, Hamada et al. introduced the wild-type *p53* gene into cervical cancer cells through the recombinant adenoviral vector Ad5CMV-*p53* to determine its effects on the growth of human cervical cancer cells *in vitro* and *in vivo* and whether the mechanism of this growth-suppressive effect is by induction of apoptosis (119). They were able to show that after six injections of Ad5CMV-*p53* to the mice model, the tumor growth suppressive effect reached 95% reduction. Their findings suggest that transfection of cervical cancer cells with the wild-type *p53* gene with Ad5CMV-*p53* is a potential novel approach to the therapy of cervical cancer.

Currently, numerous research efforts are under way in designing clinical trials of adenovirus-based gene therapy in gynecologic cancer. Tait et al. conducted a phase I trial of retroviral *BRCA1* gene therapy in ovarian cancer. *BRCA1* splice variant retroviral vector therapy was carried out through an indwelling intraperitoneal catheter (Port-a-Cath) with dose escalation. Three of 12 patients developed acute sterile peritonitis, which spontaneously resolved within 48 hours. Eight patients showed stable disease for 4 to 16 weeks, and 3 patients showed tumor reduction with diminished miliary tumor implants at reoperation and radiographic shrinkage of measurable disease. This phase I trial showed that ovarian cancer may provide an important model for retroviral gene therapy, and this approach may become an effective treatment strategy in the future (120).

SUMMARY

We need to understand the pathogenesis of gynecologic cancers on epidemiologic, biochemical, genetic, and physiologic levels. Advances in molecular genetics are emerging rapidly, leading to new insights into the origin and pathogenesis of several gynecologic cancers. The application of these advances to hereditary cancers rests on well-researched family histories that provide opportunities for investigation into the molecular basis of oncogenesis in highly selected affected and cancer-prone individuals. New discoveries about tumor cause and control that can be gleaned from the study of hereditary cases may then become applicable to their sporadic counterparts. As our knowledge of tumor biology and molecular mechanism underlying the process of carcinogenesis continues to expand, so too will the potential for intervention.

The process of tumor invasion and metastasis is a complex cascade of biochemical and genetic events that are mediated by multiple signal transduction pathways and molecular systems. Simultaneous with an improved understanding of invasion and metastasis, new discoveries have yielded insight into the role of tumor heterogeneity and the molecular events that modulate metastases.

The study of oncogenes and TSGs offers the prospect of yielding a full description of genetic elements involved in the regulation of cell growth and neoplasia. As additional genes are identified and their functions are determined, we should have a clearer understanding of these diseases. This global approach of understanding the pathogenesis of gynecologic malignancies will translate into improved diagnosis, better prevention modalities, and novel therapeutic treatments.

10 KEY POINTS

1. It is essential that we understand the pathogenesis of gynecologic malignancies on epidemiologic, biochemical, genetic, and physiologic levels.

2. Oncogenes are positive cell-cycle regulators that, when overexpressed, amplified, or genomically altered, result in malignant transformation.

3. TSGs are negative cell-cycle regulators. The loss of product results in failure of normal control of growth and thus contributes to the acquisition of the malignant phenotype.

4. Neoplasia can be viewed as a disorder of cellular communication mediated by growth factor receptors and signal transduction.

5. Cancer metastasis consists of a repetitive process of linked, sequential steps involving numerous tumor cell-host interactions such as proliferation, adhesion, proteolysis, migration, and angiogenesis.

6. Chemotherapeutic agents act primarily by disrupting some aspect of critical DNA, RNA, or protein synthesis, which is likely to be more destructive to rapidly proliferating cells.

7. The biologically important cell-cycle effects are those concerned with replication fidelity, apoptosis, accelerated senescence, and terminal differentiation.

8. Engineered monoclonal antibodies directed against tumor-associated or tumor-specific antigens can improve tumor targeting and reduce host toxicities, and they are the basis of tumor-targeting immunotherapeutics.

9. DNA testing of patients with potential hereditary cancer syndrome must be performed in the context of genetic counseling, and many complex clinical and nonclinical issues are important in this process.

10. The principles of gene therapy are based on the ability to deliver DNA or related nucleic acid derivatives into a cell as an anticancer agent that may reverse tumorigenic phenotype or may cause the cell to undergo apoptosis.

REFERENCES

1. Landis SH, Taylor M, Bolde S, et al. Cancer statistics, 1998. *CA Cancer J Clin* 1998;48:6–30.
2. Cramer DW, Hutchinson GB, Welch WR, et al. Factors affecting the association of oral contraceptives and ovarian cancer. *N Engl J Med* 1982;307:1047.
3. Greene MH, Clark JW, Blayney DW. The epidemiology of ovarian cancer. *Semin Oncol* 1984;11:209.
4. Schildkraut JM, Bastos E, Berchuck A. Relationship between lifetime ovulatory cycles and overexpression of mutant *p53* in epithelial ovarian cancer. *J Natl Cancer Inst* 1997;89:932–938.
5. Mosgaard BJ, Lidegaard O, Kjaer SK, et al. Infertility, fertillity drugs, and invasive ovarian cancer: a case-control study. *Fertil Steril* 1997;67:1005-1012.
6. National Institutes of Health Consensus Development Conference Statement. Ovarian cancer: screening, treatment, and follow-up: April 5–7, 1994. *Gynecol Oncol* 1994;55:S4-S14.
7. Easton DF, Ford D, Bishop DT. Breast and ovarian cancer incidence in *BRCA1* mutation carriers. *Am J Hum Genet* 1995;56:265–271.
8. Rubin SC, Benjamin I, Boyd J, et al. Clinical and pathological features of ovarian cancer in women with germ-line mutation of *BRCA1*. *N Engl J Med* 1996;335:1413–1416.
9. McGuire WP, Hoskins WJ, Brady MF, et al. Cyclophosphamide and cisplatin compared with paclitaxel and cisplatin in the patients with stage III and stage IV ovarian cancer. *N Engl J Med* 1996;334:1–6.

10. Barnabei VM, Miller DS, Bauer KD, et al. Flow cytometric evaluation of epithelial ovarian cancer. *Am J Obstet Gynecol* 1990;162:1584–1592.

11. Gallion HH, Pieretti M, DePriest PD, et al. The molecular basis of ovarian cancer. *Cancer* 1995;76[Suppl 10]:1992–1997.

12. Brinton LA, Berman ML, Mortel R, et al. Reproductive, menstrual, and medical risk factors for endometrial cancer: results from a case control study. *Am J Obstet Gynecol* 1992;167:1317.

13. Kurman RJ. *Blaustein's pathology of the female genital tract,* 4th ed., 441.

14. Fechner RE, Kaufman RH. Endometrial adenocarcinoma in Stein-Leventhal syndrome. *Cancer* 1974;34:444.

15. Antunes CMF, Stolley PD, Rosenshein NB, et al. Endometrial cancer and estrogen use: report of a large case-control study. *N Engl J Med* 1979;300:9.

16. Gusberg SB, Kardon P. Proliferative endometrial response to theca granulosa cell tumors. *Am J Obstet Gynecol* 1971;111:633.

17. Lynch HT, Lynch J, Conway T, et al. Familial aggregation of carcinoma of the endometrium. *Am J Obstet Gynecol* 1994;171:24–27.

18. Cancer and Steroid Hormone Study of the Centers for Disease Control and the National Institute of Child Health and Human Development. Combination oral contraceptive use and the risk of endometrial cancer. *JAMA* 1987;257:796.

19. Fisher B, Costantino JP, Redmond CK, et al. Endometrial cancer in tamoxifen-treated breast cancer patients: findings from the National Surgical Adjuvant Breast and Bowel Project (NSABP) B-14. *J Natl Cancer Inst* 1994;86:527–537.

20. Lurain JR, Rice BL, Radealer AW, et al. Prognostic factors associated with recurrence in clinical stage I adenocarcinoma of the endometrium. *Obstet Gynecol* 1991;78:63.

21. Schink JC, Rademaker AW, Miller DS, et al. Tumor size in endometrial cancer. *Cancer* 1991;67:2791–2794.

22. Coleman RL, Schink JC, Miller DS, et al. DNA flow cytometric analysis of clinical stage I endometrial carcinoma with lymph node metastases. *Gynecol Oncol* 1993;50:20–24.

23. Sherman ME, Bur ME, Kurman RJ. *p53* in endometrial cancer and its putative precursor: evidence for diverse pathways of tumorigenesis. *Hum Pathol* 1995;26:1268–1274.

24. Sherman ME, Sturgeon S, Brinton L, et al. Endometrial cancer chemoprevention: implications of diverse pathways of carcinogenesis. *J Cell Biochem Suppl* 1995;23:160–164.

25. Berchuck A, Rodriguez G, Kinney RB, et al. Overexpression of *HER-2/neu* in endometrial cancer is associated with advanced stage disease. *Am J Obstet Gynecol* 1991;164:15.

26. Rotkin ID. Adolescent coitus and cervical cancer association of related events with increased risk. *Cancer Res* 1967;27:603.

27. Winkelstein W Jr. Smoking and cervical cancer—current status: a review. *Am J Epidemiol* 1990;131:945.

28. Reeves WC, Brinton LA, Garcia M, et al. Human papillomavirus infection and cervical cancer in Latin America. *N Engl J Med* 1989;320:1437.

29. Boursnell ME, Rutherford E, Hickling JK, et al. Construction and characterization of a recombinant vaccine virus expressing human papillomavirus proteins for immunotherapy of cervical cancer. *Vaccine* 1996;14:1485–1494.

30. Wistuba II, et al. Deletions of chromosome 3p are frequent and early events in the pathogenesis of uterine cervical carcinoma. *Cancer Res* 1997;57:3154–3158.

31. Muller CY, O'Boyle JD, Fong KM, et al. Abnormalities of *FHIT* genomic and cDNAS in human cervical cancer with HPV subtype correlation. *J Natl Cancer Inst.*

32. Sozzi G, Sard L, De Gregorio L, et al. Association between cigarette smoking and *FHIT* gene alterations in lung cancer. *Cancer Res* 1997;57:2121–2123.

33. Connor JP, Miller DS, Bauer KD, et al. Flow cytometric evaluation of early invasive cervical cancer. *Obstet Gynecol* 1993;81:367–371.

34. Hilborne LH, Fu YS. Intraepithelial invasive and metastatic neoplasms of the vagina. In: Wilkinson EJ, ed. *Pathology of the vulva and vagina.* New York: Churchill Livingstone, 1987:184.

35. Herbst AL, Ulfelder H, Poskanzer DC. Adenocarcinoma of the vagina: association of maternal stilbestrol therapy with tumor appearance in young women. *N Engl J Med* 1971;284:878–881.

36. Brinton LA, Nasca PC, Mallin K, et al. Case-control study of cancer of the vulva. *Obstet Gynecol* 1990;75:859.

37. Jimerson GK, Merrill JA. Multicentric squamous malignancy involving both cervix and vulva. *Cancer* 1970;26:150.

38. Flowers LC, Wistuba II, Scurry J, et al. Allelic loss patterns demonstrate differences between human papilloma virus (HPV) negative and positive vulvar carcinoma. *J Soc Gynecol Investig* 1999;6:213–221.

39. Kurzl R, Messerer D. Prognostic factors in squamous cell carcinoma of the vulva: a multivariate analysis. *Gynecol Oncol* 1989;32:143.

40. Malfetano JH, Piren MS, Tsukada Y, et al. Univariate and multivariate analysis of 5-yr survival, recurrence and inguinal node metastases in stages I and II vulvar carcinoma. *J Surg Oncol* 1985;30:124–131.

41. Creaseman WT. New gynecologic cancer staging. *Gynecol Oncol* 1995;58:157.

42. Figge DC, Tamimi HK, Greer BE. Lymphatic spread in carcinoma of the vulva. *Am J Obstet Gynecol* 1985;152:387.

43. Bishop JM. Cellular oncogenes and retroviruses. *Annu Rev Biochem* 1983;52:301–354.

44. Heldin CH, Westermark B. Growth factors: mechanism of action and relation to oncogenes. *Cell* 1984;37:9–20.

45. Bishop JM. Viral oncogenes. *Cell* 1985;42:23–38.

46. Berchuck A, Kamel A, Whitaker R, et al. Overexpression of *HER-2/neu* is associated with poor survival in advanced epithelial ovarian cancer. *Cancer Res* 1990;50:4087–4091.

47. Bargmann CI, Hung MC, Weinberg RA. The *neu* oncogene encodes an epidermal growth factor receptor-related protein. *Nature* 1986;319:226–230.

48. Slamon DJ, Godolphin W, Jones LA, et al. Studies of the *HER-2/neu* proto-oncogene in human breast and ovarian cancer. *Science* 1989;244:707.

49. Rubin SC, Finstadt CL, Wong GY, et al. Prognostic significance of *HER-2/neu* expression in advanced epithelial ovarian cancer: a multivariate analysis. *Am J Obstet Gynecol* 1993;168:162.

50. Hetzel DJ, Wilson TO. *HER-2/neu* expression: a major prognostic factor in endometrial cancer. *Gynecol Oncol* 1992;47:179.

51. Berchuck A, Rodriguez G, Kamel A, et al. Expression of epidermal growth factor receptor and *HER-2/neu* in normal and neoplastic cervix, vulva, and vagina. *Obstet Gynecol* 1990;76:381.

52. Kiaris H, Spandidos DA. Mutations of *ras* genes in human tumors. *Int J Oncol* 1995;7:413–421.

53. Yaginuma Y, Yamashita K. *ras* oncogene product p21 expression and prognosis of human ovarian tumors. *Gynecol Oncol* 1992;46:45.

54. Mok SC, Bell DA. Mutation of K-*ras* protooncogene in human ovarian epithelial tumor of borderline malignancy. *Cancer Res* 1993;53:1489.

55. Cuatrecasas M, Villanueva A, Matias-Guiu X, et al. K-*ras* mutations in mucinous ovarian tumors: a clinicopathologic and molecular study of 95 cases. *Cancer* 1997;79:1581–1586.

56. Duggan BD, Felix JC, Muderspach LI, et al. Early mutational activation of the c-Ki-*ras* oncogene in endometrial carcinoma. *Cancer Res* 1994;54:1604.

57. Sasaki H, Nishii H, Kohler M, et al. Mutation of Ki-*ras* protooncogene in human endometrial hyperplasia and carcinoma. *Cancer Res* 1993;53:1905–1910.

58. Lee JH, Lee SK, Yang MH, et al. Expression and mutation of H-*ras* in uterine cervical cancer. *Gynecol Oncol* 1996;62:49–54.

59. Baker VV, Borst MP. C-*myc* amplification in ovarian cancer. *Gynecol Oncol* 1990;38:340.

60. Weinberg RA. Oncogenes and tumor suppressor genes. *CA Cancer J Clin* 1994;44:160–170.

61. Hollingsworth RE Jr, Hensey CE, Lee WH. Retinoblastoma protein and the cell cycle. *Curr Opin Genet Dev* 1993;3:55–62.

62. Perry ME, Levine AJ. Tumor-suppressor *p53* and the cell cycle. *Curr Opin Genet Dev* 1993;3:50–54.

63. DeCaprio JA, Ludlow JW, Lynch D, et al. The product of the retinoblastoma susceptibility gene has properties of a cell cycle regulatory element. *Cell* 1989;58:1085.

64. Knudson AG Jr. Retinoblastoma: a prototypic hereditary neoplasm. *Semin Oncol* 1978;5:57.

65. Li SB, Schwartz PE, Lee W-H, et al. Allele loss at the retinoblastoma locus in human ovarian cancer. *J Natl Cancer Inst* 1991;83:637.

66. Park TW, Fujiwara H, Wright TC. Molecular biology of cervical cancer and its precursors. *Cancer* 1995;76:1902–1913.

67. Hollstein M, Sidransky D, Vogelstein B, et al. *p53* mutations in human cancer. *Science* 1991;253:49.

68. Rotter V, Foord O, Navot N. In search of the function of normal *p53* protein. *Trends Cell Biol* 1993;3:46.

69. Marks JR, Davidoff AM, Berchuck A, et al. Overexpression and mutation of *p53* in epithelial ovarian cancer. *Cancer Res* 1991;51:2979–2984.

70. Mazars R, Pujol P, Teillet C, et al. *p53* mutations in ovarian cancers: a late event? *Oncogene* 1991;6:1685.

71. Kupryjanczyk J, Thor AD, Yandell DW, et al. *p53* gene mutations and protein accumulation in human ovarian cancer. *Proc Natl Acad Sci U S A* 1993;90:4961–4965.

72. Kohler MF, Marks JR, Wiseman RW, et al. Spectrum of mutation and frequency of allelic deletion of the *p53* gene in ovarian cancer. *J Natl Cancer Inst* 1993;85:1513–1519.

73. Kohler MF, Kerns BJM, Humphrey PA, et al. Mutation and overexpression of *p53* in early stage epithelial ovarian cancer. *Obstet Gynecol* 1993;81:643–650.

74. Zheng J, Benedict WF, Xu HJ, et al. Genetic disparity between morphologically benign cysts contiguous to ovarian carcinomas and solitary cystadenoma. *J Natl Cancer Inst* 1995;87:1146–1153.

75. Liu E, Nuzum C. Molecular sleuthing: tracking ovarian cancer progression. *J Natl Cancer Inst* 1995;87:1099–1101.

76. Neijt JP. Advances in the chemotherapy of gynecologic cancer. *Curr Opin Oncol* 1994;6:532–538.

77. Righetti SC, Torre GD, Zunino F, et al. A comparative study of *p53* gene mutations, protein accumulation, and response to cisplatin-based chemotherapy in advanced ovarian carcinoma. *Cancer Res* 1996;56:689–693.

78. Benjamin I, Saigo P, Boyd J, et al. Expression and mutational analysis of *p53* in stage IB and IIA cervical cancer. *Am J Obstet Gynecol* 1996;175:1266–1271.

79. Liu FS, Kohler MF, Berchuck A, et al. Mutation and overexpression of the *p53* tumor suppressor gene frequently occurs in uterine and ovarian sarcomas. *Obstet Gynecol* 1994;83:118–124.

80. Lynch HT, Lemon SJ, Narod S, et al. A descriptive study of *BRCA1* testing and reactions of disclosure of test results. *Cancer* 1997;79:2219–2228.

81. Easton DF, Bishop DT, Ford D, et al. Genetic linkage analysis in familial breast and ovarian cancer: result from 214 families. *Am J Hum Genet* 1993;52:678.

82. Miki Y, Swensen J, Shattuck-Eidens D, et al. A strong candidate for the breast and ovarian cancer susceptibility gene *BRCA1*. *Science* 1994;266:66.

83. Stratton JF, Gayther SA, Ponder BAJ, et al. Contribution of *BRCA1* mutation to ovarian cancer. *N Engl J Med* 1997;336:1125–1130.

84. Shattuck-Eidens D, McClure M, Simard J, et al. A collaborative survey of 80 mutations in the *BRCA1* breast and ovarian cancer susceptibility gene. *JAMA* 1995;273:535–541.

85. Rubin SC, Benjamin I, Boyd J, et al. Clinical and pathological features of ovarian cancer in women with germ-line mutation of *BRCA1*. *N Engl J Med* 1996;335:1413–1416.

86. Buick RN, Tannock IF. Properties of malignant cells. In: Tannock IF, Hill RP, eds. *The basic science of oncology*, 2nd ed. Toronto: McGraw-Hill, 1992:139.

87. Parker MF, Sausville EA, Birrer MJ. Basic biology and biochemistry of gynecologic cancer. In: Hoskins WJ, Perez CA, Young RC, eds. *Principles and practice of gynecologic oncology*, 2nd ed. Philadelphia: Lippincott–Raven, 1996:61–86.

88. Schirrmacher V. Cancer metastasis: experimental approaches, theoretical concepts, and impacts for treatment strategies. *Adv Cancer Res* 1985;43:1.

89. Alessandro R, Bicher A, Kohn E. Tumor invasion and metastases. In: Hoskins WJ, Perez CA, Young RC, eds. *Principles and practice of gynecologic oncology*, 2nd ed. Philadelphia: Lippincott–Raven, 1996:87–106.

90. Karasik A, Menczer J, Pariente C, et al. Insulin-like growth factor-I (IGF-I) and IGF-binding protein-2 are increased in cyst fluids of epithelial ovarian cancer. *J Clin Endocrinol Metab* 1994;78:271.

91. Kleinman D, Roberts CT, Leroith D, et al. Regulation of endometrial cancer cell growth by insulin-like growth factors and the luteinizing hormone-releasing hormone antagonist SB-75. *Regul Pept* 1993;48:91.

92. Cuttitta F, Carney DN, Mulshine J. Bombesin-like peptides can function as autocrine growth factors in human small cell lung cancer. *Nature* 1985;316:823.

93. Nicolson GL, Dulski K, Basson C, et al. Preferential organ attachment and invasion *in vitro* by B16 melanoma cells selected for differing metastatic colonization and invasive properties. *Invasion Metastasis* 1985;5:144.

94. Albelda SM. Role of integrins and other cell adhesion molecules in tumor progression and metastasis. *Lab Invest* 1993;68:4.

95. Beherens J, Frixen U, Schipper J, et al. Cell adhesion in invasion and metastasis. *Semin Cancer Biol* 1992;3:169.

96. Mercurio AM. Laminin: multiple forms, multiple receptors. *Curr Opin Cell Biol* 1990;2:845.

97. Saksela O, Rifkin D. Cell-associated plasminogen-activation: regulation and physiological function. *Annu Rev Cell Biol* 1988;4:93.

98. Matrisan L. The matrix-degrading metalloproteinase. *Bioessays* 1992;14:455.

99. Kohn EC, Allesandro R, Spoonster J, et al. Angiogenesis: role of calcium-mediated signal transduction. *Proc Natl Acad Sci U S A* 1995;92:1307.

100. Furcht L. Critical factors controlling angiogenesis: cell products, cell matrix, and growth factor. *Lab Invest* 1986;5:505.

101. Folkman J, Watson K, Ingber D, et al. Induction of angiogenesis during the transition from hyperplasia to neoplasia. *Nature* 1989;339:58.

102. Huang X, Molema G, King S, et al. Tumor infarction in mice by antibody-directed targeting of tissue factor to tumor vasculature. *Science* 1997;275:547–550.

103. Boente MP, Bookman M, Bast RC. In: Hoskins WJ, Perez CA, Young RC, eds. *Principles and practice of gynecologic oncology,* 2nd ed. Philadelphia: Lippincott–Raven, 1997:149–176.

104. Kutteh WH, Miller DS, Mathis JM. Immunologic characterization of tumor markers in human ovarian cancer cell lines. *J Soc Gynecol Invest* 1996;3:216–222.

105. Young RC. Principles of chemotherapy in gynecologic cancer. In: Hoskins WJ, Perez CA, Young RC, eds. *Principles and practice of gynecologic oncology,* 2nd ed. Philadelphia: Lippincott–Raven, 1997:381–397.

106. Young RC. Mechanism to improve chemotherapy effectiveness. *Cancer* 1990;65:815.

107. Mathis JM, Muller CY, von Gruenigen VE, et al. Biologic strategies in the therapy of gynecologic cancers. In: Langdon SP, Miller WR, Berchuck A, eds. *Biology of female cancers.* Boca Raton, FL: CRC Press, 1997:167–180.

108. Bast RC Jr, Feeney M, Lazarus H, et al. Reactivity of a monoclonal antibody with human ovarian cancer. *J Clin Invest* 1981;68:1331.

109. Huston JS, Levinson D, Mudgett-Hunter M, el al. Protein engineering of antibody binding sites: recovery of specific activity in a antidigoxin single chain Fv analogue produced in *Escherichia coli. Proc Natl Acad Sci U S A* 1988;85:5879.

110. Chaudhary VK, Batra JK, Gallo MG, et al. A rapid method of cloning functional variable-region antibody genes in *Escherichia coli* as single-chain immunotoxins. *Proc Natl Acad Sci U S A* 1990;87:1066.

111. Pastan I, Chaudhary V, FitzGerald DJ. Recombinant toxins as novel therapeutic agents. *Annu Rev Biochem* 1992;61:331.

112. Bookman MA, Godfrey S, Padavic K, et al. Anti-transferrin receptor immunotoxin (IT) therapy: phase-I intraperitoneal (ip) trial. *Proc Am Soc Clin Oncol* 1990;9:187.

113. Pai LH, Bookman MA, Ozols RF, et al. Clinical evaluation of intraperitoneal Pseudomonas exotoxin immunoconjugate OVB3-PE in patients with ovarian cancer. *J Clin Oncol* 1991;9:2095.

114. Stewart JA, Belinson JL, Moore AL, et al. Phase I trial of intraperitoneal recombinant interleukin-2/lmphokine-activated killer cells in patients with ovarian cancer. *Cancer Res* 1990;50:6302.

115. Burke W, Daly M, Barger J, et al. Recommendations for follow-up care of individuals with an inherited predisposition to cancer with *BRCA1* and *BRCA2. JAMA* 1997;277:997–1003.

116. Schrag D, Kuntz K, Garber JE, et al. Decision analysis—effects of prophylactic mastectomy and oophorectomy on life expectancy among women with *BRCA1* or *BRCA2* mutations. *N Engl J Med* 1997;336:1465–1471.

117. Santoso JT, Tang DC, Mathis JM, et al. Adenovirus-based *p53* gene therapy in ovarian cancer. *Gynecol Oncol* 1995;59:171–178.

118. von Gruenigen VE, O'Boyle J, Coleman R, et al. Successful adenovirus-mediated *p53* gene therapy in ovarian cancer. *Gynecol Oncol* 1998;69:197–204.

119. Hamada K, Alemany R, Mitchel MF, et al. Adenovirus-mediated transfer of a wild-type *p53* gene and induction of apoptosis in cervical cancer. *Cancer Res* 1996;56:3047–3054.

120. Tait DL, Obermiller PS, Redlin-Frazier S, et al. A phase I trial of retroviral *BRCA1*sv gene therapy in ovarian cancer. *Clin Cancer Res* 1997;3:1959–1968.

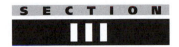

OBSTETRICS

MATERNAL PHYSIOLOGIC ADAPTATIONS TO PREGNANCY

JOYCE D. STEINFELD
JOSEPH R. WAX

Pregnancy is marked by profound physiologic adaptations, beginning early in gestation. Often, even before a woman is aware that she is pregnant, symptoms of the vast changes taking place are present. What is our first hypothesis when a reproductive-aged female has a syncopal episode, bouts of nausea and vomiting, or looks washed out and tired? She must be pregnant! The following chapter introduces the reader to many of the significant adaptations women's bodies make to accommodate pregnancy and explains the basis for many of the symptoms of gestation.

CARDIOVASCULAR SYSTEM

The enormity of the changes seen in the *cardiovascular system* is startling. It is amazing that most women make the physiologic transition to pregnancy without difficulty, and it is easy to understand why women with preexisting cardiac disease or other physical disorders can become disabled or even die trying to cope with the increased demands of gestation. One of the most remarkable things about pregnancy is that change which would usually be considered pathologic becomes physiologic. Nowhere is this overlap of physiologic findings with pathology as notable as in the cardiovascular system. Syncope, subjective dyspnea, dependent edema, and systolic murmurs are common and normal in pregnancy. In contrast, Table 24.1 lists some of the findings that signal cardiac disease in the pregnant patient.

Total maternal blood volume increases 30% to 50% in singleton gestations. The mean increase is 33% (1). Substantially greater increases are seen with larger babies and with multiple gestations (2,3). The actual presence of a fetus is not a prerequisite for maternal *hypervolemia*—it occurs even in pregnancies consisting of a hydatidiform mole (4). Volume expansion begins by 7 weeks, peaks at about 32 weeks, and is maintained until delivery. The early onset of hypervolemia may serve a protective function for the gravida, should there be pregnancy-associated bleeding, and it may also help to blunt some of the other potentially disabling physical effects of gestation (e.g., decreased venous return when rising from a seated position).

The components of volume expansion do not occur in their normal proportion and do not necessarily occur synchronously. The plasma volume increases more than the red cell mass. Water retention is marked during pregnancy by a fall in plasma osmolality (5). Numerous mechanisms contribute to a net increase in sodium resorption, which helps to maintain the increased volume. Factors that increase sodium resorption include increased renin, angiotensin, and aldosterone levels, increased deoxycorticosterone activity, and increased estrogen levels. The factors favoring increased sodium excretion—markedly increased glomerular filtration rate (GFR) and increased levels of progesterone—are outweighed by the resorptive changes (6).

Increases in prolactin, progesterone, chorionic somatomammotropin, and estrogen result in increased erythropoiesis (7,8). Because plasma volume increases disproportionately, the maternal hematocrit is lower as a result of dilution. This resulting *physiologic anemia of pregnancy* is most pronounced in the third trimester.

Structural changes occur in the heart during gestation. The dimensions and thickness of the left ventricle increase in parallel with the increasing blood volume (9). Heart size appears to increase by approximately 12% during pregnancy. As the uterus enlarges and the diaphragm becomes elevated, the heart becomes displaced upward and to the left, with the apex moved laterally. These changes account for the alterations in cardiac silhouette seen on radiographs and the left axial deviation noted on electrocardiograms during pregnancy.

Cardiac output, the product of heart rate and stroke volume, also begins to increase early in the first trimester. During a normal singleton pregnancy, an increase of 35% to 50%, or as much as 1.5 L per minute, occurs. Cardiac output reaches its maximum level by about 24 weeks and is maintained until term. Most of the increase in cardiac output is lost shortly after delivery. Absence of this normal physiologic adaptation may predispose the pregnant patient to complications such as intrauterine growth restriction (10).

Investigators disagree about the timing of the changes in heart rate and stroke volume and about which of these factors is primarily responsible for the increased cardiac

TABLE 24.1. SIGNS AND SYMPTOMS OF CARDIAC DISEASE

History
   Progressive or severe dyspnea
   Dyspnea at rest
   Paroxysmal nocturnal dyspnea
   Angina or syncope with exertion
   Hemoptysis
Physical examination
   Loud systolic murmur or click
   Diastolic murmur
   Cardiomegaly including parasternal heave
   Cyanosis or clubbing
   Persistent jugular venous distention
   Features of Marfan's syndrome
Electrocardiogram
   Dysrhythmia

From Landon MB. Heart disease. In: Gabbe SG, Niebyl JR, Simpson JL, eds. *Obstetrics: normal and problem pregnancies,* 3rd ed. New York: Churchill Livingstone, 1996, with permission.

output at any given time in gestation. The maternal resting heart rate increases as early as 7 weeks of gestation, and increases to about 15 beats per minute above nonpregnant levels by the beginning of the third trimester. The rise in stroke volume seen early in gestation may decline in the third trimester.

The distribution of maternal cardiac output changes as pregnancy progresses. Early in gestation, the uterus and breasts receive 2% to 3% and less than 1%, respectively, of the cardiac output, compared to 17% and 2% at term. Increased blood flow to the skin helps to dissipate heat produced by the increased maternal-fetal mass and cardiorespiratory work of pregnancy. The brain, kidneys, and coronary arteries receive the same fraction (but a larger absolute amount) of cardiac output throughout pregnancy. Because a greater volume of blood is available, restriction of maternal activity can be used to manipulate its distribution later in gestation. For example, a fetus suffering from suboptimal intrauterine growth may benefit from having uteroplacental blood flow maximized. If a gravida is at bedrest, some of the "discretionary" blood flow available will be shunted to the uterus; conversely, if the gravida is engaging in strenuous activity, her skeletal muscles will utilize more of what is available.

Maternal positioning during measurement can greatly alter cardiac output. The supine position can decrease cardiac output by as much as 25% (11). Compression of the venacava by the enlarged uterus results in decreased venous return; this, in turn, causes decreased stroke volume and cardiac output. If the paravertebral vessels and other vena caval collaterals are not well developed and perfused, the gravida may suffer from *supine hypotensive syndrome* (12). This consists of hypotension, bradycardia, dizziness, lightheadedness, nausea, and even syncope when the gravida remains in the supine position for too long, and it is present

in approximately 10% of pregnant women (13). The effect of supine position on cardiac output increases as gestation progresses from the midsecond trimester through the third trimester.

Decreased systemic vascular resistance (SVR) is one of the earliest maternal adjustments to pregnancy, beginning at about 5 weeks of gestation (14). SVR reaches a nadir in the second trimester and rises gradually as term is approached. To compensate for the increased cardiac output, SVR remains slightly decreased at term when compared to prepregnant levels.

The mechanisms responsible for the decrease in SVR are not completely understood. There are clearly hormonal influences on the vasculature, such as peripheral vasodilation from circulating progesterone. Prostacyclin decreases the responsiveness of the peripheral vascular bed to circulating catecholamines, which are increased during pregnancy. This desensitization helps to allow vascular relaxation. Speculation exists about other circulating arterial and venous dilating substances that may play a role, including endothelin and nitric oxide.

Blood pressure decreases in normal pregnancy, with a more marked change in diastolic than systolic values. The systolic pressure falls an average of 5 to 10 mm Hg below baseline levels and the diastolic pressure falls 10 to 15 mm Hg by 24 weeks of gestation. Values return to prepregnancy levels by term. Discussion of blood pressure is always clouded by controversies regarding methods of measurement. The position to be used is not standardized, and values are lower with gravidas in left lateral recumbent position than when they are seated or standing. Whether to measure diastolic values at Korotkoff sound IV (muffling) or V (disappearance) is another point of disagreement. The most important point clinically is consistency, not which position or sound is chosen for measurement.

An important contribution to the understanding of cardiovascular physiology in pregnancy was made by Clark and colleagues in 1989 (15). Pulmonary artery catheters were used to obtain data on basic hemodynamic parameters in normal pregnant patients carrying single fetuses in late pregnancy and then post partum. This work represented a distinct departure from the usual exclusion of pregnant women from interventional studies.

In *twin gestations,* cardiac output increases about 15% more than in singletons. The increase occurs by 20 weeks and is sustained for the remainder of the pregnancy. The augmented output beyond that seen in singleton gestations is believed primarily to result from a higher heart rate. Blood volume and left atrial size increase more in twin pregnancies, whereas mean arterial pressure and systemic vascular resistance decrease more in midtrimester. Virtually no data exist for higher-order gestations. As increasing numbers of multiple gestations occur (16), the effects of these marked stresses on maternal cardiovascular reserve will become more apparent.

Despite the magnitude of the changes that occur, the transition to pregnant cardiovascular physiology is usually accomplished quietly and seamlessly. Some patients may not make the transition well, because of the presence of preexisting maternal medical conditions. As more patients with *cardiac lesions* survive to adulthood, more become pregnant. Successful pregnancy has been reported after cardiac transplantation (17). It is possible to predict the risk of maternal complications and mortality by specific lesion. Lesions may be grouped into categories of low, moderate, or high risk of complications and mortality (Table 24.2). Data from the United States and Europe suggest that the conditions almost exclusively associated with maternal mortality are pulmonary hypertension, endocarditis, coronary artery disease, cardiomyopathy, and sudden arrhythmia (18). In general, valvular insufficiency or regurgitation is better tolerated than stenosis (19), and right-sided lesions, except those resulting from or associated with pulmonary hypertension, are better tolerated than left-sided lesions. Even in patients with corrected anatomic lesions, other complications of pregnancy (e.g., intrauterine growth restriction) may be more common (20). Some information is also available regarding the recurrence risk of a congenital cardiac abnormality in a patient's child (21,22).

Lesions associated with an increased risk of *thrombosis* (e.g., atrial fibrillation) become even more perilous because of the hypercoagulability normally associated with pregnancy. The anticoagulant of choice in the United States for pregnant patients is heparin. Heparin does not cross the placenta because of its high molecular weight and strongly negative charge. Therefore, it cannot act as a teratogen. Patients who are unable to tolerate heparin or who require coumarin anticoagulation for another reason (e.g., presence of a mechanical heart valve) must be counseled about the risks of coumarin derivatives for the fetus. First trimester exposure is associated with an embryopathy, which commonly includes nasal hypoplasia and stippled epiphyses. Other features that may be present include low birth weight, hypoplasia of the extremities, developmental delay, defects in hearing, eye abnormalities including blindness, seizures, and congenital heart disease. The critical period for exposure is between the sixth and ninth weeks of gestation. The use of coumarin derivatives is also associated with an increased risk of spontaneous abortion and stillbirth, central nervous system defects, and hemorrhage. Exposure after the first trimester is associated with central nervous system defects (23).

Marfan's syndrome is an autosomal dominant connective tissue disorder associated with lens subluxation, cardiac dysfunction, and aortic dilation. Because of changes in blood volume and cardiac output, gravidas with Marfan's syndrome are at increased risk of aortic dissection during gestation. This risk correlates with the aortic root size. In addition to the maternal morbidity and possible mortality resulting from pregnancy, the 50% risk of inheritance of the disorder for each fetus must be considered (24).

Other disease processes may negatively affect the gravida's ability to tolerate pregnancy successfully. Pregnancy is accompanied by hypertension, hemoconcentration, and poor cardiac function more often in obese patients (25). Chronic hypertension and diabetes requiring insulin therapy place the gravida at significantly increased risk of superimposed preeclampsia and early delivery (26,27).

Peripartum cardiomyopathy is a disorder of unknown origin that is unique to late pregnancy or the puerperium. It occurs in one of every 3,000 to 15,000 pregnancies and is characterized by left ventricular dysfunction and congestive heart failure (28). Patients at increased risk of the disorder include those carrying twins, older patients, and multiparas. Treatment is generally supportive, including digitalis and diuretics. Anticoagulation may be required in the presence of dilated chambers. Prognosis depends on the clinical course, including recovery of left ventricular function and persistence of chamber dilation (29). Concern has been expressed that even with return to normal ventricular dimensions and left ventricular function on echocardiogram, contractile reserve and therefore response to hemodynamic stress (as is associated with pregnancy) may be suboptimal in patients who have recovered from peripartum cardiomyopathy (30).

A careful assessment of reproductive-aged women with underlying heart disease is prudent before conception. This allows optimization of physical status, evaluation of medica-

TABLE 24.2. MATERNAL RISK ASSOCIATED WITH PREGNANCY[a]

Group I: minimal risk of complication
  Atrial septal defect
  Ventricular septae defect
  Patent ductus arteriosus
  Pulmonic or tricuspid disease
  Corrected tetralogy of Fallot
  Bioprosthetic valve
  Mitral stenosis: New York Heart Association (NYHA)
    classes I and II
  Marfan's syndrome with normal aorta
Group II: moderate risk of complications
  Mitral stenosis with atrial fibrillation
  Artificial valve
  Mitral stenosis, NYHA classes III and IV
  Aortic stenosis
  Coarctation of aorta, uncomplicated
  Uncorrected tetralogy of Fallot
  Previous myocardial infarction
Group III: major risk of complications or death
  Pulmonary hypertension
  Coarctation of aorta, complicated
  Marfan's syndrome with aortic involvement

[a]All estimates assume use of heparin, rather than warfarin, for anticoagulation.
From Clark SL. Cardiac disease. In: Clark SL, Cotton DB, Hankins GDV, et al., eds. *Critical care obstetrics,* 3rd ed. Malden, MA: Blackwell Science, 1997, with permission.

tions that may pose a teratogenic risk, and assessment of the risk of pregnancy to both mother and fetus.

HEMATOLOGIC SYSTEM

For the necessary pregnancy-associated changes to occur in the cardiovascular system, the *hematologic system* must also adapt. Without an understanding of these physiologic adaptations, improper interpretation of the gravida's laboratory values and state of health may occur.

As early as 10 weeks of gestation, *red blood cell mass* begins to increase and continues to rise until term (4). Augmented red blood cell production appears to be secondary to the effects of human placental lactogen and progesterone, which cause marrow hyperplasia. In iron-supplemented women, the red cell mass increases approximately 30% or 400 to 450 mL, whereas nonsupplemented women demonstrate an 18% or 250-mL rise (7).

However, plasma volume increases proportionately more than red cell volume and results in a decreased hematocrit (6). Anemia, therefore, is not typically diagnosed in pregnancy with hemoglobin values greater than or equal to 10 g/dL (4). Aldosterone, progesterone, and estrogen may all play roles in raising intravascular volume. Erythrocyte 2,3-diphosphoglycerate increases during gestation. This decreases the oxygen affinity of maternal red cells and thereby allows easier transplacental oxygen transfer (31).

A potential benefit of red cell and plasma volume changes is the previously noted protective effect against blood loss at delivery. Average blood loss for a singleton vaginal delivery is 500 mL, whereas a cesarean delivery or vaginal delivery of twins is associated with a 1,000-mL loss. Should a cesarean hysterectomy be required, an average blood loss of 1,500 mL is expected (4).

Normal pregnancy is associated with marked *leukocytosis,* accounted for primarily by an increased number of polymorphonuclear cells. The monocyte count also rises, but to a lesser degree. In contrast, *lymphocytes,* especially T cells, eosinophils, and basophils, decrease (32). Cognizance of these changes assists in differentiating physiologic leukocytosis of pregnancy from pathologic leukocytosis, such as that associated with sepsis.

The absolute white blood cell count begins to rise in the first trimester and reaches 5,000 to 12,000/mm^3 at term (33). During labor and delivery, and immediately post partum, leukocyte values of 25,000 to 30,000/mm^3 are not uncommon. This is not indicative of infection, and often worries the uninformed healthcare professional. These effects have been attributed to elevated estrogen and cortisol levels (32).

A steady decline in the *platelet count* is observed over the course of gestation. The average fall is approximately 20% (32). Although this phenomenon may be partially explained by hemodilution, there is also evidence of increased platelet consumption. Mean platelet volume and mean platelet volume distribution width are increased (34). The platelet count returns to early pregnancy values by 6 weeks post partum (32).

The normal pregnancy-associated decline in platelet count must be distinguished from pathologic processes. Those unique to pregnancy include preeclampsia and HELLP (hemolysis, elevated liver enzymes, and low platelet count) syndrome. A process occasionally seen in the reproductive-aged woman that is associated with thrombocytopenia is immune thrombocytopenic purpura. As always, medication exposure must be evaluated as a possible cause of thrombocytopenia. In management of the gravida with thrombocytopenia, it is critical to remember that the maternal platelet count does not correlate with the fetal platelet count.

Fibrinogen levels rise over the course of gestation and contribute to the increased erythrocye sedimentation rate noted during pregnancy. Vitamin K–dependent *clotting factors* VII to X also increase with pregnancy. No significant changes occur in the levels of factors II, V, or XII, and the bleeding time remains stable. In contrast, the levels of factors XI and XIII and the level of antithrombin III decrease. These changes, coupled with the progressive venous stasis seen in the lower extremities of the gravida, lead to the *hypercoagulable state of pregnancy.* This relative hypercoagulability peaks within 2 weeks of delivery and persists for at least 6 weeks post partum. Thus, the risk of thromboembolic phenomena should be considered to be increased over this entire time interval (6).

PULMONARY SYSTEM

The blood volume expansion and vasodilation of pregnancy result in hyperemia and edema of the *upper respiratory mucosa.* These changes predispose the gravida to nasal congestion, epistaxis, and even changes in voice. Long-term use of decongestants should be discouraged for physiologic nasal edema because they result in rhinitis medicament (35). Nonteratogenic medications are available for relief of intolerable symptoms.

Marked changes in the *chest wall and diaphragm* characterize pregnancy. With relaxation of the ligamentous attachments of the ribs, the subcostal angle increases from about 68 to 103 degrees. The transverse and anteroposterior chest diameters each increase by about 2 cm, resulting in a 5- to 7-cm expansion of the chest circumference. Although the diaphragm is elevated approximately 4 cm by the enlarging uterus, its function is not compromised, with excursion actually increased by 1 to 2 cm. Chest wall compliance, however, decreases with advancing gestation, and this change increases the work of breathing. Chest x-ray findings in normal pregnancy reveal shortening and widening of the lungs, with upward and lateral displacement of the heart (36).

TABLE 24.3. LUNG VOLUMES AND CAPACITIES IN PREGNANCY

Measurement	Definition	Change in Pregnancy
Respiratory rate (RR)	Number of breaths per minute	Unchanged
Vital capacity (VC)	Maximum amount of air that can be forcibly expired after maximum inspiration (IC + ERV)	Unchanged
Inspiratory capacity (IC)	Maximum amount of air that can be inspired from resting expiratory level (V_t + IRV)	Increased 5%
Tidal volume (V_t)	Amount of air inspired and expired with normal breath	Increased 30% to 40%
Inspiratory reserve volume (IRV)	Maximum amount of air that can be inspired at end of normal inspiration	Unchanged
Functional residual capacity (FRC)	Amount of air in lungs at resting expiratory level (ERV + RV)	Decreased 20%
Expiratory reserve volume (ERV)	Maximum amount of air that can be expired from resting expiratory level	Decreased 20%
Residual volume (RV)	Amount of air in lungs after maximum expiration	Decreased 20%
Total lung capacity (TLC)	Total amount of air in lungs at maximal inspiration (VC + RV)	Decreased 5%

From Cruikshank DP, Wigton TR, Hays PM. Maternal physiology in pregnancy. In: Gabbe SG, Niebyl JR, Simpson JL, eds. *Obstetrics: normal and problem pregnancies*, 3rd ed. New York: Churchill Livingstone, 1996, with permission.

Minute ventilation, the product of tidal volume and respiratory rate, increases by 30% to 40%, reflecting an increased tidal volume and stable respiratory rate. Expansion of the rib cage and increased respiratory drive create the larger tidal volume. Progesterone appears to play a key role in increasing respiratory drive either by decreasing the respiratory center's oxygen sensitivity or by acting as a primary respiratory stimulant.

The rise in tidal volume occurs at the expense of the functional reserve capacity, which decreases by 10% to 25%. Obesity or the recumbent position results in an even more profound diminution. Expiratory reserve and residual volumes are diminished approximately 20% (Table 24.3). No significant changes are seen in the vital capacity, inspiratory reserve capacity, 1-second forced expiratory volume (FEV_1), forced vital capacity, diffusing capacity, or lung compliance (Fig. 24.1) (37,38).

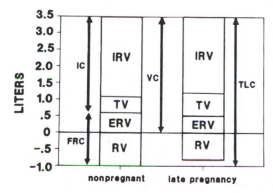

FIGURE 24.1. Lung volumes in nonpregnant and pregnant women. ERV, expiratory reserve; FRC, functional residual capacity; IC, inspiratory capacity; IR, inspiratory reserve; RV, residual volume; TLC, total lung capacity; TV, tidal volume; VC, vital capacity. (From Cruikshank DP, Wigton TR, Hays PM. Maternal physiology in pregnancy. In: Gabbe SG, Niebyl JR, Simpson JL, eds. *Obstetrics: normal and problem pregnancies*, 3rd ed. New York: Churchill Livingstone, 1996, with permission.)

Oxygen consumption increases by about 15% to 20% to support the additional maternal-fetal mass and the cardiorespiratory work of gestation. This requirement, coupled with the lower functional residual capacity, lowers the maternal oxygen reserve. It is important to consider this in the management of the gravida with chronic lung disease or when administering general anesthesia to the pregnant patient.

The increased minute ventilation facilitates *gas exchange* during pregnancy. Both the alveolar oxygen partial pressure (PAO_2) and the arterial oxygen partial pressure (PAO_2) are increased. Physiologic hyperventilation decreases arterial carbon dioxide partial pressure ($PACO_2$) and creates an increased carbon dioxide gradient from fetus to mother. There is no net change in arterial pH because of increased renal bicarbonate excretion (Table 24.4) (35,39).

Up to 60% to 70% of pregnant women with no underlying preexisting respiratory disease experience *dyspnea*. Because symptoms often begin in the first or second trimester and plateau during the third trimester, it is unlikely that the mechanical effects of the enlarging uterus play an etiologic role. Furthermore, no correlation exists between dyspnea of pregnancy and abnormal pulmonary function tests. Thus, this phenomenon may reflect heightened patient awareness of the physiologic hyperventilation of pregnancy (40,41).

Exercise during pregnancy is characterized by a compensatory rise in respiratory rate, tidal volume, and oxygen consumption (42). This adaptive response to increased respiratory work is blunted as compared with nonpregnant controls. Hence, it is advisable to recommend decreased intensity of aerobic exercise during gestation. During labor, painful uterine contractions are accompanied by a similar response, which can be attenuated by administration of analgesics (35). Resolution of pregnancy-induced respiratory changes begins within 24 to 48 hours after delivery and is essentially complete by 7 weeks post partum (36–38).

TABLE 24.4. ACID-BASE BALANCE AND BLOOD GASES

	Nonpregnant	Pregnant
P_{O_2} (mm Hg)	98–100	101–104
P_{CO_2} (mm Hg)	35–40	25–30
Arterial pH	7.38–7.44	7.40–7.45
Bicarbonate (mEq/L)	24–30	18–21
Base deficit (mEq/L)	0.07	3–4

From Myers SA, Gleicher N. Physiologic changes in normal pregnancy. In: Gleicher N, ed. *Principles and practice of medical therapy in pregnancy,* 2nd ed. Norwalk, CT: Appleton & Lange, 1992, with permission.

RENAL SYSTEM

The *genitourinary system* also distinguishes itself during pregnancy by its ability to adapt. The kidneys increase in both length and weight, and the renal pelvises and ureters dilate during gestation. The ureters both elongate and widen, with the right ureter usually more dilated than the left, because the uterus is more often dextrorotated during gestation. In addition to compression of the ureters at the bony pelvic brim, the hydronephrosis and hydroureter seen in pregnancy are promoted by increased levels of progesterone. This leads to decreased smooth muscle tone in the ureters, although this response to progesterone is not seen in the nonpregnant patient. Hyperplasia of the smooth muscle of the distal third of the ureters may decrease luminal size and may promote compensatory dilation in the upper two-thirds. All these factors result in increased urinary stasis and an increased risk of urinary tract infection during gestation (43). For this reason, aggressive treatment of asymptomatic bacteriuria is necessary in the pregnant patient because it decreases the likelihood of progression to overt urinary tract infection (44).

Numerous factors affect *renal function* during pregnancy, including increased plasma volume, GFR, increased renal plasma flow, and alterations in hormone levels, including adrenocorticotropic hormone, antidiuretic hormone, aldosterone, cortisol, thyroid hormone, and chorionic somatomammotropin. The GFR increases early in gestation to about 50% over nonpregnant values, and it remains elevated until about 20 weeks post partum. The renal plasma flow increases by 25% to 50% over nonpregnant levels by mid-pregnancy (45). Investigators disagree about whether this increase is sustained at the same level until term or whether some decrease occurs late in gestation (46).

Remarkably, in spite of the tremendously increased workload of the kidneys during gestation, the *volume of urine* provided daily is not increased. Up to 80% of the filtrate received by the kidneys is resorbed in the proximal tubules independent of hormonal control. The urinary frequency associated with pregnancy is largely a result of compression of the bladder by the enlarging uterus. The bladder is displaced upward and is flattened in anteroposterior diameter. The decreased muscle tone of the bladder during gestation actually results in an increase in bladder capacity (43).

Creatinine clearance increases markedly, peaking at about 50% above nonpregnant levels. The peak occurs at about 32 weeks of gestation, with some diminution as term is approached. Serum creatinine and urea nitrogen decrease proportionately to the increase in GFR, a finding that is important to remember when interpreting laboratory values during pregnancy. Mean serum creatinine levels, for example, decrease from 0.82 mg/dL before pregnancy to 0.73, 0.58, and 0.53 mg/dL, respectively, in the first, second, and third trimesters (47).

The increased *GFR,* coupled with impaired tubular resorption capacity for filtered glucose, results in excretion of glucose in the urine at some time during pregnancy in more than 50% of patients. Although glycosuria is a common and often physiologic finding during gestation, it may be seen in association with gestational diabetes, and it requires evaluation. Increased urinary glucose also increases susceptibility to infection.

One sees little change in *protein excretion* in healthy patients during normal pregnancies, with up to 200 to 300 mg in a 24-hour period considered physiologic. Many patients with proteinuria before gestation experience a progressive increase in the amount of protein spilled during gestation, and onset of significant proteinuria is a sign of trouble for most gravidas. It is most commonly seen with preeclampsia and is considered part of the diagnostic triad for this disorder. The quantity that is considered diagnostic of severe preeclampsia varies from 3,000 to 5,000 mg in a 24-hour collection, depending on geographic area.

Although no one has fully delineated the physiologic basis for *preeclampsia,* one of the factors responsible is a lack of the normal pregnancy response to the renin-angiotensin-aldosterone system. Renin is an enzyme produced in the kidney. Its level increases early in gestation, and it continues to increase until term. Renin acts on angiotensinogen, which is formed in the liver, to produce angiotensin I and angiotensin II. Although the levels of angiotensins I and II increase during pregnancy, healthy pregnant women do not respond with the vasoconstriction and subsequent blood pressure elevation one would expect in a nonpregnant patient. In other words, healthy pregnant women are resistant to the pressor effects of elevated levels of angiotensin II. Women with preeclamsia, however, are not resistant to these effects.

In gravidas with preeclampsia, renal filtration, resorption, and excretion of other substances also deviate from normal pregnancy levels. The creatinine clearance decreases, with a subsequent increase in serum creatinine. Blood urea nitrogen and uric acid levels are also noted to rise. In severe cases, oliguria and even acute tubular necrosis may result. Fortunately, nearly all patients return to their baseline renal function after delivery.

The population of women with *renal allografts* who have subsequently conceived continues to increase. There does not appear to be a long-term decrement in allograft function as a result of pregnancy in most patients (48,49). These patients are subject to an increased incidence of preeclampsia (about 30%) and intrauterine growth restriction, resulting in a much-increased incidence of preterm delivery. Route of delivery is generally not influenced by the presence of an allograft; these grafts are usually placed in the false pelvis and do not result in dystocia (50).

When counseling a patient with *chronic renal disease* regarding pregnancy, both maternal long-term renal function and fetal outcome must be considered. The degree of elevation of the serum creatinine and the degree of diminution of creatinine clearance provide guidelines. Patients with serum creatinine levels greater than 1.4 mg/dL have increased incidences of poor pregnancy outcomes, including preterm delivery and intrauterine growth restriction (51). Successful pregnancy outcomes are more often seen when maternal creatinine clearance is 40 mL/min/1.73 m^2 or greater. Patients with hypertension at the onset of pregnancy have poorer fetal outcomes and more frequent maternal complications than patients who are normotensive. The patient's specific disease process or histologic abnormality causing her impaired renal function can also be used for prognostic guidance (47). In general, successful pregnancy outcome and preservation of maternal renal function have become far more common over the last decade (52).

Increased numbers of pregnancies are occurring in patients receiving *hemodialysis* (53). Both peritoneal dialysis and hemodialysis have been used successfully in pregnant patients (54). Pregnant patients require different treatment parameters; it is helpful to decrease the osmotic load and azotemia to the fetus. To minimize the possibility of fetal bradycardia, it is necessary to avoid hypotension and to limit changes in volume. Later in gestation, it may be prudent to provide continuous fetal monitoring during hemodialysis.

GASTROINTESTINAL SYSTEM

"Morning sickness" that lasts all day, bizarre cravings, constipation, hemorrhoids, heartburn, and more—these are the makings of pregnancy lore. The changes experienced in appetite, digestion, and elimination, most of which result from the hormonal milieu of gestation, are among the most distressing experienced during pregnancy.

The reported incidence of *nausea and vomiting* during pregnancy varies from 50% to 90% (55). Many studies have attempted to describe which patients are more likely to develop nausea and vomiting during pregnancy. Patients who have tolerated oral contraceptive pills poorly, with symptoms such as nausea, vomiting, weight gain, depression, headache, and irregular bleeding, are more likely to experience nausea and vomiting while they are pregnant and to have these symptoms for a longer time (56). Data

are inconsistent regarding the likelihood of nausea and vomiting in primigravidas versus multiparas, although data suggest that patients who experienced the problem in a preceding pregnancy are more likely to have it recur. The disorder is virtually nonexistent in Native American, African, Inuit, and Asian (except industrialized Japanese) women. It is widely believed that psychologic and sociocultural factors are significant determinants of how a patient tolerates the nausea and vomiting of pregnancy and whether they will develop hyperemesis.

Hyperemesis gravidarum can be defined as intractable nausea and vomiting early in gestation that results in dehydration, electrolyte disturbances, or nutritional deficiencies with resultant weight loss. It occurs in up to 2% of pregnancies (57). The basic approach to nausea and vomiting in pregnancy and hyperemesis is to relieve symptoms as simply and noninvasively as possible, while allowing adequate hydration and nutrition. In addition to avoiding certain foods and odors, dispersing meals into small, frequent snacks is helpful to many patients. If dietary manipulation alone is unsuccessful, supplementation with vitamin B$_6$ and ginger has shown promise (58,59). Some relief of symptoms has been reported with the use of accupressure, hypnotherapy, and selective electrical stimulation (60–62). Numerous medications are used for symptomatic relief, with highly variable results. These include prochlorperazine, metoclopramide, and more recently, ondansetron (63), a medication used for chemotherapy-associated nausea and vomiting.

If adequate oral intake is not possible, then *intravenous hydration and hyperalimentation* may be required. Although this treatment can often be provided at home at a significantly lower cost (64), such therapy is invasive and cumbersome. Tube feedings have also been used successfully (65).

Several of the most annoying symptoms associated with pregnancy reflect the effects of progesterone on the digestive tract. Marked slowing of gastric emptying and intestinal motility combined with relaxation of the lower esophageal sphincter set the stage for heartburn, constipation, and hemorrhoids. These maladies are often responsive to simple manipulations. To avoid heartburn, gravidas are advised not to assume a recumbent position shortly after eating. Over-the-counter or prescription antacid preparations provide significant relief to many patients and are safe at any stage of pregnancy (66,67). In many patients, these measures suffice. When the uterus is unusually large, such as in multiple gestations, or with a macrosomic fetus or hydramnios, the upward displacement of the stomach may make symptoms more difficult to remedy. To combat constipation from slowed transit time and resultant hemorrhoids from straining, increased intake of fluids and high-fiber foods is recommended.

The *gallbladder* also experiences dilation and decreased motility during gestation. Bile may become thickened, with an increased likelihood of cholestasis. For reasons that are unknown, maternal cholestasis is associated with increased fetal morbidity and mortality, a finding that has led some investigators to advocate more aggressive therapy (68) than the usual diphenhydramine used to alleviate pruritus.

Cholelithiasis, cholecystitis, and gallstone pancreatitis are more frequent during pregnancy. Traditionally, treatment of the gravida with cholelithiasis has been medical and supportive, relying on elimination of oral intake, intravenous hydration, narcotic analgesics, and antibiotics as needed. In the nonpregnant patient, laparoscopic cholecystectomy is now considered the treatment of choice for symptomatic cholelithiasis. This technique has been successfully employed during all trimesters of pregnancy and continues to increase in popularity (69,70). Because of the high rate of relapse in pregnant patients with symptomatic cholelithiasis, surgery is promoted by some investigators as primary therapy (71).

Relative carbohydrate intolerance occurs in pregnancy due to a combination of factors. The placenta produces substances that antagonize the effects of insulin and make it more difficult for the gravida to cope with a carbohydrate load. Fasting euglycemia and postpartum hyperglycemia are the most common patterns in gestational diabetes. Initial treatment consists of dietary manipulation, including more even and frequent distribution of calories, and avoidance of simple sugars. If control of the condition is inadequate, insulin therapy is used. Oral hypoglycemic agents are contraindicated in pregnancy; they do not provide good glycemic control, may be teratogenic, and can result in neonatal hypoglycemia. Uncontrolled or poorly controlled gestational diabetes can result in numerous pregnancy and neonatal complications, including abnormal fetal growth, hydramnios, shoulder dystocia, and postpartal hypoglycemia. Gestational diabetes also presages the onset of type II diabetes in at least half of those who experience it (72).

10 KEY POINTS

1. Total maternal blood volume and cardiac output increase as much as 50% in singleton gestations.

2. Physiologic anemia occurs during pregnancy, because the plasma volume increases more than the red cell mass.

3. Blood pressure normally decreases during gestation and returns to prepregnancy levels by term.

4. Marked leukocytosis normally occurs during gestation.

5. The maternal platelet count falls an average of 20% during gestation.

6. Pregnancy is a hypercoagulable state and is associated with an increased risk of thromboembolic events.

7. Oxygen consumption increases 15% to 20% to cope with the increased metabolic demands of gestation.

8. Physiologic hydronephrosis and hydroureter occur during gestation and result in increased urinary stasis and risk of infection.

9. The GFR and renal plasma flow are markedly increased during gestation, with concomitant decreases in blood urea nitrogen and serum creatinine levels.

10. Increased levels of progesterone result in slower gastric emptying, decreased intestinal motility, and relaxation of the esophageal sphincter, factors that contribute to constipation, hemorrhoids, and heartburn.

REFERENCES

1. Hytten FE, Lind T. Indices of cardiovascular function. In: Hytten FE, Lind T, eds. *Diagnostic indices in pregnancy.* Basel: Documenta Geigy, 1973.
2. Hytten FE, Leitch I. *The physiology of human pregnancy,* 2nd ed. Oxford: Blackwell Scientific, 1971.
3. Rovinsky JJ, Jaffin H. Cardiovascular hemodynamics in pregnancy. I. Blood and plasma volumes in multiple pregnancy. *Am J Obstet Gynecol* 1965;93:1–15.
4. Pritchard JA. Changes in the blood volume during pregnancy and delivery. *Anesthesiology* 1965;26:393.
5. Lindheimer MD, Barron WM, Durr J, et al. Water homeostasis and vasopressin release during rodent and human gestation. *Am J Kidney Dis* 1987;9:270–275.
6. Cruikshank DP, Wigton TR, Hays PM. Maternal physiology in pregnancy. In: Gabbe SG, ed. *Obstetrics: normal and problem pregnancies,* 3rd ed. New York: Churchill Livingstone, 1996.
7. Jepson JH. Endocrine control of maternal and fetal erytfropoiesis. *Can Med Assoc J* 1968;98:844–847.
8. Ireland R, Abbas A, Thilaganathan B, et al. Fetal and maternal erythropoietin levels in normal pregnancy. *Fetal Diagn Ther* 1992;7:21–25.
9. Mone SM, Sanders SP, Colan SD. Control mechanisms for physiologic hypertrophy of pregnancy. *Circulation* 1996;94:667–672.
10. Duvekot JJ, Cheriex EC, Pieters FA, et al. Severely impaired fetal growth is preceded by maternal hemodynamic maladaption in very early pregnancy. *Acta Obstet Gynecol Scand* 1995;74:693–697.
11. Ueland K, Hansen JM. Maternal cardiovascular hemodynamics. II. Posture and uterine contractions. *Am J Obstet Gynecol* 1969;103:1–7.
12. Howard BK, Goodson JH, Mengert WF: Supine hypotensive syndrome in late pregnancy. *Obstet Gynecol* 1953;1:371.
13. Kinsella SM, Lohmann G. Supine hypotensive syndrome. *Obstet Gynecol* 1994;83:774–788.
14. Capeless EL, Clapp JF. Cardiovascular changes in early phase of pregnancy. *Am J Obstet Gynecol* 1989;161:1449–1453.
15. Clark SL, Cotton DB, Lee W, et al. Central hemodynamic assessment of normal term pregnancy. *Am J Obstet Gynecol* 1989;161:1439–1442.
16. Luke B. The changing pattern of multiple births in the United States: maternal and infant characteristics, 1973 and 1990. *Obstet Gynecol* 1994;84:101–106.
17. Kim KM, Sukhani R, Slogoff S, et al. Central hemodynamic changes associated with pregnancy in a long-term cardiac transplant recipient. *Am J Obstet Gynecol* 1996;174:1651–1653.
18. Clark SL. Cardiac disease. In: Clark SL, Cotton DD, Hankins GDV, et al., eds. *Critical care obstetrics,* 3rd ed. Malden, MA: Blackwell Science, 1997.
19. Oakley CM. Valvular disease in pregnancy. *Curr Opin Cardiol* 1996;11:155–159.
20. Lao TT, Sermer M, Colman JM. Pregnancy after the fontan

procedure for tricuspid atresia: a case report. *J Reprod Med* 1996; 41:287–290.

21. Nora JJ, Berg K, Nora AH. *Cardiovascular diseases: genetics, epidemiology and prevention.* Oxford: Oxford University Press, 1991.

22. Whittemore R, Hobbins JC, Engle MA. Pregnancy and its outcome in women with and without surgical treatment of congenital heart disease. *Am J Cardiol* 1982;50:641–651.

23. Briggs GG, Freeman RK, Yaffe SJ. *Drugs in pregnancy and lactation,* 4th ed. Baltimore: Williams & Wilkins, 1994.

24. Gordon CF 3d, Johnson MD. Anesthetic management of the pregnant patient with Marfan syndrome. *J Clin Anesth* 1993;5: 248–251.

25. Tomoda S, Tamura T, Sudo Y, et al. Effects of obesity on pregnant women: maternal hemodynamic change. *Am J Perinatol* 1996;13:73–78.

26. Rey E, Couturier A. The prognosis of pregnancy in women with chronic hypertension. *Am J Obstet Gynecol* 1994;171:410–416.

27. Greene MF, Hare JW, Krache M, et al. Prematurity among insulin-requiring diabetic gravid women. *Am J Obstet Gynecol* 1989;161:106–111.

28. Brown CS, Bertolet BD. Peripartum cardiomyopathy: a comprehensive review. *Am J Obstet Gynecol* 1998;178:409–414.

29. Lampert MB, Lang RM. Peripartum cardiomyopathy. *Am Heart J* 1995;130:860–870.

30. Lampert MB, Weinert L, Hibbard J, et al. Contractile reserve in patients with peripartum cardiomyopathy and recovered left ventricular function. *Am J Obstet Gynecol* 1997;176:189–195.

31. Bille-Brahe NE, Rorth M. Red blood cell 2,3 diphosphoglycerate in pregnancy. *Acta Obstet Gynecol Scand* 1979;58:19–21.

32. Pitkin RM, Witte DL. Platelet and leukocyte counts in pregnancy. *JAMA* 1979;242:2696–2698.

33. Efrati P, Presentey B, Margalith M, et al. Leukocytes of normal pregnant women. *Obstet Gynecol* 1964;23:429–432.

34. Fay RA, Hughes AO, Farron NT. Platelets in pregnancy: hyperdestruction in pregnancy. *Obstet Gynecol* 1983;61:238–240.

35. Elkus R, Popovich J Jr. Respiratory physiology in pregnancy. *Clin Chest Med* 1992;13:555–565.

36. Thomson KJ, Cohen ME. Studies on the circulation. II. Vital capacity observations in normal pregnant women. *Surg Gynecol Obstet* 1938;66:591–603.

37. Cugell DW, Frank R, Gaensler EA, et al. *Am Rev Tuberc* 1953; 67:568–597.

38. Alaily AB, Carroll KB. Pulmonary ventilation in pregnancy. *Br J Obstet Gynaecol* 1978;85:518–524.

39. Crapo RO. Normal cardiopulmonary physiology during pregnancy. *Clin Obstet Gynecol* 1996;39:3–16.

40. Gilbert R, Auchincloss JH. Dyspnea of pregnancy: clinical and physiologic observations. *Am J Med Sci* 1966;252:270–276.

41. Gilbert R, Epifano L, Auchincloss JH. Dyspnea of pregnancy: a syndrome of altered respiratory control. *JAMA* 1962;182:1073–1077.

42. Artal R, Wiswell R, Romem Y, et al. Pulmonary responses to exercise in pregnancy. *Am J Obstet Gynecol* 1986;154:378–383.

43. Moore PJ. Maternal physiology during pregnancy. In: DeCherney A, Pernoll ML, eds. *Current obstetric and gynecologic diagnosis and treatment,* 8th ed. Norwalk, CT: Appleton & Lange, 1994.

44. Samuels P. Renal disease. In: Gabbe SG, Niebyl JR, Simpson JL, eds. *Obstetrics: normal and problem pregnancies,* 3rd ed. New York: Churchill Livingstone, 1996.

45. Barron WM, Lindheimer MD. Effect of oral protein loading on renal hemodynamics in human pregnancy. *Am J Physiol* 1995; 269:R888–R895.

46. Sturgiss SN, Dunlop W, Davison JM. Renal haemodynamics and tubular function in human pregnancy. *Baillieres Clin Obstet Gynaecol* 1994;8:209–234.

47. Jungers P, Chaveau D. Pregnancy in renal disease. *Kidney Int* 1997;52:871–885.

48. Sturgiss SN, Davison JM. Effect of pregnancy on long-term function of renal allografts. *Am J Kidney Dis* 1992;19:167–172.

49. Sturgiss SN, Davison JM. Effect of pregnancy on the long-term function of renal allografts: an update. *Am J Kidney Dis* 1995;26:54–56.

50. Davison JM. Renal transplantation and pregnancy. *Am J Kidney Dis* 1987;9:374–380.

51. Jones DC, Hayslett JP. Outcome of pregnancy in women with moderate or severe renal insufficiency. *N Engl J Med* 1996; 335:226–232.

52. Jones DC. Pregnancy complicated by chronic renal disease. *Clin Perinatol* 1997;24:483–496.

53. Hou SH. Frequency and outcome of pregnancy in women on dialysis. *Am J Kidney Dis* 1994;23:60–63.

54. Redrow M, Cherem L, Elliott J, et al. Dialysis in the management of pregnant patients with renal insufficiency. *Medicine (Baltimore)* 1988;67:199–208.

55. Gadsby R, Barnie-Adshead AM, Jagger C. A prospective study of nausea and vomiting during pregnancy. *Br J Gen Pract* 1993; 43:245–248.

56. Jarnfelt-Samsoie A, Samsioe G, Velinder G. Nausea and vomiting in pregnancy: a contribution to its epidemiology. *Gynecol Obstet Invest* 1983;16:221–229.

57. Boyce RA. Enteral nutrition in hyperemesis gravidarum: a new development. *J Am Diet Assoc* 1992;92:733–736.

58. Erick M. Vitamin B6 and ginger in morning sickness [Letter]. *J Am Diet Assoc* 1995;95:416.

59. Vutyavanich T, Wongtra-ngan S, Ruangsri R. Pyridoxine for nausea and vomiting of pregnancy: a randomized, double-blind, placebo-controlled trial. *Am J Obstet Gynecol* 1995;173:881–884.

60. Hoo JJ. Acupressure for hyperemesis gravidarum. *Am J Obstet Gynecol* 1997;176:1395–1397.

61. Torem MS. Hypnotherapeutic techniques in the treatment of hyperemesis gravidarum. *Am J Clin Hypn* 1994;37:1–11.

62. Golaszewski TM, Frigo P, Mark HE, et al. Treatment of hyperemesis gravidarum by electrical stimulation of the vestibular system. *J Psychosom Obstet Gynaecol* 1997;18:244–246.

63. Tincello DG, Johnstone MJ. Treatment of hyperemesis gravidarum with the 5-HT3 antagonist ondansetron (Zofran). *Postgrad Med J* 1996;72:688–689.

64. Naef RW 3rd, Chauhan SP, Roach H, et al. Treatment for hyperemesis in the home: an alternative to hospitalization. *J Perinatol* 1995;15:289–292.

65. Newman V, Fullerton JT, Anderson PO. Clinical advances in the management of severe nausea and vomiting during pregnancy. *J Obstet Gynecol Neonat Nurs* 1993;22:483–490.

66. Larson JD, Patatanian E, Miner PB Jr, et al. Double-blind, placebo-controlled study of ranitidine for gastroesophageal reflux symptoms during pregnancy. *Obstet Gynecol* 1997;90:83–87.

67. Magee LA, Inocencion G, Kamboj L, et al. Safety of first trimester exposure to histamine H2 blockers: a prospective cohort study. *Dig Dis Sci* 1996;41:1145–1149.

68. Davies MH, daSilva RC, Jones SR, et al. Fetal mortality associated with cholestasis of pregnancy and the potential benefit of therapy with ursodeoxycholic acid. *Gut* 1995;37:580–584.

69. Davis A, Katz VL, Cox R. Gallbladder disease in pregnancy. *J Reprod Med* 1995;40:759–762.

70. Eichenberg BJ, Vanderlinden J, Miguel C, et al. Laparoscopic cholecystectomy in the third trimester of pregnancy. *Am Surg* 1996;62:874–877.

71. Swisher SG, Schmit PJ, Hunt KK, et al. Biliary disease during pregnancy. *Am J Surg* 1994;168:576–579, 580–581.

72. Buchanan TA, Unterman TG, Metzger BE. *Clin Perinatol* 1985; 12:625–650.

PLACENTAL PHYSIOLOGY

LESLIE MYATT

The placenta performs a remarkable number of different functions within its relatively short life span. In the adult many of these functions are handled by distinct organs. The placenta serves to transport respiratory gases and nutrients and waste products between mother and fetus. It is an extremely active endocrine gland synthesizing a wide range of peptide and steroid hormones essential for the maintenance of pregnancy and the regulation of fetal growth and maturation, and it also acts as the immune interface between the mother and the fetal allograft. In helping the placenta fulfill these roles, the trophoblast plays a pivotal role and can assume invasive, endothelial or specialized epithelial phenotypes and functions. There is a great deal of interest among obstetricians in placental function. There are several situations, such as preeclampsia and intrauterine growth restriction (IUGR), that are associated with increased perinatal morbidity and mortality and that appear to have their causes firmly linked to placental dysfunction. Placental function is critical to fetal growth and development, and there is now increasing awareness that abnormalities in placental and fetal development *in utero* may be a major determinant of long-term consequences for adult health including stroke, hypertension, and non–insulin-dependent diabetes (1).

IMPLANTATION AND EARLY PLACENTAL DEVELOPMENT

Fertilization of the ovum occurs within the fallopian tube at the ampullary-isthmic junction. As the embryo travels toward the uterus, mitosis occurs. The embryo has reached the morula stage when it reaches the uterine cornua. Four days following fertilization, blastulation has occurred and after entry into the uterus, the zona pellucida has shed, so that the outer surface of the embryo comprises trophoblast cells. Six days following fertilization, the blastocyst attaches to the uterine mucosa. The inner cell mass will form the embryo, umbilical cord, and amnion tissue, and the mesenchyme and blood vessels of the placenta. The trophoblast cells of the blastocyst will intrude between uterine epithelial cells and migrate into the stroma of the receptive endometrium (Fig. 25.1). The trophoblast cells at the forefront of

invasion process fuse to form a syncytium (syncytiotrophoblast) with an underlying single layer of progenitor cytotrophoblasts. At 8 days the embryo is still only partially embedded in endometrium, but at 10 days it is almost completely embedded and vacuoles have appeared in the syncytium that fuse to form lacunae filled with maternal blood (2). Mesoderm then invades the cores of primary chorionic villi, converting them into secondary villi, the mesenchymal core of these villi containing fibroblasts, collagen fibers, and Hofbauer cells (fetal macrophages). By the third week of gestation, the circulation of the embryo is starting to form and fetal blood vessels increasingly penetrate the cores of the villi, converting them to tertiary structures. Cytotrophoblast cells at the tips of these villi grow rapidly, break through the syncytial layer, and expand laterally as cytotrophoblast columns. The lateral expansion of the columns causes the columns to fuse so that the shell of cytotrophoblast is formed around the embryo. The syncytiotrophoblast remaining within the shell forms the fetal lining of the intervillous space (Fig. 25.1).

TROPHOBLAST INVASION

A critical aspect of successful trophoblast invasion and development is the invasion of the decidua by the trophoblast (3). In the first trimester the extravillous interstitial trophoblast erupts from the tips of anchoring villi into the decidua, forming the giant cells of the placental bed. The endovascular trophoblast travels in a retrograde manner down the spiral arteries, removing the endothelial lining and the musculature, and replacing it with trophoblast and fibrinoid, the net result being widening of the arteries to increase blood flow to the placenta, the so-called physiologic change of pregnancy (3). It is currently uncertain whether endovascular trophoblast causes the physiologic adaptation or if vessels begin to remodel prior to their invasion (4). In the early second trimester a second wave of trophoblast invasion occurs in the intramyometrial portions of the spiral arteries at a time when increasing blood flow to the placenta is required (3). This secondary wave of invasion does not occur in preeclampsia or IUGR (5), suggesting that a lack of the normal physiologic change may give rise to relative

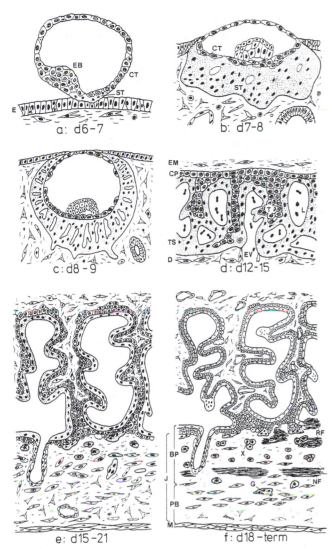

FIGURE 25.1. Early placental development. **A,B:** Prelacunar stages. **C:** Lacunar stage. **D:** Transition from lacunar to primary villous stage. **E:** Secondary villous stage. **F:** Tertiary villous stage. Note that the basal segments of the anchoring villi **(E,F)** remain merely trophoblast-forming cell columns. E, endometrial epithelium; EB, embryoblast; CT, cytotrophoblast; ST, syncytiotrophoblast; EM, extraembryonic mesoderm; CP, primary chorionic plate; T, trabeculae and primary villi; L, maternal blood lacunae; TS, trophoblastic shell; EV, endometrial vessel; D, decidua; RF, Rohr's fibrinoid; NF, Nitabuch's or uteroplacental fibrinoid; G, trophoblastic giant cell; X, X cells or extravillous cytotrophoblast; BP, basal plate; PB, placental bed; J, junctional zone. (From Benirschke K, Kaufmann P. *Pathology of the human placenta,* 3rd ed. New York: Springer-Verlag, 1995, with permission.)

placental hypoxia or ischemia, although direct evidence of this is lacking. In preeclampsia the decidual arteries of the placental bed also show a characteristic condition called acute atherosis, with fibrin deposition, platelet aggregation, and occlusion with lipid laden cells (5).

Trophoblast invasion appears to be regulated locally by a variety of growth factors and of maternal/trophoblast interactions during this period (6). Crucial to this process

appears to be the expression of integrins by trophoblast cells, the integrins then binding to extracellular matrix of decidual cells facilitating proliferation, differentiation, and migration of the trophoblast (7). Villous cytotrophoblasts express the $\alpha_6\beta_4$ integrin, a laminin receptor that polarizes cells and anchors them to the basement membrane. Some cells become nonpolarized, express $\alpha_5\beta_1$ integrin, a receptor for fibronectin, and invade the fibronectin-rich matrix of invasive cell columns losing the $\alpha_6\beta_4$ integrin but expressing $\alpha_1\beta_1$, which binds to collagen and laminin (7). Villous cytotrophoblasts also express other cell adhesion molecules including $\alpha_v\beta_5$ integrin and the adhesion molecule E-cadherin, a marker of epithelial cells. Cytotrophoblasts at the foot of the invading cell columns express $\alpha_v\beta_6$ and those of the invasive front in the placental bed express $\alpha_v\beta_3$. In an *in vitro* system, blockade of $\alpha_v\beta_3$ or $\alpha_1\beta_1$ by antibodies prevents trophoblast invasion (8), suggesting that these receptors mediate invasiveness. Trophoblasts in the placental bed also progressively lose E-cadherin but express VE-cadherin, a marker of endothelial cells, suggesting that invasive trophoblasts, particularly the endovascular trophoblast invading spiral arteries, adopt an endothelial phenotype (8). Again blockade of VE-cadherin prevents invasion. These endovascular trophoblasts also express other endothelial markers such as vascular cell adhesion molecule-1 (VCAM-1) and platelet endothelial cell adhesion molecule-1 (PECAM).

Degradation of the extracellular matrix is necessary for trophoblast invasion, and this appears to be mediated by a variety of metalloproteinases, particularly the 92-kd type IV collagenase and tissue inhibitors of metalloproteinases, which are expressed by both trophoblast and decidua (6,9). Interstitial cytotrophoblasts invade the decidua, and the endovascular cytotrophoblasts invade the blood vessels in the decidua and first third of the myometrium. The depth of cytotrophoblast invasion in the uterus may be critically regulated by the ontogeny of integrin expression of cytotrophoblast. In preeclampsia where trophoblast invasion is defective (5), significant alterations in differentiation of cytotrophoblasts, differences in the expression patterns of integrins, and expression of metalloproteinases are found (10). It appears that the integrin phenotype expressed by cytotrophoblast under these conditions may not permit the depth of invasion required to support a normal pregnancy. In the differentiating cytotrophoblast $\alpha_1\beta_1$ integrin is not expressed, the cadherin switch does not occur, and VCAM-1 and PECAM-1 are not upregulated, suggesting these defective trophoblasts do not adopt an endothelial phenotype (10).

PLACENTAL STRUCTURE AND BLOOD SUPPLY

Fetal arterial blood to the placenta comes from two arteries within the umbilical cord, and the oxygenated blood returns to the fetus by a single vein (2). Each of these vessels branches out of the chorionic plate (fetal surface of the placenta). In 96% of pregnancies, the two umbilical arteries anastomose, the vessels divide to form networks of secondary and tertiary vessels, and paired tertiary arteries and veins penetrate to the chorionic plate to enter the main stem villi of the placenta. Each stem villus forms a villous tree and divides up to five times to give second- and third-order villous stem vessels. Whereas some of these structures terminate in the cytotrophoblastic shell surrounding the placenta to form anchoring villi, the majority form freely suspended branches within the terminal villi, the exchange units of the placenta. There are 60 to 70 main stem villi within the placenta. Several stem villi may be gathered together in one fetal cotyledon, of which there are 10 to 30 within the placenta. Maternal blood entering through the basal plate from the spiral arteries comes into the central region of each cotyledon or villous tree and there are about 100 spiral arteries that supply the whole placenta.

Blood moves outward toward the edges of the intervillous space before draining into the subchorial space in the basal plate of the placenta and exits by 50 to 60 venules in the basal plate, which are arranged around the periphery of each villous tree. The stem villi of the fetal cotyledon have diameters of 900 to 3,000 μm and contain connective tissue and large fetal blood vessels. The stem villi lead to the intermediate villi, which contain loose or reticular stroma and Hofbauer cells or fetal macrophages along with the fetal blood vessels. The terminal villi arise from the intermediate villi and contain fetal capillaries early in gestation. The terminal villi are covered by the syncytiotrophoblast, which overlays a complete layer of cytotrophoblast (Langhans cells) that is set upon a basal membrane. As pregnancy continues, the cytotrophoblast cells of the Langhans' layer differentiate into syncytiotrophoblast such that at term very few cytotrophoblast cells are present in the terminal villi, and the syncytiotrophoblast is in direct contact with the basal membrane.

Whereas the artery of the stem villi is surrounded by up to three to five layers of smooth muscle and the vein by two layers, in the terminal villi there are only a single artery and vein with a thin layer of smooth muscle around them and they are accompanied by up to ten capillaries with no smooth muscle. Therefore, smooth muscle can only constrict blood vessels in regions that are proximal to the smallest stem villi and any of those with diameters of 150 μm or greater. The terminal villi contain capillaries with occasional sinusoids of diameters up to 40 to 50 μm in mature placentae and branches to form parallel loops. The lengths of capillaries in the main circulation are 3,000 to 5,000 μm, which can pass through several terminal villi in a serial fashion. The length of these capillaries and the formation of sinusoids may have evolved to reduce resistance to flow and lengthen the time available for exchange of substances between fetal and maternal circulation. Growth of the ter-

minal villi and the increase in surface area of the placenta in the third trimester is primarily due to capillary branching and growth (2).

Whereas in preeclampsia defects in cytotrophoblast differentiation may result in the failure to establish an adequate uteroplacental blood supply to the placenta, in other situations, such as IUGR, abnormal development of the fetal blood supply into the villi of the placenta may have adverse consequences for fetal growth and development. In terminal villi of growth-restricted fetuses with absent end-diastolic flow, fewer yet longer capillary loops with fewer branches per loop and a lack of coiling in the loops were observed (11). Hence, there can be maldevelopment of the vasculature of the terminal villous region consistent with an increase in vascular impedance (or a failure of the normal decrease in impedance), which may lead to defective gas and nutrient transfer and IUGR. Growth factors such as vascular endothelial growth factor (VEGF) and fibroblast growth factor may play a role in placental angiogenesis as extravillous trophoblast express the messenger RNA (mRNA) and protein for the fms-like tyrosine kinase (flt), a receptor for VEGF (12), which may allow these cells to interact with macrophages in the maternal decidua that expresses VEGF. In preeclampsia where there is reduced capillary branching in the terminal villi, reduced levels of VEGF are seen (13), suggesting VEGF may be involved in villous angiogenesis. Interestingly, although preeclampsia is thought of as a state of relative placental hypoxia, hypoxia is normally a stimulus to VEGF synthesis.

The stroma fills the volume between fetal blood vessels and trophoblasts in chorionic villi and comprises several cell types derived from mesenchymal cells of extraembryonic mesoderm. The number of mesenchymal cells declines as pregnancy proceeds and they differentiate. The main villous stromal cell at term is the reticular cell, which may further differentiate to form the large reticular cells, Hofbauer cells, and fibroblasts (2). The Hofbauer cell is a fetal macrophage of 10 to 30 μm in diameter that is highly vacuolated and contains granular cytoplasm. These cells may play an immunologic role within the placenta as they contain receptors for immunoglobulin G and they may be capable of pinocytosis.

The cytotrophoblast differentiates to form a syncytiotrophoblast, which performs endocrine, epithelial, and endothelial cell functions. The plasma membrane of the syncytiotrophoblast contains microvilli, and the basal side comes into contact with the basement membrane. At term the syncytiotrophoblast thins over the villous surface and its membranes here are very closely opposed to the fetal capillary endothelium and consequently are described as vasculosyncytial membranes (2). At this point the diffusion distance between the maternal and fetal blood is at a minimum (1 to 2 μm). The syncytiotrophoblast is highly metabolically active and it contains a high concentration of organelles including mitochondria, lysosomes, vesicles, and endoplasmic reticulum. The syncytiotrophoblast also contains pinocytotic vesicles and lamellar bodies, which may be involved in transport processes.

DETERMINANTS OF FETAL-PLACENTAL BLOOD FLOW

Fetal blood flow to the placenta is determined by fetal cardiac output and umbilical placental vascular resistance (14). At term the placenta receives approximately 40% of combined ventricular output of the fetus. Over the last third of pregnancy umbilical blood flow remains approximately constant at 110 to 125 mL/min/kg. Fetal biventricular cardiac output is approximately 450 mL/kg and again remains approximately constant over this gestational age range. In the absence of autonomic innervation, vascular resistance in the fetal placental circulation must be determined by humoral factors in blood or by local autocrine or paracrine effectors. *In vitro* investigations have shown distinct differences between the various regions of the fetal placental circulation (umbilical vasculature, chorionic plate vessels, and villous tree) in their sensitivity to various families of vasoactive autocoids (15) (Fig. 25.2). Whereas in the umbilical cord prostacyclin appears to be a more potent vasodilator than nitric oxide, in the villous tree nitric oxide appears to be more potent than prostacyclin as a vasodilator.

It is generally accepted that fetal cardiac output is maximal and the placenta is maximally vasodilated with little room for regulation. However, regulation of vascular tone in the fetal placental circulation may be important in situations such as hemorrhage, blood flow changes around parturition, and pathologic situations such as preeclampsia and IUGR. With the discovery of the active vasodilator effects of nitric oxide (endothelial-derived relaxing factor), attention has centered on the role that nitric oxide plays in the maintenance of fetal placental resistance (5). Nitric oxide appears to maintain low resistance in the fetal-placental vasculature and to attenuate the action of vasoconstrictors such as endothelin and thromboxane (16,17). The major stimulus to nitric oxide release in the placental vasculature appears to be flow or shear stress over the surface of endothelial cells (18,19). Therefore, situations that may alter flow or shear stress including viscosity of blood or diameter of blood vessels may be important determinants of resistance in this vasculature. In addition, there is considerable interest in the role that hypoxia might play in expression of the endothelial nitric oxide synthase gene, with consequent effects for regulation of fetal placental blood flow and on gas and nutrient transfer to the fetus. Many other autocoids including components of the renin angiotensin system, prostaglandins, and thromboxane have been shown to regulate human fetal-placental vascular resistance *in vitro* (15). Similarly, several peptide hormones including corticotropin-releasing hor-

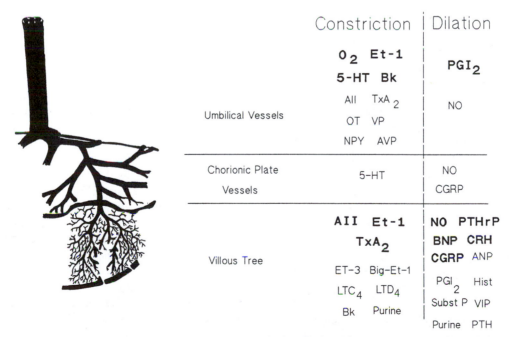

FIGURE 25.2. Regional actions of autocoids in the umbilical placental circulation. Various families of autocoids are shown, endothelin-1 (ET-1), endothelin-3 (ET-3), 5-hydroxytryptamine (5-HT), bradykinin (BK), angiotensin II (AII), thromboxane A_2 (TxA_2), oxytocin (OT), vasopressin (VP), neuropeptide Y (NPY), arginine vasopressin (AVP), leukotriene C_4 and D_4, prostacyclin (PGI$_2$), nitric oxide (NO), calcitonin gene–related peptide (CGRP), parathyroid hormone (PTH), parathyroid hormone–related peptide (PTHRP), atrial and brain natriuretic peptides (ANP, BNP), corticotropin-releasing hormone (CRH), substance P, histamine (hist), and vasoactive intestinal peptide (VIP). **Bold type** indicates predominance of action.

mone (CRH) (20) derived from trophoblast and atrial natri-uretic peptide and brain natriuretic peptide (21) from the fetal heart also appear to function as vasodilators *in vitro*. However, the interactions of these various autocoids toward the overall regulation of fetal placental blood flow during pregnancy remain to be established *in vivo*.

ABNORMAL FETAL-PLACENTAL BLOOD FLOWS

Preeclampsia and IUGR are both associated with increased fetal morbidity and mortality, and characteristically in both situations increases in fetal placental vascular impedance can be demonstrated by abnormal umbilical flow velocity waveforms (22,23). The increases in fetal placental vascular resistance may arise from alterations in vasoactive mecha-nisms, but also may be due to defects in placental angiogen-esis. As previously stated, in placentae of IUGR fetuses with absent end-diastolic flow velocity, there appears to be a failure of angiogenesis as capillary loops, which are sites of low resistance in the fetal placental circulation, are not formed, leaving the fetal placental circulation as a high-resistance circuit (11). As normalization of fetal placental vascular resistance and improvement of placental blood flow may improve the outcome of such pregnancies, many inves-tigators have examined production and action of various autocoids in the placentas of these pregnancies. It is well accepted that preeclamptic pregnancies are characterized by a relative imbalance of the thromboxane to prostacyclin ratio in the placenta, with thromboxane production and vasoconstriction being predominant (24). However, recent trials of low-dose aspirin prophylaxis, which will reduce thromboxane synthesis, in populations at low risk of devel-oping preeclampsia have failed to yield improvements in fetal outcome (25). In pregnancies complicated by pre-eclampsia and/or IUGR, an apparent paradoxical upregu-lation of endothelial nitric oxide synthase is found in the villous vasculature (26). This increased expression of nitric oxide synthase and consequent increased production of nitric oxide, measured as increased concentrations of the breakdown product, nitrate, in umbilical cord blood (27,28), may be a compensatory or adaptive response to the increased resistance seen in the placenta in these preg-nancies. The stimulus to this upregulation may be increased shear stress over the endothelial cells in the vasculature (18,19) or a response to the purported relative hypoxia experienced by the placenta. Interestingly, there are several reports that maternal administration of the nitric oxide donors nitroglycerin or isosorbidinitrate (29,30) can acutely improve the abnormal flow velocity waveforms in these pregnancies. This suggests that there may be some compo-nent of abnormal vascular reactivity in the placenta in these situations. However, in a certain proportion of such preg-nancies, administration of the nitric oxide donors was un-able to normalize the umbilical cord flow-velocity wave-forms (29).

PLACENTAL TRANSFER MECHANISMS

The placenta is responsible for transfer of the vast majority of nutrients and waste products between mother and fetus. The hemomonochorial placenta of the human is anatomi-cally the simplest, with only three layers of fetal tissue (trophoblast, villous stroma, and vascular endothelium) sep-arating maternal and fetal bloods (2). As such, it should be the most efficient in transfer of substrates and, indeed, at vasculosyncytial membranes, the syncytiotrophoblast is in direct contact with fetal vascular endothelium with a diffu-sion distance of only 1 to 2 μm between maternal and fetal blood. This is the main site of transfer of gases and water and the location of glucose carriers. Transfer across the syncytiotrophoblast may occur via the transcellular route, through the cytoplasm of the trophoblast or possibly via a paracellular route by a transtrophoblastic channel. A precise anatomic description of the paracellular route has yet to be established in the human placenta, although permeability to hydrophilic solutes suggest this pathway does exist (31). Lipophilic solutes will cross the trophoblast membrane and diffuse down a concentration gradient. However, hydro-philic solutes must interact with integral transport proteins within the trophoblast membrane. Solutes passed into the fetus must leave the syncytiotrophoblast by the basement membrane, and cross the interstitium and the capillary endothelium. Transfer across the endothelium appears to be predominantly by a paracellular pathway.

A distinction can be made between flow- and membrane-limited transport processes. Membrane limitation occurs when the passage of solute across the placental membranes is slower than the rate at which it is delivered or removed by the blood stream. When transfer across the membranes is faster than transport across the bloodstream, transport is said to be flow limited and controlled by factors that regulate maternal and fetal blood circulations. Membrane transfer by either a carrier or channel protein may involve coupling of metabolism to transport (active transport) or may occur in response to differences in concentration or electrical po-tential (facilitated diffusion). The carriers need not involve just movement of a single solute. Coupled transport may occur when two different solute molecules are simultane-ously carried, with cotransport occurring if they move in the same direction and countertransport occurring if they move in opposite directions.

Transport of Oxygen and Carbon Dioxide

Both oxygen and carbon dioxide are lipophilic molecules that cross the placenta by simple diffusion, which is regu-lated by membrane surface area thickness, diffusion coefficient of the gas in the membrane phase, and the concentration gradient of the gas across the membrane. The diffusion capacity of the placenta for oxygen is composed of the dissociation of oxygen from the hemoglobin and exit from maternal red cells, diffusion through maternal plasma, diffusion across the placental villous membrane itself, diffusion through the fetal plasma and entry into fetal red cells, and association with hemoglobin. The major contributor to resistance to oxygen diffusion in the placenta is the villous membrane itself. Supply and removal of oxygen by the placenta from maternal and fetal blood also depends on the concentration and type of hemoglobin as well as the ratio of blood flow rates (32). Fetal blood has a higher hemoglobin concentration than maternal blood and can carry 20 to 25 mL of oxygen/dL, whereas maternal blood can only carry 15.3 mL/dL. Fetal blood has greater affinity for oxygen compared to the maternal circulation due to the presence of fetal hemoglobin and fetal red cells. Both fetal and maternal oxygen association show changes associated with pH that give rise to the double Bohr effect, which facilitates transfer of oxygen from mother to fetus. The uptake of oxygen by the fetus is relatively insensitive to short-term changes in umbilical blood flow rate. As blood flow falls, there is a compensatory increase in the fractional extraction of oxygen. Long-term reductions in fetal blood flow have a greater effect; therefore, short-term alterations in blood flow such as caused by uterine contractions may not compromise the fetus, whereas more persistent reductions in blood flow may harm fetal development. Although the fetus may be able to compensate for up to a 50% reduction in placental oxygen delivery by increasing extraction and hence maintaining O_2 content, this may not be without deleterious effects as the reduction in pO_2 may affect many processes that are regulated by pO_2 rather than by oxygen content. The placenta itself has one of the highest rates of O_2 consumption at 1.2 to 2.0 μmol/min/g, equivalent to that of the brain.

Carbon dioxide is carried in blood predominantly as bicarbonate, with some bound to hemoglobin as carboxyhemoglobin. The high hemoglobin content of fetal blood compared to the mother enables it to carry more carbon dioxide with a given pH and pCO_2. As carbon dioxide is produced by fetal metabolism and raises fetal blood levels of pCO_2, the gas will diffuse across the placenta from the fetal to maternal compartments, provided that fetal pCO_2 exceeds maternal pCO_2 (32). Maternal pCO_2 falls during pregnancy by about 10 torr as a consequence of hyperventilation. A transplacental gradient of about 10 torr is maintained throughout the latter stages of pregnancy. Carbon dioxide will also bind to hemoglobin, which is not bound to oxygen. Maternal hemoglobin has a higher affinity for carbon dioxide than fetal hemoglobin, which gives rise to a double haldane effect that complements the double Bohr effect. The capacity of blood for carbon dioxide at a given pCO_2 is increased by the release of oxygen, so maternal blood will be able to bind increasing amounts of carbon dioxide for the same pCO_2 as it passes through the placenta, while the reverse occurs for fetal blood. This considerably augments the exchange of carbon dioxide across the placenta.

Water Transfer

At term approximately 80% of the weight of the intrauterine contents is water (approximately 4 L), and the unidirectional flux of water across the placenta in both directions is about 60 mL per minute, which is some 10,000 times greater than the net flux (33). The driving force for net water flux across the placenta is probably hydrostatic and osmotic pressure differences between the fetal and maternal placental circulations. Experimental observations have shown that increase in the osmotic pressure by injections of hypotonic solutions (34) or altering the hydrostatic pressure gradients between circulations (35) alters water flow across the perfused placenta. However, the *in vivo* size and direction of osmotic and hydrostatic pressure differences across the placenta are unknown. The mechanisms regulating water transfer in the human are unclear, as we are uncertain currently whether fetal plasma total osmolarity is higher than or equal to maternal plasma osmolarity, and it also appears that the estimated hydrostatic pressure in the intervillous space is lower than that in the umbilical vein (36). If these observations are applicable *in vivo*, they are incompatible with net transplacental acquisition of water by the fetus. Further, it is unclear how much of transplacental water flow is transcellular as opposed to paracellular (37).

Transport and Metabolism of Carbohydrates

The major carbohydrate transported by the placenta is glucose, the principal substrate for energy metabolism. Transport of glucose occurs by facilitated diffusion in a saturable, stereoselective, and bidirectional manner. When glucose levels in the maternal bloodstream exceed those in the fetal circulation, glucose may be transferred from mother to fetus without using metabolic energy. At term, maternal plasma levels of glucose are about 3.7 mmol/L, whereas fetal cord arterial glucose is 3.2 mmol/L. Placental glucose uptake from the maternal circulation greatly exceeds the uptake by the fetal circulation, as glucose entering the trophoblast is either oxidized or stored as glycogen.

Six members of the facilitative glucose transporter (GLUT) family have been identified to date (38). They are designated GLUT proteins 1 to 5 and 7. GLUT 6 is a pseudogene that is not expressed at the protein level. The various isoforms are expressed in a tissue-specific manner and range in size from 492 to 524 amino acids with 39% to 68% sequence homology (38). GLUT 1 is ubiquitously expressed, has a high affinity for glucose, and is probably responsible for constitutive glucose uptake, particularly in endothelial cells where it may move glucose between blood and organs. In the placenta GLUT 1 is found in capillary endothelium and erythrocytes throughout gestation and in both the apical and basal plasma membranes of syncytiotrophoblast (39). Whereas immunostaining for GLUT 1 is more intense on the apical membranes in early gestation, in later gestation immunostaining becomes more intense on the basal membranes, suggesting an ontogenic change that may be hormonally regulated. In many different cell types, growth factors and hormones such as insulin, the insulin-like growth factors (IGFs), glucose, and estrogen increase GLUT 1 expression. Insulin receptors are also found in the human placenta (40), being highly expressed on syncytiotrophoblasts in early gestation but decreasing in density throughout gestation, whereas expression in fetal endothelium increases throughout gestation. This suggests a potential autocrine/paracine effect of insulin in placental development, which may be growth-promoting on trophoblasts in early gestation together with an as yet undetermined role for insulin in the fetal-placental vasculature. GLUT 2 is the low-affinity, high-capacity transporter found in adult liver and pancreatic b cells where it may function in concert with glucokinase as a glucose-sensing system. GLUT 3 is also found in almost all tissues and may, like GLUT 1, play a role in basal transport of glucose. In the pregnant uterus GLUT 3 is found in amnion epithelial cells and on cytotrophoblasts (41). The high affinity of GLUT 3, like GLUT 1, suggests it may be able to scavenge glucose from the mother for the fetus during times of hypoglycemic stress. Available data to date (41) suggest that GLUT 4 is not expressed in the placenta.

As the levels of glucose in maternal and fetal blood are between 2 and 4 mmol/L, and glucose transport studies of placental vesicles have found Michaelis constant (K_m) values for carriers in the region of 23 to 31 mmol/L, and studies on perfused tissues have given K_m values of 13 to 17 mmol/L, the carrier appears to be far from saturated under normal physiologic conditions and hence increases in numbers of glucose carriers will not enhance glucose flux. Whereas insulin is an important regulator of membrane glucose transport, insulin appears to have no effect on transplacental movement of glucose. There is little evidence for hormonal downregulation of placental glucose transport despite the potential for regulation of the transporters. No differences have been found to date in GLUT 1 levels between the placentae of preterm or term IUGR fetuses despite the occurrence of hypoglycemia (42) nor in GLUT 1 or 3 levels between normal and gestational diabetic placentae (43).

Glucose is a metabolic fuel, its oxidation producing adenosine triphosphate (ATP). The principal metabolic pathway for glucose metabolism in trophoblasts is the Embden-Meyerhof pathway. Glucose is broken down aerobically with 2 mol of ATP generated per mole of glucose consumed. Pyruvate formed by the process is converted to lactate (an-

aerobic glycolysis) or enters the citric acid cycle (aerobic glycolysis). Conversion to lactate does not require oxygen and produces no further ATP. In the citric acid cycle, ATP is generated by oxidative phosphorylation such that 38 mol of ATP is produced for each molecule of glucose during aerobic glycolysis. Transfer to the fetus may represent only 40% to 50% of glucose taken up by the placenta (44). Placental glycolysis involves both aerobic and anaerobic pathways, with only about 20% of total glucose metabolism occurring aerobically in the placenta, the remainder being converted to lactate. The pentose phosphate pathway is also present in the placenta for glycolysis. The proportion of glucose utilized by the placenta declines toward term as fetal growth and glucose demands increase. Studies in humans suggest that at midgestation 73% of glucose retained by the placenta is metabolized by glycolysis, 10% via the pentose phosphate pathway and the remainder by lipid and glycogen synthesis. The utilization falls toward term largely as a consequence of a decline in the pentose phosphate pathway and the anabolic pathways, so that at term glycolysis accounts for 90% of all glucose utilized by the placenta.

Lactate is produced by the placentae of every species and enters the maternal and fetal circulations.

Amino Acid Transport

The majority of amino acids are transported from mother to fetus against a concentration gradient in an energy-dependent manner (45) via transporter proteins found at the microvillous membrane of the placenta. For most amino acids the fetal to maternal concentration ratio is >1.0; however, there are quantitative differences between species (46). Where the fetal to maternal concentration ratio of amino acid is <1.0, the overall transport of that amino acid may still be energy-dependent, as the concentration within the trophoblast is greater than within the maternal plasma (46). This is particularly true for taurine, glutamate, and aspartate. The energy-dependency of placental amino acid transport means that inhibition of both glycolysis and aerobic metabolism can depress placental amino acid transport. At least ten different transporter systems for amino acid uptake have been identified (47). These are divided into the sodium-dependent (designated by upper-case letters) and the sodium-independent (designated by lower-case letters) systems. Although there is a fair amount of overlap between the systems for different amino acid transport, most of the essential amino acids are transported by the alanine-serine-cystine (ASC) system. Studies employing microvesicle preparations of human placenta have shown that the A, N, $X-_{AG}$, b, y+, y+L, and I systems are found in the maternal microvillous membrane of the syncytiotrophoblast, and the A, ASC, $X-_{AG}$, y+, $b^{o,+}$, and I systems are active in the basal membrane of the trophoblast (48). As the various transporter proteins compete for the various amino acids and the capacity of the different transporters may be saturable, changes in amino acid concentration may affect the ratios of amino acids that are transported by the placenta. Additionally, some amino acids may be actively transported into trophoblasts and then moved down a concentration gradient into fetal plasma, whereas others may be actively transported out of trophoblastic tissue into fetal plasma, therefore exercising another level of control on fetal amino acid concentrations. Studies of amino acid transport in the perfused human placenta have shown bidirectional transport of many amino acids, but the kinetics are different in different directions such that transplacental transfer is greater in the maternal-fetal direction for all amino acids taken up by the placenta (49).

In addition to transferring amino acids from mother to fetus, the placenta also has a large number of enzymes that will metabolize amino acids. These will include metabolic pathways such as gluconeogenesis, glycogen synthesis, protein synthesis, amino acid oxidation, and ammoniagenesis. The placenta also requires a large amount of amino acids for synthesis of secreted peptides and proteins.

There is evidence both *in vitro* and *in vivo* that activity of amino acid transporters can be regulated. Reduction of amino acid concentrations will increase amino acid transport measured as increased B_{max} and reduced K_m mediated by synthesis of new transport proteins. In pregnancies complicated by IUGR amino acid concentrations are lower in the fetus when compared to appropriately grown fetuses (50–52). The placentas from these infants showed reductions in transport of many amino acids, particularly the essential amino acids. Further, microvillous membrane vesicle preparations of small-for-gestational-age infants showed a significant reduction in activity of the A system transporters when compared to placentas from appropriate-for-gestational-age (AGA) infants (53). A reduction in system A activity in placenta microvillous plasma membrane was reported in IUGR pregnancies with a reduction in umbilical blood flow compared to AGA pregnancies (54), suggesting system A activity is related to the severity of IUGR. There is as yet little evidence that placental amino acid transporters are regulated by hormones. However, the recent cloning of many of the amino acid transporters will lead to an expansion of knowledge in this area. Currently, there is some preliminary evidence that insulin may enhance placental amino acid uptake and transport to the fetus (55), and uptake of aminoiso butyric acid (AIB) by trophoblast cells has been shown to be enhanced by insulin, dexamethasone, glucagon, and 3′,5′-cyclic adenosine monophosphate (cAMP) (56). Both *in vitro* and *in vivo*, ethanol has been shown to inhibit placental amino acid transport, although at very high concentrations (57), and nicotine has also been shown to inhibit system A amino acid transport in the placenta (58). Currently, however, it is speculative whether placental amino acid transport is altered in the placentae of women who both smoke and drink alcohol, although

clinically this may produce growth restriction. Another drug of abuse, cocaine, which causes fetal growth restriction has also been shown to inhibit placental uptake of amino acids and binds to a high-affinity binding protein in the human placenta (59,60). The effect of cocaine on placental amino acid transport may be direct by effect on amino acid transport systems (61), or possibly indirect via reduction of uterine and umbilical blood flow, which produces generalized vasoconstriction and reduced oxygen transport to the fetus (62). We currently lack an integrated picture of overall amino acid transport into the fetus, particularly regarding the effect of one amino acid on the transport of another, and are only just beginning to utilize molecular probes to study the localization and regulation of activity of the various transporters. This will be particularly useful in determining the biologic significance of the reported variations in fetal plasma amino acid concentrations in abnormally grown fetuses (50–52). As transport of amino acids is a flow-independent process, the effects of dramatic reductions in blood flow to the placenta such as are found in severe IUGR may be less than the consequent effects of reduced fetal oxygenation and energy metabolism on amino acid transport.

Lipid Transport and Metabolism

Transport of lipids and essential fatty acids from the mother to the fetus is necessary to support fetal growth and brain development (63). In addition, the transport of nonessential lipids is necessary for accretion in fetal body fat, which then becomes an important substrate during early postnatal life (64). Species such as the human, guinea pig, and rabbit, which all possess a hemochorial placenta, the simplest form of placenta, transport the greatest amount of fatty acid during fetal life (65). In these species body fat at term represents a substantial proportion of fetal body weight (being 10% in the guinea pig and 16% in the human) and de novo fatty acid synthesis by the fetal tissues is insufficient to fulfill this demand. In species with more complex placental arrangements, with both maternal and fetal tissue layers in the placenta, such as the sheep, pig, and cat, transfer of fatty acid to the fetus is generally small in contrast to that seen in the rabbit, guinea pig, primate, and human. Fatty acids are relatively insoluble in water, and therefore are carried in the blood either as albumin-bound free fatty acids or esterified as triglycerides, phospholipids, and esterified cholesterol, which are associated with other lipids and proteins in the form of lipoproteins. These maternal free fatty acids, esterified fatty acids that are hydrolyzed at the placenta, and the unmodified lipoproteins can all be transferred to the fetal circulation (Fig. 25.3). When fatty acids are taken up by the placenta, they can subsequently be used for triglyceride synthesis, cholesterol esterification, membrane biosynthesis, oxidation, or transferred to the fetus. Probably the major determinant of fatty acid transfer into the fetus

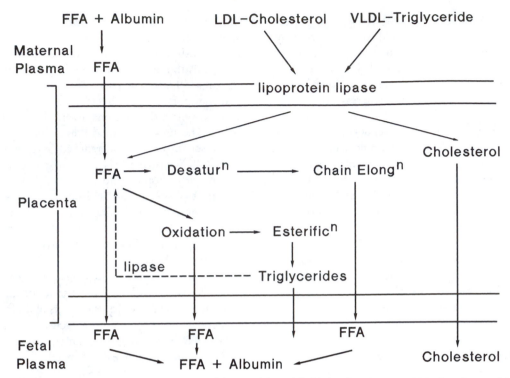

FIGURE 25.3. Transfer and metabolism of fatty acids and lipids by the placenta. FFA, free fatty acid.

is maternal plasma-free fatty acid concentration (66). Placental triglyceride concentrations are greater in women who are fasting, who deliver preterm infants, or who have diabetes mellitus or conditions in which maternal plasma-free fatty acid concentrations are increased. Manipulation of the maternal dietary fatty acid composition will lead to corresponding changes in the fatty acid composition of the fetus.

In addition to direct transport of fatty acids to the fetus across the placenta by a specific transporter, fatty acids can also undergo desaturation, elongation, and partial oxidation at the placenta before transfer to the fetus (67) (Fig. 25.3). The 20 carbon fatty acid arachidonic acid is formed by desaturation and elongation of linoleic acid in the placenta. Arachidonic acid is the precursor of prostaglandins of the two series and a variety of other eicosanoids (68). The trophoblast can also esterify fatty acids and mono- or diglycerides obtained from the maternal plasma or released from circulatory lipoproteins by placental lipoprotein lipase into di- and triglycerides and into phospholipids (69). The compounds can either be stored in the placenta or subsequently hydrolyzed by phospholipases and acylglycerol lipases to release more fatty acid into the circulation. A supply of essential fatty acids and their derivatives is necessary for the fetus to provide structural components of membranes, particularly in the developing central nervous system. Overall the concentration of free fatty acids in fetal plasma is lower than that in maternal plasma, suggesting that there is some restriction to fatty acid transfer across the placenta.

There does not seem to be any selectivity for fatty acid transfer, as both essential and nonessential free fatty acids appear to be transported using the same pathway. Overall, simple diffusion seems to be the mechanism for transfer of lipids across the placenta. Within the physiologic range, transfer of free fatty acids to the fetus correlates with maternal free fatty acid concentrations. The transfer of free fatty acids will be affected by both uterine and umbilical blood flows (66) and the concentration of fetal plasma albumin that binds the free fatty acid (70). In this manner, the increasing concentration of albumin during the third trimester in the human fetus may actually serve to increase its free fatty acid concentrations.

The source of cholesterol for the placenta is low-density lipoprotein (LDL) cholesterol, which is taken up by LDL receptors and endocytosis into the trophoblast cells and then degraded by the lysozymes. Although some cholesterol is transferred directly to the fetus, there is no correlation of fetal cholesterol concentration with maternal cholesterol blood concentration and, hence, the contribution of cholesterol from the placenta appears to be of minimal importance, as fetal liver has a high capacity for synthesis of cholesterol to meet fetal requirements (71). However, cholesterol is the major precursor of placental production of progesterone and estrogen.

Maternal plasma glycerol concentrations are elevated during late pregnancy due to the active lipolytic activity of maternal adipose tissue (72). Plasma glycerol concentrations are higher in the mother than in the fetus, and although the low molecular weight of glycerol suggests that it should cross to the fetus by simple diffusion, there is little evidence in the human that glycerol indeed does transfer to the fetus in any substantial quantity. The placenta actively converts glycerol to lactate and lipids, and this rapid metabolism may actually prevent a high fetal accumulation of glycerol (73). Also, maternal liver and kidney cortex rapidly utilizes glycerol for gluconeogenesis, hence, probably limiting the transfer to the fetus.

Ketone bodies will also cross the placenta by simple diffusion. Although the two main ketone bodies, β-hydroxybutyrate and acetoacetate, are present as the dissociated or ionized forms at pH 7.4, which theoretically should retard their diffusion across the placenta, the substantial maternal to fetal concentration gradient for ketone bodies suggests that there is relatively efficient placenta transfer (74). This transfer of maternal ketone bodies to the fetus underlies the increased stillbirth rate, increased incidence of congenital malformations, and impaired neurophysiologic development in the infant of the poorly controlled pregnant diabetic with or without acidosis where there is maternal ketonemia (75). The placenta can utilize ketone bodies as substrate for both oxidation and lipogenesis in preference to other substrates such as glucose, lactate, and amino acids. The activity of ketone bodies metabolizing enzymes in fetal tissues can be increased by conditions that result in maternal hyperketonemia such as starvation, high-fat diet, and diabetes.

Calcium, Phosphorus, and Magnesium Transport

The human fetus accumulates 28 g of calcium during pregnancy, most of which is transported during the third trimester of pregnancy (76), up to 200 mg/day. In all species the rate of maternal to fetal calcium transfer increases during the last trimester of pregnancy. The concentration of total and ionized calcium in fetal plasma is greater than that in maternal plasma, and this gradient is present as early as 20 to 26 weeks' gestation. Therefore, active transcellular mechanisms must be involved in transporting calcium across the placenta, which takes place against a concentration gradient in an energy-dependent manner and at a faster rate than would be achieved by simple diffusion. However, there is bidirectional transport of calcium across the mammalian placenta, which is considerably higher than the net flux of calcium to the fetus.

Trophoblast intracellular calcium concentration must be buffered during translocation of calcium from maternal to fetal facing surfaces of trophoblast. Uptake of calcium at the apical surface of trophoblasts occurs by passive diffusion down an electrochemical gradient via a calcium channel (77). This step may be rate limiting for transcellular calcium flux. Calcium-binding proteins that have been identified in the placenta of the rat, mouse, and human (78) may serve to transfer calcium across the cell and protect the intracellular calcium concentration from becoming too high. In the rat rapid increases in placental concentrations of calcium-binding protein have been shown to occur during the period of increased rate of fetal growth and calcium accumulation in late gestation, suggesting this protein may be involved in placental calcium transport (79). In human placental microsomal membrane vesicles, uptake of calcium is inhibited by preincubation with an antibody to human calcium-binding protein. Transfer of calcium across the basal plasma membrane of trophoblast may be via a calcium adenosine triphosphatase (ATPase). Hydrolysis of ATP would provide the energy to overcome the calcium concentration gradient. Calcium ATPase has been identified in human placental homogenates (80) and plasma membrane vesicles (81). There is little change in expression of calcium ATPase mRNA in the human (82) or rat placenta throughout gestation, suggesting this protein does not limit the rate of placental calcium transport.

Transfer of calcium to the fetus may be influenced by maternal and fetal blood flows to the placenta and the capacity of placental transport mechanisms. However, the rapidly increased transfer of calcium that occurs during the third trimester of pregnancy is far greater than could be explained by an increase in placental surface area or blood flow, and therefore transcellular active transport is probably rate limiting for placental calcium transport. Maternal plasma calcium concentrations will influence placental calcium transport. In pregnant Chinese women, dietary deficiencies associated with maternal plasma calcium concentrations as low as 1 mmol/L led to infants with congenital rickets (83). Infants born in summer months are reported to have a lower bone mineral content at birth when compared to infants born in winter. This may be related to seasonal differences in maternal and fetal calciotrophic hormone (84). There are reports of maternal vitamin D deficiencies causing neonatal rickets, consistent with the hypothesis that maternal vitamin D may be important for placental calcium transport; indeed, 1,25-dihydroxyvitamin D_3 may regulate placental calcium transport (85). Parathyroid hormone (PTH) also appears to stimulate maternal to fetal calcium transport, perhaps due to a direct action on the placental calcium transporters or alternatively by increase in fetal 1,25-dihydroxyvitamin D_3 production (86). Further PTH-related peptide (PTHrP) produced by the fetal parathyroid glands may also be capable of stimulating maternal-fetal calcium transport acting via a receptor distinct from the PTH/PTHrP receptor and that recognizes a midmolecule region of PTHrP (87).

Phosphorus is necessary for the developing fetus because of its role in intermediate metabolism and skeletal mineralization. During the latter part of gestation plasma concentrations of phosphorus in the fetus are higher than that of the mother, suggesting maternal-fetal transport of phosphorus against a concentration gradient by an active transport process. The human fetus contains approximately 16 g of phosphorus at term, the majority of which is transferred in the third trimester of pregnancy (76). Again, there is bidirectional transport of phosphorus across the placenta, with the flux in the maternal-fetal direction exceeding that in the fetal-maternal direction. The net flux in humans is about 4.5 mg/day after the fifth month of pregnancy. In the guinea pig the transcellular transport of phosphorus depends on a sodium-dependent active transport mechanism, and the transfer is reduced by anoxic conditions or addition of cyanide. In the human pH, temperature, sodium, and amino acid concentrations appear to modulate the transport of phosphorus from maternal plasma into trophoblasts (88). There is little data on mechanisms regulating phosphorus transport across the placenta, although 1,25-dihydroxyvitamin D_3 and fetal PTH may be involved.

Mechanisms regulating magnesium transport across the placenta have not been very well elucidated. Membrane proteins mediating the active transport of magnesium have not been identified but could be magnesium channels or facilitated-type carriers. The flux across the fetal facing plasma membrane is likely to be an energy-dependent process. Magnesium, however, is transported across the placenta by a distinct mechanism from that involving calcium. In diabetic pregnancies, the bone mineral content of infants is reduced by about 10% when compared to normal infants. There is an increased incidence of hypocalcemia and hypomagnesemia in infants of diabetic mothers (89). In the streptozotocin-induced diabetic rat the maternal-fetal flux of both calcium and magnesium is reduced by between 20% and 40% in the presence of the untreated maternal diabetes (90). These deficiencies in placental transport were prevented by control of diabetes with insulin. It has been found that the calcium-binding protein is reduced in the placentas of diabetic rats (91), illustrating that there may be a relationship between placental transport of calcium and the activity of calcium-binding protein.

Transfer of Immunoglobulin G

Concentration of immunoglobulin G (IgG) in cord plasma at term is reported to be higher than that in the maternal plasma, suggesting that there is active transport of IgG across the placenta (92). Indeed, transfer of IgG is greater than that of albumin despite albumin being a smaller molecule. The transfer of IgG is also greater than that of other immunoglobulin classes. There do appear to be differences between the four different subclasses of IgG, with preferential transport of IgG1 and the slowest transport of IgG2 (93). Selective transfer of IgG across the placenta confers passive immunity to the fetus (94). In other species, particularly rabbit, guinea pig, and rodent, IgG is transferred by the yolk sac placenta rather than the chorioallantoic placenta. The most likely mechanism of selected transfer is receptor-mediated endocytosis by specific FCγ receptors

in coated pits (95). Three subtypes of FCγ receptors for IgG are found on the microvillous plasma membrane of the human placenta (96) and purified coated microvesicles from human placentas contain IgG. These purified coated microvesicles also contain transferrin, and 40% also contain ferritin. The endocytotic vesicles may fuse with each other and with lysosomes and fuse with the basal plasma membrane to exocytose IgG into the extracellular space on the fetal side. Although currently poorly defined, it appears that IgG also crosses the vascular endothelium by transcytosis (97).

PLACENTAL STEROIDOGENESIS

The human placenta produces large amounts of progesterone and estrogenic steroids. The site of steroidogenesis in the placenta is the syncytiotrophoblast. As the placenta has a very limited capacity to synthesize cholesterol de novo from acetate, cholesterol has to be supplied to it in the maternal circulation. The human placenta also lacks the 17α-hydroxylase/17,20-lyase activity (P-450$_{C17}$) and thus cannot convert the C-21 steroids pregnenolone and progesterone to C-19 products, which are precursors of estrogen. Therefore, separate steroid precursors are required by the human placenta for the biosynthesis of progesterone and estrogen (Fig. 25.4).

Progesterone

Maternal cholesterol with LDL is bound to specific LDL receptors on syncytiotrophoblast, taken up by endocytosis and then hydrolyzed to free cholesterol within the lysosomes. Within the syncytiotrophoblast cholesterol is then converted to pregnenolone by the mitochondrial enzyme complex 20,22 desmolase. Pregnenolone is then converted to progesterone (98) by the 3β-hydroxysteroid dehydrogenase, Δ5-Δ4-isomerase complex, which is the rate-limiting step for progesterone biosynthesis. The majority of this progesterone (90%) is then secreted into the maternal circulation, with the other 10% being secreted into the fetal circulation where it can be used as a precursor for Δ4-3-ketosteroids. Although the fetus can synthesize pregnenolone, it lacks the ability to convert it to progesterone. Hence, progesterone synthesis by the placenta is completely independent of the fetus. Although the placenta begins to synthesize progesterone very early in gestation, prior to 35 to 47 days postovulation progesterone from the corpus luteum, or exogenous supplementation with progesterone is required to support pregnancy (99). Past this time placental progesterone production alone can support pregnancy even in the absence of an ovary. Placental production of progesterone increases steadily throughout pregnancy and reaches a maximum a few weeks prior to term at 300 mg progesterone per day (100), with maternal serum concentrations of be-

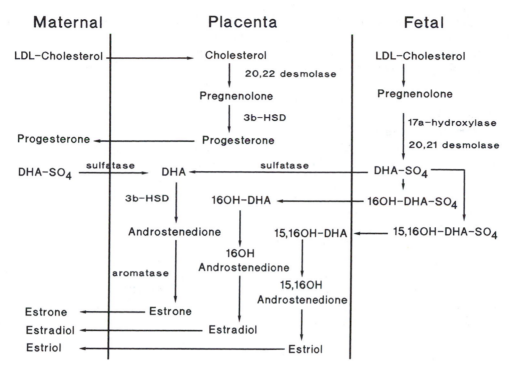

FIGURE 25.4. Synthesis of progesterone and estrogens by the human fetal-placental unit.

tween 400 and 500 nmol/L (Fig. 25.5). The major function of progesterone during pregnancy appears to be maintenance of uterine quiescence (99). Studies in small animals and sheep have clearly shown that withdrawal of progesterone at term, with the resulting switch to estrogen action, is necessary for the expression of a variety of contraction associated proteins in myometrium, which ultimately leads to labor (101). While evidence for active progesterone withdrawal at term occurring prior to the onset of parturition is lacking in humans, a large amount of indirect evidence suggests that progesterone still fulfills a role in maintenance of uterine quiescence throughout the majority of pregnancy and that some reduction in the bioactivity of progesterone is associated with the onset of labor (102).

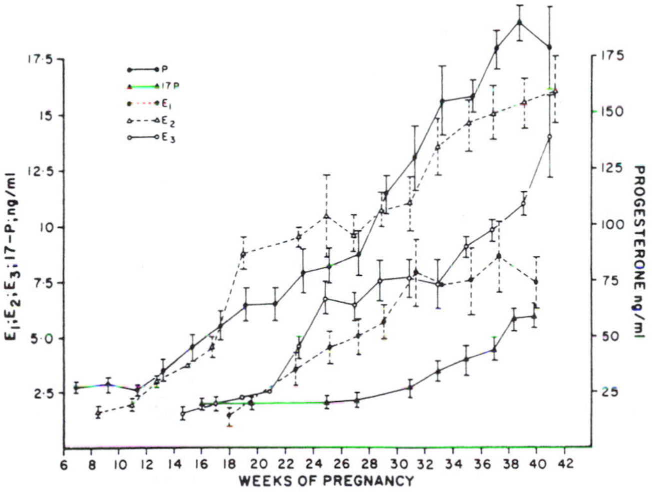

Estrogens

Estrogen production also increases dramatically during pregnancy (1,000-fold) to reach approximately 80 mg per day near term with a maternal concentration of estradiol of 100 nmol/L (100) (Fig. 25.5). The major estrogen produced by the placenta is estriol, which is a weak estrogen found in the nonpregnant individual as an hepatic metabolite of estradiol. As the placenta lacks the P-450$_{C17}$ enzyme, it cannot synthesize the C19 estrogens from the C21 precursors pregnenolone and progesterone (103). However, the fetal adrenal cortex will produce large quantities of the C19 steroid dehydroepiandrosterone sulfate (DHAS), which can then be converted to estrogen by the placenta. In the fetal adrenal zone, adrenal adrenocorticotropic hormone (ACTH) stimulates the conversion of LDL cholesterol to pregnenolone. Pregnenolone is then converted to DHAS by the actions of the fetal adrenal zone enzymes 17α-hydroxylase and 20,21-desmolase (104). The DHAS is secreted into the fetal circulation and reaches the placenta directly, or alterna-

FIGURE 25.5. Maternal plasma concentrations of progesterone (P), 17-hydroxyprogesterone (17P), estrone (E1), estradiol (E2), and estriol (E3) throughout human pregnancy. (From Tulchinsky D, Hobel CJ, Yeager E, et al. Plasma esterone, estradiol, estriol, progesterone and 17-hydroxyprogesterone in human pregnancy. I. Normal pregnancy. *Am J Obstet Gynecol* 1972;112:1095–1100, with permission.)

tively may be hydroxylated in the fetal liver at the 16α or 15α position prior to reaching the placenta. However, the sulfate must be cleaved before the placental 3β-hydroxysteroid dehydrogenase-isomerase complex can convert DHA or hydroxylated DHA to androstenedione or hydroxylated androstenedione. Both then serve as substrates for the aromatase enzyme system to yield estrone, estradiol, and estriol (105). The major pathway for estriol synthesis in the placenta involves 16α-hydroxy DHAS from the fetal liver. The placenta can also utilize DHAS secreted by maternal adrenal for estrogen biosynthesis and in the last 10 weeks of pregnancy approximately half of the estrone and estradiol produced by the placenta arises from the maternal precursor, whereas only about 10% of the estriol comes from this source. The majority of estrogens synthesized by the placenta are secreted into maternal circulation. As estrogens are predominantly formed from fetal steroidogenic precursors, measurements of estriol in the maternal circulation were used in the past as indicators for fetal well-being.

During pregnancy the high estrogen concentrations stimulate the maternal liver to produce serum cortisol, testosterone, and thyroxine-binding proteins and also increase the hepatic production of LDL and high-density lipoprotein (HDL) cholesterol. Estrogens also cause proliferation of the ductal system in the breast, while progesterone acting in concert with estrogen promotes development of the glandular tissue. Although estrogen stimulates the secretion of prolactin at the hypothalamic pituitary level, estrogen and progesterone act on the breast to inhibit milk secretion by blocking the stimulus from this prolactin. The withdrawal of estrogen and progesterone at delivery allows lactation to then be established. Estrogens also appear to mediate the uterine growth, the increasing uterine blood flow, and the onset of contractility at term in the uterus. In species such as the sheep, there is a fall in plasma progesterone concentrations at term, which is accompanied by a significant increase in estrogen synthesis by the placenta, and corresponding increase in plasma estrogen concentrations (106), which is associated with the expression of the contraction-associated proteins of myometrium, leading to parturition (101). This fall in plasma progesterone cannot be observed in humans; as the term of pregnancy approaches, however, estrogen concentrations rise constantly throughout pregnancy in the human, whereas progesterone concentrations begin to plateau toward term (102) such that at term the ratio of estrogen to progesterone begins to favor estrogen, a situation favorable for the expression of the contraction-associated proteins in the myometrium.

Glucocorticoids

During pregnancy the fetus needs to be protected from the large concentrations of glucocorticoid that may reach it. The enzyme 11β-hydroxysteroid dehydrogenase (11β-HSD) is the enzyme responsible for the interconversion of biologically active glucocorticoid and their inactive 11 ketone me-

tabolites. Two isoforms are present in mammals. The 11β-HSD1 isoform has oxoreductase activity, appears to be distributed ubiquitously, and interconverts cortisol and cortisone requiring reduced nicotinamide adenine dinucleotide phosphate (NADPH) as a cofactor (107). The 11β-HSD2 isoform has only dehydrogenase activity and is NAD dependent (108), and therefore converts cortisol to the inactive metabolite cortisone. Both species of 11β-HSD1 have been demonstrated in the human placenta (109). 11β-HSD2 is found only in the syncytiotrophoblast (110), whereas 11β-HSD1 is undetectable in placental syncytiotrophoblast but is found in the endothelium of blood vessels and umbilical cord (110). The placenta can convert cortisone to cortisol; therefore, it would appear that 11β-HSD1 is active in placenta. The reductase activity of placental tissue increases with gestational age, probably due to an increase in 11β-HSD1 activity (111). The differential distribution of 11β-HSD1 and 11β-HSD2 in the placenta may provide a coordinated mechanism whereby the amounts of maternal glucocorticoid that reach the fetus are precisely controlled. Epidemiologic studies have suggested that small babies have a high incidence of cardiovascular disease in adult life (1). It has been postulated that this may be due to excessive exposure to maternal glucocorticoid during fetal life as a result of a deficiency in placental 11β-HSD2 (112). In humans glucocorticoid has also been shown to stimulate the synthesis of CRH from the placenta and to increase levels of placental CRH mRNA expression (113). This is unlike the hypothalamus, where glucocorticoids inhibit CRH synthesis. Therefore, again, the coordinated expression of 11β-HSD1 and 11β-HSD2, which may control the bioactivity of glucocorticoids in the placenta, may influence CRH expression and release, and may subsequently affect the timing of parturition.

Errors of Placental Steroid Metabolism

Steroid sulfatase deficiency is an X-linked recessive trait that affects only males, occurring in about 1 in 5,000 births. In most cases the deficiency results from the complete deletion of the gene on the short arm of the X chromosome (Xp22.3). In the fetus the disorder is apparent as placental sulfatase deficiency that causes a decrease in placental estrogen production, particularly that of estriol, as the precursors DHEAS and 16-hydroxy DHEAS cannot be hydrolyzed (114). The pregnancies, however, appear clinically normal, though at term a small number may show failure of cervical ripening and may not progress into spontaneous labor. Postnatally the affected individuals develop the hyperkeratosis skin condition of X-linked ichthyosis within 3 months of birth.

Aromatase deficiency is a rare abnormality inherited as an autosomal-recessive trait and arises from mutation of the aromatase gene rather than from deletion of the gene (115). In an affected fetus, placental estrogen production is impaired and concentrations of estriol and other estrogens are decreased in maternal and fetal compartments. As there is no aromatase activity in the placenta, significant amounts of testosterone and androstenedione will be secreted by the placenta, which may result in virilization in the mother during late pregnancy. If the fetus is female, virilization of the external genitalia will occur. These females will then be of short stature, will not experience puberty after birth, and will exhibit signs of virilization and estrogen deficiency. Following puberty, affected males will be of tall stature with delayed bone maturation, and epiphyses will remain unclosed until exposure to estrogen.

PLACENTAL PEPTIDE HORMONE SYNTHESIS

The placenta produces a large variety of peptide and protein hormones in addition to the steroids for the maintenance of pregnancy and support of fetal growth. Many of these hormones act in an autocrine/paracrine manner on the placenta itself in addition to the well-described endocrine actions.

Human Chorionic Gonadotropin

Human chorionic gonadotropin (hCG) is a glycoprotein with a molecular weight of 36 to 40 kd, which is produced by the syncytiotrophoblast (116). It is composed of α and β subunits translated from separate mRNAs (117). The α subunit of 92 amino acids is noncovalently linked to the distinct β subunit of 145 amino acids. hCG resembles the pituitary glycoproteins luteinizing hormone (LH), follicle-stimulating hormone (FSH), and thyroid-stimulating hormone (TSH), with which it shares a common α subunit coded for by a single gene on chromosome 6. The β subunit of hCG is coded for by six genes found on chromosome 19 together with the gene for the β subunit of LH. The β subunit of hCG has 80% sequence homology with the 121 amino acid β subunit of LH but has a different 24 amino acid carboxy terminus (118). Antisera raised against this C terminal amino acid sequence of the hCG β subunit allow for its specific measurement in pregnancy tests, and the extension of the β subunit markedly increases the half-life of hCG *in vivo*. hCG has a similar luteotrophic role to LH, and therefore plays a role in the maintenance of early pregnancy. Trophoblasts will secrete hCG into the maternal circulation immediately following implantation of the blastocysts so that an increase in hCG secretion can be detected in maternal circulation by 24 hours postimplantation and subsequently increases with a doubling time of 2.11 days (119). hCG will act on the ovaries to maintain the corpus luteum, preventing degradation and stimulate secretion of progesterone and estradiol. As previously mentioned, by 6 to 8 weeks of pregnancy placental production of steroids is sufficient to take over from that of the corpus luteum (99). Maximum placental hCG production is seen around 8 to 10 weeks, after which production rapidly decreases

and remains low throughout the remainder of gestation (120). The stimulus to hCG synthesis by syncytiotrophoblasts is gonadotropin-releasing hormone (GnRH) produced by the cytotrophoblast. As estrogens can inhibit GnRH stimulation of hCG, a feedback loop is established such that as steroid production by the placenta increases throughout pregnancy, hCG production is effectively shut down.

Human Placental Lactogen

Human placental lactogen (hPL), also known as human chorionic somatomammotrophin (hCS), is a 191 amino acid single chain polypeptide with a molecular weight of 22 kd (121). hPL is 96% homologous to human growth hormone (hGH) and is encoded for by five closely related genes found on chromosome 17. hPL is also synthesized by syncytiotrophoblasts, and the amount synthesized is related to the mass of trophoblast tissue found in the placenta; therefore, concentration increases throughout pregnancy (122). It is first detectable at 5 weeks' gestation and increases to 5 to 15 mg/L at 35 weeks, when placental production is 1 g per day, being 10% of total placental protein production. The majority of hPL is secreted into the maternal circulation, where it has biologic properties very similar to that of hGH, although it is less potent. hPL will induce metabolic changes that include increasing maternal blood free fatty acids, glucose, and insulin concentrations, and increasing the extent of lipolysis and the insulin resistance (122). This will impair glucose uptake and gluconeogenesis, resulting in enhanced glucose and amino acid availability for fetal uptake. Although hPL has structural similarity to prolactin, there is no strong evidence that it is lactogenic in humans, although it may stimulate proliferation of epithelial cells in the breast. Interestingly, hPL in not essential for a successful pregnancy. Normal pregnancies and normal outcomes have been reported with gene deletions, which lead to an absolute deficiency of hPL production.

Activin and Inhibin

Activin and inhibin are members of the transforming growth factor-β superfamily of glycoproteins (123). Inhibin is a heterodimer composed of two dissimilar α and β subunits linked by disulfide bonds and has a molecular weight of 32 kd. The α subunit consists of 133 amino acids, whereas there are two distinctive β subunits, βA of 116 amino acids and βB of 115 amino acids; therefore, there are two possible forms of inhibin, inhibin A ($\alpha\beta$A) and inhibin B ($\alpha\beta$B). Activin is a homodimer of the inhibin β subunit linked by disulfide bridges and hence can exist in three forms, A, B, and AB, with molecular weights of 26 to 28 kd. The placenta synthesizes both inhibin and activin. Cytotrophoblast synthesizes the α subunit, whereas syncytiotrophoblasts can synthesize the βB subunit. The βA subunit is synthesized by both cyto- and syncytiotrophoblasts (123). Again, inhibin and activin are secreted mainly into the maternal circulation, where concentrations increase throughout pregnancy, and activin is bound to the high-affinity binding protein follistatin (124). Maternal serum activin concentrations increase significantly from 20 weeks' gestation onward, but there is a marked increase that occurs with the onset of labor both at term and preterm. As activin can stimulate prostaglandin production by human fetal membranes, it has been suggested that activin may therefore play a role in the onset of labor. Inhibin and activin may also have paracrine roles within the placenta (125). Inhibin inhibits GnRH stimulation of hCG production, whereas activin will potentiate GnRH-stimulated hCG release. Increased concentrations of inhibin A and total activin A have been found in maternal plasma of patients with preeclampsia compared to control pregnancies (126), suggesting that production by trophoblast is altered in this condition.

Corticotropin-Releasing Hormone (CRH) and ACTH

The placenta contains a local hypothalamic-pituitary axis (127,128) with a CRH-ACTH pathway whose activity is stimulated by the same factors that lead to stress-induced activation of the hypothalamic-pituitary-adrenal axis. CRH is a 41 amino acid peptide initially shown to regulate the hypothalamic-pituitary-adrenal axis, where it controls ACTH secretion by stimulation of synthesis of the precursor protein pro-opiomelanocortin from the anterior pituitary. CRH synthesis also, however, occurs in the syncytiotrophoblast, which is the source of the exponential increase in concentrations of CRH found in the maternal circulation during pregnancy, and in the placenta CRH stimulates local ACTH production (127). CRH is barely detectable in nonpregnant individuals, but in pregnancy during the second trimester serum concentrations begin to increase exponentially to term (129) (Fig. 25.6). However, they fall dramatically following delivery and are undetectable within 24 hours. Interestingly, higher concentrations are found in patients with twin pregnancies, with pregnancy-induced hypertension, or with IUGR, suggesting that increased trophoblast mass or stress may mediate CRH production by trophoblast (130). The biologic effect of CRH on the maternal pituitary to stimulate ACTH is inhibited by the binding of CRH to a CRH-binding protein (CRH-BP) in the maternal circulation (131). CRH-BP is also produced by the placenta and the maternal liver. The serum concentrations of CRH-BP remain high throughout pregnancy, effectively blocking the effects of CRH until term approaches, when the CRH-BP concentrations fall markedly; at the same time the placental production of CRH is increasing rapidly (132) (Fig. 25.6). The net result of the decrease in CHR-BP with continuing increase in CRH production is an increase in the amount of bioactive CRH available. The trigger for the fall in CRH-BP may be the amount of bioavailable CRH, as this can promote metabolic clearance of binding protein. Interestingly, this increase in bioavailable CRH at term does not lead to a dramatic increase in maternal serum ACTH, as free cortisol is also increased at this time, which may balance out the effect of increased bioavailable CRH. A

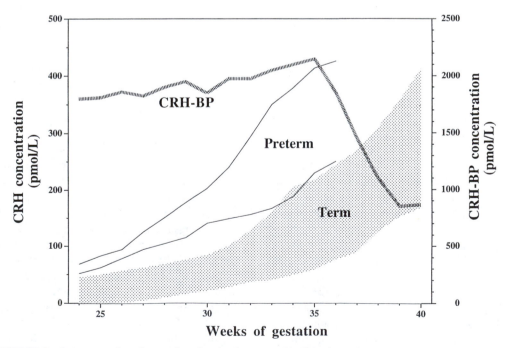

FIGURE 25.6. Ontogeny of corticotropin-releasing hormone (CRH) and CRH-binding protein (CRH-BP) throughout gestation in pregnancies that deliver at term or preterm. (From Keelan JA, Myatt L, Mitchell MD. Endocrinology and paracrinology of parturition. In: Elder MG, Lamont RF, Romero R, eds. *Preterm labor.* New York: Churchill-Livingstone 1997:457–491, with permission.)

similar increase in CRH concentrations is observed in patients prior to the development of preterm labor (133). This may give a clue as to the role of placental CRH, perhaps being important in the onset of labor.

CRH receptors have been characterized in both nonpregnant and pregnant human myometrium (134), and *in vitro* CRH has been shown to potentiate the actions of oxytocin on myometrial contractility (135). Again, *in vitro* CRH has been shown to stimulate production of prostaglandins E_2 and $F_{2\alpha}$ from amnion, chorion-decidua, and placenta (128). Therefore, indirectly CRH may stimulate uterine contractility via prostaglandins. At the hypothalamus, cortisol inhibits CRH secretion, whereas in placental cell cultures dexamethasone has actually been shown to stimulate expression of CRH (136). This may provide the link among so-called stress situations (preeclampsia, IUGR, preterm labor, and the onset of labor). The finding that placental CRH secretion was increased prior to both term and preterm labor has been interpreted to represent CRH being part of a placental clock that times the onset of parturition (137). This clock must be set early in pregnancy such that CRH concentrations increase and then exponentially rise prior to parturition. The CRH may stimulate the fetal pituitary adrenal axis to give cortisol-induced maturational changes in the fetus to prepare it for its extrauterine existence, and at the placental and fetal membrane level CRH initiates the changes in prostaglandin synthesis and action, which may bring about labor. In this hypothesis a certain proportion of preterm labors would appear to result from presetting of the clock. Obviously, however, preterm labors due to intrauterine infection with consequent cytokine production and prostaglandin synthesis occur independent of this clock. CRH from the syncytiotrophoblast may also fulfill another paracrine role in the placenta. It has been reported that CRH is a potent vasodilator in the human fetal placental circulation, being 50 times more potent than prostacyclin (20). This action has been demonstrated in the *in vitro* perfused placental cotyledon, whereas in isolated human placental vessels CRH does not appear to be a vasodilator (138). This suggests that the action of CRH may possibly be modulated by another placental component, possibly by nitric oxide release stimulated by CRH from syncytiotrophoblasts (139).

Insulin-Like Growth Factors

Insulin-like growth factors-I and -II (IGF-I and IGF-II) are synthesized by the human placenta (140). IGF-I is localized predominantly in the syncytiotrophoblast (141), which also synthesizes the binding proteins IGF-BP–I and IGF-BP–II that protect IGF from degradation but block its bioactivity. The IFG-I receptor has also been identified in the human placenta (140). The IGFs potentiate the action of epidermal growth factor (EGF), stimulate decidual prolactin production, and enhance the synthesis of progesterone but inhibit that of estrogen. The IGFs also increase the placental transport of glucose and amino acids; therefore, it is thought that they play a major role in regulation of fetal growth. Placental IGF concentrations correlate with that of growth hormone throughout pregnancy and both are decreased in IUGR (142).

Placental Proteins

Protein synthesized by the placenta will include both pregnancy associated proteins, i.e., those that are synthesized predominantly during pregnancy but can also be found in the nonpregnant state, and pregnancy-specific proteins that are only found in pregnant women (143). These proteins can fulfill a variety of regulatory and structural roles in the placenta itself but can also be secreted into the maternal circulation for endocrine and other actions. Oxvig et al. (143) defined placental proteins in four different types: (a) those that are expressed not only in placenta but in other tissues in a virtually identical manner; (b) those expressed in placenta and other tissues but that are modified posttranslationally in the placenta and in a tissue-specific manner; (c) those that are unique placental proteins that show sequence homology to proteins from other tissues and whose biologic activities are the same, resulting from alternate splicing of mRNA; and (d) unique placental proteins whose amino acid sequences are not similar to other known proteins. Over the last 20 years a whole range of placental proteins have been defined beyond the so-called classic placental proteins. Many of these have been shown to be identical to proteins found in other tissues, but a large number still remain with unknown functions. These include the pregnancy-associated plasma proteins (PAPP) A, B, C, and D (144), which were recognized by immunochemical means, the Schwangerschafts proteins 1, 2, 3, and 4 (145), the placental proteins 1 to 26 (146), and the membrane-associated placental proteins 1 to 10 (147). Some of these proteins were shown to be identical to previously identified proteins; for example, PAPP-C and PAPP-D were found to be identical to SP1 and hPL, whereas PAPP-A and PAPP-B are still believed to be unique proteins. The use of molecular techniques will enable workers to more easily determine the identities and putative roles of these placental proteins by comparison with sequences of other known proteins. Further discovery of homologues of the placental proteins in other animals will also aid in identification of their roles. The whole field of placental proteins has recently been reviewed by Oxvig et al. (143).

SUMMARY

Throughout its short life span, the placenta fulfills a remarkably diverse series of functions to optimize fetal growth, providing signals to the mother and fetus that facilitate the supply of substrate and its efficient utilization. To achieve this goal, the placenta maintains an extremely high level of metabolic activity, both supporting its own functions and supplying precursors for fetal growth and development. The placenta may also play an integral role in determining the length of gestation and the onset of parturition. Although the fetus may be apparently unaffected by mild changes in placental function, and the functional reserve of the placenta or the fetal compensatory mechanisms are still sufficient to support adequate fetal well-being, major functional defects may have profound effects on fetal growth and development. The fetus develops and matures many of its organ systems *in utero;* hence, alterations at this time can easily be seen to lay the foundations for long-term effects on structural and metabolic events that impact adult health, e.g., cardiovascular disease. Altered blood flows to the placenta can be easily recognized by ultrasound techniques. Altered maternal or fetal-placental flows may arise from different etiologies involving a failure of trophoblast invasion or a failure of villous vascular angiogenesis, respectively. While the consequences for transfer of flow-limited substances can be easily recognized, the consequences for substances that are actively transported in an energy-dependent manner and the subsequent effects on fetal growth and well-being cannot be so easily determined. Similarly, the effects of such circumstances on placental metabolism and function per se and the subsequent paracrine/endocrine effects, e.g., on the timing of parturition, are likely to be complex. The challenge for clinicians and basic scientists is to develop models or methods for elucidating such effects and applying the resultant knowledge to clinical practice to reduce perinatal morbidity and mortality.

10 KEY POINTS

1. Abnormalities in placental function and fetal development *in utero* may have long-term consequences for adult health.

2. Trophoblast invasion of the uterus is locally regulated by growth factors and by decidua/trophoblast interactions.

3. Reduced blood flow to the placenta may result from abnormal trophoblast invasion of the uterus or from a defect in angiogenesis of the villous vascular tree.

4. Fetal-placental blood flow is regulated by humoral or autocrine/paracrine factors.

5. Transport processes across the placenta may be either flow limited or membrane limited. Membrane transport occurs by active transport or facilitated diffusion.

6. Energy-dependent active transport processes, e.g., amino acid transport, may be more affected by reduced fetal oxygenation and energy metabolism than by reduced blood flows in severe IUGR.

7. The human placenta cannot convert the C21 steroids pregnenolone and progesterone to the C19 precursors of estrogens. The fetus supplies precursors for estrogen synthesis to the placenta.

8. Placental 11β-HSD may protect the fetus from maternal corticosteroids and may influence activity of the CRH-ACTH pathway in the placenta.

9. The glucocorticoid-CRH-ACTH pathway in the placenta may regulate fetal maturation and function as part of a placental clock regulating parturition.

10. The function of many placenta-specific proteins remains to be determined.

REFERENCES

1. Barker DJP. *Mothers, babies and disease in later life.* London Publishing Group, 1994.
2. Benirschke K, Kaufmann P. *Pathology of the human placenta,* 3rd ed. New York: Springer-Verlag, 1995.
3. Pijnenborg R, Robertson WB, Brosens I, et al. Trophoblast invasion and the establishment of haemochorial placentation in man and laboratory animals. *Placenta* 1981;2:71–92.
4. Craven CM, Morgan T, Ward K, Decidual sprial artery remodeling begins before cellular interaction with cytotrophoblasts. *Placenta* 1998;19:241–252.
5. Brosens IA, Robertson WB, Dixon HG. The role of the spiral arteries in the pathogenesis of preeclampsia. *Obstet Gynecol Annu* 1972;1:177–191.
6. Lala PK, Hamilton GS. Growth factors, proteases and protease inhibitors in the maternal-fetal dialogue. *Placenta* 1996;17:545–555.
7. Damsky CH, Fitzgerald ML, Fisher SJ. Distribution patterns of extracellular matrix components and adhesion receptors are intricately modulated during first trimester cytotrophoblast differentiation along the invasive pathway in vivo. *J Clin Invest* 1992;89:210–222.
8. Zhou Y, Fisher S, Janatpour M, et al. Human cytotrophoblasts adopt a vascular phenotype as they differentiate. *J Clin Invest* 1997;99:2139–2151.
9. Hurskainen T, Hoyhtya M, Tuuttila A, et al. mRNA expressions of TIMP-1, -2, -3 and 92-KD type IV collagenase in early human placenta and decidual membrane as studied by in situ hybridization. *J Histochem Cytochem* 1996;44:1379–1388.
10. Zhou Y, Damsky CH, Fisher SJ. Preeclampsia is associated with failure of human cytotrophoblasts to mimic a vascular adhesion phenotype. *J Clin Invest* 1997;99:2152–2164.
11. Krebs C, Macara LM, Leiser R, et al. Intrauterine growth restriction with absent end-diastolic flow velocity in the umbilical artery is associated with maldevelopment of the placental terminal villous tree. *Am J Obstet Gynecol* 1996;175:1534–1542.
12. Charnock-Jones DS, Sharkey AM, Boocock CA, et al. Vascular endothelial growth factor receptor localization and activation in human trophoblast and choriocarcinoma cells. *Biol Reprod* 1994;51:524–530.
13. Cooper JC, Sharkey AM, Charnock-Jones DS, et al. VEGF mRNA levels in placentae from pregnancies complicated by pre-eclampsia. *Br J Obstet Gynaecol* 1996;103:1191–1196.
14. Adamson SL, Myatt L, Byrne BMP. Regulation of umbilical blood flow. In: Polin RA, Fox WW, eds. *Fetal and neonatal physiology,* 2nd ed. Philadelphia: WB Saunders, 1998:977–988.
15. Myatt L. Control of vascular resistance in the human placenta. *Placenta* 1992;13:329–341.
16. Myatt L, Brewer A, Brockman DE. The action of nitric oxide in the perfused human fetal-placental circulation. *Am J Obstet Gynecol* 1991;164:687–692.
17. Myatt L, Brewer AS, Langdon G, et al. Attenuation of the

vasoconstrictor effects of thromboxane and endothelin in the human fetal-placental circulation. *Am J Obstet Gynecol* 1992; 166:224–230.

18. Wieczorek KM, Brewer AS, Myatt L. Shear stress may stimulate release and action of nitric oxide in the human fetal-placental vasculature. *Am J Obstet Gynecol* 1995;175:708–713.

19. Learmont JG, Poston L. Nitric oxide is involved in flow-induced dilation of isolated human small fetoplacental arteries. *Am J Obstet Gynecol* 1996;174:583–588.

20. Clifton VL, Read MA, Leitch IM, et al. Corticotropin-releasing hormone-induced vasodilatation in the human fetal placental circulation. *J Clin Endocrinol Metab* 1994;79:666–669.

21. Holcberg G, Kassenjans W, Brewer A, et al. The action of two natriuretic peptides (atrial natriuretic peptide and brain natriuretic peptide) in the human placental vasculature. *Am J Obstet Gynecol* 1995;172:71–77.

22. Giles WB, Trudinger BJ, Baird PJ. Fetal umbilical artery flow velocity waveforms and placental resistance: pathological correlation. *Br J Obstet Gynaecol* 1985;92:31–38.

23. Erskine RLA, Ritchie JWK. Umbilical artery blood flow characteristics in normal and growth-retarded fetuses. *Br J Obstet Gynaecol* 1985;92:605–610.

24. Wang Y, Walsh SW, Kay NH. Placental lipid peroxides and thromboxane are increased and prostacyclin is decreased in women with preeclampsia. *Am J Obstet Gynecol* 1992;167: 946–949.

25. Sibai BM, Caritis SN, Thom E, et al. Prevention of preeclampsia with low-dose aspirin in healthy, nulliparous pregnant women. The National Institute of Child Health and Human Development Network of Maternal-Fetal Medicine units. *N Engl J Med* 1993;329:1213–1218.

26. Myatt L, Eis Al, Brockman DE, et al. Endothelial nitric oxide synthase in placental villous tissue from normal, pre-eclamptic and intrauterine growth-restricted pregnancies. *Hum Reprod* 1997;12:167–172.

27. Lyall F, Young A, Greer IA. Nitric oxide concentrations are increased in the fetoplacental circulation in pre-eclampsia. *Am J Obstet Gynecol* 1995;173:714–718.

28. Lyall F, Greer IA, Young A, et al. Nitric oxide concentrations are increased in the feto-placental circulation in intrauterine growth restriction. *Placenta* 1996;17:165–168.

29. Giles W, O'Callaghan S, Boura A, et al. Reduction in human fetal umbilical-placental vascular resistance by glyceryl trinitrate. *Lancet* 1992;340:856.

30. Grunewald C, Kublickas M, Carlstrom K, et al. Effects of nitroglycerin on the uterine and umbilical circulation in severe preeclampsia. *Obstet Gynecol* 1995;86:600–604.

31. Sibley CP, Boyd RDH. Mechanisms of transfer across the human placenta. In: Polin RA, Fox WW, eds. *Fetal and neonatal physiology,* 2nd ed. Philadelphia: WB Saunders, 1998:77–88.

32. Meschia G. Placental respiratory gas exchange and fetal oxygenation. In: Creasy RK, Resnik R, eds. *Maternal fetal medicine. Principles and practice.* Philadelphia: WB Saunders, 1984:274–285.

33. Hutchinson DL, Gray MJ, Plenth AA, et al. The role of the fetus in the water exchange of the amniotic fluid of normal and hydramniotic patients. *J Clin Invest* 1959;38:971–980.

34. Bruns PD, Hellegers AE, Seeds AE. Effects of osmotic gradients across the primate placenta upon the fetal and placenta water contents. *Pediatrics* 1964;34:407–411.

35. Power GG, Roos PJ, Longo LD. Water transfer across the placenta: hydrostatic and osmotic forces and the control of fetal cardiac output. In: Longo LD, Reneau DD, eds. *Fetal and newborn cardiovascular physiology.* New York: Garland, 1978: 317–344.

36. Reynolds SRM, Freese VE, Bieniar ZJ, et al. Multiple simultane-

ous intervillous space pressures recorded in several regions of the hemochorial placenta in relation to functional anatomy of the fetal cotyledon. *Am J Obstet Gynecol* 1968;102:1128–1134.

37. Illsley NP, Verkman AS. Serial permeability barriers to water transport in human placental vesicles. *J Membr Biol* 1986;94: 267–278.

38. Bell GI, Burant CF, Takeda J, et al. Structure and function of mammalian facilitative sugar transporters. *J Biol Chem* 1993; 268:19161–19164.

39. Todokaro C, Yoshimoto Y, Sakata M, et al. Localisation of human placental glucose transporter 1 during pregnancy. An immunohistochemical study. *Histol Histopathol* 1996;11:673–681.

40. Desoye G, Hartmann M, Blaschitz A, et al. Insulin receptors in syncytiotrophoblast and fetal endothelium of human placenta. Immunohistochemical evidence for developmental changes in distribution pattern. *Histochemistry* 1994;101:277–285.

41. Wolf HJ, Desoye G. Immunohistochemical localization of glucose transporters and insulin receptors in human fetal membranes at term. *Histochemistry* 1993;100:379–385.

42. Jansson TS, Wennergren M, Illsley NP. Glucose transporter protein expression in human placenta throughout gestation and in intrauterine growth retardation. *J Clin Endocrinol Metab* 1993;77:1554–1562.

43. Suzuki N, et al. Protein contents of Glut-1 and Glut-3 of human placental tissue at delivery of diabetic mothers do not relate to neonatal birth weight. Proceedings of the 1st International Symposium on Diabetes and Pregnancy in the 90s, 1992:104(abst).

44. Hauguel S, Challier JC, Cedard L, et al. Metabolism of the human placenta in vitro: glucose transfer and utilization, O_2 consumption, lactate and ammonia production. *Pediatr Res* 1983;17:729–732.

45. Yudilevich DL, Sweiry JH. Transport of amino acids in the placenta. *Biochem Biophys Acta* 1985;822:169–201.

46. Battaglia FC, Meschia G. *An introduction to fetal physiology.* Orlando, FL: Academic Press, 1986.

47. Montgomery D, Young M. The uptake of naturally occurring amino acids by the plasma membrane of the human placenta. *Placenta* 1982;3:13–20.

48. Hay WW Jr. Fetal requirements and placental transfer of nitrogenous compounds. In: Polin RA, Fox WW, eds. *Fetal and neonatal physiology,* 2nd ed. Philadelphia: WB Saunders, 1998: 619–634.

49. Eaton BM, Yudilevich DL. Uptake and asymmetric efflux of amino acids at maternal and fetal sides of placenta. *Am J Physiol* 1981;241:C106–112.

50. Cetin I, Marconi AM, Bozzetti P, et al. Umbilical amino acid concentrations in appropriate and small for gestational age infants: a biochemical difference present in utero. *Am J Obstet Gynecol* 1988;158:120–126.

51. Cetin I, Corbetta C, Sereni LP, et al. Umbilical amino acid concentrations in normal and growth-retarded fetuses sampled in utero by cordocentesis. *Am J Obstet Gynecol* 1990;162: 253–261.

52. Economides DL, Nicolaides KH, Gahl WA, et al. Plasma amino acids in appropriate and small-for-gestational-age fetuses. *Am J Obstet Gynecol* 1989;161:1219–1227.

53. Mahendran D, Donnai P, Glazier JD, et al. Amino acid (system A) transporter activity in microvillous membrane vesicles from the placentas of appropriate and small for gestational age babies. *Pediatr Res* 1993;34:661–665.

54. Glazier JD, Cetin I, Perugino G, et al. Association between the activity of the system A amino acid transporter in the microvillous plasma membrane of the human placenta and severity of

fetal compromise in intrauterine growth restriction. *Pediatr Res* 1997;42:514–519.

55. Greenberg RE, Wogenrick FJ, Garcia P, et al. Fetal insulin increases placental amino acid transport. *Clin Res* 1989;37: 178A.

56. Karl PI, Alpy KL, Fisher SE. Amino acid transport by the cultured human placental trophoblast: effect of insulin on AIB transport. *Am J Physiol* 1992;262:C834–839.

57. Henderson GI, Turner D, Patwardhan RV, et al. Inhibition of placental valine uptake after acute and chronic maternal ethanol consumption. *J Pharmacol Exp Ther* 1981;216:465–472.

58. Rowell PP, Sastry BVR. The influence of cholinergic blockade on the uptake of alpha-aminoisobutyric acid by isolated human placental villi. *Toxicol Appl Pharmacol* 1978;45:79–93.

59. Ahmed MS, Zhou DH, Maulik D, et al. Characterization of a cocaine binding protein in human placenta. *Life Sci* 1990; 6:553–561.

60. Barnwell SL, Sastry BVR. Depression of amino acid uptake in human placental villus by cocaine, morphine and nicotine. *Trophoblast Res* 1983;1:101–120.

61. Dicke JM, Henderson GI. Placental amino acid uptake in normal and complicated pregnancies. *Am J Med Sci* 1988;295: 223–227.

62. Woods JR Jr, Plessinger MA, Clark KE. Effect of cocaine on uterine blood flow and fetal oxygenation. *JAMA* 1987;157: 957–961.

63. Crawford MA, Hassam AG, Williams G. Essential fatty acid and fetal brain growth. *Lancet* 1976;1:452–453.

64. Hull D. Total fat metabolism. In: Beard RW, Nathanielz G, eds. *Fetal physiology and medicine*. London: WB Saunders, 1976:105–120.

65. Widdowson EM. Chemical composition of newly born mammals. *Nature (Lond)* 1950;166:626–628.

66. Stephenson T, Stammers J, Hull D. Maternal to fetal transfer of FFA in the in situ perfused rabbit placenta. *J Dev Physiol* 1990;13:117–123.

67. Shand JH, Noble RC. Δ9 and Δ6-desaturase activities of the ovine placenta and their role in the supply of fatty acids to the foetus. *Biol Neonate* 1979;36:298–304.

68. Kuhn DC, Crawford M. Placental essential fatty acid transport and prostaglandin synthesis. *Prog Lipid Res* 1986;25:345–353.

69. Coleman RA. Placental metabolism and transport of lipid. *Fed Proc* 1986;45:2519–2523.

70. Stephenson T, Stammers J, Hull D. Placental transfer of FFA: importance of fetal albumin concentration and acid-base status. *Biol Neonate* 1993;63:273–280.

71. Belknap WM, Dietschy JM. Sterol synthesis and low density lipoprotein clearance in vivo in the pregnant rat, placenta, and fetus: sources for tissue cholesterol during fetal development. *J Clin Invest* 1988;82:2077–2085.

72. Chaves JM, Herrera E. In vivo glycerol metabolism in the pregnant rat. *Biol Neonate* 1980;37:172–179.

73. Gilbert M. Origin and metabolic fate of plasma glycerol in the rabbit and rabbit fetus. *Pediatr Res* 1977;11:95–99.

74. Kim YJ, Felig P. Maternal and amniotic fluid substrate levels during caloric deprivation in human pregnancy. *Metabolism* 1972;21:507–512.

75. Miodovnik M, Lavin JP, Harrington DJ, et al. Effect of maternal ketoacidemia on the pregnant ewe and the fetus. *Am J Obstet Gynecol* 1982;144:585–593.

76. Widdowson EM, Spray CM. Chemical development in utero. *Arch Dis Child* 1951;26:205.

77. van Kreel BK, van Dijk JP. Mechanism involved in the transfer of calcium across the isolated guinea pig placenta. *J Dev Physiol* 1983;5:155–165.

78. Tuan RS. Calcium-binding protein of the human placenta: characterization, immunohistochemical localization and functional involvement in Ca^{2+} transport. *Biochem J* 1985;227: 317–326.

79. Delorme AC, Marche P, Garel JM. Vitamin D-dependent calcium-binding protein: changes during gestation, prenatal and postnatal development in rats. *J Dev Physiol* 1979;1:181–194.

80. Miller RK, Berndt WO. Evidence for Mg^{2+}-dependent (Na^+ K^+)-activated ATPase and Ca^{2+}-ATPase in the human placenta. *Proc Soc Exp Biol Med* 1973;143:118–122.

81. Treinen KA, Kulkarni AP. High-affinity, calcium-stimulated ATPase in brush border membranes of the human term placenta. *Placenta* 1986;7:365–373.

82. Howard A, Legon S, Walters JR. Plasma membrane calcium pump expression in human placenta and small intestine. *Biochem Biophys Res Commun* 1992;183:499–505.

83. Maxwell JP. Further studies of adult rickets (osteomalacia) and fetal rickets. *Proc R Soc Med* 1935;28:265–300.

84. Namgung R, Mimouni F, Campaigne BN, et al. Low bone mineral content in summer-born compared with winter-born infants. *J Pediatr Gastroenterol Nutr* 1992;15:285–288.

85. Ross R, Care AD, Robinson JS, et al. Perinatal 1,25-dihydroxycholecalciferol in the sheep and its role in the maintenance of the transplacental calcium gradient. *J Endocrinol* 1980;87: 17P–18P.

86. Robinson NR, Sibley CP, Mughal MZ, et al. Fetal control of calcium transport across the rat placenta. *Pediatr Res* 1989;26: 109–115.

87. Kovacs CS, Lanske B, Hunzelman JL, et al. Parathyroid hormone-related peptide (PTHrP) regulates fetal-placental calcium transport through a receptor distinct from the PTH/PTHrP receptor. *Proc Natl Acad Sci USA* 1996;93:15233–15238.

88. Lajeunesse D, Brunette MG. Sodium gradient-dependent phosphate transport in the placental brush border membrane vesicles. *Placenta* 1988;9:117–128.

89. Tsang RC, Strub R, Brown DR, et al. Hypomagnesium in infants of diabetic mothers: perinatal studies. *J Pediatr* 1976;89: 115–119.

90. Husain SM, Birdsley TJ, Glazier JD, et al. Effect of diabetes mellitus on maternofetal flux of calcium, magnesium and calbindin 9k: mRNA expression in rat placenta. *Pediatr Res* 1994;35: 376–381.

91. Verhaeghe J, Thomasse TM, Brehier A, et al. 1,25 $(OH)_2D_3$ and Ca-binding protein in fetal rats: relationship to the maternal vitamin D status. *Am J Physiol* 1988;254:E505–512.

92. Pitcher-Wilmott RW, Hindocha P, Wood CB. The placental transfer of IgG subclasses in human pregnancy. *Clin Exp Immunol* 1980;41:303–308.

93. Malek A, Sager R, Kuhn P, et al. Evolution of maternofetal transport of immunoglobulins during human pregnancy. *Am J Reprod Immunol* 1996;36:248–255.

94. Brambell FWR. The transmission of immunity from mother to young and the catabolism of immunoglobulins. *Lancet* 1966; 2:1087–1093.

95. Wild AE. Endocytic mechanisms in protein transfer across the placenta. *Placenta* 1981;(suppl 1):165.

96. Kameda T, Koyama M, Matsuzaki N, et al. Localization of three subtypes of Fcγ-receptors in human placenta by immunohistochemical analysis. *Placenta* 1991;12:15–26.

97. Leach L, Eaton BM, Firth JA, et al. Immunocytochemical and labelled tracer approaches to uptake and intracellular routing of immunoglobulin-G (IgG) in the human placenta. *Histochem J* 1991;23:444–449.

98. Ryan KJ, Meigs R, Petro Z. The formation of progesterone by the human placenta. *Am J Obstet Gynecol* 1966;96:676–686.

99. Csapo AI, Pulkkinen MO, Wiest WG. Effects of lutectomy and progesterone replacement in early pregnant patients. *Am J Obstet Gynecol* 1973;115:759–765.

100. Tulchinsky D, Hobel CJ, Yeager E, et al. Plasma esterone, estradiol, estriol, progesterone and 17-hydroxyprogesterone in human pregnancy. I. Normal pregnancy. *Am J Obstet Gynecol* 1972;112:1095–1100.

101. Lefebvre DL, Piersanti M, Bai XH, et al. Myometrial transcriptional regulation of the gap junction gene, connexin-43. *Reprod Fertil Dev* 1995;7:603–611.

102. Keresztes P, Ayers JW, Menon KM, et al. Comparison of peripheral, uterine and cord estrogen and progesterone levels in laboring and non-laboring women at term. *J Reprod Med* 1988;33:691–694.

103. Albrecht ED, Pepe GJ. Placental steroid hormone biosynthesis in primate pregnancy. *Endocr Rev* 1990;11(1):124–150.

104. Benirschke K. Synthesis in vitro of steroids by human fetal adrenal gland slices. *J Biol Chem* 1959;234:1085–1089.

105. Siiteri PK, MacDonald PC. The utilization of circulating dehydroisoandrosterone sulfate for estrogen synthesis during human pregnancy. *Steroids* 1963;2:713–730.

106. Ryan KJ. Maintenance of pregnancy and the initiation of labor. In: Tulchinsky D, Ryan KJ, eds. *Maternal-fetal endocrinology*. Philadelphia: WB Saunders, 1980:297–309.

107. Monder C, Lakshmi V. Corticosteroid 11β-dehydrogenase of rat tissues: immunological studies. *Endocrinology* 1990;126:2435–2443.

108. Krozowski Z, Maguire JA, Stein-Oakley AN, et al. Immunohistochemical localization of the 11β-hydroxysteroid dehydrogenase type II enzyme in human kidney and placenta. *J Clin Endocrinol Metab* 1995;80:2203–2209.

109. Lasshmi V, Nath N, Muneyyirci-Delale. Characterization of 11β-hydroxysteroid dehydrogenase of human placenta: evidence for the existence of two species of 11β-hydroxysteroid dehydrogenase. *J Steroid Biochem Mol Biol* 1993;45:391–397.

110. Sun K, Yang K, Challis JRG. Differential expression of 11β-hydroxysteroid dehydrogenase types 1 and 2 in human placenta and fetal membranes. *J Clin Endocrinol Metab* 1997;82:300–305.

111. Giannopolous G, Jackson K, Tulchinsky D. Glucocorticoid metabolism in human placenta, decidua, myometrium and fetal membranes. *J Steroid Biochem* 1982;17:371–374.

112. Seckl JR, Benediktsson R, Lindsay RS, et al. Placental 11β-hydroxysteroid dehydrogenase and the programming of hypertension. *J Steroid Biochem Mol Biol* 1995;55:447–455.

113. Riley SC, Walton JC, Herlick JM, et al. The localization and distribution of corticotropin-releasing hormone in the human placenta and fetal membranes throughout gestation. *J Clin Endocrinol Metab* 1991;72:1001–1007.

114. Shapiro LJ. Steroid sulfatase deficiency and X-linked ichthyosis. In: Scriver CR, Beaudet AL, Sly WS, et al., eds. *The metabolic basis of inherited disease*, vol 2, 6th ed. New York: McGraw-Hill Information Services, 1989:1945–1964.

115. Conte FA, Grumbach MM, Ito Y, et al. A syndrome of female pseudohermaphrodism, hypergonadotrophic hypogonadism, and multicystic ovaries associated with missense mutations in the gene encoding aromatase (P450 arom). *J Clin Endocrinol Metab* 1994;78:1287–1292.

116. Midgley AR, Pierce GB. Immunohistochemical localization of human chorionic gonadotropin. *J Exp Med* 1962;115:289–294.

117. Vaitukaitis JL, Ross GT, Braunstein GD, et al. Gonadotropins and their subunits: basic and clinical studies. *Recent Prog Horm Res* 1976;32:289–331.

118. Jameson JL, Hollenberg AN. Regulation of chorionic gonadotropin gene expression. *Endocr Rev* 1993;14:203–221.

119. Fritz MA, Guo SM. Doubling time of human chorionic gonadotropin (hCG) in early normal pregnancy: relationship of hCG concentration and gestational age. *Fertil Steril* 1987;47:584–589.

120. Tulchinsky D, Hobel CJ. Plasma human chorionic gonadotropin, estrone, estradiol, estriol, progesterone, and 17 alpha-hydroxyprogesterone in human pregnancy. 3. Early normal pregnancy. *Am J Obstet Gynecol* 1973;117:884–893.

121. Josimovich JB, MacLaren JA. Presence in the human placenta and term serum of a highly lactogenic substance immunologically related to pituitary growth hormone. *Endocrinology* 1962;71:209–220.

122. Grumbach MM, Kaplan SL, Sciarra TT, et al. Chorionic growth hormone-prolactin: secretion, disposition, biologic activity in man, and postulated function as the "growth hormone" of the second half of pregnancy. *Ann NY Acad Sci* 1968;148:501–531.

123. Vale W, River C, Vaughan J. The role of inhibin and activin. In: Knobil E, Neill JD, eds. *The physiology of reproduction*. New York: Raven Press, 1994:1861–1878.

124. Nakamura T, Takio K, Eto Y, et al. Activin-binding protein from the rat ovary is follistatin. *Science* 1990;247:836–838.

125. Petraglia F, Florio P, Nappi C, et al. Peptide signaling in human placenta and membranes: autocrine, paracrine and endocrine mechanisms. *Endocr Rev* 1996;17:156–186.

126. Muttukrishna S, Knight PG, Groome NP, et al. Activin A and inhibin A as possible endocrine markers for pre-eclampsia. *Lancet* 1997;349:1285–1288.

127. Petraglia F, Sawchenko PE, Rivier T, et al. Evidence for local stimulation of ACTH secretion by corticotropin-releasing factor in human placenta. *Nature* 1987;328:717–719.

128. Challis JJ, Matthews SG, Van Meir C, et al. The placental corticotropin-releasing hormone-adrenocorticotropin axis. *Placenta* 1995;16:481–502.

129. Sasaki A, Shinkawa O, Margioris AN, et al. Immunoreactive corticotropin-releasing hormone in human plasma during pregnancy, labor and delivery. *J Clin Endocrinol Metab* 1986;64:224–229.

130. Perkins AV, Linton EA, Eben F, et al. Corticotrophin-releasing hormone and corticotrophin-releasing hormone binding protein in normal and pre-eclamptic human pregnancies. *Br J Obstet Gynecol* 1995;102:118–122.

131. Linton EA, Behan DP, Saphier PW, et al. Corticotropin-releasing hormone-binding protein: reduction in adrenocorticotropin-releasing activity of placental but not hypothalamic CRH. *J Clin Endocrinol Metab* 1990;70:1574–1580.

132. Perkins AV, Eben F, Wolfe CD, et al. Plasma measurements of corticotrophin-releasing hormone-binding protein in normal and abnormal human pregnancy. *J Endocrinol* 1993;138:149–157.

133. Berkowitz GS, Lapinski RH, Lockwood CJ, et al. Corticotropin-releasing factor and its binding protein: maternal serum levels in term and pre-term deliveries. *Am J Obstet Gynecol* 1996;174:1477–1483.

134. Hillhouse EW, Grammatopolous D, Milion NGN, et al. The identification of a human myometrial corticotropin-releasing hormone receptor that increases in affinity during pregnancy. *J Clin Endocrinol Metab* 1993;76:736–741.

135. Quartero HW, Noort WA, Fry CH, et al. Role of prostaglandins and leukotrienes in the synergistic effect of oxytocin and corticotropin-releasing hormone (CRH) on the contraction force in human gestational myometrium. *Prostaglandins* 1991;42:137–150.

136. Jones SA, Brooks AN, Challis JR. Steroids modulate corticotropin-releasing hormone production in human fetal membranes and placenta. *J Clin Endocrinol Metab* 1989;68:825–830.

137. McLean M, Bisits A, Davies J, et al. A placental clock controlling the length of human pregnancy. *Nature Med* 1995;1:460–463.

138. Dixon WD, Tribe RM, Palmer AM, et al. Corticotrophin-releasing hormone does not relax isolated human fetoplacental resistance arteries. *J Soc Gynecol Invest* 1996;3:225A.

139. Clifton VL, Read MA, Leitch IM, et al. Corticotropin-releasing hormone-induced vasodilatation in the human fetal-placental circulation. Involvement of the nitric oxide-cyclic guanosine $3',5'$-monophosphate-mediated pathway. *J Clin Endocrinol Metab* 1995;80:2888–2893.

140. Boehm K, Daimon M, Gordeski IG, et al. Expression of insulin-like and platelet-derived growth factor genes in human uterine tissues. *Mol Reprod Dev* 1990;27:93–101.

141. Hill DJ, Clemmons DR, Riley SC, et al. Immunohistochemical localization of insulin-like growth factors (IGFs) and IGF binding proteins -1, -2, -3 in human placenta and fetal membranes. *Placenta* 1993;14:1–12.

142. Caufriez A, Frankenne F, Englert Y, et al. Placental growth hormone as a potential regulator of maternal IGF-I during human pregnancy. *Am J Physiol* 1990;258:E1014–1019.

143. Oxvig C, Haaning J, Wagner JM, et al. Placenta proteins. In: Polin RA, Fox WW, eds. *Fetal and neonatal physiology,* 2nd ed. Philadelphia: WB Saunders, 1998:103–113.

144. Lin TM, Galbert SP, Kiefer D, et al. Characterization of four human pregnancy-associated plasma proteins. *Am J Obstet Gynecol* 1974;118:223–236.

145. Bohn H, Dati F. Placental and pregnancy-related proteins. In: Ritzmann SE, Killingsworth LM, eds. *Proteins in body fluids, amino acids, and tumor markers. Diagnostic and clinical aspects.* New York: Alan R. Liss, 1983:333–374.

146. Bohn H. Biochemistry of placental proteins. In: Bischof P, Klopper A, eds. *Proteins of the placenta.* Basel: Karger, 1985: 1–25.

147. Bohn H, Winckler W, Grundmann U. Immunologically detected placental proteins and their biological functions. *Arch Gynecol Obstet* 1991;249:107–118.

26

TECHNIQUES OF PRENATAL DIAGNOSIS

DAVID S. MCKENNA
JAY W. MOORE

Advances in biochemical, molecular, and genetic diagnostic instruments and techniques have made possible the diagnosis of numerous fetal conditions previously recognized only after delivery. The field of prenatal diagnosis has grown with these technologic advances, and a variety of techniques offer a prenatal diagnosis by earlier gestational ages. Screening tests for common birth defects and testing of at-risk individuals are now considered standard care.

Prenatal testing consists of screening and diagnostic tests, and may be applied to entire populations or limited to individuals at high risk of a congenital abnormality. Screening tests are used to identify those individuals from a large population with an increased risk for a specific disorder, so the at-risk group can be offered a diagnostic test (1). A screening test is usually applied to entire populations, is simple, inexpensive to perform, has a high sensitivity, and tests for a condition with an intervention. Table 26.1 lists representative prenatal screening tests that are commonly performed during pregnancy.

A diagnostic test is performed to confirm the presence or absence of the condition for which a patient is at risk. Diagnostic tests are more specific and expensive than screening tests, and are usually invasive. Diagnostic tests are usually preceded by a screening test that has identified an individual at risk. Genetic amniocentesis for women at risk for aneuploidy is an example of a common obstetrical diagnostic test. Table 26.2 lists indications and the respective screening tests for prenatal diagnostic testing.

Maternal or fetal tissue is utilized for screening and diagnostic testing. Biochemical, cytogenetic, traditional molecular, or molecular cytogenetic tests can be performed on the tissue. Biochemical tests determine the amount or functionality of a gene product, such as the presence or quantity of a specific protein or an enzyme activity. The maternal serum alpha-fetoprotein test (MSAFP) is an example of biochemical screening of maternal tissue, in which a fetal protein is measured in the maternal serum by a protein assay.

Cytogenetic analysis involves chromosome karyotyping to characterize the fetal chromosomal constitution by determining the number and morphology of the chromosomes. Metaphase cells are stained by a number of techniques that yield characteristic patterns. G-banding utilizes a permanent stain that lightly stains euchromatin and darkly stains heterochromatin, and is the standard stain used for numeric and structural analysis. Low-resolution g-banded karyotypes have approximately 400 bands in a haploid karyotype, while an extended high-resolution g-banded karyotype may have as many as 850 bands (2). Karyotyping is commonly performed on amniocytes from a genetic amniocentesis and is able to determine gross chromosomal changes and segmental abnormalities such as deletions involving as little as 5 megabases of DNA.

A number of new molecular genetic tests are available for prenatal diagnosis that can identify mutations as small as single base pair changes. A molecular genetic test is based on the analysis of DNA extracted from maternal or fetal cells, either by Southern blot or the polymerase chain reaction (PCR). The DNA test for cystic fibrosis mutations is an example of a molecular genetics test that will identify up to 90% of mutations within the CFTR locus. There are currently over 5,000 disorders for which specific gene loci have been established and new loci are continuously discovered. The Online Mendelian Inheritance in Man (OMIM) is an excellent resource for identifying whether a specific disorder's genetic locus has been identified and is amenable to prenatal diagnosis (3). Table 26.3 lists a sample of common disorders that may be diagnosed prenatally either by molecular linkage analysis or by direct analysis of DNA sequences. Because of the rapid development of new test procedures, one should refer to OMIM for details about molecular diagnosis of specific disorders.

Molecular cytogenetic tests use DNA probes to identify genes or gene segments isolated by molecular genetic studies at specific loci on the chromosome by hybridizing gene-specific probes to the location on the chromosome, using the procedure of *in situ* hybridization (ISH). Molecular cytogenetic techniques permit identification of the gain, loss, or rearrangement of DNA segments between 10,000 to 100,000 base pairs [10 to 100 kilobases (kb)], intermediate between those identifiable by traditional cytogenetic and molecular genetic techniques.

CLINICAL SCREENING TECHNIQUES

Neonatal Versus Prenatal Screening

Screening for congenital diseases and malformations may be performed antenatally or after delivery. The choice of

TABLE 26.1. COMMON PRENATAL SCREENING TESTS

Test	Timing
Urine culture for asymptomatic bacteruria	First prenatal appointment
Screening for sexually transmitted diseases	First prenatal appointment
Screening for cervical dysplasia/cancer by Papanicolaou smear	First prenatal appointment
Glucola for gestational diabetes	24 to 28 weeks' gestation, earlier if at risk
Maternal serum α-fetoprotein screening for neural tube and abdominal wall defects	15 to 22 weeks' gestation
Maternal serum screening for trisomy 21 and other aneuploidies (maternal age less than 35 years old at delivery)	15 to 22 weeks' gestation

when to perform the screening test depends on several factors such as the prevalence of the disease, the ability to treat antenatally, cost-effectiveness, and the family's desire to know the diagnosis. Table 26.4 lists commonly performed neonatal screens. For example, all newborns in North America and Europe are screened for phenylketonuria (PKU), an autosomal-recessive disorder with an incidence of 1/15,000 births, by blood phenylalanine determination. PKU has no clinical effect prenatally, but if untreated postnatally will lead to devastating clinical manifestations; if promptly treated after birth, affected individuals will show minimal effects. PKU could be diagnosed prenatally by molecular analysis of fetal tissue; however, this is not routinely performed as a screening test due to the significantly greater risks of antenatal screening vs. neonatal screening for PKU. Neonatal screening for PKU, although a rare disorder, is safe and inexpensive, and PKU has an effective treatment. Prenatal screening by amniocentesis for PKU in the general population, assuming a fetal loss rate of 1/300 for the procedure, would result in 50 losses of normal fetuses for each affected fetus identified. For these reasons, prenatal screening for PKU and most other genetic disorders consists of screening for parental carrier status. Prenatal diagnosis for the majority of diagnosable disorders is offered not to the general population, but only to parents with an identified increased risk (previously affected child, or personal or family history).

Major congenital anomalies are present in approximately 3% of liveborn infants (4), about 0.6% are due to chromosomal abnormalities (e.g., trisomy 21), 1% are due to single-gene mutations (e.g., cystic fibrosis), and 1% are due to multifactorial disorders (e.g., spina bifida). In addition, about 35% of first-trimester miscarriages show chromosomal abnormalities (5,6), and 7% to 21% of stillborn fetuses have an obvious major malformation (7). Due to the prevalence of congenital anomalies in the population, some degree of prenatal screening should be performed for all pregnancies.

Family History and Parental Screening

A genetic and ethnic history should be obtained from all pregnant women. A genetic family history and pedigree are usually obtained at the first prenatal or preconceptual visit, or the parents may complete a written questionnaire. A historical screen should encompass three generations and note occurrences of congenital abnormalities, spontaneous and therapeutic abortions, unexplained perinatal deaths, consanguinity, and mental retardation. A diagnostic evaluation is warranted when the initial screen identifies a pregnancy at risk.

Individuals of certain ethnic groups should be tested for heterozygosity for specific autosomal-recessive disorders. There are autosomal-recessive disorders specific to some

TABLE 26.2. INDICATIONS FOR PRENATAL DIAGNOSTIC TESTING

Prenatal Diagnostic Test	Indications	Screening Test
Fetal tissue for karyotype	1. Maternal age >35	1. History
	2. Previous aneuploid pregnancy	2. History
	3. Fetal anomaly on ultrasound	3. Prenatal ultrasound
	4. Abnormal maternal serum screening in women <35 years	4. Triple screen
	5. Parental chromosomal rearrangements	5. Parental karyotypes
Fetal tissue for molecular or biochemical studies	Personal or family history that identifies individual at risk	History and pedigree, and possibly parental biochemical or molecular screening

TABLE 26.3. REPRESENTATIVE DISEASES DIAGNOSABLE BY MOLECULAR TESTS

Sickle cell anemia
Cystic fibrosis
Duchenne's muscular dystrophy
Fragile X syndrome
Huntington's disease
Thalassemias
Tay-sachs disease
Myotonic dystrophy
Marfan syndrome
Osteogenesis imperfecta
Phenylketonuria

ethnic groups. For example, Jewish couples of Ashkenazic or Sephardic descent should be offered parental carrier testing for Tay-Sachs disease, Canavan's disease, Gaucher's disease, and cystic fibrosis, and individuals of East Asian descent are at risk for thalassemias. Other indications for diagnostic testing include having had a previous child with aneuploidy or a genetic abnormality, parental chromosomal rearrangements, and a personal or family history of a mendelian disorder or an inborn error of metabolism. In addition to screening based on history and ethnic background, counseling should be provided about current biochemical screening programs, which consist of maternal serum screening for neural tube defects (NTDs) and abdominal wall defects (AWDs) for women of all ages, and for trisomy 21 and other aneuploidies for women under the age of 35.

Prenatal Biochemical Screening

Maternal Serum Alpha Fetoprotein

Alpha fetoprotein (AFP) is a 69-kd protein, structurally similar to albumin, produced sequentially by the fetal yolk sac, gastrointestinal tract, and liver. AFP may also be produced by certain maternal ovarian or hepatic neoplasms. Fetal serum AFP levels reach a peak concentration at the end of the first trimester and decline thereafter. AFP enters the maternal circulation by transplacental passage (two thirds), and by transamniotic transfer (one third) (8). AFP

is also excreted through the fetal kidney resulting in high amniotic fluid concentrations. Maternal serum AFP concentrations continue to rise through the second trimester, and low and high MSAFP levels may be indicative of abnormal fetal conditions (1). Maternal serum AFP screening will detect 85% of all open NTDs and 90% of cases of anencephaly; in addition, abdominal wall defects (e.g., omphalocele and gastroschisis) result in and can be detected by an elevated MSAFP. Current recommendations are for all pregnant women to be offered MSAFP screening between 15 and 22 weeks' gestation and preferably between 16 and 18 weeks when the test is most accurate (1).

Maternal Serum Screening for Trisomy 21

Maternal age was the original screening test utilized for identifying women at risk of having a fetus with trisomy 21. This is based on the increased risk of aneuploidy with advancing maternal age. The a priori risk for a 35-year-old woman of having a fetus with a trisomy 21 genotype during the second trimester is approximately 1/270, similar to the risk of procedure-associated loss from traditional amniocentesis (9); 35 years was chosen by the American Medical Association (AMA) as the cutoff for "advanced" maternal age. Using the criteria of AMA as a screen for trisomy 21, all women 35 or older are currently offered amniocentesis. However, 80% of trisomy 21 infants are born to women younger than 35 years old and screening by maternal age alone identifies only a minority of trisomy 21 fetuses. Clearly another method was needed to screen for the at-risk pregnancies of women younger than 35.

In 1984, Merkatz et al. (10) reported the association between decreased MSAFP and fetal chromosomal abnormalities. MSAFP is about 20% lower in women with chromosomal abnormalities, permitting identification of 25% to 35% of trisomy 21 pregnancies in women younger than 35 years of age (11). Additional maternal serum markers are altered in pregnancies of trisomy 21 fetuses: human chorionic gonadotropin (hCG) levels are elevated, and levels of unconjugated estriol (uE$_3$) are decreased (12–14). The

TABLE 26.4. NEONATAL SCREENS COMMONLY PERFORMED IN THE UNITED STATES

Condition Screened For	Incidence (Live Births)	No. of States with Routine Screen
Phenylketonuria	1/13,000	50
Hypothyroidism	1/4,000	50
Hemoglobinopathies	1/500	45
Galactosemia	1/100,000	43
Maple syrup urine disease	<1/100,000	Less than half
Homocystinuria	<1/100,000	Less than half
Biotinidase deficiency	1/70,000	Less than half
Congenital adrenal hyperplasia	1/15,000	Less than half
Cystic fibrosis	1/2,500	Less than half

From National screening status report. *Infant Screen* 1994;17(5)120, with permission.

addition of hCG and uE$_3$ to MSAFP to form a triple screen results in detection of 55% to 60% of trisomy 21 fetuses in women younger than 35 (15,16).

Other Serum Markers for Trisomy 21 and Screening for Trisomy 18

Investigators have found maternal serum levels of a number of other placental products to be altered in trisomy 21 pregnancies. Human placental lactogen, progesterone, the free beta subunit of hCG, inhibin-A, and urinary metabolites of hCG have all been proposed as markers (17–19). The continued desire for techniques for the diagnosis of anomalies and aneuploidies in the first trimester, will undoubtedly result in refinement of current markers and the discovery of new ones.

Trisomy 18 may also be detected by multiple marker screening. In contrast to trisomy 21, all three of the triple screen analytes are decreased when the fetal karyotype is trisomy 18. Using the triple screen markers and maternal age, Palomaki et al. (20) have demonstrated that 60% of pregnancies with trisomy 18 would have been identified.

Ultrasonography

Prenatal ultrasound may be used as a screening tool to identify abnormalities in fetal structure and growth, amniotic fluid, and the placenta. Screening ultrasonography is performed in many countries including England, Norway, and Canada, but is not recommended in the United States due to lack of evidence of a favorable cost/benefit ratio for the low-risk fetus. Recently, numerous ultrasound "markers" have been proposed to identify fetuses at risk for aneuploidy.

The utility of ultrasound as a screening technique was evaluated by a large multicenter randomized study, the Routine Antenatal Diagnostic Imaging with Ultrasound (RADIUS) study, which was published in 1993 (21). The results of the RADIUS study received much attention in the scientific and lay press and have substantially influenced practice patterns. The RADIUS study randomized over 15,000 women to either a screening group or a control group. The screening group had two ultrasounds performed, one at 15 to 22 weeks and the second at 31 to 35 weeks. The control group had ultrasound examinations only when medically indicated.

The RADIUS investigators concluded that routine ultrasonographic screening did not improve perinatal outcome compared to the selective use of ultrasound. However, there were several criticisms of the RADIUS study. First, the rate of detection of anomalies was lower than expected: only 34.8% of anomalies were detected in the screening group prior to delivery, compared to detection rates of 60% to 84% in other studies of screening sonography (22–24). Also, the study did not include interventional protocols to

manage the pregnancies identified as abnormal, and the rate of induced abortion in patients with anomalies was 29% in the screening group compared to 50% in the control group. The low detection rate for anomalies and the low rate of therapeutic abortions may have resulted in an increased perinatal mortality rate. The RADIUS study despite its shortcomings is considered by many as the definitive evaluation of ultrasound as a screening tool, and many practitioners and third-party payers have based their methods on the study's conclusion.

Second-Trimester Ultrasound Screening for Aneuploidy

The use of a second-trimester genetic sonogram has been reported by Vintzileos et al. (25) as a further screening tool for trisomy 21. Women identified as being at increased risk for trisomy 21, due to AMA or abnormal maternal serum screening, underwent a genetic sonogram. In addition to standard biometry and anatomy, the following markers for trisomy 21 were evaluated for abnormalities: face, hands, heart, reduced femur and humerus length, pyelectasis, increased nuchal fold thickness, echogenic bowel, choroid plexus cysts, hypoplastic middle phalanx of the fifth digit, wide space between the first and second toes, and two vessel umbilical cord; 93% of cases of trisomy 21 were detected by this method with an amniocentesis rate of less than 20%.

Midtrimester ultrasound as a screen for aneuploidy could be complementary to serum screening and increase the sensitivity of prenatal diagnosis. In the future, the results of a genetic ultrasound may be considered along with serum markers to determine a composite risk for aneuploidy. However, there are several questions regarding the utility of genetic ultrasound, such as, Can all centers expect to obtain sensitivities of over 90% in a timely and cost-effective manner? The sensitivity of the method is operator dependent, and the time and cost of performing a genetic ultrasound is considerable. Vintzeileos et al.'s (25) study was done at a tertiary referral center, and they evaluated patients who were at increased risk of aneuploidy. Can similar results be obtained at other centers evaluating low-risk populations? These issues must first be resolved prior to recommending genetic ultrasonography as a routine procedure.

First Trimester Ultrasound Screening for Aneuploidy

Snijders et al. (26) have proposed the use of nuchal skinfold measurements to provide an age-adjusted risk for aneuploidy in the first trimester. Using the combination of maternal age and nuchal translucency thickness from transabdominal ultrasound performed at 10 to 14 weeks gestational age, over 80% of fetuses with trisomy 21 were identified. The Fetal Medicine Foundation (FMF), a registered charity, was established to avoid criticisms similar to those of the RADIUS study. The low number of anomalies found in the RADIUS study is thought to be due to inadequately trained personnel performing the majority of the ultra-sounds, and this led to the erroneous conclusions that screening ultrasound is not beneficial. The FMF provides free comprehensive training, support, and auditing for the proper implementation of the 10- to 14-week screening ultrasound. Once a center has passed the theoretical and practical examinations, the software for calculation of risks is provided for implementation.

Snijders et al. (26) reported a sensitivity for detection of trisomy 21 of over 80% using an age-adjusted risk cutoff of 1/300 in 42,000 completed singleton pregnancies that were examined by an FMF "certified" 10- to 14-week screening sonogram. Increased nuchal translucency at 10 to 14 weeks has also identified fetuses with trisomy 13, trisomy 18, and monosomy X. The nuchal translucency at 10 to 14 weeks holds promise as a new method of early ultrasound screening for aneuploidy, but is currently not routinely available in the United States. The FMP "certi-fication" process is designed to guarantee the correct application of this new technology; however, it may hamper dis-semination into clinical practice in the United States. Currently, investigators at several centers in the United States are developing their own protocols for first trimester aneuploidy screening, employing a combination of maternal serum markers and the fetal nuchal skinfold (27).

DIAGNOSTIC TECHNIQUES

Techniques in routine use to obtain fetal tissue samples for prenatal diagnosis include traditional amniocentesis, early amniocentesis, chorionic villus sampling (CVS), and fetal blood sampling. A few physicians have experience with other experimental procedures (e.g., fetoscopy, endocervical lavage), and these are performed in a limited number of centers. The trend has been to develop techniques that safely provide a diagnosis at the earliest gestational age. Different procedures are compared in terms of their accuracy and risk of pregnancy loss. Technical differences in the preparation of specimens and the fetal loss rate are gestational age dependent.

When comparing prenatal diagnostic procedures, the gestational and maternal age loss rates must be considered, and spontaneous losses, termination of abnormal pregnancies, stillbirths, and neonatal deaths should be addressed. After 8 weeks the loss rate for an ultrasonically confirmed normal pregnancy is approximately 3%, with most of these occurring in the next 2 months (28). The risk of spontaneous miscarriage in ultrasonographically normal pregnancies is also significantly increased with advancing maternal age (29). Investigators have developed several measures of safety for prenatal procedures:

1. Postprocedure fetal loss rate: the total number of pregnancy losses occurring after the procedure until full term, including spontaneous losses, procedure-associated losses, and losses and stillbirths due to other causes.
2. Procedure-associated loss rate: usually defined as losses occurring within the first 4 weeks postprocedure, and may include both procedure-related losses and spontaneous losses, as the cause of a pregnancy loss is not always clear.
3. Preprocedure loss rate: important when comparing procedures performed at different gestational ages, as it takes into account spontaneous losses that occur after the earlier procedure but prior to the later procedure.
4. Number of abnormal pregnancies terminated: may be included in the postprocedure loss data for early procedures in order to compare loss rates with later procedures. Women having an earlier procedure may electively abort an abnormal pregnancy that is destined to spontaneously abort. If the number of abnormal pregnancies terminated is not included in an earlier procedure's loss data, then the loss rate will appear to be artificially lower. However, these are not procedure-associated losses and should be listed separately.

Amniocentesis

Amniocentesis was first described by Liley (30) in 1963 for evaluation of fetuses with Rh isoimmunization. Ultrasound examination is usually performed first, noting the position of the fetus and the placenta. Next, a hollow spinal needle is inserted into the amniotic cavity under ultrasound guidance. Fluid is then withdrawn for testing. It is possible to perform biochemical assays on the amniotic fluid for diagnosis of a known disorder where the effect on the fetus results in the excretion of a biochemical marker into the amniotic fluid; however, few applications exist for biochemical testing of amniotic fluid for prenatal diagnosis. One example is the diagnosis of fetal congenital adrenal hyperplasia, which is characterized by an elevated level of amniotic fluid 17α-hydroxyprogesterone.

The greatest yield from amniocentesis is from the cellular material in the fluid, which contains fetal DNA. Amniotic fluid cells consist of fetal cells collectively called "amnio-cytes," originating from the fetal skin, respiratory, gastrointestinal, and urinary tracts, along with amnion cells from the amniotic membrane. The cells are centrifuged, washed, and resuspended in medium and cultured. The cultured cells can then be used for biochemical studies for enzymatic defects, molecular studies, and cytogenetics.

Midtrimester genetic amniocentesis (MA) became routinely available in the 1970s, and is considered the gold standard to which other prenatal diagnostic procedures are compared. Most of the data that established MA as efficacious and safe were from studies that used 16 weeks as the earliest gestational age when the procedures were done, and were performed without the aide of real-time ultrasound guidance (31). With the advent of higher quality ultrasound, MA is now routinely performed as early as 14 weeks. Early amniocentesis (EA) evolved in the 1980s as an alternative to CVS. An amniocentesis is usually considered "early" when performed between 12 and 13 completed weeks of gestation, while a few operators are performing "very early amniocentesis" at less than 12 weeks (31). The technique of EA is essentially the same as MA, which is an advantage over other sampling techniques such as CVS that require a learning curve.

When compared to MA, the proposed disadvantages of EA are an increased rate of procedure-associated pregnancy loss, increased rates of fetal deformations, failed sampling, and ambiguous results. Several large multicenter trials have been conducted to establish the safety of MA. Collectively, a 0.5% procedure-related loss rate was demonstrated. The risk of loss was found to be increased when larger gauge needles were used and when there were more than two needle insertions (32). EA has not been as extensively studied as MA. Wilson (33) reviewed 41 nonrandomized reports of experience with EA published between 1987 and 1994 and found postprocedure loss rates ranging from 0.2% to 6.5%. Sundberg et al. (34) reviewed 12 large (>100 patients) reports on experience with EA and found a postprocedure loss rate of less than 4% in almost 5,000 cases. This compares to the 3% to 5% loss rate reported in the initial MA studies (32). The retrospective studies evaluating the safety of EA and MA have not demonstrated an increase in structural defects or incidence of small-for-gestational-age infants (32).

One randomized clinical trial has compared EA to MA. The Canadian Early and Mid-Trimester Amniocentesis Trial (CEMAT) randomized 4,374 women to EA between 11 and 12 and 6/7 gestational weeks, and to MA between 15 and 16 and 6/7 weeks (35). Total pregnancy loss rates were determined by including preprocedure, postprocedure (spontaneous and therapeutic), intrauterine, and neonatal deaths. EA had a total pregnancy loss of 7.6% compared to 5.9% for MA. This difference was statistically significant. In addition, a statistically higher rate of talipes equinovarus was found in the EA group. The calculated postprocedural spontaneous loss rate, excluding intrauterine (>20 weeks) and neonatal death, was 0.8% for MA, comparable to previous series, while the postprocedural loss rate was 2.6% for EA (32). The authors were clear to point out that loss rates of the two procedures are not comparable because of differences in procedural timing (35). The CEMAT investigators are correct in not attempting to compare the procedural loss rates between MA and EA. The background loss rate (spontaneous losses after the procedure) will be higher in the group of women who had EA, simply due to there being a greater amount of time for them to have a spontaneous loss after their procedure, compared to women in the MA group. Despite the CEMAT investigators' caution regarding

comparing the two procedures' loss rates, their results have cast doubt on the future utility of early amniocentesis (36).

Potential technical difficulties in culturing of the amniocytes obtained from early amniocentesis include culture failure and maternal cell contamination. Cells obtained prior to 14 completed weeks gestation are generally of poorer quality and require longer culturing time (8 to 12 days) compared to cells obtained after 15 weeks (5 to 8 days in culture). The cell culture failure rate is dependent on the cell concentration and the proportion of viable cells. Amniotic fluid cell concentrations increase from 9 to 14 weeks, with the most rapid increase occurring after week 12 (37). Sundberg et al. (34) reported a 0.3% rate of EA culture failure compared to 0.2% for MA in their lab, and reviewed 14 cytogenetic studies of cultivation results from EA, and generally found a culture failure rate of 0% to 1.9%, pseudomosaicism in 0% to 1.9%, and mean culture days of 10 to 17 days. In the CEMAT study a chromosomal diagnosis was not made in 1.7% of EA specimens compared to only 0.2% of MA specimens (35). A technique of recirculation and filtration of amniotic fluid obtained by EA has been described (38,39). With the filter technique the authors found a significantly increased number of colonies in the amniotic fluid cultures, and in more than 400 EAs obtained at a mean gestational age of 12 weeks, there was no suggestion of increased risk of abortion compared to other published studies on EA (34). Sundberg et al. (40), in a randomized trial comparing EA with the filter technique to CVS, had only one culture failure in 548 EA procedures (0.18%), and required a mean culturing time of 9.5 days. The CEMAT study's findings of decreased efficacy and safety of EA will possibly result in many centers reconsidering their use of EA. Patients who are considering EA should be counseled on the possibility of increased risk of fetal loss, talipes, and culture failure compared to MA.

Chorionic Villus Sampling

Chorionic villus sampling (CVS) involves ultrasound-guided transcervical or transabdominal biopsy of the chorion frondosum. In most cases cytotrophoblasts contain a chromosomal complement identical to the developing fetus, and can be used as a source of tissue for prenatal diagnosis at the biochemical, molecular, and cytogenetic levels. CVS has been used for first trimester prenatal diagnosis for the past 12 years, and is most commonly performed between 10 and 13 weeks of gestational age. The safety and accuracy of CVS has been compared to both EA and MA.

Questions concerning the safety of CVS center around the fetal loss rate and fetal structural defects. The postprocedure loss rate of CVS was first compared in a randomized prospective manner to MA in the Canadian Collaborative-Amniocentesis Clinical Trial, which found no statistical difference in the loss rates between the two groups (41). Subsequent comparisons have yielded similar results (42–

44), except for the European Medical Research Council (MRC) Working Party on the Evaluation of CVS, which found a 4.6% greater loss rate for CVS compared to amniocentesis (45). It is not certain why the European study found a higher loss rate; however, operator experience may have been a contributing factor. Williams et al. (46) demonstrated the number of catheter or needle insertions was significantly higher during the first 100 procedures performed by a single operator, and the risk of fetal loss significantly increased with three or more insertions. The average number of procedures performed per site in the European trial was 52, which was significantly less than in the U.S. studies, which was 325, and the Canadian study, which was 106 (41–43,45). The American College of Obstetrics and Gynecology (ACOG) Committee on Genetics has concluded that transcervical and transabdominal CVS performed at 10 to 12 weeks' gestation are safe and acceptable alternatives to MA when performed by an experienced operator (47). CVS compared to EA at similar gestational ages has been demonstrated to have equal or lower fetal loss rates. Nicolaides et al. (48) prospectively studied 1,492 women (37% were randomized) who had either transabdominal CVS or EA at 10 to 13 weeks' gestation, and found the rate of fetal loss was significantly higher in the EA group (4.9%) compared to the CVS group (2.1%). Sundberg et al. (40) randomized 1,160 women to EA at 11 to 13 weeks' gestational age or to CVS at 10 to 12 weeks (40). There was not a statistically significant difference in total fetal loss for EA (5.4%) vs. CVS (4.8%). However, the trial was discontinued due to the increased rate of talipes equinovarus (1.7%) in the EA group.

In 1991, Firth et al. (49) reported an increased incidence of limb reduction defects (LRDs) in infants whose mothers underwent CVS. These claims were substantiated by subsequent reports (50,51). The increase in these rare fetal anomalies was primarily seen when CVS procedures were performed at less than 10 weeks' gestational age. In a case-control study conducted by the Centers for Disease Control and Prevention, there was a sixfold increased risk for transverse digital deficiency (1 per 3,000 births) (52). This is in contrast to a review that evaluated risks of CVS, and found the majority of studies have not reported an association between CVS and LRDs (53). CVS probably does carry a slightly increased risk of LRDs. The increase is most pronounced when procedures are performed prior to 10 weeks' gestation, and these should be routinely avoided. Further studies are required to establish the actual risk of LRDs after 10 weeks. Patients should be counseled that there may be an increased risk of LRDs on the order of 1/3,000 births for procedures performed after 10 weeks' gestation (47).

The inability to diagnose NTDs and AWDs by analysis of amniotic fluid alpha fetoprotein (AFAFP), and acetylcholinesterase (AChE) is a disadvantage of CVS compared to amniocentesis. Fluid obtained by MA can be sent for analysis of AFAFP and AChE, and gestational-age–specific tables exist for interpretation between 14 and 22 weeks with a sensitivity of >98%. The sensitivity of AFAFP and AChE prior to 14 weeks has not been established; however, median values of AFAFP increase to a maximum around week 13 and decrease after. Sundberg et al. (34) have suggested the use of the cutoff limit from week 14 for AFAFP and AChE for screening for NTDs and AWDs by EA.

Fetal Blood Sampling

First reported by Wladimiroff and Jahoda (54) in 1977, ultrasound-directed percutaneous umbilical vein sampling (PUBS) is an alternative to amniocentesis and CVS for obtaining fetal blood for prenatal diagnosis after 16 weeks' gestation. Typical indications for PUBS include resolution of discrepancies (e.g., mosaicism) found at the time of amniocentesis or CVS; rapid fetal biochemical, molecular, or cytogenetic testing, particularly in the third trimester; culture, immunologic, or molecular studies for infectious agents; and evaluation of isoimmunization or fetal coagulation disorders. PUBS carries a procedure-associated fetal loss rate that in experienced hands has been reported to be 0.8% to 3%, which is slightly higher than CVS or amniocentesis (55–58).

Other Procedures

Other techniques that have been used to obtain fetal tissue for prenatal diagnosis include fetal skin sampling (59), fetal muscle biopsy (60), embryoscopy by either a transcervical or transabdominal rigid endoscope (61,62), and endocervical irrigation (63). Experience with these procedures is limited, and published series have contained only small numbers of patients.

Fetal skin sampling is required for the prenatal diagnosis of a group of serious autosomal-recessive skin diseases known as genodermatoses. Skin sampling was originally performed under direct visualization using a fetoscope, with a 4% to 7% procedure loss rate (64,65). Elias et al. (59) described a technique of ultrasound-directed skin sampling with a biopsy forceps through a 14-gauge Angiocath (Deseret Medical, Sandy, UT). The biopsy forceps appears to be a safe alternative to fetoscopic biopsy with a lower fetal loss rate; however, the numbers were too small in Elias's series to ascertain the actual rate. Fetal muscle biopsy has been performed using a coring biopsy gun, usually used for kidney biopsies, under ultrasound or endoscopic guidance (60). Muscle biopsies have primarily been performed for clarification of ambiguous molecular results from CVS or amniocentesis done for diagnosis of a myopathy such as Duchenne or Becker muscular dystrophies in a family with an affected individual. Embryoscopy has been used for verification of anomalies diagnosed by other methods, and may potentially be used for fetal blood sampling and therapy (62). Endocervical irrigation is a potentially minimally invasive method to obtain first-trimester trophoblasts for prenatal diagnosis, but is still experimental at this point (63).

Prenatal Diagnosis Using Fetal Cells From Maternal Blood

The presence of fetal cells in maternal blood was first suggested in 1969 by Walknowska et al. (66), who detected male fetal XY metaphases in leukocyte cultures obtained from centrifugation of maternal blood. The hypothesis that fetal cells exist in maternal blood could not be confirmed when it was found that not all individuals carrying male fetuses showed XY metaphases, and XY metaphases were present in some women carrying female fetuses (67). Next, Herzenberg et al. (68) in 1979 identified fetal human leukocyte antigen (HLA)-A2–positive cells in maternal serum by fluorescence-activated cell sorting of maternal peripheral blood lymphocytes from HLA-A2–negative women stained for HLA-A2 antigen (68). However, when cells were flow sorted and subjected to karyotyping, fetal karyotypes could not always be detected. Unfortunately, these two techniques were not specific, and the presence of fetal cells in maternal blood could not be confirmed. By the mid-1980s few groups were actively pursuing new techniques to identify cells of fetal origin in maternal serum (69).

Interest in identifying fetal cells in maternal serum was rekindled with the development of new molecular techniques, in particular PCR, an enzyme-catalyzed biochemical reaction in which small amounts of specific DNA segments are amplified into large amounts of linear double-stranded DNA (70,71). Lo et al. (72,73) unequivocally demonstrated the presence of fetal cells in maternal blood by using PCR to amplify Y sequences. This technique was further refined by Bianchi et al. (74), who first flow-sorted cells based on the transferrin receptor (CD71) and then identified Y sequences in the sorted cells by PCR. Flow sorting has permitted the separation of an extremely small number of fetal cells ($1:10^6$ maternal cells) from maternal serum (75). The addition of PCR and fluorescent *in situ* hybridization (FISH) has allowed identification of specific DNA sequences and aneuploidies from fetal cells flow sorted from maternal serum. Specific fetal gene sequences identified in maternal blood include hemoglobin Lepore-Boston, rhesus D, and HLA-DQ alpha, and aneuploidies diagnosed by FISH include trisomy 21, trisomy 18, 47,XXY (Klinefelter syndrome), and 47,XYY (76).

The application of using fetal cells isolated from maternal blood for noninvasive prenatal diagnosis is considered experimental at this time. Currently, a multicenter (National Institute of Child Health and Human Development) clinical evaluation of this technique is being funded (77). The study's goal is to enroll 3,000 women undergoing amniocentesis or CVS for genetic indications. The enrolled women will have a sample of maternal serum obtained prior to the procedure. Fetal cells will be isolated from the maternal blood and ana-

lyzed. The results will be compared to the amniocentesis or CVS results for accuracy. It is not appropriate to offer the use of fetal cells isolated from maternal serum for prenatal diagnosis until the evaluation of this technology is complete. It is unlikely that fetal cells obtained from maternal serum will supplant amniocentesis and CVS as a diagnostic test. The most likely application will be as a screening tool, applied in a similar manner as the triple screen.

MOLECULAR CYTOGENETIC TECHNIQUES

Molecular cytogenetic testing permits identification of specific gene loci at the specific physical location upon a chromosome. *In situ* hybridization (ISH) is based on the quality of double-stranded DNA to separate into single strands when heated, or denatured, and then to recombine specifically with the complementary sequence, or hybridize, upon cooling (78). DNA from a single gene may be isolated and combined with a detection molecule, either a fluorochrome dye that can be incorporated into the gene segment, or an intermediate molecule that can combine with a visible marker; the labeled DNA segment is the gene probe. The chromosome and probe DNA are denatured and combined on the slide, incubated for 2 to 17 hours to permit sorting of complementary DNA sequences, and then cooled to permit annealing of the chromosome DNA and the probe. FISH utilizes a fluorescent dye marker to detect the probe. With FISH studies the chromosomes may be examined immediately by fluorescence microscopy, and the results are rapidly available. Detection of a probe location may also be by radioactive label autoradiography, which takes days to develop and is less specific than the fluorescent dyes, or enzyme markers that produce a permanent though diffuse signal. A variety of probes are available, each with an application that will complement cytogenetic analyses.

Types of Molecular Probes

Centromere Specific Probes

The DNA at the centromere of each chromosome contains unique arrangements of repetitive base sequences 171 bases in length, the alpha-satellite DNA. Two pairs of chromosomes are exceptions to this unique feature of centromeric DNA. Chromosomes 13/21 and 14/22, have arrangements of the alpha-satellite DNA that are so similar they cannot be distinguished. The alpha-satellite DNA centromere probes can be used for chromosome identification in metaphase cells and chromosome enumeration in metaphase cells and interphase nuclei (79).

Locus-Specific Probes

DNA segments from specific genes are inserted into cosmid BAC or YAC to provide an adequate signal for locus identification. These probes usually contain 20,000 to 80,000 base pairs (20 to 80 kb), although probes as small as 800 to 1,000 bases in length may contain sufficient label to be detected. Multicolor FISH uses combinations of probes with different fluorescent dyes for detection and will permit chromosome enumeration in interphase nuclei. Multiple probes labeled with different fluorochromes may be used, so two or three chromosomes may be detected in a single hybridization (80,81). Probes for specific loci can also be used for microdeletion identification, such as the microdeletion for Prader-Willi syndrome, or the submicroscopic deletions for DiGeorge syndrome or Williams syndrome (82–87).

Prenatal Interphase FISH Screen

Multicolor FISH using combinations of probes for chromosomes most frequently present in viable aneuploid fetuses may be used for rapid detection of aneuploidy in uncultured amniotic fluid cells (88,89). The probe mixtures include centromere probes for the X and Y chromosomes, centromere or locus-specific probes for chromosome 18, and locus-specific probes for chromosomes 21 and 13. Uncultured amniocytes from 2 to 5 mL of amniotic fluid are treated to remove most cytoplasm; the fluid is fixed and slides are prepared. FISH is performed with mixtures of two or three probes labeled with different fluorochromes using a 2- to 4-hour hybridization, and fluorescent analysis for multicolor signals are scored for 50 to 100 interphase nuclei for each probe. Over 85% of the cells should have the modal number of signals for each probe; trisomy is present when three signals are found for one probe, monosomy is present when a single signal is found, and triploidy is found when three signals are present for each probe. The advantage of this technique is that results are available in 24 to 48 hours, and normal results will provide comfort to the patient. Abnormal results must be confirmed by cytogenetic studies before any irreversible actions are taken (90). The prenatal FISH screen is limited by the specificity of the probes used for interphase studies. For example, structural abnormalities are present in nearly 50% of patients with a clinical phenotype consistent with Turner syndrome, but would not be detected by the prenatal FISH screen. Deleted chromosomes, isochromosomes, and ring and small marker chromosomes may give false-negative results, and low levels of mosaicism cannot be identified (91).

Telomere-Specific Probes

The ends of chromosomes, the telomeres, are important sites for DNA replication. The telomeres are 10 to 20 kb in length, composed of multiple copies of tandemly repeated copies of the sequence, 5′-TTAGGG-3′; the number of repeats is reduced with each DNA replication cycle. Although all chromosomes have the same telomeric sequences, the subtelomeric sequences are unique for each arm of each chromosome. Subtelomeric probes have been isolated for each chromosome (92–94). These probes are especially useful for identifying small rearrangements, called cryptic translocations, which involve chromosome segments that cannot be identified with certainty by G-banding. Cryptic translocations are one possible cause of multiple spontaneous abortions for couples with apparently normal karyotypes (95,96).

Chromosome-Specific Painting Probes

Probe combinations composed of numerous unique DNA sequences specific to a single chromosome can be used to paint chromosomes with signal along the entire length of the chromosome, although the repetitive sequences of the centromere and telomere regions are not represented (78). The whole chromosome paint (WCP) probes are especially useful for confirmation of balanced or unbalanced rearrangements including translocations, duplications, and insertions. If additional chromosome material is found in a chromosome, the paint probe will identify it as either material duplicated within the chromosome, or translocated from another chromosome. If a parent of a fetus is a known translocation carrier, the amniotic fluid cells can be studied by FISH to determine whether the fetus has a normal, balanced, or unbalanced karyotype and do not require high-resolution analysis for confirmation (97,98).

Multiple Color Karyotyping

Chromosome karyotyping can be performed rapidly and automated by using a combination of whole chromosome paint probes for each of the 24 different chromosomes. Each chromosome is identified with a different fluorescent dye, or combination of fluorochromes, and digital imaging is used to analyze the chromosomes for each specific fluorochrome. Computer imaging is used to superimpose the multiple images, with each chromosome combination being given a distinct chromosome-specific pseudocolor. Speicher and Ward (99) labeled each of the 24 chromosomes and each arm of chromosomes 3, 5, and 11, using 27 fluorochrome combinations of seven specific dyes to identify each chromosome with a detectable color, a method called multiplex FISH (M-FISH). The fluorochromes are individually analyzed using narrow band filters for each color, and the digital image is interpreted by an image analysis system. Other workers have analyzed chromosomes using a computer-driven refractometer to isolate specific colors, a technique referred to as spectral karyotyping (SKY) (100). Color karyotyping is especially useful for study of acquired rearrangements and aneuploidy in neoplastic tissues for which few metaphase preparations are available. For constitutional abnormalities, M-FISH would identify aneuploidy; balanced, unbalanced, and complex rearrangements; insertions; and marker chromosomes of unknown origin. This method may be useful in identifying cryptic translocations for couples with multiple spontaneous abortions, but the resolution of the procedure and the analysis systems need to be determined. Of all the new FISH procedures available, this method has the greatest potential for significant new applications, including automation of the karyotyping process (99).

Comparative Genomic Hybridization (CGH)

Comparative genomic hybridization is useful to identify deletions of 10 to 20 megabases and duplications of 5 to 10 megabases of chromosome material, and is especially useful for the analysis of solid tumors in which few metaphase cells are available. The procedure can also be applied to identification of marker chromosomes and unbalanced de novo translocations/insertions. DNA is isolated from the test specimen and labeled with fluorescein (green); DNA from a normal reference individual is isolated and labeled with Texas Red (red) (101). Labeled DNA from both sources are mixed and hybridized *in situ* to normal metaphases. If a chromosome region is duplicated, the metaphase cells will have an increased green/red ratio in the duplicated region; conversely, a deletion in the test specimen DNA will result in a decreased green/red ratio as determined by an image analysis system. The role of CGH to identify constitutional aneuploidy is limited by the relatively low resolution at this time, and is primarily used for tumor studies (102,103).

DIAGNOSTIC PITFALLS

Cells obtained from amniocentesis or CVS may not be entirely fetal in origin. Amniotic fluid contains cells primarily of fetal origin, but may also contain a small number of maternal blood and epidermal cells, as well as cells from the placenta and extraembryonic membranes. Trophoblast specimens from CVS are of placental origin, which may not represent the fetal genome, and from which the maternal cells must be carefully dissected. The use of tissue from extraembryonic membranes, and not directly obtained from the fetus, can result in an inaccurate or equivocal diagnosis. When an abnormal result is obtained in a portion of a sample, it is imperative that the results represent the fetus, and not the placenta, the mother, or a culture artifact.

Mosaicism in Amniotic Fluid Samples

Mosaicism occurs when cells with two or more different karyotypes are found in a cytogenetic specimen, with one karyotype aneuploid, most often trisomy. In amniotic fluid cultures, 2% to 4% of the samples studied may have at least one cell with an abnormal karyotype. Constitutional

mosaicism is confirmed in 0.3% of the cases, with significant risk of clinical abnormality, although predicting the clinical outcome is very difficult due to the great variability in mosaicism in different tissues. Pseudomosaicism is found in the remaining 2% to 3%, and is an artifact of cell culture with no clinical effect (104,105).

Cytogenetic analysis of mosaicism in amniotic fluid cultures is a significant problem. When amniotic fluid cultures are established, amniotic fluid cells are centrifuged from the fluid, and resuspended in culture medium. The cultures are established on coverslips in 35-mm Petri dishes by placing a bubble of the cell suspension on the coverslip, and incubating for 2 to 3 days until cells attach. The dishes are then flooded with complete medium, and incubated for 4 to 8 days with replenishment of the medium at 2-day intervals. During culture, colonies will form on the coverslip, with each colony formed as a clone of cells from an original amniocyte; it is estimated that three colonies will form for each milliliter of the initial amniotic fluid sample. The cultures are harvested with the colonies in place (*in situ* harvest), so multiple metaphase cells may be found in each colony. If a single cell is found in a colony with a structural or numerical abnormality, and the remaining cells are normal, the abnormality is interpreted as a culture artifact. Similarly, if cells in one colony are abnormal, but no other colonies are found with the same abnormality, the single colony is interpreted as a pseudomosaic colony. However, if colonies on two different cultures have the same abnormality, true constitutional mosaicism is confirmed.

Statistical tests to distinguish between constitutional mosaicism and pseudomosaicism involving different chromosomes have been described by Hsu et al. (106). For standard cytogenetic analyses, 20 single cells or 15 colonies are analyzed to rule out mosaicism greater than 10% (95% confidence level). Single cell mosaicism with one aneuploid cell in one colony (1/15 colonies analyzed) requires no further analysis, nor does a single colony with a balanced rearrangement or chromosome break. A moderate workup, in which 12 colonies are analyzed from other cultures, will rule out mosaicism greater than 23% (95% confidence level). A moderate workup is recommended when a single colony or multiple colonies from the same culture have the following: sex chromosome trisomy or monosomy, autosomal monosomy, a marker chromosome, balanced (multiple colonies) or unbalanced (single colony) rearrangement, or autosomal trisomy for chromosomes 2, 3, 4, 5, 6, 7, 10, 11, 16, 17, or 19. An extensive workup involves the study of 24 colonies from other cultures to rule out mosaicism greater than 12% (95% confidence level). The extensive study is recommended when a single colony or multiple colonies are found on the same culture with autosomal trisomy involving the viable trisomies for chromosomes 21, 18, 13, 8, and 9, as well as the mosaic trisomies for chromosomes 12, 14, 15, 20, and 22; multiple colonies with unbalanced rearrangements; and multiple colonies with an unidentified marker chromosome. These statistical tables have been extended by Sikkema-Raddatz et al. (107) for those situations in which too few colonies are available for analysis. If two or more colonies on two or more cultures are found with the same additional chromosome, or three colonies missing the same chromosome, true constitutional mosaicism is diagnosed. The clinical effect of each mosaic condition must be identified for the specific chromosome involved; summaries of clinical features for the rare mosaic autosomal trisomies were described by Hsu et al. (108).

Mosaicism in Chorionic Villus Sampling, and Confined Placental Mosaicism

Mosaicism is found in 6% to 8% of the chorionic villus samples studied, with 0.1% to 0.3% representing constitutional mosaicism in the fetus, 2% to 3% being mosaicism in the chorion only but not in the fetus, and 3% to 4% being pseudomosaicism (109,110). Generalized, or constitutional, mosaicism is found in the chorionic villus cells and the embryo, and is confirmed by analysis of amniotic fluid, fetal blood, or fetal tissue. In contrast, mosaicism may also be found in cells derived from the chorion but not in the embryo (a false-positive result), referred to as confined placental mosaicism (CPM) (111,112). Constitutional mosaicism may also be present in the embryo with no mosaicism detected in the villi (false-negative result).

The occurrence of mosaic aneuploidy in either the placenta or embryo is determined by (a) the mechanism of trisomy formation, (b) the time, and (c) the location at which the aneuploidy occurs. Mosaicism that is due to

failure of chromosomes to be distributed properly during mitosis in the early cleavage to morula stages of embryonic development is postzygotic mitotic nondisjunction.

The mechanism of formation of mosaicism is significant. A trisomy zygote could lose one chromosome of the trisomy chromosomes and result in mosaicism for trisomy and disomy for that chromosome. The result of this type of nondisjunction event results in "trisomic zygote rescue," permitting an otherwise lethal condition in the embryo to result in a normal disomic embryo (Fig. 26.1) (110). A second mechanism occurs when a normal disomic embryo develops an abnormal trisomic cell line by mitotic nondisjunction; nondisjunction during cleavage would result in the normal disomic cells, plus the products of nondisjunction, which would be trisomy and monosomy, with the monosomic cell line not surviving (110). Both mechanisms have been documented, with the former usually having a high ratio of trisomy to disomy, while the latter has a low incidence of trisomy to disomy. Intermediate frequencies must be investigated using chromosome-specific DNA polymorphisms to determine the mechanism involved (113).

The timing of the nondisjunction event during cleavage and morula formation is critical. If nondisjunction occurs before the third mitotic cleavage division, it is likely that generalized constitutional mosaicism will develop, with trisomic cells in both the CVS and amniotic fluid/embryonic specimens. In contrast, if nondisjunction occurs later in development when only a small number of the trophoblast cells from the inner cell mass will form the embryoblasts, it is possible that the embryo will be disomic and the chorion will be mosaic for disomy/trisomy, or the embryo will

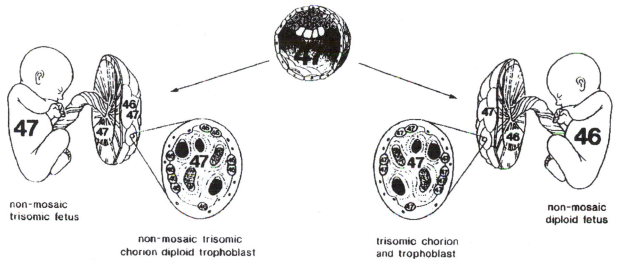

non-mosaic
trisomic fetus

non-mosaic trisomic
chorion diploid trophoblast

trisomic chorion
and trophoblast

non-mosaic
diploid fetus

FIGURE 26.1. Trisomic zygote rescue. Two variations may occur. The first is a nonmosaic diploid fetus with a trisomic chorion and trophoblast (fetus on the *right*). The second variation is a nonmosaic trisomic fetus with a trisomic chorion and diploid trophoblast (fetus on the *left*). The survival of the embryo is greatest when the chorion is diploid. (From Kalousek DK. Current topic: confined placental mosaicism and intrauterine fetal development. *Placenta* 1994;15:219–230, with permission.)

be trisomic with mosaicism in the chorion. The survival of the embryo is greatest if the embryo is disomic and the chorion mosaic, although clinically significant abnormalities are possible. CPM is reported to result in severe intrauterine growth restriction (IUGR), intrauterine fetal demise, or developmental abnormalities in 15% to 20% of cases reported, which may be related to placental insufficiency in the trisomic cells, the specific chromosome involved, or possible chromosome imprinting (114).

Confined Placental Mosaicism and Uniparental Disomy

Confined placental mosaicism has been found in 1% to 2% of CVS, in which the fetus has a normal karyotype and mosaicism is found in the placental cells. The clinical significance of CPM is the increased risk of IUGR and spontaneous abortion (110,113). In addition, the finding of mosaicism in the placenta but not in the fetus identifies one mechanism for uniparental disomy (UPD). If trisomic zygote rescue results in an embryo that has lost one copy of the extra chromosome, there is a 1:3 probability that both remaining chromosomes are from one parent (Fig. 26.2) (113). For example, since most nondisjunction events resulting in a trisomic zygote occur during maternal meiosis, if one of the trisomic chromosomes is lost, the probability is 1 in 3 that both of the remaining chromosomes are from the mother, resulting in maternal uniparental disomy (maternal UPD). If the nondisjunction event occurred at the first division of meiosis, two different maternal chromosomes would be present, resulting in maternal heterodisomy; if nondisjunction was at meiosis II, two copies from the same chromosome would be present, resulting in maternal isodisomy. If nondisjunction during mitosis resulted in a trisomic embryo from a disomic zygote, isodisomy may be maternal or paternal, as determined by the equal proba-

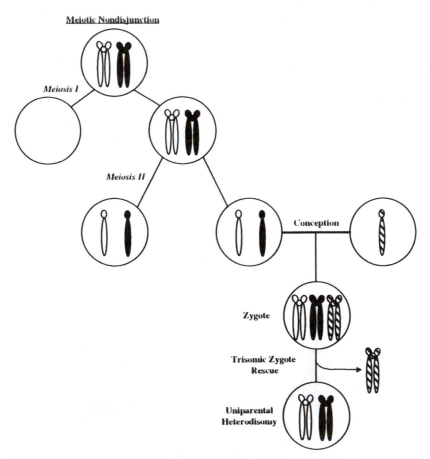

FIGURE 26.2. Uniparental disomy. Three variations may occur. The first, which is illustrated, is when nondisjunction occurs in maternal meiosis I, and results in maternal heterodisomy (two different maternal chromosomes). If the defect occurs during maternal meiosis II, then maternal isodisomy (two copies of the same maternal chromosome) would be the result. Finally, if nondisjunction during mitosis resulted in a triploid embryo from a disomic zygote, then isodisomy of either maternal or paternal origin will occur. (From Gardner RM, Sutherland GR, Bobrow M, et al. *Chromosome abnormalities and genetic counseling.* New York: Oxford University Press, 1996.)

bility of the doubling of either chromosome. A study of CPM by Robinson et al. (115) examined over 100 cases of CPM and found both trisomy resulting from mitotic nondisjunction and meiotic errors, the latter being associated with clinical abnormality, usually IUGR 110).

The phenotypic expression of the genetic conditions of Prader-Willi syndrome and Angelman syndrome are both affected by the parent of origin, and are examples of parental imprinting. Both syndromes may be caused by deletion of band 15q12; Prader-Willi syndrome involves deletion of the chromosome 15 from the father, and Angelman syndrome results from deletion of the same band on the chromosome 15 inherited from the mother. Thirty percent of the Prader-Willi syndrome patients do not have a visible deletion, but rather will inherit both chromosome 15s from the mother (maternal uniparental disomy), with no paternal chromosome 15 present (113,116,117). A significant number of these patients have maternal heterodisomy, with both chromosome 15's inherited from the mother, with the probability that the original embryo was trisomy 15; loss of one additional chromosome 15 by mitotic nondisjunction would result in a viable disomic embryo, trisomic embryo rescue, which would have no paternal chromosome 15 present and would have the Prader-Willi syndrome (118,119). In contrast, only 5% of patients with Angelman syndrome have paternal UPD, probably affected by the low frequency of nondisjunction involving the paternal gametes.

The advent of the maternal triple screen has alleviated the need for amniocentesis in many instances, and the future holds promise for additional noninvasive screening methodologies such as first-trimester ultrasound, and fetal cells obtained from maternal serum. Midtrimester amniocentesis and CVS are reasonable methods for obtaining fetal tissue for prenatal analysis, but the safety and accuracy of EA appears to be less than that of the other two. Technically, there are not considerable differences in the accuracy of MA and CVS, and the largest difference is the timing in gestation. It is important for clinicians to be trained and competent in performing diagnostic procedures, as the rate of procedure-associated fetal loss is directly related to the operator's experience.

Counseling families regarding prenatal diagnosis options is paramount to preventing misunderstanding and obtaining informed consent. A clear understanding of the limitations of screening tests and some discussion of diagnostic testing should be established when initial screens are offered. When an abnormal screen is obtained, additional counseling regarding the significance of the results and diagnostic testing is necessary. When an abnormal diagnosis is obtained, further counseling, which is often redundant, is also necessary. The general rule in prenatal diagnosis is for counseling to require considerably greater time than the actual performance of any of the tests. However, extensive counseling will benefit both families and clinicians by ensuring that expectations and wishes are satisfied.

SUMMARY

The field of prenatal testing and diagnosis has significantly expanded over the past 20 years. The number and variety of conditions that can be diagnosed antenatally is increasing daily. To keep current, a clinician must make use of computer databases and the sharing of information via the Internet. Practicing obstetricians, perinatologists, clinical geneticists, and genetic counselors should be experienced with resources such as OMIM. Screening tests should be offered and applied to the appropriate cohorts, and then followed up with diagnostic testing when indicated.

Effective prenatal diagnosis requires a team approach and rapport among the team members, which include as a minimum, a clinician, counselor (may be clinician), and molecular and cytogenetics laboratory professionals. In addition, consultation with personnel from biochemical laboratories is frequently necessary. It is important for the clinician to be current on molecular techniques: indications, accuracy of specific tests, failures, and alternative tests. Laboratory personnel should be familiar with the clinical syndromes that are being tested, the sources and types of tissue, and the type of information clinicians hope to obtain from a particular test.

10 KEY POINTS

1. The majority of tests available for prenatal diagnosis are molecular tests—a current computer database, such as OMIM, should be consulted for information about specific disorders.

2. Maternal serum screening for neural tube defects and abdominal wall defects by MSAFP should be offered to all pregnant women at between 15 and 22 weeks; maternal serum screening for trisomy 21 and other aneuploidies should be offered to all pregnant women younger than 35 years of age.

3. Genetic amniocentesis should be offered to all pregnant women aged 35 or older, and to those with a maternal serum triple screen that places them at increased risk of having an aneuploid fetus.

4. Prenatal ultrasonography is a screening test, but the sensitivity and specificity is not clearly defined due to the operator dependence.

5. The RADIUS study concluded routine ultrasound screening did not improve perinatal outcome, but the participating centers had a low rate of detection of anomalies, therapeutic abortions, and lacked interventional protocols.

6. Early amniocentesis has an increased risk of proce-

dure-associated fetal loss and talipes equinovarus, compared to midtrimester amniocentesis or chorionic villus sampling.

7. Chorionic villus sampling, when performed between 10 and 13 weeks gestational age, is a safe alternative to amniocentesis and does not carry an appreciable risk for limb reduction defects after 10 weeks.

8. The use of fetal cells obtained from maternal blood for prenatal diagnosis is currently experimental, but may provide a useful screening tool in the future.

9. Mosaicism occurs when cells are found in a cytogenetic specimen with two or more karyotypes, and must be analyzed by the laboratory to determine if it is constitutional or an artifact.

10. Confined placental mosaicism is found in 1% to 2% of CVS, and carries an increased risk of intrauterine growth retardation and spontaneous abortion.

REFERENCES

1. American College of Obstetricians and Gynecology. *Maternal serum screening.* Educational bulletin number 228. Washington, DC: ACOG, 1996.
2. Verma R, Babu A. Karyotype interpretation. In: Verma R, Babu A, ed. *Human chromosomes: principles and techniques.* New York: McGraw-Hill, 1995:345–361.
3. Online Mendelian Inheritance in Man, OMIM (TM). World Wide Web URL: http://www.ncbi.nlm.gov/Omim/. Baltimore: Johns Hopkins University and National Center for Biotechnology Information, National Library of Medicine, 1997.
4. Simpson JL. Genetic counseling and prenatal diagnosis. In: Gabbe SG, Niebyl JR, Simpson JL, eds. *Obstetrics: normal and problem pregnancies.* New York: Churchill-Livingstone, 1996: 215–248.
5. Boue J, Boue A, Lazar P. Retrospective and prospective epidemiological studies of 1500 karyotyped spontaneous abortions. *Teratology* 1975;12:11.
6. Hassold T. A cytogenetic study of repeated spontaneous abortions. *Am J Hum Genet* 1980;32:723.
7. Schauer GM, Kalousek DK, Magee JF. Genetic causes of stillbirth. *Semin Perinatol* 1992;16:341–351.
8. Los FJ, DeBruijn HWA, Van Beek Calkoen-Carpay T, et al. AFP transport across the fetal membranes in the human. *Prenat Diagn* 1985;5:277–281.
9. Hook EB, Cross PK, Schreinemachers DM. Chromosomal abnormality rates at amniocentesis and in live-born infants. *JAMA* 1983;249:2034–2038.
10. Merkatz IR, Nitowsky HM, Macri JN, et al. An association between low maternal serum alpha-fetoprotein and fetal chromosomal abnormalities. *Am J Obstet Gynecol* 1984;184:896.
11. New England Regional Genetics Group Prenatal Collaborative Study of Down Syndrome Screening. Combining maternal serum α-fetoprotein measurements and age to screen for Down syndrome in pregnant women under age 35. *Am J Obstet Gynecol* 1989;160:575.
12. Bogart MH, Pandian MR, Jones OW. Abnormal maternal serum gonadotropin levels in pregnancies with fetal chromosomal abnormalities. *Prenat Diagn* 1987;7:623.
13. Petrocik E, Wassman ER, Kelly JC. Prenatal screening for Down syndrome with maternal serum human chorionic gonadotropin levels. *Am J Obstet Gynecol* 1989;161:1168.
14. Canik JA, Knight GJ, Palomaki GE, et al. Low second trimester maternal serum unconjugated estriol in Down syndrome pregnancy. *Br J Obstet Gynaecol* 1988;95:330.
15. Haddow JE, Palomaki BS, Knight GJ, et al. Prenatal screening for Down's syndrome with use of maternal serum markers. *N Engl J Med* 1992;327:588.
16. Phillips OP, Elias S, Shulman LP, et al. Maternal serum screening for fetal Down syndrome in women less than 35 years of age using alpha-fetoprotein, hCG, and unconjugated estriol: a prospective 2-year study. *Obstet Gynecol* 1992;80:353.
17. Knight GJ, Palomaki GE, Haddow JE, et al. Maternal serum levels of the placental products hCG, hPL, SPI and progesterone are all elevated in cases of fetal Down syndrome. *Am J Hum Genet* 1989;45(suppl):263.
18. Wald NJ, Densem JW, George L, et al. Prenatal screening for Down's syndrome using inhibin-A as a serum marker. *Prenat Diagn* 1996;16:143.
19. Canick JA, Delln LH, Saller DN, et al. Second-trimester levels of maternal urinary gonadotropin peptide in Down syndrome pregnancy. *Prenat Diagn* 1995;15:739.
20. Palomaki GE, Haddow JE, Knight GJ, et al. Risk-based prenatal screening for trisomy 18 using alpha-fetoprotein, unconjugated oestriol and human chorionic gonadotropin. *Prenat Diagn* 1995;15:713.
21. Ewigman BG, Crane JP, Frigoletto FD, et al., and the RADIUS Study Group. Effect of prenatal ultrasound screening on perinatal outcome. *N Engl J Med* 1993;329:821–827.
22. Shirley IM, Bottomley F, Robinson VP. Routine radiographer screening for fetal abnormalities by ultrasound in an unselected low risk population. *Br J Radiol* 1992;65:564–569.
23. Chitty LS, Hunt GH, Moore J, et al. Effectiveness of routine ultrasonography in detecting fetal structural abnormalities in a low risk population. *Br Med J* 1992;303:1165–1169.
24. Luck C. Value of routine ultrasound scanning at 19 weeks: a four year study of 8849 deliveries. *Br Med J* 1992;304:1474–1478.
25. Vintzileos AM, Cambell WA, Rodis JF, et al. The use of second-trimester genetic sonograms in guiding clinical management of patients at increased risk for fetal trisomy 21. *Obstet Gynecol* 1996;87:948–952.
26. Snijders RJ, Johnson S, Sebire NJ, et al. First-trimester ultrasound screening for chromosomal defects. *Ultrasound Obstet Gynecol* 1996;7:216–226.
27. Krantz D, Hallahan T, Orlandi F, et al. First trimester ultrasound screening. *Am J Obstet Gynecol* 1998;178:S22(abst).
28. Simpson JL, Mills JL, Holmes LB, et al. Low fetal loss rates after ultrasound-proved viability in early pregnancy. *JAMA* 1987;258:2555–2557.
29. Wilson RD, Kendrick V, Wittman BK, et al. Risk of spontaneous abortion in ultrasonically normal pregnancies. *Lancet* 1984;2:920–921.
30. Liley AW. Intrauterine transfusion of foetus in haemolytic disease. *Br J Obstet Gynaecol* 1963;2:1107–1109.
31. Evans MI, Johnson MP, Holzgreve W. Early amniocentesis: what exactly does it mean? *J Reprod Med* 1994;39:77–78.
32. Reece EA. Early and midtrimester genetic amniocentesis. *Obstet Gynecol Clin North Am Fetal Diagn Ther* 1997;24:71–81.
33. Wilson RD. Early amniocentesis: a clinical review. *Prenat Diagn* 1995;15:1259–1273.
34. Sundberg K, Jorgensen FS, Tabor A, et al. Experience with early amniocentesis. *J Perinat Med* 1995;23:149–158.
35. Canadian Early and Mid-Trimester Amniocentesis Trial (CEMAT) Group. Randomised trial to assess safety and fetal

outcomes of early and midtrimester amniocentesis. *Lancet* 1998; 351:242–247.

36. Whittle MJ. Early amniocentesis: time for a rethink. *Lancet* 1998;351:226–227.

37. Elejalde BR, De Elejalde MM, Acuna JM, et al. Prospective study of amniocentesis performed between weeks 9 and 16 of gestation: its feasibility, risks, complications and use in early genetic prenatal diagnosis. *Am J Med Genet* 1990;35:188.

38. Sundberg K, Smidt-Jensen S, Lundsteen L, et al. Filtration and recirculation of early amniotic fluid. Evaluation of cell cultures from 100 diagnostic cases. *Prenat Diagn* 1993;13:1101.

39. Sundberg K, Smidt-Jensen S, Philip J. Amniocentesis with increased cell yield, obtained by filtration and reinjection of the amniotic fluid. *Ultrasound Obstet Gynecol* 1991;1:1.

40. Sundberg K, Bang J, Smidt-Jensen S, et al. Randomised study of risk of fetal loss related to early amniocentesis versus chorionic villus sampling. *Lancet* 1997;350:697–703.

41. Canadian collaborative CVS–Amniocentesis Clinical Trial Group. Multicentre randomised clinical trial of chorion villus sampling and amniocentesis. *Lancet* 1989;1:1–6.

42. Rhoads GG, Jackson LG, Schlesselman SE, et al. The safety and efficacy of chorionic villus sampling for early prenatal diagnosis of cytogenetic abnormalities. *N Engl J Med* 1989;320: 609–617.

43. Jackson LG, Zachary JM, Fowler SE, et al. A randomized comparison of transcervical and transabdominal chorionic-villus sampling. The U.S. National Institute of Child Health and Human Development Chorionic-Villus Sampling and Amniocentesis Study Group. *N Engl J Med* 1992;327:594–598.

44. Smidt-Jensen S, Permin M, Philip J. Sampling success and risk by transabdominal chorionic villus sampling, transcervical chorionic villus sampling and amniocentesis: a randomized study. *Ultrasound Obstet Gynecol* 1991;1:86.

45. MRC Working Party on the Evaluation of Chorionic Villus Sampling. Medical Research Council European Trial of Chorionic Villus Sampling. *Lancet* 1991;337:1491.

46. Williams J III, Wang BBT, Rubin CH, et al. Chorionic villus sampling: experience with 3016 cases performed by a single operator. *Obstet Gynecol* 1992;80:1023–1029.

47. American College of Obstetricians and Gynecologists Committee on Genetics. *Chorionic villus sampling*. Opinion number 160. Washington, DC: ACOG, 1995.

48. Nicolaides KH, de Lourdes Brizot M, Patel F, et al. Comparison of chorion villus sampling and early amniocentesis for karyotyping in 1,492 singleton pregnancies. *Fetal Diagn Ther* 1996;11: 9–15.

49. Firth HV, Boyd PA, Chamberlain P, et al. Limb abnormalities and chorion villus sampling. *Lancet* 1991;338:51.

50. Burton BK, Schulz CJ, Burd LI. Limb anomalies associated with chorionic villus sampling. *Obstet Gynecol* 1992;79:726–730.

51. Brambati B, Simoni G, Travi M, et al. Genetic diagnosis by chorionic villus sampling before 8 gestational weeks: efficiency, reliability, and risks on 317 completed pregnancies. *Prenat Diagn* 1992;12:789–799.

52. Olney RS, Khoury MJ, Alo CJ, et al. Increased risk for transverse digital deficiency after chorionic villus sampling results of the United States multistate case-control study, 1988–1992. *Teratology* 1995;51:20–29.

53. Wapner RJ. Chorionic villus sampling. *Obstet Gynecol Clin North Am Fetal Diagn Ther* 1997;24:83–110.

54. Wladimiroff JW, Jahoda MCJ. Real time scanning and transabdominal fetal blood sampling. *Lancet* 1977;1:593–597.

55. Daffos F. Fetal blood sampling. *Annu Rev Med* 1989;40:319.

56. Ghidini A, Sepulvada W, Lockwood CJ, et al. Complications of fetal blood sampling. *Am J Obstet Gynecol* 1993;168:1339.

57. Wilson RD, Farquharson DF, Wittmann BK, et al. Cordocentesis: overall pregnancy loss rate as important as procedure loss rate. *Fetal Diagn Ther* 1994;9:142.

58. Donner C, Simon P, Karioun A, et al. Experience of a single team of operators in 891 diagnostic funipunctures. *Obstet Gynecol* 1994;84:827–831.

59. Elias S, Emerson DS, Simpson JL, et al. Ultrasound-guided fetal skin sampling for prenatal diagnosis of genodermatoses. *Obstet Gynecol* 1994;83:337–341.

60. Evans MI, Hoffman EP, Cadrin C, et al. Fetal muscle biopsy: collaborative experience with varied indications. *Obstet Gynecol* 1994;84:913–917.

61. Reece EA, Goldstein I, Chatwani A, et al. Transabdominal needle embryofetoscopy: a new technique paving the way for early fetal therapy. *Obstet Gynecol* 1994;84:634–636.

62. Reece EA. Embryoscopy and early prenatal diagnosis. *Obstet Gynecol Clin North Am Fetal Diagn Ther* 1997;24:111–121.

63. Bahado-Singh RO, Kliman H, Yeng Feng T, et al. First-trimester endocervical irrigation: feasibility of obtaining trophoblast cells for prenatal diagnosis. *Obstet Gynecol* 1995;85:461–464.

64. Elias S, Esterly NB. Prenatal diagnosis of hereditary skin disorders. *Clin Obstet Gynecol* 1981;24:1069–1087.

65. Golbus MS, for the International Fetoscopy Group. Special report: the status of fetoscopy and fetal tissue sampling. *Prenat Diagn* 1984;4:79–81.

66. Walknowska J, Conte FA, Grumbeck MM. Practical and theoretical implications of fetal/maternal lymphocyte transfer. *Lancet* 1969;1119–1122.

67. Simpson JL, Elias S. Isolating fetal cells in maternal circulation for prenatal diagnosis. *Prenat Diagn* 1994;14:1229–1242.

68. Herzenberg LA, Bianchi DW, Schroder J, et al. Fetal cells in the blood of pregnant women: detection and enrichment by fluorescence-activated cell sorting. *Proc Natl Acad Sci USA* 1979;76:1453–1455.

69. Simpson JL, Elias S. Isolating fetal cells from maternal blood. *JAMA* 1993;270:2357–2361.

70. Mullis KB, Faloona FA. Specific synthesis of DNA in vitro via a polymerase-catalyzed chain reaction. *Methods Enzymol* 1987;155:335–350.

71. Mullis KB. The unusual origin of the polymerase chain reaction. *Sci Am* 1990;July:56–65.

72. Lo Y-MD, Wainscoat JS, Gilmer MDG, et al. Prenatal sex determination by DNA amplification from maternal peripheral blood. *Lancet* 1989;2:1363–1365.

73. Lo Y-MD, Pate P, Sampietro M, et al. Detection of single-copy fetal DNA sequence from maternal blood. *Lancet* 1990; 335:1463–1464.

74. Bianchi DW, Flint AF, Pizzimenti MF, et al. Isolation of fetal DNA from nucleated erythrocytes in maternal blood. *Proc Natl Acad Sci USA* 1990;87:3279–3283.

75. Bianchi DW, Shuber AP, DeMaria M, et al. Fetal cells in maternal blood: determination of purity and yield by quantitative polymerase chain reaction. *Am J Obstet Gynecol* 1994;171: 922–926.

76. Bianchi DW. Clinical trials and experience: Boston. In: Simpson JL, Elias S, eds. *Fetal cells in maternal blood: prospects for noninvasive prenatal diagnosis*. New York: Annuals of the New York Academy of Sciences, 1994:93–104.

77. de la Cruz FF, Shifrin H, Elias S, et al. Prenatal diagnosis by the use of fetal cells isolated from maternal blood. *Am J Obstet Gynecol* 1995;173:1354–1355.

78. Swiger RR, Tucker JD. Fluorescence in situ hybridization: a brief review. *Environ Mol Mutagen* 1996;27:245–254.

79. Lee C, Wevrick R, Fisher RB, et al. Human centromeric DNAs. *Hum Genet* 1997;100:291–304.

80. Divane A, Carter NP, Spathas DH, et al. Rapid prenatal diagnosis of aneuploidy from uncultured amniotic fluid cells using five-colour fluorescence in situ hybridization. *Prenat Diagn* 1994;14:1061–1069.

81. Delhanty JD, Harper JC, Ao A, et al. Multicolour FISH detects frequent chromosomal mosaicism and chaotic division in normal preimplantation embryos from fertile patients. *Hum Genet* 1997;99:755–760.

82. Driscoll DA, Spinner NB, Budarf ML, et al. Rapid publication—deletions and microdeletions of 22q11.2 in velo-cardio-facial syndrome. *Am J Med Genet* 1992;44:261–268.

83. Ewart AK, Morris CA, Atkinson D, et al. Hemizygosity at the elastin locus in a developmental disorder, Williams syndrome. *Nat Genet* 1993;5:11–16.

84. Buiting K, Saitoh S, Gross S, et al. Inherited microdeletions in the Angelman and Prader-Willi syndromes define an imprinting centre on human chromosome 15. *Nat Genet* 1995;9:395–400.

85. Zackowski JL, Nicholls RD, Gray BA, et al. Cytogenetic and molecular analysis in Angelman syndrome. *Am J Med Genet* 1993;46:7–11.

86. Cassidy SB, Knoll JH, et al. Diagnostic testing for Prader-Willi and Angelman syndromes: report of the ASHC/ACMC Test and Technology Transfer Committee. *Am J Hum Genet* 1996;58:1085–1088.

87. Cassidy SB, Forsythe M, Heeger S, et al. Comparison of phenotype between patients with Prader-Willi syndrome due to deletion 15q and uniparental disomy 15. *Am J Med Genet* 1997;68:433–440.

88. Evans MI, Ebrahim SA, Berry SM, et al. Fluorescent in situ hybridization utilization for high-risk prenatal diagnosis: a tradeoff among speed, expense, and inherent limitations of chromosome-specific probes. *Am J Obstet Gynecol* 1994;171:1055–1057.

89. Hogge WA, Surti U, Kochmar SJ, et al. Molecular cytogenetics: an essential component of modern prenatal diagnosis. *Am J Obstet Gynecol* 1996;175:352–356.

90. American College of Medical Genetics (ACMG). Prenatal interphase fluorescence in situ hybridization (FISH) policy statement. *Am J Hum Genet* 1993;53:526–527.

91. Guttenbach M, Engel W, Schmid M. Analysis of structural and numerical chromosome abnormalities in sperm of normal men and carriers of constitutional chromosome aberrations. A review. *Hum Genet* 1997;100:1–21.

92. Ning Y, Rosenberg M, Biesecker LG, et al. Isolation of the human chromosome 22q telomere and its application to detection of cryptic chromosomal abnormalities. *Hum Genet* 1996;97:765–769.

93. Ning Y, Roschke A, Smith AC, et al. A complete set of human telomeric probes and their clinical application. *Nat Genet* 1996;14:86–89.

94. Knight SJ, Horsley SW, Regan R, et al. Development and clinical application of an innovative fluorescence in situ hybridization technique which detects submicroscopic rearrangements involving telomeres. *Eur J Hum Genet* 1997;5:1–8.

95. Flint J, Wilkie AO, Buckle VJ, et al. The detection of subtelomeric chromosomal rearrangements in idiopathic mental retardation. *Nat Genet* 1995;9:132–140.

96. Senger G, Chudoba I, Friedrich U, et al. Prenatal diagnosis of a half-cryptic translocation using chromosome microdissection. *Prenat Diagn* 1997;17:369–374.

97. Cannizzaro LA. Chromosome microdissection: a brief overview. *Cytogenet Cell Genet* 1996;74:157–160.

98. van Zelderen-Bhola SL, Breslau-Siderius EJ, Beverstock GC, et al. Prenatal and postnatal investigation of a case with Miller-Dieker syndrome due to a familial cryptic translocation t (17;20) (p13.3;q13.3) detected by fluorescence in situ hybridization. *Prenat Diagn* 1997;17:173–179.

99. Speicher MR, Ward DC. The coloring of cytogenetics. *Nat Med* 1996;2:1046–1048.

100. Macville M, Veldman T, PadillaNash H, et al. Spectral karyotyping, a 24-colour FISH technique for the identification of chromosomal rearrangements. *Histochem Cell Biol* 1997;108:299–305.

101. Karhu R, Kahkonen M, Kuukasjarvi T, et al. Quality control of CGH: impact of metaphase chromosomes and the dynamic range of hybridization. *Cytometry* 1997;28:198–205.

102. Sonoda G, Palazzo J, duManoir S, et al. Comparative genomic hybridization detects frequent overrepresentation of chromosomal material from 3q26, 8q24, and 20q13 in human ovarian carcinomas. *Genes Chromosomes Cancer* 1997;20:320–328.

103. Forozan F, Karhu R, Kononen J, et al. Genome screening by comparative genomic hybridization. *Trends Genet* 1997;13:405–409.

104. Warburton D, Byrne J, Canki N, et al. *Chromosome anomalies and prenatal development: an atlas.* New York: Oxford University Press, 1991:104.

105. Hsu LY, Yu MT, Richkind KE, et al. Incidence and significance of chromosome mosaicism involving an autosomal structural abnormality diagnosed prenatally through amniocentesis: a collaborative study. *Prenat Diagn* 1996;16:1–28.

106. Hsu LY, Kaffe S, Jenkins EC, et al. Proposed guidelines for diagnosis of chromosome mosaicism in amniocytes based on data derived from chromosome mosaicism and pseudomosaicism studies. *Prenat Diagn* 1992;12:555–573.

107. Sikkema-Raddatz B, Castedo S, TeMeerman GJ. Probability tables for exclusion of mosaicism in prenatal diagnosis. *Prenat Diagn* 1997;17:115–118.

108. Hsu L, Yu MT, Neu R, et al. Rare trisomy mosaicism diagnosed in amniocytes, involving an autosome other than chromosomes 13, 18, 20 and 21: karyotype/phenotype correlations. *Prenat Diagn* 1997;17:201–242.

109. Hahnemann JM, Vejerslev LO, European Collaborative Research on Mosaicism in CVS (EUCROMIC). Fetal and extrafetal cell lineages in 192 gestations with CVS mosaicism involving single autosomal trisomy. *Am J Med Genet* 1997;70:179–187.

110. Kalousek DK. Current topic: confined placental mosaicism and intrauterine fetal development. *Placenta* 1994;15:219–230.

111. Kalousek DK, Barrett IJ, McGillivray BC. Placental mosaicism and intrauterine survival of trisomies 13 and 18. *Am J Hum Genet* 1989;44:338–343.

112. Roland B, Lynch L, Berkowitz G, et al. Confined placental mosaicism in CVS and pregnancy outcome. *Prenat Diagn* 1994;14:589–593.

113. Gardner RM, Sutherland GR, Bobrow M, et al. *Chromosome abnormalities and genetic counseling.* New York: Oxford University Press, 1996.

114. VanOpstal D, Van Den Berg C, Deelen W, et al. Prospective prenatal investigations on potential uniparental disomy in cases of confined placental trisomy. *Prenat Diagn* 1998;18:35–44.

115. Robinson WP, Barrett IJ, Bernard L, et al. Meiotic origin of trisomy in confined placental mosaicism is correlated with presence of fetal uniparental disomy, high levels of trisomy in trophoblast, and increased risk of fetal intrauterine growth restriction. *Am J Hum Genet* 1997;60:917–927.

116. Nicholls RD. Imprinting: the embryo and adult point of view. *Trends Genet* 1994;10:389.
117. Nicholls RD. Genomic imprinting and uniparental disomy in Angelman and Prader-Willi syndromes—a review. *Am J Med Genet* 1993;46:16.
118. Saitoh S, Buiting K, Cassidy SB, et al. Clinical spectrum and molecular diagnosis of Angelman and Prader-Willi syndrome patients with an imprinting mutation. *Am J Med Genet* 1997;68:195–206.
119. Sikkema-Raddatz B, Sijmons RH, Tansindhunata MB, et al. Prenatal diagnosis in two cases of de novo complex balanced chromosomal rearrangements. Three-year follow-up in one case. *Prenat Diagn* 1995;15:467–473.
120. National screening status report. *Infant Screen* 1994;17:5.

THE INITIATION AND MANAGEMENT OF NORMAL LABOR

ERROL R. NORWITZ
JULIAN N. ROBINSON
JOHN T. REPKE

The initiation and management of normal labor is a broad and complex topic. A comprehensive and exhaustive review is not within the scope of this chapter. The first half of this chapter focuses on the biochemical and physiologic mechanisms responsible for the initiation and maintenance of labor at term. The second half describes the mechanics of normal labor and subsequent clinical management. In the spirit of the overall text, emphasis has been placed on those areas of clinical management that are controversial and that have a well-defined physiologic basis, namely, the active management of labor, the effect of epidural anesthesia on the progress of labor, and the changing role of fetal birth asphyxia as an etiologic factor in subsequent neonatal neurologic injury. A more comprehensive review of labor—including such topics as the management of preterm labor, abnormal labor, operative delivery, and multiple gestation—can be found elsewhere in this text.

THE PHYSIOLOGIC BASIS OF PARTURITION

Characteristics of Labor at Term

Labor can be defined as regular uterine contractions leading to effacement and dilatation of the cervix, and ultimately to expulsion of the products of conception. It is a complex process involving fetal, placental, as well as maternal signals. The sum total of such a multifactorial system is often more than the sum of the individual parts. To facilitate understanding, it is useful to dissect out and analyze separately each of the autocrine/paracrine pathways implicated in the mechanism of labor.

The onset of labor is a clinical diagnosis encompassing three distinct elements: (a) an increase in myometrial activity or, more precisely, a switch in the myometrial contractility pattern from "contractures" (long-lasting, low-frequency activity) to "contractions" (frequent, high-intensity, high-frequency activity); (b) effacement and dilatation of the uterine cervix; and (c) rupture of the fetal membranes. Furthermore, in the majority of cases, there appears to be

a critical time-dependent relationship between these elements: the biochemical connective tissue changes in the cervix usually precede uterine contractions, which in turn precede cervical dilatation. All of these events usually precede rupture of the membranes. In only around 8% of term pregnancies will spontaneous rupture of the membranes occur prior to the onset of uterine activity (1).

Historical Perspective

The factor(s) responsible for the initiation and maintenance of labor at term remain enigmatic. However, there is considerable evidence in animals that the fetus is in control of its own destiny as regards the timely onset of labor and birth (2–4). This seems to hold true whether pregnancy is maintained by the placenta (as in the sheep) or by the corpus luteum (as in the goat and mouse).

In ruminants such as sheep and cows, activation of the fetal hypothalamic-pituitary-adrenal axis occurs 7 to 10 days prior to delivery. This results in a sharp rise in the concentration of cortisol in the fetal circulation, which acts as the trigger for labor (5). The mechanism by which fetal cortisol initiates labor in such animals has been elegantly demonstrated. It involves the activation in the ruminant placenta of a specific enzyme (17α-hydroxylase/$C_{17,20}$-lyase), thereby allowing placental metabolism of C21 steroids completely through to estrogen (Fig. 27.1). The resultant fall in circulating progesterone and rise in estrogen concentrations provide the impetus for prostaglandin (PG) F release and labor (5–7). In such animals, surgical lesions in the paraventricular region of the hypothalamus, hypophysectomy, and/or adrenalectomy of the fetus *in utero* will lead to prolonged gestation (7,8). Conversely, infusion of adrenocorticotropic hormone (ACTH) or glucocorticoid into the fetus will result in preterm labor (7,8). It is clear in such animals that the fetal hypothalamic-pituitary-adrenal axis can be activated prematurely if the intrauterine environment becomes unfavorable, as in the setting of severe hypoxemia (9). With hypoxemia, there is an increased expression of corticotropin-releasing hormone (CRH) in the fetal hypothalamus as well

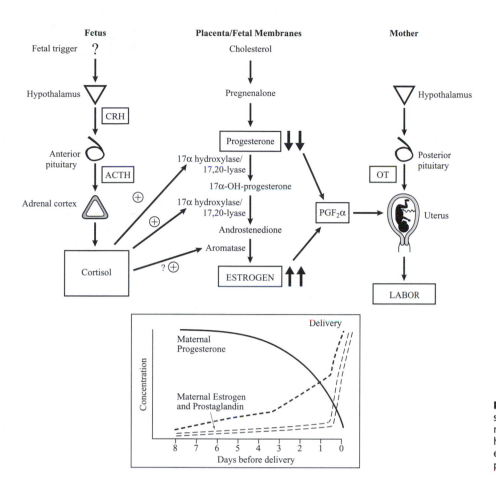

FIGURE 27.1. Mechanism of labor in sheep. ACTH, adrenocorticotropic hormone; CRH, corticotropin-releasing hormone; DHEAS, dehydroepiandrosterone sulfate; OT, oxytocin; $PGF_{2\alpha}$, prostaglandin $F_{2\alpha}$.

as an increase in pro-opiomelanocortin (POMC) in the fetal anterior pituitary gland (8,9). The end result is an elevation in circulating levels of cortisol in the fetus, which appears capable of provoking preterm labor and of stimulating the maturation of those fetal organ systems required for extrauterine life (such as the respiratory system). However, stimulation of organ system maturation is not without a detriment, namely, inhibition of cell growth. This occurs in part through cortisol-mediated suppression of insulin-like growth factors (10). These findings have prompted some authors to propose that labor and birth in such animals represent "a necessary escape of the fetus from an environment of hypercortisolism" (10).

Primate placentae, including that of the human, lack the glucocorticoid-inducible 17α-hydroxylase enzyme (6). As a result, the mechanism demonstrated for the induction of labor in ruminants does not apply. Indeed, when Novy and Walsh (11) administered steroids to their chronically catheterized pregnant rhesus monkeys, not only were they unable to initiate preterm labor, but 71% of these animals actually delivered postdates. Other differences exist as well; for example, in sheep, the switch from contractures to contractions occurs abruptly, generally at night, and progresses directly to labor and delivery. In primates, however, this

switch occurs and augments for a few hours each night until delivery occurs after several days (12). In primates, the hormonal control of parturition represents a jigsaw in which many of the pieces of scientific knowledge are still missing. A proposed mechanism for the induction of labor at term in primates is illustrated in Fig. 27.2, and will be discussed below.

Phases of Parturition

Parturition at term is perhaps best regarded physiologically as a release from the inhibitory effects of pregnancy on the myometrium, rather than as an active process mediated by uterine stimulants. However, both mechanisms appear to be important. In the human, it is useful to consider the regulation of uterine activity during the latter part of pregnancy and early puerperium as being divided into four distinct physiologic phases (Fig. 27.3) (8). During phase 0, the uterus is maintained in a state of functional quiescence through the action of one or more of a series of inhibitors. These inhibitors include progesterone, prostacyclin (PGI_2), relaxin, parathyroid hormone–related peptide (PTH-rP), and nitric oxide (NO). Other hormones that have been more recently implicated include calcitonin gene–related

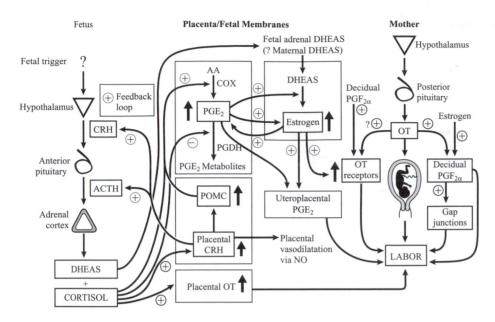

FIGURE 27.2. Proposed mechanism of labor in humans. AA, arachidonic acid; ACTH, adrenocorticotropic hormone; COX, cyclooxygenase; CRH, corticotropin-releasing hormone; DHEAS, dehydroepiandrosterone sulfate; NO, nitric oxide; OT, oxytocin; PGDH, 15-hydroxyprostaglandin-dehydrogenase; PGE_2, prostaglandin E_2; $PGF_{2\alpha}$, prostaglandin $F_{2\alpha}$; POMC, pro-opiomelanocortin.

peptide, adrenomedullin, and vasoactive intestinal peptide. Before term, the uterus undergoes a process of activation (phase 1) and stimulation (phase 2). Activation of the myometrium is brought about in response to one or more uterotopins, among which estrogen has a prominent role. It is characterized by increased expression of a series of contraction-associated proteins (including receptors for PGs and oxytocin [OT], proteins required to increase the functional activity of certain ion channels, and an increase in connexin-43 [a key component of gap junctions]). The

physiologic importance of permeable gap junctions between myometrial cells is believed to be the establishment of electrical synchrony in the myometrium. This synchrony allows for effective coordination of contractions and thereby greater force during labor. Following activation (phase 1), the "primed" uterus can then be acted upon by uterotonins and stimulated to contract (phase 2). Such uterotonins include the stimulatory PGs (predominantly PGE_2 and $PGF_{2\alpha}$) and OT. The "initiation" of parturition can be considered as the switch from quiescence to activation

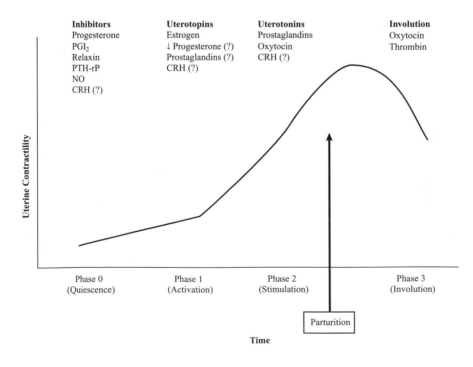

FIGURE 27.3. Regulation of uterine contractility during pregnancy and postpartum. CRH, corticotropin-releasing hormone; NO, nitric oxide; PTH-rP, parathyroid hormone–related peptide; PGI_2, prostaglandin I_2 (prostacyclin).

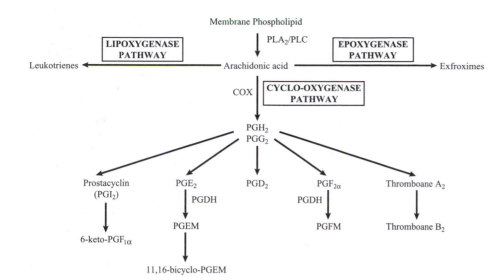

FIGURE 27.4. Pathway of arachidonic acid metabolism. COX, cyclo-oxygenase; PGDH, 15-hydroxy-prostaglandin-dehydrogenase; PG, prostaglandin; PGEM, 13,14-dihydro-15-keto-PGE$_2$; PGFM, 13,14-dihydro-15-keto-PGF$_{2\alpha}$; PLA$_2$, phospholipase A$_2$; PLC, phospholipase C.

(phase 0 to phase 1), while the "maintenance" of parturition incorporates both phases 1 and 2. Phase 3 events include uterine involution following delivery, and are mediated primarily by OT.

The Endocrine Control of Labor

In contrast to vascular smooth muscle, myometrial cells have a sparse innervation that is further reduced during pregnancy (13). The regulation of the contractile function of the uterus is therefore largely humoral and/or dependent on intrinsic factors within myometrial cells. A number of hormones have been implicated in this process. Some of these are discussed below.

Prostaglandins

The PG biosynthetic pathway is detailed in Fig. 27.4. Human uterine tissues are selectively enriched with arachidonic acid (AA), an essential fatty acid stored predominantly at the sn-2 position of membrane phospholipids. AA is the obligate precursor of PGs of the 2-series (14). The release of unesterified (free) AA is the rate-limiting step in PG biosynthesis, and is mediated by a series of phospholipase enzymes. The most important of these enzymes *in vivo* appears to be phospholipase A$_2$ (PLA$_2$). Phospholipase C (PLC) is produced mainly by bacteria and has been implicated in the mechanism of preterm labor associated with infection. PLC requires the actions of additional enzymes (mono- and diacylglycerol lipases) to release free AA. AA is then converted via the cyclooxygenase pathway to the endoperoxidase intermediates, PGG$_2$ and PGH$_2$, which are rapidly metabolized to the primary PGs. This step is mediated by the enzyme cyclooxygenase (COX), also known as PGH synthase. COX exists in two isoforms. COX-1 is coded by a constitutively expressed housekeeping gene pres-

ent in many tissues. COX-2 is the inducible form of the enzyme, which is upregulated in response to a number of inflammatory cytokines and growth factors (15). In trophoblast-derived tissues, COX-2 may also be induced by glucocorticoids (16). PGs are predominantly paracrine/autocrine hormones, meaning that they act locally at their site of production on contiguous cells. Only the primary PGs are biologically active with half-lives in the peripheral circulation of 1 to 2 minutes. They are cleared predominantly by the lungs. Degradation of the primary PGs is initiated by the enzyme, nicotinamide adenine dinucleotide (NAD)-dependent 15-hydroxy-PG-dehydrogenase (15-OH PGDH) (Fig. 27.4).

An increase in PG biosynthesis in the uterus is consistently seen in the transition into labor (14,17), and is probably common to all species (18). The first documented association between PGs and human pregnancy was in 1966 when Karim (19) identified the presence of PGs in amniotic fluid of women in the third trimester of pregnancy. It now seems likely that the final pathway for the onset of labor in women, both at term and preterm, is an increased synthesis of PGs of the E and F series within the uterine compartment, predominantly from the decidua and fetal membranes (Fig. 27.2). The evidence can be summarized briefly as follows:

1. The concentrations of PGs in amniotic fluid and in maternal plasma and urine are increased during parturition (3,14,20). Using serial transabdominal amniocentesis in a large series of patients, Romero et al. (21) were able to demonstrate that PG concentrations in amniotic fluid increase prior to the onset of myometrial concentrations.

2. The intraamniotic, intravenous, or vaginal administration of exogenous PGs, at any stage of gestation, and in all species examined, has the capacity to initiate labor (3).

3. PGs have been implicated in the three events most temporally related to the onset of labor in women:
   a. the onset of powerful, synchronous uterine contractions (22–25);
   b. cervical "ripening" (26–28); and
   c. the increase in myometrial sensitivity to OT, due to an increase in myometrial gap junction formation [a process known to be stimulated by PGs (29,30)] and/or to an increase in OT receptor concentrations [PGF$_{2\alpha}$ is capable of upgrading OT receptor levels in the rat uterus (31), but whether this is true in primates is unclear (6,32)].
4. Inhibitors of PG synthesis (including COX inhibitors such as indomethacin) are capable of suppressing myometrial contractility both *in vitro* and *in vivo,* and of prolonging the length of gestation (33,34).

Taken together, such data suggest that the increase in PG production by utero-placental tissues precedes myometrial contractility, and is not a consequence of uterine contractions. This is in keeping with detailed studies in a number of animal species (35–38). In the mouse, for example, an animal in which pregnancy is maintained by the corpus luteum, PGs were initially thought not to be necessary for parturition. The evidence put forward to support this hypothesis is based on experiments with gene null mutations and transgenic animals. COX-2 knockout mice, for example, show reduced fecundity, but did not appear to have differences as regards labor onset or gestational length (36). Similarly, COX-1 knockout mice were able to deliver spontaneously, although they appeared to have lengthy, protracted labors, and the young had poor viability (37). More recently, however, a study from Japan by Sugimoto et al. (38) demonstrated that mice lacking the gene encoding for the receptor for PGF$_{2\alpha}$ (FP-receptor) developed normally, but were unable to deliver normal fetuses at term. They did not show the normal decline in serum progesterone concentrations prior to labor onset (day 20). In addition, they were unable to respond to exogenous OT because of the lack of induction of OT receptors. Despite these observations, the FP-receptor–deficient mice showed no abnormality in the estrous cycle, ovulation, fertilization, or implantation. Ovariectomy at day 19 of gestation restored induction of OT receptors and permitted successful delivery in these FP-receptor deficient mice. These data suggest that, in the mouse, parturition is initiated when PGF$_{2\alpha}$ (presumably originating from the fetoplacental unit) acting through its receptor on the luteal cells of the ovary induces luteolysis. This once again affirms the critical role of PGs in the initiation and maintenance of labor in animals.

In humans, PG production is discretely compartmentalized within the uterus. The precise intrauterine origins of the various members of the PG family and their respective physiologic importance during pregnancy and labor remains an area of intense debate. The maternal decidua is the main source of PGF$_{2\alpha}$ in the uterus; the fetal membranes (especially the amnion) produce primarily PGE$_2$; and the myometrium produces predominantly prostacyclin (PGI$_2$) (14). Measurement of PG concentrations in the maternal circulation and/or in amniotic fluid do not necessarily reflect their concentration at the choriodecidual or myometrial interface. These limitations should be considered when examining PG metabolism in the uterus near term. Levels of PGE$_2$ and its primary metabolite 13,14-dihydro-15-keto-PGE$_2$ (PGEM) increase in fetal membranes and amniotic fluid during labor (14), but not in maternal blood (39). The chorion is selectively enriched with 15-OH PGDH unlike the amnion, which is devoid of PGDH. *In vitro* studies have demonstrated that PGE$_2$ does not transfer freely across the intact amniochorio-decidua, either before or after the onset of labor (40). These observations suggest that although PGE$_2$ appears to be a more potent uterotonic agent than PGF$_{2\alpha}$ *in vitro* (41), levels of PGE$_2$ in amnion and amniotic fluid have little or no effect on myometrial contractility *in vivo.* Conversely, levels of 13,14-dihydro-15-keto-PGF$_{2\alpha}$ (PGFM), the primary metabolite of PGF$_{2\alpha}$, do increase in maternal plasma during labor (14). PGF$_{2\alpha}$ is capable of inducing contractions in strips of myometrium both *in vitro* and *in vivo.* These data suggest that PGF$_{2\alpha}$ is more important physiologically as regards myometrial contractility. Indeed, many investigators now believe that it is the decidua that is maintained in a state of functional quiescence during pregnancy, and that spontaneous labor results from the withdrawal of the fetal-paracrine support of pregnancy with decidual activation and resultant PGF release. PGE$_2$ appears to have a more important role as regards cervical "ripening" and possibly rupture of the fetal membranes. The latter statement is supported by data showing regional differences in PGDH gene expression in fetal membranes with the onset of labor. Van Meir et al. (42) demonstrated that 15-OH PGDH activity in the fetal membranes overlying the cervical os was high in women undergoing elective cesarean section at term in the absence of labor, but was selectively decreased in women undergoing cesarean section after the onset of labor. Histologic examination of the tissues suggest that these changes are not due to loss or destruction of trophoblast cells, but appear to be directly related to alteration in transcriptional regulation of the PGDH gene (42,43). Inflammation/infection of the chorioamnion is associated with a decrease in 15-OH PGDH messenger RNA (mRNA) in the membranes (42,43). This decrease may be due to a loss of trophoblast cells, and may impair the ability of the fetal membranes to metabolize the primary PGs. This appears to upset the delicate balance set up between antagonistic PG metabolites, thereby allowing more PGE$_2$ to reach the myometrium and initiate contractions. A similar effect may be seen in patients with a deficiency of PGDH immunostaining in chorion trophoblast cells (either congenital or acquired), and such patients have been identified as being at risk for idiopathic preterm labor (42,43).

PGs act through specific binding sites (receptors) in the decidua and myometrium. These receptors have been identified and cloned. The concentration and affinity of the various PG receptors do not appear to change throughout pregnancy and labor (44,45). There are currently five known PG receptor subtypes and eight known heptahelical guanosine triphosphate-binding proteins (G proteins) (46). The PG receptor family members are classified according to the specificity of their ligand binding. Members of the PG receptor family include TP [which selectively binds thromboxane A_2 (TXA_2)], DP (PGD_2), IP (PGI_2), FP ($PGF_{2\alpha}$), and EP (PGE_2). EP receptors are further subdivided into EP_1, EP_2, EP_3, and EP_4. $PGF_{2\alpha}$ and TXA_2 are usually associated with smooth muscle contraction, vasoconstriction, and uterine contractions, whereas PGE_2, PGD_2, and PGI_2 usually cause relaxation of vascular smooth muscle and vasodilatation. This effect is probably due to differences in G-protein coupling and/or second messenger pathways, although these have not been examined in detail during pregnancy. Another potential confounder is the lack of specificity of prostanoids acting through different receptors. PGE_2 at low concentrations, for example, appears to act through EP_2 or EP_4 receptors to stimulate $G\alpha_s$ (stimulatory)-induced adenylyl cyclase activity, thereby promoting 3',5'-cyclic adenosine monophosphate (cAMP) accumulation and smooth muscle relaxation. At higher concentrations of PGE_2, however, EP_1 and EP_3 receptors may be activated with inhibition of adenyl cyclase and/or activation of PLC via $G\alpha_i$ (inhibitory) or $G\alpha_q$, resulting in increased myometrial intracellular calcium and myometrial contraction. Much is yet to be learned about the role of prostanoids in myometrial function.

Steroid Hormones

Antiprogesterone agents [such as the progesterone receptor antagonists RU-486 (Mifepristone) and ZK98299 (Onapristone)] readily induce abortion in early human pregnancy ($\leq$49 days of amenorrhea) (47,48). Such studies demonstrate conclusively that progesterone is necessary for early pregnancy maintenance. Later in pregnancy, however, progesterone receptor antagonists alone are not effective in terminating pregnancy (48). At term, progesterone withdrawal does not occur in all women before labor. Indeed, circulating progesterone levels during labor are similar to levels measured 1 week prior to labor (49), suggesting that progesterone withdrawal is not a prerequisite for labor in humans. This is in contrast to most laboratory animals in which progesterone withdrawal is an essential component of parturition (with the noted exception of the guinea pig and armadillo). However, circulating hormone levels do not necessarily reflect activity at a tissue level, and the possibility that the onset of labor in women may be preceded

by a physiologic withdrawal of progesterone activity at the level of the uterus still exists. There is as yet no agent available to suppress progesterone gene expression in the uterus in a tissue-specific, gene-specific fashion to test this hypothesis.

In primates, the placenta is an incomplete steroidogenic organ, and estrogen synthesis by the placenta has an obligate need for androgen precursor (Fig. 27.2). Estrogens do not cause myometrial contractions, but do appear to promote a variety of myometrial changes that enhance the capacity of the myometrium to generate powerful contractions. For example, they promote myometrial cell hypertrophy, improve cell-to-cell communicability by promoting gap junction formation, and upregulate uterotonin receptors including L-type calcium channels and OT receptors. Many of these stimulatory effects of estrogen are negated by progesterone. Longitudinal measurements of circulating maternal estrogen concentrations immediately prior to spontaneous labor show an increase in all primate species. Figueroa and colleagues (50) were able to induce premature contractions in chronically catheterized pregnant monkeys by administering androstenedione. In the same model, surgically induced myometrial contractions can be inhibited by the aromatase inhibitor 4-hydroxyandrostenedione (51). Furthermore, continuous infusion of androstenedione into the pregnant rhesus monkey at 0.8 of gestation has been shown to initiate labor and delivery (52). Interestingly, in the latter study, although the infusion of androgen was continuous and the increase in estrogen concentration in maternal serum was sustained over the 24-hour day, the switch from contractures to contractions occurred only around the hours of darkness. Furthermore, the switch could be abolished by the OT antagonist, $MPA^1D-Tyr(Et)^2Thr^4Orn^8$ oxytocin (Atosiban), suggesting that it may be driven by OT. A similar effect has been demonstrated using a continuous intraamniotic infusion of estrogen (11). Systemic infusion of estrogen does not precipitate labor and delivery in pregnant rhesus monkeys. These data further support a role for local paracrine actions of placental steroid hormones in the induction of labor in primates at term. Most likely, estrogens and progesterone act in concert to maintain phase 0 of parturition. Estrogens act, in part at least, by upregulating progesterone receptors directly via the estrogen response element on the progesterone receptor gene, thereby promoting progesterone responsiveness.

Oxytocin

Oxytocin is a potent endogenous uterotonic agent that is capable of stimulating uterine contractions at intravenous infusion rates of 1 to 2 mU/min at term (53). Maternally derived OT is synthesized in the hypothalamus and released from the posterior pituitary in a pulsatile fashion. Its biologic half-life is around 3 to 10 minutes, but appears to be shorter when higher doses are infused. OT is inactivated largely in the liver and kidney. During pregnancy, OT is also degraded by placental oxytocinase. The paracrine/autocrine mechanisms regulating OT and its receptor within the fetoplacental unit are central to the control of uterine contractions and parturition. Concentrations of OT in the maternal circulation do not change significantly during pregnancy or prior to the onset of labor, but do rise late in the second stage of labor (53,54). Myometrial OT receptor concentrations increase on average 100- to 200-fold during pregnancy, reaching a maximum during early labor (53–56). The increase in OT receptor concentrations is due to an increase in OT receptor gene expression. This is evidenced by a rise in OT receptor mRNA prior to the onset of labor. This increase is regulated by the sex steroids (estrogens increase and progesterone decreases OT receptor levels) and possibly by OT itself (53). This rise in receptor concentration is paralleled by an increase in uterine OT sensitivity during the second half of gestation. The avidity of the OT receptor does not change with pregnancy or labor, but there do appear to be regional differences in OT receptor distribution with large numbers of receptors in the fundal area and few receptors in the lower uterine segment and cervix (32). The genes for OT and its receptor are on human chromosomes 20 and 3, respectively (53), and the structure of the OT receptor gene was characterized by Kimura et al. (57) in 1992. An estrogen response element is not present in the human OT receptor gene, but three half-palindromic estrogen response element motifs have been identified.

Aside from the myometrium, specific high-affinity OT receptors have also been isolated from human amnion and decidua parietalis, but not decidua vera (32,53). Neither amnion nor decidual cells are contractile, and the action of OT on these tissues remains uncertain. OT in physiologic concentrations stimulates COX activity and increases $PGF_{2\alpha}$ production by decidual explants and/or dispersed decidual cells *in vitro* (32,58,59). It has been suggested that OT may play a dual role in the mechanism of parturition. It may act directly through both OT receptor-mediated and nonreceptor, voltage-mediated calcium channels to affect intracellular biochemical pathways and promote uterine contractions. It may also act indirectly through stimulation of amniotic and decidual PG production. Indeed, induction of labor at term is successful only when the OT infusion is associated with an increase in $PGF_{2\alpha}$ production in spite of seemly adequate uterine contractions in both induction failures and successes (32). High-dose OT infusions have been associated with adverse effects including fluid retention (caused by excessive binding to V_2 vasopressin receptors in the kidney) as well as natriuresis and hyponatremia (acting through specific renal OT receptors).

Studies on fetal pituitary OT production, the umbilical arteriovenous difference in plasma OT, amniotic fluid OT levels, and fetal urinary OT output demonstrate conclu-

sively that the fetus secretes OT toward the maternal side (53,60). Furthermore, the calculated OT secretion rates from the fetus suggest an increase from a baseline of 0.2 ± 1.0 mU/min prior to labor to around 3 mU/min after spontaneous labor. The latter is similar to the dose of OT that is normally administered to women to induce labor at term (2 to 8 mU/min). Using molecular biologic techniques, the amnion, chorion, decidua, and placenta have all been shown to express OT gene products (53). Therefore, although maternal serum OT levels are not increased with the onset and during the first stage of labor, OT derived from the fetus and possibly from local decidual and other uterine sources could act on the myometrial OT receptors in an endocrine/paracrine fashion to initiate and maintain effective uterine contractions. The decidual cells located closest to the myometrium (decidua parietalis) have the highest level of OT mRNA. Amniotic fluid OT (derived mainly from fetal urine) is associated with release of PGE_2 by amnion cells *in vitro,* and has been proposed as a potential fetal trigger for labor.

Corticotropin-Releasing Hormone (CRH)

Maternal plasma CRH concentrations increase progressively throughout the second and third trimesters of pregnancy, and correlate with increases in placental CRH mRNA and placental CRH content, suggesting that its origin is from placenta and/or fetal membranes (61,62). During the final 6 to 8 weeks of pregnancy, both at term and preterm, plasma levels of CRH increase in a dramatic fashion. Progesterone and NO decrease the release of CRH from placental tissue *in vitro* by interfering with CRH mRNA expression. Conversely, a number of agents such as inflammatory cytokines, catecholamines, acetylcholine, and some neuropeptides (including OT) have been shown to increase the release of CRH (8). During pregnancy, CRH bioactivity (i.e., its ability to promote ACTH release from the pituitary as well as its ability to stimulate PGE_2 release from decidual tissue) is decreased due to an increase in high-affinity CRH-binding protein (CRH-BP). In the last 3 to 5 weeks of gestation, CRH-BP concentrations fall, resulting in a rise in circulating free CRH (63,64). Furthermore, the CRH receptor has been identified in myometrium (65) and placenta (66) during pregnancy, and its avidity appears to increase late in pregnancy. Whether the actions of CRH are systemic or confined to the uterus, or both, is still uncertain. Interestingly, glucocorticoids have also been shown to increase CRH mRNA expression and CRH output by placental cells *in vitro* (67). Studies demonstrating an increase in circulating CRH (with a decrease in ACTH and cortisol) in women receiving antepartum glucocorticoids to promote fetal lung maturation suggest that this mechanism may also be operative *in vivo*. Once again, the source of the CRH in such patients appears to be the uteroplacental unit. There is evidence of markedly increased staining for immunoreactive CRH in the placentae of women treated with glucocorticoids as compared with elective cesarean section and vaginal delivery controls (67).

Glucocorticoids

Glucocorticoids are able to upregulate PGE_2 production by dispersed amnion cells *in vitro* (16,68). Whether this is by direct action on the amnion cells or indirectly through the upregulation of CRH expression by intrauterine tissues remains unclear. More recent data suggest that glucocorticoids (acting through specific glucocorticoid receptors and trophoblast-specific gene promotor regions that have been identified in amnion, chorionic trophoblast, and in decidual stromal cells) may upregulate COX-2 expression in the placenta (16). In addition, steroids are capable of decreasing 15-OH PGDH activity (and thereby PG metabolism and inactivation) in a dose-dependent fashion in dispersed trophoblast cells from both fetal membranes and placenta *in vitro* (8). The resultant increase in PGs in the fetal membranes near term may provide a mechanism whereby the maturing fetus could prepare the uterus for labor. The glucocorticoids cortisol and cortisone are interconverted by the enzyme, 11β-hydroxysteroid dehydrogenase (11β-HSD) (69). This enzyme exists as two isoforms: 11β-HSD-2 is unidirectional and predominates in the placenta where, among other functions, it prevents the transplacental passage of cortisol to the fetal compartment; 11β-HSD-1 is bidirectional and predominates in trophoblast cells in the choriodecidua, the same cells responsible for PG production in this tissue (70). An autocrine/paracrine regulatory mechanism in the placenta and fetal membranes involving glucocorticoids and PGs is proposed. Fetal pituitary-adrenal activity increases gradually over the last few weeks of gestation, and may act to fine-tune the time of onset of labor, rather than as an on/off switch as in sheep.

Parathyroid Hormone–Related Peptide (PTH-rP)

PTH-rP is a potent smooth muscle relaxant. PTH-rP mRNA is present in high levels in the myometrium in a number of species including humans, and can be stimulated in response to 17β-estradiol and myometrial stretch (71). Its role in human parturition remains unclear.

Luteinizing Hormone/Human Chorionic Gonadotropin (LH/hCG)

The heptahelical receptor for LH/hCG has been demonstrated in a number of extragonadal tissues including myometrial smooth muscle and blood vessels in the rat, rabbit, and pig. Levels of LH/hCG receptor mRNA in myometrium are greater before as compared with after the onset

of labor (8). LH/hCG acts to activate adenylyl cyclase by way of a plasma membrane receptor $G\alpha_s$-linked second messenger system to increase intracellular levels of cAMP, which favors uterine relaxation. In this way, LH/hCG may be important in maintaining uterine quiescence.

Relaxin is a member of the insulin-like growth factor family of proteins, and exists in two isoforms encoded by two separate genes (H1 and H2). Plasma levels of relaxin are greatest at 8 to 12 weeks' gestation (± 1 ng/mL), and decline thereafter to lower levels that persist to term (72). Plasma levels are thought to reflect production by the corpus luteum of the ovary (which expresses the H2 gene). Decidua and trophoblast express both H1 and H2 gene products, but their function in these tissues remains unclear. The membrane receptor for relaxin has yet to be identified. Relaxin appears to promote myometrial relaxation, and may have a role to play in cervical ripening and rupture of the fetal membranes.

Summary

Despite the volume of research, the factors responsible for the initiation and maintenance of human parturition at term remain enigmatic. It seems likely that a "parturition cascade" exists in the human (much like the "coagulation cascade"), which is responsible at term for the recruitment of interactive positive feed-forward loops and the removal of mechanisms responsible for pregnancy maintenance (Fig. 27.2). Given its teleologic importance, it is easy to envisage a parturition cascade with multiple redundant loops in order to ensure a fail-safe system to secure pregnancy success, and ultimately the preservation of the species. For example, multiple defects in estrogen synthesis have been identified (such as fetal adrenal hypoplasia, aromatase deficiency, sulfatase deficiency) in pregnancies that progress and deliver uneventfully at term, despite the proposed critical role of the steroid hormones in the mechanism of labor.

A further feature of this parturition cascade would be the ability of the fetoplacental unit to trigger labor prematurely if the intrauterine environment became hostile and threatened the well-being of the fetus. Preterm birth occurs in 7% to 10% of all deliveries, but accounts for over 85% of early neonatal morbidity and mortality (73). Such deliveries may represent a breakdown in the normal mechanisms responsible for maintaining uterine quiescence such as a functional deficiency of 15-OH PGDH that Challis and Gibb (8) believe may account for up to 15% of idiopathic preterm labor. Alternatively, such deliveries may represent a short-circuiting or overwhelming of the normal parturition cascade. For example, the release of large amounts of PGE_2 in the setting of intrauterine infection may overwhelm the 15-OH PGDH metabolizing capacity of the choriodecidua, thereby allowing PGE_2 to pass to the myometrium and initiate contractions. Preterm labor probably represents a *syndrome* rather than a diagnosis since the etiologies are varied.

A better understanding of the physiologic mechanisms responsible for the induction of labor at term would allow for the development of more appropriate and successful screening and treatment protocols for preterm labor. Research is focused primarily on understanding the interaction between these various hormones in the primate model.

THE CLINICAL MANAGEMENT OF NORMAL LABOR

Stages and Mechanics of Normal Labor at Term

Labor is the physiologic process by which the products of conception are passed from the uterus to the outside world. For clinical purposes, labor is divided into three stages. The first stage entails cervical dilatation in preparation for passage of the fetus. The second stage commences when the cervix achieves full dilatation (10 cm) and ends with delivery of the fetus. The third stage entails delivery of the placenta and fetal membranes.

Stages of Labor

The first stage of normal labor is further divided into phases according to the rate of cervical dilatation. The latent phase is characterized by slow cervical dilatation, whereas the active phase is associated with a greater rate of cervical dilatation. The active phase is further subdivided into an acceleration phase, a phase of maximum slope, and a deceleration phase (Fig. 27.5). These were originally described in the primigravida by Friedman (74) in 1955. He described

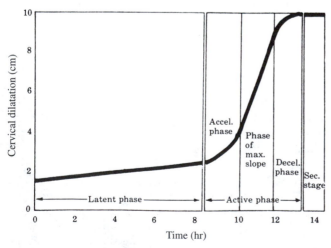

FIGURE 27.5. Composite of the average cervical dilatation curve for nulliparous labor. (From Friedman EA. *Labor: clinical evaluation and management*, 2nd ed. New York: Appleton-Century-Crofts, 1978, with permission.)

averages and a statistical maximum (2 standard deviations greater than the mean) for each phase. From the normal profile produced by Friedman, it is possible to identify the abnormal patterns of a prolonged latent phase, primary dysfunctional labor, and secondary arrest. A prolonged latent phase is characterized by a latent phase of ≥20 hours in the nulliparous patient or ≥14 hours in the multiparous patient (75). By definition, a diagnosis of primary dysfunctional labor is made when the active phase is entered and the rate of cervical dilatation is less than 2 standard deviations from the mean (i.e., ≤1.2 cm/hour for the primigravida, or ≤1.5 cm/hour for the multipara). Secondary arrest is defined as arrest of cervical dilatation after a period of normal active phase dilatation. The difficulty in identifying abnormal labor, as evident from these definitions, is that the diagnosis is retrospective. Therefore, the clinician managing the labor has to exercise vigilance, and have a mental image of the standard labor curve at all times when assessing the first stage. In clinical management, this task can be facilitated by the use of the partogram (76). The partogram is a graphical representation of the normal labor curve against which a patients' progress is plotted, so that a patient who is "falling off the curve" can easily be identified and appropriate measures taken. A hypothetical "action line" has been proposed by Studd (76) that attempts to define labor dystocia in primigravid patients. In the setting of adequate uterine contractions, a delay in cervical dilatation of ≥2 hours over that expected suggests labor dystocia and requires further evaluation.

The second stage of labor is characterized by descent of the presenting part through the maternal pelvis. This is assessed clinically by the position of the presenting part relative to the ischial spines. The mother can assume a more active role in the second stage, using maternal effort to aid descent of the fetus. In modern obstetric practice, the nulliparous patient is recommended to push for a maximum of 3 hours with regional anesthesia or 2 hours without regional anesthesia. The multiparous patient is recommended to push for a maximum of 1 hour without regional anesthesia or 2 hours with regional anesthesia (77). In reality, the achievement of full cervical dilatation is not a prerequisite for descent of the presenting part, and descent can commence in the first stage. However, no active intervention (either maternal expulsive efforts or obstetric maneuvers) should be attempted until full cervical dilatation has been achieved. The third stage of labor usually lasts less than 10 minutes, but up to 30 minutes may be allowed for delivery of the placenta and fetal membranes before active intervention is considered, as long as blood loss is not excessive.

Mechanics of Normal Labor at Term

The ability of the fetus to successfully negotiate the pelvis and deliver is dependent on the complex interaction of a number of variables. In classical obstetric teaching, this complex lexicon has been reduced to three main concepts: the powers, the passenger, and the passage. The powers consist of the forces generated by the uterine musculature, the passenger is the fetus, and the passage consists of the bony pelvis and the resistance provided by the soft tissues.

The Powers

Uterine activity is the most apparent mechanism of labor, and as such has been the subject of much study and analysis. Assessment of uterine activity has included simple observation, manual palpation, external objective assessment techniques (such as external guard-ring tocodynometry), and direct measurement of intrauterine pressure (using either internal manometry or pressure transducers). Uterine activity can be characterized by the frequency, amplitude, and duration of contractions. The introduction of intrauterine pressure transducers has enabled objective measurement and recording of uterine activity. Various units have been devised to objectively measure uterine activity. Montevideo units (the strength of contractions in millimeters of mercury multiplied by the frequency per 10 minutes), for example, measure frequency and average amplitude above basal tone (78). Alexandria units measure frequency, amplitude, and duration (79).

Despite technologic improvements in the measurement of intrauterine pressure, the definition of "adequate" uterine activity during normal labor remains unclear. Some practitioners rely on simple clinical techniques such as counting uterine contractions in any given time period. Classically, three to five contractions in 10 minutes has been used to define adequate labor, and this contraction pattern is seen in around 95% of women in spontaneous labor. In the active management of labor protocols, seven contractions in 15 minutes is judged as adequate (80). If an intrauterine pressure monitor is being used, 150 to 200 Montevideo units is deemed adequate (78). Perhaps the ultimate barometer of uterine activity, however, is the rate of cervical dilatation and descent of the presenting part that accompanies the contractions. In the setting of absolute cephalopelvic disproportion (CPD), worsening caput and molding of the fetal head without cervical effacement and dilatation suggests that the uterine contractions are probably sufficient to effect vaginal delivery if it were possible.

Despite being one of the simplest variables in labor to measure and manipulate, uterine activity has been subject only to simplistic scientific scrutiny. Investigators and observers of labor have, in general, focused on achieving "adequate" intensity of uterine activity with little regard to how this single variable interacts in the complex equation of normal labor. The classical lexicon of powers, passenger, and passage seems to imply a passive process, where uterine contractions push a rigid object through a fixed aperture. As such, the lexicon can be interpreted to suggest that

the more optimal the powers, the more likely a successful outcome. Indeed, the American College of Obstetricians and Gynecologists (ACOG) has recommended using the terms *hypotonic* and *hypertonic* to define patterns of labor (81). These designations, too, suggest that a relationship exists between uterine activity and progress in labor. There is no scientific data to support this inference (82). The concept of active management of labor has been based on the premise that optimizing uterine contractions in a nulliparous labor will improve the progress of labor and subsequent outcome. This premise will be reviewed in further detail below.

The Passenger

For the singleton fetus, there are two main variables that influence the course of normal labor: attitude of the presenting head (i.e., degree of flexion and/or extension) and absolute fetal size. Both of these variables may contribute to relative or absolute CPD. Flexion of the fetal head is important to facilitate engagement in the maternal pelvis. When the fetal chin is optimally flexed onto the chest, the suboccipitobregmatic diameter (9.5 cm) presents at the pelvic inlet. This is the smallest possible presenting diameter in the cephalic presentation. As the head deflexes (extends), the diameter presenting to the pelvic inlet progressively increases even before the malpresentations of brow and face are encountered, and may contribute to failure to progress in labor. Increased uterine activity in the early stages of labor may correct deflexion. Absolute fetal size may also contribute to failure to progress in labor. Fetal size can be estimated either clinically or with real-time ultrasound, but both are subject to a large degree of error. The assessment of fetal size and pelvic capacity, and prediction of success in labor based on such estimates, is at best an inexact science. Progress in labor is the best test of whether a vaginal delivery can be effected or not.

The size, presentation, and lie of the fetus can be assessed by abdominal palpation. The *lie* of the fetus refers to the longitudinal axis of the fetus relative to the longitudinal axis of the uterus, and can be longitudinal, transverse, or oblique. Fetal *presentation* can be either cephalic or breech, referring to the pole of the fetus that overlies the pelvic inlet. The *position* of the fetus is the relationship of a nominated site of the presenting part to a denominating location on the maternal pelvis, and can be assessed most accurately on bimanual examination. In a cephalic presentation, the nominated site is the occiput (e.g., right occiput anterior, ROA); in the breech, the nominated site usually the sacrum (e.g., right sacrum anterior, RSA). The various positions of a cephalic presentation are illustrated in Fig. 27.6. The *station* refers to the level of the presenting part in relation to the maternal pelvis. The ischial spines are taken as the denominator in the pelvis, and the presenting part is assessed in relation to these in centimeters, with above nominated as negative and below as positive.

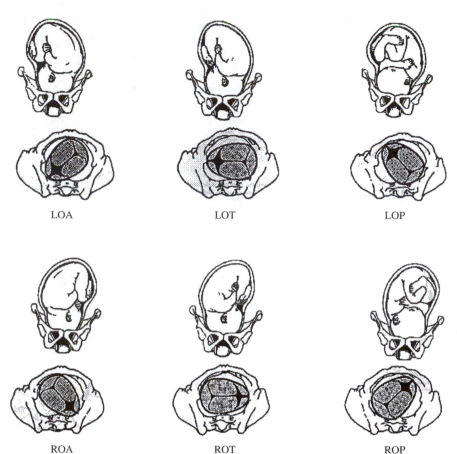

LOA   LOT   LOP

ROA   ROT   ROP

FIGURE 27.6. Fetal presentations and positions in labor. LOA, left occiput anterior; LOT, left occiput transverse; LOP, left occiput posterior; ROA, right occiput anterior; ROT, right occiput transverse; ROP, right occiput posterior.

The Passage

The bony pelvis is composed of the sacrum, ilium, ischium, and pubis. The pelvis is divided into the greater and lesser pelvis by the pelvic brim, which is demarcated by the sacral promontory, the anterior ala of the sacrum, the arcuate line of the ilium, the pectineal line of the pubis, and the pubic crest culminating in the symphysis. The pelvic inlet is largest in its transverse diameter (usually ≥12 cm). The obstetric conjugate (the distance from the sacral promontory to the inferior margin of the symphysis pubis as assessed on bimanual examination) is a clinical representation of the anteroposterior diameter of the pelvic inlet. This is the smallest diameter of the inlet, and usually measures around 10 to 11 cm. The true conjugate of the pelvic inlet is the distance from the sacral promontory to the superior aspect of the symphysis pubis. This measurement cannot be made clinically, but can be estimated by subtracting 1.5 to 2.0 cm from the obstetric conjugate. The limiting factor in the midpelvis is the diameter between the ischial spines, which is usually the smallest diameter of the pelvis but should be greater than 10 cm. The pelvic outlet is rarely of clinical significance. The anteroposterior diameter from the coccyx to the symphysis pubis is usually around 13 cm, and the transverse diameter between the ischial tuberosities around 8 cm.

The shape of the pelvis can be classified into one or more of four broad categories: gynecoid, android, anthropoid, and platypelloid. These were initially described by Caldwell and Moloy (83) in 1933. The gynecoid pelvis is the classical female shape with an oval-shaped inlet, diverging midpelvic side walls, and far-spaced ischial spines. The android pelvis is male in pattern with a heart-shaped inlet, prominent sacral promontory and ischial spines, shallow sacral hollow, and converging midpelvic side walls. The anthropoid pelvis has an exaggerated oval shape to the inlet with the largest diameter being anteroposterior, and with limited anterior capacity to the pelvis. The platypelloid pelvis is a broad flat pelvis with the inlet again an exaggerated oval shape, but with the largest diameter being the transverse diameter.

Pelvic soft tissues may provide resistance in both the first and second stages of labor. In the first stage, resistance is offered primarily by the cervix; in the second stage, it is the muscles of the pelvic floor. Despite the first stage of labor being dedicated to observation of cervical effacement and dilatation, the concept that the cervix may provide resistance to the progress of labor has not been widely popularized. However, as far back as 1975, Crawford (84) suggested that rapid labors may result from low pelvic resistance rather than from high myometrial activity. It has also been observed that intrauterine pressures are lower when the cervix has been softened with PGs rather than when OT alone is used to augment labor (85). It is thought that, in the second stage of labor, the resistance of the pelvic musculature plays an important role in the rotation and movement of the presenting part through the pelvis. Excessive resistance, however, may contribute to failure to progress in labor.

Cardinal Movements in Labor

The mechanics of labor can be divided into seven discrete cardinal movements: engagement, descent, flexion, internal rotation, extension, external rotation, and expulsion. The presenting part is said to be engaged when the widest diameter has entered the pelvic inlet. In the cephalic presentation, the widest diameter is the biparietal diameter; in the breech, it is the bitrochanteric diameter. Engagement of the presenting part can be assessed abdominally or vaginally. With a cephalic presentation, engagement is achieved when only two fifths of the fetal head are palpable abdominally, or when the presenting part is at zero station on bimanual examination (i.e., at the level of the ischial spines). Descent refers to the downward passage of the presenting part through the pelvis, which classically begins during the deceleration phase of the first stage of labor and continues throughout the second stage. Flexion of the fetal head occurs passively with descent due to the shape of the bony pelvis and the resistance offered by the soft tissues of the pelvic floor. The result of flexion is to present the smallest diameter of the fetal head (the suboccipitobregmatic diameter) for optimal passage through the pelvis. Internal rotation refers to rotation of the presenting part from the transverse to the anteroposterior diameter as it passes through the true pelvis. This is again a passive movement resulting from the shape of the pelvis and the pelvic floor musculature. Due to the angle of inclination between the maternal lumbar spine and pelvic inlet, the fetal head engages in an asynclitic fashion (i.e., with one parietal eminence lower than the other). With uterine contractions, the leading parietal eminence descends and is first to engage the pelvic floor. As the uterus relaxes, the pelvic floor musculature causes the fetal head to rotate until it is no longer asynclitic. Extension is the continued movement of the presenting part under the symphysis pubis. In the cephalic presentation, this is achieved by full extension of the fetal head. External rotation, also referred to as restitution, is the return of the fetal head to the correct anatomic position in relation to the fetal torso. This can occur to either side depending on the orientation of the fetus. This again is a passive movement dependent on the tone of the fetal musculature. Expulsion refers to delivery of the rest of the fetus.

Clinical Assistance at Delivery

When the fetal head crowns and delivery is imminent, pressure from the accoucheur's hand is used to hold the head flexed and to control delivery, thereby preventing precipitous expulsion, which has been associated with perineal tears as well as intracranial trauma. If there is a delay in delivery of the fetal head, a modified Ritgen maneuver may be attempted. Using a sterile towel, the fetal chin is palpated through the perineum or rectum, and upward pressure is applied. Once the fetal head is delivered, the mouth and pharynx can be gently suctioned. Care should be taken not to suction too vigorously as posterior pharyngeal stimulation can cause a vagal response and fetal bradycardia. If a nuchal cord is present, it should be reduced at this time. If too tight for reduction, the umbilical cord can be double clamped and cut.

Following external rotation, a hand is placed on each parietal eminence and the anterior shoulder is delivered with the next contraction by downward traction toward the mother's sacrum. In this way, the anterior shoulder is encouraged to slip under the pubis. The posterior shoulder is then delivered by upward traction. These movements should be performed with as little downward or upward force as possible to avoid perineal injury and/or traction injuries to the brachial plexus. Once the shoulders are delivered, expulsion of the torso invariably occurs without difficulty. The infant should be supported at all times. The umbilical cord should be double clamped and cut. The third stage of labor can be managed either passively or actively. Passive management is characterized by patiently awaiting the signs of placental separation; namely, apparent lengthening of the umbilical cord, a "separation" bleed, and a change in the shape and consistency of the uterine fundus. In active management, OT can be administered (either intramuscularly, intravenously, or infused into the umbilical vein) to shorten the stage and reduce blood loss. The placenta can be delivered using the Brandt-Andrews maneuver of controlled cord traction in which an abdominal hand secures the uterine fundus, thereby preventing uterine inversion, while the other hand exerts sustained downward traction on the umbilical cord. At the end of the third stage, the placenta and membranes should be examined to ensure that they are complete, and the number of blood vessels in the umbilical cord should be recorded.

The routine use of episiotomy in obstetric practice to enlarge the soft tissue outlet is discouraged. In selected instances, however, such as prevention of an imminent extensive tear, to expedite delivery in the setting of fetal distress in the second stage, and in association with an instrumental delivery, episiotomy may be useful. Median episiotomies are preferred in the United States, but have been associated with a paradoxical increased incidence of fourth-degree lacerations (i.e., rectal injuries) (86). Mediolateral episiotomies are favored in Europe, and do appear to decrease the number of fourth-degree extensions. Chronic complications such as unsatisfactory anatomic results and inclusions within the scar may be more common with medi-

TABLE 27.1. PATIENT ASSESSMENT PRIOR TO INDUCTION OF LABOR

Confirm indication for induction
Review for contraindications to labor and/or vaginal delivery
Confirm gestational age
Estimate fetal weight (clinically or by ultrasound)
Determine fetal position
Assess shape and adequacy of bony pelvis (clinical pelvimetry)
Assess cervical exam (Bishop score)
Confirm fetal well-being
Assess need for documentation of fetal lung maturity
Review risks and benefits of induction of labor with patient

olateral episiotomies, as is the blood loss at the time of procedure. Although it is often said that mediolateral episiotomy causes more pain in the postpartum period than medial episiotomy, and that it is associated with prolonged dyspareunia, the literature does not support this statement (87).

Cervical Ripening and Induction of Labor at Term

The goal of induction of labor is to eliminate the maternal or fetal risks from continuation of the pregnancy, while minimizing the chance of an operative delivery. The risks and benefits of induction should be weighed carefully against the chance of a successful vaginal delivery. A firm indication for delivery is a prerequisite for induction. With recent technologic advances, the therapeutic armamentarium available to the obstetrician has increased, as has the temptation to intervene. In the absence of a clear indication, intervention may not be in the best interest of the mother or fetus. A number of factors should be documented prior to induction of labor (Table 27.1).

The appropriate timing for induction of labor is the point at which the benefits to the mother and/or the fetus are greater if the pregnancy is interrupted than if the pregnancy is continued, and is gestational-age dependent. Indications and contraindications for induction of labor at term are detailed in Tables 27.2 and 27.3, respectively. Having made the decision to induce labor, the choice of induction technique should be individualized. A single technique is rarely effective on its own, and a combination of maneuvers may be required. The options available are reviewed in Table 27.4.

The success of an induction attempt is determined, in part, by the initial state of the cervix. When induction of labor is attempted against an unfavorable cervix, the likelihood of a successful outcome is reduced (88,89). In 1964, Bishop (90) designed a scoring system for cervical evaluation at elective induction of labor. This scoring system is based on the properties of the cervix that change with "ripening," namely, dilatation, effacement, station, consistency, and position (Table 27.5). Bishop demonstrated that when the cervical score exceeded 8, the incidence of vaginal delivery subsequent to induction was similar to that for spontaneous labor. ACOG has since recommended that a Bishop's score of ≥6 be deemed favorable and likely to result in a successful induction of labor (Table 27.6) (91). It would therefore seem logical that enhancement of cervical maturation would be an appropriate first step toward induction of labor when the cervix is unfavorable. Cervical maturation or "ripening" describes the complex series of hormonally mediated biochemical events that alter both cervical collagen and ground substance, resulting in a softer and more pliable cervix prior to and during labor (Table 27.7).

TABLE 27.2. INDICATIONS FOR INDUCTION OF LABOR AT TERM

Absolute Indications	Relative Indications
Maternal indications	
Preeclampsia/eclampsia	Chronic hypertension
Pregnancy-induced hypertension	Gestational diabetes
Maternal medical problems	Logistic factors
Diabetes mellitus	Risk of rapid labor
Chronic renal disease	Distance from the hospital
Chronic pulmonary disease	Psychosocial indications
Fetal indications	
Chorioamnionitis	Premature rupture of membranes
Abnormal antepartum testing	Fetal macrosomia
Intrauterine growth restriction	Fetal demise
Postterm pregnancy (>42 weeks)	Previous stillbirth
Isoimmunization	Fetus with a major congenital anomaly
Uteroplacental indications	
Placental abruption	Unexplained oligohydramnios

TABLE 27.3. CONTRAINDICATIONS FOR INDUCTION OF LABOR AT TERM

Absolute Contraindications	Relative Contraindications
Maternal contraindications	
Active genital herpes	Cervical carcinoma
Serious chronic medical conditions	Pelvic deformities
Fetal contraindications	
Malpresentation	Fetal macrosomia
Extreme fetal distress	
Uteroplacental contraindications	
Cord prolapse	Low-lying placenta
Placenta previa	Unexplained vaginal bleeding
Vasa previa	Cord presentation
Prior high vertical hysterotomy ("classical" cesarean section)	Myomectomy involving the uterine cavity

A number of agents are available to facilitate this maturation (Table 27.4).

Prostaglandins

The use of PGs to induce cervical ripening in cases where the cervical score is unfavorable (Bishop's score <6) would seem appropriate to mimic the events that occur in spontaneous labor. The introduction of PGs to promote cervical ripening occurred in the 1970s, and initial studies were favorable. Calder et al. (92) reported on the use of a gel preparation of PGE_2 (240 to 280 μg) administered extraamniotically to ripen the cervix 1 day prior to induction. In their series, the rate of failed inductions (defined as the inability to establish labor) was 0.8%. Other investigators reported on the use of a 500-μg dose of PGE_2 placed endocervically 1 day prior to induction, and reported a failed induction rate of 6.3% (93). O'Herlihy and MacDonald (94) used a 2-mg PGE_2 gel preparation and reported a failed induction rate of 1.5%. Similarly, in an early trial using 3 mg of PGE_2 in lipid vaginal pessaries repeated in 12 hours, a failure of induction in 5.5% of cases was reported (95). The failed inductions seen in the setting of an unfavorable cervix may be due to an insensitivity of the cervix to PGs, or to inadequate delivery of PGs to their target organs. In a recent meta-analysis of all randomized, placebo-controlled trials on the effect of PGs on preinduction cervical ripening and on subsequent induction success, Keirse (96) demonstrated that PGs administered by any route improved the rate of spontaneous vaginal delivery, and decreased the rate of both cesarean section and operative vaginal delivery.

TABLE 27.4. METHODS OF CERVICAL RIPENING AND INDUCTION OF LABOR AT TERM

Techniques for Preinduction Cervical Ripening	Initiation and/or Augmentation of Myometrial Contractility
Hormonal techniques	Amniotomy
Prostaglandins	
PGE_2 (dinoprostone)	Hormonal techniques
PGE_1 (misoprostol)	Oxytocin
Oxytocin	Prostaglandins
Estrogen	$PGF_{2\alpha}$ (dinoprost)
RU-486 (mifepristone) (?)	PGE_2
Relaxin (?)	PGE_1 (misoprostol) (?)
DHEAS (?)	RU-486 (mifepristone) (?)
Membrane stripping	
Mechanical dilators	
Hygroscopic dilators (laminaria, lamicel, dilapan)	
Balloon catheter (alone, with traction, with infusion)	
Amniotomy	

DHEAS, dehydroepiandrosterone sulfate; PG, prostaglandin.

TABLE 27.5. ASSESSMENT OF CERVICAL STATUS BY MODIFIED BISHOP SCORE

	Score			
	0	1	2	3
Dilatation (cm)	0	1–2	3–4	≥5
Effacement (%)	0–30	40–50	60–70	≥80
Station	−3	−2	−1 or 0	≥1+
Consistency	Firm	Medium	Soft	
Cervical position	Posterior	Midposition	Anterior	

TABLE 27.7. HORMONAL AND BIOCHEMICAL CHANGES CHARACTERIZING CERVICAL RIPENING

Decreased	Collagen production and content
	Dermatan and chondroitin sulfate in cervical ground substance
	Progesterone
Increased	Collagenase and other proteolytic enzyme activity
	Collagen degradation
	Proteoglycan production
	Hyaluronic acid in ground substance
	Phospholipase activity and prostaglandin E_2 production
	17β-Estradiol
	Relaxin (?)

Most of the initial research on cervical ripening focused on PGE_2, which was known to be more potent than $PGF_{2\alpha}$ in this regard (97,98). Gastrointestinal side effects from PGE_2 were reported with all routes of administration, but appeared to be minimized with vaginal administration. The most commonly used PGE_2 preparation is 0.5 mg dinoprostone gel (Prepidil), which received Food and Drug Administration (FDA) approval for this indication in the United States in 1992. Local application of PGE_2 gel has now become the "gold standard" for cervical ripening in clinical practice. Whether such agents should be placed intracervically or in the posterior fornix of the vagina is debated. It has been suggested that PGE_2 will have its optimal effect if administered in the cervical canal since this is its primary site of action (99). A large multicenter randomized trial with 285 participants was carried out in Europe to compare the endocervical and vaginal routes of administration (100). The findings showed that, while the endocervical PGE_2 had a more marked effect on cervical ripening, there was no significant difference in labor or delivery outcomes. This decision is therefore best left to the discretion of the individual practitioner. In 1995, a sustained release preparation of PGE_2 (Cervidil) was approved by the FDA. The advantage of this preparation is that, unlike the gel, it can be easily removed if clinical complications such as tachysystole or uterine hypertonus ensue (101).

More recent attention has been focused on the use of the PGE_1 analogues, such as misoprostol (Cytotec), for cervical ripening. Although such preparations are FDA approved only for the treatment of peptic ulcer disease and have not received approval for use during pregnancy, they have been used for induction of labor. They can be adminis-

TABLE 27.6. POTENTIAL BENEFITS OF PREINDUCTION CERVICAL RIPENING

Fewer failed inductions
Fewer serial inductions
Better timing of delivery
Shorter hospital stay
Lower fetal and maternal morbidity
Lower medical costs
Lower cesarean section rates (?)

tered either vaginally [50 μg every 3 hours to a maximum of six doses (102), or 25 μg every 3 hours to a maximum of eight doses (103)] or orally [50 μg every 4 hours (104)]. To date, there has been no evidence of fetotoxic, teratogenic, or carcinogenic effects in animal studies (105). Results of clinical trials suggest that misoprostol is as effective as PGE_2 for cervical ripening and labor induction (102–104), and at least two groups have found it to be more effective than PGE_2 (106,107). In addition, the cost of misoprostol is a fraction of that of any of the PGE_2 preparations. The optimal dosage regimen for PGE_1 has yet to be determined. However, the less-frequent, higher-dosage schedules appear to be associated with shorter intervals to delivery, less requirement for OT infusion, and fewer failed inductions (108). On a cautionary note, the authors would like to emphasize that this drug is not approved for use in pregnancy, and that a higher prevalence of tachysystole and meconium passage has been reported with its use (102).

Until recently, induction of labor had been undertaken exclusively on an inpatient basis with close and continuous monitoring of both mother and fetus. However, as newer and safer pharmacologic agents have been developed, consideration has been given to outpatient management. Indeed, outpatient low-dose PGE_2 gel has been shown to be both effective and safe for initiating labor in patients with an unfavorable cervix at term (109). With increasing attention being given to issues of cost-containment in clinical practice, and with the increasing availability of low-dose and oral PG preparations, it is likely that this approach will be seen with increasing frequency in the future.

The rate of cesarean birth in the United States rose from 5.5% in 1970 to 24.7% in 1988 (110,111). More recently, a modest decrease has been noted with a reported national cesarean section rate of 22.8% in 1993 (111). This decrease has been attributed, in part at least, to more liberal use of the practice of vaginal birth after cesarean (VBAC). The primary risk associated with VBAC is uterine rupture. Despite anecdotal reports in the literature of uterine rupture in association with PG gel (112,113), the precise incidence of this complication remains unclear. To address this question, MacKenzie et al. (114) carried out a large prospective trial of 143 consecutive patients with previous cesarean section undergoing induction of labor with vaginal PGE$_2$ gel. In this series, 76% of patients delivered vaginally including 68% of cases with an unfavorable cervix. There were no cases of uterine rupture. The authors conclude that the use of local PGs for induction of labor in women with a previous cesarean section and unfavorable cervix is a safe and viable alternative to elective repeat cesarean section.

Oxytocin

Continuous low-dose (1 to 4 mU/min) OT infusion has been shown to be effective in preinduction cervical ripening (115,116). This approach may be as effective as PGE$_2$ gel (117), although at least one study has shown it to be less effective (118). A number of different low-dose OT protocols have been investigated. Blakemore et al. (119) studied the effect of hourly versus quarter-hourly incremental increases (0.5 mU/min) in OT infusion on labor progress and outcome. This study suggested that a slow rate of increase in OT administration was as effective for inducing labor as a fast rate of increase, while at the same time minimizing OT requirements. Some investigators have tried to mimic the physiologic pulsatile nature of OT secretion. Willcourt et al. (120) reported on a prospective trial in which 310 nulliparous women were randomized to continuous intravenous OT (either low-dose or "aggressive" administration) or pulsatile infusion regulated by a computer-controlled pump. The efficacy of labor induction and the perinatal outcome were similar in all three groups. However, the group receiving pulsatile OT required only 20% of the dosage required by the women receiving continuous infusion. The advantages of OT lie in its cost and familiarity for the clinician. However, its use necessitates continuous fetal monitoring and an intravenous infusion, both of which increase ancillary and staffing requirements. As for adverse effects, maternal water intoxication is exceedingly unlikely at this dosage, but the incidence of neonatal hyperbilirubinemia has been shown to be higher with the use of OT than with PGs (121). Overall, PGE$_2$ gel is probably a better agent for preinduction cervical ripening than OT, being equally if not more effective, simpler to administer, and possibly safer for the fetus. However, the use of either continuous low-dose or pulsatile OT is still considered safe, and is a reasonable treatment alternative in most circumstances.

Progesterone Receptor Antagonists

RU-486 (Mifepristone) is a steroid receptor antagonist that affects the action of both progesterone and glucocorticoids. ZK98299 (Onapristone) is a more selective progesterone receptor antagonist. RU-486 has been shown to cause uter-

ine contractions and cervical dilatation (122–124). In a randomized, double-blind study of 94 patients comparing RU-486 with placebo for induction of labor in the setting of third trimester intrauterine fetal demise, RU-486 successfully induced labor in 63% of cases as compared with 17.4% in the placebo group (125). RU-486 induction may also lower the cesarean section rate (124). In 1992, Frydman et al. (126) randomized 120 women, all of whom had singleton pregnancies of ≥37.5 weeks' gestation and one or more firm indications for induction of labor, to receive either RU-486 (200 mg) or placebo on days 1 and 2 of a 4-day observation period prior to planned induction on day 4. Eight patients developed fetal distress within the observation period and were excluded from the analysis; 41 of the remaining 112 women (36.6%) went into spontaneous labor, 31 in the RU-486–pretreated group and 10 in the placebo group ($p < .001$). In addition, of those women who delivered vaginally, women in the RU-486–pretreated group needed lower doses of OT during labor. The authors conclude that RU-486 is a safe and effective agent for the initiation of labor at term. More recently, RU-486 has been studied as an agent for labor induction after cesarean section in a placebo-controlled fashion (127). In this study, significantly more women went into spontaneous labor with RU-486, and their OT requirements in labor were again less. There were no differences in terms of mode of delivery or neonatal outcome. Progesterone receptor antagonists may therefore have a role to play in cervical ripening and/or induction of labor at term. More clinical studies are awaited.

Nonpharmacologic Methods

In the past, the use of physical techniques for cervical ripening was referred to as accouchement forcé. A number of such agents are still in use (Table 27.4). When compared with no preinduction ripening, an intracervical balloon catheter has been shown to significantly shorten the induction to delivery interval and to increase the rate of vaginal delivery (128). More recently, a randomized comparison between intracervical PGE$_2$ gel and intracervical Foley catheter for cervical ripening at term showed them to be equally effective. In addition, there was no difference in side effect profile, intrapartum complications, or mode of delivery (129). Hygroscopic dilators—including laminaria (desiccated seaweed), Dilapan (polyacrilonitrile), and lamicel (magnesium sulfate in polyvinyl alcohol)—rely on absorption of water to swell and forcibly dilate the cervix, and have also been found to be effective when compared with PGE$_2$ gel (130). A significant disadvantage of mechanical dilators, however, is patient discomfort, both at the time of insertion and with progressive cervical dilatation. With equally efficacious pharmacologic agents available, there is no obvious advantage in the routine use of mechanical dilators. However, in specific clinical situations (such as asthma, glaucoma, or hepatic, pulmonary, or renal disease, where PGs should be avoided) or where other products are unavailable due to reasons of supply or cost, mechanical dilators can be used both safely and effectively.

Amniotomy

Artificial rupture of the membranes (low amniotomy) is another nonpharmacologic method of labor induction. Since a degree of cervical dilatation is necessary to perform the procedure, amniotomy can only be carried out once the cervix is favorable. Despite its wide acceptance, there is a paucity of scientific literature on this topic (131). Keirse and Chalmers (132) suggest that amniotomy alone is often insufficient to induce labor, but may be more effective if used in combination with OT. However, other investigators have demonstrated that amniotomy alone is adequate to induce labor, that the interval to delivery is shortened by around 0.8 to 2.3 hours, and that it may be more acceptable to the patient than other forms of labor induction (6,131,133). Amniotomy does not appear to lower the rate of cesarean section (131,133). There are a small number of controlled trials in the literature comparing amniotomy alone to combined amniotomy and OT (131,133–136). All of these trials report a shorter induction to delivery time with combined amniotomy and OT. However, as the most recent of these studies (136) points out, the differences between these two regimens are minimal with no apparent difference in safety profile. Contraindications to amniotomy include human immunodeficiency virus (HIV) and active perineal herpes simplex infection, and possibly viral hepatitis. Low amniotomy does not increase the likelihood of umbilical cord prolapse (137).

Sweeping of Fetal Membranes

Sweeping or stripping of the fetal membranes (i.e., digital separation of the chorioamniotic membranes from the lower uterine segment) is a suggested method of inducing labor at term, and was first described in 1810 (138). It is believed to work by releasing endogenous PGs. Several trials have suggested benefit of this procedure (139–141), but the majority of these studies are flawed in terms of their study design and/or analysis. More recent studies suggest no significant increase in the proportion of women going into spontaneous labor within 7 days (142).

Augmentation of Labor at Term

There are two established methods of managing labor at term: traditional management and active management. The major differences between these two approaches are in the definition of failure to progress and in the OT protocol chosen for labor augmentation if progress is deemed to be unsatisfactory. Traditional management uses a lower-dose OT regimen as compared with active management protocols, with longer intervals between dose increments. Low-dose OT infusion was first described by Seitchik and Castillo (143) in 1982. In this study, the low-dose OT regimen (starting at an infusion rate of 1 mU/min and increasing by 1 to 2 mU/min at intervals of not less than 30 minutes) significantly shortened the interval from initiation of OT augmentation to full dilation as compared with physician-directed regimens. The most significant difference was the rate of increment of OT infusion. This low-dose OT protocol has subsequently been endorsed by ACOG (144). Further work by Seitchik and colleagues (145) described the pharmacokinetics of OT and its effect on uterine contractility. They found that around 40 minutes was required for OT to reach a steady state in the plasma, and that this corresponded to maximal uterine contractility, irrespective of dose. However, more recent investigation has revealed that peripheral plasma levels of OT may reflect only the rate and dose of OT infusion, and may not accurately reflect uterine activity or progress in labor (146).

There has been considerable debate as to whether a low-dose or high-dose OT protocol is more effective for augmentation of labor at term, but there are few publications that directly compare these two protocols. In 1995, Xenakis et al. (147) published a comparison of 310 women randomized to either low-dose or high-dose OT for labor augmentation at term. They found that high-dose OT (starting at an infusion rate of 4 mU/min and increasing by 4 mU/min every 15 minutes "until adequate uterine contractility was obtained") shortened the length of labor and lowered the rate of cesarean section in both nulliparous and multiparous patients. However, as will be discussed below, there is considerable debate as to whether the OT regimen chosen actually changes obstetric outcome or whether it merely produces the same outcome but in a shorter period of time.

Active Management of Labor

Active management of labor describes a pragmatic protocol of clinical management that focuses on the first stage of labor. It is based on the premise that efficient uterine action is the key to success in labor, that by foreshortening the first stage of labor the outcome of the second stage can be improved (80). Active management protocols apply specifically to nulliparous patients in spontaneous labor with a cephalic presentation. They are not applicable to the multiparous patient, to patients undergoing induction of labor, or the management of patients with a prior cesarean section. The popularized view of the active management of labor is that of a high-dose OT regimen. However, there are many other important components to this approach of management. These components can be broadly classified into medical and logistic elements. The medical components consist of two main cornerstones of management: the diagnosis of labor, and the early diagnosis of inefficient uterine activity. The definition of labor is based on the presence of regular, painful contractions in conjunction with at least one further finding of either complete cervical effacement or bloody show, and/or rupture of the fetal membranes. The early diagnosis of inefficient uterine activity is made if the patient does not achieve and maintain a cervical dilatation rate of ≥ 1.0 cm/hour. If the diagnosis of inefficient uterine activity is made, augmentation with OT is instituted at a rate of 6 mU/min, and increased by the same amount every 15 minutes until a uterine contraction frequency of seven contractions per 15 minutes is achieved or the maximum OT infusion rate of 40 mU/min is reached. The logistic component of the active management protocol aims to allay patient fear and anxiety. Emphasis has been placed on antenatal education with a view to realistic expectations for the patient, close supervision by a senior obstetrician, and one-on-one nursing care. An emphasis on peer review of all cesarean sections was highlighted in the original protocol.

Although the initial objective with active management was to shorten the length of nulliparous labor, it has attracted much attention for its apparent ability to lower the cesarean section rates. The National Maternity Unit in Dublin, Ireland, which pioneered this method of labor management in 1968, has maintained a low cesarean section rate, with statistics from 1980 reporting an overall cesarean section rate of 5.5% for nulliparous women (148). Since the introduction of this management protocol, institutions around the world have implemented a similar style of management, some of which have reported a decrease in cesarean births (149–153). However, in terms of the effect of this protocol on cesarean section rates, there have been only two randomized trials comparing the active management of labor with preexisting management strategies (152,153). In 1992, Lopez-Zeno et al. (152) reported a controlled trial carried out in the United States in which 705 nulliparous, term, singleton pregnancies were randomized to either active management or to a more traditional management protocol. The active management protocol was similar to that carried out in previous trials with strict criteria for the diagnosis of labor, amniotomy within an hour of labor onset, augmentation when cervical dilatation was not maintained at ≥ 1.0 cm/hour, and a nearly identical OT regimen to that detailed above (initial infusion rate of 6 mU/min, which was increased by the same amount every 15 minutes, except that the maximum OT infusion rate was 36 mU/min). Less emphasis was placed on antenatal education and individualized obstetric nursing care than in the original Dublin studies. Results of this trial suggested that the active management group had a 26% reduction in the rate of cesarean sections when compared with controls [10.5% vs. 14.1%; odds ratio, 0.57; 95% confidence interval (CI), 0.36 to 0.95]. The length of labor was also decreased by an average of 1.66 hours in the active management group, and there was a decrease in maternal infectious

morbidity. There was no other difference in maternal or neonatal morbidity.

The second randomized trial, that of Frigoletto et al. (153) in 1995, adhered more strictly to the logistic concerns of the active management protocol as detailed above, with greater patient participation, antenatal classes, improved patient education, and individualized nursing. The OT augmentation protocol was slightly different from the study by Lopez-Zeno et al., with a starting rate of 4 mU/min and a 4 mU/min incremental rate every 15 minutes to a maximum of 40 mU/min. The studies were otherwise almost identical. A total of 1,934 nulliparous, low-risk women were randomly assigned to either active management or usual care prior to 30 weeks' gestation. Outcome data included cesarean section rates, as well as measures of maternal and neonatal morbidity and mortality. Results showed that the cesarean section rates were similar between the two groups (19.4% vs. 19.5%) (153). Again, the length of labor and infectious morbidity were decreased with active management.

The evidence regarding cesarean section rates and active management of labor is therefore contradictory. Multivariate analysis by the Oxford Collaborative Group (154) aimed at distinguishing the individual components of the active management of labor strategy showed that OT augmentation (either on its own or in combination with amniotomy) did not reduce the rate of cesarean delivery. The authors did find, interestingly, that psychological support during labor was associated with a decrease in operative delivery, but only when the patient's partner was not present. In support of the argument that active management does not decrease the cesarean section rate, attention has been drawn to centers with similar cesarean section rates to those reported in the original active management studies using a minimal intervention management style (155,156).

Regardless of the effect on cesarean section rates, the active management strategy is associated with a shortening in the duration of labor. The reason for this is unclear. It may be due to the influence of a supportive "doula" or midwife-like figure, to the lower incidence of epidural anesthesia, to the more aggressive OT augmentation protocol, or simply to delayed diagnosis of labor. It has also been suggested that the aggressive introduction of high-dose OT may overcome early (and subclinical) labor dystocia before uterine infection and fatigue make it less responsive to augmentation (157).

Intrapartum Fetal Monitoring

Fetal morbidity and mortality can occur as a consequence of labor, regardless of the risk status of the mother. This observation has led to the development of techniques of intrapartum surveillance in an attempt to minimize poor obstetric outcome. Intrapartum fetal surveillance may range from simple bedside observation to the use of highly sophisticated technology (Table 27.8).

Intrapartum Fetal Cardiotocography

Early techniques concentrated on observation of the fetal heart rate. The first documentation of the fetal heart rate was reported by Jean Alexandre Le Jumeau in a paper entitled "Mémoir sue l'Auscultation Appliquée l'Étude de la Grossesse" presented to the Royal Academy of Medicine in Paris in 1822. In 1833, Kennedy (158), a Dublin obstetrician, recorded in detail the characteristic features of the fetal heart rate in his landmark publication, *Observations on Obstetric Auscultation.* Originally, observation was limited to documentation of fetal cardiac activity and estimation of baseline heart rate. However, with the development of electronic devices to produce a continuous graphic recording of fetal heart rate, analysis was increased in sophistication. A fetal electrode for the continuous monitoring of fetal heart rate was introduced by Hon in 1963 (159). Doppler technology, which was developed shortly thereafter, made external fetal heart analysis possible. The less invasive nature of Doppler technology led to its more widespread use. By 1979, an estimated 60% of American obstetricians believed that continuous electronic fetal monitoring should be used during labor (160). Today, this practice is almost universal in the United States.

Characteristics of Intrapartum Fetal Heart Rate

Various characteristics of the fetal heart rate are observed and used in clinical interpretation. The fetal heart rate does not exist in isolation, and interpretation of the fetal heart rate tracing should always take into account the underlying clinical risk factors and drug therapy (Table 27.9). Baseline fetal heart rate refers to the dominant reading usually taken over a period of ≥10 minutes. The normal baseline fetal heart rate is 110 to 160 beats per minute (bpm) (161). Bradycardia is a baseline rate that is less than 110 bpm

for ≥10 minutes (162). A rate of 100 to 109 bpm for this period of time (mild bradycardia) in the absence of other abnormality is acceptable. Moderate bradycardia is defined as 80 to 100 bpm, and severe bradycardia is less than 80 bpm for ≥3 minutes (161). Tachycardia is a baseline rate above 160 bpm, and can be classified into mild (161 to 180 bpm) and severe (≥181 bpm) (161). Baseline variability is divided into two types. Short-term variability (also known as beat-to-beat variability) is the fluctuation of the heart rate baseline over short intervals. Normal short-term variability is an excursion of ≥5 bpm from the baseline (20). Long-term variability is the fluctuation over longer intervals (conventionally ≥2 minutes). Normal long-term variability is defined as three to five cycles per minute (163). Accelerations are periodic, transient increases in the baseline fetal heart rate of at least 15 bpm for ≥15 seconds (161), and are often associated with fetal activity or uterine contractions. Decelerations are periodic, transient decreases in the fetal heart baseline rate that are associated with uterine contractions. They can be further classified by their timing in relation to the contraction. An early deceleration coincides with a uterine contraction and rarely falls below 20 to 30 bpm below the baseline (162). A late deceleration is a symmetrical decrease in the fetal heart rate that begins at or after the peak of a contraction (161). Variable decelerations are variable in both timing and depth, and are considered significant only when they are repetitive (i.e., occurring with more than 50% of contractions) and severe (defined as decreasing to less than 70 bpm and last for ≥60 seconds) (161).

Interpretation of Intrapartum Fetal Heart Rate Patterns

For clinical use, the above various descriptive characteristics of fetal heart rate pattern are integrated in a collective fashion to give an overall clinical impression. Such a clinical impression varies from reassuring to unreassuring. The terms used to describe these patterns vary from reactive

TABLE 27.8. ASSESSMENT OF FETAL WELL-BEING[a]

Antepartum	Intrapartum	Postpartum
Fetal cardiotocography (NST) External monitor (Doppler)	Fetal cardiotocography (NST) External monitor (Doppler) Internal (scalp electrode)	Clinical response (seizures, poor feeding, abnormal movements, HIE)
Biophysical profile	Vibroacoustic stimulation	Apgar score
Vibroacoustic stimulation	Contraction stress test	Umbilical cord pH
Contraction stress test	Fetal scalp stimulation	Meconium
Fetal movement charts ("kickcharts")	Biophysical profile (?)	
Fetal startle response (?)	Fetal startle response (?)	
Doppler ultrasound (?)	Fetal pulse oximetry (?) Fetal EKG (?)	

[a] Tests should be interpreted in light of gestational age, and the presence or absence of congenital anomalies.
EKG, electrocardiogram; HIE, hypoxic ischemic encephalopathy; NST, nonstress test.

TABLE 27.9. DRUGS AFFECTING INTRAPARTUM FETAL HEART RATE TRACING

Effect on Fetal Heart Rate Tracing	Drug
Fetal tachycardia	Adrenalin
	Atropine
	β-Agonists (ritodrine, terbutaline)
Fetal bradycardia	Antithyroid agents (including propothiouracil)
	β-Blockers (such as propranolol)
	Epidural anesthesia (regardless of the agent used)
	Methergine (contraindicated prior to delivery)
	Oxytocin (if associated with excessive uterine activity)
Sinusoidal heart rate pattern	Narcotic analgesics (especially alphaprodine, butorphanol, and/or meperidine)
Diminished variability	Atropine (rate-related decrease in variability)
	Anticonvulsants (but not phenytoin)
	β-Blockers
	Betamethazone
	Ethanol
	General anesthesia
	Hypnotics (including diazepam)
	Insulin (if associated with hypoglycemia)
	Magnesium sulfate
	Narcotic analgesics (including meperidine)
	Promethazine (Phenergan)

(defined as two accelerations in 20 minutes, and considered reassuring), to suspicious or equivocal (indeterminate), and finally to ominous or agonal (unreassuring). Fetal heart rate interpretation is to some degree subjective. Reassuring elements of the fetal heart rate include normal baseline, normal variability, and the presence of accelerations. Unreassuring elements include the absence of accelerations, decreased variability, bradycardia, tachycardia, and/or repetitive severe variable or late decelerations. Unreassuring fetal heart rate patterns of some form or another are seen in up to 60% of all labors, suggesting that these changes are not specific to hypoxia (164). The significance of such an observation therefore needs to be assessed in terms of the overall clinical setting, and in terms of changes in the fetal heart rate pattern with time.

The development of hypoxemia and/or acidosis in the fetus depends to a large degree on the physiologic reserve of the fetus, which can be deduced in part from the clinical setting. Fetuses that are premature and/or growth restricted are less likely to tolerate episodes of decreased placental perfusion and hypoxia. In terms of fetal heart rate patterns, a loss of baseline variability over time (in the absence of narcotic analgesics or other medications that can interfere with heart rate variability) suggests a fetus with diminishing physiologic reserve. Such fetuses may be more prone to acidosis if tachycardia or repetitive late decelerations develop (165). A review of the literature suggests that the positive predictive value of repetitive late decelerations (i.e., the ability of such a fetal heart rate pattern to predict poor fetal outcome) is only around 40% (166). Although the predictive values of other unreassuring fetal heart rate patterns are equally low, current standards of care would suggest that some form of intervention is indicated.

In a recent meta-analysis (167) of 12 prospective, controlled clinical trials involving more than 59,000 infants worldwide in which women in labor were randomized to either continuous electronic fetal heart rate monitoring or intermittent auscultation, there did appear to be a decrease in the incidence of neonatal seizures in the continuous monitoring group [relative risk (RR), 0.5; 95% CI, 0.30 to 0.82]. There was also a decreased incidence in 1-minute Apgar scores ≤4 in the same group (RR, 0.82; 95% CI, 0.65 to 0.98) but only in studies performed outside the United States, and there was no apparent difference in 5-minute Apgar scores ≤7. There were no other differences in measures of short-term perinatal morbidity or in perinatal mortality. Furthermore, the increase in neonatal seizures did not translate into differences in long-term morbidity such as cerebral palsy, mental retardation, or seizures after 28 days of life. There was a significant increase in obstetric intervention (including operative vaginal delivery and cesarean section) in the continuous monitoring group. Other investigators have shown that severely abnormal fetal heart rate patterns are uncommon, occurring in only 0.3% of all fetal heart rate tracings (168), and this incidence justifies aggressive obstetric management.

A baseline fetal heart rate that is described as saltatory (i.e., one in which there are large oscillations of the baseline rate) is of unclear clinical significance. Some investigators have suggested that it is indicative of cord occlusion (169), but this is not widely accepted. The lambda pattern is an acceleration followed by a deceleration, and is attributed to fetal movement. It is not felt to be of pathologic significance (170). A sinusoidal heart rate pattern is one with normal baseline, decreased variability, and a cyclic sinusoidal pattern with a frequency of two to five cycles per minute and an amplitude of 5 to 15 bpm (171). It has been associated most strongly with fetal anemia, but may also be seen with fetal distress and impending fetal demise, chorioamnionitis, maternal drug administration, and as an incidental finding.

Fetal Scalp Blood Sampling

From the discussion above, it is apparent that interpretation of the fetal heart trace may be complex and difficult. The pH of fetal capillary blood, which lies between that of fetal arterial and venous blood (Table 27.10), may be useful in selected cases where there is difficulty in interpreting the fetal heart trace. The technique of fetal blood sampling was introduced by Saling (172) in 1961. A simple protocol has been developed in clinical practice for the management of fetal scalp sample pH (173). If the pH is greater than 7.25, expectant management may be instituted. If the pH is between 7.20 and 7.25, the measurement is repeated at intervals of 20 to 30 minutes. If the pH is less than 7.20, prompt delivery is advised. In recent years, there has been a move away from the practice of fetal scalp sampling in labor. Accurate interpretation of the fetal heart rate tracing has been shown to be superior to the fetal scalp sample in predicting a noncompromised fetus: a reactive fetal nonstress test predicts delivery of a fetus with a 5-minute Apgar score of ≥7 with an accuracy of 99% (174) as compared with a 85% to 90% prediction with a scalp pH >7.20 (175,176). However, as seen in the above section on the interpretation of fetal heart rate tracing, an unreassuring pattern is poor in predicting a compromised fetus. It is for this latter clinical scenario that the use of fetal scalp sampling may be of value.

Intrapartum Fetal Monitoring and Subsequent Neurologic Impairment

Intrapartum monitoring is carried out in an attempt to reduce peripartum morbidity and mortality. In recent times, poor perinatal outcome has become synonymous with suboptimal obstetric care. Since birth injury is rare, attention has focused on cerebral palsy and more subtle forms of mental retardation as potential markers of obstetric error. In the past three decades, assessment of fetal well-being has focused primarily on birth asphyxia and subsequent hypoxemia and/or acidosis as evidence of peripartum fetal compromise. Various tests have been developed to assess the condition of the fetus at birth, including clinical measures, such as the Apgar score (Table 27.11), and biochemical measurements, such as fetal cord pH. Such measurements are often used, rightly or wrongly, to speculate as to the probability of future developmental problems. For a considerable period of time, the reliability of intrapartum monitoring to predict asphyxia as well as the validity of asphyxia as an indicator of fetal condition have been questioned.

In 1983, Paneth and Stark (177) reported that 50% of children with cerebral palsy had no demonstrable depression at birth, and concluded that mental retardation should not be attributed to birth asphyxia. In 1981, Nelson and Ellenberg (178) showed that it was not until the Apgar score was severely depressed for a prolonged period of time (less than 3 for ≥20 minutes) that significant long-term neurologic handicap was likely. Further work by these same investigators reinforced the finding that hypoxia is not a common cause of cerebral palsy (179,180). Other investigators have examined acidosis at birth. Dennis et al. (181) found that severe acidosis at birth was not predictive of poor outcome at 4 1/2 years of age; indeed, their data suggested that the outcome might even be improved. The finding of a poor predictive value of fetal cord pH at birth for subsequent developmental outcome has now been reported by a number of investigators (182–185). Acidemia

TABLE 27.10. NORMAL FETAL ACID-BASE VALUES AT TERM

	pH	Po$_2$ (mm Hg)	Pco$_2$ (mm Hg)	Bicarbonate (mEq/L)	O$_2$ saturation (%)
Umbilical vein[a]	7.35 ± 0.05	29.2 ± 5.9	38.2 ± 5.6	20.4 ± 2.1	70
Umbilical artery[a]	7.28 ± 0.05	18.0 ± 6.2	49.2 ± 8.4	22.3 ± 2.5	28
Fetal scalp blood[b]					
Early first stage	7.33 ± 0.03	21.8 ± 2.6	44.0 ± 4.05	20.1 ± 1.2	
Late first stage	7.32 ± 0.02	21.3 ± 2.1	42.0 ± 5.1	19.1 ± 2.1	
Second stage	7.29 ± 0.04	16.5 ± 1.4	46.3 ± 4.2	17.0 ± 2.0	

[a]From American College of Obstetricians and Gynecologists. *Assessment of fetal and newborn acid-base status.* ACOG technical bulletin no. 127. Washington, DC: American College of Obstetricians and Gynecologists, 1989, with permission.
[b]From Huch R, Huch A. In: Beard RW, Nathanielsz PW, eds. *Fetal physiology and medicine.* New York: Marcel Dekker, 1984, 366, with permission.

TABLE 27.11. APGAR SCORING SYSTEM

	Score		
	0	1	2
Appearance	Blue, pale	Pink body, blue extremity	Pink all over
Heart rate (beats per min)	Absent	<100	≥100
Grimace	No response	Some response	Cry, cough
Activity	Limp	Some flexion	Active motion
Respiratory effort	Absent	Slow	Strong cry

with anaerobic glycolysis may be a normal physiologic response to hypoxia. If the hypoxemic stress is prolonged, then fetal reserves may limit the acidotic response (186). The National Institutes of Health (187) stated, "The causes of severe mental retardation are primarily genetic, biochemical, viral, and developmental, and not related to birth events."

Attention has more recently turned to hypoxic ischemic encephalopathy (HIE) as a marker of birth asphyxia and predictor of long-term outcome. HIE is a clinical condition that develops within the first hours or days of life. It is characterized by abnormalities of tone and feeding, alterations in consciousness, and convulsions. To attribute such a clinical state to birth asphyxia, ACOG (188) has four requirements, all of which need to be fulfilled: (a) profound metabolic or mixed acidemia (pH <7.00) on an umbilical cord arterial blood sample, if obtained; (b) an Apgar score of 0 to 3 for longer than 5 minutes; (c) neonatal neurologic manifestations (e.g., seizures, coma, or hypotonia); and (d) multisystem organ dysfunction (e.g., cardiovascular, gastrointestinal, hematologic, pulmonary, or renal system). HIE is classified as mild, moderate, or severe. In the absence of moderate or severe HIE, intrapartum hypoxia is unlikely to be causally related to long-term outcome (189). The outcomes related to HIE have been reported to be unrelated to Apgar scores or acidemia at birth (190). Indeed, only 3% to 20% of cases of cerebral palsy in infants born at term can be attributed to HIE (191). In a review by Nelson et al. (191) of 473 term singleton infants with birth weight ≥2,500 g born from 1983 through 1985 in four California counties (95 infants who subsequently developed cerebral palsy and 378 controls), only 27% of children with cerebral palsy had evidence of severely abnormal intrapartum fetal heart rate tracings. These infants represented only 0.19% of deliveries with such fetal-monitoring findings, for a false-positive rate of 99.8%. The lack of evidence linking fetal asphyxia and hypoxia to neonatal outcome has led one author to recommend the abandonment of the term *birth asphyxia* (192).

As dissatisfaction with birth asphyxia as a causal event in the etiology of mental retardation and cerebral palsy has grown, other possible causes for these developmental abnormalities have been considered (Table 29.12). Exposure to maternal or placental infection may be associated with increased risk of cerebral palsy (193–195). Maternal fever exceeding 38°C in labor as well as a clinical diagnosis of chorioamnionitis in the absence of maternal fever have been associated with increased risk of cerebral palsy in children of normal birth weight (odds ratio, 9.3; 95% CI, 2.7 to 31.0) (196). The odds ratio for spastic quadriplegia in the presence of placental infection was 31.0 (95% CI, 7.9 to 109). In this series, maternal infection was also linked to low Apgar scores, need for resuscitation, and neonatal seizures, all of which are signs also commonly attributed to birth asphyxia. It is accurate to say that our current understanding of the causes of cerebral palsy and mental retardation is limited. Furthermore, intrapartum monitoring and preventative strategies developed to date appear to be unreliable and ineffective.

Pain Control During Labor

The techniques available for pain control during labor are outlined in Table 27.13. These range from noninvasive techniques (such as drug administration) to more invasive regional nerve blocks. Noninvasive techniques include fringe techniques such as hypnosis, aromatherapy, and acupuncture. Such techniques do have a place in practice if desired by the patient and practitioner; however, their efficacy remains to be proven. Medical noninvasive techniques include transcutaneous electrical nerve stimulation (TENS) and inhalational analgesia. Neither is currently used widely

TABLE 27.12. CAUSES OF IRREVERSIBLE NEONATAL CEREBRAL INJURY

Congenital abnormalities (including chromosomal disorders)
Intracerebral hemorrhage
Hypoxic ischemic encephalopathy
Infection
Drugs
Trauma
Metabolic derangements (such as hypoglycemia, thyroid dysfunction)
Hypotension/shock

TABLE 27.13. PAIN RELIEF IN LABOR

Pharmacologic methods	
Systemic analgesia[a]	Opioid agonists
	Morphine/diamorphine
	Meperidine (pethidine)
	Sufentanil
	Alfentanil
	Fentanyl (?)
	Partial opioid agonist/antagonists
	Buprenorphine
	Butorphanol
	Nalbuphine
	Pentazocine
	Meptazinol
Local anesthesia[b]	Field block (local infiltration)
	Paracervical block
	Pudendal block
Regional anesthesia[b]	Epidural block
	Spinal block
	Combined spinal-epidural block
	Caudal block (saddle block)
Inhalational anesthesia	Ether (historic interest only)
	Chloroform (historic interest only)
	Nitrous oxide (alone, with air, with oxygen [Entenox])
Nonpharmacologic methods	Transcutaneous nerve stimulation (TENS)
	Acupuncture
	Continuous presence and support of a midwife
	Emotional support of a "doula-like" figure
	Hot baths, back rubbing, massage, relaxation
	Aromatherapy (?)
	Hypnosis (?)

[a] Can be given intramuscularly and/or intravenously; may be more effective if given along with an effective and nonsedating antiemetic such as promethazine (Phenergan) or metoclopramide.
[b] Local anesthetic agents include bupivacaine, lidocaine, chloroprocaine, ropivacaine (prilocaine is not recommended because of the possibility of methemoglobinemia).

in the United States. The former has little evidence of efficacy in the scientific literature. However, patient-controlled inhalation of nitrous oxide is widely used in other countries in the Western hemisphere, with good patient satisfaction.

Drug Administration for Pain Relief in Labor

Intramuscular or intravenous drug administration can be used for the control of pain in labor. The most popular group of drugs in this regard are the opiate agonists. These drugs have good analgesic and sedative properties, but delay gastric emptying and can cause neonatal sedation and respiratory depression. They should therefore always be given along with an agent to reduce gastric acidity in the event general anesthesia becomes necessary. A reversal agent (such as naloxone) should always be available in case of maternal or neonatal respiratory depression. Partial opioid agonists (such as nalbuphine) have been developed to minimize unwanted side effects including neonatal respiratory depression. However, the reduction in unwanted side effects is often accompanied by a reduction in efficacy. Despite these shortcomings, drug therapy continues to play a major role

in pain relief during labor, especially in the early stages, due to its availability and ease of administration.

More Invasive Techniques for Pain Relief in Labor

The use of local anesthetic, in its simplest form, involves local infiltration of the nerve endings in the vulva and labia (known as a field block). This is most often used just prior to performing an episiotomy or repairing a perineal laceration. A pudendal nerve block is a regional block, and involves local infiltration of the two or three branches of the pudendal nerve as they exit Alcock's canal and circumnavigate the ischial spines. This procedure anesthetizes the perineal area (sacral nerve roots S2, S3, and S4), and is useful for outlet manipulations in the second stage of labor. A paracervical block can be performed by infiltrating the sensory nerves leaving the uterus through the cardinal ligaments. This is most useful to provide anesthesia for the latter part of the first stage of labor. More invasive techniques include the regional blockade of sensory nerves as they enter the spinal cord, such as spinal, epidural, and caudal blocks. Combinations of these procedures can also be used. Spinal anesthesia involves a once-only injection of local anesthetic into the subarachnoid space. For epidural anesthesia, a cannula is inserted and left in place in the peridural fat, and enables bolus injections and continuous infusions of local anesthetic agents to achieve effective analgesia. The caudal block (or saddle block) is a localized epidural through the sacral hiatus.

The Effect of Pain Management on the Progress of Labor

It has long been a matter of controversy as to whether the administration of epidural analgesia prolongs the length of labor and increases the incidence of operative delivery or not. Published retrospective studies and randomized trials have not clearly resolved this issue, which is compounded by the complexity of obstetric management and the high degree of variability in individual labor patterns. Is epidural analgesia more likely to be used when the labor is long or difficult and more likely to have obstetric intervention, or does epidural analgesia causally contribute to that clinical situation? There have been three randomized, prospective trials addressing this issue (197–199). Chestnut et al. (197) examined the effect of epidural anesthesia on 150 nulliparous women in active labor already receiving OT augmentation in which the use of epidural was randomized to early (<5-cm cervical dilatation) or late (≥5 cm). Their results suggest that early epidural placement did not increase the length of labor, nor did it increase the frequency of instrumental vaginal delivery or cesarean section as compared with late placement (cesarean section rates of 18% vs. 19%, respectively).

In a second publication, Chestnut et al. (198) examined the effect of epidural analgesia on 334 nulliparous women in spontaneous labor. In this trial, the authors found that the use of an epidural did not increase the length of labor or the incidence of OT augmentation as compared with women who did not receive epidural anesthesia. Similarly, epidural administration did not increase the incidence of malposition, instrumental delivery, or cesarean section (10% vs. 8%, respectively). No adverse effects were noted on the fetus. The lower cesarean section rate noted in the second paper was probably due to the study design in that all women in the second trial were in spontaneous labor, whereas a large proportion of women in the first trial were undergoing induction of labor. These results are in contrast with an earlier study by Thorp et al. (199), in which 93 nulliparous women were randomized to receive either epidural anesthesia or intravenous opioid analgesia for pain relief in spontaneous labor. In this study, patients who were randomized to receive epidural analgesia experienced prolongation of both the first and second stages of labor, more frequent OT augmentation, and an increase in cesarean section rate as compared with women receiving opioids (25% vs. 2.2%, respectively). In addition, the authors argue

that the increase in cesarean section may be related to epidural placement early in the latent phase of labor since the incidence of cesarean birth appeared to correlate with cervical dilatation at the time of catheter placement. The reported incidence of cesarean section was 50% if the epidural was placed at 2 cm, 33% if placed at 3 cm, 26% if placed at 4 cm, and 0% if placed at ≥5 cm. The small patient numbers, concerns over the randomization protocol, and the absence of any cesarean births in the 13 women with cervical exams of ≥5 cm at the time of epidural placement make it unclear whether the data in this study support the conclusions.

In addition to the above prospective trials, there have been a number of retrospective reports addressing the issue of epidural anesthesia and progress in labor, again with conflicting findings. In a large retrospective review of 1,733 low-risk, nulliparous patients in spontaneous labor at term, Lieberman et al. (200) reported a cesarean section rate of 17% in those women receiving epidural as compared with 4% in those not. The greatest increase in risk for cesarean section was noted when the epidural was sited in early labor. However, there was an increased incidence of cesarean delivery throughout labor irrespective of the timing of placement.

Regardless of whether or not epidural analgesia has a deleterious effect on the length of labor, on the incidence of dystocia, or on the incidence of operative deliveries, its use in routine obstetric practice is well established. Its efficacy in terms of pain management during labor is unparalleled. Pain, no matter how short lived, represents significant maternal morbidity. The potential deleterious effects of epidural analgesia should therefore be balanced against the benefits of pain relief and the apparent negligible effect on perinatal morbidity. The mode of pain relief during labor should be individualized, and is a decision that is best left in the hands of the patient and her care provider. However, the patient should be well informed about the potential risks and benefits, many of which are only now coming to the fore. For example, one association with epidural analgesia in labor is that of maternal fever (201,202). Fever can be a marker for infection that could adversely affect both mother and fetus. A retrospective review by Lieberman et al. (202) of 1,657 nulliparous women who were afebrile on admission in labor revealed that an intrapartum fever of ≥38°C (or ≥100.4°F) occurred in 14.5% of women receiving an epidural, but in only 1% of those not receiving an epidural. This resulted in neonates of mothers who received epidurals being more often evaluated for sepsis (34% vs. 9.8%, respectively). Given this association, the criteria for neonatal sepsis evaluation may need to be reconsidered.

SUMMARY

We have outlined the basic obstetric principles that are essential for the understanding and effective management of normal labor at term. In addition, we have highlighted specific areas of clinical management that are of current interest, namely, the active management of labor, the effect of epidural anesthesia on the progress of labor, and the changing role of fetal birth asphyxia as an etiologic factor in subsequent neonatal neurologic injury. From this review, it is apparent that the clinical management of labor has evolved under the guidance of the clinician rather than the scientist. Consequently, only fragments of the available scientific knowledge regarding the physiologic basis of parturition have been incorporated into clinical practice. It is also apparent that our understanding of the many hormonal pathways involved in the initiation and maintenance of labor is at best rudimentary. It is logical to assume that if the physiologic basis of parturition can be clarified, and if this knowledge can be integrated into clinical practice, the effective management of labor may be optimized. As such, future changes in clinical practice may lie in the hands of the parturition endocrinologist.

10 KEY POINTS

1. Labor is a clinical diagnosis encompassing three distinct elements: uterine contractions, effacement and dilatation of the cervix, and rupture of the fetal membranes.

2. Although the factors responsible for the initiation and maintenance of labor at term remain unclear, it is likely that the fetus is in control of the timing of labor and birth.

3. Parturition at term is perhaps best regarded physiologically as a release from the inhibitory effects of pregnancy on the myometrium, rather than as an active process mediated by uterine stimulants. However, both mechanisms appear to be important.

4. Prostaglandins (especially $PGF_{2\alpha}$ derived from the maternal decidua) appear to have a central role to play in human parturition. Other hormones that have been implicated in this regard include steroid hormones, oxytocin, corticotropin-releasing hormones, glucocorticoids, parathyroid hormone–related peptide, luteinizing hormone/human chorionic gonadotropin, and relaxin.

5. Although uterine activity is the most visible element of labor to the observer, there is no good scientific evidence relating its quantity or quality to obstetric outcome.

6. Cervical ripening by any method will improve the outcome of induction of labor in the presence of an unfavorable cervix.

7. Oxytocin can be used to augment labor in either a low-dose or high-dose protocol. Both protocols appear to be equally effective.

8. The active management of labor decreases the duration of labor, but an improvement in obstetric outcome has yet to be conclusively demonstrated.

9. The ability of intrapartum monitoring to predict asphyxia is limited. The scientific validity of birth asphyxia as the major cause of long-term neurologic injury is becoming less tenable.

10. Epidural analgesia appears to increase the incidence of operative vaginal delivery and possibly cesarean section. However, given its unparalleled efficacy in controlling the pain of labor and delivery, the choice of pain relief in labor should belong to the patient.

REFERENCES

1. Duff P, Huff RW, Gibbs RS. Management of premature rupture of membranes and unfavorable cervix in term pregnancy. *Obstet Gynecol* 1984;63:697–702.
2. Liggins GC. The onset of labour: an overview. In: McNellis D, Challis JRG, MacDonald PC, et al., eds. *The onset of labour: cellular and integrative mechanisms.* A National Institute of Child Health and Human Development Research Planning Workshop (November 29–December 1, 1987). Ithaca, NY: Perinatology Press, 1988:1–3.
3. Casey LM, MacDonald PC. The initiation of labour in women: regulation of phospholipid and arachidonic acid metabolism and of prostaglandin production. In: Creasy RK, Warshaw JB, eds. *Seminars in perinatology,* vol 10. Orlando, Florida: Irvine & Stratton, 1986:270–275.
4. Thorburn GD, Challis JRG, Robinson JS. The endocrinology of parturition. In: Wynn RM, ed. *Cellular biology of the uterus.* New York: Plenum Press, 1977:653–732.
5. Flint APF, Anderson ABM, Steele PA, et al. The mechanism by which fetal cortisol controls the onset of parturition in the sheep. *Biochem Soc Trans* 1975;3:1189–1194.
6. Liggins GC. Initiation of labor. *Biol Neonate* 1989;55:366–394.
7. Liggins BJ, Fairclough RJ, Grieves SA, et al. The mechanism of initiation of parturition in the ewe. *Recent Prog Horm Res* 1973;29:111–159.
8. Challis JRG, Gibb W. Control of parturition. *Prenat Neonat Med* 1996;1:283–291.
9. Matthews SG, Challis JRG. Regulation of the hypothalamo-pituitary-adreno-cortical axis in fetal sheep. *Trends Endocrinol Metab* 1996;4:239–246.
10. Li J, Saunders JC, Gilmour RS, et al. Insulin like growth factor-II messenger ribonucleic acid expression in fetal tissues of the sheep during late gestation: effect of cortisol. *Endocrinology* 1993;132:2083–2089.
11. Novy MJ, Walsh SW. Dexamethasone and estradiol treatment in pregnant rhesus macaques: effects on gestational length, maternal plasma hormones, and fetal growth. *Am J Obstet Gynecol* 1983;145:920–931.
12. Nathanielsy PW. A time to be born. In:Nathanielsy PW, ed. *Life before birth: the challenges of fetal development.* New York: WH Freeman, 1996:162–181.
13. Pauerstein CJ, Zauder HL. Autonomic innervation, sex steroids and uterine contractility. *Obstet Gynecol Surv* 1970;25(suppl):617–630.
14. Keirse MJNC. Endogenous prostaglandins in human parturition. In: Keirse MJNC, Anderson ABM, Bennebroek-Gravenhorst J, eds. *Human parturition.* Leiden: Leiden University Press, 1979:101–142.
15. Hla T, Neilson K. Human cyclooxygenase-2 cDNA. *Proc Natl Acad Sci USA* 1992;89:7384–7388.
16. Economopoulos P, Sun M, Purgina B, et al. Glucocorticoids stimulate prostaglandin H synthase type 2 (PGHS-2) in the

fibroblast cells in human amnion cultures. *Mol Cell Endocrinol* 1996;117:141–147.

17. Casey ML, MacDonald PC. Biomolecular processes in the initiation of parturition: decidual activation. *Clin Obstet Gynecol* 1988;31:533–551.

18. Liggins GC. Initiation of parturition. In: Novy MJ, Resko JA, eds. *Fetal endocrinology*. New York: Academic Press, 1981:211–238.

19. Karim SMM. Identification of prostaglandins in human amniotic fluid. *J Obstet Gynaecol Br Commonw* 1966;73:903–908.

20. Keirse MJNC, Turnbull AC. Prostaglandins in amniotic fluid during late pregnancy and labour. *J Obstet Gynaecol Br Commonw* 1973;80:970–973.

21. Romero R, Munoz H, Gomez R, et al. Increase in prostaglandin bioavailability precedes the onset of human parturition. *Prostaglandins Leukotrienes Essent Fatty Acids* 1996;54:187–191.

22. Karim SM, Hillier K. Prostaglandins in the control of animal and human reproduction. *Br Med Bull* 1979;35:173–180.

23. Garrioch DB. The effect of indomethacin on spontaneous activity in the isolated human myometrium and on the response to oxytocin and prostaglandin. *Br J Obstet Gynaecol* 1978;85:47–52.

24. Zuckerman H, Reiss U, Rubinstein I. Inhibition of human premature labor by indomethacin. *Obstet Gynecol* 1974;44:787–792.

25. Wiqvist N, Lundstrom V, Green K. Premature labor and indomethacin. *Prostaglandin* 1975;10:515–526.

26. Golichowski AM. Biochemical basis of cervical maturation. In: Huszar G, ed. *The physiology and biochemistry of the uterus in pregnancy and labour*. Boca Raton, FL: CRC Press, 1986:261–280.

27. Ellwood DA, Mitchell MD, Anderson ABM, et al. The in vitro production of prostanoids by the human cervix during pregnancy: preliminary observations. *Br J Obstet Gynaecol* 1980;87:210–214.

28. Hillier K, Wallis RM. Prostaglandins, steroids and the human cervix. In: Ellwood DA, Anderson ABM, eds. *The cervix in pregnancy and labour: clinical and biochemical investigations*. Edinburgh: Churchill-Livingstone, 1981:144–162.

29. Garfield RE, Kannan MS, Daniel SS. Gap junction formation in myometrium: control by estrogens, progesterone and prostaglandins. *Am J Physiol* 1980;238:81–89.

30. Verhoeff A, Garfield RE. Ultrastructure of the myometrium and the role of gap junctions in myometrial function. In: Huszar G, ed. *The physiology and biochemistry of the uterus in pregnancy and labour*. Boca Raton, FL: CRC Press, 1986:73–91.

31. Chan WY. Enhanced prostaglandin synthesis in the parturient rat uterus and its effect on myometrial oxytocin receptor concentration. *Prostaglandin* 1987;34:889–902.

32. Fuchs A-R. The role of oxytocin in parturition. In: Huszar G, ed. *The physiology and biochemistry of the uterus in pregnancy and labour*. Boca Raton, FL: CRC Press, 1986:163–183.

33. Wiqvist N, Lundstrom V, Green K. Premature labor and indomethacin. *Prostaglandins* 1975;10:515–526.

34. Garrioch DB. The effect of indomethacin on spontaneous activity in the isolated human myometrium and on the response to oxytocin and prostaglandin. *Br J Obstet Gynaecol* 1978;85:47–52.

35. Guillette LJ Jr, Dubois DH, Cree A. Prostaglandins, oviductal function, and parturient behavior in nonmammalian vertebrates. *Am J Physiol* 1991 260(5):854–861.

36. Morham SG, Langenbach R, Loftin CD, et al. Prostaglandin synthase 2 gene disruption causes severe renal pathology in the mouse. *Cell* 1995;83:473–482.

37. Langenbach R, Morham SG, Tiano HF, et al. Prostaglandin synthase 1 gene disruption in mice reduces arachidonic acid-induced inflammation and indomethacin-induced gastric ulceration. *Cell* 1995;83:483–492.

38. Sugimoto Y, Yamasaki A, Segi E, et al. Failure of parturition in mice lacking the prostaglandin F receptor. *Science* 1997;277:681–683.

39. Mitchell MD, Ebenhack K, Kraemer DL, et al. A sensitive radioimmunoassay for 11-deoxy-13,14-dihydro-15-keto-11,16-cyclo-prostaglandin E_2: application as an index of prostaglandin E_2 biosynthesis during human pregnancy and parturition. *Prostaglandin Leukotriene Med* 1982;9:549–557.

40. Roseblade CK, Sullivan MH, Kahn H, et al. Limited transfer of prostaglandin E_2 across the fetal membrane before and after labor. *Acta Obstet Gynecol Scand* 1990;69:399–403.

41. Word RA, Kamm KE, Casey ML. Contractile effects of prostaglandins, oxytocin, and endothelin-1 in human myometrium in vitro: refractoriness of myometrial tissue of pregnant women to prostaglandin E_2 and F_2 alpha. *J Clin Endocrinol Metab* 1992;75:1027–1032.

42. van Meir CA, Sangha RK, Walton JC, et al. Immunoreactive 15-hydroxyprostaglandin dehydrogenase (PGDH) is reduced in fetal membranes from patients at preterm delivery in the presence of infection. *Placenta* 1996;17:291–297.

43. Sangha RK, Walton JC, Ensor CM, et al. Immunohistochemical localization, mRNA abundance and activity of 15-hydroxyprostaglandin dehydrogenase in placenta and fetal membranes during term and pre-term labor. *J Clin Endocrinol Metab* 1994;78:982–989.

44. Hofman GE, Rao CV, De Leon FD, et al. Human endometrial prostaglandin E_2 binding sites and their profiles during the menstrual cycle and in pathological states. *Am J Obstet Gynecol* 1985;151:369–375.

45. Wakeling AE, Wyngarden LJ. Prostaglandin receptors in the human, monkey and hamster uterus. *Endocrinology* 1974;95:55–64.

46. Negishi M, Sugimoto Y, Ichikawa A. Molecular mechanisms of diverse actions of prostanoid receptors. *Biochim Biophys Acta* 1995;1259:109–120.

47. Peyron R, Aubény E, Targosz V, et al. Early termination of pregnancy with mifepristone (RU 486) and the orally active prostaglandin misoprostol. *N Engl J Med* 1993;328:1509–1513.

48. Spitz IM, Bardin CW. Mifepristone (RU 486)—a modulator of progestin and glucocorticoid action. *N Engl J Med* 1993;329:404–412.

49. Turnbull AC. The endocrine control of labour. In: Turnbull AC, Chamberlain G, eds. *Obstetrics*. London: Churchill-Livingstone, 1989:189–204.

50. Figueroa JP, Honnebier MBOM, Binienda Z, et al. Effect of 48 hour intravenous delta 4-androstenedione infusion on pregnant rhesus monkeys in the last third of gestation: changes in maternal plasma estradiol concentrations and myometrial contractility. *Am J Obstet Gynecol* 1989;161:481–486.

51. Nathanielsy PW, Fame JD, Winter JA, et al. Local paracrine effects of estradiol are central to parturition in the rhesus monkey. *Nat Med* 1998;4:456–459.

52. Mecenas CA, Giussani DA, Owiny JR, et al. Production of premature delivery in pregnant rhesus monkeys by androstenedione infusion. *Nature Med* 1996;2:443–448.

53. Zeeman GG, Khan-Dawood FS, Dawood MY. Oxytocin and its receptor in pregnancy and parturition: current concepts and clinical implications. *Obstet Gynecol* 1997;89:873–883.

54. Fuchs A-R, Fuchs F. Endocrinology of human parturition: a review. *Br J Obstet Gynaecol* 1984;91:948–967.

55. Fuchs AR, Fuchs F, Husslein P, et al. Oxytocin receptors and human parturition: a dual role for oxytocin in the initiation of labor. *Science* 1982;215:1396–1398.

56. Fuchs AR, Fuchs F, Husslein P, et al. Oxytocin receptors in the human uterus during pregnancy and parturition. *Am J Obstet Gynecol* 1984;150:734–741.

57. Kimura T, Tanizawa O, Mori K, et al. Structure and expression of a human oxytocin receptor. *Nature* 1992;356:526–529.

58. Husslein P, Fuchs A-R, Fuchs F. Oxytocin and the initiation of human parturition. I. Prostaglandin release during induction of labor with oxytocin. *Am J Obstet Gynecol* 1981;141:688–693.

59. Fuchs A-R, Husslein P, Fuchs F. Oxytocin and the initiation of human parturition. II. Stimulation of prostaglandin production in human decidua by oxytocin. *Am J Obstet Gynecol* 1981;141:694–697.

60. Dawood MY, Wang CF, Gupta R, et al. Fetal contribution to oxytocin in human labor. *Obstet Gynecol* 1978;52:205–209.

61. Campbell EA, Linton E, Wolfe CDA, et al. Plasma corticotropin-releasing hormone concentrations during pregnancy and parturition. *J Clin Endocrinol Metab* 1987;64:1054–1059.

62. Sasaki A, Shinkawa O, Margioris AN, et al. Immunoreactive corticotropin-releasing hormone in human plasma during pregnancy, labor and delivery. *J Clin Endocrinol Metab* 1987;64:224–229.

63. Petraglia F, Benedetto C, Fioro P, et al. Effect of corticotropin-releasing factor binding protein on prostaglandin release from cultured maternal decidual decidua and on contractile activity of human myometrium in vitro. *J Clin Endocrinol Metab* 1965;80:3073–3076.

64. Polter E, Behan DP, Fischer WH, et al. Cloning and characterization of the cDNA's for human and rat corticotropin-releasing factor binding-protein. *Nature* 1991;349:423–426.

65. Hillhouse EW, Grammatopooulos D, Milton NGN, et al. The identification of a human myometrial corticotropin-releasing hormone receptor that increases in affinity during human pregnancy. *J Clin Endocrinol Metab* 1993;76:736–741.

66. Clifton VL, Owens PC, Robinson PJ, et al. Identification and characterization of a corticotropin-releasing hormone receptor in human placenta. *Eur J Endocrinol* 1995;133:591–597.

67. Robinson BG, Emanuel RL, Frim DM, et al. Glucocorticoid stimulates expression of corticotropin-releasing hormone gene in human placenta. *Proc Natl Acad Sci USA* 1988;85:5244–5249.

68. Potestio F, Zakar T, Olson DM. Glucocorticoids stimulate prostaglandin synthesis in human amnion cells by a receptor-mediated mechanism. *J Clin Endocrinol Metab* 1988;67:1205–1210.

69. Brown RW, Chapman KE, Edwards CR, et al. Human placental 11β-hydroxysteroid dehydrogenase: evidence for and partial purification of a distinct NAD-dependent isoform. *Endocrinology* 1993;132:2614–2621.

70. Sun K, Yang K, Challis JRG. Differential expression of 11β-hydroxysteroid dehydrogenase type 1 and 2 in human placenta and fetal membranes. *J Clin Endocrinol Metab* 1997;82:300–305.

71. Thiede MA, Harm SC, Hasson DM, et al. In vivo regulation of PTH-rP messenger ribonucleic acid in the rat uterus by 17β-estradiol. *Endocrinology* 1991;128:2317–2323.

72. MacLennan AH, Nicholson R, Green RC. Serum relaxin in pregnancy. *Lancet* 1986;2:241–243.

73. Rush RW, Keirse MJNC, Howat P, et al. Contribution of preterm delivery to perinatal mortality. *Br Med J* 1976;2:965–968.

74. Friedman EA. Primigravid labor: a graphicostatistical analysis. *Obstet Gynecol* 1955;6:567–587.

75. Friedman EA, Sachtelben MR. Dysfunctional Labor. I. Prolonged latent phase in the nullipara. *Obstet Gynecol* 1961;17:135–148.

76. Studd J. Partograms and nomograms of cervical dilatation in the management of primigravid labour. *Br Med J* 1973;4:451–455.

77. American College of Obstetricians and Gynecologists. *Operative vaginal delivery.* ACOG technical bulletin no. 196. Washington, DC: American College of Obstetricians and Gynecologists, 1994.

78. Caldyro-Barcia R, Sica-Blanco Y, Poseiro JJ, et al. A quantitative study of the action of synthetic oxytocin on the pregnant human uterus. *J Pharmacol Exp Ther* 1957;121:18–31.

79. El Shawi SE, Gaafr AA, Toppozada HK. A new unit for the evaluation of uterine activity. *Am J Obstet Gynecol* 1967;98:900–903.

80. O'Driscoll K, Meagher D. Induction. In: O'Driscoll K, Meagher D, eds. *Active management of labour,* 2nd ed. Eastbourne, UK: Bailliere Tindall, 1986:96–99.

81. American College of Obstetricians and Gynecologists. *Dystocia and the augmentation of labor.* ACOG technical bulletin no. 218. Washington, DC: American College of Obstetricians and Gynecologists, 1995.

82. Schifrin SC, Cohen WR. Labor's dysfunctional lexicon. *Obstet Gynecol* 1989;74:121–124.

83. Caldwell WE, Moloy HC. Anatomical variations in the female pelvis and their effect in labor with a suggested classification. *Am J Obstet Gynecol* 1933;26:479–505.

84. Crawford JW. Computer monitoring of fetal heart rate and uterine pressure. *Am J Obstet Gynecol* 1975; 21:342–350.

85. Lamont RF, Neave S, Baker AC, et al. Intrauterine pressures in labours induced by amniotomy and oxytocin or vaginal prostaglandin gel compared with normal labour. *Br J Obstet Gynaecol* 1991;98:441–447.

86. Helwig JT, Thorp JM Jr, Bowes WA Jr. Does midline episiotomy increase the risk of third- and fourth-degree lacerations in operative vaginal deliveries? *Obstet Gynecol* 1993;82:276–279.

87. Coates PM, Chan KK, Wilkins M, et al. A comparison between midline and mediolateral episiotomies. *Br J Obstet Gynaecol* 1980;87:408–412.

88. Friedman EA, Niswander KR, Bayonet-Rivera NP, et al. Relation of prelabor evaluation in inducibility and the course of labor. *Obstet Gynecol* 1966;28:495–501.

89. Calder AA, Embery MP, Hillier K. Extra-amniotic prostaglandin E$_2$ for induction of labor at term. *Br J Obstet Gynaecol* 1974;81:39–46.

90. Bishop EH. Pelvic scoring for elective induction. *Obstet Gynecol* 1964;24:266–268.

91. American College of Obstetricians and Gynecologists. *Induction of labor.* ACOG Technical Bulletin no. 217. Washington, DC: American College of Obstetricians and Gynecologists, 1995.

92. Calder AA, Embery MP, Tait T. Ripening of the cervix with extra-amniotic prostaglandin E$_2$ in viscous gel before induction of labor. *Br J Obstet Gynaecol* 1977;84:264–268.

93. Ulmsten U, Wingerup L, Belfrage P, et al. Intracervical application of prostaglandin gel for induction of term labor. *Obstet Gynecol* 1982;59:336–339.

94. O'Herlihy C, MacDonald HN. Influence of pre-induction prostaglandin E$_2$ gel on cervical ripening and labour induction. *Obstet Gynecol* 1979;54:708–710.

95. Sheperd JH, Pearce JMF, Sims C. Induction of labor using prostaglandin E$_2$ pessaries. *Br Med J* 1979;2: 108–110.

96. Keirse MJNC. Prostaglandins in preinduction cervical ripening: meta-analysis of world wide clinical experience. *J Reprod Med* 1993;38:89–100.

97. MacKenzie IZ, Embery MP. A comparison of PGE$_2$ and PGF$_{2\alpha}$ vaginal gel for ripening the cervix before induction of labor. *Br J Obstet Gynaecol* 1979;85:657–661.

98. Neilson DR, Prins RP, Bolton RN, et al. A comparison of

prostaglandin E$_2$ gel and prostaglandin PGF$_{2\alpha}$ gel for pre-induction cervical ripening. *Am J Obstet Gynecol* 1983;146:526–530.

99. Ekman G, Forman A, Marsal K, et al. Intravaginal versus intracervical application of prostaglandin E$_2$ in viscous gel for cervical priming and induction of labor at term in patients with an unfavourable cervical state. *Am J Obstet Gynecol* 1983;147:657–661.

100. Keirse JNC, de Koning Gans HJ. Randomized comparison of the effects of endocervical and vaginal prostaglandin E$_2$ gel in women with various degrees of cervical ripeness. *Am J Obstet Gynecol* 1995;173:1859–1864.

101. Rayburn WF, Wapner RJ, Barss VA, et al. An intravaginal controlled release prostaglandin E$_2$ pessary for cervical ripening and initiation of labor at term. *Obstet Gynecol* 1992;79:374–379.

102. Wing DA, Jones MM, Rahall A, et al. A comparison of prostaglandin E$_2$ gel for preinduction cervical ripening and labor induction. *Am J Obstet Gynecol* 1995;172:1804–1810.

103. Wing DA, Rahall A, Jones MM, et al. Misoprostol: an effective agent for cervical ripening and labor induction. *Am J Obstet Gynecol* 1995;172:1811–1816.

104. Windrin R, Bennet K, Mundle W. Oral administration of misoprostol for labor induction: a randomized controlled trial. *Obstet Gynecol* 1997;89:392–397.

105. Garris RE, Kirkwood CF. Misoprostol: a prostaglandin E$_1$ analogue. *Clin Pharm* 1989;8:627–644.

106. Varaklis K, Gumina R, Stubblefiel PG. Randomized controlled trial of vaginal misoprostol and intracervical prostaglandin E$_2$ gel for induction of labor at term. *Obstet Gynecol* 1995;86:541–544.

107. Chuck FJ, Huffaker BJ. Labor induction with intravaginal misoprostol versus intracervical prostaglandin E$_2$ gel: randomized comparison. *Am J Obstet Gynecol* 1995;173:1137–1142.

108. Wing DA, Paul RH. A comparison of differing dosing regimens of vaginally administered misoprostol for preinduction cervical ripening and labor induction. *Am J Obstet Gynecol* 1996;175:158–164.

109. O'Brien JM, Mercer BM, Cleary NT, et al. Efficacy of outpatient induction with low-dose intravaginal prostaglandin E$_2$: a randomized double-blind, placebo-controlled trial. *Am J Obstet Gynecol* 1995;173:1855–1859.

110. Flamm BL. Once a cesarean, always a controversy. *Obstet Gynecol* 1997;90:312–315.

111. Centers for Disease Control. Rates of cesarean delivery—United States, 1993. *MMWR* 1995;44:303–307.

112. Bennet MJ, Laurence DT. Induction of labour with prostaglandin E$_2$ vaginal pessaries in high risk pregnancies. *J Obstet Gynaecol* 1981;2:71–73.

113. Fay RA, Fraser IS. Vaginal prostaglandins and scar rupture. *Am J Obstet Gynaecol* 1983;4:139–140.

114. MacKenzie IZ, Bradley S, Embery MP. Vaginal prostaglandins and labor induction for patients previously delivered by caesarean section. *Br J Obstet Gynaecol* 1984;91:7–10.

115. Baxi LV, Petrie RM. Pharmacological effects on labor: effects of drugs on dystocia, labor and uterine activity. *Clin Obstet Gynecol* 1987;30:19–32.

116. Valentine BV. Intravenous oxytocin and oral prostaglandin E$_2$ for ripening the unfavourable cervix. *Br J Obstet Gynaecol* 1977;84:846–854.

117. Magann EF, Perry KG, Dockery JR, et al. Cervical ripening before medical induction of labor: a comparison of prostaglandin E$_2$ gel, estradiol and oxytocin. *Am J Obstet Gynecol* 1995;172:1702–1708.

118. Pollnow DM, Broekhuizen FF. Randomized, double-blind trial of prostaglandin E$_2$ intravaginal gel versus low-dose oxytocin for cervical ripening before induction of labor. *Am J Obstet Gynecol* 1996;174:1910–1916.

119. Blakemore KJ, Qin N, Petrie RH, et al. A prospective comparison of hourly and quarter hourly oxytocin increase intervals for the induction of labor at term. *Obstet Gynecol* 1990;75:757–761.

120. Willcourt RJ, Pager D, Wendel J, et al. Induction of labor with pulsatile oxytocin by a computer-controlled pump. *Am J Obstet Gynecol* 1994;170:603–608.

121. Chew WC. Neonatal hyperbilirubinaemia: a comparison between prostaglandin E$_2$ and oxytocin inductions. *Br Med J* 1977;2:679–680.

122. Johnson N, Bryce FC. Could antiprogesterones be used as alternative cervical ripening agents? *Am J Obstet Gynecol* 1990;162:688–690.

123. Swahn ML, Brydgeman M. The effect of the antiprogestin mifepristone on uterine contractility and sensitivity to prostaglandin and oxytocin. *Br J Obstet Gynaecol* 1988;95:126–134.

124. Sanchez-Ramos L, Kaunitz AM, Wears RL, et al. Misoprostol for cervical ripening and labor induction: a meta-analysis. *Obstet Gynecol* 1997;89:633–642.

125. Cabrol D, Dubois C, Cronje H, et al. Induction of labor with mifepristone (RU486) in intrauterine fetal death. *Am J Obstet Gynecol* 1990;163:540–542.

126. Frydman R, Lelaidier C, Baton-Saint-Mleux C, et al. Labor induction in women at term with mifepristone (RU486): a double-blind, randomized, placebo-controlled study. *Obstet Gynecol* 1992;80:972–975.

127. Lelaidier C, Baton C, Benifla JL, et al. Mifepristone for labor induction after caesarean section. *Br J Obstet Gynaecol* 1994;101:501–503.

128. Embery MP, Mollison BC. The unfavourable cervix and the induction of labor using a cervical balloon. *J Obstet Gynaecol Br Commonw* 1967;74:44–48.

129. Onge RD, Connors GT. Preinduction cervical ripening: a comparison of intracervical prostaglandin E$_2$ gel versus the Foley catheter. *Am J Obstet Gynecol* 1995;172:687–690.

130. Sanchez-Ramos L, Kaunitz AM, Connor PM. Hygroscopic cervical dilators and prostaglandin E$_2$ gel for preinduction cervical ripening. *J Reprod Med* 1992;37:355–359.

131. Brisson-Carroll G, Fraser W, Bréart G, et al. The effect of routine early amniotomy on spontaneous labor: a meta-analysis. *Obstet Gynecol* 1996;87:891–896.

132. Keirse MJNC, Chalmers I. Methods for inducing labour. In: Chalmers I, Enkin M, Keirse MJNC, eds. *Effective care in pregnancy and childbirth.* Oxford: Oxford University Press, 1989:1057–1079.

133. Fraser WD, Marcoux S, Moutquin J-M, et al. Effect of early amniotomy on the risk of dystocia in nulliparous women. *N Engl J Med* 1993;328:1145–1149.

134. Patterson WM. Amniotomy, with or without simultaneous oxytocin infusion. *J Obstet Gynaecol Br Commonw* 1971;78:310–316.

135. Saleh YZ. Surgical induction of labor with and without oxytocin infusion. *Aust NZ J Obstet Gynaecol* 1975;15:80–83.

136. Moldin PG, Sundell G. Induction of labour: a randomised clinical trial of amniotomy versus amniotomy with oxytocin infusion. *Br J Obstet Gynaecol* 1996;103:306–312.

137. Roberts WE, Martin RW, Roach HH, et al. Are obstetric interventions such as cervical ripening, induction of labor, amnioinfusion, or amniotomy associated with umbilical cord prolapse? *Obstet Gynecol* 1997;176:1181–1185.

138. Kerr JMM, Johnstone RW, Phillips MH. *Historical review of British obstetrics and gynaecology, 1800–1950.* London: E&S Livingston, 1954:34.

139. Swann RO. Induction of labor by stripping membranes. *Obstet Gynecol* 1958;11:74–78.

140. Wiriyasirivaj B, Vutyavanich T, Ruangsri RA. A randomized

controlled trial of membrane stripping at term to promote labor. *Obstet Gynecol* 1996;87:767–770.

141. Berghella V, Rogers RA, Lescale K. Stripping of membranes as a safe method to reduce prolonged pregnancies. *Obstet Gynecol* 1996;87:927–931.

142. Crane J, Bennett K, Yound D, et al. The effectiveness of sweeping membranes at term: a randomized trial. *Obstet Gynecol* 1997;89:586–590.

143. Seitchik J, Castillo M. Oxytocin augmentation of dysfunctional labor. I. Clinical data. *Am J Obstet Gynecol* 1982;144:899–905.

144. American College of Obstetricians and Gynecologists. *Induction and augmentation of labor.* ACOG technical bulletin no. 110. Washington, DC: American College of Obstetricians and Gynecologists, 1987.

145. Seitchik J, Amico J, Robinson AG, et al. Oxytocin augmentation of dysfunctional labor. *Am J Obstet Gynecol* 1984;150:225–228.

146. Perry RL, Saatin AJ, Barth WH, et al. The pharmacokinetics of oxytocin as they apply to labor induction. *Am J Obstet Gynecol* 1996;174:1590–1603.

147. Xenakis EMJ, Langer O, Conway D, et al. Low-dose versus high-dose oxytocin augmentation of labor: a randomized trial. *Am J Obstet Gynecol* 1995;173:1874–1878.

148. O'Driscoll K, Foley M, MacDonald D. Active management of labour as an alternative to cesarean section for dystocia. *Obstet Gynecol* 1984;63:485–490.

149. Turner MJ, Brassil M, Gordon H. Active management of labor associated with a decrease in the cesarean section rate in nulliparas. *Obstet Gynecol* 1988;71:150–154.

150. Akoury HA, Brodie G, Caddick R, et al. Active management of labor and operative delivery in nulliparous women. *Am J Obstet Gynecol* 1988;158:255–258.

151. Boylan P, Frankowski R, Roundtree R, et al. Effect of active management of labor on the incidence of cesarean section for dystocia in nulliparas. *Am J Perinatol* 1991;8:373–379.

152. Lopez-Zeno JA, Peaceman AM, Adashek JA, et al. A controlled trial of a program for the active management of labor. *N Engl J Med* 1992;326:450–454.

153. Frigoletto FD, Lieberman E, Lang JM, et al. A clinical trial of active management of labor. *N Engl J Med* 1995;333:745–750.

154. Thornton JG, Lilford RJ. Active management of labour: current knowledge and research issues. *Br Med J* 1994;309:366–369.

155. Rockenschaub A. Technology-free obstetrics at the Semmelweiss clinic. *Lancet* 1990;335:977–978.

156. van Alten D, Eskes M, Treffers PE. Midwifery in the Netherlands. The Wormerveer study: selection, mode of delivery, perinatal mortality and infant morbidity. *Br J Obstet Gynaecol* 1989;96:656–662.

157. Satin AJ, Mayberry MC, Leveno KJ, et al. Chorioamnionitis: a harbiger of dystocia. *Obstet Gynecol* 1992;79:913–915.

158. Kennedy E. *Observations on obstetric ausculatation.* Dublin, Ireland: Hodges & Smith, 1833.

159. Hon EH. Instrumentation of the fetal heart rate and fetal electrocardiography. II. A vaginal electrode. *Am J Obstet Gynecol* 1963;86:772–784.

160. Banta HD, Thacker SB. Assessing the costs and benefits of electronic fetal monitoring. *Obstet Gynecol Surv* 1979;34:627–642.

161. American College of Obstetricians and Gynecologists. *Intrapartum fetal heart rate monitoring.* ACOG technical bulletin no. 132. Washington, DC: American College of Obstetricians and Gynecologists, 1989.

162. Freeman RK, Garite TH, Nageotte MP. *Fetal heart rate monitoring,* 2nd ed. Baltimore: Williams & Wilkins, 1991.

163. Paul RH, Suidon AK, Yeh SH. Clinical fetal monitoring. VII. The evaluation of the intrapartum baseline FHR variability. *Am J Obstet Gynecol* 1975;123:206–210.

164. Ingemarsson E, Ingemarsson I, Solum T, et al. A one year study of routine fetal heart rate monitoring during the first stage of labour. *Acta Obstet Gynecol Scand* 1980;59:297–300.

165. Beard RW, Filshie GM, Knight CA, et al. The significance of the changes in the continuous fetal heart rate in the first stages of labour. *J Obstet Gynaecol Br Commonw* 1971;78:865–881.

166. Spencer JAD. Clinical overview of cardiotocography. *Br J Obstet Gynaecol* 1993;100:4–7.

167. Thacker SB, Stroup DF, Peterson HB. Efficacy and safety of electronic fetal monitoring: an update. *Obstet Gynecol* 1995; 86:613–620.

168. Umstad MP, Permezel M, Pepperell RJ. Intrapartum cardiotocography and the expert witness. *Aust NZ J Obstet Gynecol* 1994;34:20–23.

169. Leveno KJ, Quirk JG, Cunningham FG, et al. Prolonged pregnancy: observations concerning the causes of fetal distress. *Am J Obstet Gynecol* 1984;150:465–473.

170. Brubaker K, Garite TJ. The lambda fetal heart rate pattern: an assessment of its significance in the intrapartum period. *Obstet Gynecol* 1988;72:881–885.

171. Mondanlou H, Freeman RK. Sinusoidal fetal heart pattern: its definition and clinical significance. *Am J Obstet Gynecol* 1982; 142:1033.

172. Saling E. Neue Untersuchungsmöglichkeiten des Kindes und der Geburt. *Zentralbl Gynakol* 1961;83:1906–1908.

173. Zalar RW, Quilligan EJ. The influence of scalp sampling on the cesarean section rate for fetal distress. *Am J Obstet Gynecol* 1979;135:239–246.

174. Schifrin BS, Dame L. Fetal heart rate patterns: prediction of Apgar score. *JAMA* 1972;219:1322–1325.

175. Beard RW, Morris ED, Clayton SG. pH of fetal capillary blood as an indicator of the condition of the fetus. *J Obstet Gynaecol Br Commonw* 1967;74:812–817.

176. Bowe ET, Beard RW, Finster M, et al. Reliability of fetal blood sampling. *Am J Obstet Gynecol* 1979; 133:762–768.

177. Paneth N, Stark R. Cerebral palsy and mental retardation in relation to indicators of perinatal asphyxia. *Am J Obstet Gynecol* 1983;147:960–966.

178. Nelson KB, Ellenberg JH. Apgar scores as predictors of chronic neurological disability. *Pediatrics* 1981;68:36–44.

179. Nelson KB, Ellenberg JH. Antecedents of cerebral palsy—multivariate analysis of risk. *N Engl J Med* 1986;315:81–86.

180. Freeman JM, Nelson KB. Intrapartum asphyxia and cerebral palsy. *Pediatrics* 1987;82:240–249.

181. Dennis J, Johnson A, Mutch L, et al. Acid-base status at birth and neurodevelopmental outcome at four and one half year. *Am J Obstet Gynecol* 1989;161:213–220.

182. Dijxhorn MJ, Visser GHA, Touwen BCL, et al. Apgar score, meconium and acidaemia at birth in small for gestational age infants born at term, and their relation to neonatal neurological morbidity. *Br J Obstet Gynaecol* 1987;94:873–879.

183. Ruth VJ, Raivio KO. Perinatal brain damage: predictive value of metabolic acidosis and the Apgar score. *Br Med J* 1988; 297:24–27.

184. Winkler CL, Hauth JC, Tucker JM, et al. Neonatal complications at term as related to the degree of umbilical artery acidemia. *Am J Obstet Gynecol* 1991;164:637–641.

185. Goodwin TM, Belai I, Hernandez P, et al. Asphyxial complications in the term newborn with severe umbilical acidemia. *Am J Obstet Gynecol* 1992;167:1506–1512.

186. Umstad P, Permezel M, Pepperell RJ. Litigation and the intrapartum cardiotocograph. *Br J Obstet Gynaecol* 1995;102:89–91.

187. Hall DB. National Institutes of Health report on causes of mental retardation and cerebral palsy, 1985. Birth asphyxia and cerebral palsy. *Pediatrics* 1989;299:279–282.

188. American College of Obstetricians and Gynecologists. *Use and*

abuse of the Apgar score. ACOG Committee opinion no. 174. Washington, DC: American College of Obstetricians and Gynecologists, 1996.

189. Levene MI, Sands C, Grindulis H, et al. Comparison of two methods of predicting outcome in perinatal asphyxia. *Lancet* 1986;1:67–69.

190. Robertson C, Finer N. Term infants with hypoxic ischemic encephalopathy. *Dev Med Child Neurol* 1985;27:473–485.

191. Nelson KB, Dambrosia JM, Ting TY, et al. Uncertain value of electronic fetal monitoring in predicting cerebral palsy. *N Engl J Med* 1996;334:613–618.

192. Clark RB, Quirk JG. What is birth asphyxia? *Am J Obstet Gynecol* 1990;163:1367–1368.

193. Nelson KB, Ellenberg JH. Predictors of low and very low birth rates and the relation of these to cerebral palsy. *JAMA* 1985; 254:1473–1479.

194. Cooke RWI. Cerebral palsy in very low birth weight infants. *Arch Dis Child* 1990;65:201–206.

195. Murphy DJ, Sellers S, MacKenzie IZ, et al. Case-control study of antenatal and intrapartum risk factors for cerebral palsy in very preterm singleton babies. *Lancet* 1995;346:1449–1454.

196. Gether JK, Nelson KB. Maternal infection and cerebral palsy in infants of normal birth weight. *JAMA* 1997;278:207–211.

197. Chestnut DH, Vincent RD, McGrath JM, et al. Does early administration of epidural analgesia affect obstetric outcome in nulliparous women who are receiving intravenous oxytocin? *Anesthesiology* 1994;80:1193–1200.

198. Chestnut DH, McGrath JM, Vincent RD, et al. Does early administration of epidural analgesia affect obstetric outcome in nulliparous women who are in spontaneous labor? *Anesthesiology* 1994;80:1201–1208.

199. Thorp JA, Hu DH, Albin RM, et al. The effect of intrapartum epidural analgesia on nulliparous labor: a randomized controlled, prospective trial. *Am J Obstet Gynecol* 1993;169:851–858.

200. Lieberman E, Lang JM, Cohen A, et al. Association of epidural analgesia with cesarean delivery in nulliparas. *Obstet Gynecol* 1996;88:993–1000.

201. Fusi L, Steer PJ, Maresh MJA, et al. Maternal pyrexia associated with the use of epidural in labour. *Lancet* 1989;1:1250–1252.

202. Lieberman E, Lang JM, Frigoletto F, et al. Epidural analgesia, intrapartum fever, and neonatal sepsis evaluation. *Pediatrics* 1997;99:415–419.

MOLECULAR EFFECTORS OF HUMAN PRETERM PARTURITION

DOUGLAS A. KNISS
JAY D. IAMS

The act of giving birth to a new child remains one of the great mysteries of modern biology. Few areas of reproductive research have received so much investigation in the last three decades as the control of uterine contractility or cervical changes culminating in expulsion of the human fetus. Yet, we are no closer today than 30 years ago in affecting the clinical consequences of an unwanted preterm delivery. To affect the prenatal side of the preterm birth equation significantly will require continuing research to understand the biologic basis for normal parturition as well as preterm labor.

Throughout the reproductive years of a woman's life, a monthly cycle of endometrial proliferation, secretion, and preparation for implantation of a fertilized ovum occurs with great regularity. However, this cycle is frequently interrupted by union of gametes, resulting in a conceptus and the requirement for a novel biologic program characterized by receptivity of the uterus. In this chapter, we attempt to codify the information regarding the endocrine and paracrine mediators of human parturition.

ENDOCRINE ASPECTS OF PARTURITION

Inasmuch as the central nervous and endocrine systems influence many peripheral organs and physiologic processes in the adult organism, it is not surprising that the hypothalamic (central nervous system), pituitary (endocrine), and adrenal (endocrine) axes are vital to the development of the fetus and its successful emergence from the uterus into the new world. Laboratory rodents, domestic sheep, and nonhuman primates provide convenient experimental paradigms in which many of the details of endocrine influences on the fetoplacental unit have been elegantly defined. However, whereas many of the features of endocrine control of gestation and parturition are similar in the human female, some of the fine details vary markedly among species. Thus, results from animal models can often be deceiving, albeit they provide experimental approaches that frequently are not achievable in human female reproductive medicine. Before the explosion in paracrine biology (i.e., cytokines, polypeptide growth factors, autacoids), investigators thought that female gonadal steroids were the chief orchestrators of the events in late gestation defined as *parturition.* This concept was based in part on the absolute quantities of these two steroids produced by the placenta during pregnancy and, secondarily, on the results obtained from the rat and sheep models of mammalian pregnancy. Debate persists about the mechanisms that govern uterine activity (or lack thereof) during pregnancy; that is, is the uterine myometrium under tonic forces working against the generation of expulsive contractions that must be extinguished before the onset of parturition, or does uterine smooth muscle remain in a passive state of quiescence, requiring one or more uterotonins to produce active labor? Despite statements to the contrary, this controversy is not yet resolved completely. Studies in several laboratories indicate that ovarian steroids play a role in preparing the intrauterine microenvironment for the earliest events of parturition and also play at least an indirect, if not a central, role in human parturition.

Placental Steroidogenesis

Investigators have long appreciated that, in many species, the fetoplacental compartment imparts significant influences over the timing of parturition. Historically, this was thought to involve chiefly steroid hormones synthesized in the placenta (1). Later, investigators hypothesized that other autacoids (e.g., platelet-activating factor, PAF; prostaglandins, PGs) may also exert direct and indirect uterotonic actions (2–4). Although it was recognized previously that the mammalian fetus contributed to placental steroid biosynthesis, Casey and MacDonald et al. were among the first to codify the so-called fetal organ communication system in which endocrine or paracrine influences emanating from the fetal compartment (kidney, adrenal gland, or lung) could exert a positive impact on the initiation of early parturition events at term (5,6). Although the topic of placental production of estrogens and progestins during pregnancy has been reviewed in detail previously (7), a few unique features of this synthetic pathway in the human female deserve mention here.

As gestation advances in several species, there is a concomitant increase in the biosynthetic capacity for steroid hormones in the placenta, including estrogens, progesterone, and glucocorticoids. The work of Siiteri and MacDonald demonstrated a complex relationship between the fetal adrenal axis and the placental unit, in that androgens (dehydroepiandrosterone sulfate and androstenedione) produced within the fetal adrenal cortex are delivered to the placental trophoblast as primary substrates for subsequent estrogen biosynthesis (8).

In many adult endocrine tissues that synthesize steroids (i.e., estrogens, progestins, glucocorticoids, and mineralocorticoids), the enzyme systems are present locally to use low-density lipoprotein cholesterol as the principal precursor for hormone biosynthesis. In those cases, the side-chain enzyme hydrolyzes the side chain at C_{22} from the cholesterol moiety by the rate-limiting enzyme cytochrome P_{450}^{scc} (9,10). This reaction yields pregnenolone, which serves as the precursor for subsequent steroid production, including progesterone and androgens (dehydroepiandrosterone and androstenedione) (9,11). However, because the human placenta essentially is devoid of 17α-hydroxylase and $17\text{-}\rightarrow$ 20-desmolase activities, this tissue cannot use C_{21} steroids

(progesterone or pregnenolone) to produce C_{19} steroids (androgens) for estrogen biosynthesis (11,12). Thus, alternative pathways evolved in the human fetoplacental unit to supply the necessary substituents for the complete spectrum of steroids required for pregnancy maintenance.

A fascinating and dynamic relationship exists among the placental trophoblast, the maternal circulation, and the fetal adrenal cortex that provides the biochemical substrates for placental steroidogenesis (Fig. 28.1.) Because the placenta does not synthesize appreciable amounts of cholesterol *de novo* from acetate, the major contribution of cholesterol and of its immediate reaction product pregnenolone is derived from the maternal circulation (11). Pregnenolone is then converted through 3β-hydroxysteroid dehydrogenase to progesterone (11). Placental progesterone is the major substrate for fetal adrenal synthesis of glucocorticoids and mineralocorticoids, although much of the fetal cortisol that is produced derives from circulating low-density lipoprotein cholesterol of hepatic origin (7). The fetal adrenal zone produces prodigious amounts of pregnenolone and dehydroepiandrosterone. Because the fetus essentially lacks 3β-hydroxysteroid dehydrogenase/Δ (4–5) isomerase activity, it must use progesterone produced in the placenta as its principal source of substrate for corticosteroid production (11,12).

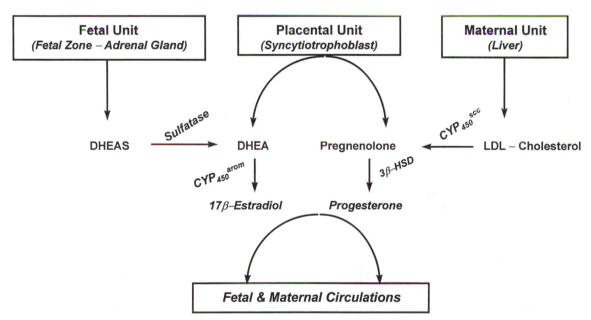

FIGURE 28.1. Interrelationship among the fetal-maternal units for placental steroidogenesis. Fetal androgen (dehydroepiandrosterone sulfate, DHEAS) derived from the fetal zone of the fetal adrenal cortex supplies precursors for trophoblast estrogen biosynthesis by aromatase (CYP$_{450}^{arom}$). Low-density lipoprotein cholesterol derived principally from the maternal circulation supplies the precursor for progesterone production by the intermediate formation of pregnenolone by the action of cytochrome P$_{450}$-side chain cleavage enzyme (CYP$_{450}^{scc}$); 3β-hydroxysteroid dehydrogenase (3β-HSD) catalyzes the formation of progesterone in the trophoblast.

Role of Estradiol and Progesterone in Parturition

Progesterone produced by the placenta subserves several functions for pregnancy maintenance (11,13). First, progesterone, derived initially from the corpus luteum and later from the trophoblast, appears to be a requirement for early pregnancy events such as successful implantation and placentation, because disruption of its action by the receptor antagonist RU-486 (mifepristone) is a potent abortifacient (14,15). Second, progesterone elicits several biochemical actions that contribute to uterine myometrial quiescence, including a decrease in spontaneous electrical activity (16), a decrease in the number of gap junctions among myometrial smooth muscle cells (17), and an inhibition of PG biosynthesis (18–21). Thus, in the progesterone-dominant state, uterine inactivity predominates, whereas in the estrogen-primed condition, a condition of hyperactivity within the myometrium and cervix prevails (16). Although this model is likely simplistic and is too linear to reflect accurately all the complex interactions that exist during parturition, the general precepts of the paradigm nonetheless appear to be supported by experimental investigations.

PARACRINE ASPECTS OF PARTURITION

Within endocrine tissues, hormones and other bioactive molecules are manufactured and emanate to distal sites of action through the circulation. The concept that biomolecules can be produced locally and can be secreted to have their actions within the tissues in which they were synthesized is a relatively recent idea. This dichotomy of biologic activities (i.e., local versus distal) has prompted many investigators to attempt to measure potentially relative bioactive substances from peripheral plasma or serum. Such measurements are often hampered by intersubject variability, interfering binding proteins that result in lower bioavailability of a given analyte, or extensive metabolism of the parent compounds under study. Thus, although peripheral levels of certain paracrine factors can be instructive, these data must be interpreted with caution and with the knowledge that plasma or serum concentrations of particular analytes may not accurately reflect their actual tissue levels.

Salient examples of the potential pitfalls of assaying peripheral levels of molecules that act in an autocrine or paracrine manner are the measurements of certain polypeptide growth factors (e.g., insulin-like growth factors, IGFs), PAF, and many eicosanoids (e.g., prostacyclin, PGI_2, PGE_2, and $PGF_{2\alpha}$). For example, IGF-I circulates in plasma bound to several IGF-binding proteins (22,23). The free, bioavailable IGF-I in blood represents a minute percentage of the total circulating IGF-I (24,25). PAF is an ether phospholipid that contains an acetate residue in the sn-2 position of the triglyceride backbone that is absolutely required for

bioactivity (4,26,27). Active PAF is short-lived, because PAF acetylhydrolase found in many tissues and plasma rapidly hydrolyzes the acetyl group and renders the molecule biologically inert (4,28). Other examples of discrepancies between local tissue levels of bioactive molecules and circulating plasma levels are eicosanoids (cyclooxygenase and lipoxygenase metabolites). Several bioactive PGs (e.g., PGE_2 and $PGF_{2\alpha}$) are rapidly degraded intracellularly or in the immediate extracellular microenvironment by 15-hydroxy-prostaglandin dehydrogenase (29,30). Moreover, PGI_2 and thromboxane A_2 are both degraded nonenzymatically within seconds of their release into the extracellular milieu to inactive 6-keto $PGF_{2\alpha}$ and thromboxane B_2, respectively (29). Thus, measuring peripheral plasma levels of arachidonic acid metabolites typically underrepresents the bioavailable tissue levels of these potent biomediators. Within the kidney, many eicosanoids are converted to their inactive dinor metabolites and are excreted in the urine (31). As such, measuring the primary active metabolites of arachidonic acid in urine dramatically underestimates the tissue concentrations of many eicosanoids.

Thus, tissue levels of substances acting in a paracrine manner must be obtained if relevant biologic interpretations are to be ascribed to a given mediator. Alternatively, when considering the eicosanoids, it is possible to measure concentrations of various inactive metabolites in peripheral blood (e.g., dehydrogenated metabolites) or urine (e.g., dinor metabolites), to provide a window into the approximate tissue levels of the primary active PGs and thromboxanes (31).

Cytokines and Chemokines

Interleukin-1α and Interleukin-1β

Interleukin-1 (IL-1) occupies a central role in the proinflammatory cascade that underlies myriad systemic clinical conditions, including septic shock, adult respiratory distress syndrome, and rheumatoid arthritis (32), as well as experimental granulomatous diseases (33). IL-1 is a pleiotypic cytokine existing in two homologous but genetically distinct isoforms (i.e., IL-1α and IL-1β) that mediates a variety of biologic and pathophysiologic activities in mammalian tissues, including stimulation of arachidonic acid metabolism, elevation of basal body temperature, hypotension, neutrophilia, increased acute-phase reactants, increased turnover of extracellular matrix components, enhanced antibody production, increased cytokine expression (e.g., IL-2 to IL-7, IL-10, and IL-12), increased expression of cell surface IL-2 receptors on T lymphocytes, increased expression of cell adhesion molecules (e.g., intercellular adhesion molecule-1, endothelial-leukocyte adhesion molecule-1, and vascular cell adhesion molecule-1), and enhancement of cell proliferation (e.g., fibroblasts, vascular smooth muscle cells, renal mesangial cells) (34). The precursors IL-1α and

IL-1β, approximately 31 kd, are processed to bioactive 17-kd polypeptides by an IL-1–converting enzyme (35).

Furthermore, voluminous experimental evidence provided by Romero and colleagues as well as other investigators demonstrated a critical role of this cytokine in parturition, especially in the preterm setting complicated by maternal gram-negative bacterial infections (36,37). Initially, Romero et al. demonstrated that both IL-1α and IL-1β were elevated in the amniotic fluid of women presenting to labor and delivery services with preterm uterine contractions in association with intrauterine bacterial infections (37,38). Subsequently, Romero's group discovered that uterine decidua was an abundant source of bioactive IL-1 measured by a sensitive and specific bioassay and that decidual IL-1 was a potent stimulus for PGE$_2$ biosynthesis in human amnion (39,40). Albert et al. and Kennard et al. then demonstrated that IL-1β was able to trigger PGE$_2$ production in human amnion-derived WISH cells and in primary cultures of human decidua, respectively, and that the increased PG synthesis was correlated with upregulation of cyclooxygenase-2 (41,42).

Molnar et al. demonstrated that direct application of IL-1β to myometrial cells grown *in vitro* led to the turnover of arachidonic acid in membrane phospholipids because of activation or induction of PLA$_2$ (43). Mitchell and colleagues reported that, in addition to its ability to enhance PG biosynthesis, IL-1β also stimulated the expression of messenger RNA (mRNA) encoding IL-6 and the release of IL-6 immunoreactive protein (44). Rouru et al. demonstrated that amniochorion membranes produced IL-1β and offered the possibility that the fetal membranes are also a paracrine source of IL-1 that drive PG formation in preparation for or during parturition (45).

Most of the studies cited previously were performed *in vitro* using primary cultures of human intrauterine tissues or continuous cell lines maintained from such tissues. Moreover, much of the earlier work on the putative role of IL-1 in parturition employed amniotic fluid samples collected at the time of amniocentesis to rule out suspected intraamniotic colonization. More recent evidence using a murine model of endotoxin-elicited preterm birth has demonstrated a more direct role of IL-1 in triggering uterine activity culminating in expulsion of the fetus before term (36). Hirst et al. subsequently reported that lipopolysaccharide-induced preterm birth was associated with *de novo* expression of cyclooxygenase-2 in the uterus and placenta (46).

Interleukin-1 Receptor Antagonist

Proinflammatory cytokines are frequently produced in the context of natural receptor blockers (e.g., IL-1 receptor antagonist [IL-1ra] and soluble tumor necrosis factor [TNF] and IL-6 receptors). Investigators have hypothesized that the IL-1ra evolved as part of the IL-1 family by a process of gene duplication that occurred early in the evolution of

the entire gene family (47). Nucleotide and amino acid sequence analyses have revealed that the human IL-1ra shares homology with both human IL-1α and IL-1β and also with the murine and rat sequences, findings indicating a clear evolutionary link likely the result of duplication of an ancestral gene (47). However, the amino terminal portion of the IL-1ra protein apparently was derived from a region of genomic DNA that was distinct from IL-1α or IL-1β, and this difference may explain the diverse biologic actions of the IL-1 agonist versus the IL-1ra (47).

Evidence from a variety of experimental and clinical models suggests that IL-1ra neutralizes many of the proinflammatory properties of IL-1 by competitively binding to the type I IL-1 receptor (48,49). Roessler and colleagues reported that transduction of a complementary DNA encoding IL-1ra could attenuate IL-1–induced rheumatoid arthritis provided a direct link for the antagonistic action of IL-1ra in IL-1–induced inflammation (50). Furthermore, several groups have shown that IL-1ra can inhibit systemic shock or lethality from gram-negative bacterial infections by using experimental paradigms (51).

Romero et al. examined the role of endogenous IL-1ra within the uterine microenvironment in altering the response of the myometrium to IL-1 actions in infection-mediated premature labor. For example, Romero et al. reported that administration of IL-1ra to pregnant mice attenuated IL-1–induced preterm birth *in vivo* (52). Fidel et al. later demonstrated that IL-1ra was expressed within intrauterine tissues after induction of premature labor in the fetal membranes (amniochorion) and decidua (53), a finding that lends further support for an endogenous role of IL-1ra in modulating the molecular events of preterm parturition. Baergen et al. subsequently reported that IL-1 and IL-1ra were synthesized within the placenta and may have a role in the induction of parturition at term (54). Based on these early findings of IL-1ra blockade of IL-1 actions in the context of preterm parturition, investigators postulated that IL-1ra may serve as a natural tocolytic agent within the uterine microenvironment and could possibly be exploited as an exogenous pharmacologic agent in the setting of preterm labor (52,53,55). At high concentrations (approximately 500 to 1,000 ng/mL), IL-1ra may have partial agonist activity, a finding calling into question the utility of this cytokine antagonist as a realistic tocolytic drug (56).

Tumor Necrosis Factor-α

TNF-α is a central proinflammatory cytokine mediating myriad biologic activities in almost every cell type (57). In 1975, TNF was originally identified as a factor isolated from the sera of endotoxin-treated rabbits that induced the necrotic death of certain tumors (58). It was then characterized independently as a molecule that contributed to the wasting syndrome (i.e., cachexia) observed in patients with malignant cancers and was hence named cachectin (59). In reality, the bioactivity of TNF had been described in the 1890s as Coley's toxin, a material that caused the partial regression of tumors in humans (60).

IL-1 and TNF-α are nearly interchangeable cytokines mediating many of the same functions in the context of parturition, both term and preterm. Both cytokines stimulate the synthesis of the other; for example, TNF-α induces IL-1α production in cultured fibroblasts (61). Moreover, Baggia and associates demonstrated that infusion of IL-1α into pregnant rhesus monkeys elicited the production of TNF-α (62). As an example of this apparent cytokine redundancy, investigators demonstrated experimentally that IL-1ra can protect mice against the lethality of exogenously administered TNF-α (63).

The molecular and biologic attributes of TNF-α have been the subject of several comprehensive reviews, and, therefore, only those aspects of TNF action directly related to pregnancy and parturition are dealt with in this chapter (64,65). However, it is important to understand some of the salient details of TNF synthesis and release. TNF-α is actually a member of a family of cytokines that includes TNF-β, lymphotoxin-α, lymphotoxin-β, FAS ligand, and CD40 ligand (64). TNF-α is synthesized as a 26-kd precursor molecule that is membrane bound and is then processed to a 17-kd moiety through a TNF-converting enzyme analogous to IL-1–converting enzyme (66). The mature TNF-α molecule is a homotrimer of a relative molecular mass of approximately 51 kd (64).

In many experimental paradigms of human infectious or inflammatory disease, TNF-α has been shown to be a central participant in the host response to a homeostatic challenge. Bacterial endotoxin has been reported to elicit enhanced TNF-α release, which may contribute to the deleterious consequences of infection. From a perinatal perspective, elevated levels of TNF-α immunoreactivity have been detected in the plasma of neonates manifesting overt sepsis, a finding suggesting that vertical transmission of bacterial colonization can elicit a fetal immune response to infectious insults (67).

TNF-α immunoreactivity has been detected in normal pregnancy, both in the amniotic fluid and at the maternal-fetal interface (68,69). Romero et al. reported increased TNF-α immunoreactivity and bioactivity in amniotic fluid of women presenting with preterm uterine contractions associated with intraamniotic bacterial colonization (70). This group also demonstrated that human uterine decidua is the likely source of TNF-α within the amniotic cavity (71). In experimental models of preterm parturition, TNF-α was shown to be a potent stimulus for fetal demise or premature labor (72). For example, Fidel et al. demonstrated the *de novo* expression of TNF-α immunoreactivity in pregnant mice induced to undergo preterm parturition with a single injection of *Escherichia coli* endotoxin (36). The placental production of TNF-α, among other proin-

flammatory cytokines, has been shown to contribute to spontaneous fetal abortion in a murine model (73).

As has been shown in other disease states (e.g., rheumatoid arthritis, bacterial infections, septic shock), in the setting of immune-mediated pregnancy complications, TNF-α has been reported to work alone or in concert with IL-1β to generate a series of bioactive mediators that lead to deleterious clinical symptoms, including direct cellular cytotoxicity, exacerbated PG biosynthesis and uterine hypercontractility (e.g., fetal membrane PG biosynthesis or myometrial arachidonic acid liberation), or enhanced degradation of extracellular matrix components (activation of matrix metalloproteinases) within the fetal membranes or cervix leading to the premature onset of parturitional events (43,62,74–77). For TNF-α to be an effective mediator of the events of parturition, TNF receptors must be present within those tissues producing bioactive substances that drive myometrial contractions and cervical maturation. Indeed, this is the case, because both type I (p55-60) and II TNF (p75-80) receptors have been localized to certain intrauterine tissues, including placental trophoblast and amniochorion membranes (78).

The recognition that many tissues and plasma contain soluble forms of the TNF receptor has prompted a reappraisal of the role of circulating TNF-binding proteins (e.g., extracellular portions of the TNF receptor) in modulating TNF-α actions. For example, using *in situ* hybridization, Fortunato et al. found that soluble type I TNF receptor mRNA (p55) was expressed in amniochorion membranes (79). Baumann and Romero et al. showed that soluble TNF receptors are part of the host response to intraamniotic infection in women with premature labor (80). Similar to the findings described earlier for IL-1ra and soluble type II IL-1 receptors, recombinant soluble TNF receptors have been shown to protect mice from the lethal effects of endotoxin, a finding suggesting that the receptor may neutralize the biologic actions of lipopolysaccharide-elicited circulating TNF-α (81).

Soluble TNF receptors are roughly analogous to the type II IL-1 receptor in that these circulating binding proteins may serve to modulate that portion of the total plasma TNF that is bioavailable to activate TNF-responsive cells (82). Soluble TNF receptors either produced *de novo* or shed from the surface of cells have been measured under various clinical circumstances, including cancer, bacterial sepsis, infection with human immunodeficiency virus, and inflammatory or autoimmune disorders (82). Aderka et al. suggested that soluble TNF receptors may actually augment the biologic actions of TNF-α by stabilizing the cytokine in plasma and preventing its clearance or degradation (83). The precise biologic role of the soluble forms of TNF receptors must await additional investigations, but many of these circulating soluble receptors are elevated in the setting of human disease and notably in pregnancies complicated by premature uterine contractility (80).

Interleukin-6

IL-6 has been the subject of myriad studies in reproductive medicine and inflammation biology (84,85). IL-6, a primary proinflammatory cytokine (originally identified as interferon-β_2), is a 26-kd highly glycosylated and phosphorylated polypeptide secreted by a variety of cell types (84). IL-6 elicits diverse biologic functions, including induction of acute-phase reactants within the liver (e.g., C-reactive protein, serum amyloid protein, serum amyloid A, mannose-binding protein) that are ancient innate immune mechanisms (84). IL-6 also plays a central role in nearly all acute inflammatory responses to either infectious or foreign body invaders such as activation of complement, opsonization of bacteria, mobilization of neutrophils, elevation of basal body temperature, and activation of T and B lymphocytes (84).

Inasmuch as many of the immune responses cited earlier occur in pregnancies complicated by preterm labor, premature rupture of membranes, or premature cervical ripening, several investigators studied the potential role of IL-6, especially in association with intrauterine bacterial colonization. In this regard, Romero's research group contributed many important observations on the putative role of IL-6 in infection-mediated or inflammation-mediated onset of parturition. For example, Gomez et al. demonstrated a strong correlation among amniotic fluid IL-6 concentrations, white blood cell counts in amniotic fluid specimens, and invasion of the amniotic cavity with gram-negative microorganisms in term pregnancies (86). Greig et al. showed that IL-6 levels in amniocentesis specimens also correlated with histologically demonstrable chorioamnionitis in preterm labor with intact fetal membranes (87). More recently, investigators reported that elevated amniotic fluid IL-6 levels and the accumulation of stable metabolites of nitric oxide (NO) were present in the setting of intraamniotic infection by microorganisms (88).

Many studies *in vitro* have shown that intrauterine tissues (e.g., endometrium, decidua, amnion, chorion, placenta) synthesize and release IL-6 into the extracellular milieu (44,89–92). Tabibzadeh reported that endometrium devoid of epithelial cells, endothelial cells, and lymphocytes is an active site of IL-6 biosynthesis that is highly inducible by IL-1 (89). Dudley et al. demonstrated that human decidua, when exposed to IL-1, secreted immunoreactive IL-6 into the culture medium (93,94). Dudley's group also showed that stimulation of uterine decidua with endotoxin elicited IL-6 secretion (72). Finally, Casey and MacDonald et al. hypothesized that IL-6 production is part of a generalized mechanism of decidual activation in preparation for parturition (6,95).

Although IL-6 production appears to be an early response to inflammatory challenge, new concepts are arising that suggest that IL-6 may play a role as an antiinflammatory mediator to limit the degree of tissue injury that would occur in its absence. For example, Tilg and colleagues

demonstrated that IL-6 can induce the increased production of IL-1ra and the soluble 55-kd form of the TNF receptor in a manner that ultimately contributes to neutralization of IL-1 and TNF-α signals (96). Moreover, Xing et al. used IL-6 knockout mice (IL-6$^{-/-}$) to show that aerosol instillation of endotoxin in murine lungs led to the synthesis of TNF-α, macrophage inhibitory protein-1, and neutrophilic infiltrates into the lung (97). However, in wild-type mice (IL-6$^{+/+}$), there was a more enhanced inflammatory response in the lung, a finding indicating that endogenous IL-6 likely plays a role in dampening cytokine release and white blood cell infiltration into sites of tissue injury (97).

Interleukin-8 and Other Chemokines

IL-8 and the entire family of chemokines are a relatively recently discovered group of cytokine mediators principally involved in infiltration of leukocytes into injured tissues (98). *Chemokines,* as their name implies, are a superfamily of cytokines involved in the chemoattraction and infiltration of many types of inflammatory cells (e.g., neutrophils, monocyte-macrophages, lymphocytes, mast cells, and eosinophils) into sites of acute tissue injury (98,99). These small polypeptides (approximately 7 to 10 kd) are categorized into three separate groups, based on the position and number of cysteine residues in their amino termini (100). The CXC subfamily of chemokines contains two terminal cysteine residues separated by an unconserved amino acid (100). Members of this subfamily include IL-8, growth-related oncogenes (*GRO-α, GRO-β,* and *GRO-γ*), platelet factor 4, regulated upon activation, normal T expression, presumably secreted (RANTES), and IP-10 (induced protein-10) (100). Other subfamilies of the chemokines have since been discovered, but they have not yet been investigated in the context of human parturition and thus are beyond the scope of this chapter.

The first chemokine to be evaluated in pregnancy was IL-8 (neutrophil attractant-activating peptide-1). Romero et al. discovered that IL-8 levels in the amniotic fluid of women presenting with preterm labor correlated with the concentration of neutrophils invading the amniotic cavity (101). This finding also showed a positive correlation with bacterial colonization of the intrauterine microenvironment and histologic chorioamnionitis and suggested that IL-8 may provide a stimulus for leukocyte attraction of neutrophils into the uterus in the presence of infection (101). In a similar type of study, Romero and colleagues reported that macrophage inhibitory protein-1α was elevated in amniotic fluids associated with infection-mediated preterm labor (102). Dudley et al. reported similar findings in patients with group B β-streptococcal infections or gram-negative infections (103). In an *in vitro* investigation, Laham et al. demonstrated that gestational tissues (fetal membranes, decidua, placenta) were capable of synthesizing IL-8 (104).

A few studies have addressed the potential role of IL-8 in ripening of the uterine cervix in preparation for parturition. Barclay et al. demonstrated IL-8 immunoreactivity in the human cervix at the time of parturition (105). These investigations postulated that IL-8 may serve as a potent stimulus for infiltration into the uterus of neutrophils, which are responsible for remodeling of the cervical extracellular matrix through elastase and collagenase activities (106).

Prostaglandins

Clinical and basic science investigations have provided nearly incontrovertible evidence that PGs (principally PGE_2 and $PGE_{2\alpha}$) modulate, if not directly mediate, myometrial contractions and biochemical changes within the uterine cervix that culminate in labor (16,107–110). Early work by Okazaki and MacDonald and colleagues had demonstrated that human parturition was associated with increased activity of phospholipase A_2 and the biosynthesis of PGs (111,112). Yet some investigators have suggested that PG biosynthesis is the mere consequence and not the cause of initial parturition events (113). Other investigators have challenged this notion by demonstrating a continuous increase in amniotic fluid PG levels before the onset of overt uterine contractions (114,115).

In this section, we consider separately the data supporting a role for PGs in driving uterine myometrial contractility and changes in the cervix leading to complete dilatation and effacement. In some cases, the data used to support the contention of PG regulation of parturition are less than completely direct. However, given the nature of human reproductive medicine, unequivocal cause-and-effect experimental relationships are essentially impossible to establish, but the volume of correlative data is compelling.

Early work reported principally by Okazaki and MacDonald and associates demonstrated a concomitant increase in the level of free arachidonic acid within amniotic fluid and the production of PGE_2 by isolated fetal membranes (amniochorion) (111). This finding suggested that mobilization of arachidonic acid from intrauterine tissues (amnion, chorion, or decidua vera) by phospholipase A_2 liberated free arachidonate and thus provided sufficient substrate for PG biosynthesis. At the time these data were presented, it was thought that a single cyclooxygenase isoform, constitutively present in cells, was responsible for PG production (111, 116–118). However, observations made by Casey et al. indicated that exogenously applied agents (e.g., epidermal growth factor) were capable of inducing *de novo* expression of cyclooxygenase and thus regulating, at a potentially molecular level, the production of PGs (119). These data suggested that the model of PG biosynthesis in which phospholipase A_2–liberated arachidonic acid was readily converted to

bioactive eicosanoids was simplistic and that more complex regulation was responsible for the massive increase in PGE_2 and $PGF_{2\alpha}$ levels in amniotic fluid and plasma seen in the setting of active parturition (120–122).

As further evidence that PGs are direct mediators of parturition, a PGF receptor murine knockout model has been reported that manifests impaired or delayed labor and delivery (123). Pregnant mice carrying the null mutation for the PGF receptor failed to respond to $PGF_{2\alpha}$ by labor onset, but they progressed to birth when they administered oxytocin (123).

Cyclooxygenase-2

In the early 1990s, several laboratories reported on the molecular cloning of a second isoform of cyclooxygenase from a variety of species, including mouse, rat, and human. Thus, for the first time, regulation of arachidonic acid metabolism was envisaged to involve the expression of increased copies of cyclooxygenase enzyme (cyclooxygenase-2) that used free arachidonate for PG biosynthesis (124,125,126). Today, the picture of PG production is clearer. For example, a constitutively expressed isoform of cyclooxygenase (cyclooxygenase-1) present in most tissues in the body mediates the formation of low levels of various eicosanoids (PGE_2, PGI_2, thromboxane A_2, PGD_2) for normal physiologic requirements, such as gastrointestinal cytoprotection, renal blood flow, and platelet aggregation (125–127). This isoenzyme undergoes only subtle modulation during inflammatory responses. In contrast, cyclooxygenase-2 is typically not present in appreciable quantities in most normal tissues, but it is rapidly and transiently upregulated after myriad inflammatory stimuli (41,42,128–130). These two isoenzymes carry out nearly identical biochemical reactions, including the cyclooxygenation of arachidonic acid to PGG_2, followed by the peroxidative reduction of PGG_2 to the highly reactive PGH_2 (29,131). PGH_2 is then rapidly converted into one of several PGs or thromboxane A_2, depending on the tissue.

Investigators have begun to examine the potential role of cyclooxygenase-1 and cyclooxygenase-2 in human or animal reproductive tissues (46,116,132). For example, several groups, including our own, have reported that cyclooxygenase-2 is rapidly induced in fetal membrane cells (amnion, chorion laeve), myometrium, uterine endometrium and pregnant decidua, and trophoblast (42,46,74,130,133–136). Upregulation of cyclooxygenase-2 is thought to be responsible for the prodigious amounts of PGE_2 and $PGF_{2\alpha}$ that are detected in the amniotic fluid compartment or plasma during preterm or term parturition (115,137). This work is also supported by the findings of Hirst and Olson and co-workers who measured increased catalytic activity of cyclooxygenase in fetal membranes and uterine decidua obtained from women in active labor (46,133).

Using experimental animal models, the expression of

cyclooxygenase-2 was further examined after the stimulation of preterm delivery using endotoxin. Swaisgood et al. (138) demonstrated that endotoxin elicited a rapid and robust onset of cyclooxygenase-2 expression *de novo* in fetal membranes and uterine tissues that correlated with the preterm delivery of mice (137). Similar results have also been reported by Mitchell and colleagues (139). Thus, although the exact mechanisms governing PG formation during parturition are not yet completely elucidated, accumulating evidence implicates cyclooxygenase-2 induction as a key control point in the initiation or maintenance of labor.

Although overwhelming experimental evidence points to a critical role for cyclooxygenase-2 in the onset and maintenance of labor, at least in the preterm setting, the exact role played by cyclooxygenase-1 has been less well established. Nelson and collaborators reported that transgenic mice harboring a null mutation for cyclooxygenase-1 (cyclooxygenase-1$^{-/-}$) exhibit impaired normal labor at full term (140). Thus, both isoforms of cyclooxygenase likely cooperate in the full onset of parturition, although this has not been unequivocally established in women.

Platelet-Activating Factor

PAF is a proinflammatory phospholipid that has been implicated in a variety of pathophysiologic processes (31). Work in the early 1980s suggested that PAF was a potential fetal signal for the onset of labor. Johnston et al. showed that human amniotic fluid contained demonstrable levels of PAF that appeared as macromolecular lamellar bodies, a finding indicating that they were derived from surfactant shedding from the fetal lung (4). PAF was also shown to be a weak activator of myometrial contractions and PGE_2 synthesis in human amnion cells, a finding further implicating this autacoid in parturition (4).

Nitric Oxide

NO is a free radical gaseous substance produced by the catalytic abstraction of the guanidino nitrogen from L-arginine by NO synthase (NOS) using tetrahydrobiopterin and the reduced form of nicotinamide-adenine dinucleotide phosphate as cofactors (141–146). Three genetically separate isoforms make up the NOS gene family, including endothelial NOS (*eNOS*) (147), inducible NOS (*iNOS*) (148), and neuronal NOS (*nNOS*) (142,149). Originally described as endothelium-dependent relaxation factor, NO causes relaxation in a variety of smooth muscle cell types, including vascular smooth muscle, penile erectile tissue and visceral smooth muscle (e.g., myometrium).

Although each isoform of NOS catalyzes identical reactions to produce NO, the quantitative differences between eNOS or nNOS and iNOS are striking. Thus, eNOS and nNOS produce picomolar amounts of NO that act locally on vascular smooth muscle cells for vasorelaxation (150,

151) or platelets for antiaggregation (151), and nNOS acts postsynaptically in neuromodulation (152). Moreover, both these isoforms are expressed constitutively and are activated by changes in intracellular calcium concentration (142,147,149). In contrast, iNOS is not typically expressed under basal conditions, but it is rapidly upregulated in response to inflammatory stimuli to mediate the synthesis of micromolar quantities (148,153), and it is cytotoxic in the context of innate immune cell killing of microorganisms, viruses, parasites, and tumor cells (148,154–158). Given its potent muscular relaxant properties, investigators have begun to explore the role of NO in uterine contractile function and the potential for this agent to be used pharmacologically as a tocolytic drug (159). Lees et al. used glyceryl trinitrate patches to demonstrate that NO donors could prolong gestation in women experiencing preterm labor (158). These initial observations prompted researchers to study the expression of NOS activity and protein expression within uterine tissues of experimental animal models of pregnancy. Several studies have shown the existence of eNOS immunoreactivity and mRNA within intrauterine tissues, including endometrium, placental trophoblast, decidua, and amniochorion (160–167).

Based on its actions in the vascular smooth muscle, many investigators have postulated that NO mediates myometrial relaxation and results in uterine quiescence (160,168,169). This finding would suggest that NOS is an excellent target for tocolytic therapy by enhancing the levels of NO using exogenous pharmacologic means and thereby creating uterine quiescence (158,170). However, the story is not so simple. Our group demonstrated that iNOS is part of a proinflammatory cascade linking iNOS-generated biosynthesis to the *de novo* expression of cyclooxygenase-2 during endotoxin-driven preterm labor in a murine model of pregnancy (138). Moreover, this investigation also showed that blockade of iNOS activity using aminoguanidine (a selective inhibitor) completely prevented lipopolysaccharide-induced upregulation of cyclooxygenase-2 and partially, but not completely, delayed preterm delivery (138). Currie's group et al. demonstrated a direct effect of NO on cyclooxygenase catalytic activity using *in vivo* and *in vitro* systems (171–173). This paradigm was confirmed by Davidge et al., who showed that NO accentuated the production of eicosanoids in endothelial cells (174).

Thus, although the experimental evidence from vascular smooth muscle and myometrium suggests that NO is a potent mediator of relaxation (especially as an endogenous uterine relaxant), it must also be appreciated that several isoforms of NOS exist, that they are expressed under myriad physiologic and pathologic circumstances, and that they produce either low levels or prodigious quantities of NO. It is far too early in the study of NO action to conclude that NOS is either an appropriate target for tocolytic therapy or a major mediator of the proinflammatory cascade leading to preterm labor and parturition.

Antiinflammatory Cytokines

Traditionally, investigators envisaged that immune cells were classified according to their specific molecular and cellular functions. Thus, B lymphocytes produce antigen-specific antibodies, whereas T lymphocytes carry out a variety of functions such as cytotoxic, helper, and suppressor activities. In recent years, a novel concept has evolved in immunology that postulates the existence of subsets of T-helper cells categorized according to the profile of cytokines they secrete (175–178). T_H1 lymphocytes secrete as their prototypic cytokines IL-2, interferon-γ, granulocyte-macrophage colony-stimulating factor (GM-CSF), and TNF-α among others, whereas T_H2 cells manufacture IL-4, IL-5, IL-10, IL-13, and transforming growth factor-β.

In general, T_H1 cells secrete cytokines that mediate cell-mediated immune responses, whereas T_H2 lymphocytes produce cytokines that trigger humoral responses (179). Although exceptions to this model have been noted, these principles appear to hold for most T-cell–driven immunity (175,176,180). Another feature of this dual T-cell paradigm is the apparently reciprocally antagonistic nature of these two T-lymphocyte subsets (180,181). That is, T_H1-cell–derived cytokines tend to inhibit the release of T_H2 cytokines and vice versa (180,182). Investigators have postulated that T_H1 responses are classically proinflammatory, whereas T_H2 responses tend to be directed toward antiinflammatory actions (183).

As investigators have described the cytokine profiles that appear at the maternal-fetal interface or within the intrauterine milieu during parturition, patterns of cytokine synthesis have emerged that allow the initial characterization of paracrine-autocrine cytokine biology during gestation and in the setting of overt labor (either term or preterm). For example, Hunt and Jones et al. reviewed the expression of cytokines within the uteroplacental microenvironment and concluded that both T_H1 (e.g., type I interferons, IL-2, TNF-α, GM-CSF) and T_H2 (transforming growth factor-β) types are present (179,184). The success or failure of pregnancy (i.e., spontaneous abortion, preterm labor and birth, or normal parturition) likely results from induced shifts in the delicate balance of cytokines within these tissues (uterus, placenta, fetal membranes) that result in a proinflammatory milieu (183,184).

10 KEY POINTS

1. The principal precursors for estrogen biosynthesis in the placental trophoblast are androgens derived largely from the fetal adrenal gland.

2. The human placenta lacks 17α-hydroxylase and therefore cannot use progesterone or pregnenolone for androgen precursors.

3. Proinflammatory cytokines (IL-1 and IL-6 and TNF-α) are elevated in the amniotic fluid of women in the setting of infection-mediated preterm labor.

4. Most of the biologic activities are shared between IL-1 and TNF-α.

5. TNF-α was originally discovered as a substance that caused the regression of certain types of malignant tumors.

6. IL-6 is a proinflammatory cytokine that orchestrates the production of several acute-phase reactants from the liver, including serum amyloid A, C-reactive protein, mannose-binding protein, and serum amyloid protein.

7. Chemokines, of which IL-8 is an example, are cytokines that serve principally to attract leukocytes into sites of acute or chronic inflammation.

8. PGs, derived from the essential fatty acid arachidonate, are the chief biomediators of uterine contractility and cervical dilatation.

9. Increasing experimental evidence implicates cyclooxygenase-2 as a critical enzyme in the cascade of events culminating in preterm labor.

10. NO is a pleiotropic biomediator of both uterine relaxation and proinflammatory activities, depending in part on the timing and magnitude of its production.

REFERENCES

1. Tabibzadeh S. Cytokines and the hypothalamic-pituitary-ovarian-endometrial axis. *Hum Reprod Update* 1994;9:947–967.
2. McGregor JA. Prevention of preterm birth: new initiatives based on microbial-host interactions. *Obstet Gynecol Surv* 1988;43:1.
3. Bienkiewicz A, Pajszczyk-Kieszkiewicz T, Kus E, et al. The effect of platelet activating factor antagonist (BN 52021) on pregnancy duration and collagen content in the pregnant rat uterus and cervix. *Endocr Res* 1994;20:387.
4. Johnston JM, Maki N, Angle MJ, et al. Regulation of the arachidonic acid cascade and PAF metabolism in reproductive tissues. In: Mitchell MD, ed. *Eicosanoids in reproduction*. Boca Raton, FL: CRC Press, 1990:5–37.
5. Casey ML, MacDonald PC. Decidual activation: the role of prostaglandins in labor. In: McNellis D, Challis JRG, MacDonald PC, et al., eds. *The onset of labor: cellular and integrative mechanisms*. Ithaca, NY: Perinatology Press, 1988:141–156.
6. MacDonald PC, Koga S, Casey ML. Decidual activation in parturition: examination of amniotic fluid for mediators of the inflammatory response. *Ann N Y Acad Sci* 1991;622:315.
7. Pepe GJ, Albrecht ED. Actions of placental and fetal adrenal steroid hormones in primate pregnancy. *Endocr Rev* 1995;16:608.
8. Siiteri PK, MacDonald PC. Utilization of circulating dehydroepiandrosterone sulfate for estrogen synthesis during human pregnancy. *Steroids* 1963;2:713.
9. Robel P. Steroidogenesis: the enzymes and regulation of their genomic expression. In: Thibault C, Levasseur M-C, Hunter RHF, eds. *Reproduction in mammals and man*. Paris: Ellipses, 1993:135–142.
10. Simpson AE. The cytochrome P450 4 (CYP4) family. *Gen Pharmacol* 1997;28:351.
11. Speroff L, Glass RH, Kase NG. *Clinical gynecologic endocrinology and infertility*. Baltimore: Williams & Wilkins, 1994:251–289.
12. Conley AJ, Bird IM. The role of cytochrome P450 17α-hydrox-

ylase and 3β-hydroxysteroid dehydrogenase in the integration of gonadal and adrenal steroidogenesis via the delta5 and delta4 pathways of steroidogenesis in mammals. *Biol Reprod* 1997; 56:789.

13. Challis JRG, Lye SL. Parturition. In: Knobil E, Neill JD, eds. *The physiology of reproduction.* New York: Raven, 1994:985–1031.

14. Spitz IM, Croxatto HB, Robbins A. Antiprogestin: mechanism of action and contraceptive potential. *Annu Rev Pharmacol Toxicol* 1996;36:47.

15. Bygdeman M, Swahn ML, Gemzell-Danielsson K, et al. Mode of action of RU486. *Ann Med* 1993;25:61.

16. Wray S. Uterine contraction and physiological mechanisms of modulation. *Am J Physiol* 1993;264:C1.

17. Garfield RE, Ali M, Yallampalli C, et al. Role of gap junctions and nitric oxide in control of myometrial contractility. *Semin Perinatol* 1995;19:41.

18. Salamonsen LA, Hampton AL, Clements JA, et al. Regulation of gene expression and cellular localization of prostaglandin synthase by oestrogen and progesterone in the ovine uterus. *J Reprod Fertil* 1991;92:393.

19. Brennand JE, Leask R, Kelly RW, et al. Changes in prostaglandin synthesis and metabolism associated with labour, and the influence of dexamethasone, RU 486 and progesterone. *Eur J Endocrinol* 1995;133:527.

20. Hedin L, Eriksson A. Prostaglandin synthesis is suppressed by progesterone in rat preovulatory follicles *in vitro. Prostaglandins* 1997;53:91.

21. Wu WX, Ma XH, Zhang Q, et al. Regulation of prostaglandin endoperoxide H synthase 1 and 2 by estradiol and progesterone in nonpregnant ovine myometrium and endometrium *in vivo. Endocrinology* 1997;138:4005.

22. Clemmons DR. Insulin-like growth factor binding protein control secretion and mechanisms of action. In: Raizada MK, LeRoith D, eds. *Molecular biology and physiology of insulin and insulin-like growth factors.* New York: Plenum, 1991:113–123.

23. Clemmons DR. Insulin-like growth factor binding proteins. In: LeRoith D, ed. *Insulin-like growth factors: molecular and cellular aspects.* Boca Raton, FL: CRC Press, 1991:151–179.

24. Bach LA, Rechler MM. Insulin-like growth factors and diabetes. *Diabetes Metab Rev* 1992;8:229.

25. Bell SC, Jackson JA, Ashmore J, et al. Regulation of insulin-like growth factor-binding protein-1 synthesis and secretion by progestin and relaxin in long term cultures of human endometrial stromal cells. *J Clin Endocrinol Metab* 1991;72:1014.

26. Braquet P, Rola-Pleszcynski M. Platelet-activating factor and cellular immune responses. *Immunol Today* 1987;8:345.

27. Braquet P, Touqui L, Shen TY, et al. Perspectives in platelet-activating factor research. *Pharmacol Rev* 1987;39:97.

28. Tjoelker LW, Wilder C, Eberhardt C, et al. Anti-inflammatory properties of a platelet-activating factor acetylhydrolase. *Nature* 1995;374:549.

29. Needleman P, Turk J, Jakschik BA, et al. Arachidonic acid metabolism. *Annu Rev Biochem* 1986;55:69.

30. Van Meir CA, Sangha RK, Walton JC, et al. Immunoreactive 15-hydroxyprostaglandin dehydrogenase (PGDH) is reduced in fetal membranes from patients at preterm delivery in the presence of infection. *Placenta* 1996;17:291.

31. Campbell WB, Halushka PV. Lipid-derived autacoids: eicosanoids and platelet-activating factor. In: Hardman JG, Limbird LE, Molinoff PB, et al., eds. *Goodman and Gilman's pharmacologic basis of therapeutics.* New York: McGraw-Hill, 1996:601–616.

32. Dinarello CA. Role of interleukin-1 and tumor necrosis factor in systemic responses to infection and inflammation. In: Gallin JI, Goldstein IM, Snyderman R, eds. *Inflammation: basic principles and clinical correlates.* New York: Raven, 1992:211–232.

33. Appleton I, Tomlinson A, Colville-Nash PR, et al. Temporal and spatial immunolocalization of cytokines in murine chronic granulomatous tissue: implications for their role in tissue development and repair processes. *Lab Invest* 1993;69:405.

34. Dinarello CA. Biological basis for interleukin-1 in disease. *Blood* 1996;87:2095.

35. Ayala JM, Yamin T-T, Egger LA, et al. IL-1α–converting enzyme is present in monocytic cells as an inactive 450kDa precursor. *J Immunol* 1994;153:2592.

36. Fidel PL, Romero R, Wolf N, et al. Systemic and local cytokine profiles in endotoxin-induced preterm parturition in mice. *Am J Obstet Gynecol* 1994;170:1467.

37. Romero R, Brody DT, Oyarzun E, et al. Infection and labor. III. Interleukin-1: a signal for the onset of parturition. *Am J Obstet Gynecol* 1989;160:1117.

38. Romero R, Mazor M, Brandt F, et al. Interleukin-1 alpha and interleukin-1 beta in preterm and term human parturition. *Am J Reprod Immunol* 1992;27:117.

39. Romero R, Wu YK, Brody DT, et al. Human decidua: a source of interleukin-1. *Obstet Gynecol* 1989;73:31.

40. Romero R, Durum S, Dinarello CA, et al. Interleukin-1 stimulates prostaglandin biosynthesis by human amnion. *Prostaglandins* 1989;37:13.

41. Albert TJ, Su H-C, Zimmerman PD, et al. Interleukin-1α regulates the inducible cyclooxygenase in amnion-derived WISH cells. *Prostaglandins* 1994;48:401.

42. Kennard EA, Zimmerman PD, Friedman CI, et al. Interleukin-1β induces cyclooxygenase-2 in cultured human decidual cells. *Am J Reprod Immunol* 1995;34:65.

43. Molnar M, Romero R, Hertelendy F. Interleukin-1 and tumor necrosis factor stimulate arachidonic acid release and phospholipid metabolism in human myometrial cells. *Am J Obstet Gynecol* 1993;169:825.

44. Mitchell MD, Branch DW, Lundin-Schiller S, et al. Immunologic aspects of preterm labor. *Semin Perinatol* 1991;15:210.

45. Rouru J, Anttila L, Koskinen P, et al. Serum leptin concentrations in women with polycystic ovary syndrome. *J Clin Endocrinol Metab* 1997;82:1697.

46. Hirst JJ, Mijovic JE, Zakar T, et al. Prostaglandin endoperoxide H synthase-1 and -2 mRNA levels and enzyme activity in human decidua at term labor. *J Soc Gynecol Invest* 1998;5:13.

47. Eisenberg SP, Brewer MT, Verderber E, et al. Interleukin 1 receptor antagonist is a member of the interleukin 1 gene family: evolution of a cytokine control mechanism. *Proc Natl Acad Sci U S A* 1991;88:5232.

48. Dinarello CA, Thompson RC. Blocking IL-1: interleukin 1 receptor antagonist *in vivo* and *in vitro. Immunol Today* 1991; 12:404.

49. Dinarello CA. Interleukin-1 and interleukin-1 antagonism. *Blood* 1991;77:1627.

50. Roessler BJ, Hartman JW, Vallance DK, et al. Inhibition of interleukin-1–induced effects in synoviocytes transduced with the human IL-1 receptor antagonist cDNA using an adenoviral vector. *Hum Gene Ther* 1995;6:307.

51. Wakabayashi G, Gelfand JA, Burke JF, et al. A specific receptor antagonist for interleukin 1 prevents *Eschericia coli*–induced shock in rabbits. *FASEB J* 1991;5:338.

52. Romero R, Tartakovsky B. The natural interleukin-1 receptor antagonist prevents interleukin-1–induced preterm delivery in mice. *Am J Obstet Gynecol* 1992;167:1041.

53. Fidel PL Jr, Romero R, Ramirez M, et al. Interleukin-1 receptor antagonist (IL-ra) production by human amnion, chorion, and decidua. *Am J Reprod Immunol* 1994;32:1.

54. Baergen R, Benirschke K, Ulich TR. Cytokine expression in

the placenta: the role of interleukin 1 and interleukin 1 receptor antagonist expression in chorioamnionitis and parturition. *Arch Pathol Lab Med* 1994;118:52.

55. Romero R, Gomez R, Galasso M, et al. The natural interleukin-1 receptor antagonist in the fetal, maternal, and amniotic fluid compartments: the effect of gestational age, fetal gender, and intrauterine infection. *Am J Obstet Gynecol* 1994;171:912.

56. Kniss DA, Zimmerman PD, Garver CL, et al. Interleukin-1 receptor antagonist blocks interleukin-1–induced expression of cyclooxygenase-2 in endometrium. *Am J Obstet Gynecol* 1997; 177:559.

57. Beutler B, van Huffel C. Unraveling function in the TNF ligand and receptor families. *Science* 1994;264:667.

58. Old LJ. Tumor necrosis factor (TNF). *Science* 1985;230:630.

59. Beutler B, Greenwald D, Hulmes JD, et al. Identity of tumor necrosis factor and the macrophage-secreted factor cachectin. *Nature* 1985;316:542.

60. Coley WB. The treatment of malignant tumours by repeated inoculations of erysipelas: with a report of ten original cases. *Am J Med Sci* 1893;105:487.

61. Le J, Weinstein D, Gubler U, et al. Induction of membrane-associated interleukin 1 by tumor necrosis factor in human fibroblasts. *J Immunol* 1987;138:2137.

62. Baggia S, Gravett MG, Witkin SS, et al. Interleukin-1β intra-amniotic infusion induces tumor necrosis factor-α, prostaglandin production, and preterm contractions in pregnant rhesus monkeys. *J Soc Gynecol Invest* 1996;3:121.

63. Everaerdt B, Brouckaert P, Fiers W. Recombinant IL-1 receptor antagonist protects against TNF-induced lethality in mice. *J Immunol* 1994;152:5041.

64. Tracey KJ, Cerami A. Tumor necrosis factor: a pleiotropic cytokine and therapeutic target. *Annu Rev Med* 1994;45:491.

65. Vassalli P. The pathophysiology of tumor necrosis factors. *Annu Rev Immunol* 1992;10:411.

66. Jue DM, Sherry B, Luedke C, et al. Processing of newly synthesized cachectin/tumor necrosis factor in endotoxin-stimulated macrophages. *Biochemistry* 1990;29:8371.

67. de Bont ESJ, Martens A, van Raan J, et al. Tumor necrosis factor-α, interleukin-1β, and interleukin-6 plasma levels in neonatal sepsis. *Pediatr Res* 1993;33:380.

68. Opsjon S-L, Wathen NC, Tingulstad S, et al. Tumor necrosis factor, interleukin-1, and interleukin-6 in normal human pregnancy. *Am J Obstet Gynecol* 1993;169:397.

69. Vince G, Shorter S, Starkey P, et al. Localization of tumour necrosis factor production in cells at the materno/fetal interface in human pregnancy. *Clin Exp Immunol* 1992;88:174.

70. Romero R, Manogue KR, Mitchell MD, et al. IV. Cachectin-tumor necrosis factor in the amniotic fluid of women with intraamniotic infection with preterm labor. *Am J Obstet Gynecol* 1989;161:336.

71. Romero R, Mazor M, Manogue K. Human decidua: a source of tumor necrosis factor. *Eur J Obstet Gynecol Reprod Biol* 1991; 41:123.

72. Dudley DJ, Chen C-L, Branch DW, et al. A murine model of preterm labor: inflammatory mediators regulate the production of prostaglandin E$_2$ and interleukin-6 by murine decidua. *Biol Reprod* 1993;48:33.

73. Cerami A. Inflammatory cytokines. *Clin Immunol Immunopathol* 1992;62:S3.

74. Perkins DJ, Kniss DA. Tumor necrosis factor-α promotes sustained cyclooxygenase-2 expression: attenuation by dexamethasone and NSAIDs. *Prostaglandins* 1997;54:727.

75. So T, Ito A, Sato T, et al. Tumor necrosis factor-α stimulates the biosynthesis of matrix metalloproteinases and plasminogen activator in cultured human chorionic cells. *Biol Reprod* 1992; 46:772.

76. Pollard JK, Thai D, Mitchell MD. Mechanism of cytokine stimulation of prostaglandin biosynthesis in human decidua. *J Soc Gynecol Invest* 1994;1:31.

77. Norwitz ER, Lopez Bernal A, Starkey PM. Tumor necrosis factor-alpha selectively stimulates prostaglandin F$_{2α}$ production by macrophages in human term decidua. *Am J Obstet Gynecol* 1992;167:815.

78. Yelavarthi KK, Hunt JS. Analysis of p60 and p80 tumor necrosis factor-α receptor messenger RNA and protein in human placentas. *Am J Pathol* 1993;143:1131.

79. Fortunato SJ, Menon R, Swan KF II. Expression of TNF-α and TNFR p55 in cultured amniochorion. *Am J Reprod Immunol* 1994;32:188.

80. Baumann P, Romero R, Berry S, et al. Evidence of participation of the soluble tumor necrosis factor receptor I in the host response to intrauterine infection in preterm labor. *Am J Reprod Immunol* 1993;30:184.

81. Lesslauer W, Tabuchi H, Gentz R, et al. Recombinant soluble tumour necrosis factor receptor proteins protect mice from lipopolysaccharide-induced lethality. *Eur J Immunol* 1991;21: 2883.

82. Aderka D. The potential biological and clinical significance of the soluble tumor necrosis factor receptors. *Growth Factor Cytokine Rev* 1996;7:231.

83. Aderka D, Engelman H, Maor Y, et al. Stabilization of the bioactivity of tumor necrosis factor by its soluble receptors. *J Exp Med* 1992;175:323.

84. Van Snick J. Interleukin-6: an overview. *Annu Rev Immunol* 1990;8:253.

85. Heinrich PC, Rose-John S. Interleukin-6. In: Sim E, ed. *The natural immune system: humoral factors.* Oxford: IRL Press, 1993:47–63.

86. Gomez R, Romero R, Galasso M, et al. The value of amniotic fluid interleukin-6, white blood cell count, and Gram stain in the diagnosis of microbial invasion of the amniotic cavity in patients at term. *Am J Reprod Immunol* 1994;32:200.

87. Greig PC, Ernest JM, Teot L, et al. Amniotic fluid interleukin-6 levels correlate with histologic chorioamnionitis and amniotic fluid cultures in patients in premature labor with intact membranes. *Am J Obstet Gynecol* 1993;169:1035.

88. Hsu C-D, Meaddough E, Hong S-F, et al. Elevated amniotic fluid nitric oxide metabolites and interleukin-6 in intra-amniotic infection. *J Soc Gynecol Invest* 1998;5:21.

89. Tabibzadeh S. Human endometrium: an active site of cytokine production and action. *Endocr Rev* 1991;12:272.

90. Mitchell MD, Dudley DJ, Edwin SS, et al. Interleukin-6 stimulates prostaglandin production by human amnion and decidual cells. *Br J Pharmacol* 1991;192:189.

91. Dudley DJ, Trautman MS, Edwin SS, et al. Biosynthesis of interleukin-6 by cultured human chorion laeve cells: regulation by cytokines. *J Clin Endocrinol Metab* 1992;75:1081.

92. Kameda T, Matsuzaki N, Sawal K, et al. Production of interleukin-6 by normal human trophoblasts. *Placenta* 1990;11:205.

93. Dudley DJ, Trautman MS, Araneo BA, et al. Decidual cell biosynthesis of interleukin-6: regulation by inflammatory cytokines. *J Clin Endocrinol Metab* 1992;74:884.

94. Dudley DJ, Edwin SS, Mitchell MD. Macrophage inflammatory protein-1α regulates prostaglandin E$_2$ and interleukin-6 production by human gestational tissues *in vitro. J Soc Gynecol Invest* 1996;3:12.

95. Semer D, Reisler K, MacDonald PC, et al. Responsiveness of human endometrial stromal cells to cytokines. *Ann N Y Acad Sci* 1991;622:99.

96. Tilg H, Trehu E, Atkins MB, et al. Interleukin-6 (IL-6) as an anti-inflammatory cytokine: induction of circulating IL-1

receptor antagonist and soluble tumor necrosis factor receptor p55. *Blood* 1994;83:113.

97. Xing Z, Gauldie J, Cox G, et al. IL-6 is an antiinflammatory cytokine required for controlling local or systemic acute inflammatory responses. *J Clin Invest* 1998;101:311.

98. Baggiolini M, Dewald B, Walz A. Interleukin-8 and related chemotactic cytokines. In: Gallin JI, Goldstein IM, Snyderman R, eds. *Inflammation: basic principles and clinical correlates.* New York: Raven, 1992:247–263.

99. Taub DD. Chemokine-leukocyte interactions: the voodoo that they do so well. *Growth Factor Cytokine Rev* 1996;7:355.

100. Schluger NW, Rom WN. Early responses to infection: chemokines as mediators of inflammation. *Curr Opin Immunol* 1997;9:504.

101. Cherouny PH, Pankuch GA, Romero R, et al. Neutrophil attractant/activating peptide-1/interleukin-8: association with histologic chorioamnionitis, preterm delivery, and bioactive amniotic fluid leukoattractants. *Am J Obstet Gynecol* 1993;169:1299.

102. Romero R, Gomez R, Galasso M, et al. Macrophage inflammatory protein-1 alpha in term and preterm parturition: effect of microbial invasion of the amniotic cavity. *Am J Reprod Immunol* 1994;32:108.

103. Dudley DJ, Edwin SS, Dangerfield A, et al. Regulation of cultured human chorion cell chemokine production by group B streptococci and purified bacterial products. *Am J Reprod Immunol* 1996;36:264.

104. Laham N, Brennecke SP, Rice GE. Interleukin-8 release from human gestational tissue explants: the effects of lipopolysaccharide and cytokines. *Biol Reprod* 1997;57:616.

105. Barclay CG, Brennaud JE, Kelly RW, et al. Interleukin-8 production by the human cervix. *Am J Obstet Gynecol* 1993;169:625.

106. El Maradny E, Kanayama N, Halim A, et al. Interleukin-8 induces cervical ripening in rabbits. *Am J Obstet Gynecol* 1994;171:77.

107. Olson DM, Mijovic JE, Sadowsky DW. Control of human parturition. *Semin Perinatol* 1995;19:52.

108. Ferre F. Molecular mechanisms of parturition. *Infect Dis Obstet Gynecol* 1997;5:98.

109. Maltier J-P, Legrand C, Breuiller M. Parturition. In: Thibault C, Levasseur M-C, Hunter RHF, eds. *Reproduction in mammals and man.* Paris: Ellipses, 1993:481–502.

110. Keirse MJNC, Mitchell MD, Hicks BR, et al. Increase of the prostaglandin precursor, arachidonic acid, in amniotic fluid during spontaneous labour. *Br J Obstet Gynaecol* 1977;84:937.

111. Okazaki T, Casey ML, Okita JR, et al. Initiation of human parturition. XII. Biosynthesis and metabolism of prostaglandins in human fetal membranes and uterine decidua. *Am J Obstet Gynecol* 1981;139:373.

112. Okazaki T, Okita JR, MacDonald PC, et al. Initiation of human parturition. X. Substrate specificity of phospholipase A₂ in human fetal membranes. *Am J Obstet Gynecol* 1978;130:432.

113. MacDonald PC, Casey ML. The accumulation of prostaglandins (PG) in amniotic fluid is an after effect of labor and not indicative of a role for PGE₂ or PGF₂ₐ in the initiation of human parturition. *J Clin Endocrinol Metab* 1993;76:1332.

114. Romero R, Baumann P, Gonzalez R, et al. Amniotic fluid prostanoid concentrations increase early during the course of spontaneous labor at term. *Am J Obstet Gynecol* 1994;171:1613.

115. Romero R, Munoz H, Gomez R, et al. Increase in prostaglandin bioavailability precedes the onset of human parturition. *Prostaglandins Leukot Essent Fatty Acids* 1996;54:187.

116. Olson DM, Zakar T, Smieja Z, et al. A pathway for the regulation of prostaglandins and parturition. In: Drife JO, Calder AA, eds. *Prostaglandins and the uterus.* London: Springer-Verlag, 1992:149–160.

117. Irvine RF. How is the level of free arachidonic acid controlled in mammalian cells? *Biochem J* 1982;204:3.

118. Liggins GC, Wilson TW. Phospholipases in the control of human parturition. *Am J Perinatol* 1989;6:153.

119. Casey ML, Korte K, MacDonald PC. Epidermal growth factor stimulation of prostaglandin E₂ biosynthesis in amnion cells: induction of prostaglandin H₂ synthase. *J Biol Chem* 1988;263:7846.

120. Habenicht AJR, Goerig M, Grulich J, et al. Human platelet-derived growth factor stimulates prostaglandin synthesis by activation and by *de novo* synthesis of cyclooxygenase. *J Clin Invest* 1985;75:1381.

121. Mitchell MD. Current topic: the regulation of placental eicosanoid biosynthesis. *Placenta* 1991;12:557.

122. Keirse MJNC. Eicosanoids in human pregnancy and parturition. In: Mitchell MD, ed. *Eicosanoids in reproduction.* Boca Raton, FL: CRC Press, 1990:199–222.

123. Sugimoto Y, Yamasaki A, Segi E, et al. Failure of parturition in mice lacking the prostaglandin F receptor. *Science* 1997;227:681.

124. Smith WL, Garavito RM, DeWitt DL. Prostaglandin endoperoxide H synthases (cyclooxygenases)-1 and -2. *J Biol Chem* 1996;271:33157.

125. Smith WL, DeWitt DL. Prostaglandin endoperoxide H synthases-1 and -2. *Adv Immunol* 1996;62:167.

126. Williams CS, Dubois RN. Prostaglandin endoperoxide synthase: why two isoforms? *Am J Physiol* 1996;270:G393.

127. Riese J, Hoff T, Nordhoff A, et al. Transient expression of prostaglandin endoperoxide synthase-2 during mouse macrophage activation. *J Leukoc Biol* 1994;55:476.

128. O'Sullivan MG, Chilton FH, Huggins EM Jr, et al. Lipopolysaccharide priming of alveolar macrophages for enhanced synthesis of prostanoids involves induction of a novel prostaglandin H synthase. *J Biol Chem* 1992;267:14547.

129. Perkins DJ, Kniss DA. Rapid and transient cyclo-oxygenase 2 induction by epidermal growth factor. *Biochem J* 1997;321:677.

130. Smith WL, Marnett LJ. Prostaglandin endoperoxide synthase: structure and catalysis. *Biochim Biophys Acta* 1991;1083:1.

131. Bennett P, Slater D. COX-2 expression in labour. In: Vane J, Botting J, Botting R, eds. *Improved non-steroidal anti-inflammatory drugs: COX-2 enzyme inhibitors.* London: Kluwer Academic, 1996:167–188.

132. Teixeira FJ, Zakar T, Hirst JJ, et al. Prostaglandin endoperoxide-H synthase (PGHS) activity and immunoreactive PGHS-1 and PGHS-2 levels in human amnion throughout gestation, at term, and during labor. *J Clin Endocrinol Metab* 1994;78:1396.

133. Hirst JJ, Teixeira FJ, Zakar T, et al. Prostaglandin endoperoxide-H synthase-1 and -2 messenger ribonucleic acid levels in human amnion with spontaneous labor onset. *J Clin Endocrinol Metab* 1995;80:517.

134. Slater D, Berger L, Newton R, et al. The relative abundance of type 1 and type 2 cyclo-oxygenase mRNA in human amnion at term. *Biochem Biophys Res Commun* 1994;198:304.

135. Imseis HM, Zimmerman PD, Samuels P, et al. Tumour necrosis factor-α induces cyclo-oxygenase-2 gene expression in first trimester trophoblasts: suppression by glucocorticoids and NSAIDs. *Placenta* 1997;18:521.

136. Bennett PR, Slater D, Sullivan M, et al. Changes in amniotic arachidonic acid metabolism associated with increased cyclo-oxygenase gene expression. *Br J Obstet Gynaecol* 1993;100:1037.

137. Swaisgood CM, Zu H-X, Perkins DJ, et al. Coordinate expression of inducible nitric oxide synthase and cyclooxygenase-2 genes in uterine tissues of endotoxin-treated pregnant mice. *Am J Obstet Gynecol* 1997;177:1253.

138. Silver RM, Edwin SS, Trautman MS, et al. Bacterial lipopolysaccharide-mediated fetal death: production of a newly recognized form of inducible cyclooxygenase (COX-2) in murine decidua in response to lipopolysaccharide. *J Clin Invest* 1995;95:725.

139. Tanaka S, Kunath T, Hadjantonakis A-K, et al. Promotion of trophoblast stem cell proliferation by FGF4. *Science* 1998;282:2072.

140. Gross GA, Imamura T, Luedke C, et al. Opposing actions of prostaglandins and oxytocin determine the onset of murine birth. *Proc Natl Acad Sci USA* 1998;95:11875–11879.

141. Lowenstein CJ, Dinerman JL, Snyder SH. Nitric oxide: a physiologic messenger. *Ann Intern Med* 1994;120:227.

142. Drapier J-C, Hibbs JB Jr. Differentiation of murine macrophages to express nonspecific cytotoxicity for tumor cells results in L-arginine–dependent inhibition of mitochondrial iron-sulfur enzymes in the macrophage effector cells. *J Immunol* 1988;140:2829.

143. Mills CD. Molecular basis of "suppressor" macrophages: arginine metabolism via the nitric oxide synthetase pathway. *J Immunol* 1991;146:2719.

144. Knowles RG, Moncada S. Nitric oxide synthesis in mammals. *Biochem J* 1994;298:249–258.

145. Moncada S. The L-arginine: nitric oxide pathway. *Acta Physiol Scand* 1992;145:201.

146. Knowles RG, Moncada S. Nitric oxide as a signal in blood vessels. *Trends Biochem Sci* 1992;17:399.

147. Nathan C. Nitric oxide as a secretory product of mammalian cells. *FASEB J* 1992;6:3051.

148. Wang Y, Marsden PA. Nitric oxide synthase: gene structure and regulation. In: Ignarro L, Murad F, eds. *Nitric oxide: biochemistry, molecular biology, and therapeutic implications.* San Diego: Academic Press, 1995;71–90.

149. Azadzoi KM, Kim N, Brown ML, et al. Endothelium-derived nitric oxide and cyclooxygenase products modulate corpus cavernosum smooth muscle tone. *J Urol* 1992;147:220.

150. Gude NM, King RG, Brennecke SP. Role of endothelium-derived nitric oxide in maintenance of low fetal vascular resistance in placenta. *Lancet* 1990;336:1589.

151. Van de Voorde J, Vanderstichele H, Leusen I. Release of endothelium-derived relaxing factor from human umbilical vessels. *Circ Res* 1987;60:517.

152. Karupiah G, Xie Q-W, Buller RML, et al. Inhibition of viral replication by interferon-gamma–induced nitric oxide synthase. *Science* 1993;261:1445.

153. Nathan C, Brukner L, Kaplan G, et al. Role of activated macrophages in antibody-dependent lysis of tumor cells. *J Exp Med* 1980;152:183.

154. Nathan C, Cohn Z. Role of oxygen-dependent mechanisms in antibody-induced lysis of tumor cells by activated macrophages. *J Exp Med* 1980;152:198.

155. Karupiah G, Xie Q-W, Buller RM, et al. Inhibition of viral replication by interferon-gamma–induced nitric oxide synthase. *Science* 1993;261:1445.

156. Nathan C. Natural resistance and nitric oxide. *Cell* 1995;82:873.

157. Yallampalli C, Dong Y-L, Gangula PR, et al. Role and regulation of nitric oxide in the uterus during pregnancy and parturition. *J Soc Gynecol Invest* 1998;5:58.

158. Lees C, Campbell S, Jauniaux E, et al. Arrest of preterm labour and prolongation of gestation with glyceryl trinitrate, a nitric oxide donor. *Lancet* 1994;343:1325.

159. Yallampalli C, Garfield RE, Byam-Smith M. Nitric oxide inhibits uterine contractility during pregnancy but not during delivery. *Endocrinology* 1993;133:1899.

160. Jones GD, Poston L. The role of endogenous nitric oxide synthesis in contractility of term or preterm human myometrium. *Br J Obstet Gynaecol* 1997;104:241.

161. Norman J. Nitric oxide and the myometrium. *Pharmacol Ther* 1996;70:91.

162. Telfer JF, Lyall F, Norman JE, et al. Identification of nitric oxide synthase in human uterus. *Hum Reprod* 1995;10:19.

163. Dong YL, Gangula PRR, Yallampalli C. Nitric oxide synthase isoforms in the rat uterus: differential regulation during pregnancy and labor. *J Reprod Fertil* 1996;107:249.

164. Sladek SM, Magness RR, Conrad KP. Nitric oxide and pregnancy. *Am J Physiol* 1997;272:R441.

165. Ramsay B, Sooranna SR, Johnson MR. Nitric oxide synthase activities in human myometrium and villous trophoblast throughout pregnancy. *Obstet Gynecol* 1996;87:249.

166. Buhimschi I, Ali M, Jain V, et al. Differential regulation of nitric oxide in the rat uterus and cervix during pregnancy and labour. *Hum Reprod* 1996;11:1755.

167. Yallampalli C, Izumi H, Byam-Smith M, et al. An L-arginine–nitric oxide-cyclic guanosine monophosphate system exists in the uterus and inhibits contractility during pregnancy. *Am J Obstet Gynecol* 1994;170:175.

168. Reece MS, McGregor JA, Allen KG, et al. Prostaglandins in selected reproductive tissues in preterm and full-term gestations. *Prostaglandins Leukot Essent Fatty Acids* 1996;55:303.

169. Salvemini D, Misko TP, Masferrer JL, et al. Nitric oxide activates cyclooxygenase enzymes. *Proc Natl Acad Sci U S A* 1993;90:7240.

170. Salvemini D, Seibert K, Masferrer JL, et al. Endogenous nitric oxide enhances prostaglandin production in a model of renal inflammation. *J Clin Invest* 1994;93:1940.

171. Salvemini D, Manning PT, Zweifel BS, et al. Dual inhibition of nitric oxide and prostaglandin production contributes to the antiinflammatory properties of nitric oxide synthase inhibitors. *J Clin Invest* 1995;96:301.

172. Davidge ST, Baker PN, McLaughlin MK, et al. Nitric oxide produced by endothelial cells increases production of eicosanoids through activation of prostaglandin H synthase. *Circ Res* 1995;77:274.

173. Swain SL, Bradley LM, Croft M, et al. Helper T-cell subsets: phenotype, function and the role of lymphokines in regulating their development. *Immunol Rev* 1991;123:115.

174. Coffman RL, Varkila K, Scott P, et al. Role of cytokines in the differentiation of CD4+ T-cell subsets *in vivo. Immunol Rev* 1991;123:189.

175. Cherwinski HM, Schumacher JH, Brown KD, et al. Two types of mouse helper T cell clone. III. Further differences in lymphokine synthesis between Th1 and Th2 clones revealed by RNA hybridization, functionally monospecific bioassays, and monoclonal antibodies. *J Exp Med* 1987;166:1229.

176. Mosmann TR, Cherwinski H, Bond MW, et al. Two types of murine helper T cell clone. I. Definition according to profiles of lymphokine activities and secreted proteins. *J Immunol* 1986;136:2348.

177. Hunt JS. Cytokine networks in the uteroplacental unit: macrophages as pivotal regulatory cells. *J Reprod Immunol* 1989;16:1.

178. Fiorentino DF, Bond MW, Mosmann TR. Two types of mouse T helper cell. IV. Th2 clones secrete a factor that inhibits cytokine production by Th1 clones. *J Exp Med* 1989;170:2081.

179. Oswald IP, Caspar P, Jankovic D, et al. IL-12 inhibits Th2 cytokine responses induced by eggs of *Schistosoma mansoni. J Immunol* 1994;153:1707.

180. Fiorentino DF, Zlotnik A, Vieria P, et al. IL-10 acts on the

antigen-presenting cell to inhibit cytokine production by Th1 cells. *J Immunol* 1991;146:3444.

181. Abbas AK, Murphy KM, Sher A. Functional diversity of helper T lymphocytes. *Nature* 1996;383:787.

182. Jones CA, Finlay-Jones JJ, Hart PH. Type-1 and type-2 cytokines in human late-gestation decidual tissue. *Biol Reprod* 1997; 57:303.

183. Wegmann TG, Guilbert LJ. Immune signalling at the maternal-fetal interface and trophoblast differentiation. *Dev Comp Immunol* 1992;16:425.

184. Wegmann TG, Lin H, Guilbert L, et al. Bidirectional cytokine interactions in the maternal-fetal relationship: is successful pregnancy a TH2 phenomenon? *Immunol Today* 1993;14: 353.

29

MULTIPLE GESTATION

JOHN RODIS

The accident of more than one birth at a single confinement should be anything but a matter of usual amazement and chagrin to the physician, astonishment and dismay to the parents and amusement to everybody else.

Hirst, 1939

Although multifetal gestations account for only 2.4% of births in the United States, they account for approximately 10% of neonatal intensive care admissions and, most important, approximately 14% of neonatal deaths (1,2). In this chapter, I review the physiology of twinning and describe the differences between monozygotic and dizygotic twins. Moreover, I review how multiple gestation influences pregnancy and discuss in detail specific complications of multifetal gestation. I also discuss high-order multifetal gestation, because these situations are increasing in frequency throughout the world with the greater availability of assisted reproductive technologies.

ETIOLOGY AND INCIDENCE OF TWINNING

Twins may either be monozygotic or dizygotic. *Monozygotic twins* result from fertilization of a single ovum by a single sperm. The single zygote ultimately divides either before or after implantation into the uterus. Depending on when division occurs, the placentation may be diamniotic dichorionic, diamniotic monochorionic, or monochorionic monoamniotic. Figure 29.1 illustrates the relationship between the timing of monozygotic twin formation and the type of placentation. *Dizygotic twins,* conversely, are the result of two ova fertilized by two sperm. Thus, their placentation is always dichorionic diamniotic, although the placentas may be fused. In general, approximately two-thirds of twins are dizygotic and one-third are monozygotic, although the percentage of dizygotic twins may be increasing as a result of the use of ovulation-inducing medications, as well as assisted reproductive technologies, including *in vitro* fertilization. Placentation in higher-order multiples can be any combination of monozygotic and dizygotic twins; for example, a triplet gestation may consist of monozygotic

twins and another single fetus, and as such may have a dichorionic triamniotic placentation.

Monozygotic twins occur with a frequency of approximately 4 per 1,000 births, a frequency that is relatively constant throughout the world. The rate does not appear to vary with maternal age, parity, or ethnic or racial differences. Although it was once believed that ovulation-inducing agents did not alter the frequency of monozygotic twinning, more recent evidence suggests that the incidence doubles after ovulation induction (3). In contrast to monozygotic twins, the frequency of dizygotic twins varies markedly throughout the world. The highest incidence is found in western Nigeria, with a frequency of 45 per 1,000 births, and it is lowest in Asian populations, in whom twins may represent only 6 per 1,000 births (4).

In general, the worldwide incidence of twins is approximately 1 in 80 pregnancies; in the United States, the incidence is 12 per 1,000 births. In the United States, the incidence is higher in women of African-American descent and lower in Asian-American women. The incidence of dizygotic twinning also varies with maternal age (5). The incidence of dizygotic twins in 20-year-old women is approximately 3 per 1,000; this rises to approximately 14 per 1,000 in 35- to 40-year-old women. Thereafter, the rate appears to decline. Moreover, the multifetal rate increases with maternal parity.

As noted previously, the incidence of multifetal gestation is increasing, particularly since the availability of ovulation-induction agents (3,6). The incidence of multiple gestations in anovulatory patients treated with clomiphene citrate ranges from 6% to 17%. Patients treated with gonadotropins have an even higher incidence of multiple births, ranging from 18% to 53%. *In vitro* fertilization and embryo transfer may be associated with an even further increased incidence. Approximately 90% of multifetal gestations arising from these modalities are twins, whereas 10% involve three fetuses or more.

PLACENTATION

As depicted in Fig. 29.1, the *placentation* in monozygotic twins depends on the time in which the zygote divides

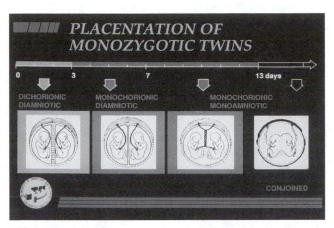

FIGURE 29.1. The relationship between the timing of monozygotic twinning and the resulting placentation.

(7). If twinning occurs during the first 2 to 3 days after fertilization, before the inner cell mass or morula is formed and before complete chorion formation, dichorionic diamniotic twins will result. Hence, each twin has its own placenta and amniotic sac. The membrane appears thickened on ultrasound and histologically has chorion between two layers of amnion (Fig. 29.2). This type of placenta is found in 30% of monozygotic twins. If twinning occurs between the third and eighth day after fertilization, after chorion formation but before complete amnion formation, the result will be a monochorionic diamniotic placenta. This is the most common form of placentation in monozygotic twins, and it accounts for almost 70% of cases. When division occurs between 8 and 13 days, after both chorion and amnion have formed, the result is monochorionic monoamniotic placentation. Fortunately, this only occurs in 1% of monozygotic twins. If division occurs beyond the thirteenth day after fertilization, after the embryonic disc is formed, division will be incomplete, resulting in conjoined

twins. The placentation in conjoined twins is always monochorionic monoamniotic. Each type of placentation and the complications particular to it are discussed in greater detail later in this chapter.

With the exceptions of postterm gestation, macrosomia, and shoulder dystocia, all other obstetric complications are increased in multifetal gestations. Table 29.1 lists these complications and their relative increased risk associated with multiple gestations. In general, these risks are even further increased in high-order multiple gestations. Obviously, other obstetric complications such as death of one twin, twin-twin transfusion syndrome (TTS), conjoined twins, cord entanglement, acardiac twin, and discordant fetal growth are unique to multiple gestations. Each of these issues is addressed in greater detail later in this chapter. However, the first step in the management of a twin gestation is accurate prenatal diagnosis.

PRENATAL DETECTION OF MULTIFETAL GESTATION

In the 1970s, only 50% of twins were detected before delivery. Today, with the widespread use of prenatal ultrasound, as well as maternal serum screen for birth defects that detects many multiple gestations, it is unusual for twins not to be detected before labor. The clinical signs of a multifetal gestation include a uterus that is larger than expected for dates, clinical evidence of hydramnios, unexplained maternal anemia, auscultation of more than one heart, pregnancy resulting from ovulation induction or assisted reproductive technology, or elevated maternal serum α-fetoprotein levels. Approximately 50% of twins have a maternal serum α-fetoprotein level greater than 2.0 multiples of the median, and 30% have elevations greater than 2.5 multiples of the median (8).

TABLE 29.1. COMPLICATIONS OF TWIN PREGNANCIES AND THEIR RELATIVE INCREASED RISK

Complication	Relative Risk	Investigator (Reference)
Spontaneous abortion	2–3×	Grobman (91)
Major congenital abnormalities	2–3×	Spellacy (92), Doyle (93)
Chromosomal abnormalities	2×	Rodis (13)
Preterm birth (<37 wk)	5×	Alexander (1)
Very preterm birth (<32 wk)	9×	Kiely (5)
Low birth rate (<2,500 g)	8×	Alexander (1)
Very low birth weight (<1,500 g)	9×	Alexander (1)
Small size for gestational age (<10th percentile)	4×	Alexander (1)
Severe handicaps	1.7×	Luke (94)
Cerebral palsy	10×	Petridou (95)
Cesarean delivery	2–3×	Senat (96)
Preeclampsia	2–3×	Santema (97), Chaim (98)
Postpartum hemorrhage	3–4×	Stones (99), Combs (100)
Maternal mortality	2–3×	Senat (96)

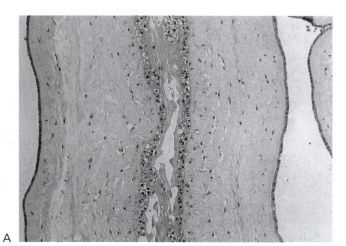
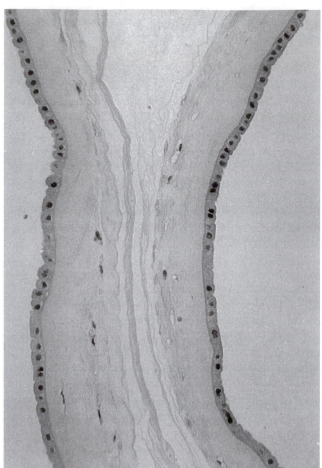

FIGURE 29.2. **A:** T section of a diamniotic dichorionic placenta illustrating two layers of chorion between two layers of amnion. **B:** T section of a diamniotic monochorionic placenta illustrating two layers of amnion connected by loose connective tissue and no intervening layers of chorion.

Diagnosis and Evaluation Using Ultrasound

Multifetal gestation should be readily diagnosed using real-time *ultrasound*. Using transabdominal, high-resolution ultrasound, two separate sacs should be seen by 6 weeks' gestation, and an embryo within each sac should be noted by 7 weeks' gestation. Distinct fetal heartbeats should be noted between 7 and 8 weeks' gestation. Using transvaginal ultrasound, all these findings may be detected approximately 1 to 2 weeks earlier. Although the merits of routine ultrasound studies in all pregnancies are still debated in the United States, routine early ultrasound screening of multiple pregnancies has been shown to be effective in improving perinatal outcome (9). The initial step in ultrasonic evaluation of multifetal gestation should be to ensure the exact number of fetuses and their viability and to discern their placentation.

Ultrasonic diagnosis of twin placentation or chorionicity can be best ascertained by first detecting the number of placentas, the thickness or thinness of the dividing amniotic membrane, and the sexes of the fetuses (10). Figure 29.3 is a flow chart that can be used to ascertain the chorionicity and zygocity (when possible) using ultrasound. Approximately 35% of twins are of the opposite sex and thus are dizygotic and dichorionic. In the remaining 65%, which are of the same sex, a single placenta with a thin dividing membrane (Fig. 29.4) is noted in approximately one-third. The remaining two-thirds are like-sex twins with two placentas, approximately 80% dizygotic and 20% monozygotic. Zygocity in these cases cannot be determined before birth using ultrasound alone; it can be established after delivery or prenatally using invasive modalities (i.e., amniocentesis, chorionic villus sampling, or cordocentesis) by fetal blood typing, detection of different blood group antigens, human leukocyte antigen haplotypes, and further DNA testing. The dichorionic diamniotic placentas may be apart (Fig. 29.5) or fused. In either case, the dividing amniotic membrane appears thick. In the latter case, dichorionicity can be established by visualizing the chorion near the site at which the membranes attach to the placenta (Fig. 29.6). This has been called the *twin peak sign,* (11) and it is

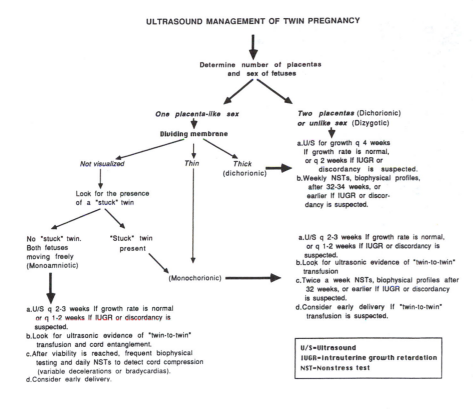

ULTRASOUND MANAGEMENT OF TWIN PREGNANCY

Determine number of placentas
and sex of fetuses

One placenta–like sex

Dividing membrane

Not visualized — *Thin* — *Thick* (dichorionic)

Look for the presence
of a "stuck" twin

No "stuck" twin.
Both fetuses
moving freely
(Monoamniotic)

"Stuck" twin
present

(Monochorionic)

a.U/S q 2-3 weeks If growth rate is normal
or q 1-2 weeks If IUGR or discordancy is
suspected.
b.Look for ultrasonic evidence of "twin-to-twin"
transfusion and cord entanglement.
c.After viability is reached, frequent biophysical
testing and daily NSTs to detect cord compression
(variable decelerations or bradycardias).
d.Consider early delivery.

Two placentas (Dichorionic)
or unlike sex (Dizygotic)

a.U/S for growth q 4 weeks
If growth rate is normal,
or q 2 weeks If IUGR or
discordancy is suspected.
b.Weekly NSTs, biophysical profiles,
after 32-34 weeks, or
earlier If IUGR or discordancy is suspected.

a.U/S q 2-3 weeks If growth rate is normal,
or q 1-2 weeks If IUGR or discordancy is
suspected.
b.Look for ultrasonic evidence of "twin-to-twin"
transfusion
c.Twice a week NSTs, biophysical profiles after
32 weeks, or earlier If IUGR or discordancy
is suspected.
d.Consider early delivery If "twin-to-twin"
transfusion is suspected.

U/S=Ultrasound
IUGR=Intrauterine growth retardation
NST=Nonstress test

FIGURE 29.3. Flow chart demonstrating the role of ultrasound in the establishment of chorionicity and a management scheme for twin pregnancies.

associated with dichorionic diamniotic placentas. Conversely, as shown in Fig. 29.4, monochorionic diamniotic placentas have no intervening layers of chorion between the layers of amnion at the site of attachment of the membranes to the placenta, and this can be confirmed histologically (Fig. 29.2B).

Chorionicity can be established using ultrasound relatively easily and accurately, particularly in the first and second trimesters (9,11). I believe that chorionicity and amnionicity should be established so appropriate counseling can be provided to the patient. For example, there is a high perinatal

mortality rate in monoamniotic twins and a much lower complication rate in dizygotic dichorionic twin gestations.

PHYSIOLOGIC ADAPTATION TO MULTIPLE GESTATIONS

Numerous alterations to maternal physiology occur in multiple gestations. These include an increase in weight gain compared with singleton gestation. For example, whereas an ideal weight gain is suggested to be between 11 and 16

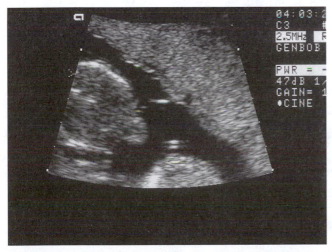

FIGURE 29.4. Ultrasound image of a diamniotic monochorionic twin placenta. Note the one common placenta (P) with a thin membrane (*arrow*) attached to it.

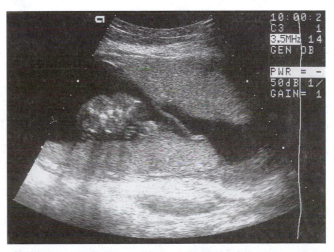

FIGURE 29.5. Ultrasound image of diamniotic dichorionic twin placentas. The placentas are separated, one anterior and one posterior, and the dividing membrane appears thick.

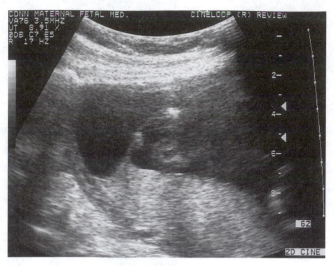

FIGURE 29.6. Ultrasound image of a diamniotic dichorionic twin placenta with a twin peak sign at the insertion of the membranes into the placenta.

kg (25 and 35 lb) in a singleton gestation, for twins it is suggested to be 18 to 20 kg (40 to 45 lb), and in triplets 23 to 25 kg (50 to 55 lb) (12). One sees an increase in red cell volume and an even greater increase in plasma volume, resulting in increased hemodilution effect in multiple gestations. The fibrinogen level is also significantly increased. One sees a greater fall in diastolic blood pressure in the second trimester and a greater rise in diastolic blood pressure before delivery. As noted previously, maternal complications of pregnancy such as preeclampsia and gestational diabetes are increased in multiple gestations. There also appears to be an increased incidence of urinary tract infections in pregnancies complicated by multiple gestation.

CONGENITAL AND CHROMOSOMAL ABNORMALITIES

The incidence of *congenital anomalies* is increased in multiple gestations and ranges from 1.5 to 3.5 times that seen in singletons. Although there is frequently discordance for these anomalies, both twins are affected in 15% of cases. Whereas all congenital anomalies may be increased in multiple gestations, some defects particularly increased in frequency include sirenomelia, holoprosencephaly, anencephaly, and other open neural tube defects. Acardiac twinning is another form of congenital malformation unique to multiple gestation. One may also note skeletal deformations, rather than malformations, as a result of intrauterine crowding. Because of the increased incidence of congenital abnormalities in multifetal gestations, I recommend that all patients with multifetal gestations undergo a targeted ultrasound examination between 16 and 20 weeks' gestation to rule out major congenital malformations. Moreover, be-

cause most twins are dizygotic, and each ovum or sperm has a chance for an abnormal chromosomal complement, there appears to be an increased frequency of *chromosomal abnormalities* in twin gestations (13). Table 29.2 describes the estimated incidence of chromosome abnormalities in twin gestations in comparison with singleton gestations at the time of genetic amniocentesis. As noted, at a maternal age of 32 to 33 years, the likelihood that at least one twin is affected by a major chromosomal abnormality is comparable to that of the risk for a 35-year-old woman with a singleton gestation.

PRENATAL DIAGNOSIS IN MULTIPLE GESTATIONS

Prenatal diagnosis in multifetal gestation should be approached in a manner similar to that of a singleton gestation. The *serum screen* for birth defects, with parameters such as maternal serum α-fetoprotein level, β-human chorionic gonadotropin, and estriol, is effective in identifying some cases of Down's syndrome in multifetal gestation, as well as the defects associated with elevated α-fetoprotein, such as open neural tube defects, gastroschisis, omphalocele, and death of a twin. As mentioned previously, targeted ultrasound examinations performed by experienced examiners using high-resolution ultrasound equipment should be able to ascertain the placentation or chorionicity in the multifetal gestation and to detect most major congenital malformations. Prenatal diagnostic tests, including amniocentesis and chorionic villus sampling, have been performed safely in multifetal gestations and do not appear to have higher risks than in singleton gestations, although large series are lacking.

The serum screen for birth defects, or *triple screen*, has a screen-positive rate for Down's syndrome across all ages of approximately 6.5% in a multiple gestation (14). The detection rate for chromosome abnormalities in monozygotic twins is greater than 70% because, obviously, both fetuses are affected in these cases. The detection rate of chromosomal abnormalities in dizygotic twins, conversely, is slightly greater than 40%. If the zygosity is unknown, as is frequently the case, the detection rate for Down's syndrome is greater than 50%. Unfortunately, insufficient data are available to ascertain the detection rate of chromosomal abnormalities in one or more of a triplet gestation. The risk of trisomy 18, of which approximately half can be detected in singleton gestations by serum screening, is not calculated in multifetal gestations by most laboratories.

Chorionic villus sampling has been used safely in multifetal gestations including twins and triplets. In the hands of an experienced operator, chorionic villus sampling appears to be at least as safe and effective as amniocentesis (15). Some controversy exists regarding the risks of amniocentesis in twin gestations. Some reports suggest amniocentesis-related pregnancy loss rates of 4.9% to 16.7% (16). However, data

TABLE 29.2. ESTIMATED RATE OF DOWN'S SYNDROME OR ANY CHROMOSOMAL ANEUPLOIDY IN TWIN GESTATIONS AT AMNIOCENTESIS

Maternal Age (yr)	Down's Syndrome			All Chromosomal Aneuploidies		
	Singleton[a]	Twins		Singleton[a]	Twins	
		One or Both	Both Affected		One or Both	Both Affected
29	1/850	1/472	1/4230	1/750	1/417	1/3730
30	1/720	1/400	1/3580	1/540	1/300	1/2680
31	1/620	1/345	1/3080	1/370	1/206	1/1830
32	1/520	1/289	1/2580	1/280	1/156	1/1380
33	1/420	1/234	1/2080	1/220	1/122	1/1080
34	1/320	1/178	1/1580	1/170	1/95	1/830
35	1/250	1/139	1/1230	1/140	1/78	1/681
36	1/190	1/106	1/930	1/100	1/56	1/481
37	1/150	1/84	1/731	1/80	1/45	1/381
38	1/110	1/61	1/531	1/60	1/34	1/281
39	1/90	1/50	1/431	1/50	1/28	1/231
40	1/70	1/39	1/331	1/40	1/22	1/182
41	1/50	1/28	1/231	1/30	1/17	1/132
42	1/40	1/22	1/182	1/25	1/14	1/108
43	1/30	1/17	1/132	1/20	1/11	1/83
44	1/25	1/14	1/108	1/15	1/9	1/59
45	1/20	1/11	1/83	1/12	1/7	1/45
46	1/15	1/9	1/59	1/9	1/5	1/31
47	1/12	1/7	1/45	1/7	1/4	1/22
48	1/9	1/5	1/31	1/6	1/4	1/18
49	1/7	1/4	1/22	1/4	1/3	1/10

[a]From Hook.

Rodis, JF, Egan JF, Craffey A, et al. Calculated risk of chromosome abnormalities in twin gestations. *Obstet Gynecol* 1990;76:1037–1041, with permission.

are difficult to analyze because of the increased spontaneous pregnancy loss rate in multifetal gestations. Other investigators have concluded that second trimester amniocentesis in twin gestations is not associated with excess pregnancy loss (17). Whatever modality of invasive prenatal testing is performed, each specimen must be labeled with appropriate identifiers (e.g., twin A, maternal left side, posterior placenta) in case a chromosomal abnormality is identified and selective termination is an option.

Selective Termination

When one twin of the pair has a major chromosomal or congenital abnormality, *selective termination* of the abnormal fetus can be considered. Occasionally, this may be indicated even when the anomaly is lethal, as in the example of anencephaly, in which polyhydramnios in the anencephalic twin can lead to preterm birth and, thus, prematurity of the normal co-twin. In general, the procedure is performed under ultrasonic guidance with the insertion of a fine-gauge needle into the thorax of the abnormal fetus, and potassium chloride is injected until cardiac asystole is noted. Air embolism and fetal exsanguination were used in the past. Evans et al. reported the experience and efficacy of second trimester selective termination from the world's largest centers (18). The overall spontaneous loss rate before 24 weeks for the entire group was 13%. In general, preg-

nancy losses occur less frequently when potassium chloride is used, when the procedures are performed before 20 weeks' gestation, and when the twins are dichorionic.

PRETERM BIRTH

The single biggest contributor to perinatal mortality and morbidity in multiple gestations is *preterm delivery*, which may be a consequence of preterm labor or may occur as a result of pregnancy complications, such as premature rupture of the amniotic membranes or preeclampsia. Preterm labor may be the result of increased uterine distention, increased uterine tone, increased intraamniotic pressure, or uteroplacental insufficiency. All have been implicated as factors resulting in preterm delivery.

Approximately 50% of twins are delivered before 37 completed weeks, and approximately 10% of twins weigh less than 1,500 g at birth (5). The average age of delivery in triplet gestations is 33 weeks, with 90% born before 37 weeks. The average gestational age for quadruplets is 29 weeks, and essentially all are born preterm. As noted previously, approximately 14% of all perinatal deaths are related to multiple gestations. Thus, antenatal care in multiple gestations is aimed primarily at reducing the incidence of preterm birth.

Prevention of Preterm Birth in Multiple Gestations

Prevention of preterm birth in multiple gestations relies first on accurate prenatal diagnosis using ultrasound. Once prenatal diagnosis is made, the patient should be educated regarding the frequency of preterm birth, as well as the signs and symptoms of preterm labor. Numerous strategies have been employed to prevent preterm birth, with largely disappointing results. Modalities to prevent preterm birth of unproved value include bed rest, cervical cerclage, cervical examinations, prophylactic tocolytics, and progesterone.

Although earlier studies suggested that increased *bed rest* in a multiple gestation can improve perinatal outcome, by either increasing the gestational age at delivery or by increasing birth weight (9,19,20), more recent prospective trials failed to show an improvement in perinatal outcome with bed rest (21–23). Whereas decreasing the workload and decreasing physical activity are frequently advocated by some investigators, no randomized clinical trials are available. However, available case-control data suggest that prolonged work in the standing position is associated with an increased rate of preterm delivery (24). Moreover, a population-based study from France found that when all twin mothers were advised to reduce their physical effort after 22 weeks' gestation, and when leave was prescribed to those women who were employed, the proportion of twins delivering before 32 weeks was 5.4%, in comparison with 11% in the United States without such a policy during a comparable period (25). Alternatively, Newman and Ellings in the United States recommended a 2-hour rest period three times a day (morning, afternoon, and evening), as part of a comprehensive, "twin clinic" approach to prenatal care in multiple gestations (26).

Prophylactic *cervical cerclage* has been used in observational as well as controlled studies to prevent preterm birth and to prolong pregnancy duration in multifetal gestations (27,28). However, this approach resulted in an even higher incidence of preterm births.

Newman et al. used weekly digital *cervical examination* (29), and Neilson et al. used a single digital examination at 32 weeks to predict the risk of preterm labor in multiple gestations (30). However, both studies found a low sensitivity as well as a low specificity. Furthermore, Crowther et al. showed no improvement in pregnancy outcome in patients hospitalized for cervical dilatation (21). More recently, transabdominal and transvaginal ultrasound has been used to determine cervical length. Moreover, other signs such as funneling of the cervix have been evaluated. Although most of the studies to date have involved singleton gestations, a multicenter trial revealed that cervical length less than or equal to 2.5 cm at 24 weeks was the best predictor of spontaneous preterm birth in twin pregnancies (31).

Numerous controlled studies have evaluated the routine prophylactic use of *betamimetic therapy* in the third trimester of multiple gestations. The data available suggest that the prophylactic use of these agents does not decrease the incidence of preterm birth. Moreover, mothers with multifetal pregnancies are far more likely to develop pulmonary edema. However, tocolytic therapy may be helpful for short-term use (48 hours), so antenatal steroids can be administered (32).

Although *home uterine activity monitoring* may have some value in higher-order multiple gestations, results of trials in twin gestations have been disappointing and inconclusive. Whereas investigators have shown that in multiple gestations uterine activity is significantly increased during the 24 hours before the diagnosis of labor. Peaceman et al. had comparable pregnancy outcomes in high-order multiples without home uterine monitoring (33). In a collaborative study that included 215 multifetal pregnancies, there was no difference in the incidence of preterm labor (as expected), clinical dilation at the time of diagnosis, or number of preterm deliveries between the monitored group and the group receiving sham monitoring (34). On the other hand, Knuppel et al. and Dyson et al. showed that preterm labor was diagnosed earlier in the group receiving home uterine activity monitoring, with the majority of patients presenting at less than 2 cm dilated (35,36). Colton et al. performed a metaanalysis of randomized trials on home uterine activity monitoring and concluded that monitoring alone results in the earlier diagnosis of preterm labor, prolonged pregnancy, a decreased risk of spontaneous delivery, and a reduction in neonatal intensive care admissions (37).

Antenatal Steroids

Although most authors suggest the use of *antenatal steroids* to promote fetal lung maturity in high-risk multiple gestations as well as in all high-order multiple gestations, randomized trials confirming efficacy are lacking. Moreover, no data are available suggesting what dose of prenatally administered glucocorticoid would be effective in reducing the frequency of hyaline membrane disease in newborns in multiple gestations. Despite these limitations, the United States National Institutes of Health sponsored the Consensus Development Conference on Corticosteroids for Fetal Maturation in 1994 that recommended treatment for women with multiple gestations and impending delivery (38).

Premature Rupture of Membranes

Premature rupture of membranes is more likely to occur in a multifetal gestation. Premature rupture of membranes, when it occurs, almost always involves the presenting sac. As with singletons, intraamniotic infection is present in 10% to 30% of cases. Thus, amniocentesis to rule out intraamniotic infection should be strongly considered in the ruptured sac. However, if amniocentesis cannot be performed in the ruptured sac because of oligohydramnios or fetal position, the unruptured sac can be sampled because intraamniotic infection may be detected in it. Whenever elective preterm delivery of a multiple gestation is entertained, consideration should be given to performing amniocentesis in both sacs. In general, a close correlation exists in twins between the lecithin-to-sphingomyelin (L/S) ratios obtained by amniocentesis (39). I have found concordance for maturity or immaturity in approximately 90% of cases. However, if only a single sac can be sampled, a lecithin-to-sphingomyelin ratio greater than 2.5 should be associated with little risk of hyaline membrane disease in either newborn.

FETAL GROWTH

Discordance in fetal growth occurs in approximately one-fourth to one-third of twin gestations and more frequently in high-order multiples (39,40). Because fundal height measurements have low sensitivity to detect discordant fetal growth in a multiple gestation, ultrasound is the most reliable method. In general, the rate of growth in twin gestations is comparable to that of singleton gestations until about 30 to 32 weeks' gestation, at which time the rates of growth slow significantly. Discordant fetal growth may occur more frequently at earlier gestational ages in monozygotic twins with monochorionic placentas complicated by TTS. Definitions of twin discordancy range from 15% to 25% difference in birth weight, as calculated by the weight of the larger infant minus the weight of the smaller infant, divided by the weight of the larger, times 100%: (large − small/ large × 100).

Unfortunately, studies are lacking correlating birth rate discordancy with perinatal outcome. Although most authors consider 20% discordancy as significant, smaller differences may be important when there is an arrest of fetal growth in one fetus. Discordance of growth may be suspected when the difference in fetal biparietal diameters is greater than 6 mm. However, a more sensitive marker for discrepancy would be differences in abdominal circumference of approximately 2 cm, or estimated fetal weight differences of 20% or greater. Ultrasonic estimation of fetal weight has been shown to have the greatest sensitivity and positive predictive value in identifying discordancy (41,42).

My colleagues and I recommend that serial ultrasound examinations to assess fetal growth be performed every 3 to 4 weeks in multiple gestations or more frequently in twins with monochorionic placentas if one suspects TTS. Moreover, if discordant fetal growth is detected, even in dichorionic twins, the frequency of ultrasound examinations should be increased. I prefer to obtain baseline measurements of fetal growth at approximately 18 weeks' gestation, along with the targeted ultrasound examination of the fetuses to rule out major congenital anomalies. I suggest that during serial ultrasound examinations, rates of fetal growth be plotted on growth curves so a visual assessment of fetal growth can be obtained. Moreover, I prefer that the growth be plotted on curves generated for twin gestations, as opposed to curves derived for singleton gestations (43). If one uses curves derived for singleton gestations, an erroneous diagnosis of intrauterine growth restriction or small for gestational age may be reached (44). Attention should be paid on each ultrasound examination to identify each fetus accurately (e.g., by position, gender, placental location), so each fetus' growth can be plotted longitudinally. When significant discordant fetal growth is noted in a monochorionic placenta, the index of suspicion for TTS should be raised. This is particularly true if one also sees a marked disparity in the amniotic fluid volume in the two sacs, with the larger twin exhibiting polyhydramnios and the smaller twin exhibiting oligohydramnios. However, because most twins are dizygotic and, thus, dichorionic, most cases of discordant fetal growth are merely the result of intrauterine growth restriction in one fetus of the pair.

My colleagues and I found, in a series of 24 pairs of discordant twins, that the fetal growth rate of the larger twin in the pair mirrored the growth rates noted from a cohort of 60 pairs of concordant twins (43). The smaller twin of the discordant pair, conversely, frequently exhibited demonstrable differences in estimated fetal weight and fetal abdominal circumference as early as 20 weeks' gestation. Fetal growth rates in these cases declined significantly, particularly after 32 weeks. Thus, I recommend that serial ultrasound examinations be continued throughout gestation until delivery. When discordant fetal growth is suspected, ultrasonic surveillance should be performed more frequently, at least every 2 weeks. When twins are noted to be growing concordantly and both exhibit growth within the normal range for twin gestations, the interval between ultrasonic examinations can be every 3 to 4 weeks. If intrauterine growth restriction is identified, antenatal fetal testing should be initiated. If no fetal growth is identified in either or both fetuses over a 2-week interval, delivery should be considered, particularly in pregnancies beyond 32 weeks' gestation. Antenatal steroids can be administered and delivery delayed for 48 hours if fetal rate monitoring or fetal biophysical profile testing is reassuring.

COMPLICATIONS UNIQUE TO TWIN GESTATIONS

Twin-Twin Transfusion Syndrome

TTS occurs in fetuses with monochorionic placentation. Although placental vascular anastamoses are seen in virtually 100% of monochorionic placentas, TTS occurs in only 5% to 30%. TTS is believed to result from an imbalance of net blood flow across the placental vascular communication. Studies by Bajoria and colleagues suggested that whereas superficial anastamoses are present in essentially all monochorionic twin placentas, the deep anastamoses, rather than the superficial ones, are most frequently associated with TTS (45). Thus, a single cotyledon may be supplied by the artery of one fetus (donor) and drained by the vein of the co-twin (recipient); hence, one fetus becomes a chronic blood donor to its co-twin. This frequently causes the donor twin to become anemic and growth restricted at birth, and it may become hydropic owing to high-output cardiac failure secondary to severe anemia or low-output cardiac failure secondary to myocardial ischemia. The recipient fetus, conversely, may have polycythemia or polyhydramnios and is frequently ruddy and plethoric in appearance at birth. Hyaline membrane disease is more common in the recipient fetus, and congestive cardiac failure because of circulatory overload may result. Moreover, thrombosis of peripheral vessels may develop because of hyperviscosity secondary to polycythemia. Velamentous cord insertions have been noted more frequently in cases of TTS, usually involving the cord of the smaller, donor twin. The precise diagnosis of TTS may be difficult to make. In a newborn, it is classically made by discordance in birth weight of greater than 20% and a hemoglobin difference of greater than 30%. However, neither one of these conditions is necessarily present. Ultrasonographic diagnosis is generally based on the findings of polyhydramnios in one sac and severe oligohydramnios in the donor sac. There is frequently, but not always, discordance in the fetal weight, with the recipient fetus in the polyhydramniotic sac the larger of the two.

When one fetus appears to be stuck to the uterine wall in an amniotic sac with severe oligohydramnios, the term *stuck-twin syndrome* has been applied. Although stuck-twin syndrome is frequently the result of TTS, it may also result from congenital abnormalities such as renal agenesis in one fetus. Thus, all cases of suspected TTS should have a targeted high-resolution ultrasound performed by an experienced sonographer. TTS syndrome must be differentiated from a twin pregnancy with a normally grown twin and a growth retarded co-twin. In general, in the latter cases, the normally grown twin has a normal amount of surrounding amniotic fluid, whereas the smaller fetus may have oligohydramnios. Twin growth curves are helpful in making this distinction because the larger twin in the normally grown case usually exhibits a normal longitudinal rate of growth, whereas the larger twin in TTS complicated by discordant fetal growth may exhibit an accelerated rate of growth.

Umbilical arterial Doppler studies have been used to aid in the diagnosis and management of TTS, with mixed results. Farmakides et al. suggested that simultaneous observation of high- and low-resistance systolic-to-diastolic ratio is highly suggestive of the diagnosis (46). However, Giles et al. found no difference in umbilical arterial S/D ratio (47). Pretorius et al. found no consistent pattern, although they concluded that absent or reversed diastolic flow invariably predicted a poor outcome (48). Hecher et al. used color Doppler imaging to identify communicating vessels in TTS (49).

Perinatal mortality in TTS has been reported to be as high as 80% to 100% (45). The prognosis depends on gestational age at diagnosis; those cases diagnosed earlier have a worse prognosis. Severe polyhydramnios may require therapeutic amniocentesis to prevent maternal respiratory compromise. Fetal hydrops carries a poor prognosis.

Numerous treatment strategies have been used in management of TTS. These include selective feticide (50), umbilical cord ligation (51), serial amniocentesis (52), and laser coagulation of placental vessels (53,54). Selective feticide was considered after the observation that in some cases after the spontaneous death of one twin, the process seemed to reverse itself, and the surviving co-twin resumed a normal rate of growth and developed a normal amount of amniotic fluid. Thus, some authors suggested that performing selective feticide could improve the prognosis because the mortality had been reported up to 100% before any therapeutic intervention. Umbilical cord ligation using fetoscopy was also suggested by some authors, although this can be technically difficult, and only a few investigators have any experience with it. Umbilical cord occlusion may be indicated in an acardiac or in a monochorial placenta in which selective termination of one twin is indicated. However, there appears to be little indication for selective feticide or umbilical cord occlusion today, because effective alternative therapies exist.

Serial amniocentesis has become the standard treatment for TTS complicated by polyhydramnios-oligohydramnios sequence. By removing the excess amniotic fluid from the large sac, the process may reverse itself. Indeed, survival rates exceeding 70% have been reported with this treatment (52,55). Although numerous authors have suggested different strategies regarding the amount of fluid obtained at a single visit and the rate at which it is removed, no controlled clinical trials are available. Some authors have determined intraamniotic pressures using a water manometer in normal twin pregnancies, as well as those complicated by TTS, and have suggested that amniotic fluid be removed from the polyhydramniotic sac until the intraamniotic pressure is normal (56,57). In general, I remove amniotic fluid until the amount remaining appears to be in the normal range, with resulting maximum vertical depth pockets of 4 to 7 cm. I suggest weekly assessment of amniotic fluid volume once serial amniocentesis is initiated. If the maximum amniotic fluid pocket becomes greater than 8 cm in maximum vertical depth, if the maternal abdomen is clinically tense, or if there is persistent severe oligohydramnios around the stuck twin, the procedure is repeated. Patients may require one to seven amniocenteses.

Endoscopic laser coagulation of the placenta has been performed to treat TTS (53,54), and 53% survival rates have been reported. However, numerous reports using therapeutic amniocentesis have comparable, if not better, survival rates. Endoscopic laser coagulation could be considered in cases failing to respond to therapeutic amniocentesis. Unfortunately, there is a higher risk of preterm birth secondary to preterm labor after endoscopic surgery in pregnancy. In my experience, pregnancies complicated by TTS are at high risk of antepartum and intrapartum fetal distress, and frequent antepartum surveillance is recommended. Moreover, cesarean delivery rates are higher in these cases.

Monoamniotic Twin Gestations

When twinning occurs between the eighth and thirteenth day after conception, the result is *monochorionic monoamniotic* placentation in which both fetuses lie within a single amniotic cavity. Earlier studies suggested that this condition is associated with up to 50% perinatal mortality, primarily because of fetal cord entanglement (58). In general, monoamniotic twins account for approximately 1% to 2% of monozygotic twins; thus, the incidence is approximately 1 per 10,000 to 1 per 25,000 pregnancies. However, several more recent studies suggested that the perinatal mortality may be much lower. Indeed, my colleagues and I reported a series of 13 pairs of monoamniotic twins with 92% perinatal survival (59), even though all cases were complicated by cord entanglement (Fig. 29.7). We suggested that frequent fetal testing in the form of daily nonstress tests improved perinatal survival. Specifically, in 8 of 13 cases, the indication for delivery was nonreassuring fetal heart rate testing. Moreover, in an extensive review of the literature, many of the perinatal deaths reported occurred between 24 and 40 weeks' gestation, a finding thus supporting a possible role for antepartum heart rate monitoring. Moreover, we found that an accurate prenatal diagnosis was associated with higher perinatal survival.

Our protocol for management of monoamniotic twins is as follows. We suggest that serial ultrasound studies be performed to confirm the diagnosis because it may be difficult to visualize an extremely thin dividing membrane in some cases of monochorionic diamniotic twin gestations. We recommend weekly antenatal steroid administration beginning at 24 weeks' gestation and daily fetal heart rate testing beginning at 28 weeks. Other investigators have suggested that umbilical arterial Doppler imaging of each

fetus may be helpful to identify at risk monoamniotic twin fetuses, particularly if there is a marked discordance in the umbilical arterial Doppler velocity (60). We have found color-flow Doppler imaging to be helpful in identification of umbilical cord entanglement, although this may be of limited clinical utility because cord entanglement is universally present in monoamniotic gestations. We suggest elective cesarean delivery at 35 to 36 weeks' gestation once fetal lung maturity has been documented by amniocentesis. Obviously, the amniocentesis specimen reflects an average of the two fetuses' lung profiles. In our experience, a mature lung profile in these settings is not associated with respiratory distress in either fetus. Delivery should be undertaken earlier if evidence of nonreassuring fetal heart rate testing is noted or if other pregnancy complications such as preeclampsia develop. We recommend elective cesarean delivery in all cases to avoid the reported complication of a tight nuchal cord around twin A having to be cut to facilitate delivery, with subsequent realization that the severed cord was that of twin B. This catastrophic complication has been associated with intrapartum death of twin B. All placentas from suspected monoamniotic twin gestations should be inspected in the delivery room to confirm the diagnosis. Although some authors have suggested that TTS does not occur in monoamniotic twins, that is not our experience. Numerous cases appear in the published literature, and we had 1 case in our series of 13 sets. Obviously, in a monoamniotic gestation, the findings of polyhydramnios in one sac and oligohydramnios in the other are impossible to visualize because no dividing membrane is present. However, the findings in our case and others reported suggesting TTS include markedly discordant fetal growth as well as marked differences in hematocrit, with the higher hematocrit in the larger twin. Moreover, in these settings, the larger, polycythemic twin may exhibit evidence of fluid overload and respiratory distress syndrome.

Acardiac Twins

One of the more unusual types of monochorionic twin gestations is the *acardiac twin*. It has occurred in one fetus of monozygotic twins, triplets, or even quintuplets. The incidence is 1 per 30,000 deliveries. The acardiac twin fetus usually has no heart (*holoacardia*) or has only some rudimentary cardiac tissue (*pseudocardia*). Acardiac twins always have monochorial placentas that sustain the life of the acardiac twin. Several theories exist on the causation of acardiac twins (61). One such theory is that reversal of flow through the acardiac twin secondary to at least one artery-to-artery and vein-to-vein connection in the placenta leads to twin reversed arterial perfusion (TRAP) sequence. Other theories suggest that acardiac twins result from a primary defect in cardiac development. Probably, both events must occur to have an acardiac twin.

On ultrasound examination, the acardiac twin appears

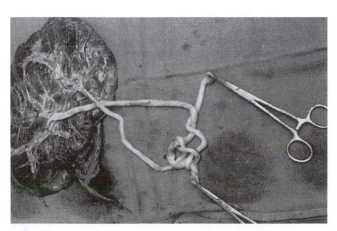

FIGURE 29.7. Monoamniotic monochorionic twin placenta with umbilical cord entanglement.

to be an amorphous mass with pulsation but no obvious cardiac activity. The mass may have some features of a normal fetus including fetal long bones, although in general it is clear that this does not represent a normal fetus (Fig. 29.8). Over time, the acardiac twin exhibits growth, and the otherwise normal co-twin may develop nonimmune hydrops. In such cases, death of the normal co-twin as a result of nonimmune hydrops has occurred. The only effective treatment in such cases of nonimmune hydrops in the normal co-twin is either delivery, if the pregnancy is at or beyond 32 weeks' gestation, or umbilical cord occlusion of the cord to the acardiac twin. This latter procedure has been performed using fetoscopy or ultrasonically guided hooking of the umbilical cord and tying an extracorporeal knot in it by pulling it through a small incision in the maternal abdominal and uterine wall. Each of these procedures has been associated with successful reversal of nonimmune hydrops in the normal co-twin and pregnancy prolongation to term. Obviously, such procedures should be performed by experienced operators.

Conjoined Twins

Conjoined twins result when twinning is initiated after the embryonic disc and amniotic sac have formed, which occurs approximately 13 days after fertilization. If division of the embryonic disc is incomplete, conjoined twins result. The twins can be joined at numerous body sites. If they are joined at the chest, the term *thoracopagus* applies, and when they are joined at the head, the term *craniopagus* is used. Ultrasound can and has been used to diagnose conjoined twins reliably (62). Most important, whenever monoamniotic twins are suspected, an effort should be made to be sure that each fetus is moving independently within the amniotic

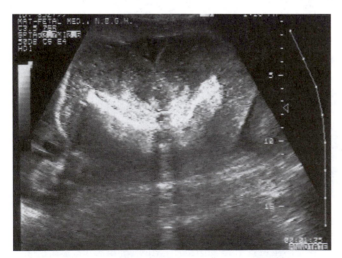

FIGURE 29.8. Ultrasound image of an acardiac twin presenting as an intraamniotic amorphous mass without a heart, but separate from its twin, with some features of "normal" structures, such as long bones.

sac. If the fetuses lie extremely close to each other and do not appear to move independently, conjoined twins should be suspected. A precise incidence of conjoined twins is difficult to obtain because this is an exceedingly rare complication, and most of these twins likely undergo spontaneous abortion. The most famous conjoined twins were Chang and Eng Bunker, the so-called Siamese twins, who were brought to America from Thailand (formerly Siam) in the mid-19th century and toured the world in P.T. Barnum's "Greatest Show on Earth." Unfortunately, there is an exceedingly high mortality with conjoined twins because many share vital structures such as the brain, heart, and liver. Surgical separation may be successful when essential organs are not shared. Planned delivery and separation of conjoined twins should be undertaken only at regional referral centers with experience, because the logistics of an operative delivery of the mother followed by establishing airways and surgical separation of the twins is technically challenging.

Death of a Twin

The true incidence of multiple gestations conceived is probably much higher that the live-born data would suggest. Thirty percent of all pregnancies are estimated to be lost before the mother is aware that she is pregnant (63), so-called *chemical pregnancies*. Another 20% to 33% of twins die in the first or early second trimester after documentation of fetal hearts by ultrasound (64,65). The twin's "disappearance" has led to the term *vanishing twin syndrome*. When death of one twin occurs early in pregnancy, absorption of the missed abortion occurs, and major pregnancy complications are infrequent, although vaginal bleeding may occur. When the pregnancy is beyond 7 weeks, a fetal pole may be seen without a heartbeat, and over time the amniotic fluid around this fetus will diminish markedly and the fetus will be compressed against the uterine side wall. The result at delivery is a small, nonviable *fetus papyraceus,* which has undergone flattening, necrosis, atrophy, and mummification.

When fetal death occurs in a twin later in gestation, there is significant morbidity and mortality in the survivor. Fetal death of one twin occurs from 0.5% to 7% of twin gestations in the second and third trimesters (66). The incidence is even higher in monochorial placentation and is higher yet in monoamniotic gestations. When fetal death occurs in one twin before term, the risks of prematurity with delivery in the surviving twin must be weighed against the risks to both mother and fetus if left undelivered. Prematurity and neonatal death rates among surviving fetuses are high. Monochorionic placentation is associated with a risk of fetal disseminated intravascular coagulopathy, as well as twin embolization syndrome. *Twin embolization syndrome* probably results when thromboplastic material from the dead fetus is shunted to the surviving fetus through vascular communications in the monochorial placenta. The predominant features of twin embolization syndrome are renal cortical necrosis and cerebral necrosis manifested by multicystic encephalomalacia in the surviving twin. Other lesions associated with thromboembolism or possibly secondary to hypotension and hypoxia in the surviving twin include gastrointestinal lesions, pulmonary anomalies, facial anomalies, aplasia cutis, and limb aplasia. Fortunately, twin embolization appears to be uncommon, occurring in fewer than 5% of cases after fetal death in one twin.

Another complication of death of a twin in monochorionic placentas is the so-called *twin reverse arterial perfusion syndrome, or TRAP sequence*. This results when after death of the donor fetus, blood flow from the surviving, high-pressure, high-volume fetus to the now low-pressure, dead, previously donor fetus is reversed. Thus, the larger fetus, who had been the recipient fetus, may exsanguinate into its dead sib. Thus, when death of a twin occurs, close fetal surveillance is indicated in the surviving fetus. Fetal tests of well-being may include nonstress tests, ultrasound, fetal biophysical profiles, and Doppler velocimetry.

As with all cases of fetal death, the cause should be sought. If a significant maternal condition has led to the fetal death, such as poorly controlled diabetes or a severe hypertensive disorder of pregnancy, expeditious delivery in the surviving fetus at or near term should be undertaken after maternal stabilization. Conversely, if the death appears to result from congenital abnormalities or severe intrauterine growth restriction with oligohydramnios in a dichorionic twin gestation, conservative management with frequent antepartum heart rate surveillance should be undertaken. In such cases, when delivery does not occur within 4 weeks of fetal death, the mother will be at risk of developing disseminated intravascular coagulation. Thus, in all cases of fetal death of a twin when expectant management is to be followed or the time of fetal death is not known, serial weekly fibrinogen levels should be obtained. If hypofibrinogenemia (serum fibrinogen less than 100 mg/dL) develops, treatment consists either of correction of the coagulopathy with fresh frozen plasma or cryoprecipitate and delivery of the patient or, in cases remote from term in which pregnancy prolongation is desired, anticoagulation with intravenous heparin, which has been shown to reverse the hypofibrinogenemia successfully (67–69). Romero et al. were able to extend one pregnancy as many as 8 weeks after hypofibrinogenemia developed (69). They found that when heparin was discontinued after fibrinogen values had returned to normal, hypofibrinogenemia recurred. Fortunately, this condition was reversed again by anticoagulating the mother. These findings suggest that anticoagulation should be continued with full-dose heparin until delivery is planned, at which time the heparin can be discontinued, and the effects of the heparin can be reversed with protamine sulfate before delivery. Other investigators have reported spontaneous resolution of hypofibrinogenemia without the use of heparin (70,71).

In general, the prognosis for the surviving twin is correlated to the cause of death of the first twin, the degree of shared fetal circulation, the gestational age, and the time between the death of one twin and the delivery of the other. Management depends on the viability of the surviving twin. Expectant management until approximately 34 weeks' gestation using fetal biophysical profile assessment, antepartum heart rate testing, and serial ultrasound examinations should be performed. Delivery should be undertaken at or after 34 weeks' gestation, after documentation of fetal lung maturity.

Death in one twin is also associated with profound and complex *emotional issues* for the parents. For example, subsequent birthdays in the surviving twin will be associated with a sense of loss as well. Some parents have found it comforting to have a memorial service the day before the birthday or on the day fetal death occurred, to separate the two events temporally and emotionally. Caregivers should be sensitive to the possibility that after delivery of the live twin, the parents' primary emotional response may be grief. It is not unusual for the mother in such cases to have difficulty and lack of desire to bond with the surviving infant. In general, she should not be pressured to do so, and gentle supportive care is indicated. The parents need immediate and long-term support.

Multifetal Pregnancy Reduction

With the advent of ovulation-induction agents and assisted reproductive technology, the incidence of high-order multiple gestations is rising precipitously. As a result, many patients are encountered with triplets, quadruplets, or even greater numbers of fetuses. Pregnancies complicated by higher-order multiples beyond triplets are at extremely high risk of extremely preterm birth, and the likelihood of taking home intact infants is small. Moreover, the numerous social and financial implications of raising high-order multiple pregnancies can be formidable for most families. Thus, *multifetal pregnancy reduction* was developed to offer patients an option to reduce the number of fetuses (71). In most cases, the procedure involves reducing the total number of fetuses to 2, although occasionally reduction to a single fetus is performed. Evans et al. reported on the international experience with multifetal pregnancy reduction in almost 2,000 patients (73). The authors reported overall loss rate before 24 weeks of 17%, with a range as low as 8% when triplets were reduced to twins to a rate as high as 23% when sextuplets or greater were reduced. In general, as with selective reduction, the earlier the procedures are performed, the better the prognosis. Most clinicians prefer to perform this procedure between 10 and 12 weeks' gestation. The procedure is performed using ultrasonic guidance with injection of potassium chloride into the fetal thorax through a small-gauge needle, introduced either through the maternal abdomen or transvaginally. In general, pregnancies reduced from triplets or quadruplets to twins can be expected to achieve greater gestational age and greater birth weight with decreased morbidity and mortality in the live born infants. Several excellent reviews of the ethical considerations of multifetal reduction (74), as well as of the long-term psychologic reaction in patients undergoing the procedure (75), have been published.

Delivery of Twin Fetuses

As noted previously, essentially all *obstetric complications* are increased in multiple gestations, and those that occur during the intrapartum and postpartum periods are no exception. Specifically, premature labor, preterm premature ruptured membranes, dysfunctional uterine labor, malpresentation, prolapse of the umbilical cord, placental abruption, and postpartum hemorrhage are more likely to occur in multifetal gestations. The key to a successful outcome is to have adequate preparation and assistance available. Most important, an experienced obstetrician and anesthesiologist, as well as appropriate health care providers skilled in resuscitation of newborns, should be present or immediately available. Ideally, each fetus should have two people available for resuscitation. It is most helpful to have two skilled obstetricians available as well. Intravenous access should be established, and continuous fetal monitoring should be used. Care should be taken to ensure that each fetus is monitored adequately and simultaneously.

The *mode of delivery* depends on the gestational age, positions of the fetuses, and the skill and experience of the obstetrician. Because of all the potential complications and the rate of malpresentations, it is not surprising that the overall cesarean section rate in the United States for multiple gestations is approximately 50%. When both fetuses are in a cephalic presentation, which is the case in approximately 40% of cases, most clinicians advise attempts at vaginal delivery. Obviously, this applies only when no other contraindications exist to labor, such as fetal distress or placenta previa. When women with twin pregnancies present in labor, ultrasound examination should be performed to determine fetal presentations accurately. If the fetal heart rate tracings are reassuring, labor can be allowed to progress. Twin A can be managed as any singleton pregnancy and delivered as needed, either spontaneously or operatively using forceps or vacuum. An episiotomy should be performed as needed. After delivery of twin A, the position and station of twin B can be determined manually, and as soon as the head is comfortably applied to the cervix, amniotomy can be performed to expedite the delivery. Care should be taken that the head is indeed applied to the cervix so artificial rupture of membranes does not result in umbilical cord prolapse. It is not unusual after delivery of twin A for uterine activity to abate, and we have found it helpful to initiate oxytocin in a continuous infusion if uterine activity does not resume within 10 to 15 minutes of delivery of twin A. Although in the past some authors

suggested that delivery of the second twin should occur within 15 to 30 minutes of the first twin, more recent studies have suggested that as long as the fetal heart retracing is reassuring, this interval can be longer (76,77). Indeed, in some cases, several hours or even days may pass between the delivery of the twins (78). On average, however, most second twins deliver within 30 minutes of the sib. Again, as with twin A, delivery of twin B may be spontaneous, or operative, using forceps, vacuum, or cesarean section as needed.

Significant controversy exists regarding the delivery of twin gestation in which the presentation of the first twin is cephalic and the second twin is noncephalic. Although randomized trials to help resolve the role of vaginal delivery versus elective cesarean section for noncephalic second twins are few (79), numerous authors advocate different approaches (80–84). One approach, perhaps the simplest, is for elective cesarean section in all cases of twins in which the second twin is noncephalic. This approach is associated with the increased maternal morbidity and mortality of cesarean delivery, including hemorrhage, infection, and anesthesia complications. Another approach is to attempt an assisted vaginal delivery of twin B if it is in breech presentation. The obstetrician should be comfortable with vaginal breech deliveries, and adequate assistance should be available as with all breech deliveries. Moreover, an anesthesiologist should be present during the delivery in all such cases. As long as the second twin is not significantly larger than the first twin, successful vaginal delivery can be anticipated by experienced obstetricians. Alternatively, rather than wait for an assisted vaginal breech delivery, total breech extraction can be performed electively for delivery of the second twin. Indeed, numerous authors advocate this management for cephalic-noncephalic twins (81,82). If umbilical cord prolapse occurs with rupture of membranes of the second twin, options include total breech extraction or cesarean delivery.

Another option to consider when twins present in cephalic-breech or cephalic-transverse position is vaginal delivery of the first twin with ultrasonic guidance of the second twin and possible external cephalic version, to deliver both twins as cephalic (84). Ultrasound equipment should be available in the delivery room, and an experienced person should visualize the second twin as twin A is delivering. Frequently, when the second twin is in a transverse lie, gentle external pressure applied to the cephalic region can ensure that the fetus will present in a cephalic manner. When the second twin presents as a breech after delivery of the first twin, external cephalic version can frequently be performed successfully because there is more than adequate room in the distended uterus. Adequate analgesia and anesthesia are required. Ultrasound is used to ensure that the forces are applied to the appropriate fetal parts and also to visualize the fetal heart during the procedure. Once the fetus is rotated to cephalic presentation and adequate descent has occurred, artificial rupture of membranes can be performed, and delivery can proceed. If version is unsuccessful, either vaginal breech delivery or cesarean delivery may be performed.

When the presenting twin is in breech or transverse presentation, as occurs in 5% to 10% of twins, most authors advocate cesarean delivery. One potential complication of breech-cephalic twin presentation is the phenomenon of *locked twins.* This occurs when the chin of the presenting breech fetus "locks" in the neck and chin of the second cephalic fetus with descent of the presenting infant. Although this complication is exceedingly rare (85), it is also potentially devastating for both infants as well as the mother; thus, cesarean section is advised in these cases. Case reports have described external cephalic version of a breech twin A in breech-cephalic presentation (86).

Thus, numerous ways exist for the safe delivery of twin fetuses, and the method chosen clearly depends on the sizes of the fetuses, the maternal pelvis, the experience of the operator, and the availability of assistants and ultrasound equipment. Obviously, if the operator is not experienced in vaginal breech deliveries or internal podalic version, external cephalic version or cesarean delivery is safest, whereas internal podalic version or vaginal breech delivery of noncephalic second twins may be a reasonable alternative with an obstetrician experienced in such modes of delivery.

Whatever mode of delivery is chosen, it is important to monitor both fetuses until they are delivered, to have adequate anesthesia and an anesthesiologist available, and to have assistance for the obstetrician and adequate personnel to resuscitate both infants if necessary. Moreover, the team should be prepared to perform an emergency cesarean delivery if needed. The mode of delivery should be determined by the skill and experience of the operator.

When three or more fetuses are present, my preference is for elective cesarean delivery in all cases. However, several reports have documented successful vaginal delivery of triplet gestation using numerous modalities (87,88). These include internal podalic version, breech extraction, and external cephalic version. The opportunities for umbilical cord prolapse, premature separation of the placentas, intrapartum fetal distress, and complications of malpresentation are high in such cases (89–100). Thus, I prefer elective cesarean delivery.

If cesarean delivery is undertaken for multiple gestations, the surgeon must make an incision in the skin and in the uterus that will allow adequate room for maneuvers necessary to deliver the infants safely. In general, the fetuses should be delivered expeditiously. Patients with multiple gestations are particularly prone to supine hypotension, and, thus, it is important to preload the mother with adequate intravenous fluids before administration of anesthesia and to maintain a left lateral tilt during surgery. Epidural, spinal, or general anesthesia can be used. In all cesarean deliveries for multiple gestations, the obstetrician and anesthesiologist should be prepared for uterine atony because of uterine overdistention, and appropriate uterotonic agents should be readily available. Moreover, whether delivery is vaginal or by cesarean section, one should inspect the placenta to ensure its completeness.

In conclusion, multiple gestations are increasing in frequency and can be complicated pregnancies. However, with accurate prenatal diagnosis, close fetal and maternal surveillance, and a well-equipped and prepared team in the delivery room, a successful pregnancy outcome can be achieved in most cases.

10 KEY POINTS

1. Multiple pregnancies are increasing in frequency, largely because of the more widespread use and availability of ovulation induction and assisted reproductive technologies.

2. Although multiple gestations account for only 2.4% of all live births, they represent 14% of neonatal deaths.

3. All dizygotic twins have dichorionic placentas, whereas monozygotic twin placentas may be dichorionic in 20% to 30%, monochorionic in 60% to 70%, or monoamniotic in 1% to 2%, depending on when division occurs.

4. TTS, a complication of monozygotic twins with monochorionic placentation and deep vascular anastamoses, can be treated with therapeutic amniocentesis.

5. Serum screening for birth defects is helpful in twin pregnancies; most open neural tube defects and approximately 50% of cases of Down's syndrome can be identified.

6. Although essentially all obstetric complications are increased in multiple gestations, preterm birth is the single biggest contributor to the increased perinatal mortality.

7. All patients with multiple pregnancies should have a targeted ultrasound examination to rule out the major congenital abnormalities more frequent in multiple pregnancies, to establish chorionicity, and to obtain baseline growth parameters.

8. Serial ultrasound studies are the only reliable way to assess fetal growth in a multiple gestation, and parameters should be plotted on curves generated for twins.

9. Monoamniotic twins represent a rare and extremely high-risk group of multiple pregnancies, but with accurate prenatal diagnosis, intensive fetal surveillance, and planned early abdominal delivery, successful pregnancy outcomes can usually be expected.

10. Numerous strategies exist for the delivery of the cephalic-noncephalic twin pregnancy, and the choice depends on the skill and experience of the operator, as well as on adequate assistance, available ultrasound equipment, adequate anesthesia, and the capability to perform a cesarean delivery in a timely manner if vaginal delivery fails.

REFERENCES

1. Alexander GR, Kogan M, Martin J, et al. What are the fetal growth patterns of singletons, twins, and triplets in the United States? *Clin Obstet Gynecol* 1998;41:115–125.
2. National Center for Health Statistics. *1991 birth cohort linked birth/infant death data set.* CD-ROM series 20, No. 7. Hyattsville, MD: United States Public Health Service, 1996.
3. Derom C, Derom R, Vlietinick R, et al. Increased monozygotic twinning rate after ovulation induction. *Lancet* 1987;1:1236–1238.
4. MacGillivray I. Epidemiology of twin pregnancy. *Semin Perinatol* 1986;10:4–8.
5. Kiely JL. What is the population-based risk of preterm birth among twins and other multiples? *Clin Obstet Gynecol* 1998;41:3–11.
6. Jewell SE, Yip R. Increasing trends in plural births in the United States. *Obstet Gynecol* 1995;85:229–232.
7. Benirschke K. The placenta in twin gestation. *Clin Obstet Gynecol* 1990;33:18–31.
8. Knight GJ, Palomaki GE. Maternal serum alpha-fetoprotein and the detection of open neural tube defects. In: Elias S, Simpson JL, eds. *Maternal serum screening for fetal genetic disorders.* New York: Churchill Livingstone, 1992:41–58.
9. Persson PH, Grennert L, Gennser G, et al. On improved outcome of twin pregnancy. *Acta Obstet Gynaecol Scand* 1979;58:3–7.
10. Mahony BS, Filly RA, Callen PW. Amnionicity and chorionicity in twin pregnancies: prediction using ultrasound. *Radiology* 1985;155:205–209.
11. Findberg H. The twin peak sign: reliable evidence of dichorionic twinning. *J Ultrasound Med* 1992;11:571–577.
12. Luke B. What is the influence of maternal weight gain on the fetal growth of twins? *Clin Obstet Gynecol* 1998;41:57–64.
13. Rodis JF, Egan JF, Craffey A, et al. Calculated risk of chromosomal abnormalities in twin gestations. *Obstet Gynecol* 1990;76:1037–1041.
14. Neveux LM, Palomaki GE, Knight GJ, et al. Multiple marker screening for Down syndrome in twin pregnancies. *Prenat Diagn* 1996;16:29–34.
15. Wapner RJ. Genetic diagnosis in multiple pregnancies. *Semin Perinatol* 1995;19:351–362.
16. Pruggmayer M, Baumann P, Schutte H, et al. Incidence of abortion after genetic amniocentesis in twin pregnancies. *Prenat Diagn* 1991;11:637–640.
17. Ghidini A, Lynch L, Hicks C, et al. The risk of second trimester amniocentesis in twin gestations: a case-control study. *Am J Obstet Gynecol* 1993;169:1013–1016.
18. Evans MI, Goldberg JD, Dommergues M, et al. Efficacy of second-trimester selective terminations for fetal abnormalities: international collaborative experience among the world's largest centers. *Am J Obstet Gynecol* 1994;171:90–94.
19. Komaromy B, Lampe L. The value of bed rest in twin pregnancy. *Int J Gynaecol Obstet* 1977;15:262–266.
20. Jeffrey RJ, Bowes WA, Delaney JJ. Role of bed rest in twin gestation. *Obstet Gynecol* 1974;43:822–825.
21. Crowther CA, Verkuyl DA, Neilson JP, et al. The effects of hospitalization for rest on fetal growth, neonatal morbidity and length of gestation in twin pregnancy. *Br J Obstet Gynaecol* 1990;97:872–877.
22. Goldenberg RL, Cliver SP, Bronstein J, et al. Bed rest in pregnancy. *Obstet Gynecol* 1994;84:131–136.
23. Gilstrap LC, Hauth JC, Hankins GD, et al. Twins: prophylactic hospitalization and ward rest at early gestational age. *Obstet Gynecol* 1987;69:578–581.
24. Luke B, Mamelle N, Keith LG, et al. The association between occupational factors and preterm birth: a US Nurses' study. *Am J Obstet Gynecol* 1995;173:849–862.
25. Papiernik E, Richard A, Tafforeau J, et al. Social groups and prevention of preterm births in a population of twin mothers. *J Perinat Med* 1996;24:669–676.
26. Newman RB, Ellings JM. Antepartum management of the multiple gestation: the case for specialized care. *Semin Perinatol* 1995;19:387–402.
27. Dor J, Shalev J, Mashiach S, et al. Elective cervical suture of twin pregnancies diagnosed ultrasonically in the first trimester following induced ovulation. *Gynecol Obstet Invest* 1982;13:55–60.
28. Grant A. Cervical cerclage to prolong pregnancy. In: Chalmers I, Enkin M, Keirse MJ, eds. *Effective care in pregnancy and childbirth.* New York: Oxford University Press, 1991.
29. Newman RB, Godsey RK, Ellings JM. Assessment of cervical change. In: Keith LG, Papiernik E, Keith DM, et al., eds. *Multiple pregnancy: epidemiology, gestation and perinatal outcome.* London: Parthenon, 1995:453–470.
30. Neilson JP, Verkuyl DA, Crowther CA, et al. Preterm labor in twin pregnancies: prediction by cervical assessment. *Obstet Gynecol* 1988;72:719–723.
31. Goldenberg RL, Iams J, Miodovnik M, et al. The preterm prediction study: risk factors in twin gestations. National Institute of Child Health and Human Development Maternal-Fetal Medicine Units Network. *Am J Obstet Gynecol* 1996;175:1047–1053.
32. Roberts WE, Perry KG, Naef RW, et al. The irritable uterus: a risk factor for preterm birth? *Am J Obstet Gynecol* 1995;172:138–142.
33. Peaceman AM, Dooley SL, Tamura RK, et al. Antepartum management of triplet gestations. *Am J Obstet Gynecol* 1992;167:1117–1120.
34. The Collaborative Home Uterine Monitoring Study (CHUMS) Group. A multicenter randomized controlled trial of home uterine monitoring: active versus sham device. *Am J Obstet Gynecol* 1995;173:1120–1127.
35. Knuppel RA, Lake MF, Watson DL, et al. Preventing preterm birth in twin gestation: home uterine activity monitoring and perinatal nursing support. *Obstet Gynecol* 1990;76:24S–27S.
36. Dyson DC, Crites YM, Ray DA, et al. Prevention of preterm birth in high risk patients: the role of education and provider contact versus home uterine activity monitoring. *Am J Obstet Gynecol* 1991;164:756–762.
37. Colton T, Kayne HL, Zhang Y, et al. A metaanalysis of home uterine activity monitoring. *Am J Obstet Gynecol* 1995;173:1499–1505.
38. The effect of antenatal steroids for fetal maturation on perinatal outcomes. NIM consens statement 1994, 12(2), 1–24.
39. Leveno KJ, Quirk JG, Whalley PJ, et al. Fetal lung maturation in twin gestation. *Am J Obstet Gynecol* 1984;148:405–411.
40. Reece EA, Yarkoni S, Abdalla M, et al. A prospective longitudinal study of growth in twin gestations compared with growth in singleton pregnancies. *J Ultrasound Med* 1991;10:445–450.
41. Rodis JF, Vintzileos AM, Campbell WA, et al. Intrauterine fetal growth in concordant twin gestations. *Am J Obstet Gynecol* 1990;62:1025–1029.
42. Storlazzi E, Vintzileos AM, Campbell WA, et al. Ultrasonic diagnosis of discordant fetal growth in twin gestations. *Obstet Gynecol* 1987;69:363–367.
43. Rodis JF, Vintzileos AM, Campbell WA, et al. Intrauterine fetal growth in concordant twin gestations. *Am J Obstet Gynecol* 1990;162:1025–1029.

44. Alexander GR, Kogan M, Martin J, et al. What are the growth patterns of singleton, twins and triplets in the United States? *Clin Obstet Gynecol* 1998;41:115–125.

45. Bajoria R, Wigglesorth J, Fisk NM. Angioarchitecture of monochorionic placenta in relation to the twin-twin transfusion syndrome. *Am J Obstet Gynecol* 1995;172:856–863.

46. Farmakides G, Schulman H, Saldana LR, et al. Surveillance of twin pregnancy with umbilical arterial velocimetry. *Am J Obstet Gynecol* 1985;153:789–792.

47. Giles WB, Trudinger BJ, Cook CM. Umbilical waveforms in twin pregnancy. *Acta Genet Med Gemellol (Roma)* 1985;34:233–237.

48. Pretorius DM, Manchester D, Barkin S, et al. Doppler ultrasound of twin transfusion syndrome. *J Ultrasound Med* 1989;8:531–532.

49. Hecher K, Ville Y, Nicolaides KH. Color Doppler ultrasonography in the identification of communicating vessels in twin-twin transfusion syndrome and acardiac twins. *J Ultrasound Med* 1995;14:37–40.

50. Bebbington MW, Wilson RD, Machan L, et al. Selective feticide in twin transfusion syndrome using ultrasound-guided insertion of thrombogenic coils. *Fetal Diagn Ther* 1995;10:32–36.

51. Quintero RA, Romero R, Reich H, et al. *In utero* percutaneous umbilical cord ligation in the management of complicated monochorionic multiple gestations. *Ultrasound Obstet Gynecol* 1996;8:16–22.

52. Saunders NJ, Snijders RJ, Nicolaides KH. Therapeutic amniocentesis in twin-twin transfusion appearing in the second trimester of pregnancy. *Am J Obstet Gynecol* 1992;166:820–824.

53. De Lia JE, Kuhlman RS, Harstad TW, et al. Fetoscopic laser ablation of placental vessels in severe previable twin-twin transfusion syndrome. *Am J Obstet Gynecol* 1995;172:1202–1211.

54. Ville Y, Hyett J, Hecher K, et al. Preliminary experience with endoscopic laser surgery for severe twin-twin transfusion syndrome. *N Engl J Med* 1995;332:224–227.

55. Urig MA, Clewell WH, Elliot JP. Twin-twin transfusion. *Am J Obstet Gynecol* 1990;163:1522–1526.

56. Meagher S, Tippett C, Renou P, et al. Twin-twin transfusion syndrome: intraamniotic pressure measurement in the assessment of volume reduction at serial amniocentesis. *Aust N Z J Obstet Gynaecol* 1995;11:176–180.

57. Ville Y, Sideris I, Nicolaides KH. Amniotic fluid pressure in twin-twin transfusion syndrome: an objective prognostic factor. *Fetal Diagn Ther* 1996;11:176–180.

58. Rodis JF, Vintzileos AM, Campbell WA, et al. Antenatal diagnosis and management of monoamniotic twins. *Am J Obstet Gynecol* 1987;157:1255–1257.

59. Rodis JF, McIlveen PF, Egan JFX, et al. Monoamniotic twins: improved perinatal survival with accurate prenatal diagnosis and antenatal fetal surveillance. *Am J Obstet Gynecol* 1997;177:1046–1049.

60. Aisenbrey GA, Catanzarite VA, Hurley TJ, et al. Monoamniotic and pseudoamniotic twins: sonographic diagnosis, detection of cord entanglement, and obstetric management. *Obstet Gynecol* 1995;86:218–222.

61. Van Allen MI, Smith DW, Shepard DH. Twin reversed arterial perfusion (TRAP) sequence: a study of 14 twin pregnancies with acardius. *Semin Perinatol* 1983;7:285–293.

62. van den Brand SF, Nijhuis JG, van Dongen PW. Prenatal ultrasound diagnosis of conjoined twins. *Obstet Gynecol Surv* 1994;49:656–662.

63. Miller JF, Williamson E, Glue J, et al. Fetal loss after implantation. *Lancet* 1980;2:554–556.

64. Seoud MA, Toner JP, Kruithoff C, et al. Outcome of twin, triplet, and quadruplet *in vitro* fertilization pregnancies: the Norfolk experience. *Fertil Steril* 1992;57:825–834.

65. Landy HJ, Weiner S, Corson AL, et al. The "vanishing" twin: ultrasonographic assessment of fetal disappearance in the first trimester. *Am J Obstet Gynecol* 1986;155:14–19.

66. Enbom JA. Twin pregnancy with intrauterine death of one twin. *Am J Obstet Gynecol* 1985;152:424–429.

67. Jimenez JM, Prichard JA. Pathogenesis and treatment of coagulation defects resulting from fetal death. *Obstet Gynecol* 1968;32:449.

68. Skelly H, Marivate M, Norman R, et al. Consumptive coagulopathy following fetal death in a triplet pregnancy. *Am J Obstet Gynecol* 1982;142:595–596.

69. Romero R, Duffy TP, Berkowitz RL, et al. Prolongation of a preterm pregnancy complicated by death of a single twin *in utero* and disseminated intravascular coagulation: effects of treatment with heparin. *N Engl J Med* 1984;310:772–774.

70. Hypovolemic shock and disseminated intravascular coagulation. In: Cunningham FG, MacDonald PC, Gant NF, et al., eds. *Williams obstetrics,* 20th ed. Stamford, CT: Appleton & Lange, 1997:790.

71. Chescheir NC, Seeds JW. Spontaneous resolution of hypofibrinogenemia associated with death of a twin *in utero:* a case report. *Am J Obstet Gynecol* 1988;159:1183–1184.

72. Berkowitz RL, Lynch L, Chitkara U, et al. Selective reduction of multifetal pregnancies in the first trimester. *N Engl J Med* 1988;318:1043–1047.

73. Evans MI, Dommergues M, Wapner RJ, et al. International collaborative experience of 1,789 patients having a multifetal pregnancy reduction: a plateauing of risks and outcomes. *J Soc Gynecol Invest* 1996;3:23–26.

74. Simpson JL, Carson SA. Multifetal reduction in high-order gestations: a non-elective procedure? *J Soc Gynecol Invest* 1996;3:1–2.

75. Schreiner-Engel P, Walther VN, Mindes J, et al. First trimester multifetal pregnancy reduction: acute and persistent psychological reactions. *Am J Obstet Gynecol* 1995;172:541–547.

76. Rayburn WF, Lavin JP, Miodovnik M, et al. Multiple gestation: time interval between delivery of the first and second twins. *Obstet Gynecol* 1984;63:502–506.

77. Saacks CB, Thorp JM, Hendricks CH. Cohort study of twinning in an academic health center: changes in outcome and management over forty years. *Am J Obstet Gynecol* 1995;173:432–437.

78. Chervenak FA, Johnson RE, Youcha S, et al. Intrapartum management of twin gestation. *Obstet Gynecol* 1985;65:119–124.

79. Rabinovici J, Barkai G, Reichman B, et al. Randomized management of the second nonvertex twin: vaginal delivery or cesarean section. *Am J Obstet Gynecol* 1987;156:52–56.

80. Cetrulo C. The controversy of mode of delivery in twins: the intrapartum management of twin gestation. Part I. *Semin Perinatol* 1986;10:39–43.

81. Gocke Se, Nageotte MP, Garite T, et al. Management of the nonvertex second twin: primary cesarean, external version, or primary breech extraction. *Am J Obstet Gynecol* 1989;161:111–114.

82. Chauhan SP, Roberts WE, McLaren RA, et al. Delivery of the nonvertex second twin: breech extraction versus external cephalic version. *Am J Obstet Gynecol* 1995;173:1015–1020.

83. Houlihan C, Knuppel RA. Intrapartum management of multiple gestation. *Clin Perinatol* 1996;23:91–116.

84. Chervanak FA. The optimum route of delivery. In: Keith LG, Papiernik E, Keith DM, et al., eds. *Multiple pregnancy: epidemiology, gestation, and perinatal outcome.* London: Parthenon, 1995:491–501.

85. Cohen M, Kohl SG, Rosenthal AH. Fetal interlocking complicating twin gestation. *Am J Obstet Gynecol* 1965;91:407.

86. Bloomfield MM, Philipson EH. External cephalic version of twin A. *Obstet Gynecol* 1997;89:814–815.

87. Dommergues M, Mahieu-Caputo D, Mandelbrot L, et al. Delivery of uncomplicated triplet pregnancies: is the vaginal route safer? *Am J Obstet Gynecol* 1995;172:513–517.

88. Wildschut HI, van Roosmalen J, van Leeuwen E, et al. Planned abdominal delivery compared with planned vaginal birth in triplet pregnancies. *Br J Obstet Gynaecol* 1995;102:292–296.

89. Feingold M, Cetrulo C, Peters M, et al. Mode of delivery in multiple birth of higher order. *Acta Genet Med Gemellol* (*Roma*) 1988;37:105–109.

90. Itzkowic D, A survey of 59 triplet pregnancies. *Br J Obstet Gynaecol* 1979;86:23–28.

91. Grobman WA, Peaceman AM. What are the rates and mechanisms of first and second trimester pregnancy loss in twins? *Clin Obstet Gynecol* 1998;41:37–45.

92. Spellacy WN, Handler A, Ferre CD. A case-control study of 1253 twin pregnancies from a 1982–1987 perinatal data base. *Obstet Gynecol* 1990;75:168–171.

93. Doyle PE, Beral V, Botting B, et al. Congenital malformations in twins in England and Wales. *J Epidemiol Community Health* 1990;45:43–48.

94. Luke B, Keith LG. The contribution of singletons, twins, and triplets to low birth weight, infant mortality, and handicap in the United States. *J Reprod Med* 1992;37:661–666.

95. Petridou E, Koussouri M, Toupadaki, et al. Risk factors for cerebral palsy: a case-control study in Greece. *Scand J Soc Med* 1996;24:14–26.

96. Senat MV, Ancel PY, Boubier-Colle MH, et al. How does multiple pregnancy affect maternal mortality and morbidity? *Clin Obstet Gynecol* 1998;41:79–83.

97. Santema J, Koppelaar I, Wallenburg H. Hypertensive disorders in twin pregnancies. *Eur J Obstet Gynecol Reprod Biol* 1995;58: 9–13.

98. Chaim W, Fraser D, Mazor M, et al. Hypertensive disorders in twin pregnancies. *Acta Genet Med Gemellol* (*Roma*) 1995;44: 31–39.

99. Stones RW, Paterson CM, Saunders NJ. Risk factor for major obstetric hemorrhage. *Eur J Obstet Gynecol Reprod Biol* 1993; 48:15–18.

100. Combs CA, Murphy E, Laros RK. Factors associated with postpartum hemorrhage with vaginal birth. *Obstet Gynecol* 1991;77:69–76.

MATERNAL AND FETAL HEMATOLOGY

JEFFREY R. JOHNSON
PHILIP SAMUELS

Mature *blood cells* are derived from undifferentiated stem and progenitor cells in a complex series of maturation and divisional steps, which are not yet completely understood (Fig. 30.1). Between 1 to 5×10^9 erythrocytes and 1 to 5×10^6 white blood cells are produced each hour of the day during a person's lifetime. In addition to the normal maturation process, there must be a system included that is able to respond acutely to stress such as blood loss or infection, in addition to maintenance of the pool of undifferentiated cells from which mature cells are derived. In addition, mature blood cells must function in anatomic locations widely separated from the bone marrow, which is where most cells arise. Any disturbances, even small ones, during the enormous production process of hematopoietic stem cells can cause large abnormalities in blood production.

Most blood precursors arise in the bone marrow. During hematopoietic cell production, hematopoietic stem cells give rise to morphologically distinguishable daughter cells, called *precursors*. The differentiation of stem cells to precursor cells is under hormonal and cytokine control. Blood cell formation results from a series of successive cell divisions, resulting in mature blood cells (Fig. 30.2). This compartment is made up of rare primitive cells that are multipotential (able to maintain the capacity to give rise to all lineages of blood cells) and have a high self-renewal capacity (able to give rise to "identical" daughter stem cells). One characteristic of the stem cell compartment is that most stem cells are mitotically quiescent (1). *Commitment* is a process that involves the transition from pluripotential self-renewing cells in the stem cell compartment to the progenitor cell compartment. This process is not well understood, but it is characterized by a restriction in the stem cell proliferative capacity. Progenitor cells are composed mainly of cells with the capacity to differentiate along one lineage (unipotential progenitors) with lower frequencies of multipotential primitive cells. Commitment therefore involves the acquisition of specific growth factor receptors and loss of others. Progenitor cells are generally defined functionally by the capacity of these cells to form colonies. They demonstrate little self-renewal capacity. Mitotically active cells are far more frequent in the progenitor cell compartment when compared with the stem cell compartment.

Precursor cells make up most cells in the bone marrow

and exhibit easily recognized nuclear and cytoplasmic characteristics that are used to classify the lineage of future development of the precursor cell. For example, a myeloblast has distinguishing morphologic characteristics that allow classification into the lineage of cells destined to be white blood cells. Little self-renewal capacity exists in this compartment, but because of the high number of precursor cells and the high mitotic activity, considerable amplification in cell numbers occurs within this compartment. Early cells have the capacity to give rise to large numbers of progeny cells because of cloning during the transition from stem cell to differentiated cell (Fig. 30.2).

Human precursor hematopoietic stem cells are purified by using expression of the CD34 antigen, lack of human leukocyte antigen–DR expression, and lack of specific antigens that are expressed on more differentiated progenitors (2). Development of progenitor cells is stimulated by exposure to growth factors and causes the expression of cell-specific surface proteins. These growth factors somehow affect the transcription in genetic material by a process that is not yet completely understood. The CD34 antigen is a primitive cell surface protein that is specific for immature stem cells. As the immature stem cell becomes more differentiated, the expression of the CD34 antigen is lost. Other cell surface proteins that are specific for a particular type of cell gradually replace it (3).

The factors that regulate hematopoietic cell proliferation and differentiation remain unknown. Theories of stem cell behavior include the *stochastic model*, which considers stem cell renewal versus differentiation to be based on probability, and the *hematopoietic interactive environment theory*, which links commitment to local environmental signals. The microenvironment of the bone marrow is a complex organ in which stromal cells are responsible for providing factors as required for the orderly development of hematopoietic stem cells. Stromal cells are both mesenchymal and hematopoietic in origin and include osteoblasts, fibroblasts, adipocytes, myocytes, endothelial cells, and macrophages. Adipocytes are probably responsible for providing nutrition to the developing cells, as well as possibly providing certain growth factors. The degree of cellular development can be ascertained by the amount of fat present within the bone marrow. Conditions that lead to decreased cellular production lead to

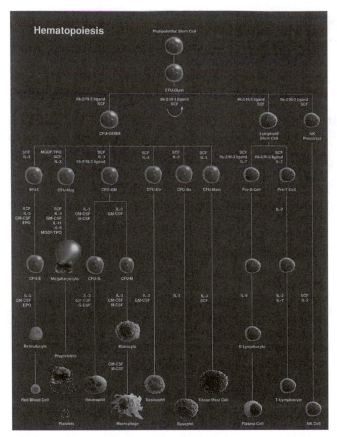

FIGURE 30.1. Flow chart for development of all hematopoietic stem cell lineages from precursor cell to adult cell stage. (From Amgen, Inc., Thousand Oaks, California, with permission.)

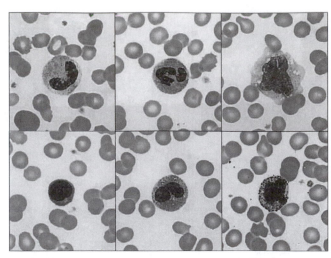

FIGURE 30.3. Peripheral blood smear. Normal leukocytes. *Top left to right:* band neutrophil, segmented neutrophil, monocyte. *Bottom left to right:* lymphocyte, eosinophil, basophil (Wright-Giemsa, 100×).

increased amounts of fat within the bone marrow, whereas increases in cellular production lead to replacement of fat cells with immature stem cell precursors (3).

When bone marrow is examined microscopically, hematopoietic cells in different stages of maturation can be found within distinct areas throughout the bone marrow space (Figs. 30.3 to 30.5). Cells with immature morphology can be found lining the subendosteal region in close proximity of osteoblasts. More clearly differentiated progenitors and precursors of the myeloid, erythrocyte, and megakaryocytic lineages are located throughout the marrow. The apparent association of lineage-specific progenitors and the more clearly differentiated precursors in cellular islands suggest

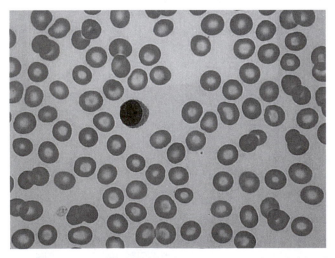

FIGURE 30.2. Peripheral blood smear. Normal red blood cell (RBC) morphology. Erythrocyte diameter approximates that of the nucleus of a normal lymphocyte (Wright-Giemsa, 100×).

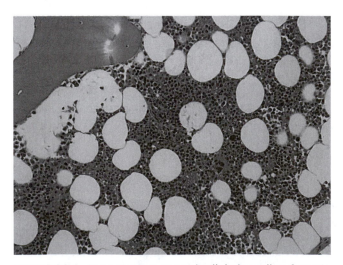

FIGURE 30.4. Bone marrow. Normal cellularity, cell-to-fat ratio approximately 50% (hematoxylin and eosin, 40×).

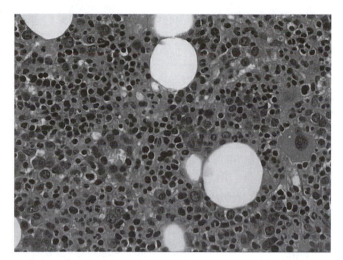

FIGURE 30.5. Bone marrow. Hypercellular marrow, cell-to-fat ratio approximately 90% (hematoxylin and eosin, 40×).

that differentiation into a lineage-specific cellular type may depend on specialized progenitor–stromal cell interactions. Such interactions would consist of specialized stromal cells that produce extracellular matrix components and *hematopoietic supporter cytokines* conducive to the commitment and differentiation of progenitor cells at a specific stage of development (4,5).

EXTRACELLULAR MATRIX

Extracellular matrix components are produced by stromal cells and are required for the regulation of myelopoiesis. Some examples of extracellular matrix components include several types of collagen, laminin, fibronectin, thrombospondin, proteoglycans, and hemonectin. Although the exact role of extracellular matrix components on myelopoiesis is unknown, they serve to localize progenitor cells and stem cells in the bone marrow microenvironment. Adhesion of stem cells to the extracellular matrix may affect proliferation and differentiation of progenitors directly, or it may alter the response of progenitors to cytokines within the microenvironment. Proteoglycans may play an additional role by concentrating, protecting, and presenting cytokines to the developing cells.

Fibronectin

Fibronectin is a large, 450-kd glycoprotein composed of two similar subunits joined by a pair of disulfide bonds in a series of globular domains separated by regions of flexible polypeptide chains. Fibronectin is abundantly present in normal adult bone marrow, where it is produced by endothelial cells and fibroblasts (6). Fibronectin is found in almost all tissues, and the various domains of the fibronectin

molecule interact with different types of cell surface receptors. Adhesion to fibronectin influences the growth of cells by increasing the sensitivity of cells to soluble cytokines, and the adhesive interaction itself between cells and fibronectin may affect cell survival and proliferation. Interaction with fibronectin is required for the terminal differentiation of erythroid progenitors and for the survival and differentiation of B-cell lymphoid progenitors. In addition, fibronectin may play an important role in homing of stem cells. Because fibronectin is universally present, specificity and selectivity for the adhesion to fibronectin of different cell types that are at different stages of maturation are provided by tissue-specific expression of various forms of fibronectin, as well as by differential expression of multiple fibronectin surface receptors on developing cells (7).

Thrombospondin

Thrombospondin is a 450-kd glycoprotein produced by platelets, endothelial cells, and fibroblasts. Several thrombospondin domains have been identified that bind to other cellular components, such as glycosaminoglycans, fibronectin, or other surface receptors. Specific cell surface receptors and CD36 bind to different sites on thrombospondin as well (8). Thrombospondin is present in the bone marrow microenvironment in abundant quantities, and it is localized to megakaryocytes, fibroblasts, and the part of the extracellular matrix associated with active hematopoiesis. Thrombospondin serves as a ligand for committed progenitors, and the interaction of progenitor cells and thrombospondin may constitute some signal that modulates the response of progenitors to cytokines within the microenvironment. Thrombospondin has been shown to amplify the response to soluble cytokines such as interleukin-3 (IL-3) and granulocyte-macrophage colony-stimulating factor (GM-CSF) (9).

Proteoglycans

The bone marrow is rich in *proteoglycans,* which include heparins, dermatan, and hyaluronic acid. Proteoglycans consists of a core protein to which at least one glycosaminoglycan is attached. *Glycosaminoglycans* are long, negatively charged, unbranched polysaccharide chains composed of repeating sulfated polysaccharide units. The type of the sugar residues, the type of linkage between these residues, and the quantity and location of sulfated groups are important for the interaction of glycosaminoglycans with extracellular matrix components, cells, and growth factors, and this interaction provides specificity for the function of glycosaminoglycans (10). Heparan sulfate glycosaminoglycans secreted by hematopoietic supportive stromal cells play an important role in the maintenance and expansion of immature hematopoietic stem cells (11).

Collagen

Collagen is a fibrous protein found in the extracellular space. The most common types of collagen in marrow are types I, II, III, and IV. Collagen types I to III are assembled in collagen fibers and constitute the structural backbone of the extracellular space, seen as "reticulin" fibers on bone marrow biopsy (12). Collagen type IV is not assembled into large fibers but rather into a sheetlike mesh that constitutes a major portion of the basal membrane. A specific role for collagen in the process of localization, nonproliferation, or differentiation of hematopoietic progenitors in the bone marrow microenvironment has not been defined. Passage of mature hematopoietic cells from the bone marrow into the blood requires passage of the cells through the collagen-rich basal membrane of the endothelium (12). Whether a specific interaction occurs between mature cells and collagen is not known.

GROWTH FACTORS

The bone marrow has a remarkable capacity to respond to environmental stimuli in ways that protect the host from the hazards of each stimulus. The discussion of the various types of hematopoiesis would not be complete without a discussion of *growth factors, cytokines*, and their ability to modulate the process of hematopoiesis. The responsiveness of each line within the hematopoietic system results from coordinated increases in the production and the functional activity of specific hematopoietic cell types, without expansion of those cell types that are not relevant to adaptation. For example, a person at high altitude develops a specific expansion of the erythroid bone marrow and subsequent red cell production (Fig. 30.6), but the bone marrow does

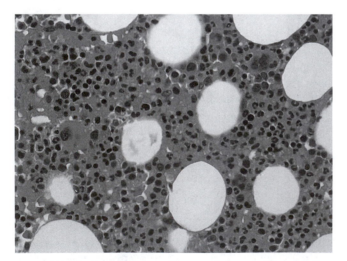

FIGURE 30.6. Bone marrow. Normocellular marrow showing megakaryocytes (*white arrow*), myeloid elements (*gray arrow*), and erythroid precursors (*yellow arrow*) (hematoxylin and eosin, 100×).

not increase production of neutrophils, myocytes, eosinophils, or platelets. This response is specific for protection against hypoxia. All lineage-specific responses of hematopoietic cells in the steady state and under conditions of environmental stress depend on the availability of proteins within hematopoietic tissues that stimulate or inhibit production, differentiation, or traffic of mature blood cells or progenitors. Hematopoietic growth factors and the genes that code for their receptors have become available, and this knowledge helps to explain the interactions between structure and function. As the genes become better characterized, additional functions for existing cytokines are discovered, and new growth factors and circulating substances are identified. Hematopoietic growth factors have been assigned to one of three groups: those that function as a supporter of a specific lineage, those with an effect on multipotential hematopoietic stem cells encouraging differentiation, and those that regulate hematopoiesis indirectly by inducing the expression of direct-acting growth factor genes in auxiliary cells.

Cytokines

The production of red blood cells involves at least nine different *cytokines*. Factors involved in production of red cells include IL-3, IL-9, IL-11, thrombopoietin (TPO), GM-CSF, and erythropoietin (EPO). Other factors may play a role as well, including angiotensin II (13). None of these factors can induce erythroid cellular proliferation in the absence of the lineage-specific factor EPO, which is the pivotal humoral factor that functions to prevent programmed cell death of the most committed erythroid progenitor cells and their progeny. EPO is encoded by a gene on the long arm of chromosome 7, is 18 kd, and is expressed by cells in the liver in embryonic life, the kidney, and to a lesser extent liver in adult life and certain hepatoma cell lines. EPO production is induced by hypoxia in a mechanism that involves the initial activation of proteins that stimulate EPO gene expression. EPO stimulates growth, survival, and differentiation of erythroid progenitor cells and stimulates proliferation, RNA synthesis and erythroid precursor maturation. EPO has also been shown to suppress programmed cell death in erythroid progenitor cells, and it induces the release of reticulocytes from bone marrow (14). EPO induces globin synthesis in erythroid precursor cells, and it may function as a mitogen in neonatal cardiac myocytes.

EPO was the first hematopoietic growth factor to be identified experimentally, and the use of a commercially available form has been shown to be effective in the management of anemia associated with renal failure. Other clinical indications for EPO include use in patients with anemia related to cancer therapy (15), use in patients who refuse blood transfusion (16), and use in patients with anemia related to acquired immunodeficiency syndrome (AIDS)

(17). The effects of EPO on aprogenitor cell proliferation are optimal in the presence of steel factor (see below), a highly glycosylated protein encoded by a gene on chromosome 12. EPO has been shown to be safe for use in pregnancy (18), because it is a highly charged molecule and therefore does not cross the placenta. The optimal dose is one vial subcutaneously three times per week. If the anemia results from renal failure, the dose may be modified to 100 U/kg body weight.

Steel Factor

Steel factor (also known as stem cell factor) is elaborated in both membrane-bound and soluble forms, the latter resulting from cleavage of an exon within the expressed gene. Steel factor promotes the proliferation and differentiation of the most primitive hematopoietic progenitor cells into committed progenitor cells, also known as multipotential colony burst-forming units, erythroid burst-forming units, granulocyte-macrophage colony burst-forming units, and megakaryocyte colony-burst forming units. Steel factor itself has no intrinsic colony-stimulating activity but acts synergistically with IL-3, GM-CSF, and EPO to produce the previously mentioned burst-forming units (19). In addition, steel factor is a chemoattractant for mast cells and enhances the release of mast cell mediators such as histamine. Steel factor administration induces a profound expansion in the compartment of committed hematopoietic progenitor cells as well as inducing a striking mast cell hyperplasia. Curiously, appropriately regulated steel factor expression is necessary for normal melanocyte development and for gametogenesis (19).

Insulin-like Growth Factors

Insulin-like growth factors I and II (IGF-I and IGF-II) are small peptides, which are homologues of proinsulin. The primary site of IGF production is in the liver; these factors exert their effects on a variety of cells, and their receptors are found ubiquitously throughout the body. The exact role of IGF-II in hematopoiesis is unclear at this time. The activity of IGF-I is largely mitogenic and is known to regulate the growth of both normal and malignant cells (20). Heterozygous deletion of IGF-I results in severely growth-restricted fetuses, neurologic defects, and prenatal mortality. Homozygous deletion of IGF-I has not been described and is likely lethal. IGF-I causes erythroid progenitor cells to form erythroid colonies, even in the absence of EPO. The combination of EPO and IGF-I results in greater growth of colony formation than does each factor alone. In addition, patients with polycythemia vera were more than two standard deviations more sensitive to IGF-I than were hematologically normal patients (21). The production and release of IGF are induced by growth hormone (20).

Immune Cell Production

The production of *white blood cells* begins from a common stem cell precursor known as a colony-forming unit granulocyte-eosinophil-macrophage-mast cell unit (CFU-GEMM). The differentiation from this stem cell to progenitor cell is under the control of multiple growth factors, including steel factor, GM-CSF, and granulocyte colony-stimulating factor (G-CSF). G-CSF is a necessary for neutrophil production. Melanocyte colony-stimulating factor is necessary for myocyte production. IL-5 is a strong growth and survival factor for eosinophils. The production of basophils and mast cells is less well understood, but mast cell deficiency is found with steel factor deficiency, a finding indicating that steel factor is necessary for the process of formation and differentiation of mast cell growth.

Granulocyte-Macrophage Colony-Stimulating Factor

GM-CSF is a glycoprotein weighing 14 to 35 kd, with various degrees of glycosylation, and it is coded on the long arm of chromosome 5. GM-CSF stimulates the clonal growth of CFU-GEMM, granulocyte-macrophage colony-forming unit, and eosinophil colony-forming unit (22). GM-CSF induces auxiliary cells to release neutrophil-specific growth factors. GM-CSF activates the functional activity of neutrophils, macrophages, and eosinophils, a finding indicating that lineage-specific growth factors frequently activate the function of terminally differentiated progeny. In GM-CSF deficiency, the major morbidity results from the absence of normal phagocytic function rather than from a failure to produce granulocytes (23), and when this factor is administered therapeutically, it enhances the production of neutrophils, myocytes, and eosinophils. It has been shown to induce colony growth; however, GM-CSF by itself does not induce neutrophil differentiation in the absence of G-CSF. Indirect evidence indicates that GM-CSF induces the expression of other factors, especially IL-1, which, in turn, induces the expression of G-CSF by a variety of cell types (24).

G-CSF is an 18-kd protein encoded on the long arm of chromosome 17 that stimulates the proliferation of granulocyte progenitor cells and activates neutrophil function. G-CSF is produced by a variety of mesenchymal cells under the influence of inductive factors such as IL-1, endotoxin, and tumor necrosis factor-α (22). The most notable defect in G-CSF deficiency is neutropenia, and recombinant G-CSF is widely used in clinical practice. It has been shown to mobilize stem cell traffic in the peripheral blood and to support stem cell transplantation. G-CSF also reduces the duration of neutropenia and is approved for use to prevent infectious complications. Therapy with recombinant G-CSF has been shown to have a faster neutrophil recovery rate. However, such therapy did not reduce the rate of hospitalization for febrile episodes, prolong survival, reduce the number of culture-positive infections, or reduce the cost of supportive care even when it was given prophylactically or to treat active neutropenic fever (25).

Mononuclear phagocytes are the most primitive elements of the blood, and a complete deficiency of mononuclear phagocytes is probably incompatible with life. The development of myocytes is regulated by *macrophage colony-stimulating factor* (M-CSF), which is a glycoprotein encoded on the short arm of chromosome 1. M-CSF stimulates macrophage proliferation and increases secretion of cytokines and phagocytotic function. M-CSF also regulates the genesis of osteoclasts and seems to regulate tissue remodeling and placental function (26). M-CSF is an essential regulatory protein for hematopoietic cells of many lineages, and M-CSF factor deficiency routinely is associated with bone marrow failure. Consequently, M-CSF augments cell survival and permits cells to respond to internal and external cues for differentiation (26).

Platelet Production

Megakaryocyte production is influenced by IL-3, IL-6, IL-11, steel factor, and EPO. However, the most profound effect on platelet count is exerted by TPO, a 36-kd protein coded by a gene on the long arm of chromosome 3 and produced by a variety of organs including hepatocytes, renal tubules, bone marrow stromal cells, muscle, brain, and spleen (27). Hepatocytes are the primary source of serum TPO in humans. Serum TPO is inversely related to the megakaryocyte mass, but the increase in TPO levels seen with thrombocytopenia is not caused by an increase in its production, but rather results from a decrease in TPO binding by megakaryocytes (28).

TPO stimulates the growth and differentiation of immature and mature megakaryocytes into proplatelets (Fig. 30.7). Megakaryocytes grown in the presence of TPO have increased nuclear material and prime mature platelets to respond to aggregation-inducing stimuli such as adenosine, epinephrine, and thrombin (29). The addition of TPO to bone marrow cultures increases clonal growth of all progenitor cells in combination with steel factor, IL-3, IL-6, and EPO by as much as 80% (29). The primary effect of TPO on these primitive progenitors seems to be maintaining viability and suppressing apoptosis (28).

TPO has been used in a limited number of human clinical trials (30). Treatment with a single dose or with daily doses results in a dose-dependent increase in platelet count associated with an increase in bone marrow megakaryocytes. It does not appear to have any effect on red cell or white cell counts. Data on the effect of TPO on bone marrow progenitors are conflicting, but treatment does cause mobilization of hematopoietic progenitors. Several clinical studies to date have suggested possible clinical uses for TPO. Most studies have been in patients with radiation-

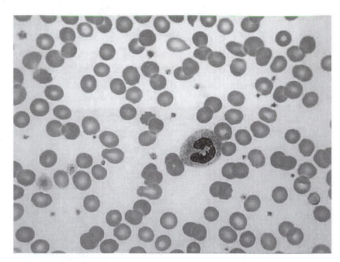

FIGURE 30.7. Peripheral blood smear. Normal platelet count with occasional giant platelet (*arrow*) (Wright-Giemsa, 100×).

or chemotherapy-induced thrombocytopenia or patients undergoing bone marrow transplantation (31). No studies to date have shown any use in pregnancy. However, studies are under way to measure TPO levels in preeclampsia and to determine whether measuring TPO levels has any clinical utility for the prediction of thrombocytopenia. No studies have examined the clinical utility of TPO in the setting of immune thrombocytopenic purpura. A theoretic concern in the clinical use of TPO is the potential for peripheral blood platelet activation and thromboembolic complications. The literature shows a low incidence (less than 5%) of thrombotic complications in TPO-treated patients with cancer (30); however, this does suggest a need for further studies to define risk factors for the thromboembolic side effects of TPO usage. In addition, TPO may induce myelofibrosis and megakaryocyte hyperplasia, although these effects have not been seen with short-term therapy (31).

Interleukins

IL-11 is a cytokine with growth and stimulatory effects on lymphoid and myeloid cells. IL-11 stimulates megakaryocyte hematopoiesis, increases peripheral platelet and neutrophil counts, and increases the numbers of all classes of committed hematopoietic progenitor cells (32). IL-11 deficiency does not lead to any hematologic defects, but outside the hematopoietic system, it stimulates hepatic production of acute-phase reactant proteins, suppresses adipogenesis, and stimulates neuronal differentiation. It is also able to stimulate the recovery of gastrointestinal endothelial cells after cytotoxic therapy.

The growth and development of lymphoid cells from the common lymphoid progenitors occur in a variety of locations and are influenced by numerous factors. Multiple growth factors have been shown to influence the differentiation of T and B lymphocytes, but natural killer cell development is less clear.

IL-7 is a true lymphopoietic factor. It is coded on chromosome 8 and is produced by bone marrow stromal cells and intestinal epithelial cells. The biologic activity of IL-7 induces the clonal growth of normal pre-B cells, pre-T cells, and various neoplastic lymphoid cells. It enhances the differentiation of T cells to the $CD8^+$ subset, and it augments the development of primitive B cells into plasma cells. In addition, a major function of IL-7 is to prevent apoptosis of lymphoid cells, and deficiency of IL-7 results in lymphocytic precursor-depleted bone marrow and profound lymphopenia (33).

IL-2 is produced by T lymphocytes, which have been stimulated by mitogens, antigens, certain antibodies, and lectins. IL-2 has an autocrine function, in that it stimulates growth and activation of T lymphocytes, as well as B lymphocytes and natural killer cells. Paradoxically, IL-2 also acts as an immunomodulator in that it inhibits the differentiation of lymphocytes from developing into the $CD4^+$ subset. Indeed, a deficiency of IL-2 causes generalized inflammation and severe colitis from overgrowth of the $CD4^+$ subset of lymphocytes, and it disrupts the immune system of "self-tolerance" (34).

IL-4 is an 18-kd protein, produced by T lymphocytes, that induces the proliferation and differentiation of B lymphocytes, T lymphocytes, mast cells, and fibroblasts. It upregulates its own receptor in B and T lymphocytes, induces isotype switching from immunoglobulin G (IgG) to IgE antibody production (35) in activated B cells, suppresses IL-2–induced B-cell proliferation, and suppresses IgM secretion (36).

FETAL RED CELL SYNTHESIS

The blood cell system derives from the mesenchymal embryonic layer (37), which originates from the cytotrophoblast surrounding the egg. Embryonic *red cells* are the first to appear, developed in blood islands of the yolk sac at around 19 days' gestation. The vascular system originates from the same area of the yolk sac and may derive from the same progenitor cells. The embryonic red cells are known as *hematocytoblasts,* which become free-floating cells within the lumen of the primitive vascular tree, and they form red blood cells. The islets of red cells eventually become connected within the yolk sac and give rise to the vitelline vessels. At day 22, similar vascular islets form in the mesenchyme of the chorion and form the chorioallantoic network, the future umbilical vessels. Between 6 and 8 weeks' gestation, the intraluminal hematopoiesis network regresses, and stem cell production migrates to the liver, where production is entirely located by 12 to 15 weeks' gestation.

Visceral (extramedullary) hematopoiesis begins in the liver around 5 to 6 weeks' gestation and is entirely functional by 9 weeks. Nests of hematopoiesis appear in the hepatic sinusoids, remaining extravascular. The red cells originating in the liver are more similar morphologically to erythroid precursors than that of yolk sac progenitors. Granulocytes and platelets are found in the circulation by 12 weeks' gestation, but 50% of the hematopoietic action of the liver is production of red blood cells. From 9 to 12 weeks, some hematopoietic activity can be found in the spleen, kidney, thymus, and lymph nodes, each organ contributing a small portion of visceral hematopoiesis. The yolk sac is fibrotic by 11 weeks' gestation. Hepatic erythropoiesis is maximal by the fifth to sixth month, then it gradually regresses until delivery, disappearing by the first to second week of life. Disease or infection may increase extramedullary hematopoiesis.

Medullary hematopoiesis begins in the fourth month with the formation of medullary spaces within the cartilaginous spaces of the long bones. These spaces form by resorption of cartilage along the central inner core. Erythropoietic tissues multiply rapidly and reach peak production around 30 weeks. The volume of red cell production continues to rise until delivery, but each lineage is present within the marrow. During the last 3 months of gestation, the marrow is the majority producer of red cells and is also active in the rest of cellular production.

The red cell count gradually increases from 2.8×10^6 to 3.8×10^6 with a proportional increase in fetal hemoglobin. Conversely, the mean corpuscular volume decreases from 131 to 115 fl.

FETAL NONERYTHROCYTE DEVELOPMENT

Leukocytes first develop within the wall of the yolk sac, with few granulocytes circulating during the first few weeks of life (38). At 8 weeks, some immature granulocytes are seen, but mature granulocytes do not appear until 12 weeks. Lymphopoiesis begins in the lymphoid tissue after 8 weeks and spreads to the thymus in the ninth week, then to lymph nodes from the third month onward. The thymus is the principal site of T-cell formation, whereas B cells are initially produced in the splenic red pulp and shift to the bone marrow during postnatal life.

The percentage of basophils, monocytes, and eosinophils remains relatively constant from 18 weeks' gestation to delivery. However, the percentage of lymphocytes at 18 to 21 weeks is 88% and decreases to around 68% by the third trimester, whereas the percentage of neutrophils increases from 6% at 18 weeks to 25% in the third trimester (37).

Megakaryocytes can be found in the wall of the yolk sac from 5 to 6 weeks and then in the liver along with red cell migration. Megakaryocytes persist in the liver until after delivery, at which time platelet production moves to the bone marrow by 3 months of life. The platelet count remains relatively constant throughout embryonic life at 250,000/mm³.

The current theory of embryonic hematopoiesis is that cells arise from a pluripotential cell, the colony-forming unit, from which all cellular lineages arise. These stem cells arise on the wall of the yolk sac and multiply in intravascular and extravascular locations, then migrate to the liver (the second generation) for continued extramedullary hematopoiesis (37). With each succeeding migration, the stem cells become increasingly differentiated and become more like the adult stem cell population. The third generation of stem cells arises from migration from the visceral sites to the primitive marrow, again becoming more differentiated. It appears that the process is more of a spectrum of differentiation with each succeeding migration, and no specific stages of differentiation have been found.

IRON-DEFICIENCY ANEMIA

Iron deficiency denotes a deficit in total body iron resulting from iron requirements that exceed the iron supply (Figs. 30.8 and 30.9). The two stages of iron deficiency may be characterized first by a decline in iron storage without a decline in the level of functional iron compounds. After iron stores are exhausted, lack of iron causes decreased production of hemoglobin and other metabolically active compounds that require iron as a cofactor, and iron-deficiency anemia develops. The effect on hemoglobin production may be insufficient to be detected. Further decreases in total body iron stores produce overt iron-deficiency anemia.

Iron deficiency is the most common cause of anemia, both in the United States (39) and worldwide (40). In the United States, the amounts of iron in the diet, together with fortifications of many foods and the widespread use of iron supplements, has reduced the overall prevalence and

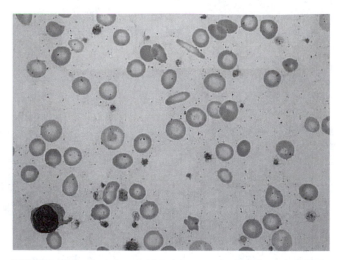

FIGURE 30.9. Peripheral blood smear. Severe iron-deficiency anemia. Microcytic, hypochromic red blood cells with occasional elliptocytes (*arrows*) (Wright-Giemsa, 100×).

severity of iron deficiency. However, iron nutrition remains a problem in some categories, such as toddlers, adolescent girls, and women of childbearing age (39). Without iron supplementation, most women would be deficient in iron during pregnancy (41).

The most common cause of increased iron requirements that lead to iron deficiency is blood loss (39). In women who are postmenopausal or in girls who have not yet begun to menstruate, iron deficiency almost invariably signifies gastrointestinal blood loss. A partial differential diagnosis includes gastritis, duodenitis, peptic ulcer disease, cholelithiasis, inflammatory bowel disease, hemorrhoids, and adenomatous polyps. Iron deficiency is often the first sign of an occult gastrointestinal malignant disease. In addition, long-term ingestion of drugs such as alcohol, aspirin, nonsteroidal antiinflammatory agents, and steroids may cause or contribute to blood loss. Some infectious complications may also lead to gastrointestinal blood loss. In women of childbearing age, menstruation is often responsible for increased iron requirements. Menstrual iron loss tends to be decreased with the use of oral contraceptives, but it may be increased with the use of intrauterine contraceptive devices (41). Other causes of the genitourinary bleeding include uterine malignant diseases, fibroids, renal stones, malignant diseases of the urinary tract, and chronic hemoglobinuria with chronic nocturnal hemoglobinuria or chronic renal stones. In rare cases, Goodpasture's syndrome may lead to the sequestration of iron in pulmonary macrophages.

At birth, the iron stores of the infant are primarily determined by birth weight and hemoglobin concentration. Mild to moderate maternal iron deficiency usually does not restrict iron delivery to the fetus, but severe iron deficiency anemia in the mother can result in both a decreased hemoglobin concentration and lower birth weight in the neonate. Premature infants with a lower birth weight and more rapid

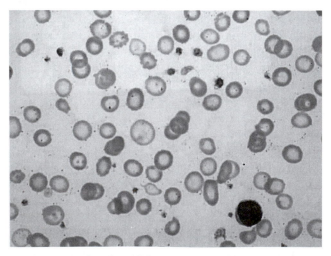

FIGURE 30.8. Peripheral blood smear. Severe iron-deficiency anemia (Wright-Giemsa, 100×).

postnatal growth rate have a higher risk of iron deficiency unless they are given iron supplementation. During the first year of life, when the body weight normally triples, iron requirements are at a high level. Iron requirements decline as growth slows during the second year of life and into childhood, but they rise again during adolescence (41).

Iron Processing During Pregnancy

Pregnancy entails the net loss of the equivalent of 1,200 to 1,500 mL of blood. On average, 270 mg of iron is donated to the fetus, an additional 90 mg is contained in the umbilical cord and placenta, and 150 mg is present in the lochia, with slightly more than 500 mg of iron lost at delivery. During pregnancy, the red cell mass increases by more than one-third, requiring almost another 500 mg of iron, which is returned to the iron stores after delivery. During breastfeeding, a lactating patient requires approximately 0.5 to 1 mg of iron per day. Women who have experienced multiple pregnancies with inadequate spacing between pregnancies have a much greater risk of iron deficiency.

Impaired absorption of iron infrequently produces iron deficiency. Intestinal malabsorption of iron may occur as a manifestation of more generalized syndromes that are related to gastrointestinal disease or diffuse enterocolitis. Atrophic gastritis may impair iron absorption because of achlorhydria. In persons of all ages, but particularly in pregnant women and children, *pica*, the compulsive chewing or ingestion of food or nonfood substances, may contribute to iron deficiency if the material consumed inhibits iron absorption. Iron deficiency also may complicate gastric surgery or gastric bypass surgery. Despite impaired absorption of iron from the gastrointestinal tract, therapeutic preparations of iron salts are well absorbed. In patients with ulcer disease and gastrointestinal blood loss, antacid abuse may exacerbate iron deficiency, because antacids interfere with dietary iron absorption.

The clinical presentation of iron deficiency may be highly specific, or the patient may exhibit no signs of iron deficiency at all (42). Common clinical manifestations include pallor, palpitations, headache, irritability, tinnitus, weakness, dizziness, and easy fatigability. The prominence of these signs depends both on the degree of the condition and on the rate of development of anemia. Because iron deficiency is often insidious and prolonged, adaptive circulatory and respiratory responses may minimize these manifestations, and the patient may manifest a surprising tolerance to extremely low hemoglobin concentrations. With a greater severity of anemia, the patient becomes increasingly debilitated as work capacity and tolerances of physical exertion are diminished and may even eventually have cardiorespiratory failure and die.

Determining whether gastric atrophy is the cause or consequence of iron deficiency can be perplexing, particularly in older patients. In some patients, pernicious anemia

and iron deficiency may coexist. Changes in the lingual or buccal mucosa have been suggested as factors contributing to the pica that develops in many patients with iron deficiency. The combination of glossitis, dysphagia, and iron deficiency is called the *Plummer-Vinson syndrome.* The prevalence of this condition seems to vary geographically, which suggests that some environmental or genetic factor may also be involved. *Koilonychia*, characterized by fingernails that are thin, friable and brittle, with the distal half in a concave or "spoon" shape, results from impaired nail bed endothelial growth and is virtually pathognomonic of iron deficiency. *Blue sclerae* were recognized in 1908 by Osler as associated with iron deficiency and are both highly specific and sensitive as indicators of iron deficiency. The bluish tinge is thought to result from thinning of the sclerae, which makes the choroid visible, and it is postulated to be the result of impaired collagen synthesis from the iron deficiency. Epithelial tissues have high iron requirements because of rapid rates of growth and turnover, and they are thin and fragile in many patients with chronic iron deficiency.

Iron deficiency shows a spectrum of laboratory findings (43). Initially, iron requirements exceed the available supply of iron, iron stores are mobilized, and iron absorption is increased. If the amount of iron available from body reserves and absorption is inadequate, depletion of storage iron follows. Bone marrow shows absence of hemosiderin and iron, the serum ferritin falls, and the total iron-binding capacity rises. Exhaustion of iron reserves results in an inadequate supply of iron to the developing erythroid cell, and iron-deficiency anemia commences. Plasma transferrin receptor concentrations increase as the total body mass of tissue receptor expands. The plasma ferritin decreases to less than 12 μg/L, reflecting the absence of storage iron, and the total iron-binding capacity continues to rise. As the plasma iron declines, and in combination with the increase in total iron-binding capacity, the transferrin saturation falls to less than 16%. Bone marrow examination shows a decrease in the proportion of erythroblasts because too little iron is available to support granule formation. The erythrocytes' zinc proportion progressively increases with reduction of the amount of iron available for hemoglobin formation.

The red cells under microscopic examination show a microcytic hypochromic population. Red cell indices such as mean corpuscular volume, mean corpuscular hemoglobin, and measures of the distribution of red cell volumes change gradually over time (Table 30.1). Chronic longstanding iron-deficiency anemia may produce pale, distorted red cells and dramatic reductions in the mean corpuscular volume and mean corpuscular hemoglobin.

The goal of therapy for iron-deficiency anemia is to provide the hemoglobin supply sufficient iron to correct the global deficit and to replenish the storage of iron. Oral iron is the treatment of choice for almost all patients because of its effectiveness, safety, and economy. Rarely, red cell

TABLE 30.1. LABORATORY FINDINGS WITH FOLATE DEFICIENCY

Increased percent saturation of transferrin
Decreased reticulocyte count
Increased bilirubin (up to 2 mg/dL)
Decreased haptoglobin
Increased lactate dehydrogenase, often >1,000 units/nL
Decreased circulating life span of red blood cells
Peripheral smear
  Increased mean corpuscular volume
  Nuclear hypersegmentation of polymorphonuclear leuko-
    cytes (PMNs) (one PMN with six lobes of 5% with five
    lobes)
  Thrombocytopenia
  Leukoerythroblastic morphology (from extramedullary hema-
    topoiesis)
Bone marrow aspirate
  Increased cellularity
  Abnormal erythropoiesis
  Abnormal leukopoiesis
  Abnormal megakaryocytopoiesis

transfusions are needed to prevent cardiac or renal failure in severe anemia or to support patients whose rate of iron loss exceeds the rate of replenishment possible. Therapy should begin with a ferrous iron salt taken apart from meals in three or four divided doses, which supply a daily total of 150 to 200 mg of elemental iron in adults. Simple ferrous preparations are the best absorbed and are the least expensive. Administration between meals maximizes absorption. In patients with a hemoglobin of less than 10 g/dL, this regimen will initially provide about 40 to 60 mg of iron per day for erythroid formation and will permit red cell production to increase to two to four times normal and the hemoglobin concentration to rise by about 0.2 g/L per day. For milder anemia, a single daily dose of about 60 mg iron is adequate. After the anemia has been fully corrected, oral iron should be continued to replenish body iron stores for an additional 4 to 6 months or until the plasma ferritin concentration exceeds 50 μg/L.

Up to 10% to 20% of patients may have symptoms attributable to the side effects of oral iron. The most common side effects are upper gastrointestinal tract symptoms and include gastric discomfort, nausea, and vomiting. Another common side effect is constipation. These side effects generally occur within 1 hour of iron ingestion, and the symptoms may be alleviated by a change to a smaller dose or by taking the medication with meals. After a period at a lower dose, patients may be able subsequently to tolerate higher doses of iron. Constipation may be relieved either by using stool softeners or by increasing the amount of iron the patient takes. Excess iron remains in the gastrointestinal tract and acts as a cathartic helping to increase the frequency of bowel movements. Iron preparations with enteric coating or in sustained-release form do not appear to offer any

advantage over plain ferrous iron and are considerably more expensive.

Parenteral therapy, with the risk of adverse reactions, should be reserved for patients who remain intolerant to oral therapy, who have iron needs that cannot be met by oral therapy because of uncontrollable bleeding, or who malabsorb iron (44). A screening test for iron malabsorption is the administration of 100 mg of ferrous sulfate in liquid form to a fasting patient, followed by measurements of the plasma iron 1 to 2 hours later. In an iron-deficient patient with an initial plasma iron concentration of less than 50 μg/dL, an increase of 200 to 300 μg/dL is expected. An increase in plasma iron of less than 100 mg/dL suggests malabsorption and is an indication for a small bowel biopsy (43).

The most widely used parenteral preparation is iron dextran containing 50 mg/mL of elemental iron in a colloidal suspension of oxyhydroxide and low-molecular-weight dextran. The preparation may be given intramuscularly or intravenously in the dose calculated from the deficit of total body iron. The most serious risk is life-threatening anaphylaxis and is seen in 0.5% to 1% of patients when the preparation is given either intramuscularly or intravenously. Later, reactions resembling serum sickness may develop in a substantial proportion of patients, with symptoms of fever, urticaria, adenopathy, myalgias, and arthralgias. Iron dextran may exacerbate arthritis in some patients with rhematoid arthritis. With intramuscular administration, local reactions include skin staining, muscle necrosis, phlebitis, and persistent pain at the injection site. Before every administration of iron dextran, the manufacturer recommends that a 0.5-mL test dose be given at least 1 hour before the therapeutic injection. Parenteral iron should be administered only in facilities with medical expertise for managing anaphylactic reactions should they occur. The maximum intravenous or intramuscular daily dose should not exceed 100 mg of iron or the equivalent of 2 mL of undiluted iron dextran. Despite these risks and restrictions, parenteral iron therapy is still preferred for those patients whose condition cannot be managed with oral iron, owing to the hazards and expense of long-term red cell transfusions.

Mild reticulocytosis begins within 3 to 5 days, is maximal by days 8 to 10, and then declines. The hemoglobin concentration begins to increase after the first week and usually returns to normal within 6 weeks. Complete recovery from microcytosis may take up to 4 months. Although the endothelial abnormalities begin to improve promptly with treatment, resolution of glossitis and koilonychia may take several months. The overall prognosis depends on the underlying disorder responsible for iron deficiency. Coexisting conditions such as other nutritional deficiencies, hepatic or renal disease, or infectious, inflammatory, or malignant disorders may slow recovery, and inadequate response to oral iron therapy after 2 to 4 weeks necessitates a search for other potential causes of the anemia (43).

FOLATE DEFICIENCY

Folates are widely distributed in nature and are found in green leafy vegetables, such as spinach, broccoli, lettuce, and beans, as well as in some fruits such as bananas, melons, and lemons. Folate is also found in mushrooms, yeast, liver, and kidney. Folate is thermolabile, and boiling foods for longer than 15 minutes destroys folate. The minimum daily requirements are 3 μg/kg per day (adults, 100 μg; children, 50 μg; pregnant women, 500 μg; and lactating women, 300 μg). The brush border of the jejunum easily absorbs most sources of folate. Peak plasma levels are reached 1 to 2 hours after oral administration. It is rapidly cleared from the blood (more than 95% within 3 minutes), and there is a large enterohepatic circulation of folate (90 μg per day). In the plasma, one-third of folate is free, and two-thirds is nonspecifically bound to serum proteins. Movement of folate into cells may be through specific folate receptors within cellular membranes, by folate carriers, or by passive diffusion. The primary mechanism of transplacental folate passage is by a reduced carrier transport system, with passive diffusion making up the remainder of folate passage (45–47).

Folate deficiency is manifested in many ways (Table 30.1). Defective DNA synthesis is seen by numerous chromosomal breaks, exaggerated centromere winding, and excessive DNA lengthening. Moreover, weakening of DNA around methylation sites causes a larger than normal proportion of cells to become arrested in the G_2 phase or prophase of mitosis of the cell cycle. Thus, many cells have 2N or 4N of DNA complement.

In folate deficiency, all proliferating cells exhibit megaloblastosis, including epithelial cells of the gastrointestinal tract (buccal mucosa, tongue, small intestine), cervix, vagina, and uterus. Ineffective hematopoiesis extends into the bone marrow, especially the long bones, and biopsy specimens show hypercellularity. Erythroid hyperplasia reduces the myeloid-to-erythroid ratio from a normal 3:1 ratio to 1:1. The nucleus of the immature reticulocytes is eccentrically placed, with bizarre-shaped nuclei, and the chromatin appears stippled, reticular, or sievelike. Eighty percent to 90% of proerythroblasts die in the bone marrow, and macrophages scavenge dead or partially disintegrated megaloblasts. This process forms the basis for *ineffective hematopoiesis*. The earliest sign of megaloblastosis and ineffective hematopoiesis is an increase in the mean corpuscular volume. Cells containing DNA remnants (Howell-Jolly bodies) and nonhemoglobin iron (Cabot rings) may be seen under light microscopy. With severe ineffective hematopoiesis, extramedullary hematopoiesis may be seen, with overall leukopenia.

If iron deficiency is also present, the mean corpuscular volume may be normal, and iron therapy will unmask megaloblasts and will enable one to make the diagnosis of folate deficiency. In thalassemias, the erythrocyte morphology may

be normal, but abnormal leukocyte development is still present.

Leukopoiesis is also ineffectual, with an absolute increase in proleukocytes and stippled chromatin. Nuclear hypersegmentation of DNA in polymorphonuclear cells strongly suggests folate deficiency. The nuclei may become so immense that the cell is unable to traverse the marrow sinuses to be released into the circulation. Cytoplasmic granule formation is unaffected.

Megakaryocytes may be unaffected by folate deficiency, or they may be increased in numbers, with hypersegmentation and release of giant platelets into the circulation. The net output of platelets is decreased, and abnormal platelet function may be seen, as demonstrated by abnormal bleeding times.

PERNICIOUS ANEMIA

Pernicious anemia is a disease of unknown origin, in which the fundamental defect is atrophy of parietal cells within the gastric mucosa and which decreased hydrochloric acid secretion, leading eventually to absence of intrinsic factor (IF). IF is required for normal absorption (especially from the terminal ileum) and metabolism of folate. Congenital IF deficiency may be transmitted as an autosomal recessive trait and is characterized by pure IF deficiency without other gastric abnormalities. The development of pernicious anemia may have a genetic disposition, with an average age of onset at 60 years. Persons with a family history of pernicious anemia have an up to 20 times higher likelihood of developing the disease, and there is concordance of pernicious anemia among identical twins. In addition, an association between pernicious anemia and other autoimmune diseases exists, such as Graves' disease, Hashimoto's thyroiditis, vitiligo, Addison's disease, idiopathic hypoparathyroidism, and adult hypogammaglobulinemia. Ninety percent of patients have antiparietal IgG antibodies directed toward the hydrogen, potassium adenosine triphosphatase enzyme found on the membrane of parietal cells. Eight percent of the hematologically normal population also have these antibodies, and up to 60% of patients with simple atrophic gastritis also test positive. Anti-IF antibodies are found in 60% of patients with pernicious anemia and are diagnostic of this condition.

When assessing the patient for pernicious anemia, the clinician should be aware that certain drugs may interfere with IF absorption, especially histamine (H_2) antagonists (but not omeprazole). Therapy consists of discontinuing these agents and of administering oral folate therapy. The usual dose is 1 to 5 mg per day, even in patients with defective IF or malabsorption. The response is rapid, with reversal to normal hematopoiesis within 48 hours. Patients usually have a dramatic improvement in neurologic function, appetite, and sense of well-being. With the dramatic increase in hematopoiesis, a rapid decline in serum iron and potassium is seen, and potassium repletion is essential to prevent fatal arrhythmias. The reticulocyte count increases on the second or third day and peaks by day 8 (the degree of reticulocytosis is proportional to the degree of preexisting anemia).

FOLATE, PREGNANCY, AND INFANCY

Pregnancy and lactation are associated with significantly higher folate requirements (300 to 400 μg per day) for growth of the fetus, placenta, breast, and maternal red blood cell mass. The placenta has many folate receptors, a feature that facilitates the binding and transport of folate across the placenta, even with maternal folate deficiency (46). Folate deficiency can lead to small placentas, prematurity, and low birth weight. A recent trend has been the recognition of folate-sensitive hyperhomocysteinemia as a risk factor for women with unexplained pregnancy loss, placental abruption, and premature parturition. Hyperhomocysteinemia is discussed elsewhere in this chapter.

Transport across the placenta is a two-part, energy-requiring process, concentrating against a gradient (46,47). Higher maternal folate levels enhance this ability. The key to this mechanism is the placenta, which actively binds 5-methyltetrahydrofolate (5-MTHF) to a specialized placental folate receptor. The 5-MTHF is concentrated in the placenta and is displaced by additional folate within the maternal circulation. As the 5-MTHF is displaced by additional folate from the serum, it is able to flow down a concentration gradient to the fetus, the second part of folate transport across the placenta.

From studies on preconceptional folate supplementation, folate is necessary for the developing fetal nervous system (48). In newborns with congenital folate malabsorption syndrome, ingestion of adequate amounts of folate by pregnant women can reduce the prevalence of mental retardation, cerebral calcifications, seizures, and peripheral neuropathy.

HEMOGLOBINOPATHIES

Sickle Cell Disease

Sickle cell disease is an inherited disorder that features chronic hemolytic anemia and recurrent painful episodes. The primary disorder of this disease results from the mutant sickle cell hemoglobin (hemoglobin S). The syndromes (and genotypes) that make up sickle cell disease are mainly sickle cell anemia (hemoglobin SS), sickle cell β-thalassemia, and SC disease (hemoglobin SC). Sickle cell trait (hemoglobin AS) is not associated with anemia and recurrent pain, a feature that distinguishes it from sickle cell disease.

The first modern description of hemoglobin SS began in 1910 with a report by Dr. James Barrett of Chicago on recurrent pain, anemia, and the sickled appearance of red blood cells of a dental student from Granada (49). Disease manifestations had long been recognized in Africa, where sickle cell disease is thought to confer a protective effect against the malarial parasite. The sickling of red cells (Fig. 30.10) resulting from deoxygenation was first described in 1927. Deoxygenation increasing the viscosity of red blood cells was also described. Hemoglobin SS was first described in 1950 using gel preparations of deoxygenated hemoglobin SS solutions. In 1957, the substitution of valine for glutamic acid at the sixth amino acid position in the β-globin chain was discovered.

The prevalence among African Americans of sickle cell disease is 8% to 10% among newborns, with approximately 4,000 to 5,000 pregnancies a year at risk (50). The incidence of the sickle cell gene in the United States is 5% to 10% in African-Americans, but it as high as 25% to 30% in western Africa, with an estimated annual birth of 120,000 babies with sickle cell disease. Evolutionary pressures and transmission of the gene through trade routes and slavery influenced the distribution and frequency of the sickle cell gene in different areas of the world.

Oxygenated hemoglobin SS is as soluble as hemoglobin A, but because of the valine substitution at the sixth amino acid position, there is decreased solubility of the deoxygenated hemoglobin molecule. Intermolecular bonding of the hemoglobin SS polymers generates polymer filaments that associate into bundles. During periods of deoxygenation, these bundles coalesce into organized linear fibers. As the fibers collate during prolonged deoxygenation, the cell membrane is pulled inward irregularly, thus causing the classic sickle shape. It appears that hemoglobin F protects against polymerization and sickling (51). Cells that become irreversibly sickled have lower concentrations of fetal hemoglobin (hemoglobin F). Cells become irreversibly sickled as

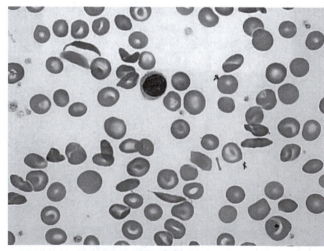

FIGURE 30.10. Peripheral blood smear. Sickle cell anemia. Note the sickled red blood cells, Howell-Jolly body (*lower right*), polychromasia, and occasional target cells (Wright-Giemsa, 100×).

they age, because of the constant sickling and unsickling during the life span of red blood cells (52). These cells are removed and destroyed by the reticuloendothelial system, especially the spleen. During times of oxidative stress or dehydration, damaged red blood cells are seen by light microscopy as they pass through the reticuloendothelial system and are "attacked" by macrophages. During steady state or relative quiescence, the proportion of irreversibly sickled cells remains the same.

With increased sickling, the red blood cells are less deformable and distensible and therefore cannot pass through the small blood vessels easily. The primary site of vasoocclusion is the prearteriolar sphincter. As capillary beds are deprived of blood flow and oxygen by the sludging and plugging of the prearteriolar vessels, patients have increased pain from ischemia and anaerobic metabolism.

Destruction of sickled erythrocytes occurs both intravascularly and extravascularly. Extravascular hemolysis results from abnormalities of the sickle cell membrane and leads to destruction by macrophages within the reticuloendothelial system. Oxidative damage from "attacks" by macrophages (Fig. 30.11) allows the binding of IgG, along with impaired complement inactivation on sickled cell surfaces, which facilitates destruction by macrophages. Elevation of free plasma hemoglobin suggests that one-third of red blood cell destruction occurs intravascularly, and the primary mechanism of intravascular hemolysis appears to result from complement binding to the surface of the sickled cell, causing fragmentation and destruction by circulating polymorphonuclear leukocytes and macrophages.

Immune System

Immune deficit is also characteristic of sickle cell disease. Splenic function is impaired by autoinfarction from sequestration of abnormal cells, decreased serum-opsonizing capacity, and an increased susceptibility to encapsulated organisms such as *Streptococcus pneumoniae*. Vaccination against *S. pneumoniae* is recommended for all persons with sickle cell disease.

Clinical Manifestations

The clinical manifestations of sickle cell disease are varied; some patients do not have crises, whereas others have frequent crises. The typical course is a relatively normal life with occasional crises and chronic anemia. The life expectancy of a person with sickle cell disease has increased dramatically, with the average going from 14.3 years in 1973 to 48 years in 1994. This improvement has been attributed to advances in transfusion medicine, aggressive hydration during crises, and prophylactic penicillin to prevent pneumococcal disease during a crisis.

Acute pain is the first manifestation of a crisis in 25% of patients, with painful episodes peaking between the ages of 19 and 39 years. Cold, dehydration, infection, menses, and alcohol consumption may precipitate pain, but most patients have no identifiable cause. The common sites of pain are the chest, abdomen, and hips and extremities. In some cases, fever, tachypnea, swelling, tenderness, and hypertension may manifest during a crisis. Ophthalmologic examinations are important because of the risk of anterior chamber infarction during vasoocclusive crises. In severe cases, multiorgan failure results from severe vasoocclusive disease. Any organ system may be affected, but the most common conditions are hepatic, renal, and cardiac failure. Multiorgan failure usually is avoided by aggressive hydration and transfusion therapy.

Other cornerstones of therapy include pain control, but many clinicians are wary of overuse of narcotics in these patients. Many patients with sickle cell disease become tolerant of narcotics over time and may require high doses. However, adequate pain control is critical for these patients, because the pain is chronic and at times severe. Narcotics are clearly indicated for good pain control during a crisis. Transfusions are also used liberally to keep the amount of hemoglobin SS to less than approximately 40% to 50% and to improve the oxygen-carrying capacity (53). Bloodborne infections such as with hepatitis B and C and human immunodeficiency virus (HIV) are a concern, but the blood supply in the United States is carefully screened and is considered safe. Other transfusion-related complications may include iron overload and alloimmunization. Hydroxyurea has been used to increase the synthesis of hemoglobin F through an unknown mechanism. The number and duration of pain crises were lower, and an increase in reticulocytosis occurred, as well as a decrease in the total number of units of blood transfused to patients who received hydroxyurea. This therapy is contraindicated in pregnancy because of the potential for miscarriage.

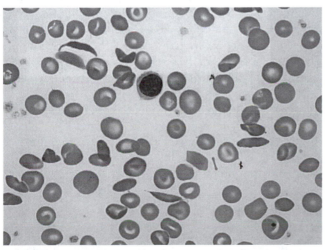

FIGURE 30.11. Peripheral blood smear. Microangiopathic hemolytic anemia, with frequent schistocytes, severe thrombocytopenia (Wright-Giemsa, 100×).

Obstetric and Gynecologic Manifestations

Women with sickle cell disease experience delayed menarche, dysmenorrhea, ovarian cysts, pelvic infections, and fibrocystic disease of the breast. The primary concern, however, is pregnancy. Fetal complications result from impaired placental blood flow, which can cause miscarriage, intrauterine growth restriction, intrauterine fetal demise late in pregnancy, preeclampsia, low birth weight, and prematurity. Pregnancy is also complicated by an increase in the frequency of painful crises, severe anemia, and infectious complications. Better pregnancy outcomes have been observed over the past 3 decades, because of better hematologic and obstetric care. An unresolved issue has been the role of transfusion therapy during pregnancy. Some investigators have advocated prophylactic transfusions during pregnancy to maintain the percentage of hemoglobin SS at less than 40% to 50%. A large randomized study showed no improvement in fetal outcome from this management approach (54). No indication for cesarean delivery exists other than the usual obstetric indications.

Variant Sickle Cell Syndromes

Sickle cell syndromes that result from inheritance of sickle cell genes heterozygously or that occur in combination with other mutant β-globin chain genes are generally milder clinically.

Sickle cell trait (SST) affects 8% to 10% of African Americans, with the hemoglobin AS phenotype. SST is benign, but the affected person is a carrier for the abnormal sickle gene. Red cell morphology, red cell indices, and reticulocyte counts are normal. Sickle cell forms are not seen in peripheral smears. The proportion of hemoglobin A to hemoglobin S is approximately 60:40 because of the greater affinity of α-globin chains for the normal hemoglobin A globin over the hemoglobin S globin. The most common manifestation of SST is hematuria and impaired urinary concentrating ability. The incidence of urinary tract infections is also slightly increased over the general population. Splenic infarction, although extremely rare, occurs more commonly in whites than in those of African ancestry, and only at high altitudes.

Hemoglobin SC Disease

The gene for *hemoglobin SC* is one-fourth as frequent among African Americans as the sickle gene (55). Deoxygenated hemoglobin SC forms crystals, but it does not participate in polymerization with deoxygenated hemoglobin S molecules (Fig. 30.12). Red cell desiccation resulting from potassium chloride cotransport sustained by hemoglobin SC increases the intracellular concentration of hemoglobin S that supports polymerization, sickling, and clinical symptoms. Compound heterozygosity for hemoglobin S and C results

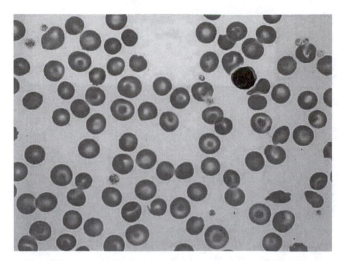

FIGURE 30.12. Peripheral blood smear. Target cells from a patient with hemoglobin SC disease (Wright-Giemsa, 100×).

in a milder clinical spectrum than sickle cell disease. Circulating hemoglobin SC cells have a longer circulating life than hemoglobin SS cells (27 versus 17 days), with less anemia and reticulocytosis. The average life span of a person with hemoglobin SC is 2 decades longer, with fewer infectious complications. There is, however, a higher risk of infection with *S. pneumoniae* and *Haemophilus influenzae*. There is also a higher risk of peripheral retinopathy than with sickle cell disease, and ophthalmologic examination is crucial.

Thalassemias

Thalassemias are characterized by defective production of one or more of the hemoglobin chains. The different forms of thalassemias are classified according to the defective globin chain produced when compared with the normal globin chains. Defective hemoglobin synthesis is the result of deletion of one or more of the hemoglobin genes within DNA, or it may be the result of a partial deletion or rearrangement that results in premature termination of DNA translation. The two major types of thalassemias involve either impaired production of the α-peptide chains or the β-peptide chains. α-Thalassemias are found predominantly in Asians, whereas β-thalassemias are predominantly Mediterranean in origin, with a slightly increased incidence in Africans (55). Molecular DNA analysis can diagnose the type of deletions present, and prenatal diagnosis should be offered for patients whose fetuses are determined to be at risk after genetic counseling.

α-Thalassemias

The inheritance of *α-thalassemia* is more complicated because there are two α-globin genes (56). Four primary clinical syndromes are associated with α–thalassemia based on the clustering of α-globin gene deletions and the amount of α-hemoglobin present. In most hematologically normal populations, the α-globin gene loci are duplicated on chromosome 16. The normal diploid genotype is αα/αα. The two main types of deletions of the α-globin gene are α-null and α-+ thalassemia. The α-null variety is expressed as −−/αα, whereas the α−+ thalassemia is characterized by deletion from a single locus from one chromosome and may be heterozygous (−α/αα) or homozygous (−α/−α) with loss from both loci. The α-null thalassemias may be of the deletion or nondeletion types.

Three phenotypes have been described based on the amount of α-hemoglobin present. The first is homozygous α-thalassemia in which all four α-hemoglobin genes have been deleted, expressed as (−−/−−). Because α-hemoglobin makes up fetal hemoglobin in conjunction with the γ-hemoglobin chain, the fetus is affected. Without the production of α-hemoglobin chains, the fetus produces hemoglobin with four γ-chains (Bart hemoglobin) or with four β-chains (hemoglobin H). Hemoglobin Bart has a much higher affinity for oxygen, and the fetus demonstrates nonimmune hydrops. The fetus dies either *in utero* or shortly after birth. Hemoglobin Bart is a common cause of hydrops and stillbirth in Asia; 65% to 98% of cases of nonimmune hydrops were caused by hemoglobin Bart in one study.

The compound heterozygous state for either α-null or α-+ thalassemia results in the deletion of three of the four genes (−−α), leaving only one functional-α hemoglobin gene per diploid genome. This state is known as *hemoglobin H disease* and is compatible with life. The red cells contain a mixture of hemoglobin Bart, hemoglobin H, and hemoglobin A. Hemolytic anemia develops after infancy once hemoglobin Bart is replaced by hemoglobin H as the fetal γ-hemoglobin production declines. Hemoglobin H disease is characterized by hemolytic anemia of varying severity, and anemia generally becomes worse during pregnancy and requires multiple transfusions because of the increased hemolysis. The risk of intrauterine growth restriction is also increased.

α-Thalassemia minor is a result of deletion of two genes and is characterized by minimal to moderate hypochromic microcytic anemia. This condition may result from α-null or α-+ thalassemia traits with the genotype −α/−α or −−αα. This disorder often goes unrecognized, with a normal to slightly decreased mean corpuscular hemoglobin concentration. Hemoglobin Bart is present at birth, but as γ-chain production decreases, it is replaced with two α-chains. Hemoglobin H is not present. Women with α-thalassemia minor tolerate pregnancy well. The single gene deletion (−α/αα) is a silent carrier state, with no clinical abnormalities evident.

α-Thalassemia minor, hemoglobin H disease, and hemoglobin Bart disease are all found among Asians, whereas in Africans, α-thalassemia minor is found in about 2% of people, hemoglobin H disease is rare, and hemoglobin Bart has not been reported. The reason for these differences is

that Asians have α-null thalassemia minor with both gene deletions from the same chromosome (−−/αα), and Africans have α-+ thalassemia minor with the gene deletions from two separate chromosomes (−α/−α).

β-Thalassemia

β-Thalassemia is a complex disorder resulting from the impaired production of the β-globin chain (56). More than 100 point mutations in the β-globin chain gene have been described. Most are single nucleotide substitutions that produce transcription defects, RNA modifications, or highly unstable hemoglobin. The β-globin gene is located on chromosome 11. In β-thalassemia, decreased β-chain production causes overproduction of α-chains. These α-chains precipitate within the red cells and cause membrane damage. With most thalassemias, hemoglobin A_2 levels are elevated.

In *β-thalassemia major,* also known as Cooley's anemia, β-globin chains are absent. There is a homozygous deletion of the β-globin chain, but it is compatible with life. The neonate is generally healthy at birth, but as fetal hemoglobin (γ-chain production) declines, the infant becomes severely anemic and fails to thrive. Children survive by receiving frequent transfusions, but life expectancy is shortened. Iron chelation therapy is an essential component because of iron overloading commonly encountered with chronic transfusions. Females are generally sterile, and few case reports of successful pregnancy outcomes exist.

In *β-thalassemia minor,* the hemoglobin A_2 (two α- and two α-globin chains) is increased beyond 3.5% and hemoglobin F (two α- and two γ-globin chains) is increased to more than 2%. The red cells are hypochromic and microcytic (Fig. 30.13), but the anemia is mild. The average hemoglobin concentration is generally decreased, to 8 to 10 g/dL. Pregnancy poses little problem in patients with

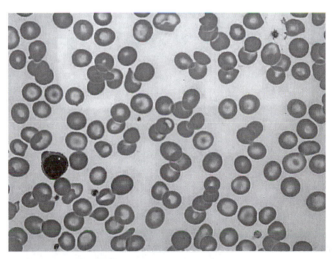

FIGURE 30.13. Peripheral blood smear. Target cells and microcytic, hypochromic anemia resulting from β-thalassemia minor (Wright-Giemsa, 100×).

β-thalassemia minor, but iron and folate supplementation are recommended.

β-*Thalassemia intermedia* is a clinical spectrum of disease attributed to β-thalassemia disease less severe than β-thalassemia major but more severe than β-thalassemia minor. This spectrum results from unusually high levels of persistent hemoglobin F synthesis, hereditary persistence of hemoglobin F production, co-inheritance of α-thalassemia, or inheritance of extra α-globin genes. The degree of anemia and of hemolysis depends on the underlying cause of disease, as do the clinical course and the potential for pregnancy outcomes.

ERYTHROCYTE MEMBRANE DEFECTS

Erythrocytes are shaped like biconcave discs with a redundancy of membrane surface area in relation to cell volume. This allows the red cell to reversibly deform and to withstand the shear forces as the cells are forced through small capillaries and splenic slits. Several red cell membrane defects cause the loss of lipids from the membrane surface and poorly deformable cells resulting in accelerated destruction.

Hereditary Spherocytosis

Hereditary spherocytosis is a syndrome resulting from several erythrocyte membrane protein defects (57). Most are an autosomally dominant spectrin deficiency; others may be autosomally recessive and caused by ankyrin or protein 4.2 deficiency or some combination of these.

Hereditary spherocytosis is characterized by varying degrees of hemolysis of microspherocytic red cells (Fig. 30.14), with resulting anemia and jaundice (57). Diagnosis is made by demonstrating spherocytes on peripheral smear, in-

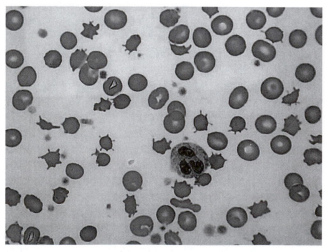

FIGURE 30.14. Peripheral blood smear. Spur cell anemia. Acanthocytes lack central pallor and have spikelike projections with knobby ends (*arrows*) (Wright-Giemsa, 100×).

creased reticulocytosis, and increased osmotic fragility. Splenectomy greatly reduces hemolysis and jaundice, although it does not correct the underlying defect in red cell membranes. Accelerated destruction, as the result of infection or dehydration or decreased production, or both, can result in "crisis" with pain to the degree seen in sickle cell anemia, but with more hyperbilirubinemia and jaundice as a consequence of the rapid hemolysis. Crisis is seen only in those patients with an intact spleen, and transfusion, aggressive hydration, and possible splenectomy are the treatment modalities. Pregnancy is well-tolerated (58), with no increase in intrauterine growth restriction. The neonate with inherited spherocytosis has a variable course, with hemolysis and hyperbilirubinemia seen in conjunction with infections.

RED CELL ENZYME DEFECTS

Red cell enzymes are required for the anaerobic utilization of glucose by the cells. Most deficiencies of red cell enzymes cause nonspherocytic anemia, and they are inherited as autosomal recessive traits. Glucose-6-phosphate dehydrogenase deficiency (G6PD) is a common defect and is actually X-linked (59). In the homozygous deficiency, both X chromosomes are affected, and women are markedly affected. This condition is seen in 2% of African-American women and is known as A-variant G6PD. The heterozygous form is more common, seen in up to 15% of African-American women, and has one X chromosome affected and one X chromosome unaffected. Random X-chromosome inactivation explains the variable clinical sequelae, and the condition confers some protection against malarial infection. Infections and several oxidizing drugs can precipitate hemolysis, and removal of the inciting agent is often curative. Young erythrocytes contain more G6PD than older cells, and maintenance of the bone marrow is essential through iron and folate therapy. Transfusions are generally reserved for when the hematocrit falls to less than 20% or in patients with evidence of heart failure or hypoxia.

ANTIPHOSPHOLIPID ANTIBODY SYNDROME

Antiphospholipid antibody syndrome (APLAS) is a disorder in which antibodies are directed against negatively charged phospholipids in cell membranes (60). These antibodies were initially named *lupus anticoagulant* (LA) because they were primarily found in patients with systemic lupus erythematosus. As many as 40% of patients with systemic lupus erythematosus will test positive for antiphospholipid antibodies (APLA); 6% to 24% will have LA, and 40% will have anticardiolipin antibody (ACLA). Paradoxically, these autoantibodies cause an increased propensity to form clots, primarily arterial, rather than to inhibit coagulation. The misnomer derives from the observation in 1952 by Conley in which plasma with LA caused an isolated increase in the prothrombin time (55), and it was not corrected with the addition of normal plasma. The two general categories of APLA recognized to date are LA and ACLA. Laboratory diagnosis for the detection of LA varies greatly from laboratory to laboratory, because there is currently no international agreement for detection of LA. Three major criteria are generally accepted for laboratory identification of LA: abnormal phospholipid-dependent clotting reaction; the abnormal clotting reaction resulting from an inhibitor of clotting, not a factor deficiency; and the recognition that the inhibitor activity is directed at phospholipids and not at specific coagulation proteins. The detection of ACLA is by standard radioimmunoassays, and these are reported as negative, low-positive, medium-positive, and high-positive, as well as in quantitative terms for both IgG and IgM. Low-positive IgG or isolated IgM titers without the presence of LA are considered false-positive and likely have little clinical significance. Approximately 79% of patients with LA will also test positive for ACLA, and higher levels of ACLA generally correspond to positivity for LA (60).

Patients with APLAS must have at least one abnormal laboratory feature twice when they are tested at least 8 weeks apart. The clinical features of APLAS are as follows: thrombosis, generally arterial, and possibly in unusual locations not commonly associated with thrombosis; recurrent pregnancy loss; unexplained stillbirth; preeclampsia; unexplained oligohydramnios; hemolytic anemia; and livedo reticularis. Patients with APLAS should have at least one clinical feature at some point during their disease for the diagnosis.

The prevalence APLAS has been reported to be between 0.3% and 2% of the general population, based on studies done in otherwise healthy pregnant women (61). More than 80% of cases of ACLA positivity in normal pregnant women were in the low-positive range, with 0.2% of IgG or IgM in the clinically significant range. Routine testing is not advocated based on this low prevalence, but if recurrent pregnancy loss or unexplained stillbirth has occurred, testing is generally recommended, because the incidence of APLAS in these patients may be as high as 10%. Other indications for APLA testing include systemic lupus erythematosus or other autoimmune disease, unexplained thrombocytopenia, unexplained pulmonary embolism, unexplained stroke or other unusual arterial vascular occlusion, false-positive syphilis test, unexplained abnormal prothrombin test, and early-onset preeclampsia (62).

The pathophysiology of pregnancy loss appears to be necrotizing vasculopathy of the maternal-placental interface, characterized by fibrinoid necrosis (63). Other features may include *atherosis*, which is the infiltration of the vessel wall with a clear or foamy cytoplasm, and a perivascular infiltrate of mononuclear and polymorphonuclear cells. The placenta is also generally noted to be small for gestational age at delivery and calcified. More consecutive pregnancy losses confer a worse prognosis for carrying a pregnancy to term, and 90% of patients with APLAS as the cause of recurrent pregnancy loss experience at least one midpregnancy loss.

Therapy is generally initiated in patients with symptomatic autoimmune disease and in patients who have had one or more pregnancy losses in the presence of APLAS. To date, the mainstay of therapy is heparin and low-dose aspirin (64,65). Many studies have concluded that the most favorable outcomes are with this combination, best begun early in the first trimester or before pregnancy is undertaken. The dose of heparin is started at 5,000 U twice daily in the first trimester and is increased to 10,000 and 15,000 U twice daily in the second and third trimesters, respectively. Full anticoagulation is generally not necessary unless the patient has a history of pulmonary embolism or recent deep venous thrombosis. Many studies have attempted to evaluate the efficacy of steroids (65,66) in combination with heparin, both with and without aspirin. Investigators have clearly demonstrated that the perinatal outcome is worse with steroid therapy in combination with heparin, regardless of aspirin therapy. Also under scrutiny has been intravenous immunoglobulin (IVIG) therapy (67), and although results are not conclusive because of the small sample sizes, this approach does not appear to have any benefit. In addition, IVIG is extremely expensive and is in short supply in the United States.

Pregnancy Outcome

Despite intensive monitoring during pregnancy, many women experience adverse outcomes. Possible complications of therapy include maternal thrombocytopenia, chorea gravidarum, early-onset preeclampsia, intrauterine growth restriction, and thrombotic episodes. Basic guidelines for monitoring of maternal and fetal well-being include monitoring maternal platelet count once per trimester, monitoring maternal blood pressure and surveillance for urinary protein at each visit, and review of any unusual maternal symptoms at each visit. Growth scans for the fetus should be performed at least every 4 weeks, or more frequently if indicated, beginning around 28 weeks' gestation. Amniotic fluid volume assessment is performed on a weekly basis. Fetal movement counts should also begin around this time. Controversial, although accepted, is serial nonstress testing beginning around 32 weeks' gestation, performed twice per week. Doppler ultrasonic measurement of umbilical artery flow is not predictive of adverse perinatal outcome, unless there is absence or reversal of end-diastolic flow. However, by this time, there are generally other findings as well, such as decreased fetal movement or decreased amniotic fluid volume. As such, routine use of Doppler flow for assessment of fetal well-being is not warranted. Despite these interventions, most women with APLAS experience premature birth of their children because of some complication of pregnancy, and it is generally iatrogenic (68). Follow-up with a rheumatologist post partum is essential.

Rh DISEASE

Red blood cells express a wide variety of antigens on their surface. Most of these antigens are determined genetically, whereas others are a result of exposure to other antigenic or immunogenic compounds (55). However, none have been so important to the field of obstetrics as the *Rh antigen group*. The Rh group is composed of several membrane surface antigens: D, C, c, E, and e. The D antigen was initially described on the surface of the red blood cell of the rhesus monkey in 1940, in an attempt to improve transfusion medicine and decrease the incidence of transfusion hemolytic reactions. The exact function of the Rh antigens is not known, but those rare persons who are Rh null, who lack any Rh antigens, have defective red blood cell membranes and suffer from mild to moderate hemolytic anemia (55). The incidence of Rh disease has dramatically declined, but it is still an important cause of hemolytic disease of the newborn. Other antibodies are increasing in importance as a cause of hemolytic disease, only because of the decrease in Rh disease.

Fetal hemolysis was first ascribed to Rh immunization in 1941 after the discovery of red blood cell antigens. The frequency of some combinations of antigens is more common than others, but the D antigen is primarily discussed. The term *Rh positive* refers to the presence of the D antigen, and *Rh negative* refers to the absence of the D antigen; there is no d antigen as such. Rh positivity follows a Mendelian autosomal dominant pattern, and Rh negativity is primarily a white trait. In most white populations, the incidence of Rh negativity is 15%, but in the Basque population, it is as high as 35%. The Rh antigens are fully expressed on the fetal red blood cell membranes by 30 days' gestation.

The primary immune response to the Rh antigen occurs after exposure of fetal Rh-positive red blood cells to an Rh-negative mother, and it generally occurs at delivery. Small fetal-maternal hemorrhages at delivery are commonplace. Other causes of fetal-maternal hemorrhages are external version, abdominal trauma, manual placenta extraction, abruption, and abortion. The primary response is slow to develop, generally requiring 6 to 12 weeks, but it may be as long as 6 months before it appears. The initial or sensitizing pregnancy is not severely affected, but the amnesic response with future pregnancies can cause severe fetal hemolysis. The initial response is through IgM, followed rapidly by an IgG response. The IgG antibodies are readily able to cross the placenta and coat Rh-positive fetal red blood cells. Fetal-maternal blood passage as small as 0.3 mL may cause Rh immunization, and 1% of women have 5 mL of fetal blood passage at the time of delivery. The development of primary Rh disease depends on the antigen dose; 15% of

patients develop disease after 1 mL of exposure to Rh-positive cells, 33% after 10 mL, and 65% after 50 to 250 mL. A secondary immune response may develop with as little as 0.05 mL of Rh positive cells. The degree of hemolytic disease is determined by the maternal IgG titer, with increasing risk beyond a titer of 1:16. Also important are the binding constant for maternal antibody to the red blood cell membrane and the ability of the fetus to keep up with hemolysis without becoming hydropic.

The red blood cells are destroyed in the fetal spleen, because IgG-coated red blood cells cannot fix complement. The resulting anemia stimulates EPO and causes increased red blood cell production in the bone marrow. The liver and spleen become enlarged with increasing extramedullary hemolysis, with a marked increase in reticulocytes and normoblasts within the fetal circulation. Islets of red cell production replace hepatic cords, obstruct portal venous return, and cause *in utero* portal hypertension. Placental hypertrophy is also a common finding with moderate or severe hemolysis.

About one-third of neonates do not require any treatment, one-third have mild hemolytic disease with kernicterus, and one-third develop hydrops fetalis (Fig. 30.15), with anasarca and congestive heart failure (69). Monitoring of pregnancies begins with maternal antibody testing at the first prenatal visit. The father should also be tested for Rh status. If the Rh-negative mother has no Rh antibodies, she is unlikely to develop Rh disease during the pregnancy, and no further testing is required. If the father is homozygous for Rh negativity, then the fetus has no likelihood of being Rh positive. ABO blood typing should also be carried out, and if ABO incompatibility exists, then the risk of developing Rh disease is also decreased, even if the fetus is Rh positive. ABO antibodies are IgM and therefore do not cross the placenta. In addition, fetal red blood cells do not

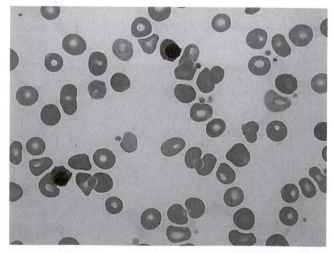

FIGURE 30.15. Umbilical cord blood. Erythroblastosis fetalis. Erythrocytes show polychromasia and circulating nucleated precursors (Wright-Giemsa, 100×).

strongly express ABO antibodies and are weaker antigenic stimuli.

If the risk of Rh disease exists, maternal antibody titers should be obtained at 18 weeks' gestation and monthly thereafter. Ultrasound should also be used to monitor for the development of hydrops. Middle cerebral artery Doppler assessment of peak blood flow has been used successfully as a means of noninvasive testing of fetal hemoglobin status (70). The peak flow through the middle cerebral artery depends on gestational age, and tables that compare the peak flow for a given gestational age and the degree of anemia have been published. In our experience, if there is the slightest hint of ascites or hydrops, then these tables are no longer predictive of fetal hemoglobin status.

The mainstay of monitoring fetal well-being is the *Liley curve*, which plots the δ optic density (OD) 450-nm wavelength of amniotic fluid against gestational age. The degree of hemolysis is reflected in the amount of bilirubin (heme breakdown products) in the amniotic fluid. Queenan et al. and Kaufman and Paidas modified the curve in 1993 to earlier gestational ages (71,72), to reflect the lower limits of viability. Serial amniocenteses are performed during pregnancy, generally beginning around 24 weeks' gestation, because this is as early as the modified Liley curve goes. The δ OD at 450-nm wavelength of light is plotted against gestational age and falls into one of four zones. Repeat amniocentesis is performed at intervals determined by the result of the Liley curve. This is an invasive method of monitoring fetal hemoglobin status and obviously makes the potential of monitoring middle cerebral artery peak velocity that much more attractive as a noninvasive means of following fetal well-being.

Fetal blood sampling by *cordocentesis* (or percutaneous umbilical blood sampling) is the most accurate method of monitoring fetal hemoglobin (72). This is generally performed once the Liley curve has reached the zone IIB or III level. Under direct ultrasound guidance, a needle is placed through the maternal abdomen into the fetal umbilical cord, and the blood sample is sent for hemoglobin and hematocrit levels, mean corpuscular volume, and reticulocyte count. The reticulocyte count should be performed manually, because most normal fetal red blood cells are nucleated, a feature that falsely elevates the reticulocyte count in most automated Coulter cell counters. If the fetal hemoglobin is low, beginning around 10 gm/dL, blood transfusions are carried out through the umbilical cord. This is generally done at the time of fetal blood sampling to decrease the number of funipunctures. The amount of blood transfused is calculated using a standard formula (Fig. 30.16), based on fetal weight determined by ultrasound, hemoglobin of the donor blood, and the current and "ideal" hemoglobin level of the fetus. Intraperitoneal transfusions are generally no longer performed (72), because of the time needed for fetal absorption of hemoglobin, lower volumes able to be transfused by this method, and the relative safety

Volume to be transfused =

$$\frac{\text{(desired final hematocrit - initial fetal hematocrit)}}{\text{Donor hematocrit}} \text{(X 150)(X fetal wt. In Kg.)}$$

FIGURE 30.16. Formula for determining volume of packed red blood cells through cordocentesis in Rh isoimmunization.

of funipuncture. Steroid therapy should be avoided during monitoring and therapy of an Rh-affected fetus, because steroids alter the results of the Liley curve and make it unreliable. Delivery can be considered after 32 to 34 weeks' gestation or after documentation of fetal lung maturity. Prematurity is the most common outcome in this group of patients because of a decline in fetal well-being during gestation. Suitable blood for transfusion should be type O, missing the antigens to which the mother is sensitized. The mother may donate her own blood for transfusion if she and the fetus are type compatible. The blood may be irradiated to destroy leukocytes and to prevent engraftment or graft-versus-host disease, although there have been no case reports of these complications. The blood should be concentrated to a hematocrit of 85 to 90 g/dL, with the goal to transfuse blood with the highest hematocrit and lowest volume possible.

Rhogam

The incidence of Rh disease has dramatically decreased in the past 30 years since the use of *RhIG* (*Rhogam*). RhIG is a concentration of Rh antibodies collected from Rh-sensitized donors that act as blocking antibodies. These prevent the Rh-negative host from developing her own host immune response to Rh-negative cells in the circulation. The usual dose is 300 μg given at 28 weeks' gestation, to prevent the development of disease from small fetal-maternal hemorrhages that are common late in pregnancy, during labor, and at delivery. A second dose is given within 72 hours of delivery if the neonatal blood is Rh incompatible. This dose is protective against 30 mL (about 15 g/dL) of fetal blood. Larger fetal-maternal hemorrhages, as determined by Kleihauer-Betke testing, require proportionally larger doses of RhIG. If Rh sensitization has already occurred, RhIG administration is useless. Prophylactic RhIG should also be given to a nonsensitized mother after amniocentesis, after external version, or after a bleeding episode. If the dose is given because of bleeding during pregnancy, the dose may be repeated every 12 weeks until delivery. RhIG is also indicated after therapeutic or spontaneous abortion. A smaller dose of 50 μg is available for first trimester abortions. There is no indication for use for RhIG before 30 days of gestation because there are no Rh antigens expressed before this gestational age.

IMMUNE THROMBOCYTOPENIC PURPURA

Immune thrombocytopenic purpura is the most commonly diagnosed thrombocytopenic condition during pregnancy (73). Immune thrombocytopenic purpura is now more commonly referred to as *autoimmune thrombocytopenic purpura* (ATP). In adults, this disorder is seen more commonly in women than in men, with a ratio of approximately 3:1. It presents in the second to third decade of life, with the clinical symptoms of easy bruising, bleeding, petechiae, ecchymosis, or menorrhagia. These symptoms are the result of a decreased number of platelets, but the platelets that remain in circulation are normal in function.

ATP is a disorder of increased platelet destruction resulting from autoantibodies that are directed against platelet surface antigens. Increased destruction of megakaryocytes within the marrow may also be seen with this disorder, and the result is relative marrow failure. On bone marrow biopsy, a normal to slightly increased number of megakaryocytes is typically seen.

The clinical diagnosis is based on four parameters: (a) a platelet count persistently less than $100,000/mm^3$; (b) a bone marrow biopsy that shows increased numbers or size of megakaryocytes; (c) exclusion of other conditions that may cause thrombocytopenia, including use of drugs associated with low platelet counts; and (d) the absence of splenomegaly. The prothrombin time and activated partial thromboplastin times are normal. The bleeding time may be normal or increased, depending on the platelet count.

The presence of antiplatelet antibodies is not required for the diagnosis, but it is confirmatory. Autoantibodies that react with the major platelet antigens are seen in about 80% of patients with ATP (74). The most common target is platelet membrane glycoproteins IIb/IIIa, IIIa, and Ib. Other sites for antibody targeting include platelet antigens Ib/V/IX, glycoprotein Ia/IIa, and glycoprotein IV. Most antibodies react with more than one platelet antigen. Most antibodies function as opsonins, and the reticuloendothelial system clears affected platelets. In unusual cases, antibodies bind to platelet antigens that are critical for platelet function, with normal platelet count, but with decreased platelet function. This results in the same bleeding symptoms mentioned earlier. This can be confusing, because the clinical picture may be worse than the platelet count would indicate.

Nonautoimmune conditions that may be associated with thrombocytopenia may include lymphoproliferative disorders, and viral syndromes including cytomegalovirus infection, and HIV disease, and these must be excluded before establishing the diagnosis of ATP. Many patients with ATP may have positive serum titers for antinuclear antibody, but few of these patients develop clinically evident systemic lupus erythematosus. Thrombocytopenia can be the initial symptom of HIV, a manifestation of AIDS-related complex, or a complication of full-blown AIDS.

True thrombocytopenia, regardless of cause, must be distinguished from a spuriously low platelet count resulting from clumping, which occurs in 0.1% of normal pregnancies (75). Mild thrombocytopenia occurs in 6% to 8% of normal pregnancies, with a platelet count generally higher than $80,000/mm^3$.

Antibodies can be detected on platelets by many mechanisms; however, because of the complexity of platelet membranes, the precise identification and measurement of antibodies have been difficult. Three types of assays are used to measure platelet-associated antibodies. Variations of these assays are based on method and on the chronologic time at which each test was developed and clinically introduced. Each assay has its own sensitivity and specificity, in other words, its own advantages and pitfalls.

Antibody testing in the diagnosis of ATP may be helpful, but it is not required for diagnosis or management. Antibody tests for platelets are often performed, but only about 80% of patients with ATP actually express some form of antibody. Several possible explanations exist for this finding. The first is that not all the potential antibodies directed against platelets have been discovered or described. Therefore, a person may have some antibody against platelets, but the test is not able to detect the presence of a particular antibody. Second, the antibody produced may be directed against an internal structure of the platelet, but it is internalized and not expressed on the surface of the platelet membrane. The management of ATP is the same regardless of platelet antibody presence or the amount of antibody. Many centers today do not test for the presence or amount of antiplatelet antibody.

The *treatment* of ATP is directed by the patient's age and the severity of disease. Patients who are discovered to have mild thrombocytopenia should be followed expectantly. Platelet counts higher than $50,000/mm^3$ are rarely associated with clinically significant bleeding. The cornerstone of therapy, when indicated, is glucocorticoid administration, most commonly intravenous methylprednisone in the initial dose of 1 mg per kilogram body weight. Platelet counts generally increase to more than $50,000/mm^3$ with glucocorticoid therapy within the first week. Most patients suffer a relapse after discontinuation of therapy, especially if the taper is too rapid. Therefore, most patients continue to take oral steroids after discontinuation of intravenous therapy. The oral dose is individualized to keep platelets at an acceptable level with the lowest possible dose, to minimize potential side effects.

In general, adults are more susceptible to intracranial bleeding than children, but platelet transfusion in adults is generally reserved for actively bleeding patients and those with platelet counts less than $20,000/mm^3$. Platelet transfusions are purely a temporizing measure, because transfused platelets will be affected by the same pathologic condition that caused the initial thrombocytopenia. Hemorrhage can also be controlled in most cases with glucocorticoids. In refractory cases, patients with hemorrhage or severe thrombocytopenia may require plasmapheresis to remove circulating antibody and antibody-antigen complexes. Other potential treatment modalities include IVIG therapy, which has also been used with success in neonatal alloimmune thrombocytopenia, the platelet analogue to Rh disease (76). Phagocytic action may be blocked temporarily by administration of IVIG through nonspecific binding to platelet receptors, thereby blocking the binding of pathologic antibodies to these same receptors. The usual dose of IVIG is 0.4 g/kg per day for 3 to 5 days. The dose may be increased up to 1.0 g/kg per day if required.

Splenectomy is the next course of action for those patients not responsive to glucocorticoid or IVIG therapy. Prolonged steroid therapy can also increase the morbidity associated with splenectomy. Patients who are refractory to steroids paradoxically are more likely to respond to splenectomy. Moreover, those patients who are steroid responsive but who are dependent on steroids are also more likely to respond to splenectomy. Seventy percent of steroid-dependent patients will have a normal platelet count within 1 week following splenectomy. However, selection of the proper candidate for splenectomy is important, because patients with HIV present a special problem. The administration of chronic steroids or splenectomy in HIV patients may increase the susceptibility to opportunistic infections. Splenectomy has been shown to be safe and effective in HIV patients before the onset of symptomatic AIDS. Immunization with *S. pneumoniae* vaccine 2 weeks before splenectomy is warranted.

Those patients who are still thrombocytopenic despite glucocorticoid therapy or splenectomy may benefit from the administration of immunosuppressive drugs. These include azathioprine, cylcophosphamide, vincristine, and vinblastine. More recently, the androgen danazol has been used with some success. Vincristine and danazol rarely produce a complete remission, and antibody levels do not decrease with these therapies. The mechanism of action is by decreasing phagocytotic action. Dapsone, a drug used to treat *Mycobacterium leprae*, was used in several small case series of ATP with platelet counts less than 30,000/mm³ and clinical bleeding (5). Response was noted in 40% of patients, and therapy was well tolerated. Until larger studies are carried out with dapsone, this treatment must be considered experimental.

Patients who remain refractory to all therapeutic modalities should be evaluated for accessory spleens, which are found in as many as 10% of patients (73). Accessory splenism may be found by the presence of asplenic red cell morphology (e.g., Howell-Jolly bodies). Further surgical intervention may be warranted.

The natural clinical course of adult ATP without treatment has not been extensively studied, because of the large proportion of patients who are treated early with glucocorticoids. Approximately 25% of patients treated with glucocorticoids will have complete response to treatment, defined as a platelet count higher than 100,000/mm³ for the duration of steroid therapy. Once steroids are discontinued, many patients suffer a relapse of disease. Approximately 5% of patients have disease refractory to steroids, and these patients are a heterogeneous group. Some patients have severe bleeding, but most have chronic, minor purpura. The risk of serious bleeding and death increases with increasing age. In addition, approximately 5% of patients will have complete remission of disease after discontinuation of steroid therapy.

Pregnancy

The management of ATP in *pregnancy* poses a challenge because of the theoretic risk of bleeding not only in the mother, but also in the fetus (73). The management of ATP in pregnancy is still controversial in regard to antenatal fetal platelet testing and the best route for delivery. Most obstetricians manage ATP expectantly and treat the mother only if the platelet count decreases to less than 50,000/mm³ or if spontaneous bleeding develops.

The autoantibodies in ATP are of the IgG class, and these antibodies cross the placenta readily. Therefore, the fetus may be severely affected, despite relatively mild maternal thrombocytopenia. The range of profound fetal thrombocytopenia (platelet counts of less than 50,000/mm³) is 4% to 15%. Noninvasive predictors of the degree of neonatal thrombocytopenia are notoriously inaccurate. Therefore, one must rely on invasive measurement of fetal platelet count before delivery. Fetal platelet counts determined by scalp sampling require that the patient be in labor, with ruptured membranes, and the samples are difficult to obtain without contamination by amniotic fluid, which is a powerful procoagulant. In addition, the capillary tubes used to collect the specimen are lined with heparin, causing platelet clumping. If clumping of platelets is seen after scalp sampling, the platelet count is generally regarded as being higher than 20,000/mm³, and the platelets are considered to be normally functioning. Under these circumstances, vaginal delivery is probably safe.

The other method of determining fetal platelet count is cordocentesis. This method is accurate for platelet counts, but drawbacks are that the procedure must be carried out in specialized centers, and if the platelet count is indeed low, there is a small risk of fetal exsanguination from the puncture site in the umbilical cord. Although these complications are rare, more investigation is warranted to determine the safety of umbilical cord sampling in this setting. In one case report, the twins of a mother affected with ATP had significantly disparate platelet counts (77). As such, both fetuses of a twin gestation should be tested.

The best mode of delivery is generally determined by obstetric factors alone. Because the risk of neonatal thrombocytopenia is low, and the risk for serious bleeding in the neonate is even less, the risk of abdominal delivery in a mother affected by ATP is regarded as being higher. Unless a fetal platelet count is documented as being less than 20,000/mm³, or if no platelet clumping is seen after scalp platelet sampling, then a cesarean delivery may be considered. Under most circumstances, however, vaginal delivery may be considered safe.

The cornerstone of therapy for ATP in pregnancy is glucocorticoids. Prednisone is well tolerated in pregnancy, with the most commonly reported side effects of sleeplessness, acne, striae, and increased appetite. Occasionally, glucose intolerance is seen, and serum glucose measurements should be taken after 24 to 26 weeks' gestation and again in the third trimester. Prednisone is generally begun once platelet counts fall to less than 50,000/mm³ or if the bleeding time is longer than 20 minutes. Splenectomy may be undertaken safely after 14 to 16 weeks' gestation, when the risk of miscarriage associated with general anesthesia and abdominal surgery is lowest. Splenectomy is successful in raising platelet counts in 75% of cases. IVIG has been used in pregnancy, but it is less well studied for this disorder. This therapy has been shown to be safe, but it is expensive and requires repeated dosing every 2 to 4 weeks. Duration of benefit is highly variable, and the best timing in relation to delivery is not entirely clear, so it should be individualized. An alternative to long-term steroid therapy and IVIG may be high-dose pulsed prednisone. In this regimen, prednisone is used in doses of 40 mg to 60 mg per day for 5 days when the platelet count drops to less than 30,000/mm³, and it is then discontinued. Therapy with immunosuppressive drugs such as vincristine, azathioprine, and cylcophosphamide are relatively contraindicated in pregnancy, because of risks to the fetus, which include intrauterine growth restriction, fetal immunosuppression, maternal and fetal neutropenia, and opportunistic infections. These drugs are considered absolutely contraindicated in the first trimester because of the theoretic risk of teratogenesis during organogenesis. If immunosuppressive drugs are used during pregnancy, the benefits must clearly outweigh the risks, and the patient must be made aware of the risks. Danazol is contraindicated in pregnancy, but it may be used safely in the postpartum period.

Cerebral hemorrhage in the fetus is exceedingly rare, but it is the most feared complication. It has been reported in the literature only in sporadic case reports or anecdotally. No antepartum prognostic factors to date can accurately assess fetal risk. Although knowing the fetal platelet count may not affect the mode of delivery, it may play a role in the management of such pregnancies. An obstetrician who knows that the fetus has a platelet count less than 50,000/mm³ may choose to avoid a fetal scalp electrode or instrumental delivery. Delivery in a tertiary institution should be considered under these circumstances for intensive pediatric care. Women who have had splenectomy before pregnancy are just as likely to have an affected pregnancy, because the circulating antibodies are still present. Maternal platelet counts may be normal in these cases, with a severely thrombocytopenic fetus, and, in fact, may be associated with a higher risk of neonatal thrombocytopenia. In addition, infants born to mothers with ATP may often develop neonatal thrombocytopenia several hours to days after delivery. This is important today because of incentives to release patients increasingly earlier from the hospital after delivery. Some degree of thrombocytopenia of the newborn is seen in up to 70% of children born to mothers with ATP. This fall in platelet counts is generally mild and peaks 4 to 6 days after delivery. The platelet count rises as the passively acquired antiplatelet antibody levels fall. Breast-feeding by affected mothers has also been associated with neonatal thrombocytopenia because antiplatelet IgG is passed through the colostrum. Breast-feeding in these patients must be individualized.

VON WILLEBRAND'S DISEASE

Von Willebrand's disease (vWD) is a genetically and clinically heterogeneous disorder caused by a deficiency or dysfunction of *von Willebrand factor* (vWF), an adhesive glycoprotein in plasma, platelets, and endothelial cells (78). The interaction of platelets with vessel walls is defective and thus impairs primary hemostasis. vWD is the most common bleeding disorder, more common than hemophilia A or B. vWD is inherited as an autosomal dominant disorder, with a population prevalence of 1.5%. Heterozygous carriers often manifest some clinical form of the disease, but penetrance is variable.

Laboratory diagnosis of vWD consists of five tests: vWF activity, vWF antigen, factor VIII activity, vWF multimeric analysis, and bleeding time (Fig. 30.17). vWF multimeric analysis is required to classify the vWD subtype accurately. The diagnosis is established by finding reduced plasma levels of vWF activity, vWF antigen, or factor VIII, and a prolonged bleeding time. When only factor VIII is low, the diagnosis may be confused with hemophilia A, and if only the bleeding time is prolonged, a platelet disorder may be mistakenly diagnosed. Ideally, all four tests are abnormal, thus making the diagnosis obvious. Normal values do not exclude the diagnosis because some variability exists within the same patient as a result of blood type, pregnancy, and stress, and testing should be repeated several weeks later. A familial pedigree is essential to determine pat-

	vWD	Hemophilia	Platelet Dysfunction
Factor VIII	low or normal	low	normal
vWF	low or normal	normal	normal
vWF:Ag	low or normal	normal	normal
Bleeding Time	increased	normal	increased

FIGURE 30.17. Laboratory tests in von Willebrand's disease.

terns of inheritance. X-linked inheritance leads in the direction of hemophilia, and autosomal dominance suggests vWD.

Classification of vWD is divided into three types, with several subtypes based on molecular analysis of the von Willebrand protein. In *type I vWD*, there is a partial quantitative deficiency of vWF. This is the most common type of vWD and accounts for 70% of cases (79). All multimers are present in plasma, but in reduced quantity, and they vary on different occasions in the same patient. Plasma levels of factor VIII and vWF antigen may be concordantly reduced, or they may be normal, and the bleeding time is also variable. *Platelet-low type I vWD* is caused by defective production of vWF, whereas *platelet-normal type I vWD* results from impaired release of vWF from cellular stores. The bleeding time in platelet-normal patients is near normal, and these patients have a better response to 1-desamino-8-D-arginine vasopressin (DDAVP). This finding suggests that platelet levels of vWF correlate more strongly with function of vWF and bleeding tendencies.

Type II vWD is characterized by a qualitative abnormality of vWF and accounts for 15% to 30% of cases (79). *Type IIa vWD* refers to a defective platelet-vWF interaction with the absence of high- and middle-molecular-weight vWF multimers in plasma. Hemostasis is adversely affected by the absence of large-molecular-weight vWF protein required for platelet binding to endothelium. Two mechanisms account for the absence of large multimeric vWF: abnormal cellular assembly and increased susceptibility to proteolysis. *Type IIb vWD* is caused by an increased affinity of vWF for its binding site on platelets, glycoprotein Ib. There is an absence of the highest-molecular-weight multimer, secondary to an abnormally high turnover of these multimers because of the increased affinity for platelet glycoprotein Ib. These patients also exhibit mild thrombocytopenia. *Type IIM vWD* refers to a form characterized by decreased platelet interaction with vWF not caused by the absence of highest-molecular-weight multimer. The multimers are, in fact, larger than normal, a feature that causes decreased binding to platelet glycoprotein Ib. *Type IIN vWD* is caused by a defective interaction of vWF with factor VIII. These patients have reduced levels of factor VIII by 5% to 15%, with normal levels of vWF and normal bleeding times. The binding region of vWF to factor VIII is abnormal, causing reduced complexing of vWF to factor VIII, and as a result the half-life of factor VIII in the plasma is markedly reduced. This form of vWD is phenotypically expressed only if the person is homozygous for the defective vWF–factor VIII binding site.

Type III vWD is the severe type (79), with complete absence of vWF. VWF activity and vWF antigen are nearly undetectable, and factor VIII is reduced to less than 10% of normal. The bleeding time is prolonged to more than 20 minutes.

Clinical Manifestations

Clinical manifestations of vWD are variable, depending on the type of disease. Patients with type I and II have mild bleeding tendencies from mucous membranes. Epistaxis, easy bruising, and gastrointestinal bleeding are common. Menorrhagia is the most common manifestation in women, out of proportion to other symptoms. Pregnancy is generally well tolerated because of the natural increase in factor VIII and vWF during gestation. Affected newborns also have normally elevated factor VIII and vWF immediately after delivery, a finding that makes the diagnosis difficult. Type III vWD results in severe, often life-threatening hemorrhages. Dental procedures may result in severe hemorrhage and may require transfusion therapy. Deep hematomas and joint hemorrhages are also common.

Patients with vWD have angiodysplasia, which is characterized by small telangiectases in the wall of the small intestine and colon, more commonly in persons older than 50 years and in type III vWD. Bleeding is intermittent and rarely is life-threatening, but it can lead to chronic anemia. Surgery is rarely indicated unless recurrent bleeding sites are identified or hemorrhage is life-threatening. Estrogen therapy may be effective in controlling symptoms. vWD may be acquired by an IgG-mediated mechanism. Antibodies are directed against vWF that interfere with binding to platelets, and patients may also exhibit mild thrombocytopenia.

Therapy is aimed at correcting vWF and factor VIII levels (80). DDAVP is a synthetic vasopressin analogue that causes release of vWF from intracellular storage sites, but it has less than 1% of the pressor effects of vasopressin. DDAVP is available in intravenous, subcutaneous, and intranasal spray forms. The intravenous preparation may be given intravenously or subcutaneously with roughly equivalent responses. The dose is 0.2 to 0.3 μg/kg body weight. The subcutaneously administered dose must be less than 1.5 mL volume per injection site, and a single treatment may require several sites. Correction of bleeding time is seen in 20 to 30 minutes. The concentrated form of the intranasal DDAVP is effective (the dilute preparation is for use in diabetes insipidus and is not effective for vWD) at a dose of 150 μg (75 μg per nostril). DDAVP causes hyponatremia and should not be administered more than once a day. Serum sodium must be measured if DDAVP is administered on consecutive days. Treatment of type II (except possibly IIA) and type III vWD with DDAVP is not effective (55). Patients with type IIA should have a trial of DDAVP to determine whether it is effective. DDAVP potentiates the response of patients with type III vWD to cryoprecipitate, and it may be used in emergency situations.

Infusion of plasma clotting factors may be required in many instances. Two commercially available forms of factor VIII concentrates are available that contain some high-molecular-weight multimers. Other factor VIII preparations may contain only low- and middle-molecular-weight multimers and are not effective in the treatment of vWD. Cryoprecipitate is a plasma fraction that contains factor VIII, vWF, fibrinogen, and fibronectin. It is obtained by collecting the precipitate that forms when frozen plasma is warmed to 4°C. The yield of factor VIII and vWF can be increased fivefold by administration of DDAVP to the donor before collection. The full range of vWF multimers is found in cryoprecipitate. There is a risk of transmission of hepatitis B and C as well as HIV in cryoprecipitate, because there is no viral inactivation step after collection. As such, all donors must be screened carefully, or collection may be from other nonaffected family members. Each bag of cryoprecipitate contains 100 U of factor VIII and 100 U of vWF. Persons with type O blood have lower levels of vWF, and donors with blood types A, B, and AB are preferred (81).

Cryoprecipitate is the treatment of choice in patients with type II and III vWD (except perhaps type IIa). Other treatments have been tried with variable success, such as hemostatic agents such as microfibrillar collagen (Avitene) or fibrin glue. The type IIb subset of vWD presents additional complexity because of a progressive decrease in platelet count that accompanies pregnancy-associated increased synthesis of this variant form of vWF. The appearance of thrombocytopenia during pregnancy necessitates the consideration of this type of vWD, because the interaction of the abnormal form of vWF and platelets results in thrombocytopenia. Because of this abnormal platelet-vWF interaction, DDAVP is contraindicated because it will exacerbate thrombocytopenia. Factor VIII concentrates adequately treat type IIb vWD, although many patients have had normal vaginal deliveries despite moderate to severe thrombocytopenia.

Pregnant patients should have a planned delivery, with administration of appropriate therapy timed before delivery. Cesarean section should be reserved for typical obstetric indications. Repeat dosing of DDAVP may be required for the first 2 to 3 days post partum, and serum sodium must be carefully monitored under these circumstances because of the risk of water intoxication. The pediatrician should test the newborn when appropriate.

HERITABLE COAGULOPATHIES IN PREGNANCY

Several causes of *coagulopathies* in pregnancy are inheritable. Most of these conditions are autosomal dominant, although variable penetrance is often observed. Inherited coagulopathies are responsible for an eightfold increased risk of thromboembolism. Unusual sites of thrombosis are often observed and include sagittal sinus thrombosis and mesenteric and portal vein thrombosis. There is also a fourfold increased risk of stillbirth, intrauterine growth restriction,

and severe preeclampsia. The most common types of autosomal dominant coagulopathies include activated protein C resistance (factor V Leiden), antithrombin III deficiency, protein C deficiency, protein S deficiency, hyperhomocysteinemia, prothrombin[G20210A] mutation, dysfibrinogenemia, and hyperfibrinogenemia. Dysfibrinogenemia and hyperfibrinogenemia are rare and promote both thrombosis and hemorrhage.

Protein C and Protein S

Protein C and *protein S* are both produced in the liver and are vitamin K–dependent factors in the fibrinolytic system (Figs. 30.18 and 30.19). Protein S is a cofactor that protein C requires to deactivate factor Va or factor VIIIa. Any conditions that decrease the normal levels of protein C or protein S increase the likelihood of forming clots resulting from uninhibited activated factors V or VIII. Circulating protein S exists in both free (40%) and bound (60%) forms. Protein S binds to its carrier protein C4b-BP, and this complex interacts with protein C. Pregnancy, inflammation, and surgery decrease circulating C4b-BP, reduce protein S activity, and increase the risk of clotting (82).

Protein C Deficiency

The prevalence of protein C deficiency is 0.2% to 0.5%, and the lifetime risk of thromboembolism is more than 50%. Mutations either reduce transcription of DNA into RNA or generate abnormal protein C structure. Type I deficiency causes concomitant reductions in protein C and functional levels, and type II deficiency causes normal pro-

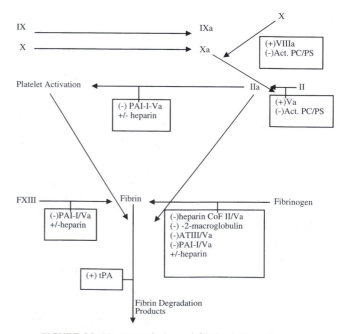

FIGURE 30.18. Hemolytic and fibrinolytic pathways.

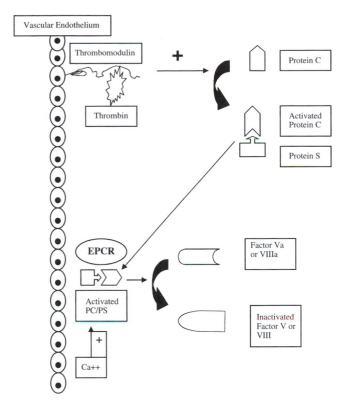

FIGURE 30.19. Thrombomodulin and protein C and protein S activities.

tein C levels, but reduced functional ability. The risk of thromboembolism is 5% to 10% during pregnancy and up to 20% in the puerperium. There is also a moderately increased risk of pregnancy loss in the third trimester, approximately twice as high as in the healthy population. Testing for protein C deficiency in pregnancy can be accurate, but it is probably best deferred until after pregnancy.

Factor V Leiden

Factor V Leiden mutation is the most common heritable coagulopathy, with a prevalence of 5% to 9% in European populations (83). It is relatively rare in Asian and African populations. The primary mutation is a guanine for arginine substitution in the gene's tenth exon, and the resultant amino acid substitution affects activated protein C and impairs the ability of activated protein C–protein S complex to inactivate factor Va. The risk of thrombosis is 5- to 10-fold higher in heterozygotes and 100-fold greater in homozygotes with this mutation (55). Factor V Leiden accounts for 20% to 40% of thromboembolic diseases. Factor V Leiden is also responsible for recurrent miscarriage, placental infarcts, and cerebral palsy (from cerebrovascular accidents). Testing for factor V Leiden mutation is easily done in pregnancy, because it is performed by polymerase chain reaction DNA testing for the mutation. Pregnancy is associated with increased resistance to activated protein

C because of lower protein S and factor VIII, and testing for protein S deficiency during pregnancy can lead to false-positive results.

Antithrombin III Deficiency

Antithrombin III deficiency is an autosomal dominant disorder resulting from numerous point mutations, deletions, or insertions (84). These mutations generate either abnormal DNA transcription or abnormal protein structure. Type I antithrombin III deficiency results from reductions in both protein levels and protein function. Type II deficiency is divided into several subclassifications. Type II RS is a reactive site mutation, HBS or heparin binding site. Pleiotropic functional defects are seen with type II PE deficiency. There is a 70% to 90% lifetime risk of thromboembolism, because it is the most thrombogenic of the inherited coagulopathies (55). Antithrombin III has a relatively low prevalence, with an incidence of 1 in 600 to 1 in 5,000. Therefore, it accounts for 1% of all thromboembolic diseases. The risk of thromboembolism during pregnancy is 15% to 60%, with a fivefold increased risk of third trimester pregnancy loss.

Hyperhomocysteinemia

Hyperhomocysteinemia has generated much interest because of the easily treatable nature of this disorder. Homocysteine is generated by metabolism of methylenetetrahydrofolate to a dihydrofolate form by the enzyme methylenetetrahydrofolate reductase (MTHFR). The cause for increased homocysteine is a mutation in the MTHFR enzyme (Fig. 30.20) in the form of a missense mutation at nucleotide 677, causing a substitution of cytosine to thymine and leading to a

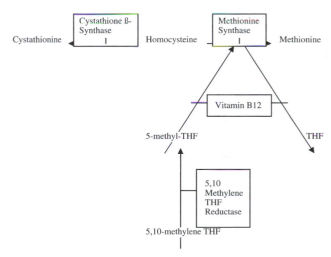

FIGURE 30.20. Homocysteine metabolism. Defects in methionine synthase, cystatione β-synthase, or 5,10-methylenetetrahydrofolate reductase activities in combination with deficient folate results in excess homocysteine levels.

defective protein by substituting valine for alanine. This causes decreased metabolism by the MHTFR enzyme and increased levels of homocysteine (85,86). Hyperhomocysteinemia may also be seen with low levels of folic acid, vitamin B_6, or vitamin B_{12}. Mild hyperhomocysteinemia is a risk factor for atherosclerosis and vascular disease, and half the vascular complications are venous. Two hypotheses have been generated in an attempt to explain how elevated levels of homocysteine can cause venous thrombosis. One hypothesis is that high levels of homocysteine have a toxic effect on vascular endothelial cells that causes cellular degeneration and exposes the basement membrane. This increases platelet aggregation, activation of the clotting cascade, and reduced fibrinolysis. The alternate hypothesis is that hyperhomocysteinemia reflects abnormal methionine metabolism that affects the methylation of DNA and cell membranes. The treatment of hyperhomocysteinemia is with supplementation of folate, and vitamins B_6 and B_{12}, although it has not been proven that supplementation decreases the risk of thrombosis.

Prothrombin[G20210A] Mutation

A *defect in the prothrombin gene* causing extremely high levels of prothrombin has been shown to increase the risk of venous thrombosis threefold. This genetic variation in the untranslated region of the prothrombin gene is caused by a guanine to adenine transition at position 20210 and is known as the prothrombin[G20210A] mutation. This mutation is equally distributed among males and females, and it may have a hereditary association with homocysteinuria, factor V Leiden mutation, and the risk of thrombosis. The exact risk of thrombosis and the association with these other heritable conditions are currently under study.

Management of Inherited Coagulopathies in Pregnancy

Diagnosis

Testing should be undertaken in those patients with a history of deep venous thrombosis occurring when they are less than 45 years of age and patients with unusual sites of thrombosis, such as mesenteric or splenic thrombosis. A family history of thrombosis is also an indication for genetic testing. Patients with a history of stillbirths, abruption, and intrauterine growth restriction, as well as of recurrent severe preeclampsia, require testing. If the patient is not pregnant, then one may test directly for levels of protein C, protein S, antithrombin III, and the factor V Leiden mutation. Fasting levels of homocysteine should be obtained. If the patient is pregnant, then a total and free protein S may be obtained and corrected for pregnancy, although this method is inaccurate. Protein C determinations may be obtained during pregnancy, but they are also inaccurate. Testing for

both protein S and protein C is best left until after pregnancy. A normal thrombin time rules out dysfibrinogenemia.

Treatment

Treatment consists of infusions either of the missing factor, as with antithrombin III, or of *heparin*. Prophylactic versus "therapeutic" or full-dose heparin therapy is determined by several factors. Prophylactic heparin is used in pregnancy in patients with a coagulopathy (except antithrombin III, see below) and those who have a history of thromboembolism antedating pregnancy by at least 6 months. Heparin is a complex glycosaminoglycan that potentiates the antithrombin effects of antithrombin III. It increases the level of factor Xa inhibitor and also inhibits platelet aggregation. Heparin does not cross the placenta because it is a large, highly charged molecule. It is therefore the anticoagulant of choice in pregnancy. Warfarin should be avoided in the first trimester because of its embryopathy, and it is best avoided in the second and third trimester as a result of its association of abnormal neuronal migration in the central nervous system. Warfarin does cross the placenta and may theoretically anticoagulate the fetus, a process leading to intraventricular hemorrhage.

The side effects of heparin include hemorrhage, especially when it is used in conjunction with aspirin, although this risk is less than 5%. There is a risk of heparin-induced thrombocytopenia caused by either prophylactic or therapeutic doses of heparin (73). This risk is around 3%, and the disorder has two basic forms. The first is an early-onset, transient form that causes inhibited platelet aggregation. The second type is IgG mediated and leads to severe thrombocytopenia. The second type occurs within 2 weeks of initiation of therapy and mandates the cessation of heparin use. Another potential side effect is osteoporosis, occurring in up to 10% of patients with long-term use. The risk increases with increasing doses greater than 15,000 units per day over 6 months of treatment. Calcium supplementation along with weight-bearing exercise should be initiated if heparin doses are greater that 15,000 units per day for greater than 6 months. Bone densitometry is safe during pregnancy to assess the degree of osteoporosis.

Pregnant patients with a heritable coagulopathy (except antithrombin III) and a history of adverse pregnancy outcomes are also candidates for prophylactic heparin. Prophylactic heparin may also be used in patients without a history of thromboembolism or adverse pregnancy outcomes, but who have been incidentally found to have a heritable coagulopathy, although some clinicians advocate that prophylaxis is not warranted. However, most would use prophylaxis in these patients, because pregnancy is also a hypercoagulable state. The usual doses are 5,000 U heparin subcutaneously, with the dose increased by 2,500 U each trimester.

Therapeutic heparin is reserved for those patients who

have a thromboembolism during pregnancy or who have antithrombin III deficiency (87) and are not candidates for antithrombin III infusions. The goal of therapy is to maintain the activated partial thromboplastin time between 1.5 and 2.5 times control. Several regimens are used to calculate the total dose of heparin required. One is a weight-based formula, but it becomes less accurate in the obese patient because of erratic absorption. A second method is to admit the patient to the hospital and to begin heparin therapy intravenously. Once the total amount of heparin is calculated within a 24-hour period to maintain the activated partial thromboplastin time between 1.5 and 2.5 times normal, this dose is divided equally into three daily doses. A third method is to begin 10,000 U three times daily and to titrate until a therapeutic dose has been achieved after measurement of the activated partial thromboplastin time 4 to 6 hours after the morning dose.

Low-molecular-weight heparin (LMWH) has gained in popularity as an alternate to unfractionated heparin (88). LMWH is a purified heparin, with a longer half-life (89). The advantages of LMWH are reduced risks of thrombocytopenia and osteoporosis. Because of its stability and predictable absorption, LMWH does not require laboratory monitoring outside of pregnancy. The dose may need to be adjusted during pregnancy as LMWH is finally cleared, and the GFR in pregnancy increases. If monitoring is performed, anti–factor Xa levels are used. This is a specialized laboratory test that many laboratories do not perform, and it is expensive. Prophylactic LMWH is given in one to two divided doses daily, according to the brand of LMWH prescribed. Therapeutic LMWH is administered by weight-based dosing according to the manufacturer's recommendations. Several case reports of epidural hematomas in conjunction with use of LMWH have been published (90,91). This risk occurs mainly in elderly women who have undergone major joint replacement. In pregnant women, it is prudent to discontinue LMWH 12 to 24 hours before anticipated delivery, so the patient may undergo regional anesthesia. LMWH may be restarted 12 to 24 hours after epidural catheter removal. No reversal agent for LMWH exists at this time.

10 KEY POINTS

1. Many growth factors are involved in the normal development of the hematopoietic system.

2. The most common cause of anemia in the United States and worldwide is iron deficiency.

3. The basic workup of anemia begins with a complete blood count, and red cell indices, to determine the type of anemia.

4. Other causes of anemia should be sought if iron supplementation does not resolve anemia.

5. Counseling, hemoglobin electrophoresis, and genetic testing should be carried out if a hemoglobinopathy is suspected.

6. Fetal red cell synthesis begins early in gestation in the yolk sac, moves to extramedullary sites in the second trimester, and eventually occurs in the bone marrow by delivery.

7. Red cell antigens are expressed on fetal red cells by 6 weeks' gestation.

8. Gestational thrombocytopenia and immune thrombocytopenic purpura result in low morbidity for both mother and fetus; alloimmune throbocytopenia in the fetus can result in increased neonatal morbidity.

9. Hypercoagulable states in pregnancy often result in increased maternal morbidity and fetal morbidity and mortality. Heparin prophylaxis should be considered during pregnancy in patients with a hypercoagulable condition, and heparin therapy is reserved for those with a thromboembolic event in pregnancy or with antithrombin III deficiency.

10. Blood disorders are often complex, and hematologic and maternal-fetal medicine specialists should be consulted in patient management.

REFERENCES

1. Dexter TM, Allen TD, Lajtha LG. Conditions controlling the proliferation of hematopoietic cells *in vitro. J Cell Physiol* 1977;91:335–339.
2. Bernstein ID, Andrews RG, Zsebo KM. Recombinant human stem cell factor enhances the formation of colonies by CD34 and CD34 lin− cells, and the generation of colony-forming cell progeny from CD34 lin− cells cultured with interleukin-3, granulocyte colony-stimulating factor, or granulocyte-macrophage colony-stimulating factor. *Blood* 1991;77:2316.
3. Li J, Sensebe L, Herve P, Charbord P. Nontransformed colony-derived stomal cell lines from normal human marrows: the maintenance of hematopoiesis from CD34 cell populations. *Exp Hematol* 1997;25:582.
4. Waller EK, Olweus J, Lund-Johansen F, et al. The "common stem cell" hypothesis reevaluated: human fetal bone marrow contains separate populations of hematopoietic and stromal progenitors. *Blood* 1995;85:2422.
5. Breems DA, Blokland EA, Neben S, et al. Frequency analysis of human primitive haematopoietic stem cell subsets using a cobblestone area forming assay. *Leukemia* 1995;8:1095.
6. Potts JR, Campbell ID. Fibronectin structure and assembly. *Curr Opin Cell Biol* 1994;6:648.
7. Weinstein R, Riordan MA, Wemc K, et al. Dual role of fibronectin in hematopoietic differentiation. *Blood* 1989;73:111.
8. Bornstein P. Thrombospondins: structure and regulation of expression. *FASEB J* 1992;6:3290.
9. Asch AS, Tepler J, Silbiger S, et al. Cellular attatchment to thrombospondin: cooperative interactions between receptor systems. *J Biol Chem* 1990;266:1740.
10. Wright TN, Kinsella MG, Keating A, et al. Proteoglycans in human long-term bone marrow cultures: biochemical and ultrastructural analyses. *Blood* 1986;67:1333.
11. Siczkowski M, Clarke D, Gordon MY. Binding of primitive hematopoietic progenitor cells to marrow stromal cells involves heparan sulfate. *Blood* 1992;80:912.

12. Engvall E. Structure and function of basement membranes. *Int J Devel Biol* 1995;39:781.

13. Stohlman FJ, Ebbe S, Morse B. Regulation of erythropoiesis: kinetics of red cell production. *Ann N Y Acad Sci* 1968;149:156.

14. Lodish HF, Hilton DJ, Klingmuller U. The erythropoietin receptor: biogenesis, dimerization, and intracellular signal transduction. *Cold Spring Harb Symp Quant Biol* 1995;60:93.

15. Henry DH. Recombinant human erythropoietin treatment of anemic cancer patients. *Cancer Pract* 1996;4:180.

16. Bennet DR, Shulman IA. Practical issues when confronting the patient who refuses blood transfusion therapy. *Am J Clin Pathol* 1997;107:S23.

17. Henry DH, Beall GN, Benson CA. Recombinant human erythropoietin in the treatment of anemia with human immunodeficiency virus (HIV) infection and zidovudine therapy: overview of four clinical trials. *Ann Intern Med* 1992;117:739.

18. McGregor E, Stewart G, Junor BJR, et al. Successful use of recombinant erythropoietin in pregnancy. *Nephrol Dial Transplant* 1991;6:292.

19. Williams DE, deVries P, Namen AE. The steel factor. *Dev Biol* 1992;151:368.

20. Stewart CEH, Rotwein P. Growth, differentiation, and survival: multiple physiological functions for insulin-like growth factors. *Physiol Rev* 1998;76:1005.

21. Correa PN, Eskinazi D, Axelrad AA. Circulating erythroid progenitors in polycythemia vera are hypersensitive to insulin-like growth factor I *in vitro*: studies in an improved serum-free medium. *Blood* 1994;83:99.

22. Migliaccio G, Migliaccio AR, Adamson JW. *In vitro* diferentiation of human granulocyte/macrophage and erythroid progenitors: comparative analysis of the influence of recombinant human erythropoietin, G-CSF, GM-CSF, and IL-3 in serum-supplemented and serum-deprived cultures. *Blood* 1988;72:248.

23. Fleischmann J, Golde DW, Weisbart RH, et al. Granulocyte-macrophage colony-stimulating factor enhances phagocytosis of bacteria by human neutrophils. *Blood* 1986;68:708.

24. Ohara A, Suca T, Saito M. Effect of recombinant human granulocyte colony-stimulating factor on hematopoetic cells in serum-free culture. *Exp Hematol* 1987;15:695.

25. Hartmann LC, Tschetter LK, Habermann TM. Granulocyte colony-stimulating factor in severe chemotherapy-induced afebrile neutropenia. *N Engl J Med* 1997;336:1776.

26. Stanley ER, Berg KL, Einstein DB. Biology and action of colony-stimulating factor-1. *Mol Reprod Dev* 1997;46:4.

27. Chang M, Suen Y, Meng G. Differential mechanisms in the regulation of endogenous levels of thrombopoietin and interleukin-11 during thrombocytopenia: insight into the regulation of platelet production. *Blood* 1996;85:981.

28. Nagata Y, Shozaki Y, Nagahisa H. Serum thrombopoietin level is not regulated by transcription but by the total counts of both megakaryocytes and platelets during thrombocytopenia and thrombocytosis. *Thromb Haemost* 1997;77:808.

29. Kobayashi M, Laver JH, Kato T. Thrombopoietin supports proliferation of human primitive hematopoietic cells in synergy with steel factor/and or interleukin-3. *Blood* 1996;88:429.

30. Vadhan-Raj S, Murray LJ, Bueso-Ramos C. Stimulation of megakaryocyte and platelet production by a single dose of recombinant human thrombopoietin in patients with cancer. *Ann Intern Med* 1997;126:673.

31. Kaushansky K. Thrombopoietin. *N Engl J Med* 1998;339:11.

32. Paul SR, Schendel P. The cloning and biological characterization of recombinant human interleukin-11. *Int J Cell Cloning* 1992;10:135.

33. Goodwin RG, Lupton S, Schmierer A. Human interleukin-7: molecular cloning and growth factor activity on human and murine B-lineage cells. *Proc Natl Acad Sci U S A* 1989;86:302.

34. Smith KA. Interleukin-2: inception, impact, and implications. *Science* 1988;240:1169.

35. Del Prete G, Maggi E, Parronchi P. IL-4 is an essential factor for the IgE synthesis induced by *in vitro* human T cell clones and their supernatants. *J Immunol* 1988;140:4193.

36. Jelinek DF, Lipsky PE. Inhibitory influence of IL-4 on human B cell responsiveness. *J Immunol* 1988;141:164.

37. Forestier F, Daffos F, Catherine N, et al. Developmental hematopoiesis in normal human fetal blood. *Blood* 1991;77:2360.

38. Zanjani ED, Ascensao JL, Tavassoli M. Liver-derived fetal hematopoietic stem cells selectively and preferentially home to the fetal bone marrow. *Blood* 1993;81:399.

39. Looker AC, Dallman PR, Carroll MD. Prevalence of iron deficiency anemia in the United States. *JAMA* 1997;277:973.

40. Cook JD, Skikne BS, Baynes RD. Iron deficiency: the global perspective. *Adv Exp Med Biol* 1994;356:219.

41. Hallberg L, Hulthen L, Bengtsson C. Iron balance in menstruating women. *Eur J Clin Nutr* 1995;49:200.

42. Oski FA. Iron deficiency in infancy and childhood. *N Engl J Med* 1993;329:190.

43. Brittenham GM. Red blood cell function, disorders of iron metabolism, and iron deficiency. In: Dale DD, ed. *Scientific American medicine*, vol 5, sect II. New York: Scientific American, 1996.

44. Swain RA, Kaplan B, Montgomery E. Iron deficiency anemia: when is parenteral therapy warranted? *Postgrad Med* 1996;100:181.

45. Cooper BA. Folate nutrition in man and animals. In: Blakely RL, Whitehead VM, eds. *Folates and pterins: nutritional, pharmacological, and physiological aspects*, vol 3. New York: Wiley Interscience, 1986.

46. Selhub J. Folate binding proteins: mechanisms for placental and intestinal uptake. In: Allen L, King J, Lonnerdahl B, eds. *Nutrient regulation during pregnancy, lactation, and infant growth*. New York: Plenum, 1994.

47. Henderson GI, Perez T, Schenker S. Maternal-to-fetal transfer of 5-methyltetrahydrofolate by the perfused human placenta cotyledon: evidence for a concentrative role by placental folate receptors in fetal folate delivery. *J Lab Clin Med* 1995;126:184.

48. Botto L, Moore CA, Khoury MJ, et al. Neural-tube defects. *N Engl J Med* 1999;341:20.

49. Savitt TL, Goldberg MF. Barrett's 1910 case report of sickle cell anemia: the rest of the story. *JAMA* 1989;261:266.

50. Motulsky AG. Frequency of sickling disorders in US blacks. *N Engl J Med* 1972;288:31.

51. Sewchand LS, Johnson CS, Meiselman HJ. The effect of fetal hemoglobin on the sickling dynamics of SS erythrocytes. *Blood Cells* 1983;9:147.

52. Brittenham GM, Schechter AN, Noguchi CT. Hemoglobin S polymerization: primary determination of the hemolytic and clinical severity of the sickling syndromes. *Blood* 1985;65:283.

53. Wayne AS, Kevy SV, Nathan DG. Transfusion management of sickle cell disease. *Blood* 1993;81:1109.

54. Davies SC, Roberts-Harewood M. Blood transfusion in sickle cell disease. *Blood Rev* 1997;11:57.

55. Embury SH, Vichinsky EP. Sickle cell disease. In: Hoffman R, Benz E, Shattil S, et al., eds. *Hematology: basic principles and practice*, 3rd ed. New York: Churchill Livingstone, 2000.

56. Bunn HF. Disorders of hemoglobin. In: Isselbacher KJ, Braunwald E, Wilson JD, et al., eds. *Harrison's principles of internal medicine*, 13th ed. New York, McGraw-Hill, 1994.

57. Agre P. Hereditary spherocytosis. *JAMA* 1989;262:2887.

58. Maberry MC, Mason RA, Cunningham FG, et al. Pregnancy complicated by hereditary spherocytosis. *Obstet Gynecol* 1992;79:735.

59. Beutler E. Glucose-6-phosphate dehydrogenase deficiency. *N Engl J Med* 1991;324:169.

60. Hughes GRV. The antiphospholipid antibody syndrome: ten years on. *Lancet* 1993;342:341.
61. Derksen RHWM, Bruinse HW, deGroot PG, et al. Pregnancy in systemic lupus erythematosus: a prospective study. *Lupus* 1994;3:149.
62. Harris EN, Spinnato JA. Should anticardiolipin tests be performed in otherwise healthy pregnant women? *Am J Obstet Gynecol* 1991;165:1272.
63. Hanly JG, Gladman DD, Rose TH, et al. Lupus pregnancy: a prospective study of placental changes. *Arthritis Rheum* 1988; 31:358.
64. Cekleniak N, Hirshberg J, Leiva MC, et al. Heparin therapy reduces the risk of fetal death and IUGR and is effective in the treatment of the antiphospholipid antibody syndrome and of repeated pregnancy losses. *Am J Obstet Gynecol* 1996;174:392.
65. Cowchock FS, Reece EA, Balaboan D, et al. Repeated fetal losses associated with antiphospholipid antibodies: a collaborative randomized trial comparing prednisone with low-dose heparin treatment. *Am J Obstet Gynecol* 1992;166:1318.
66. Silver RK, MacGregor SN, Sholl JS, et al. Comparative trial of prednisone plus aspirin versus aspirin alone in the treatment of anticardiolipin antibody positive obstetric patients. *Am J Obstet Gynecol* 1993;169:6.
67. Spinnato JA, Clark AL, Pierangeli SS, et al. Intravenous immunoglobulin therapy for the antiphospholipid syndrome in pregnancy. *Am J Obstet Gynecol* 1995;172:690.
68. Johnson MJ, Petri M, Witter FR, et al. Evaluation of preterm delivery in a systemic lupus erythematosus pregnancy clinic. *Obstet Gynecol* 1995;86:396.
69. Millard DD, Gidding SS, Socol ML, et al. Effects of intravascular, intrauterine, transfusion on prenatal and postnatal hemoysis and erythropoiesis in severe fetal isoimmunization. *J Pediatr* 1990; 117:447.
70. Mari G, for the Collaborative Group for Doppler Assessment of the Blood Velocity in Anemic Fetuses. Noninvasive diagnosis by Doppler ultrasonography of fetal anemia due to maternal red-cell alloimmunization. *N Engl J Med* 2000;342:1.
71. Queenan JT, Tomai TP, Ural SH, et al. Deviation in amniotic fluid optical density at a wavelength of 450 nm in Rh isoimmunized pregnancies from 14 to 40 weeks gestation: a proposal for clinical management. *Am J Obstet Gynecol* 1993;168:1370.
72. Kaufman GE, Paidas MJ. Rhesus sensitization and alloimmune thrombocytopenia. *Semin Perinatol* 1994;18:4.
73. Johnson JR, Samuels P. Review of autoimmune thrombocytopenia: pathogenesis, diagnosis, and management in pregnancy. *Clin Obstet Gynecol* 1999;42:2.
74. Warner M, Kelton JG. Laboratory investigation of immune thrombocytopenia. *J Clin Pathol* 1997;50:5.
75. Harrington W, Minnich V, Hollingsworth JW, et al. Demonstration of a thrombocytopenic factor in the blood of patients with thrombocytopenic purpura. *J Lab Clin Pathol* 1951;38:1.
76. Bussel JB, Zabusky MR, Berkowitz RL, et al. Maternal IVIG in neonatal alloimmune thrombocytopenia. *N Engl J Med* 1997; 337:22.
77. Moise KJ, Cotton DB. Discordant fetal platelet counts in a twin gestation complicated by idiopathic thrombocytopenic purpura. *Am J Obstet Gynecol* 1987;156:1141–1145.
78. Miller CH, Graham JB, Goldin LR, et al. Genetics of classic von Willebrand disease: phenotypic variation within families. *Blood* 1979;54:117.
79. Sadler JE. A revised classification of von Willebrand disease. *Thromb Haemost* 1994;71:520.
80. Lethagen S, Harris AS, Sjorin E, et al. Intranasal and intravenous administration of desmopressin: effect on factor VIII/vWF, pharmacokinetics and reproducibility. *Thromb Haemost* 1987;58: 1033.
81. Gill JC, Endres-Brooks J, Bauer PJ. The effect of ABO blood group on the diagnosis of von Willebrand disease. *Blood* 1987;69: 1691.
82. Faught W, Garner P, Johnes G, et al. Changes in protein C and protein S in normal pregnancy. *Am J Obstet Gynecol* 1995;172: 147.
83. Svensson PJ, Dahlback B. Resistance to activated protein C as a basis for venous thrombosis. *N Engl J Med* 1994;330:517.
84. Conard J, Horellou MH, Van Dreden P, et al. Thrombosis and pregnancy in congenital deficiencies of AT III, protein C or protein S: study of 78 women. *Thromb Haemost* 1990;63:319.
85. Den Heijer M, Brouwer IA, Bos, G, et al. Vitamin supplementation reduces blood homocysteine levels: a controlled trial in patients with venous thrombosis and healthy volunteers. *Arterioscler Thromb Vasc Biol* 1998;18:3.
86. Den Heijer M, Koster T, Blom H, et al. Hyperhomocysteinemia as a risk factor for deep-vein thrombosis. *N Engl J Med* 1996; 334:12.
87. Toglia MR, Weg JG. Venous thromboembolism during pregnancy. *N Engl J Med* 1996;335:108.
88. Gillis S, Shushan A, Eldor A. Use of low molecular weight heparin for prophylaxis and treatment of thromboembolism in pregnancy. *Int J Gynecol Obstet* 1992;39:297.
89. Hirsh J, Foster V. Guide to anticoagulant therapy. I. Heparin. *Circulation* 1994;89:1449.
90. Horlocker TT, Wedel DJ. Neuraxial block and low-molecular-weight heparin: balancing perioperative analgesia and thromboprophylaxis. *Reg Anesth Pain Med* 1998;23[Suppl 2]:6.
91. Horlocker TT, Wedel DJ. Spinal and epidural blockade and perioperative low molecular weight heparin: smooth sailing on the *Titanic*. *Anesth Analg* 1998;86:1153–1156.

METABOLISM OF MATERNAL FUELS IN PREGNANCY

E. ALBERT REECE
CAROL J. HOMKO

Alterations in maternal metabolism are necessary to meet the demands of the rapidly growing and developing fetus throughout pregnancy. Major changes in both energy expenditure and fat mass accumulation have been documented (1). Fat deposition occurs during the first half of pregnancy and reaches a plateau before the thirtieth week of gestation (2). It accounts for approximately 4.0 kg of the average 13 kg of weight gained during pregnancy (3,4). In contrast, only minor changes in the maternal basic metabolic rate are noted during early pregnancy. However, late pregnancy is characterized by dramatic changes in energy expenditure with increases of approximately 400 kcal higher than baseline in the metabolic rate (1,5).

In addition, late gestation has also been characterized by a progressive increase in insulin resistance (6–8). Longitudinal studies have shown that insulin-stimulated glucose disposal declines by approximately 50% in lean women (9) and by 40% in obese women (10) by the end of the third trimester of pregnancy. Increased maternal plasma levels of progesterone, human placental lactogen, free cortisol, and prolactin have all been implicated in this process. Human placental lactogen levels rise steadily during the first and second trimesters and then reach a plateau in the last 4 weeks of pregnancy. The diabetogenic effect of human placental lactogen results in the mobilization of lipids as free fatty acids (FFAs). These FFAs serve as a maternal energy source and thereby make glucose and amino acids available to the fetus (11,12). Cortisol levels also increase during pregnancy. Cortisol stimulates endogenous glucose production and glycogen storage and decreases glucose use, thereby reducing the effectiveness of insulin (13). Prolactin, which is increased 5- to 10-fold during late pregnancy, has a significant influence on insulin secretion by pancreatic islet cells, especially during late gestation (14). The administration of gestational hormones has been shown to increase insulin release and to produce elevated insulin-to-glucose ratios (15–17).

This chapter reviews alterations in carbohydrate, protein, and fat metabolism throughout normal gestation and describes how these processes differ in women with diabetes during pregnancy (Table 31.1). Investigations using quantitative measurements of gestational energy metabolism with stable, nonradioactive isotopes and clamp techniques are highlighted.

MATERNAL GLUCOSE HOMEOSTASIS IN THE FASTING STATE

During pregnancy, reductions in fasting blood glucose levels after an overnight fast have been reported. Lind and Aspillaga demonstrated that fasting glucose concentrations reach their nadir at about the twelfth week of gestation and remain at this level until delivery (18). Felig and Lynch reported decreases of 15 mg/dL in fasting glucose levels (19), whereas Metzger and colleagues reported reductions in fasting plasma glucose concentrations of approximately 10 mg/dL in pregnant as compared with nonpregnant women (20). Buchanan and colleagues reported a similar decline in women with gestational diabetes mellitus (GDM) during the third trimester of pregnancy (21). They observed an abrupt fall in endogenous glucose production after approximately 15 hours of fasting.

During late gestation, fasting insulin levels increase from 5 to 8 mU/L (22). However, little change is seen in fasting insulin levels during the first and second trimesters when the glucose values reach their nadir, thus precluding a cause and effect relationship. Kuhl and Holst also demonstrated that the insulin-to-glucagon ratio in pregnancy increases significantly as compared with that in the nonpregnant state (23).

RESPONSE TO GLUCOSE LOAD

Suppression of endogenous glucose production and acceleration of glucose utilization are normally seen after a carbohydrate-containing meal. In nonpregnant persons, plasma glucose load levels reach their peak 30 minutes after the ingestion of a glucose load and return to baseline in approximately 1 hour. However, during the third trimester of pregnancy, peak glucose levels are higher and are not reached until approximately 60 minutes after carbohydrate inges-

TABLE 31.1. FUEL METABOLISM AND ITS EFFECTS IN NORMAL AND DIABETIC PREGNANCIES

	Normal Pregnancy	Diabetic Pregnancy	Implications
Carbohydrate metabolism			
Fasted state	Glucose levels reduced by ~10–15 mg/dL as compared with nonpregnant state (18–20)	Fasting hyperglycemia secondary to relative or absolute deficiency of endogenous insulin (1,22,55)	Excess delivery of substrates to fetus cause of fetal hyperinsulinemia and adverse pregancy outcomes (i.e., macrosomia) (22,31,53,65)
Response to glucose load	Increased glucose utilization and reduced endogenous glucose production (1,5–7,22)	Reduced glucose utilization and increased endogenous glucose production (1,22,55)	Excess delivery of substrates to fetus cause of fetal hyperinsulinemia and adverse pregancy outcomes (i.e., macrosomia) (22,31,53,65)
Changes in insulin sensitivity	Peripheral insulin sensitivity decreased by ~40–50% during late gestation; hepatic insulin resistance also present (9,10,28,30,32,33)	Unchanged in type 1 diabetes; insulin resistance in gestational diabetes mellitus may be comparable or increased (9,21,33,60)	Inverse relationship between maternal insulin sensitivity and birth weight (74); insulin requirements increase two- to threefold during pregnancy (22)
Lipid metabolism	Accelerated lipolysis and ketogenesis (1,22,47)	Increased free fatty acids and triglyceride concentrations in diabetes as compared with nondiabetic pregnancies	Physiological adaptation to provide fatty acids to mother and spare carbohydrates for fetus (36,47); women with type 1 diabetes at increased risk for diabetic ketoacidosis (22)
Protein metabolism	Concentrations of most amino acids are reduced in maternal plasma (51)	Fasting and postprandial hyperaminoacidemia; normalization with good glucose control (55)	Correlation between maternal plasma amino acid profiles and birth weight (69)

tion. The decline to baseline is also slower, and fasting levels are not regained for about 2 hours (22,24,25).

Insulin response is also altered in pregnancy. Insulin levels reach their peak at about 1 hour after ingestion of a glucose load when glucose values are also peaking. Insulin levels decline slowly and are still not back to baseline at 2 hours. For any given glucose challenge, the pregnant woman is stimulated to produce additional insulin, but her blood glucose levels remain elevated for a longer period (22). This finding led to the concept of *insulin resistance* in pregnancy, which is believed to be mediated at the postreceptor level (26).

CHANGES IN INSULIN SENSITIVITY

Insulin resistance during pregnancy is a well-recognized phenomenon (27–29). Changes in insulin sensitivity during gestation have been examined by a variety of techniques, which include the calculation of insulin-to-glucose ratios (30), as well as minimal model analysis of intravenous glucose tolerance tests (31). These studies have universally demonstrated that the second half of pregnancy is associated with increasing insulin resistance (1,28,30,32). More recently, hyperinsulinemic-euglycemic clamping has been used to quantify the changes in insulin sensitivity.

Ryan and co-workers used this technique to compare insulin sensitivity between nonpregnant women and women in the third trimester of pregnancy with normal glucose tolerance (33). These investigators found a 33% decrease in insulin sensitivity in the pregnant women as compared with the nonpregnant controls. Catalano and colleagues assessed longitudinal changes in insulin sensitivity in lean glucose-tolerant women throughout gestation with the clamp technique (9). These investigators performed hyperinsulinemic-euglycemic clamp studies before conception, at 12 to 14 weeks' gestation, and at 34 to 36 weeks' gestation. They found a decrease of approximately 50% in peripheral insulin sensitivity from early to late gestation. In addition, they observed a 30% increase in basal hepatic glucose output despite elevated serum insulin levels, a finding indicating hepatic insulin resistance.

Sivan and co-workers performed similar studies in nondiabetic obese women during and after pregnancy (10). Six glucose-tolerant women were studied during the second and third trimesters of pregnancy and again 3 or more months post partum using the euglycemic-hyperinsulinemic clamp technique. These investigators found no significant changes with respect to the action of insulin on rates of glucose disappearance, carbohydrate oxidation, or endogenous glucose production when the second trimester of pregnancy was compared with the nonpregnant state. The third trimester, however, was characterized by reductions in insulin-stimulated glucose disposal and carbohydrate oxidation when compared with either the second trimester or postpartum state (Fig. 31.1). In addition, insulin suppression of endogenous glucose production was also significantly reduced. Glucose-tolerant obese women develop peripheral

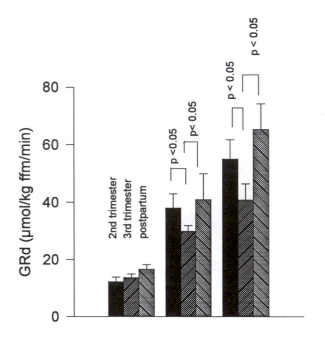

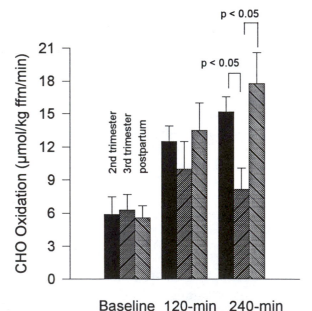

FIGURE 31.1. Rates of whole-body glucose disappearance (GRd) and carbohydrate oxidation (CHO) in six obese healthy women before (baseline) and after 120 and 240 minutes of euglycemic-hyperinsulinemic clamping during the second and third trimesters of pregnancy and postpartum. Shown are mean plus or minus standard error. Data are expressed per kilogram of fat-free mass (FFM). (From Sivan E, Chen XC, Homko CJ, et al. A longitudinal study of carbohydrate metabolism in healthy, obese pregnant women. *Diabetes Care* 1997;20:1470–1475, with permission of the American Diabetes Association.)

insulin resistance and hepatic insulin resistance during late gestation, conditions that are reversed after delivery. These alterations appear to be an adaptive mechanism to cope with the increased demand for glucose of the growing fetus. The development of peripheral and hepatic insulin resistance after midpregnancy can be seen as an effort by obese women to adapt to the fuel needs of the rapidly growing fetus. During the third trimester of pregnancy, glucose uptake by the fetus has been estimated to be 33 μmol/kg/min (34). To satisfy this additional need, obese women have sharply increased peripheral insulin resistance, thus reducing maternal glucose utilization. They also have increased hepatic insulin resistance, which probably results in the increased production of glucose. By decreasing terminal carbohydrate oxidation, these women shunt much of the glucose entering muscle into either glycogen or into lactate and thus make it available to be recycled into glucose through the Cori cycle (35).

Whereas resistance to the action of insulin on glucose transport has been established (9,10,33), information on the action of insulin on lipid metabolism during pregnancy is limited. Sivan and colleagues examined the effects of physiologic hyperinsulinemia on release, oxidation, and reesterification of FFAs throughout pregnancy and during the postpartum period (36). Seven healthy, glucose-tolerant, overweight pregnant women were studied during the second and third trimesters of pregnancy and again in the postpartum period. Four-hour euglycemic-hyperinsulinemic clamps were performed in combination with infusion of stable isotopes (^{2}H$_5$-glycerol) for measurement of rates of lipolysis and indirect calorimetry for estimation of rates of fatty acid oxidation.

Basal rates of FFA release, oxidation, and reesterification were similar during the second and third trimesters of pregnancy and during the postpartum period (Fig. 31.2). However, in response to the same degree of hyperinsulinemia, the rate of lipolysis declined by 51% (from 8.4 ± 0.6 to 4.1 ± 0.9 μmol/kg/min) in the second trimester; by 30% (from 7.0 ± 0.9 to 4.9 ± 0.9 μmol/kg/min) in the third trimester and by 51% (from 8.5 ± 1.1 to 4.2 ± 0.6 μmol/kg/min) in the postpartum period (36). Fat oxidation was not inhibited at all (from 3.5 ± 0.3 to 3.6 ± 0.5 μmol/kg/min) during the third trimester but was suppressed by 51% during the second trimester and by 38% post partum (36).

Thus, the inhibitory effect of insulin on the rate of lipolysis was significantly reduced during the third trimester of pregnancy as compared with either the second trimester or post partum (36). Hence, there was resistance during late gestation with regard to the effect of insulin on lipid and carbohydrate turnover (10). This increase in insulin resistance parallels the increases in blood levels of human placental lactogen and several other hormones found in late gestation. The parallel development of insulin resistance and increases in blood levels of human placental lactogen and placental growth hormone, both of which have strong

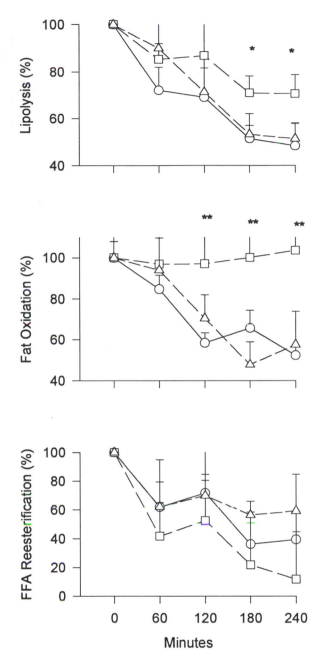

FIGURE 31.2. Changes in rates of lipolysis, fat oxidation, and free fatty acid reesterification before and during 4 hours of euglycemic-hyperinsulinemic clamping during the second (*circles*) and third (*squares*) trimesters of pregnancy and postpartum (*triangles*) in healthy women (*$p < .05$, **$p < .01$ comparing postpartum with second and third trimesters). (From Sivan E, Homko CJ, Chen X, et al. The effect of insulin on fat metabolism during and after normal pregnancy. *Diabetes* 1999;48:834–838, with permission of the American Diabetes Association.)

lipolytic and antiinsulin actions (37–40), suggests that these and perhaps other diabetogenic hormones, including cortisol, progesterone, and estrogens, may be responsible for much of the observed insulin resistance (41–45). Furthermore, although hyperinsulinemia lowered plasma FFA levels during the third trimester by 53%, fat oxidation did not decrease. The unchanged rate of fat oxidation at lower

plasma FFA concentrations indicated an increase in fractional oxidation of FFA. This could be caused by a fall in intracellular malonyl coenzyme A concentrations as a result of impaired stimulation of acetyl coenzyme A carboxylase by insulin, in addition to decreased glucose uptake during late gestation (9,10,35). Malonyl coenzyme A is known to control FFA oxidation by inhibiting carnitine palmitoyl transferase 1, the rate-limiting enzyme for transport of FFA across mitochondrial membranes (46).

In summary, these data provide further support for the concept of accelerated starvation in late gestation, that is, an earlier-than-normal switch from carbohydrate to fat utilization. The excess release of FFA is likely to contribute to the development of peripheral insulin resistance and to decreased maternal glucose utilization, thus promoting the use of lipids as a maternal energy source while preserving carbohydrates for the fetus.

LIPID METABOLISM

Accelerated fat metabolism and ketone body formation are well documented in pregnancy, particularly after long periods of starvation. The reduction in circulating glucose concentrations and acceleration of lipolysis and ketogenesis were labeled "accelerated starvation" by Freinkel (47).

All three lipoprotein fractions—very low-density lipoproteins, low-density lipoproteins, and high-density lipoproteins—increase during normal pregnancy. Very low-density lipoprotein cholesterol increases slowly, whereas low-density lipoprotein increases rapidly throughout pregnancy. High-density lipoprotein concentrations reach their peak during the second trimester and then decline near term. Although the rise in low-density lipoprotein cholesterol can be blunted by a low-cholesterol diet, it cannot be eliminated, a finding indicating a possible tendency to increased efficiency of cholesterol absorption during pregnancy (18,22,48). Triglyceride concentrations decrease during early gestation, but they steadily increase from the eighth week onward and reach concentrations of 2 to 3 mg/dL by term (49). Levels of total phospholipids increase from approximately 2.0 to 2.5 mg/dL during gestation. The fatty acid composition of the phospholipids may also change, with an increase in palmitic and oleic acids and a decrease in linoleic and arachidonic acids (1,18).

Investigators have postulated that the increased plasma concentrations of FFAs may be at least partially responsible for the development of insulin resistance during late gestation. Sivan and colleagues performed euglycemic-hyperinsulinemic clamp studies in seven glucose-tolerant women during the early second trimester of pregnancy to test this hypothesis (50). On consecutive days, women received either lipid and heparin or saline-glycerol infusions. Rates of total body glucose disposal and of carbohydrate and fat oxidation were determined using indirect calorimetry. The lipid-heparin insulin was found to inhibit insulin-stimulated

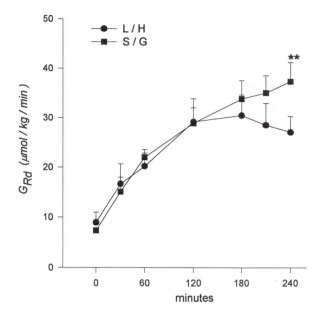

FIGURE 31.3. Glucose disappearance during euglycemic-hyperinsulinemic clamping with lipid/heparin (L/H) or saline/glycerol (S/G) infusions ($p < .01$, comparing L/H with S/G). (From Sivan E, Homko CJ, Whittaker PG, et al. Free fatty acids and insulin resistance during pregnancy. *J Clin Endocrinol Metab* 1998;83:2338–2342, with permission of the American Endocrine Society.)

total body glucose disposal by 28% as compared with the saline-glycerol insulin (Fig. 31.3). Furthermore, the lipid infusion was found to increase fat oxidation and decrease carbohydrate oxidation (Fig. 31.4). Endogenous glucose production was decreased equally. These data demonstrate that elevating plasma FFA levels during early pregnancy inhibit total body glucose uptake and oxidation. The elevation in plasma FFA observed during late pregnancy appears to contribute to the peripheral insulin resistance seen in late gestation (35). The development of insulin resistance during late pregnancy is a normal physiologic adaptation that shifts maternal energy metabolism from carbohydrate to lipid oxidation and thus spares glucose for the growing fetus.

PROTEIN METABOLISM

Information concerning *protein metabolism* during gestation is limited. It is generally believed that the concentrations of most amino acids are lower in maternal plasma during pregnancy than in the postpartum period. Young reported decreases in the plasma level of total α-amino nitrogen from 3.0 mmol in the nonpregnant state to 2.3 mmol during pregnancy (51). Additional data from animal experiments have shown that the gluconeogenic amino acids (alanine, serine, glutamine, and glutamates) are decreased during fasting in the pregnant state (26,44,52).

METABOLISM DURING DIABETIC PREGNANCY

Diabetes mellitus is a metabolic syndrome of diverse causes, characterized by abnormalities of glucose, fat, and protein metabolism. These alterations in fuel metabolism result from either a relative or an absolute deficiency of insulin leading to fasting and postprandial hyperaminoacidemia, hyperlipidemia, and hyperglycemia. These effects are further escalated in pregnancy by the placental hormones, which are known to be insulin antagonists (22). The resulting excessive delivery of substrates to the fetus leads to fetal hyperinsulinemia, which contributes to the adverse preg-

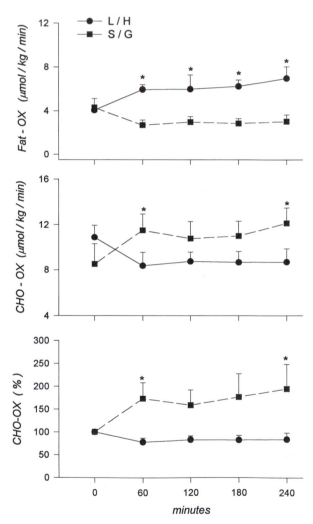

FIGURE 31.4. Rates of fat (*top*) and carbohydrate (CHO) (*middle*) oxidation during euglycemic-hyperinsulinemic clamping with lipid/heparin (L/H) or saline/glycerol (S/G) infusions. In the *bottom panel*, CHO oxidation was normalized by setting baseline values (0 minutes) at 100% ($p < .05$, comparing L/H with S/G). (From Lind T, Billewicz W, Brown G. A serial study of changes occurring in the oral glucose tolerance test during pregnancy. *J Obstet Gynaecol Br Commonw* 1973;80:1033–1039, with permission.)

nancy outcomes associated with poorly controlled diabetes (53,54).

Reece and colleagues conducted metabolic studies in 7 healthy control subjects and in 15 pregnant women with type 1 diabetes who were treated with intensive insulin regimens, either multiple daily insulin injections or continuous subcutaneous insulin infusion pumping (55). Both groups of women were able to achieve near-normal glycemic control. However, despite euglycemia, their plasma insulin profiles differed substantially from those observed in nondiabetic pregnant women. The patients with diabetes demonstrated a delayed and markedly prolonged rise in plasma insulin levels when compared with nondiabetic women. As a result, the integrated insulin area was significantly increased in women with diabetes in contrast to those who did not have diabetes.

Insulin, alanine, branched-chain amino acids, triglycerides, FFAs, and ketones were measured every 15 to 30 minutes before a standardized breakfast and for 150 minutes after the meal. Women with diabetes were studied on their usual insulin dosages. The meal studies were performed each trimester: between 10 and 12 weeks' gestation, between 26 and 28 weeks' gestation, and again between 34 and 36 weeks' gestation.

Most of the women with diabetes had the disease well controlled, with glycosylated hemoglobin levels close to or within the range of normal. Nondiabetic women reached plasma insulin concentrations between 60 and 75 U/mL 30 minutes after a meal, and they returned to baseline levels by 150 minutes. However, in women with diabetes, insulin levels rose gradually after their premeal insulin bolus and remained higher than the basal level for more than 150 minutes (55).

Despite differences in plasma insulin levels, the basal and postprandial levels and the branched-chain amino acids were similar in women with insulin-dependent diabetes mellitus and in nondiabetic women during each trimester. Fasting concentrations of cholesterol and triglycerides were also measured in both groups. Cholesterol and triglyceride levels rose significantly, but no significant difference was noted between the two groups for either of these lipid fractions. Fasting ketone levels did not differ between the groups or from baseline values within each group during pregnancy.

In summary, although type 1 diabetes is associated with maternal hyperinsulinemia, intensive insulin therapy results in near-normal glucose levels while not completely suppressing other insulin-sensitive metabolites. The infants in this study were free of the complications (i.e., macrosomia) that commonly result from poor metabolic control during pregnancy. These data support the hypothesis that improved metabolic control and the resulting normalization of amino acid, lipid, and glucose metabolism may play a role in the improved perinatal outcomes seen with intensive insulin therapy.

CARBOHYDRATE METABOLISM UNDER HYPOGLYCEMIC CONDITIONS

An increased frequency of severe *hypoglycemic episodes* has been reported among pregnant as compared with nonpregnant women with type 1 diabetes who follow both intensive and conventional insulin treatment regimens. Studies in nonpregnant patients with diabetes suggest that intensive insulin therapy is associated with a suppression of counterregulatory responses to hypoglycemia that appear to result from a lowering of the plasma glucose level that triggers these responses.

Diamond et al. and Reece and co-workers evaluated maternal and fetal responses to hypoglycemia (56,57). Ten intensively treated pregnant women with insulin-dependent diabetes were studied during an insulin-induced gradual, controlled fall in plasma glucose levels (51). Plasma glucose levels were lowered from a mean of about 100 mg/dL in 10 mg/dL decrements every 40 minutes until symptoms appeared or a level of 45 mg/dL was reached. In contrast to nonpregnant control women, reductions in glucose to 44 ± 2 mg/dL in pregnant diabetic patients failed to elicit an increase in glucagon levels. Epinephrine release during hypoglycemia was also markedly suppressed in pregnant women with diabetes (106 ± 32 versus 327 ± 52 mg/dL in controls; $p < .01$). Furthermore, the plasma glucose level at which epinephrine and growth hormone were released was 5 to 10 mg/dL lower in the pregnant diabetic women ($p < 0.05$) (Fig. 31.5). The basal fetal heart rate remained unchanged and continued to manifest accelerations during the hypoglycemic state (57).

In summary, these data clearly demonstrate that the counterregulatory hormone response to hypoglycemia is impaired in pregnant women with type 1 diabetes. Thus, intensive metabolic regulation of such patients is associated with frequent hypoglycemic episodes not only because of the effect of insulin itself, but also because of derangement of compensatory hormonal secretion.

CARBOHYDRATE METABOLISM IN GESTATIONAL DIABETES MELLITUS

Gestational diabetes mellitus (GDM) is defined as *carbohydrate intolerance* of variable severity with onset or first recognition during pregnancy (58). This definition applies whether or not the diabetes remains after delivery and whether or not insulin therapy is required for management (Table 31.2). Occasionally, therefore, GDM can include women with preexisting type 1 and type 2 diabetes. Typically, however, GDM develops during the second half of pregnancy and parallels the development of insulin resistance. Nevertheless, insulin resistance alone cannot be the sole cause of GDM because all women become insulin resistant during late gestation but only approximately 5%

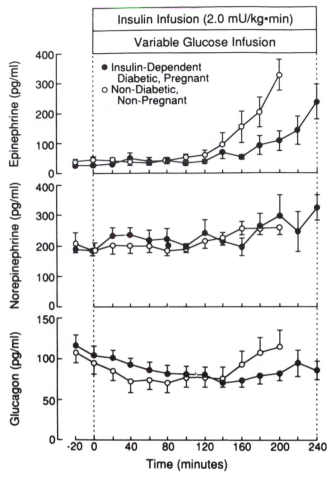

FIGURE 31.5. Epinpehrine, norepinephrine, and glucagon responses to hypoglycemia in pregnant, intensively treated insulin-dependent diabetic women, and nonpregnant, nondiabetic control women. (From Diamond MP, Reece EA, Caprio S, et al. Impairment of counterregulatory hormone responses to hypoglycemia in pregnant women with insulin-dependent diabetes mellitus. *Am J Obstet Gynecol* 1992;166:74, with permission.)

develop GDM (59). This finding suggests that women destined to develop GDM may also have a defect in insulin secretion or action.

Insulin resistance in GDM has been reported to be either comparable to or increased as compared with glucose-tolerant pregnant control subjects. For instance, Buchanan and colleagues reported similar degrees of peripheral insulin resistance in women with GDM and nondiabetic control subjects in the third trimester of pregnancy (21). In contrast, Ryan and co-workers found 40% more insulin resistance during the second trimester in women with GDM than in nondiabetic women in the third trimester of pregnancy (33); and Catalano and colleagues reported a decrease in insulin-stimulated glucose uptake in late gestation in GDM compared with nondiabetic women (9,60).

Other investigators have shown that women with GDM exhibit impaired pancreatic β-cell function. Kuhl and colleagues found that women with GDM exhibit an increased

insulin response to oral glucose and amino acids during pregnancy as compared with the postpartum period (61). In addition, the fasting insulin-to-glucagon ratio was increased in both normal pregnancies and those in women with GDM. These investigators also found an enhanced glucagon response to amino acid ingestion in pregnant women with GDM as compared with nondiabetic women, but oral triglycerides did not affect glucagon secretion. Buchanan and co-workers reported that first-phase insulin secretion in response to intravenous glucose was significantly decreased in women with GDM during the third trimester of pregnancy compared with nondiabetic women (21). Kuhl also reported that insulin responses to oral and intravenous glucose and to mixed meals were delayed and reduced during late pregnancy in GDM compared with nondiabetic pregnant women (32). Catalano and colleagues, however, found no differences in insulin concentrations in response to an oral glucose load in a comparison of patients with GDM and nondiabetic pregnant women (9,60). Kautzky-Willer and colleagues evaluated β-cell secretion and glucose metabolism in lean women with GDM using kinetic analysis of glucose, insulin, and C-peptide plasma concentrations during oral and intravenous glucose tolerance tests (62). These investigators found that lean women with GDM had inadequate insulin secretion that persisted after delivery. Moreover, Bowes and co-workers (63), using a minimal model analysis, reported that overweight women with GDM had an impaired ability to increase insulin secretion in response to glucose.

Homko and co-workers recently assessed insulin secretion, clearance, and action during and after pregnancy in both healthy pregnant women and women with GDM (64). Insulin secretion rates were determined with individual kinetic C-peptide parameters and deconvolution analysis of plasma C-peptide concentrations. The glucose clamp technique was used to ensure comparable hyperglycemic conditions (160 mg/dL) among all subjects in the study.

Eight healthy obese pregnant, glucose-tolerant women and seven women with GDM were studied during the third trimester of pregnancy and again 3 months post partum. Basal insulin secretion rates were significantly increased to more than the postpartum state during pregnancy in both patients with GDM and nondiabetic control subjects. However, during hyperglycemic clamping in late gestation, women with GDM had lower insulin secretion rates than healthy controls (720.5 ± 25.6 versus 839 ± 24.2 pmol/min; $p < .05$). The difference disappeared in the postpartum period, when insulin secretion rates were comparable between the women with GDM and the nondiabetic control subjects (373 ± 70 versus 356 ± 53 pmol/kg/min). In summary, these investigators found that during late pregnancy, women with GDM had normal basal but impaired glucose-stimulated insulin secretion, which normalized in the postpartum period. These data support the concept that

TABLE 31.2. DETECTION OF GESTATIONAL DIABETES

Screening
- Universal screening: all pregnant women.
- Alternative approach: selective screening: all pregnant women meeting one or more of the following criteria should be screened for diabetes:
  - ≥25 years of age
  - <25 years of age and obese (i.e., ≥20% over desired body weight of body mass index ≥27 kg/m²)
  - Family history of diabetes in a first-degree relative
  - Member of an ethnic/racial group with a high prevalence of diabetes (e.g., Hispanic American, Native American, Asian American, African American, or Pacific Islander)
- Screening should be performed between 24 and 28 weeks' gestation. However, women with risk factors may benefit from earlier screening.
- A 50-g oral glucose load is administered without regard to time of day or prandial state; a venous plasma glucose level is measured 1 hour later. A value of ≥140 mg/dL indicates need for 3-hour oral glucose tolerance test. However, to increase the sensitivity of the test, a cutoff of 130 mg/dL is utilized at many centers.

Diagnosis
- 100 g oral glucose load is administered in morning after an overnight fast of 8 to 14 hours and at least 3 days of an unrestricted diet (≥150 g carbohydrate and physical activity)
- Venous plasma glucose is measured fasting and at 1, 2, and 3 hours. Women should remain seated and not smoke throughout the test.
- Two or more of the venous plasma concentrations outlined below must be met or exceed for a positive diagnosis. These plasma values represent two theoretic conversions of O'Sullivan's original thresholds in whole blood. Both sets of conversions are currently utilized.

	NDDG Conversion	Carpenter/Coustan Conversion
Fasting	105 mg/dL	95 mg/dL
1 hr	190 mg/dL	180 mg/dL
2 hr	165 mg/dL	155 mg/dL
3 hr	145 mg/dL	140 mg/dL

- Women who meet or exceed only one value on the oral glucose tolerance test are at increased risk for fetal macrosomia and are treated at many centers

Alternative approach (to the two-step approach outlined above):
- One-step approach utilizing a 75-g, 2-hr oral glucose tolerance test

Fasting blood sugar	95 mg/dL
1 hr	180 mg/dL
2 hr	155 mg/dL

Based on recommendations of the American Diabetes Association, the Diabetes in Pregnancy Study Group of North America and the American College of Obstetricians and Gynecologists. ACOG Technical Bulletin No. 200. *Diabetes and pregnancy.* Washington, DC: ACOG, 1994; American Diabetes Association. Gestational diabetes mellitus. *Diabetes Care* 1999;22[Suppl 1]:S74–76; Metzger BE, Coustan DR. Summary and recommendations of the fourth international workshop-conference of gestational diabetes mellitus. *Diabetes Care* 1998;21[Suppl 2]:B161–B167; Gabbe SG. Unresolved issues in screening and diagnosis of gestational diabetes mellitus. *Prenat Neonat Med* 1998;3:523–525, with permission.

GDM is the result of both increased insulin resistance and reduced insulin secretory capacity (35).

Effect of Metabolism on Fetal Growth

The consequence of the metabolic abnormalities in the pregnancy complicated by diabetes is an increase in perinatal complications. Of major concern is excessive *fetal growth,* which augments the risk of birth trauma and maternal morbidity from operative delivery by facilitated diffusion. *Macrosomia* is defined as excessive birth weight (greater than 90%) for gestational age or as a birth weight of more than 4,000 g. Increased adiposity is the primary cause of the increased birth weight seen in the children of diabetic women. The infants tend to have almost twice as much body fat as infants of nondiabetic mothers, and their fat cells are increased both in size and number. Organomegaly is also present, as well as considerable disproportionality between head and shoulder size (65–67). Genetic factors are the major contributors controlling fetal growth during the first half of gestation, whereas other factors become more influential during the last trimester. These include nutritional, hormonal, metabolic, and environmental factors. In the case of the pregnancy complicated by diabetes, the fetus is most susceptible to alterations in fetal growth during the third trimester. Numerous studies have established a relationship between the level of maternal glucose control and macrosomia (65–67). The hyperglycemia-hyperinsulinemia hypothesis of Pederson has traditionally been used to explain macrosomia in pregnancies complicated by diabetes (53). In poorly controlled diabetes, hyperglycemia characteristically exists because of relative hypoinsulinemia. Glucose crosses the placenta by facilitated diffusion. In hyperglycemia, the carbohydrate surplus available to the fetus leads to increased insulin secretion and fetal hyperinsulinemia. Because insulin serves as the growth factor of the fetus, macrosomia develops (53).

Fetal macrosomia, however, can occur even with the achievement of maternal euglycemia. Menon et al. examined the hypothesis that macrosomia may be caused by insulin transferred to the fetus from the mother as an insulin-antibody complex (68). These investigators found the concentration of insulin antibody present in the umbilical cord serum to correlate with the maternal concentration of antiinsulin antibody. Human insulin and total insulin concentrations were higher in the cord serum of infants with macrosomia than in those without, and total insulin concentrations correlated with the degree of macrosomia. These investigators concluded that the formation of antibody to insulin in the mother is a determinant of fetal outcome independent of maternal blood glucose levels.

Kalkhoff et al. studied the relationship between maternal plasma amino acid and birth weight in infants of both diabetic and nondiabetic mothers (69). These investigators found no relationship between blood glucose control and plasma amino acid profiles. However, total plasma amino acids and six individual amino acids did correlate with neonatal birth weight. This finding supports the hypothesis that substrates other than glucose and other than those regulated by insulin also influence fetal weight. Furthermore, normalization of amino acid and lipid metabolism may influence the improved perinatal outcomes observed with stringent glycemic control.

Still other investigators have examined the role of circulating insulin-like growth factor I (IGF-I) in fetal growth. Whittaker and colleagues investigated maternal serum IGF-I levels throughout pregnancy in healthy women and those with insulin-dependent diabetes (70). The women with diabetes had significantly lower serum IGF-I concentrations than the healthy women. These investigators concluded that the physiologic changes in maternal serum IGF-I in diabetic women do not appear to be related to fetal macrosomia. In contrast, Reece and colleagues and Wiznitzer and colleagues found a direct correlation, in normal pregnancy, between neonatal levels of IGF-I and neonatal birth weight among infants appropriate for gestational age (71,72). Furthermore, that same group found a positive relationship between neonatal serum levels of IGF binding protein 3 and IGF-I and macrosomia in nondiabetic children.

Leptin concentrations have also been examined as a regulator of fetal growth. Sivan and colleagues measured plasma leptin concentrations in umbilical cord blood of 114 newborn infants (73). They found that leptin was present in all infants in concentrations comparable to those found in adults. Moreover, plasma leptin concentrations in cord blood of infants correlated with birth weight, with the strongest association in larger infants. This finding is not surprising because leptin levels have been shown to correlate closely with adiposity, and increased adiposity is characteristic of macrosomia.

Most recently, investigators have undertaken studies to examine the effect of maternal carbohydrate metabolism on fetal body composition. Catalano and associates demonstrated an inverse relationship between birth weight and maternal insulin sensitivity in both healthy control subjects and women with GDM (74). From their data, it appears that maternal insulin sensitivity is crucial for regulation of nutrient availability for the fetus. However, the exact mechanisms by which alterations in maternal nutrient metabolism affect fetal growth are unknown.

In summary, therefore, fetal growth is considered to be the result of an interaction between the genetic drive to grow and constraints provided by limitations on substrate availability or maternal metabolism. Macrosomia probably results in facilitated anabolism leading to cell hypertrophy. The regulation of fetal growth remains poorly understood, and further research is needed.

SUMMARY

In conclusion, alterations in maternal metabolism are necessary to meet the demands of the rapidly growing and developing fetus. These changes, which include fasting hypoglycemia, accelerated fat catabolism, and progressive insulin resistance, are to a large extent mediated by the placental hormones. The development of insulin resistance during late gestation is a normal physiologic adaptation that shifts maternal energy metabolism from carbohydrate to lipid oxidation and thus spares glucose for the growing fetus. In women with diabetes, pregnancy makes control of blood glucose concentrations more difficult, and the consequence of the ensuing metabolism abnormalities is an increase in perinatal complications.

10 KEY POINTS

1. Major changes occur in both energy expenditure and fat mass accumulation throughout gestation. Fat deposition occurs during the first half of pregnancy, whereas late pregnancy is characterized by an increased metabolic rate.

2. During pregnancy, plasma blood glucose concentrations are reduced after an overnight fast.

3. Accelerated fat metabolism and ketone body forma-

tion are well documented in pregnancy after long periods of starvation. In addition, the inhibitory effect of insulin on lipolysis is significantly reduced during the third trimester of pregnancy as compared with either the second trimester or the postpartum period.

4. Information concerning protein metabolism is limited, but the concentrations of most amino acids in maternal plasma are reduced.

5. Late pregnancy is characterized by a progressive increase in insulin resistance. Studies have demonstrated that insulin-stimulated glucose disposal declines by approximately 40% to 50% by the third trimester of pregnancy. This increase in insulin resistance parallels increases in blood levels of human placental lactogen and other placental hormones.

6. The development of insulin resistance during late pregnancy is a normal physiologic adaptation that shifts maternal energy metabolism from carbohydrate to lipid oxidation and thus spares glucose for the growing fetus.

7. In women with type 1 diabetes, improved metabolic control and the resulting normalization of energy metabolism may play a role in the improved perinatal outcomes seen with intensive insulin therapy.

8. The counterregulatory hormone response to hypoglycemia is impaired in pregnant women with type 1 diabetes.

9. Women with GDM have impaired pancreatic β-cell function. However, insulin resistance in GDM has been reported to be either comparable to or increased as compared with glucose-tolerant pregnant controls.

10. Fetal growth is a result of the interactions among the genetic drive to grow, the activity of *in utero* growth promoters, and constraints provided by limitations on substrate availability or maternal metabolism.

REFERENCES

1. Boden G. Fuel metabolism in pregnancy and in gestational diabetes mellitus. *Obstet Gynecol Clin North Am* 1996;23:1–10.
2. Taggart NR, Holliday RM, Billewicz WZ, et al. Changes in skinfolds during pregnancy. *Br J Nutr* 1967;21:439–451.
3. Hytten FE, Chamberlain GVP. *Clinical physiology in obstetrics.* Oxford: Blackwell, 1980.
4. Hytten FE, Leitch I. Components of weight gain: changes in the maternal body. In: *The physiology of human pregnancy,* 2nd ed. Oxford: Blackwell, 1971:333–369.
5. Durnin JVGA. Energy requirements of pregnancy. *Diabetes* 1991; 40[Suppl 2]:152–156.
6. Fischer PM, Hamilton PM, Sutherland HW, et al. The effect of gestation on intravenous glucose tolerance in women. *J Obstet Gynaecol Br Commonw* 1974;81:285.
7. Lind T, Billewicz WZ, Brown G. A serial study of changes occurring in the oral glucose tolerance test during pregnancy. *J Obstet Gynaecol Br Commonw* 1973;80:1033.
8. Marliss EB, Nakhood A, Hanna AK. Insulin glucagon and amino acid profiles during glycemic control by closed-loop artificial pancreas. *Diabetes* 1979;28:377.
9. Catalano PM, Tyzbir ED, Roman NM, et al. Longitudinal changes in insulin release and insulin resistance in non-obese pregnant women. *Am J Obstet Gynecol* 1991:165;1667.
10. Sivan E, Chen XC, Homko CJ, et al. A longitudinal study of carbohydrate metabolism in healthy, obese pregnant women. *Diabetes Care* 1997;20:1470–1475.
11. Knopp RH, Saudek CD, Arky RA, et al. Two phases of adipose tissue metabolism in pregnancy: maternal adaptations for fetal growth. *Endocrinology* 1973;92:984.
12. Samaan N, Yen SCC, Gonzalez D, et al. Metabolic effects of placental lactogen (HPL) in man. *J Clin Endocrinol Metab* 1968; 28:485.
13. Burke CW, Roulet F. Increased exposure of tissues to cortisol in late pregnancy. *BMJ* 1970;1:657.
14. Gustafson AB, Banasiak MF, Kalkhoff RK, et al. Correlation of hyperprolactinemia with altered plasma insulin and glucagon: similarity to effects of late human pregnancy. *J Clin Endocrinol Metab* 1980;51:242.
15. Costrini NV, Kalkhoff RK. Relative effects of pregnancy, estradiol, and progesterone on plasma insulin and pancreatic islet insulin secretion. *J Clin Invest* 1971;50:992–997.
16. Burke CW, Roulet F. Increased exposure of tissues to cortisol in late pregnancy. *BMJ* 1970;1:657–659.
17. Rushakoff RJ, Kalkhoff RK. Effects of pregnancy and sex steroid administration on skeletal muscle metabolism in the rat. *Diabetes* 1981;30:545–550.
18. Lind T, Aspillaga M. Metabolic changes during normal and diabetic pregnancies. In: Reece EA, Coustan DR, eds. *Diabetes mellitus in pregnancy: principles and practice.* New York: Churchill Livingstone, 1988.
19. Felig P, Lynch V. Starvation in human pregnancy: hypoglycemia, hypoinsulinemia, and hyperketonemia. *Science* 1970;170:990.
20. Metzger BE, Ravnikar V, Vileisis R, et al. "Accelerated starvation" and the skipped breakfast in late normal pregnancy. *Lancet* 1982;1:588–592.
21. Buchanan TA, Metzger BE, Freinkel N, et al. Insulin sensitivity and β-cell responsiveness to glucose during late pregnancy in lean and moderately obese women with normal glucose tolerance or mild gestational diabetes. *Am J Obstet Gynecol* 1990;162: 1008–1014.
22. Reece EA, Homko C, Wiznitzer A. Metabolic changes in diabetic and nondiabetic subjects during pregnancy. *Obstet Gynecol Surv* 1994;49:64–71.
23. Kuhl C, Holst JJ. Plasma glucagon and insulin: glucagon ratio in gestational diabetes. *Diabetes* 1976;25:16.
24. Cousins L, Rigg L, Hollingsworth D, et al. The 24-hour excursion an diurnal rhythm of glucose, insulin and C-peptide in normal pregnancy. *Am J Obstet Gynecol* 1980;136:483–488.
25. Lind T. Changes in carbohydrate metabolism during pregnancy. *Clin Obstet Gynecol* 1975;2:395.
26. Metzger BE, Hare JW, Freinkel N. Carbohydrate metabolism in pregnancy. IX. Plasma levels of gluconeogenic fuels during fasting in the rat. *J Clin Endocrinol Metab* 1971;33:869.
27. Bleicher SJ, O'Sullivan JB, Freinkel N. Carbohydrate metabolism in pregnancy. *N Engl J Med* 1964;271:866–872.
28. Lind T, Billewicz W, Brown G. A serial study of changes occurring in the oral glucose tolerance test during pregnancy. *J Obstet Gynaecol Br Commonw* 1973;80:1033–1039.
29. Cousins L, Rigg L, Hollingsworth D, et al. The 24-hour excursions and diurnal rhythm of glucose insulin and C-peptide in normal pregnancy. *Am J Obstet Gynecol* 1980;136:483–488.
30. Spellacy W, Goetz F. Plasma insulin in normal late pregnancy. *N Engl J Med* 1963;268:988–999.
31. Hollingsworth DR. Maternal metabolism in normal pregnancy and pregnancy complicated by diabetes mellitus. *Clin Obstet Gynecol* 1985;28:457–472.

32. Kuhl C. Insulin secretion and insulin resistance in pregnancy and GDM. *Diabetes* 1991;40[Suppl 2]:18–24.

33. Ryan EA, O'Sullivan MJ, Skyler JS. Insulin action during pregnancy: studies with the euglycemic clamp technique. *Diabetes* 1985;34:380–389.

34. Crenshaw C Jr. Fetal glucose metabolism. *Clin Obstet Gynecol* 1970;13:579–585.

35. Homko CJ, Sivan E, Reece EA, et al. Fuel metabolism during pregnancy. *Semin Reprod Endocrinol* 1999;17:119–125.

36. Sivan E, Homko CJ, Chen X, et al. The effect of insulin on fat metabolism during and after normal pregnancy. *Diabetes* 1999;48:834–838.

37. Beck P, Daughaday WH. Human placental lactogen: studies of its acute metabolic effects and disposition in normal man. *J Clin Invest* 1967;46:103–110.

38. Turtle JR, Kipnis DM. The lipolytic action of human placental lactogen in isolated fat cells. *Biochim Biophys Acta* 1967;144:583–593.

39. Fielder PJ, Talamantes F. The lipolytic effects of mouse placental lactogen II, mouse prolactin and mouse growth hormone on adipose tissue from virgin and pregnant mice. *Endocrinology* 1967;121:493–497.

40. Frankenne F, Scippo ML, Van Beeumen J, et al. Identification of placental human growth hormone as the growth hormone-V gene expression production. *J Clin Endocrinol Metab* 1990;71:15–18.

41. Burke CW, Roulet F. Increased exposure of tissues to cortisol in late pregnancy. *BMJ* 1970;1:657–659.

42. Costrini NV, Kalkhoff RK. Relative effects of pregnancy, estradiol, and progesterone on plasma insulin and pancreatic islet insulin secretion. *J Clin Invest* 1971;50:992–997.

43. Kalkhoff RK, Richardson BL, Beck P. Relative effects of pregnancy, human placental lactogen and prednisolone on carbohydrate tolerance in normal and subclinical diabetic subjects. *Diabetes* 1969;18:153–163.

44. Rushakoff RJ, Kalkhoff RK. Effects of pregnancy and sex steroid administration of skeletal muscle metabolism in the rat. *Diabetes* 1981;30:545–550.

45. Shamoon H, Felig P. Effects of estrogen on glucose uptake by rat muscle. *Yale J Biol Med* 1974;47:227–233.

46. Declercq PE, Falck JR, Kuwajima M, et al. Characterization of the mitochondrial carnitine plamitoyltransferase enzyme system. I. Use of Inhibitors. *J Biol Chem* 1987;262:9812–9821.

47. Freinkel N. 1980 Banting lecture: of pregnancy and progeny. *Diabetes* 1980;29:1023–1035.

48. McMurry MP, Connor WE, Goplerud CP. The effects of dietary cholesterol upon the hypercholesterolemia of pregnancy. *Metabolism* 1981;30:869.

49. Darmady JM, Postle AD. Lipid metabolism in pregnancy. *Br J Obstet Gynaecol* 1982;89:211.

50. Sivan E, Homko CJ, Whittaker PG, et al. Free fatty acids and insulin resistance during pregnancy. *J Clin Endocrinol Metab* 1998;83:2338–2342.

51. Young M. The accumulation of protein by the fetus. In: Beard RW, Nathanielsz PW, eds. *Fetal physiology and medicine.* Philadelphia: WB Saunders, 1976:59.

52. Metzger BE, Freinkel N. Regulation of maternal protein metabolism and gluconeogenesis in the fasted state. In: Camerini-Davalos RA, Cole HS, eds. *Early diabetes in early life.* New York: Academic Press, 1974:303.

53. Pederson J. *The pregnant diabetic and her newborn: problems and management,* 2nd ed. Baltimore: Williams & Wilkins, 1977:211–220.

54. Berkus MD, Langer O. Glucose tolerance test: degree of glucose abnormality correlates with neonatal outcome. *Obstet Gynecol* 1993;81:344–348.

55. Reece EA, Coustan DR, Sherwin RS, et al. Does intensive glycemic control in diabetic pregnancies result in normalization of other metabolic fuels? *Am J Obstet Gynecol* 1991;165:126.

56. Diamond MP, Reece EA, Caprio S, et al. Impairment of counter-regulatory hormone responses to hypoglycemia in pregnant women with insulin-dependent diabetes mellitus. *Am J Obstet Gynecol* 1992;166:74.

57. Reece EA, Hagay Z, Roberts AB, et al. Fetal behavioral responses during induced hypoglycemia in pregnant women using the insulin clamp technique. *Am J Obstet Gynecol* 1995;172:151–155.

58. Metzger B, Coustan DR. Summary and recommendations of the fourth international workshop-conference on gestational diabetes mellitus. *Diabetes Care* 1998;21[Suppl 2]:B161–B167.

59. Englgau MM, Herman WH, Smith PJ, et al. The epidemiology of diabetes and pregnancy in the US, 1988. *Diabetes Care* 1995;18:1029–1033.

60. Catalano PM, Tyzbir ED, Wolfe RR, et al. Carbohydrate metabolism in control subjects and women with gestational diabetes. *Am J Physiol* 1993;264:E60–E67.

61. Kuhl C, Hornnes PJ, Anderson O. Review: etiology and pathophysiology of gestational diabetes mellitus. *Diabetes* 1985;34[Suppl 2]:66–70.

62. Kautzky-Willer A, Prager R, Waldhausl W, et al. Pronounced insulin resistance and inadequate β-cell secretion characterize lean gestational diabetes during and after pregnancy. *Diabetes Care* 1997;20:1717–1723.

63. Bowes SB, Hennessy TR, Umpleby AM, et al. Measurement of glucose metabolism and insulin secretion during normal pregnancy and pregnancy complicated by gestational diabetes. *Diabetologia* 1996;39:976–983.

64. Homko CJ, Sivan E, Chen X, et al. Insulin secretion, clearance and action during and after pregnancy in women with gestational diabetes mellitus (GDM). *Diabetes* 1999;8[Suppl 2]:A53 (*abst*).

65. Berk MA, Mimouni F, Miodovnik M, et al. Macrosomia in infants of insulin-dependent diabetic mothers. *Pediatrics* 1989;86:1029–1034.

66. Willman SP, Leveno KJ, Guzick DS, et al. Glucose threshold for macrosomia in pregnancy complicated by diabetes. *Am J Obstet Gynecol* 1986;154:470–475.

67. Modanlou HD, Corchester WL, Thorosian A, et al. Macrosomia: maternal, fetal and neonatal implications. *Obstet Gynecol* 1980;55:420.

68. Menon RK, Cohen RM, Sperling MA, et al. Transplacental passage of insulin in pregnant women with insulin-dependent diabetes mellitus. *N Engl J Med* 1990;323:309.

69. Kalkhoff RK, Kandaraki E, Morrow PG, et al. Relationship between neonatal birth weight and maternal plasma amino acid profiles in lean and obese nondiabetic women and in type I pregnant women. *Metabolism* 1988;37:234.

70. Whittaker PG, Stewart MO, Taylor A, et al. Insulin-like growth factor I and its binding protein I during normal and diabetic pregnancies. *Obstet Gynecol* 1990;76:223.

71. Reece EA, Wiznitzer A, Le E, et al. The relation between human fetal growth and fetal blood levels of insulin-like growth factors I and II, their binding proteins, and receptors. *Obstet Gynecol* 1994;84:88–95.

72. Wiznitzer A, Reece EA, Homko C, et al. Insulin-like growth factors, their binding proteins and fetal macrosomia in offspring of non-diabetic women. *Am J Perinatol* 1998;12:23–28.

73. Sivan E, Lin WM, Homko CJ, et al. Leptin is present in human cord blood. *Diabetes* 1997;46:917–919.

74. Catalano PM, Drago NM, Amini SB. Maternal carbohydrate metabolism and its relationship to fetal growth and body composition. *Am J Obstet Gynecol* 1995;172:464–470.

INTRAUTERINE GROWTH RESTRICTION

ROSEMARY E. REISS

Pediatricians first recognized more than 50 years ago that human newborns could be stunted because of poor growth *in utero* (1–3). With the development of obstetric ultrasound during the past 25 years, obstetricians have acquired a tool to identify fetuses whose growth was slower than normal. Identification of these fetuses that are small for gestational age (SGA) is important because they have perinatal mortality rates almost tenfold higher than their normally grown counterparts (4). Survivors are at increased risk of short-term neonatal morbidity such as hypoxia, meconium aspiration syndrome, and hypoglycemia, as well as long-term complications including neurodevelopmental delay, cerebral palsy, and, possibly, type 2 diabetes mellitus and hypertension (5–9).

Fetuses or infants classified as SGA form a heterogeneous group. About two-thirds are constitutionally small but healthy. Causes of restricted growth among the rest include intrinsic fetal problems such as aneuploidy or mendelian disorders, acquired problems including fetal infections, exposure to toxins, or inadequate maternal nutrition, and, most commonly, abnormalities of the placenta and the placental bed.

Once intrauterine growth restriction (IUGR) has been detected, selection of appropriate clinical interventions should be based on an understanding of the underlying cause. This chapter examines common causes of fetal growth impairment, presents what is understood about their mechanisms, and discusses diagnostic and management strategies.

DEFINITIONS AND DIAGNOSTIC CRITERIA

Newborns weighing less than 2500 g are characterized as having low birth weight (LBW) by the World Health Organization and have long been recognized as being at increased risk of perinatal morbidity and mortality. About one-third of LBW newborns are SGA rather than premature (3). Obstetric ultrasound makes it possible to estimate gestational age accurately and to obtain serial information about fetal growth, so it is easier to distinguish among these causes of LBW and to identify SGA fetuses before delivery. Serial measurement of fetal size also permits the observation that growth can plateau, even when fetal weight itself is within

normal range for gestational age, and this finding is also correlated with increased morbidity (10).

Sigmoidal growth curves have been constructed from cross-sectional observations of birth weights in well-dated pregnancies (11,12) (Fig. 32.1), as well as from biometric measurements of fetuses performed with ultrasound. Using regression models, fetal weight can be estimated from combinations of measurements of fetal head, abdomen, and long bones (13,14). Using these models, the neonatal weight can be predicted with an error of approximately 10%. Detailed analysis of the statistical and other problems of applying cross-sectional population data to diagnose growth restriction in an individual fetus has been undertaken by several authors and has been well reviewed by Sparks et al. (10).

Growth curves generated from populations from different ethnic groups or living at different altitudes are not identical, although overall they are more similar than different. Male fetuses tend to be larger than females at the same gestational age. Despite these caveats, comparisons of ultrasound estimates of fetal size and weight to expected size and weight have proved clinically useful in the identification of fetal growth restriction.

In the United States, fetuses weighing less than the tenth percentile are considered growth restricted, whereas in Europe, the fifth percentile is a more usual cutoff point. Perinatal morbidity and mortality rates among fetuses labeled as growth restricted obviously differ depending on whether the fifth or the tenth percentile is chosen as the criterion. Choosing the more stringent fifth percentile diminishes the number of constitutionally small, well fetuses unnecessarily identified for increased antenatal surveillance, but it increases the risk that fetuses at risk for *in utero* demise will be overlooked. An awareness of this unavoidable trade-off between sensitivity and specificity is important when interventions such as early delivery are considered.

Clinically, SGA infants can be classified as *symmetrically small* or *asymmetrically small*. The asymmetrically small infant has normal or near-normal length and head circumference (HC), but small abdominal circumference (AC) and low weight. For the symmetrically small infant, both weight and length are low, as are both head circumference (HC) and abdominal circumference (AC). The degree of asymmetry can be quantified as a *ponderal index* formulated as

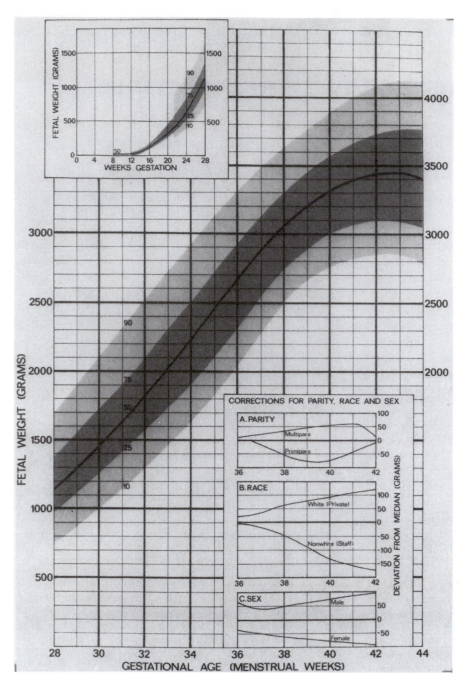

FIGURE 32.1. Plot of fetal weight versus gestational age indicating tenth, twenty-fifth, seventy-fifth, and ninetieth percentiles. Effects of parity, race, and fetal sex are also plotted. (From Brenner WE, Edelman DA, Hendricks CH. A standard of fetal growth for the United States of America. *Am J Obstet Gynecol* 1976;126:555–564, with permission.)

birth weight in grams $\times$ 100/(crown $-$ heel length in centimeters)^3 (15). A ponderal index below the tenth percentile for gestational age indicates that asymmetric growth suggests placental insufficiency. In newborns weighing more than 2500 g, a low ponderal index also suggests that *in utero* growth may have been impaired. The ponderal index is less than the tenth percentile in about 12% of SGA infants and in about 1% of infants with weights appropriate for gestational age (AGA) (16).

The concepts of symmetric growth and asymmetric growth have also been applied to ultrasound biometry, but

they must be considered in light of normal fetal growth patterns. Early in the third trimester, the fetal head is normally large relative to fetal length and girth. After 28 weeks' gestation, fetal abdominal growth accelerates as the fetus begins to store liver glycogen and adipose tissue. By about 34 weeks' gestation, the AC and HC should be approximately equal. In symmetric IUGR, HC, AC, and femur length (FL) are all smaller than expected. In asymmetric IUGR, HC continues to grow appropriately for gestational age, whereas AC and FL lag. This asymmetry becomes more pronounced after 28 weeks, when abdominal growth normally accelerates. In asymmetrically grown fetuses, the HC/AC ratio is higher than normal for gestational age. Although HC, AC, and FL all depend on gestational age, the ratio of FL to AC (FL/AC) remains constant after 25 weeks, with .24 representing the upper limit of normal (17). This makes the FL/AC a useful tool to detect IUGR in pregnancies in which accurate dating is not available. However, only about two-thirds of SGA fetuses have elevated FL/AC ratios. In a well-dated pregnancy, the most sensitive ultrasound indicator of IUGR is the AC, which is low in all types of fetal growth restriction.

Awareness that restriction of fetal growth can be either symmetric or asymmetric is important, for example, to avoid mistaking symmetrically small fetuses for more premature ones. However, although asymmetric growth suggests placental insufficiency, both symmetric IUGR and asymmetric IUGR are etiologically heterogeneous disorders.

ETIOLOGY

Detection of slow fetal growth does not really make a diagnosis; rather, it raises more questions. Small fetal size is a common manifestation of diverse disorders (Table 32.1). Abstractly, the factors controlling fetal growth are fuel composition and delivery, as well as the ability to distribute and metabolize fuels. Each of these can be influenced by the

TABLE 32.1. CONDITIONS ASSOCIATED WITH FETAL GROWTH DEFICIENCY

Uteroplacental insufficiency
Multiple gestations
Maternal malnutrition
Exposure to environmental toxins
   Medications
   Tobacco
   Alcohol
Congenital infections
   Cytomegalovirus
   Rubella
   Toxoplasmosis
Chromosomal abnormalities
   Trisomy 18, trisomy 13, trisomy 21, trisomy 22
   Triploidy
   Partial trisomy or monosomy
   Ring chromosomes
   Uniparental disomy
Genetic disorders and syndromes
   Bloom syndrome
   De Lange syndrome
   Fanconi pancytopenia syndrome
   Pallister-Hall syndrome
   Russell-Silver syndrome
   Seckel syndrome
   Skeletal dysplasias
Congenital anomalies
   Anencephaly
   Gastroschisis

genetic makeup of the mother and the fetus, by acquired disorders of mother or fetus, and by environmental factors. Although unavoidable for organizing book chapters, the traditional categorization of causes as maternal, placental, or fetal or as anatomic, genetic, or infectious is simplistic.

Normal growth and development depend on subtle interactions between genetic programming and environmental stimuli and among the embryo/fetus, the placenta, and the mother, so it is not surprising that the cause of disturbed growth may overlap categories. For example, aneuploidy produces abnormal placental function as well as abnormalities in fetal tissue growth and differentiation. Maternal viral infection may cause both fetal infection and placentitis, both of which impair growth. Maternal malnutrition may affect both placental fuel consumption and patterns of fetal blood flow by reducing insulin-like growth factor I (IGF-I) (18). As our understanding of the molecular processes involved in placentation expand, "genetic" causes for IUGR may encompass placental insufficiency as well as fetal aneuploidy or maternal phenylketonuria. Already, investigators have hinted that the abnormal placentation seen in preeclampsia may be related to mutations in genes controlling processes of trophoblastic invasion or decidual bed vessel response (19–21). Although we are still a long way from clinical applications of these exciting new possibilities, eventually they will provide tools for earlier diagnosis, better predictors of recurrence, and better therapies.

ABNORMALITIES OF THE PLACENTA AND THE PLACENTAL BED

The fetus depends on the placenta for its supply of nutrients and its exchange of respiratory gases. The placenta is also metabolically active, consuming as well as transmitting nutrients, producing hormones that affect growth, and metabolizing potential teratogens. Slow fetal growth is attributable clinically to placental insufficiency in about 15% of SGA infants.

Normal placental exchange relies on three components: normal uterine blood flow to the placental bed, a normal villous interface between fetal and maternal blood, and normal fetoplacental circulation (22). Although these components are interdependent, with disturbances at one site causing deterioration at another, an attempt is made to discuss them individually.

Abnormalities of the Uteroplacental Circulation

As pregnancy advances, uteroplacental blood flow normally increases progressively and reaches a level of approximately 500 mL per minute at term (23). This increase in flow is largely the result of vessel remodeling and vasodilatation.

In normal pregnancy, there is a dramatic increase in the diameter of the spiral arteries, the end arteries of the placental bed (24). Classically, this increase is considered to be the result of replacement of the endothelium and the internal elastic lamina and smooth muscle of the media in myometrial portions of the spiral arteries by advancing trophoblast (25). The remodeling of the spiral arteries decreases resistance to blood flow into the intervillous space. This effect is reflected in changes in the characteristics of blood flow in the uterine arteries that can be demonstrated in humans by examining Doppler flow velocimetry waveforms in the uterine arteries. Before pregnancy, the uterine waveform has a large dicrotic notch and little end-diastolic flow. In a normal pregnancy, end-diastolic flow increases with advancing gestational age, and the notch is lost by about 26 weeks' gestation (26–28).

Multiple lines of evidence show that abnormalities of the uteroplacental circulation can produce fetal growth retardation. In animal models, embolization (29,30) or ligation of the uteroplacental circulation (31,32) produces an increase in placental vascular resistance, impaired delivery of nutrients and oxygen, and fetal stunting. Umbilical blood flow and uterine blood flow decline after embolization of the ovine uterine circulation (30). In human pregnancies with IUGR, histologic examination of the placental bed sometimes shows abnormalities in the decidual vessels with abnormal persistence of the muscular layer in the myometrial portion of the spiral arteries (33–38). Some arterioles in the placental bed of patients with preeclampsia and IUGR may also display acute atherosis. The media of the affected vessels contains lipid-laden foam cells and amorphous material that narrow the lumen and may progress to vessel obliteration and focal infarction. Whereas these abnormalities were originally described as characteristic of preeclampsia, they are also observed in some normotensive women whose pregnancies are characterized by IUGR. Many investigators believe IUGR and preeclampsia to be manifestations of the same underlying disorder, both resulting from placental bed hypoxia caused by inadequate remodeling of the spiral arteries (22,36). This hypothesis is consistent with the clinical observation that fetal growth lag may precede the onset of hypertension or proteinuria in some pregnant women with preeclampsia.

Doppler velocimetry demonstrates the persistence of high resistance in the uterine arteries and their branches in some pregnancies complicated by IUGR (28,38–42). In these cases, the postsystolic notch does not disappear, and end-diastolic velocities do not increase normally with advancing gestation (Fig. 32.2). When Doppler abnormalities suggesting abnormal uterine artery impedance were present

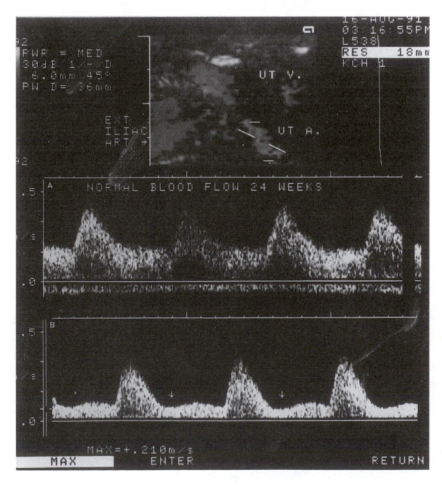

FIGURE 32.2. Uterine artery flow velocity waveforms obtained by pulsed Doppler at 24 weeks' gestation. The pattern in **A** is normal, whereas **B** illustrates an end-systolic notch predictive of intrauterine growth restriction and pregnancy-induced hypertension. (From Harrington KF, Campbell S, Bewley S, et al. Doppler velocimetry studies of the uterine artery in the early prediction of preeclampsia and intrauterine growth retardation. *Eur J Obstet Gynecol Reprod Biol* 1991;42:S14–S20, with permission.)

in pregnancies complicated by IUGR, placental bed biopsies showed absence of physiologic spiral artery remodeling in 60% and atherosis in an additional 20% (38). In a prospective study in which a general population was screened with late second trimester uterine artery Doppler velocimetry, 67% of patients with abnormal resistance indices developed either IUGR or preeclampsia, or both (41).

Abnormalities of the Fetoplacental Circulation

Doppler ultrasound techniques have also made the human fetal and umbilical circulation accessible to study. In normal pregnancies, as gestation advances, one sees a gradual decrease in umbilical artery resistance as the placenta and its vascular tree grow, manifested in Doppler velocimetry studies by an increase in end-diastolic flow velocity relative to peak systolic velocity (43) (Fig. 32.3). In some pregnancies in which the fetus is SGA, umbilical artery diastolic flow

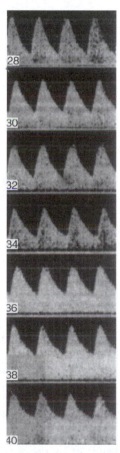

FIGURE 32.3. Serial studies of Doppler flow velocity waveforms from the umbilical artery of a normal fetus. The end-diastolic flow increases relative to systolic flow as gestation advances. (From Trudinger BJ, Giles WB, Cook CM, et al. Fetal umbilical artery flow velocity waveforms and placental resistance: clinical significance. *Br J Obstet Gynaecol* 1985;92:23–30, with permission.)

is reduced, or even reversed, a finding suggesting increased placental resistance (Fig. 32.4).

The correlation between decreased umbilical end-diastolic flow assessed by Doppler velocimetry and increased resistance in the placental circulation has been validated with invasive studies in animals. The reduction in umbilical artery diastolic flow characteristic of IUGR can be reproduced in sheep by embolization of the umbilical-placental circulation with 15- or 50-μm microspheres, a finding suggesting that obliteration of either stem villous vessels or capillaries could produce a change in Doppler indices (44,45). Progressive embolization led eventually to absent, and then to reversed end-diastolic (44), findings, mimicking changes seen in umbilical artery Doppler waveforms in severe IUGR in humans.

Several investigators have reported a reduction in the number of small arterial vessels in placentas from human SGA pregnancies with abnormal Doppler velocimetry (46–48). Pregnancies characterized by SGA with normal umbilical artery velocimetry showed villous artery counts no different from those of well-grown fetuses. These findings led Giles and co-workers to hypothesize that gradual villous small vessel obliteration is responsible for the rise in Doppler resistance indices observed as the third trimester advances in some pregnancies characterized by IUGR (46). Alternatively, failure in the development of terminal villi and their capillaries, whose volume normally increases exponentially between 31 and 36 weeks' gestation, could account for reduced umbilical artery end-diastolic flow. Histometric evidence to support this hypothesis comes from studies that found reduced terminal villi volumes and surface areas in placentas from IUGR fetuses (49–51). The effect was especially pronounced when placentas of preterm IUGR pregnancies in which end-diastolic flow in the umbilical arteries had been absent were compared with those of gestational age–matched controls that were AGA. These authors did not observe luminal obliteration of villus arteries (51). It is likely that more than one mechanism can produce both abnormal umbilical artery velocimetry and the placental insufficiency that it reflects. Whatever its mechanism, perinatal mortality and short-and long-term neonatal morbidity are much higher in SGA fetuses with elevated end-diastolic resistance than in those with normal Doppler findings (43,52,53). Doppler studies of the umbilical artery are probably the best widely available tool to distinguish those SGA fetuses at risk of perinatal asphyxia from those that are merely constitutionally small.

Fetal Circulatory Adaptation to Placental Insufficiency

Slowed growth is one of the ways in which the fetus adapts to the hypoxic stress caused by placental insufficiency. The fetus uses its limited supply of oxygen and nutrients to maintain fetal heart, brain, and adrenal function at the expense of musculoskeletal growth and glycogen or fat stor-

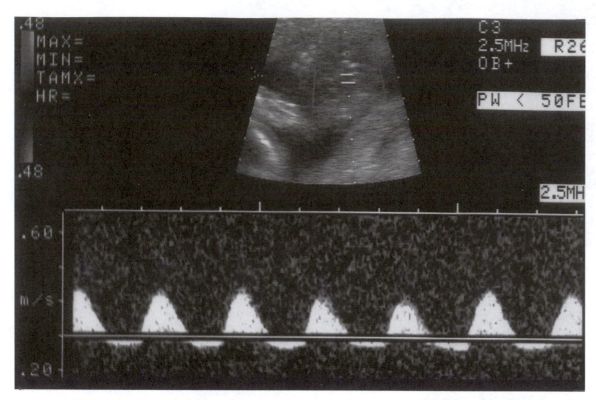

FIGURE 32.4. Flow velocity waveform displaying reversed end-diastolic flow from the umbilical artery of a growth-restricted fetus at 28 weeks. The mother presented with preeclampsia.

age. This is achieved by selectively increasing blood flow to vital organs while decreasing flow to the hepatic circulation and the rest of the body (54,55). When fuel is plentiful, about 50% of the most highly oxygenated blood returning from the placenta passes into the portal circulation and allows the liver to extract nutrients for storage, while the rest returns directly to the heart through the ductus venosus (56). Autoregulation in the venous circulation allows the fetus to divert more of this highly oxygenated blood to the heart, and thus to bypass the liver, during periods of hypoxia. Both these phenomena, originally observed in animal models (57–59), have been confirmed in SGA human fetuses using pulsed Doppler evaluation of cerebral (60–62), myocardial (63), and ductus venosus flow (64). Redistribution of flow leads to sparing of fetal brain growth, and it explains the asymmetric phenotype often seen in IUGR resulting from placental insufficiency. However, when hypoxia and acidemia have early onset or are prolonged, brain growth is also impaired.

Placental Structural and Histologic Abnormalities

Fetal growth is related to placental morphology. The weight and surface area of the placenta are correlated with fetal size (65). The normal ratio between birth weight and placental weight is about 1:7, and it is fairly constant in normal

pregnancies. This observation could indicate either that placental size determines fetal size or that fetal genetic factors program both placental size and fetal growth rate. Placental abnormalities that predispose to poor implantation, reduced umbilical flow, or decreased surface area available for nutrient exchange are associated with SGA infants (66,67). These abnormalities include placenta previa, circumvallate placenta, velamentous insertion of the cord into the placenta, and abnormalities associated with multiple gestations. Single umbilical arteries are also associated with SGA fetuses (68). Retroplacental bleeding, which causes chronic placental separation (*chronic abruption*) and produces areas of secondary infarction, is strongly associated with poor fetal growth (69).

Only a brief summary of the complex variety of histologic lesions identified in the placentas of SGA fetuses is presented here, because several excellent discussions are available elsewhere (69–71). The diversity of findings in part reflects the diversity of causes of growth impairment. The vascular pathology of the placental bed that is seen in association with growth restriction and preeclampsia has already been discussed. Many findings are thought to be caused by transient or chronic ischemia or by the reparative responses to these insults that reflect the abnormalities of the maternal blood supply. Examples of these secondary effects may include proliferation of cytotrophoblast out of proportion to syncytiotrophoblast, perivillous and subchorionic fibrin deposition, fibrinoid necrosis, and fetal arteriolar vasculopathy (69,71).

Immunologic mechanisms may also play a role in the placental lesions associated with IUGR. Villous vascular changes sometimes resemble the vasculitic lesions seen in autoimmune disease in other organs (69). Deposits of immunoglobulin M (IgM) and the complement component C_3 can be found in the walls of placental bed vessels with atherosis (72). *Chronic villitis*, the infiltration of villous stroma by lymphocytes, is often seen in placentas from pregnancies characterized by IUGR in the absence of infection (73–76). Chronic villitis is less diffuse than the villitis seen with viral infection, and it is not accompanied by inflammatory changes in the membranes and umbilical cord (71). The infiltrating inflammatory cells have been shown to be T lymphocytes of maternal origin, whereas in villitis from infection, the infiltrating cells are predominantly macrophages (74). Maternal serum levels of CH50 complement are lower than in women without villitis (77). These findings suggest that chronic villitis may represent a maternal immune response against fetal antigens.

Confined Placental Mosaicism

Chromosomal abnormalities confined to the placenta (*confined placental mosaicism* or CPM) have been identified in some cases of otherwise unexplained IUGR. Although the embryo and the placenta arise from the same zygote, postzygotic events can lead to karyotypic disparities between them. A growing body of evidence suggests that placental chromosomal abnormalities may impair growth of a chromosomally normal fetus (78–81).

Initially, CPM seems to be an experiment of nature that provides an opportunity to evaluate the effects of isolated placental chromosomal abnormalities on fetal growth. However, placental mosaicism may arise in several ways, and fetuses in some of these pregnancies may not truly be karyotypically normal. One possibility is for a mitotic error to arise in an extraembryonic cell from an originally diploid conceptus, to produce an abnormal cell line present only in the placental tissue (82). Alternatively, a diploid cell line could result from an early corrective loss of a chromosome from a trisomic conceptus, with trisomic cells persisting only in the placenta (83). In the latter case, the diploid embryo either could be karyotypically normal or could have uniparental disomy, if the lost chromosome was derived from the normal gamete. Fetal growth could be impaired either by metabolic dysfunction caused by significant numbers of karyotypically abnormal cells in the placenta or because the fetus had uniparental disomy. This would not be apparent from routine karyotyping. Molecular studies have confirmed both these mechanisms (84).

Experience with first trimester chorionic villus sampling for prenatal diagnosis shows that CPM is not uncommon, occurring in 1% to 2% of samples (79,85,86). However, placental chromosomal abnormalities lead to IUGR in only a minority of cases. A large British collaborative study of outcomes of 8,004 pregnancies karyotyped by first trimester chorionic villus sampling found CPM in 73 (79). In only 5 (8%) of the 62 ongoing pregnancies for which complete data were available were birth weights below the tenth percentile. Although this incidence of growth restriction was significantly higher than in their controls, this study shows that the relationship between CPM and fetal growth is complex, because some placental aneuploidy can be tolerated without noticeable effects.

Fetal and placental karyotypes were also studied by Wolstenholme et al. in 108 pregnancies in which IUGR was detected in the second or third trimester. These investigators found 7 (6.5%) displaying CPM. In all cases, IUGR was severe, with birth weights lower than the third percentile. Three of the placentas were mosaic for trisomy 16, 3 for other autosomes, and 1 for a structural rearrangement in chromosome 13 (79). Wilkins-Haug et al. compared the frequency of CPM in placentas from 12 IUGR infants to that in 24 gestational-age matched AGA controls (81). CPM was present in 3 (25%) of the IUGR placentas and in 2 (8.3%) of the controls. Fluorescence *in situ* hybridization demonstrated more widely distributed mosaic cells in the affected placentas of the IUGR fetuses.

The impact of CPM on fetal growth depends on interactions among the level of mosaicism, the presence or absence of uniparental disomy, and the specific chromosomes involved. Aneuploidy for chromosomes carrying genes for growth factors or proteins involved in placental transport or metabolism would be expected to have the greatest impact. Curiously, one study found decidual vasculopathy in association with CPM, but not in the euploid placentas of other SGA fetuses in the study (81). A paucity of villous arterioles has also been reported in the placentas of trisomic fetuses (87,88). Abnormal umbilical artery Doppler velocimetry has been described in some aneuploid pregnancies, with onset earlier in gestation than the placental insufficiency associated with maternal vascular disease (88).

FETAL CHROMOSOMAL ABNORMALITIES AND CONGENITAL MALFORMATIONS

Fetal aneuploidy can produce fetal growth restriction and should always be considered when growth delay is early in onset. More than half of all fetuses with trisomy 13 and trisomy 18 are growth restricted, and fetuses with trisomy 21 or Turner's syndrome can also be SGA (89). Although chromosomally abnormal fetuses are usually thought of as symmetrically small, triploidy typically produces severe asymmetric IUGR. Growth impairment is probably caused by abnormalities of cell replication and reduced cell number because of fetal aneuploidy, as well as by metabolic and vascular abnormalities of the aneuploid placenta, as already discussed.

Fetuses with congenital abnormalities but normal karyotypes can also display slow growth. Anomalies commonly associated with slow fetal growth include cardiac defects, renal agenesis, gastroschisis, skeletal dysplasias, and anencephaly (90,91). The mechanisms for the slowed slow growth seen in these settings undoubtedly vary with the disorder; for gastroschisis, impairment of umbilical arterial or venous flow is probably a factor, whereas for anencephaly, pituitary dysfunction may play a role.

MATERNAL MALNUTRITION

Adequacy of fetal nutrition can be impaired by inadequate maternal intake as well as by poor placental transfer. In humans, maternal weight, height, and weight gain during pregnancy are correlated with their infants' birth weight (92,93). Studies showed a reduction in mean birth weights of infants born during periods of famine (94–96), as compared with controls in the same population during periods of plenty. Inadequate calorie intake before pregnancy appears to magnify the effect of malnutrition during pregnancy itself (93,96). Short intervals between pregnancies are also associated with lower birth weight in infants; part of this effect may be nutritional. Poor intake of specific nutrients, such as folic acid (97) or zinc (98,99), has been suggested to impair fetal growth, although in humans it is difficult to control for effects of overall diet and for cofactors such as smoking.

Although one cannot extrapolate directly among species, evidence from animal models suggests mechanisms by which alterations in maternal nutrition could influence embryonic and fetal fuel uptake and utilization for growth. These mechanisms shed light not only on IUGR caused by maternal malnutrition, but also on fetal deprivation resulting from placental insufficiency. Some pertinent human data are available from sampling blood from the umbilical cord blood of IUGR fetuses by cordocentesis or at birth.

The primary source of fuel may differ among fetal organs within the same species. For example, studies in fetal sheep suggest that glucose is the main fuel for the brain, lung, and the rest of the body, except the kidney, heart, liver, and gut, for which lactic acid is the main fuel (10). Lactate may also serve as a fuel for the human fetus. It is tempting to speculate that these differences could contribute to the asymmetry of growth seen in some IUGR fetuses. In addition, the placenta itself has a high rate of oxidative metabolism and consumes as well as transfers fuels. For example, in sheep, the placenta consumes about 60% of the glucose extracted from the maternal circulation, and the proportion may increase with fasting (100). IGF-I may play a role

in regulating the balance between fetal and placental fuel consumption during maternal starvation (8).

Transport of nutrients to the fetus across the placenta depends on concentrations of nutrients in maternal blood, adequacy of uterine blood flow to the intervillous space, properties of the intervening membranes, and actions of transport proteins. Transport mechanisms vary among nutrients. Because mechanisms are nutrient specific, alterations in placental blood flow or maternal nutritional status may affect nutrient transport differentially, depending on whether the particular nutrient crosses by simple diffusion (e.g., water), by facilitated diffusion by membrane-bound carriers (e.g., glucose), or by active transport by transport proteins (e.g., some amino acids, calcium). Interspecies differences occur in nutrient transport and metabolism. The placenta's role in interconversion of amino acids also varies among species.

Both nutritional status and umbilical blood flow probably play a role in fetal glucose levels. Glucose crosses the placenta along its concentration gradient by facilitated diffusion. Although one study did not find a reduction in glucose levels in fetuses with IUGR (101), another (102) found that the gradient between maternal and fetal glucose was increased in IUGR, with greater differences as impairment of umbilical blood flow increased.

Amino acid transport proteins are present both on the apical ("maternal-facing") and the basal ("fetal-facing") membranes, and their production is regulated (103,104). Because of active transport, concentrations of many amino acids are higher in the fetus than in the mother (104–106). In the rat, production of some placental amino acid transplant proteins is normally upregulated during the last third of gestation when fetal growth is fastest (107). Whether this upregulation is a primary event promoting growth or a response to increased delivery of substrate in late gestation is not clear. When rats were fed a calorically adequate diet low in protein, maternal, fetal, and placental weights were all reduced significantly compared with those in animals fed an isocaloric diet with normal protein content (104). Fetal concentrations of most amino acids were found to be low. Amino acid transport and messenger RNA (mRNA) for transport proteins were reduced in both apical and basal membrane vesicles derived from the placental trophoblast. Because maternal amino acid concentrations were maintained in normal range, the authors speculated that the mechanism for downregulation of amino acid transport proteins was hormonal.

Evidence also shows decreased uptake of amino acids in human growth restriction (105,106,108). When umbilical cord blood samples were obtained at delivery from SGA and AGA infants, total α-amino nitrogen concentrations were significantly lower in the SGA infants (105). The difference resulted mostly from lower levels of the branched-chain amino acids valine, leucine, and isoleucine, which share a common transport system. Comparison of umbilical artery and venous levels suggested reduced placental uptake of amino acids. Findings in membrane vesicles isolated from human placentas are also consistent with these reports (108). Similar reductions in amino acid levels have been found in SGA fetuses sampled by cordocentesis (106,109).

Evidence from several species, including humans, indicates that IGF-I plays a significant role in fetal growth. It may mediate the effects of nutritional inadequacy whether from maternal starvation (110) or from placental insufficiency (111). In a sheep model, maternal starvation was associated with cessation of fetal growth and a rapid decline in fetal IGF-I (110). Glucose infusion restored IGF-I concentration, whereas amino acid infusion did not, a finding suggesting that either glucose or insulin may be involved in regulation of fetal IGF-I production in sheep (112). Infusion of IGF-I into the circulation of fetal lambs enhanced placental uptake of amino acids, increased fetal substrate uptake, and decreased fetal protein catabolism (113). In mice, fetal levels of IGF-I correlated with size, and mice homozygous for a mutation disrupting the IGF-I gene or its receptors were severely growth deficient (114). Levels of IGF-I concentrations in cordocentesis samples from second and third trimester human fetuses also correlate with size and are reduced in IUGR (115,116). However, the range of individual values is too wide for cord blood IGF-I levels to be useful diagnostically. Probably, in most cases, the low IGF-1 levels are a response to a low nutrient supply rather than the primary cause of growth restriction. However, it is certainly conceivable that mutations in the IGF-I gene could be responsible for some IUGR in humans as in mice. The fetal role of IGF-I and of other growth factors, an area of active research, has been reviewed (18,117,118).

FETAL INFECTION

Infection of the fetus or placenta is responsible for 5% to 10% of cases of IUGR (67). Although many organisms have been implicated, only rubella, cytomegalovirus (CMV) infection, and toxoplasmosis have been clearly shown to cause IUGR directly (119). Syphilis has also been cited in case reports as a cause of IUGR, but this was not confirmed in a quantitative morphometric autopsy study (120).

Cytomegalovirus Infection

In the United States, the organism most commonly implicated in IUGR is *CMV*, a ubiquitous DNA virus of the herpes family (121). Maternal primary infection during pregnancy usually does not produce a clinically apparent maternal illness, but 40% to 50% of the time it leads to transmission of the virus to the fetus (122,123). Fifty per-

cent of infants with symptomatic congenital CMV infection display IUGR (124). CMV causes lysis of infected cells that impairs growth by reducing cell number and causing focal necrosis in various organs. CMV can also cause vasculitis by infection of vascular endothelium (67,125).

Severity of fetal injury is greatest when the primary infection occurs before 20 weeks' gestation (126). Congenital CMV infection can cause hepatosplenomegaly, ascites, jaundice, thrombocytopenia, microcephaly, and chorioretinitis, as well as impairment of overall fetal growth. About 30% of severely infected infants die in the neonatal period. Secondary infection or reactivation can also transmit virus to the infant. These infections do not produce overt neonatal symptoms, although late sequelae, including hearing loss and other neurologic impairments, can develop (123).

If CMV infection is suspected as a cause of IUGR, maternal CMV IgG and IgM should be assayed. The presence of IgM without IgG indicates recent primary infection. When both IgG and IgM are present, it is difficult to distinguish late primary infection from reactivation. If no baseline titers were obtained, it may be possible to recover serum obtained at the time of initial routine prenatal laboratory studies for comparison titers. When fetal infection is suspected, it can be confirmed by demonstrating the presence of virus or viral DNA in fluid obtained by amniocentesis (127–129).

Currently, no effective means of fetal treatment is available. Ganciclovir has proved effective in treating immunocompromised adults with serious CMV infections and may prove useful in affected fetuses or neonates. However, because congenital CMV is unlikely to be detected before fetal growth and development has been impaired, treatment *in utero* at best may offer limited palliative effects.

Toxoplasmosis

IUGR can also be seen in fetuses infected with *Toxoplasma gondii*, a parasite that can be transmitted to humans by cats and undercooked meats, and between humans transplacentally, through breast milk or in blood transfusions in which white cells are present (130). About 6% of infected fetuses are growth restricted. Other features of severe fetal infection identifiable prenatally include neurologic damage, reflected in hydrocephalus, microcephaly, or intracranial calcifications, and occasionally ascites (131,132). Prenatal diagnosis is of value either to allow initiation of therapy or to give families the option of pregnancy termination. Treatment *in utero* has been shown to ameliorate the severity of congenital infection, although it does not eradicate the parasite (133).

The first step in evaluating a growth-restricted fetus for suspected congenital toxoplasmosis is to demonstrate the presence of maternal *Toxoplasma*-specific IgM antibodies. Because cross-reactivity with other antibodies can occur, positive IgM findings should be confirmed by an experienced reference laboratory, and serial titers may be useful. If acute maternal infection is confirmed, maternal treatment with spiramycin should be initiated while fetal evaluation is begun (133).

Methods for diagnosis of fetal toxoplasmosis are evolving. Originally, fetal blood was obtained by cordocentesis and was assayed for liver function tests and for *Toxoplasma*-specific IgA and IgM. Fetal blood and amniotic fluid were both used to inoculate mice or tissue cultures from which the parasite could then be recovered (133). Newer, polymerase chain reaction–based techniques to amplify toxoplasma DNA now allow more rapid and sensitive assays for its presence in amniotic fluid (134,135). Used in combination with amniotic fluid inoculation of tissue culture or mice, these techniques appear to have sensitivity and specificity comparable to those of the previous protocols. Investigators have suggested that cordocentesis, with its attendant higher risks of fetal loss, can probably be abandoned (135–137).

If fetal infection is confirmed, and the family chooses to continue the pregnancy, then a regimen of pyramethamine, sulfadiazine, and leukovorin is begun (130–133).

Rubella

Rubella is thought to restrict fetal growth by damaging capillary endothelium during organogenesis, thereby resulting in a decreased number of cells of normal size (138). In particular, the growth of the adrenal glands, thymus, and brain is restricted in newborns with congenital rubella. This produces a symmetric form of growth restriction.

First trimester maternal infection with rubella leads to infection of 20% of exposed fetuses, with transmission rates declining from 50% if exposure occurs during the first month to 10% when it occurs in the third month. In addition to its effects on fetal growth, rubella can cause cataracts, patent ductus arteriosus, and deafness (139). Now that use of rubella vaccine is widespread, congenital rubella is rare in the United States. Although the vaccine contains live, attenuated rubella virus, no cases of congenital rubella syndrome have been reported in infants born to mothers who conceived shortly after receiving the vaccine (140).

DRUGS AND OTHER ENVIRONMENTAL TOXINS

Drugs and Medications

Medications prescribed for the treatment of chronic maternal conditions can impair fetal growth either by acting on the fetus directly or, less commonly, by decreasing uteroplacental blood flow. *Drugs of abuse* including cocaine, opiates, and amphetamines are also associated with IUGR (141). The effects of individual agents may be difficult to assess because of concomitant use of several drugs or of alcohol

or tobacco. Commonly used drugs suspected of causing IUGR are listed in Table 32.2.

Tobacco

Maternal smoking is one of the most common causes of slow fetal growth. In a national study of LBW infants in the United States, most of whom were born at term, smoking was a factor in more than one-third (142). The likelihood and degree of growth restriction correlate with the number of cigarettes smoked and the duration of smoking during the pregnancy (143–145). Cessation of tobacco use by the end of the second trimester reduces the risk of growth impairment (145,146). Fetal growth lag resulting from smoking is usually symmetric (147,148). Overall, infants of smokers have higher rates of perinatal mortality than infants of nonsmokers, but whether this is caused by the effect of tobacco use on fetal growth or by independent effects is not clear (149).

Growth restriction probably results from combined effects of carbon monoxide and nicotine. Carbon monoxide readily crosses the placenta and binds to hemoglobin; this reduces hemoglobin's oxygen-carrying capacity (150), and it increases hemoglobin's affinity for oxygen and thereby further decreases oxygen release to fetal tissues (142,151). Nicotine readily crosses the placenta, and fetal levels exceed maternal levels in several species, including humans (152). In an ovine model, uterine blood flow was reduced after nicotine infusion, probably as the result of increased catecholamines (153). Doppler velocimetry has been used to examine the effects of nicotine and carbon monoxide on human fetal and uterine circulations, with conflicting re-

TABLE 32.2. DRUGS ASSOCIATED WITH FETAL GROWTH RESTRICTION

Drugs of abuse
  Opiates
  Cocaine
  Amphetamines
  Phencyclidine
Anticonvulsants
  Phenylhydantoin
  Carbamazepine
  Trimethadione
β-Blocking agents
  Atenolol
  ?Inderol
Immunosuppressants
  Prednisone
  Azathioprine
Folic acid antagonists
  Methotrexate
  Aminopterin
Others
  Warfarin
  Antimetabolites

sults. Baseline umbilical artery and uterine artery resistance indices do not appear to be higher in smokers than in nonsmokers, even when birth weights and placental weights are lower (154).

Administration of nicotine or smoking a single cigarette increased maternal blood pressure and maternal and fetal heart rates in all studies. Bruner and Forouzan found a significant decrease in umbilical artery end-diastolic flow after smoking or nicotine gum chewing only in current smokers, not in nonsmokers or former smokers, and these investigators found no changes in uterine artery waveforms in any group (155). Castro et al. surprisingly found a decrease in uterine artery resistance indices when chronic smokers smoked two cigarettes in succession (156). Tulzer et al. found no changes in uterine artery resistance after smoking in normal pregnancies, but they did note a marked rise in one patient with labile hypertension (157). Swedish investigators studying the fetal circulation found no significant changes in flow velocity waveforms from the umbilical artery or the fetal descending aorta after gravid smokers chewed gum containing 4 mg of nicotine (158). However, smoking one cigarette did produce a decrease in end-diastolic velocity in the fetal descending aorta, a finding they attributed to the rise in fetal heart rate (159). Administration of nicotine to pregnant smokers produced dose-dependent increases in fetal aortic and umbilical venous flow and decreases in pulsatility indices from aorta and umbilical artery waveforms, whereas carbon monoxide had no effect (160). These findings appear to indicate that nicotine produces changes in the fetal central circulation, but not in peripheral resistance.

Smoking probably also affects fetal growth through other mechanisms. Maternal weight gain is decreased in smokers (154), a finding implying an altered nutrient supply. Nicotine may directly affect placental nutrient transport (104).

Alcohol

Jones et al. first described a syndrome of growth deficiency, mental retardation, and abnormal facies in children born to mothers with *chronic alcohol ingestion* (161). Central nervous system and cardiac defects are also more common in exposed children (90). The full-blown syndrome is usually seen in children of women with heavy alcohol use (3 ounces or more of absolute ethanol daily during pregnancy), but more subtle effects and moderate growth lag can occur at lower levels of exposure (162–164). Symmetric growth lag begins *in utero* but continues postnatally. Head growth may lag behind body growth. Human and animal studies show a dose-dependent reduction in growth, which remains significant after adjusting for smoking, maternal weight gain, and level of education (142,164,165). IUGR is not seen in women with brief early first trimester alcohol exposure (163). In women who have consumed alcohol on a long-term basis, reduction of alcohol use during the preg-

nancy may lessen the risk of fetal growth impairment (166–167).

Alcohol crosses the placenta readily, and fetal blood levels equal maternal levels. Alcohol levels in amniotic fluid rise and fall more slowly. For detoxification, the fetus relies on maternal alcohol dehydrogenase, because the level of this enzyme is extremely low in the fetal liver (142). In animals, ethanol has been shown to impair placental transfer of amino acids, folic acid, and glucose (168–173), and it interferes with protein synthesis (174,175). Many other metabolic disturbances have also been proposed to explain the growth restriction seen with alcohol exposure (142).

MANAGEMENT OF PREGNANCIES WITH FETAL GROWTH RESTRICTION

Detection

Some screening for fetal growth restriction is built into routine prenatal care. Careful assessment of menstrual history at the first prenatal visit, verification of dating with ultrasound in the first or second trimester, and systematic measurement of fundal growth and maternal weight gain at each prenatal visit are adequate surveillance methods for pregnancies without risk factors. In these low-risk pregnancies, ultrasound biometry is indicated when measured fundal height lags behind expected height by 3 cm or when there is a plateau in fundal growth regardless of measurement. Women with risk factors for IUGR resulting from placental insufficiency (Table 32.3), or obese women in whom fundal growth assessment is not accurate, warrant

TABLE 32.3. MATERNAL RISK FACTORS FOR FETAL GROWTH RESTRICTION

Low maternal weight or height
Poor maternal nutrition
Maternal medical disorders
  Chronic hypertension
  Chronic renal failure
  Systemic lupus erythematosus
  Hemoglobinopathies
  Cyanotic heart disease
  Pulmonary insufficiency
  Thyrotoxicosis
  Phenylketonuria
Tobacco, alcohol, or drug abuse
Occupation requiring heavy exertion or long periods of standing
Obstetric history
  Prior IUGR infant
  Preeclampsia in prior pregnancy
Current pregnancy complications
  Elevated maternal serum AFP
  Bleeding in pregnancy
  Multiple gestation
  Pregnancy-induced hypertension, preeclampsia
  Fetal anomalies

AFP, α-fetoprotein; IUGR, intrauterine growth retardation.

screening for IUGR as part of their routine care, beginning with an ultrasound scan to assess fetal growth and amniotic fluid volume at 26 to 28 weeks' gestation. Screening Doppler studies of the umbilical and uterine arteries should also be considered in a patient at risk for placental insufficiency, and abnormal results suggest that increased surveillance of fetal growth and well-being is indicated.

At a minimum, ultrasound biometry for suspected IUGR should include biparietal diameter, HC, AC, and FL. Fetal weight may be estimated from these measurements (13,14). However, the sensitivity of ultrasound biometry to detect IUGR is less than 50% in prospective studies in low-risk populations, and the false-positive rate is at least 10% (176). In addition to assessing whether fetal weight falls below the tenth percentile, indices of symmetry of growth (HC/AC, FL/AC) should be evaluated. Although one cannot reliably determine the cause of IUGR from the growth pattern, asymmetric growth is rarely seen in constitutionally small, well fetuses.

Evaluation

When an SGA fetus has been identified, the cause of the lagging growth should be explored. Maternal medical history, past obstetric history, family history of genetic disorders, use of drugs and medications, and exposures to infectious agents should all be reviewed. Evidence of preeclampsia should be sought, because IUGR can be its earliest presenting sign. Maternal anemia or nutritional deficits should be corrected, and use of substances such as tobacco or alcohol should be discontinued. If prescribed medications for chronic maternal disorders are thought responsible, alternatives can be considered, although discontinuation of the medication rarely produces catch-up growth once IUGR has been diagnosed.

Ultrasound can be used to obtain a detailed survey of fetal and placental anatomy, in addition to obtaining fetal measurements. Amniotic fluid index should be assessed. Oligohydramnios strongly suggests placental insufficiency, and it may be an indication for delivery. Doppler velocimetry, with assessment of umbilical, fetal, and uterine artery resistance indices, may confirm a diagnosis of compromised placentation if results are abnormal. Mild placental insufficiency can be present with initially normal Doppler findings, and aneuploidy can produce abnormal umbilical resistance indices.

The earlier the onset of growth lag, the more likely there is to be a fetal problem such as trisomy or fetal infection. Although at present our ability to treat fetal causes of IUGR effectively is limited, identifying congenital infections or malformations as the cause of growth restriction is important. Interventions directed at uteroplacental insufficiency—Doppler studies, nonstress tests, bed rest, or early delivery—are burdensome, expensive, and unhelpful if an intrinsic fetal abnormality is present. Counseling about recurrence risks and about management of future pregnancies is also altered once a diagnosis of a fetal anomaly or infection is made. When fetal infection is suspected, maternal serum for IgG and IgM titers to rubella, toxoplasmosis, and CMV should be obtained. If titers suggest recent infection, amniotic fluid should be cultured or assayed using polymerase chain reaction for infectious agents. Amniocentesis or cordocentesis to obtain a karyotype should be offered, depending on the gestational age. If umbilical cord blood is to be sampled for more rapid karyotyping, a fetal blood gas determination should also be obtained. However, cordocentesis simply to obtain a blood gas determination is rarely indicated because noninvasive testing can usually provide similar information (177–181), and cord blood sampling may precipitate bradycardia or fetal demise, especially in fetuses with already compromised circulations (182).

Delivery Timing and Tests of Fetal Well-Being

If no intrinsic fetal abnormality can be documented, and if dating of the pregnancy appears to be accurate, a working hypothesis that uteroplacental insufficiency is the cause of the slowed growth can be made, and fetal surveillance can be instituted to avoid stillbirth. Timely delivery, balancing the morbidity associated with prematurity against the risk of fetal demise, is the mainstay of management for the IUGR pregnancy. This balance tilts increasingly in the direction of delivery as gestation advances or as the severity of IUGR or fetal hypoxia increases. However, about two-thirds of fetuses with weights less than the tenth percentile will be constitutionally small and not at jeopardy.

Much investigative effort has been invested in finding a noninvasive test to determine accurately whether the intrauterine environment has become so inhospitable that delivery is indicated. Doppler velocimetry of the umbilical artery is useful to distinguish those fetuses with significantly increased placental resistance from those that may be constitutionally small. SGA fetuses with elevated umbilical artery resistance indices have been well demonstrated to have increased rates of stillbirth, nonreassuring fetal heart rate tracings in labor, and neonatal morbidity and mortality as compared with SGA fetuses with normal velocimetry (183). Including the results of umbilical artery Doppler studies in the management protocols of IUGR fetuses reduces perinatal mortality (52). Near term, fetuses discovered to have absent or reversed end-diastolic flow should be delivered. Remote from term, other tests reflecting more acute changes in fetal status are needed, because some fetuses with absent end-diastolic flow are not hypoxic (177). An ideal test would be noninvasive, with both high positive and high negative predictive values.

To assess acute fetal status, the nonstress tests and the

biophysical profile are commonly used in the United States. Both the nonstress test (177,178) and the biophysical profile (179,180) have been correlated with fetal cord blood gases, and both show good negative predictive abilities, although they have significant false-positive rates. Other modalities not yet in wide use, such as computerized assessment of fetal heart rate variability and Doppler assessment of the umbilical venous or intrafetal circulation, may prove better able to pinpoint the appropriate time for delivery for SGA fetuses remote from term.

Computer-aided assessment of short-term heart rate variability or *variation* has been shown to be a more sensitive and more specific indicator of fetal asphyxia than the traditional nonstress test. Reduction of computer-assessed fetal heart rate variation has been consistently associated with hypoxemia and acidemia on cordocentesis (179). Serial studies of computer-assessed short-term heart rate variation in IUGR fetuses have demonstrated a gradual decrease in fetal heart rate variation that precedes the appearance of decelerations (184,185). A prospective study is under way to determine the level at which reduced fetal heart rate variation should become an indication for delivery (182).

Pulsed Doppler assessment of fetal redistribution of blood flow and fetal echocardiography may also provide more refined assessment of degrees of fetal compromise than umbilical velocimetry alone. Because they require sophisticated sonography and expensive ultrasound equipment not readily available to most obstetricians, these tools are not yet widely used clinically.

Other Interventions

Aside from timely delivery, no interventions for uteroplacental insufficiency have yet been shown to improve growth or to reduce morbidity in SGA human fetuses. Suggested treatments, including novel approaches such as intraamniotic nutritional supplements, maternal hyperoxygenation, and intermittent abdominal "decompression," have been reviewed (186,187). A few of the therapies more commonly offered for the amelioration or prevention of IUGR resulting from placental insufficiency are discussed here.

Aspirin

Because of its potential to inactivate cyclooxygenase and thereby to decrease synthesis of the vasoconstrictor thromboxane relative to the vasodilator prostacyclin, aspirin was thought to have potential to treat or to prevent IUGR. Aspirin's ability to reduce platelet aggregation could also be beneficial (188). Initially, several small randomized trials of low-dose aspirin suggested a beneficial effect, with higher birth weights and a lower incidence of IUGR in the treated women. One group of investigators compared aspirin with placebo used prophylactically beginning in the second trimester in women with prior histories of IUGR or preeclampsia (189). Another group randomized patients after uteroplacental insufficiency was diagnosed, based on elevated umbilical artery resistance indices (190).

In response to these promising results, several larger trials were implemented that did not show a statistically significant benefit. Newnham and colleagues (191), in a study with a design similar to that of the study reported by Trudinger et al., randomized 51 patients but found no differences in birth weight, ponderal index, or neonatal morbidity between treated patients and control pregnancies. Several large multicenter trials enrolled patients at increased risk of IUGR or gestational hypertension for randomization to placebo or low-dose aspirin at a wide range of gestational ages and also failed to demonstrate a significant reduction in IUGR (192,193). The National Institute of Child Health and Development Maternal-Fetal Medicine network trial of prophylactic low-dose aspirin begun in the second trimester in low-risk women also found no significant differences (n = 3,135); the incidence of IUGR was 5.8% in the placebo group and 4.6% in the treated group (194). These large trials had broad enrollment criteria, differing aspirin doses, and differing gestational ages at treatment onset. Their negative results do not exclude the possibility that low-dose aspirin may benefit selected patients at risk of IUGR, for example, patients with hypercoaguable conditions. One metaanalysis of 13 randomized trials published since 1985 found a significant reduction in IUGR (odds ratio 0.35; 95% confidence interval, 0.21 to 0.58) among women whose aspirin treatment began before the seventeenth week of gestation (195). Development of cyclooxygenase inhibitors more selective than aspirin is under way, but it will take many years to see whether these agents will prove more effective.

Maternal Nutritional Supplementation

Supplementing maternal diets with a balanced increase in protein and calories may have a beneficial effect on fetal growth, especially in underprivileged populations (186). However, one study of the effects of high-protein supplementation surprisingly showed an increase in the rate of SGA infants (196). Dietary enrichment of specific nutrients may promote fetal growth. For example, in a small randomized controlled study, zinc supplementation of women with at-risk pregnancies significantly decreased the incidence of SGA infants in the treated group (197). Another interesting proposed nutritional intervention to promote fetal growth is the consumption of fish oil, which may decrease levels of thromboxane relative to prostacyclin in the uteroplacental or fetal circulations (198). Although the use of various dietary supplements has produced larger birth weights or fewer SGA fetuses in controlled trials, no evidence indicates that maternal nutritional supplementation can reverse IUGR once it is established.

Bed Rest

Based on the hypothesis that rest in lateral recumbent position promotes uteroplacental blood flow, bed rest is commonly prescribed when IUGR is suspected. Data to support the beneficial effects of this approach are lacking, but few studies have been undertaken (187). One trial found no benefit in 107 patients randomized to hospital bed rest versus outpatient management in the third trimester after ultrasound diagnosis of IUGR (199).

INTRAPARTUM MANAGEMENT

In idiopathic IUGR, delivery is indicated once fetal lung maturity can be expected to be present, or when fetal testing is no longer reassuring. Although vaginal delivery can often be achieved, continuous intrapartum monitoring is necessary. If placental reserve is lacking, the fetus may decompensate rapidly when uterine contractions further decrease intervillous flow. When amniotic fluid is low or when end-diastolic flow in the umbilical arteries is absent or reversed, the fetus is likely to be hypoxemic and acidemic, and a cesarean section is often necessary (43,177).

SUMMARY

Clinically detectable growth delay is a late sequela of earlier pathologic processes. The diagnosis of growth restriction is always made long after these processes begin, and it is often impossible to pinpoint the cause. Doppler velocimetry has improved our ability to identify placental insufficiency and fetal compensatory mechanisms. Because more than half of fetuses smaller than the tenth percentile are constitutionally small and are otherwise healthy, and because ultrasound estimates of fetal weight are not always accurate, many fetuses labeled IUGR do not need any intervention. When the cause is placental insufficiency, fetal surveillance and early delivery decrease the incidence of stillbirth. Data to determine whether early elective delivery substantially reduces long-term morbidity continue to be limited. Interventions to promote better growth of the fetus still *in utero* remain experimental.

10 KEY POINTS

1. IUGR has heterogeneous causes; appropriate interventions and perinatal outcomes vary with the cause. Clinically detectable growth delay is often a late consequence of early pathologic processes that are difficult to reverse by the time they can be identified.

2. Although perinatal mortality rates for SGA infants are higher than for infants of normal size, most infants with weights less than the tenth percentile are constitutionally small and require no intervention.

3. Fetal chromosomal abnormalities, mendelian disorders, malformations, and congenital infections can slow fetal growth and should be sought, especially when fetal growth lags before 28 weeks' gestation.

4. Perinatal mortality is high when fetal abnormalities cause IUGR, but obstetric interventions have little effect on outcome in these cases.

5. Impaired nutrient and oxygen delivery to the fetus (placental insufficiency) is the most common cause of stillbirths associated with IUGR, and it is present in about 15% of pregnancies characterized by slow fetal growth. When placental insufficiency is present, timely delivery may prevent stillbirth and may allow catch-up growth *ex utero*.

6. Abnormalities in blood vessel number and caliber are found in the placental bed and the villous vascular tree in pregnancies with placental insufficiency.

7. The fetus compensates for hypoxia and nutritional deprivation by altering the distribution of flow of oxygenated blood to favor vital organs such as the heart, brain, and adrenal glands at the expense of growth of the rest of the body and fuel storage in the liver and subcutaneous fat.

8. Both placental abnormalities and compensatory fetal circulatory changes can be detected using Doppler velocimetry, the results of which may be abnormal before growth lag is present.

9. Abnormal placental implantation predisposes to preeclampsia as well as to IUGR; when one is found, the other should be sought.

10. IUGR may recur in subsequent pregnancies or within families, a finding suggesting genetically determined predisposing factors that are beginning to be elucidated.

REFERENCES

1. McBurney RD. The undernourished full term infant: case report. *West J Surg* 1947;55:363.
2. Warkany JB, Monroe BB, Sutherland BS. Intrauterine growth retardation. *Am J Dis Child* 1961;102:249–279.
3. Gruenewald P. Chronic fetal distress and placental insufficiency. *Biol Neonate* 1963;5:215.
4. Wolfe HM, Gross TL. Increased risk to the growth retarded fetus. In: Gross TM, Sokol RJ eds. *Intrauterine growth retardation.* Chicago: Year Book, 1989:111.
5. Low JA, Boston RW, Pancham SR. Fetal asphyxia during the intrapartum period in intrauterine growth-retarded infants. *Am J Obstet Gynecol* 1972;113:351–357.
6. Barker DJP, Osmond C, Golding J, et al. Growth *in utero*, blood pressure in childhood and adult life, and mortality from cardiovascular disease. *BMJ* 1989;298:564–567.

7. Barker DJP, Gluckman PD, Godfrey KM, et al. Fetal nutrition and cardiovascular disease in adult life. *Lancet* 1993;341:938–941.

8. Gluckman PD, Harding JE. Fetal growth retardation: underlying endocrine mechanisms and postnatal consequences. *Acta Paediatr Suppl* 1997;422:69–72.

9. Kjellmer I, Liedholm M, Sultan B, et al. Long-term effects of intrauterine growth retardation. *Acta Paediatr* 1997;422:83–84.

10. Sparks JW, Ross JC, Cetin I. Intrauterine growth and nutrition, In: Polin RA and Fox WW, eds. *Fetal and neonatal physiology*, 2nd ed. Philadelphia: WB Saunders, 1998:267–290.

11. Lubchenco LO, Hansman C, Dressler M, et al. Intrauterine growth as estimated from liveborn birthweight data at 24 to 42 weeks of gestation. *Pediatrics* 1963;32:793.

12. Brenner WE, Edelman DA, Hendricks CH. A standard of fetal growth for the United States of America. *Am J Obstet Gynecol* 1976;126:555–564.

13. Shepard MJ, Richards VA, Berkowitz RL, et al. An evaluation of two equations for predicting fetal weight by ultrasound. *Am J Obstet Gynecol* 1982;142:47–54.

14. Hadlock FP, Harrist RB, Carpenter RJ, et al. Sonographic estimation of fetal weight. *Radiology* 1984;150:535–540.

15. Miller HC, Hassanein K. Diagnosis of impaired fetal growth in newborn infants. *Pediatrics* 1971;48:511–522.

16. Villar J, de Onis M, Kestler E, et al. The differential neonatal morbidity of the intrauterine growth retardation syndrome. *Am J Obstet Gynecol* 1990;163:151–157.

17. Hadlock FP, Deter RL, Harrist RB, et al. A date-independent predictor of IUGR: femur length:abdominal circumference ratio. *Am J Roentgenol* 1983;141:979–984.

18. Gluckman PD, Harding JE. The physiology and pathophysiology of intrauterine growth retardation. *Horm Res* 1997;48 [Suppl 1]:11–16.

19. Zhou Y, Damsky CH, Chiu K, et al. Preeclampsia is associated with abnormal expression of adhesion molecules by invasive cytotrophoblasts. *J Clin Invest* 1993;91:950–960.

20. Inoue I, Rohrwasser A, Helin C, et al. A mutation of angiotensinogen in a patient with preeclampsia leads to altered kinetics of the renin-angiotensin system. *J Biol Chem* 1995;270:11430–11436.

21. Morgan T, Craven C, Nelson L, et al. Angiotensinogen T235 expression is elevated in decidual spiral arteries. *J Clin Invest* 1997;100:1406–1415.

22. Ghidini A. Idiopathic fetal growth restriction: a pathophysiologic approach. *Obstet Gynecol Surv* 1996;51:376–382.

23. Cunningham FG, MacDonald PC, Gant NF, et al. Maternal adaptations to pregnancy. In: Cunningham FG, MacDonald PC, Gant NF, et al., eds. *Williams obstetrics,* 20th ed. Stamford CT: Appleton & Lange, 1997:191–225.

24. Ramsay E, Harris HWS. Comparison of uteroplacental vasculature and circulation in the rhesus monkey and man. In: *Contributions to embryology*, no. 261. Washington, DC: Carnegie Institution of Washington, 1966;38:59.

25. Brosens I, Robertson WB, Dixon HG. The role of the spiral arteries in the pathogenesis of preeclampsia. *Obstet Gynecol Annu* 1972;1:171–191.

26. Campbell S, Griffin DR, Pearce JM, et al. New Doppler technique for assessing uteroplacental blood flow. *Lancet* 1983;1:675–677.

27. Campbell S, Bewley S, Cohen-Overbeek TC. Investigation of the uteroplacental circulation by Doppler ultrasound. *Semin Perinatol* 1987;11:362–368.

28. Fleischer A, Schulman H, Farmakides G, et al. Uterine artery Doppler velocimetry in pregnant women with hypertension. *Am J Obstet Gynecol* 1986;154:806–813.

29. Creasy RK, Barrett CT, de Swiet M, et al. Experimental intra-

30. uterine growth retardation in the sheep. *Am J Obstet Gynecol* 1972;112:566–573.

30. Clapp JF, Szeto HH, Larrow R, et al. Umbilical blood flow response to embolization of the uterine circulation. *Am J Obstet Gynecol* 1980;138:60–67.

31. Cohn HE, Jackson BT, Piasecki GJ, et al. Fetal cardiovascular responses to asphyxia induced by decreased uterine perfusion. *J Dev Physiol* 1985;7:289–297.

32. Ogata ES, Bussey ME, Finley S. Altered gas exchange, limited glucose and branched chain amino acids, and hypoinsulinism retard fetal growth in the rat. *Metabolism* 1986;35:970–977.

33. Brosens I, Dixon HG, Robertson WB. Fetal growth retardation and the arteries of the placental bed. *Br J Obstet Gynaecol* 1977;84:656–663.

34. De Wolf F, Brosens I, Renaer M. Fetal growth retardation and the maternal arterial supply of the human placenta in the absence of sustained hypertension. *Br J Obstet Gynaecol* 1980;87:678–685.

35. Sheppard BL, Bonnar J. An ultrastructural study of uteroplacental spiral arteries in hypertensive and normotensive pregnancy and fetal growth retardation. *Br J Obstet Gynaecol* 1981;88:695–705.

36. Gerretsen G, Huisjes HJ, Elema JD. Morphological changes of the spiral arteries in the placental bed in relation to preeclampsia and fetal growth retardation. *Br J Obstet Gynaecol* 1981;88:876–881.

37. Khong TY, De Wolf F, Robertson WB, et al. Inadequate maternal vascular response to placentation in pregnancies complicated by preeclampsia and by small for gestational age infants. *Br J Obstet Gynaecol* 1986;93:1049–1059.

38. Olofsson P, Laurini RN, Marsal K. A high uterine pulsatility index reflects a defective development of placental bed spiral arteries in pregnancies complicated by hypertension and fetal growth retardation. *Eur J Obstet Gynecol Reprod Biol* 1993;49:161–168.

39. Trudinger BJ, Giles WB, Cook CM. Uteroplacental blood flow velocity-time waveforms in normal and complicated pregnancy. *Br J Obstet Gynaecol* 1985;92:39–45.

40. Trudinger BJ, Giles WB, Cook CM. Flow velocity waveforms in the maternal uteroplacental and fetal umbilical placental circulations. *Am J Obstet Gynecol* 1985;152:155–163.

41. Bewley S, Cooper D, Campbell S. Doppler investigation of uteroplacental blood flow resistance in the second trimester: a screening study for pre-eclampsia and intrauterine growth retardation. *Br J Obstet Gynaecol* 1991;98:871–879.

42. Harrington KF, Campbell S, Bewley S, et al. Doppler velocimetry studies of the uterine artery in the early prediction of pre-eclampsia and intrauterine growth retardation. *Eur J Obstet Gynecol Reprod Biol* 1991;42:S14–S20.

43. Trudinger BJ, Giles WB, Cook CM, et al. Fetal umbilical artery flow velocity waveforms and placental resistance: clinical significance. *Br J Obstet Gynaecol* 1985;92:23–30.

44. Morrow RJ, Adamson SL, Bull SB, et al. Effect of placental embolization on the umbilical arterial velocity waveform in fetal sheep. *Am J Obstet Gynecol* 1989;161:1055–1060.

45. Trudinger BJ, Stevens D, Connelly A, et al. Umbilical artery flow velocity waveforms and placental resistance: the effects of embolization of the umbilical circulation. *Am J Obstet Gynecol* 1987;157:1443–1448.

46. Giles WB, Trudinger BJ, Baird PJ. Fetal umbilical artery flow velocity waveforms and placental resistance: pathological correlation. *Br J Obstet Gynaecol* 1985;92:31–38.

47. McCowan LM, Mullen BM, Ritchie K. Umbilical artery flow velocity waveforms and the placental vascular bed. *Am J Obstet Gynecol* 1987;157:900–902.

48. Bracero LA, Beneck D, Kirshenbaum N, et al. Doppler velo-

cimetry and placental disease. *Am J Obstet Gynecol* 1989;161: 388–393.

49. Teasdale F. Idiopathic intrauterine growth retardation: histomorphometry of the human placenta. *Placenta* 1984;5:83–92.

50. Hitschold T, Weiss E, Beck T, et al. Low target birthweight or growth retardation? Umbilical Doppler flow velocity waveforms and histometric analysis of the fetoplacenta vascular tree. *Am J Obstet Gynecol* 1993;168:1260–1264.

51. Jackson M, Walsh AJ, Morrow RJ, et al. Reduced placental villous tree elaboration in small-for-gestational-age pregnancies: relationship with umbilical artery Doppler waveforms. *Am J Obstet Gynecol* 1995;172:518–525.

52. Alfirevic Z, Neilson JP. Doppler ultrasonography in high risk pregnancies: systematic review with meta-analysis. *Am J Obstet Gynecol* 1995;172:1371–1387.

53. Ley D, Laurin J, Marsal K. Abnormal fetal aortic velocity waveform and minor neurological dysfunction at 7 years of age. *Ultrasound Obstet Gynecol* 1996;8:152–159.

54. Cohn HE, Sacks EJ, Heymann MA, et al. Cardiovascular responses to hypoxemia and acidemia in fetal lambs. *Am J Obstet Gynecol* 1974;120:817–824.

55. Peeters LLH, Sheldon RE, Jones MD, et al. Blood flow to fetal organs as a function of arterial oxygen content. *Am J Obstet Gynecol* 1979;135:637–646.

56. Teitel DF. Physiologic development of the cardiovascular system in the fetus. In: Polin RA, Fox WW, eds. *Fetal and neonatal physiology,* 2nd ed. Philadelphia: WB Saunders, 1998:827–836.

57. Behrman R, Lee MH, Peterson EN, et al. Distribution of the circulation in the normal and asphyxiated fetal primate. *Am J Obstet Gynecol* 1970;108:956–969.

58. Thornburg KL. Fetal response to intrauterine stress. In: The childhood environment and adult disease. *CIBA Found Symp* 1997;156:17–37.

59. Sukumar M, Morin FC. Response of the fetal circulation to stress. In: Polin RA, Fox WW, eds. *Fetal and neonatal physiology,* 2nd ed. Philadelphia: WB Saunders, 1998:1014–1022.

60. Wladimiroff JW, Tonge HM, Stewart PA. Doppler ultrasound assessment of cerebral blood flow in the human fetus. *Br J Obstet Gynaecol* 1986;93:471–475.

61. Vyas S, Nicolaides KH, Bower S, et al. Middle cerebral artery flow velocity waveforms in fetal hypoxemia. *Br J Obstet Gynaecol* 1990;97:797–803.

62. Mari G, Deter RL. Middle cerebral artery flow velocity waveforms in normal and small-for-gestational-age fetuses. *Am J Obstet Gynecol* 1992;166:1262–1270.

63. Baschat AA, Gembruch U, Reiss I, et al. Demonstration of fetal coronary blood flow by Doppler ultrasound in relation to arterial and venous flow velocimetry waveforms and perinatal outcome: the "heart-sparing effect." *Ultrasound Obstet Gynecol* 1997;9: 162–172.

64. van Splunder P, Stijnen T, Wladimiroff JW. Fetal atrioventricular, venous, and arterial waveforms in the SGA fetus. *Pediatr Res* 1997;42:765–775.

65. Boyd PA, Scott A. Quantitative structural studies on human placentas associated with pre-eclampsia, essential hypertension, and intrauterine growth retardation. *Br J Obstet Gynaecol* 1985; 92:714–721.

66. Varma TR. Fetal growth and placental function in patients with placenta previa. *J Obstet Gynaecol Br Commonw* 1973;80: 311–315.

67. Creasy RK, Resnik R. Intrauterine growth restriction. In: Creasy RK, Resnik R, eds. *Maternal-fetal medicine: principles and practice,* 3rd ed. Philadelphia: WB Saunders, 1994:558–574.

68. Cantazarite VA, Hendricks SK, Maida C. Prenatal diagnosis of the two-vessel cord: implications for patient counselling and

obstetric management. *Ultrasound Obstet Gynecol* 1995;5:98–105.

69. Rushton DI. Pathology of the placenta. In: Wigglesworth JS, Singer DB, eds. *Textbook of fetal and perinatal pathology,* vol 1. Boston: Blackwell Scientific, 1991:161–219.

70. Benirschke K, Kaufmann P. *Pathology of the human placenta.* New York: Springer Verlag, 1990.

71. Redline RW. Placental pathology: a neglected link between basic disease mechanisms and untoward pregnancy outcome. *Curr Opin Obstet Gynecol* 1995;7:10–15.

72. Labarrere C, Manni J, Salas P, et al. Intrauterine growth retardation of unknown etiology. I. Serum complement and circulating immune complexes in mothers and infants. *Am J Reprod Immunol Microbiol* 1985;8:87–93.

73. Labarrere C, Althabe O, Telenta M. Chronic villitis of unknown aetiology in placentae of idiopathic small for gestational age infants. *Placenta* 1982;3:309– 317.

74. Redline RW, Patterson P. Villitis of unknown etiology is associated with major infiltration of fetal tissue by maternal inflammatory cells. *Am J Pathol* 1993;143:473–479.

75. Redline RW, Patterson P. Patterns of placental injury: correlations with gestational age, placental weight, and clinical diagnosis. *Arch Pathol Lab Med* 1994;118:698–701.

76. Salafia CM, Ernst LM, Pezzullo JC, et al. The very low birthweight infant: maternal complications leading to preterm birth, placental lesions, and intrauterine growth restriction. *Am J Perinatol* 1985;12:106–110.

77. Labarrere C, Althabe OH. Intrauterine growth retardation of unknown etiology. II. Serum complement and circulating immune complexes in maternal sera and their relationship with parity and chronic villitis. *Am J Reprod Immunol Microbiol* 1986; 12:4–6.

78. Kalousek DK, Howard-Peebles PN, Olson SB, et al. Confirmation of CVS mosaicism in term placentae and high frequency of intrauterine growth retardation association with confined placental mosaicism. *Prenat Diagn* 1991;11:743–750.

79. Wolstenholme J, Rooney DE, Davison EV. Confined placental mosaicism, IUGR, and adverse pregnancy outcome: a controlled retrospective U.K. collaborative survey. *Prenat Diagn* 1994;14: 345–361.

80. Bennett P, Vaughan J, Henderson D, et al. Association between confined placental trisomy, fetal uniparental disomy, and early intrauterine growth retardation. *Lancet* 1992;340:1284–1285.

81. Wilkins-Haug L, Roberts DJ, Morton CC. Confined placental mosaicism and intrauterine growth retardation: a case control analysis of placentas at delivery. *Am J Obstet Gynecol* 1995; 172:44–50.

82. Crane JP, Cheung SW. An embryonic model to explain cytogenetic inconsistencies observed in chorionic villi versus fetal tissue. *Prenat Diagn* 1988;8:119–129.

83. Kalousek DK, Langlois S, Barrett I, et al. Uniparental disomy for chromosome 16 in humans. *Am J Hum Genet* 1993;52:8–16.

84. Robinson WP, Barrett IJ, Bernard L, et al. Meiotic origin of trisomy in confined placental mosaicism is correlated with presence of fetal uniparental disomy, high levels of trisomy in trophoblast, and increased risk of fetal intrauterine growth restriction. *Am J Hum Genet* 1997;60:917–927.

85. Schwinger E, Seidl E, Klink F, et al. Chromosome mosaicism of the placenta: a cause of developmental failure of the fetus? *Prenat Diagn* 1989;9:639–647.

86. Schreck RR, Falik-Borenstein Z, Hirata G. Chromosomal mosaicism in chorionic villus sampling. *Clin Perinatol* 1990;17:867–868.

87. Kuhlmann RS, Werner AL, Abramowicz J, et al. Placental histology in fetuses between 18 and 23 weeks gestation with abnormal karyotype. *Am J Obstet Gynecol* 1990;163:1264–1270.

88. Rochelson B, Kaplan C, Guzman E, et al. A quantitative analysis of placental vasculature in the third trimester fetus with autosomal trisomy. *Obstet Gynecol* 1990;75:59–63.

89. Eydoux P, Choiset A, Le Porrier N, et al. Chromosomal prenatal diagnosis: study of 936 cases of intrauterine abnormalities after ultrasound assessment. *Prenat Diagn* 1989;9:255–269.

90. Jones KL. *Smith's recognizable patterns of human malformations,* 5th ed. Philadelphia: WB Saunders, 1997.

91. Crawford RA, Ryan G, Wright V, et al. The importance of serial biophysical assessment of fetal well-being in gastroschisis. *Br J Obstet Gynaecol* 1992;99:899–902.

92. Institute of Medicine Committee on Nutritional Status during Pregnancy and Lactation, National Academy of Sciences. *Nutrition during pregnancy.* Washington, DC: National Academy Press, 1990.

93. Abrams B, Newman V. Small for gestational age birth: maternal predictors and comparison with risk factors of spontaneous preterm delivery in same cohort. *Am J Obstet Gynecol* 1991; 164:785–790.

94. Antonov AN. Children born during the seige of Leningrad in 1942. *J Pediatr* 1947;30:250.

95. Stein Z, Susser M. The Dutch famine, 1944–1945, and the reproductive process. I. Effects on six indices at birth. *Pediatr Res* 1975;9:70–75.

96. Stein Z, Susser M. The Dutch famine, 1944–1945, and the reproductive process. II. Interrelations of caloric rations and six indices at birth. *Pediatr Res* 1975;9:76–83.

97. Goldenberg RL, Tamura T, Cliver SP, et al. Serum folate and fetal growth retardation: a matter of compliance? *Obstet Gynecol* 1992;79:719–722.

98. Meadows NJ, Ruse W, Smith MF, et al. Zinc and small babies. *Lancet* 1981;2:1135–1137.

99. Wells JL, James DK, Luxton R, et al. Maternal leucocyte zinc deficiency at start of third trimester as a predictor of fetal growth retardation. *BMJ* 1987;294:1054–1056.

100. Sparks JW, Hay WW, Meschia G, et al. Partition of maternal nutrients to the placenta and fetus in the sheep. *Eur J Obstet Gynaecol Reprod Biol* 1983;14:331–340.

101. Bozzetti P, Ferrari MM, Marconi AM, et al. The relationship of maternal and fetal glucose concentrations in the human from midgestation until term. *Metabolism* 1988;37:358–363.

102. Marconi AM, Paolini C, Buscaglia M, et al. The impact of gestational age and fetal growth on the maternal-fetal glucose concentration difference. *Obstet Gynecol* 1996;87:937–942.

103. Moe AJ. Placental amino acid transport. *Am J Physiol* 1995; 268:C1321–1331.

104. Malandro MS, Beveridge MJ, Kilberg MS, et al. Effect of low-protein diet-induced intrauterine growth retardation on rat placental amino acid transport. *Am J Physiol* 1996;271:C295–C303.

105. Cetin I, Marconi AM, Bozzetti P, et al. Umbilical amino acid concentrations in appropriate and small for gestational age infants: a biochemical difference present *in utero. Am J Obstet Gynecol* 1988;158:120–126.

106. Economides DL, Nicolaides KH, Gahl WA, et al. Plasma amino acids in appropriate and small-for-gestational age fetuses. *Am J Obstet Gynecol* 1989;161:1219–1227.

107. Malandro MS, Beveridge MJ, Kilberg MS, et al. Ontogeny of cationic amino acid transport systems in rat placenta. *Am J Physiol* 1994;267:C804–C811.

108. Dicke JM, Henderson GI. Placental amino acid uptake in normal and complicated pregnancies. *Am J Med Sci* 1988;295: 223–227.

109. Cetin I, Corbetta C, Sereni LP, et al. Umbilical amino acid concentrations in normal and growth retarded fetuses sampled *in utero* by cordocentesis. *Am J Obstet Gynecol* 1990;162: 253–261.

110. Bassett NS, Oliver MH, Breier BH, et al. The effect of maternal starvation on plasma insulin-like growth factor I concentrations in the late gestation ovine fetus. *Pediatr Res* 1990;27:401–404.

111. Jones CT, Gu W, Harding JE, et al. Studies on the growth of the fetal sheep: effects of surgical reduction in placental size, or experimental manipulation of uterine blood flow on plasma sulphation promoting activity and on the concentration of insulin-like growth factors I and II. *J Dev Physiol* 1988;10:179–189.

112. Oliver MH, Harding JE, Breier BH, et al. Glucose but not a mixed amino acid infusion regulates IGF-I concentrations in fetal sheep. *Pediatr Res* 1993;34:62–65.

113. Harding JE, Liu L, Evans PC, et al. Insulin-like growth factor-1 alters feto-placental protein and carbohydrate metabolism in fetal sheep. *Endocrinology* 1994;134:1509–1514.

114. Liu JP, Baker J, Perkins AS, et al. Mice carrying null mutations of the genes encoding insulin-like growth factor I (IGF-I) and type I IGF receptor (IGF-IR). *Cell* 1993;75:59–72.

115. Lassare C, Hardouin S, Daffos F, et al. Serum insulin-like growth factors and insulin-like growth factor binding proteins in the human fetus: relationships with growth in normal subjects and in subjects with intrauterine growth retardation. *Pediatr Res* 1991;29:219–225.

116. Leger J, Oury JF, Noel M, et al. Growth factors and intrauterine growth retardation. I. Serum growth hormone, IGF I, IGF-II and IGF binding protein 3 levels in normally grown and growth-retarded human fetuses during the second half of gestation. *Pediatr Res* 1996;40:94–100.

117. Alsat E, Marcotty C, Gabriel R, et al. Molecular approach to intrauterine growth retardation: an overview of recent data. *Reprod Fertil Dev* 1995;7:1457–1464.

118. Levitt-Katz LE, Cohen P. Growth factor regulation of fetal growth. In: Polin RA, Fox WW, eds. *Fetal and neonatal physiology,* 2nd ed. Philadelphia: WB Saunders, 1998.

119. Klein JO, Remington JS. Current concepts of infections of the fetus and newborn infant. In: Remington JS, Klein JO, eds. *Infectious disease of the fetus and newborn infant,* 4th ed. Philadelphia: WB Saunders, 1995:1–19.

120. Naeye RL. Fetal growth with congenital syphilis. *Am J Clin Pathol* 1971;55:228–231.

121. Gibbs RS, Sweet RL. Maternal and fetal infections: clinical disorders. In: Creasy RK, Resnik R, eds. *Maternal-fetal medicine: principles and practice,* 3rd ed. Philadelphia: WB Saunders, 1994: 639–703.

122. Stagno S, Pass RF, Dworsky ME, et al. Congenital cytomegalovirus infection: the relative importance of primary and recurrent maternal infection. *N Engl J Med* 1982;306:945–949.

123. Fowler KB, Stagno S, Pass RF, et al. The outcome of congenital cytomegalovirus infection in relation to maternal antibody status. *N Engl J Med* 1992;326:663–667.

124. Boppana S, Pass RF, Britt WS, et al. Symptomatic congenital cytomegalovirus infection: neonatal morbidity and mortality. *Pediatr Infect Dis* 1992;11:93–99.

125. Naeye RL. Cytomegalovirus disease: the fetal disorder. *Am J Clin Pathol* 1967;47:738–744.

126. Stagno S, Pass RF, Cloud G, et al. Primary cytomegalovirus infection in pregnancy: incidence, transmission to fetus, and clinical outcome. *JAMA* 1986;256:1904–1908.

127. Grose C, Weiner CP. Prenatal diagnosis of congenital cytomegalovirus infection: two decades later. *Am J Obstet Gynecol* 1990; 163:447–450.

128. Lynch L, Daffos F, Emmanuel D, et al. Prenatal diagnosis of fetal cytomegalovirus infection. *Am J Obstet Gynecol* 1991;165: 714–718.

129. Lamy ME, Mulongo KN, Gadisseux JF, et al. Prenatal diagnosis

of fetal cytomegalovirus infection. *Am J Obstet Gynecol* 1992; 166:91–94.

130. Remington J, McLeod R, Desmonts G. Toxoplasmosis. In: Remington JS, Klein JO, eds. *Infectious disease of the fetus and newborn infant,* 4th ed. Philadelphia: WB Saunders, 1995:140–265.

131. Couvreur J, Desmonts G, Tournier G, et al. Etude d'une série homogène de 210 cases de toxoplamose congenitale chez des nourrisons agé de 0 de 11 mois et depistes de façon prospective. *Ann Pediatr (Paris)* 1984;31:815–819.

132. Hohlfeld P, MacAleese J, Capella-Pavlovski M, et al. Fetal toxoplasmosis: ultrasonographic signs. *Ultrasound Obstet Gynecol* 1991;1:241–244.

133. Daffos F, Forestier F, Capella-Pavlovsky M, et al. Prenatal management of 746 pregnancies at risk for congenital toxoplasmosis. *N Engl J Med* 1988;31:271–275.

134. Grover CM, Thulliez P, Remington JS, et al. Rapid prenatal diagnosis of congenital toxoplasmosis infection using polymerase chain reaction and amniotic fluid. *J Clin Microbiol* 1990; 28:2297–2301.

135. Hohlfeld P, Daffos F, Costa J-M, et al. Prenatal diagnosis of congenital toxoplasmosis with a polymerase chain reaction test on amniotic fluid. *N Engl J Med* 1994;331:695–699.

136. Hezard N, Marx-Chemla C, Foudrinier F, et al. Prenatal diagnosis of congenital toxoplasmosis in 261 pregnancies. *Prenat Diagn* 1997;17:1047–1054.

137. Fricker-Hidalgo H, Pelloux H, Muet F, et al. Prenatal diagnosis of congenital toxoplasmosis: comparative value of fetal blood and amniotic fluid using serologic techniques and cultures. *Prenat Diagn* 1997;17:831–835.

138. Cooper LZ, Preblud SR, Alford CA. Rubella. In: Remington JS, Klein JO eds. *Infectious disease of the fetus and newborn infant,* 4th ed. Philadelphia: WB Saunders, 1995:268–311.

139. Mann JM, Preblud SR, Hoffman RE, et al. Assessing risks of rubella infection. *JAMA* 1981;245:1647–1652.

140. Bart SW, Stetler HC, Preblud SR, et al. Fetal risk associated with rubella vaccine: an update. *Rev Infect Dis* 1985;7:S95–S102.

141. Briggs GG, Freeman RK, Yaffe SJ. *Drugs in pregnancy and lactation: a reference guide to fetal and neonatal risk,* 5th ed. Baltimore: Williams & Wilkins, 1998.

142. Andres RL, Jones KL. Social and illicit drug use in pregnancy. In: Creasy RK, Resnik R, eds. *Maternal-fetal medicine: principles and practice,* 3rd ed. Philadelphia: WB Saunders, 1994:182–198.

143. Meyer MB, Jonas BS, Tonascia JA. Perinatal events associated with maternal smoking during pregnancy. *Am J Epidemiol* 1976; 103:464–476.

144. Abell TD, Baker LC, Ramsey CN. The effects of maternal smoking on infant birthweight. *Fam Med* 1991;23:103–107.

145. Lieberman E, Gremy I, Lang JM, et al. Low birthweight at term and the timing of fetal exposure to maternal smoking. *Am J Public Health* 1994;84:1127–1131.

146. MacArthur C, Knox EG. Smoking and pregnancy: effects of stopping at different stages. *Br J Obstet Gynaecol* 1988;95:551–555.

147. Miller HC, Hassanein K. Maternal smoking and fetal growth of full-term infants. *Pediatr Res* 1974;8:960–963.

148. Wen SW, Goldenberg RL, Cutter GR, et al. Smoking, maternal age, fetal growth and gestational age at delivery. *Am J Obstet Gynecol* 1990;162:53–58.

149. English PB, Eshkenazi B. Reinterpreting the effects of maternal smoking on infant birthweight and perinatal mortality: a multivariate approach to birthweight standardization. *Int J Epidemiol* 1992;21:1097–1105.

150. Astrup P. Some physiological and pathological effects of moderate carbon monoxide exposure. *BMJ* 1972;4:447–452.

151. Longo LD. The biological effects of carbon monoxide on the pregnant woman, fetus and newborn. *Am J Obstet Gynecol* 1977; 129:69–103.

152. Luck W, Nau H, Hansen R, et al. Extent of nicotine and cotinine transfer to the human fetus, placenta, and amniotic fluid of smoking mothers. *Dev Pharmacol Ther* 1985;8:384–395.

153. Resnik R, Brink GW, Wilkes M. Catecholamine-mediated reduction in uterine blood flow after nicotine infusion in the pregnant ewe. *J Clin Invest* 1979;63:1133–1136.

154. Newnham JP, Patterson L, James I, et al. Effects of maternal cigarette smoking on ultrasonic measurements of fetal growth and on Doppler flow velocity waveforms. *Early Hum Dev* 1990; 24:23–36.

155. Bruner JP, Forouzan I. Smoking and buccally administered nicotine: acute effect on uterine and umbilical artery Doppler flow velocity waveforms. *J Reprod Med* 1991;36:435–440.

156. Castro LC, Allen R, Ogunyemi D, et al. Cigarette smoking during pregnancy: acute effects on uterine flow velocity waveforms. *Obstet Gynecol* 1993;81:551–555.

157. Tulzer G, Bsteh M, Arzt W, et al. Acute effects of cigarette smoking on fetal cardiovascular and uterine Doppler parameters. *Geburtshilfe Frauenheilkd* 1993;53:689–692.

158. Lindblad A, Marsal K. Influence of nicotine chewing gum on fetal blood flow. *J Perinat Med* 1987;15:13–19.

159. Sindberg-Eriksen P, Marsal K. Circulatory changes in the fetal aorta after maternal smoking. *Br J Obstet Gynaecol* 1987;94:301–305.

160. Lindblad A, Marsal K, Andersson KE. Effect of nicotine on human fetal blood flow. *Obstet Gynecol* 1988;72:371–382.

161. Jones KL, Smith DW, Ulleland CN, et al. Patterns of malformation in offspring of chronic alcoholic mothers. *Lancet* 1973;1:1267–1271.

162. Hanson JW, Streissguth AP, Smith DW. The effects of moderate alcohol consumption during pregnancy on fetal growth and morphogenesis. *Pediatrics* 1978;92:457–460.

163. Jacobson JL, Jacobson SW, Sokol RS, et al. Prenatal alcohol exposure and neurobehavioral function in infancy: evidence for threshold and differential vulnerability. *Am J Obstet Gynecol* 1992;166:346.

164. Mills JL, Graubard BI, Harley EE, et al. Maternal alcohol consumption and birth weight: how much drinking during pregnancy is safe? *JAMA* 1984;252:1875–1879.

165. Virji SK. The relationship between alcohol consumption during pregnancy and infant birthweight. *Acta Obstet Gynecol Scand* 1991;70:303–308.

166. Rosett HL, Weiner L, Lee A, et al. Patterns of alcohol consumption and fetal development. *Obstet Gynecol* 1983;61:539–546.

167. Halmesmaki E. Alcohol counselling of 85 pregnant problem drinkers: effect on drinking and fetal outcome. *Br J Obstet Gynaecol* 1988;95:243–245.

168. Fisher SE, Atkinson M, Holzman I, et al. Effect of ethanol upon placental uptake of amino acids. *Prog Biochem Pharmacol* 1981;18:216–223.

169. Fisher SE, Inselman LS, Duffy L, et al. Ethanol and fetal nutrition: effect of chronic ethanol exposure on rat placental growth and membrane-associated folic acid receptor binding activity. *J Pediatr Gastroenterol Nutr* 1985;4:645–649.

170. Marquis SM, Leichter J, Lee M. Plasma amino acids and glucose levels in the rat fetus and dam after chronic maternal alcohol consumption. *Biol Neonate* 1984;46:36–43.

171. Gordon BH, Streeter ML, Rosso P, et al. Prenatal alcohol exposure: abnormalities in placental growth and fetal amino acid uptake in the rat. *Biol Neonate* 1985;47:113–119.

172. Snyder AK, Singh SP, Pullen GL. Ethanol-induced intruterine

growth retardation: correlation with placental glucose transfer. *Alcohol Clin Exp Res* 1986;10:167–170.

173. Karl PI, Fisher SE. Chronic ethanol exposure inhibits insulin and IGF-1 stimulated amino acid uptake in cultured human placental trophoblasts. *Alcohol Clin Exp Res* 1994;18:942–946.

174. Dreosti IE, Ballard FJ, Belling GB, et al. The effects of ethanol and acetaldehyde in DNA synthesis in growing cells and on fetal development in the rat. *Alcohol Clin Exp Res* 1981;5:357–362.

175. Inselman LS, Fisher SE, Spencer H, et al. Effects of intrauterine ethanol exposure on fetal lung growth. *Pediatr Res* 1985;19: 12–14.

176. David C, Tagliavini G, Pilu G, et al. Receiver operator characteristic curves for the ultrasonographic prediction of small-for-gestational-age fetuses in low-risk pregnancies. *Am J Obstet Gynecol* 1996;174:1037–1042.

177. Pardi G, Cetin I, Marconi AM, et al. Diagnostic value of blood sampling in fetuses with growth retardation. *N Engl J Med* 1993; 328:692–696.

178. Visser GHA, Sadovsky G, Nicolaides KH. Antepartum heart rate patterns in small for gestational age third trimester fetuses: correlation with blood gas values obtained at cordocentesis. *Am J Obstet Gynecol* 1990;162:698–703.

179. Ribbert LSM, Snijders RJM, Nicolaides KH, et al. Relation of fetal blood gases and data from computerized assisted analysis of fetal heart rate patterns in small for gestational age fetuses. *Br J Obstet Gynaecol* 1991;98:820–823.

180. Manning FA, Snijders R, Harman CR, et al. Fetal biophysical profile score. VI. Correlation with antepartum umbilical venous pH. *Am J Obstet Gynecol* 1993;169:755–763.

181. Yoon BH, Romero R, Roh CR, et al. Relationship between the fetal biophysical profile score, umbilical artery Doppler velocimetry, and fetal blood acid-base status determined by cordocentesis. *Am J Obstet Gynecol* 1993;169:1586–1594.

182. Snijders R, Hyett J. Fetal testing in intra-uterine growth retardation. *Curr Opin Obstet Gynecol* 1997;9:91–95.

183. Trudinger BJ, Cook CM, Giles W, et al. Umbilical artery flow velocity waveforms in high risk pregnancy: randomised controlled trial. *Lancet* 1987;1:188–190.

184. Snijders RJM, Ribbert LSM, Visser GHA, et al. Numeric analysis of heart rate variation in intrauterine growth-retarded fetuses: a longitudinal study. *Am J Obstet Gynecol* 1992;166:22–27.

185. Weiner Z, Farmakides G, Schulman H, et al. Central and peripheral hemodynamic changes in fetuses with absent end diastolic velocity in the umbilical artery: correlation with computerized fetal heart rate pattern. *Am J Obstet Gynecol* 1994; 170:509–515.

186. Gülmezoglu M, de Onis M, Villar J. Effectiveness of interventions to prevent or treat impaired fetal growth. *Obstet Gynecol Surv* 1997;52:139–149.

187. Pollack RN, Yaffe H, Divon MY. Therapy for intrauterine growth restriction: current options and future directions. *Clin Obstet Gynecol* 1997;40:825–842.

188. Louden KA, Pipkin FB, Symonds EM, et al. A randomized placebo-controlled study of the effect of low-dose aspirin on platelet reactivity and serum thromboxane B_2 production in nonpregnant women, in normal pregnancies, and in gestational hypertension. *Br J Obstet Gynaecol* 1992;99:371–376.

189. Uzan S, Beaufils M, Breart G, et al. Prevention of fetal growth retardation with low-dose aspirin: findings of the EPREDA trial. *Lancet* 1991;337:1427–1431.

190. Trudinger BJ, Cook CM, Thompson RS, et al. Low-dose aspirin therapy improves fetal weight in umbilical placental insufficiency. *Am J Obstet Gynecol* 1988;159:681–685.

191. Newnham JP, Godfrey M, Walters BJ, et al. Low-dose aspirin for the treatment of fetal growth restriction: a randomized controlled trial. *Aust N Z J Obstet Gynaecol* 1995;35:370–374.

192. CLASP Collaborative group. CLASP: a randomized trial of low-dose aspirin for the prevention and treatment of preeclampsia among 9364 pregnant women. *Lancet* 1994;343:619–629.

193. Italian Study of Aspirin in Pregnancy. Low-dose aspirin in the prevention and treatment of intrauterine growth retardation and pregnancy-induced hypertension. *Lancet* 1993;341:396–400.

194. Sibai BM, Caritis SN, Thom E, et al. Prevention of preeclampsia with low-dose aspirin in healthy, nulliparous women. *N Engl J Med* 1993;329:213–1218.

195. Leitich H, Egarter C, Husslein P, et al. A meta-analysis of low dose aspirin for the prevention of intrauterine growth retardation. *Br J Obstet Gynaecol* 1997;104:450–459.

196. Rush D, Stein Z, Susser M. Diet in pregnancy: a randomized controlled trial of nutritional supplements. *Birth Defects* 1980;16:1–197.

197. Simmer K, Lort-Phillips L, James C, et al. A double-blind trial of zinc supplementation in pregnancy. *Eur J Clin Nutr* 1991;45:139–144.

198. Sorensen JD, Olsen SF, Pedersen AK, et al. Effect of fish oil supplementation in the third trimester of pregnancy on prostacyclin and thromboxane production. *Am J Obstet Gynecol* 1993;168:915–922.

199. Laurin J, Persson PH. The effect of bedrest in hospital on fetal outcome in pregnancies complicated by intruterine gowth retardation. *Acta Obstet Gynecol Scand* 1987;66:407–411.

INFECTIOUS COMPLICATIONS OF PREGNANCY: MATERNAL AND FETAL

ERNEST M. GRAHAM

CYTOMEGALOVIRUS

Cytomegalovirus (CMV) is the most common cause of intrauterine infection, and congenital infection occurs in 0.5% to 2.0% of all babies delivered. Even though inclusion-bearing cells were first identified in 1881, it was not until 1956 that human CMV was isolated (1). Before isolation of the virus, inclusion-bearing cells were considered to be pathognomonic, and this condition was referred to as "generalized salivary gland virus infection," "inclusion disease," and "cytomegalic inclusion disease."

CMV is a large, double-stranded DNA virus that is a member of the family Herpesviridae. The Herpesviridae family also includes herpes simplex virus, varicella-zoster virus, and Epstein-Barr virus. As with other herpesviruses, primary CMV infection is usually followed by latency and reactivation. CMV is the largest member of this family of viruses, and its 240-kb genome codes for more than 100 proteins. The viral genome is surrounded by an icosahedral protein composed of 162 capsomeres. A lipid envelope surrounds the nucleocapsid and gives the mature viral particle a diameter of about 200 nm (2). Different strains of CMV have been identified using restriction endonuclease digestion of purified viral DNA and detection of repetitive sequences in variable regions of the genome using the polymerase chain reaction (PCR) and Southern blot techniques (2).

CMV is not highly contagious, and close personal contact is required for transmission to occur. Horizontal transmission occurs by droplets, sexual contact, receipt of an infected organ, and contact with contaminated saliva, urine, or blood. Vertical transmission can occur by transplacental passage of the virus, exposure to contaminated genital tract secretions during delivery, and breast-feeding. The incubation period for CMV ranges from 28 to 60 days, with a mean of 40 days (3).

Maternal Infection

Eighty-five to 90% of CMV infections in adults (primary and recurrent) are asymptomatic. In the 15% of CMV cases that are symptomatic, patients have findings suggestive of mononucleosis. The clinical manifestations are mild and include malaise, fever, chills, lymphadenopathy, and myalgias. Patients may have lymphopenia or lymphocytosis with a high number of atypical lymphocytes on peripheral blood smear, thrombocytopenia, and mildly elevated transaminases (4). CMV can be differentiated from infectious mononucleosis by the mildness of the pharyngitis, minimal lymphadenopathy, and the absence of hepatosplenomegaly and jaundice. The diagnosis of CMV infection is confirmed by the isolation of virus in tissue culture, with the highest concentration of virus in urine, seminal fluid, saliva, and breast milk. Serologic methods are helpful in establishing the diagnosis, but the reference laboratory must be skilled in performing these tests. In the acute phase of the infection, CMV-specific immunoglobulin M (IgM) is present in serum and declines rapidly over a period of 30 to 60 days. An acute and convalescent titer that shows at least a fourfold increase in the viral-specific IgG (an increase of two dilutions) indicates a recent infection (5). Recurrent infection usually is not accompanied by IgM antibody production.

Approximately 50% of girls in the United States and Europe are susceptible to CMV by the time they reach reproductive age. The highest rate of seroconversion occurs between the ages of 15 and 35 years, and around 2% of susceptible women acquire primary CMV infection during pregnancy. Past exposure to CMV relates to sociocultural factors and sexual behavior; 50% of higher-income women are susceptible to acute CMV infection, whereas only 15% of low-income women are (6). Although CMV infection is ubiquitous, it produces serious illness only in fetuses, immunodeficient persons, and patients receiving immunosuppressive therapy.

Fetal Infection

Congenital CMV infection (*cytomegalic inclusion disease*) results from hematogenous dissemination of virus across the placenta. Congenital CMV infection causes a syndrome that includes low birth weight, microcephaly, intracranial calcifications, chorioretinitis, mental and motor retardation, sensorineural deficits, hepatosplenomegaly, jaundice, hemolytic anemia, and thrombocytopenic purpura (blueberry muffin appearance) (Fig. 33.1). The most frequent labora-

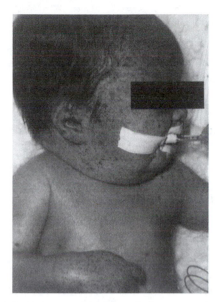

FIGURE 33.1. Neonate with congenital cytomegalovirus infection. (From Stanberry LR, Glasgow LA. Viral infections of the fetus and newborn. In: Stringfellow DA, ed. *Virology.* Kalamazoo, MI: Upjohn, 1983, with permission.)

tory abnormalities are thrombocytopenia, hyperbilirubinemia, and elevated transaminases.

Congenital infection may result from a maternal primary infection, reinfection, or reactivation of a latent infection. Primary CMV infection does not produce lasting immunity. The virus becomes latent, and periodic reactivation occurs, with viral shedding despite the presence of serum antibody. The site of latent CMV infection is unknown, but it may include monocytes, bone marrow, and kidney tissue. Congenital infections can occur after either primary or recurrent maternal infection. Of women who are immune, around 1% may have infants with congenital infection. The birth of one congenitally infected infant does not preclude the possibility that a subsequent baby may become infected *in utero.* Because most infections during pregnancy are recurrent, most congenitally infected neonates are born to women with recurrent infection. Fortunately, perinatal infections that result from recurrent maternal infection are considerably milder and are less often associated with neonatal sequelae.

Neurologic involvement in preterm infants has more diverse clinical findings, and this encephalopathic process can be progressive. CMV infection should be considered in any preterm infant with an abnormal neurologic examination (7). The overall risk of congenital infection is greatest when maternal infection occurs in the third trimester, but the probability of severe fetal injury is highest when maternal infection occurs in the first trimester.

Of fetuses with congenital infection, approximately 10% are symptomatic at birth. Approximately 30% of severely infected infants die, and 80% of the survivors have severe neurologic morbidity, ocular abnormalities, or sensorineural hearing loss (8). Interest has shifted from the 10% of infants who are obviously diseased at birth to the prognosis of the 90% of congenitally infected neonates who appear normal at birth. Of these infants, 85% to 95% develop normally, and 5% to 15% develop sequelae such as hearing loss, chorioretinitis, or mental defects within the first 2 years of life (Fig. 33.2). A classic tetrad of findings has been described among infants who have survived fulminant, clinically

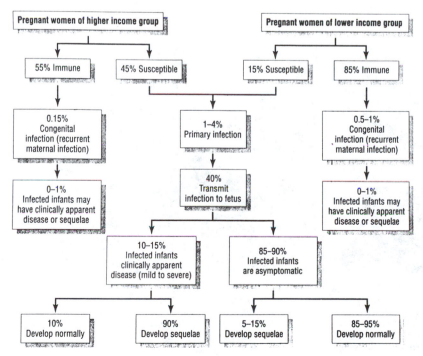

FIGURE 33.2. Characteristics of cytomegalovirus infection in pregnancy. (From Stagno S, Whitley RJ. Herpesvirus infections in pregnancy. II. Herpes simplex virus and varicella-zoster virus infections. *N Engl J Med* 1985;313:1327, with permission.)

apparent infection: (a) mental retardation, (b) chorioretinitis, (c) cerebral calcifications, and (d) microcephaly or hydrocephaly. The cerebral calcifications are characteristically periventricular in the subependymal region (Fig. 33.3).

Pregnant women with recurrent CMV infection are much less likely to transmit infection to the fetus. In a study of 125 women with primary CMV infection and 64 women with recurrent infection, investigators found that in the group with primary infection, 18% of infants were symptomatic at birth, and an additional 7% developed at least one major sequela within 5 years of follow-up (9). Of the infants with primary infection, 2% died, 15% had sensorineural hearing loss, and 13% had a measured intelligence quotient lower than 70. Among the infants born to mothers with recurrent infections, none were symptomatic at birth; however, 8% developed at least one sequela, the most common being hearing loss, but none developed multiple defects.

In addition to hematogenous spread of the virus across the placenta during the antepartum period, CMV infection may occur during delivery as a result of exposure to infected genital tract secretions. CMV can be cultured from the cervix and urine in approximately 10% of women at the time of delivery, and 20% to 60% of exposed fetuses may subsequently shed virus in their pharynx or urine. Whereas infants infected congenitally excrete CMV for an average of 4 years, those acquiring CMV at the time of birth excrete it for 2 years. Postpartum infection may also occur as a result of breast-feeding or from an infected blood transfusion. In addition to the 0.5% to 2.5% of infants who are infected congenitally, 3% to 5% of liveborn infants are infected by exposure to intrapartum or postpartum events. These infants have an initial urine culture that is negative, but excretion of CMV is demonstrated several weeks to months after delivery. Thirty to 50% of neonates whose mothers have genital CMV infection at the time of birth will acquire the virus.

Prenatal Diagnosis

Various different methods to diagnose fetal CMV infection have been studied. The virus has been cultured from amniotic fluid and fetal serum, total IgM in fetal serum may be increased after infection, anti-CMV IgM in fetal serum has been identified, and infected fetuses may have elevated transaminases and thrombocytopenia. Amniotic fluid culture of CMV is the best method to diagnose congenital infection.

The first successful diagnosis of congenital CMV infection by fetal blood sampling was reported in 1982 (10). Cordocentesis was performed on a hydropic 25-week fetus. The total IgM concentration was normal, but the fetal blood smear showed severe erythroblastosis, and CMV-specific IgM antibody was identified by radioimmunoassay.

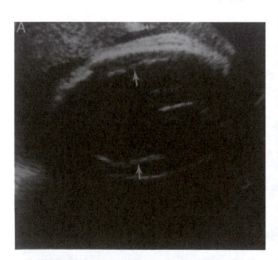
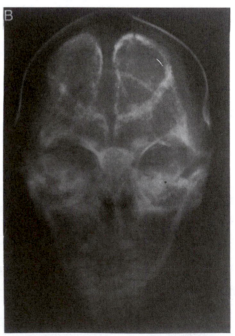

FIGURE 33.3. A: Axial sonogram through a fetal head at 35 weeks' gestational age shows echogenic walls (*arrows*) of the dilated lateral ventricles suggesting calcification. The head was also microcephalic, consistent with 23 weeks by biparietal diameter. **B:** Skull radiograph after delivery shows dense periventricular calcifications. (From Nyberg DA, Pretorius DH. Cerebral malformations. In: Nyberg DA, Mahony BS, Pretorius DH, eds. *Diagnostic ultrasound of fetal anomalies: text and atlas.* St. Louis: Mosby–Year Book, 1990, with permission.)

A subsequent study was done of 15 women with primary CMV infection during pregnancy (11). Of these 15 women, 8 had infected fetuses, and all cases of fetal infection were correctly identified by detection of viral antigen in amniotic fluid within 24 hours by the shell viral assay. For all cases in which viral antigen was identified prenatally, neonatal viral culture was positive. Four of the 8 infected fetuses (50%) had increased total IgM and elevated transaminases. Two fetuses had thrombocytopenia, and no infected fetus had a positive blood culture for CMV. A negative amniotic fluid culture was 100% specific in predicting the absence of congenital infection.

In a series of 12 patients, 7 with serologically confirmed primary CMV infection and 5 evaluated for abnormal sonographic findings, 11 underwent amniocentesis and cordocentesis (12). Of the 7 patients with primary CMV infection, 1 was infected. This patient's fetus had a positive amniotic fluid culture and an elevated γ-glutamyl transferase; however, the fetal hematocrit and platelet count were normal, and no CMV-specific IgM was identified. The 5 fetuses with abnormal sonographic findings were all infected with CMV. Four of the 5 had positive amniotic fluid cultures, but none had a positive blood culture. Four had elevated total IgM, 3 had elevated γ-glutamyl transferase, and 1 had thrombocytopenia.

The largest and most recent series involved the prenatal diagnosis of 52 pregnancies at risk for congenital CMV infection (13). The procedures used for prenatal diagnosis were ultrasound, amniocentesis, and fetal blood sampling. Specific tests for CMV infection included CMV IgM, viral culture of amniotic fluid and fetal blood, and amplification of CMV DNA by PCR. Nonspecific tests included white blood cell count, hemoglobin, hematocrit, platelets, and γ-glutamyl transferase determination. This combination of tests allowed an antenatal diagnosis of CMV in 13 of the 16 infected fetuses (sensitivity, 81%). CMV culture and PCR of amniotic fluid allowed the diagnosis in 12 of the 13 antenatally diagnosed cases. The sensitivity of CMV IgM detection in fetal blood was 69%. Fetal blood culture for CMV was not positive in any of the infected fetuses. Thrombocytopenia was present in 6 of the 16 infected cases, and abnormal ultrasound findings, which included cerebral ventriculomegaly, fetal growth restriction, and hyperechogenic areas in the fetal abdomen, were present in only 5 cases. All 4 infected neonates with no CMV detected in the amniotic fluid were asymptomatic at birth and during follow-up. These investigators concluded that amniotic fluid is the best sample to diagnose CMV infection. When examining their study in conjunction with other published reports, these investigators concluded that prenatal diagnosis of congenital CMV infection is possible with a sensitivity of 81% to 100% and a specificity close to 100%. At present, ultrasound and nonspecific tests on fetal blood are not sufficiently discriminatory to diagnose severe fetal infection. Fetal infection is demonstrated by the detection of virus in the amniotic fluid or the presence of CMV-specific IgM in fetal blood, but neither of these findings has prognostic value for the development of serious disease or severe sequelae. Cordocentesis may provide additional information about the condition of the fetus. Elevated alanine aminotransferase levels and thrombocytopenia are the most frequent laboratory abnormalities in symptomatic neonates, each seen in 80% of cases (14). Viral load may be important as a prognostic factor. Viral load has been shown to be particularly high in fetuses with ultrasonographic brain abnormalities (15). Low viral load could account for false-negative amniotic fluid cultures and for less severe infection.

Management

No effective therapy exists for maternal CMV infection. Antiviral agents such as ganciclovir, foscarnet, and cidofovir have some activity against CMV, but their use is limited primarily to treatment of life- or sight-threatening infections in immunocompromised patients. Adenosine arabinoside and cytosine arabinoside have been used for neonates with severe neonatal infection, but these drugs are toxic, and although they temporarily suppress the excretion of the virus, shedding resumes when the drugs are stopped. Ganciclovir has been shown to be tolerated reasonably well in infants with congenital CMV disease, and treatment has resulted in decreased viral shedding during administration (16). Anecdotal evidence suggests some efficacy of ganciclovir in the treatment of selected critically ill newborns with CMV (17,18). Results have been good when ganciclovir is used to treat serious CMV infection in patients with acquired immunodeficiency syndrome and as a prophylactic agent to prevent CMV disease after organ transplantation. Ganciclovir cannot be recommended for routine treatment of infants with congenital CMV disease until controlled trials prove its efficacy. Currently, a multicenter study sponsored by the National Institutes of Health is being conducted to evaluate ganciclovir in the treatment of infants with symptomatic congenital CMV disease and central nervous system involvement. A multicenter trial is also under way to evaluate the efficacy of a CMV-specific monoclonal antibody preparation in treating infants with symptomatic congenital CMV disease who demonstrate no central nervous system involvement.

Because no treatment exists for CMV infection, physicians should focus their attention on educating patients about preventive measures. CMV is a sexually transmitted disease, and sexual promiscuity significantly increases a person's risk of acquiring infection. People with multiple sexual partners should be counseled that latex condoms are an effective barrier to transmission of CMV. Health care workers, day care workers, elementary school teachers, and mothers of young children should be aware of the importance of simple infection control measures such as hand washing and proper cleansing of environmental surfaces. CMV seronegative women should practice good hygiene, especially if they are routinely exposed to young children at home or in the workplace, such as at child day care centers. Pregnant women should wash hands well after diaper changes, they should avoid kissing on the mouth, and they should not share food, eating utensils, and drinking utensils (19). Only CMV-negative blood should be given to fetuses, neonates, pregnant women, and immunocompromised patients. Organ donors and sperm donors should be screened for CMV. The principle of universal precautions should be strictly adhered to by all health care workers when they are in contact with patients or any body fluids.

The development of a CMV vaccine has been suggested as a means of preventing congenital infection. However, an anti-CMV vaccine is unlikely to offer fetal protection for several reasons. CMV is a member of the herpesvirus family, which has a latent stage, and the virus persists even in the presence of high levels of specific maternal antibody. Existing maternal antibody does not completely protect against infection; even though the fetus is more likely to become infected with a primary maternal infection, fetal infection can still occur with recurrent maternal infections.

Because neither antiviral chemotherapy nor immunoprophylaxis is available to protect the fetus or neonate, routine prenatal screening for CMV infection is not recommended. Screening should be limited to those with mononucleosis-like symptoms suggestive of acute CMV, women with occupations likely to cause exposure such as health care workers and day care workers, and immunocompromised women.

TOXOPLASMA

Toxoplasma gondii is an intracellular protozoan parasite that causes illness in many mammalian species. However, the life cycle of *T. gondii* depends on wild and domestic cats, which are the only hosts for the oocyst. The life cycle of the parasite has three distinct forms (Fig. 33.4):

1. *Oocyst*. This is found only in the intestinal tract of cats and is shed for approximately 2 weeks after a primary infection. The oocyst is shed in cat feces into the litter box or onto the ground, and humans come into contact with it by changing the cat litter box or gardening. The oocyst can also be ingested by other animals such as cows, sheep, pigs, or chickens, which are later eaten by humans.

2. *Trophozoite*. The oocyst is disrupted in the human, cow, or sheep intestine after being ingested, and the invasive trophozoite is thus released. This is the actively replicating and invasive form found in blood, body fluids, and tissue during primary infection.

3. *Tissue cyst*. This dormant form, which is found in tissues, especially the brain and retina, during chronic in-

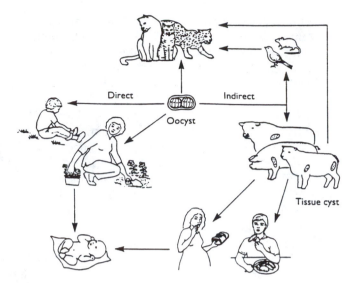

FIGURE 33.4. Life cycle of *Toxoplasma gondii* and routes of transmission to humans. (From Hall SM. Congenital toxoplasmosis. *BMJ* 1992;305:291, with permission.)

fection is capable of reactivation in an immunocompromised host.

In addition to acquiring the parasite by manual contact with cat feces or eating undercooked meat containing tissue cysts, *Toxoplasma* can also be transmitted by food contaminated by insect vectors. Unwashed hands can serve as vehicles for transporting oocysts from the soil or cat litter box into the mouth. Oocysts from cat feces can become aerosolized and inhaled. The oocysts excreted in cat feces remain infectious for months, and transmission can occur through contact with infected dirt. Infected animals shed *Toxoplasma* in milk, and this can be a route of transmission. At least one waterborne outbreak of toxoplasmosis has been recognized (20). Transmission can occur by eating raw infected eggs, by transfusion of infected blood or blood products, by heart or kidney transplants from seropositive donors to seronegative recipients, or by accidental self-inoculaton of laboratory workers who are in contact with infected animals, needles, or glassware (21). Singling out cat ownership as the major determinant of whether to offer antenatal testing is unreasonable.

In the United States, approximately 20% of women have antibody to *Toxoplasma,* and the frequency of seroconversion during pregnancy is 5% or less. The risk of fetal infection is estimated to be between 1 per 1,000 and 1 per 8,000 live births in the United States (22). A prospective study was conducted in New Hampshire and Massachusetts in 1986 to 1988 in which all newborns were screened for congenital toxoplasmosis using blood routinely collected on filter-paper cards for mandatory metabolic screening with a sensitive IgM immunoassay (23). In all, 635,000 infants were screened, and the incidence of congenital toxoplasmosis was found to be 1 per 12,000 births. Toxoplasmosis is more common in France, where approximately 80% of women of childbearing age have antibody to *T. gondii,* and the incidence of congenital toxoplasmosis is about twice that of the United States (24).

In immunocompetent adults, toxoplasmosis is asymptomatic in 80% to 90% of cases. In symptomatic cases, it usually presents as a mononucleosis-like illness with fever, fatigue, sore throat, maculopapular rash, muscle pain, and lymphadenopathy of the head and neck areas, most commonly involving a single lymph node. When clinically evident, this disease is often thought to be the flu. *T. gondii* causes 1% to 5% of cases of mononucleosis and should be suspected in patients with negative heterophile antibody test results (21). In healthy adults, toxoplasmosis is mild and self-limited, but in immunosuppressed patients, it can lead to devastating central nervous system and pulmonary involvement. Because immunity to *T. gondii* is cell mediated, patients with human immunodeficiency virus infection or those receiving long-term immunosuppressive therapy after organ transplantation are particularly susceptible to new or reactivated infection. In immunosuppressed patients, toxoplasmosis can lead to encephalitis, meningoencephalitis, and intracerebral mass lesions. It can also lead to pneumonitis, myocarditis, and generalized lymphadenopathy. Latent toxoplasmosis is reactivated only in advanced immunodeficiency. Pregnant women with CD4 cell counts less than $200/\mu$L should be considered for prophylactic therapy with trimethoprim-sulfamethoxazole (Bactrim DS), one tablet per day (25).

Diagnosis

The diagnosis of acute maternal toxoplasmosis is most often made using serologic laboratory tests. *Toxoplasma*-specific IgM antibodies usually become positive within 1 to 2 weeks of infection and persist for months or years, especially when extremely sensitive assays are used. The development of highly sensitive methods to detect anti-*Toxoplasma* IgM has confused the determination of acute infection because some persons remain IgM seropositive for as long as 12 years (26). Therefore, the detection of *Toxoplasma*-specific IgM antibodies should not be considered unequivocal proof that the infection is acute. If anti-*Toxoplasma* antibody, as determined by the Sabin-Feldman dye test or indirect florescence on enzyme-linked immunosorbent assay, is present in low titers, this probably represents previously acquired immunity. The *Sabin-Feldman dye test* requires live parasites and usually becomes positive within 1 to 2 weeks of infection; it does not differentiate between anti-*Toxoplasma* IgG and IgM antibodies. A fourfold or greater rise in serum antibody titers in parallel specimens collected 3 to 4 weeks apart can be used to confirm recent infection. If *Toxoplasma*-specific IgM *antibody titers* are initially high in conjunction with high IgG titers of more than 1:512 by the Sabin-Feldman dye test (or indirect fluorescent antibody), this is suggestive,

but not definitive evidence, of recent infection (27). *Toxoplasma*-specific IgE antibodies are also markers of acute maternal infection.

T. gondii recovered from infected tissues such as infected amniotic fluid, blood, cerebrospinal fluid, or homogenized placenta or brain can be innoculated onto tissue culture or into the peritoneal cavity of mice. Tissue cultures take about 1 week and mouse inoculation takes 6 weeks, but neither method is readily available (21). Tachyzoites can be seen in tissue sections or smears of body fluids, and their presence indicates acute infection. A lymph node or brain biopsy specimen is the best tissue for identification of *T. gondii.*

PCR tests are now commercially available that detect *T. gondii* by amplifying genes specific to the parasite (P30 or B1). These tests allow direct detection of *T. gondii* DNA in amniotic fluid (28). PCR testing can provide results within hours, as opposed to tissue cultures, which take 1 to 6 weeks.

Congenital Toxoplasmosis

Congenital toxoplasmosis occurs when a mother has a primary infection during pregnancy. Chronic or latent infection is unlikely to cause fetal injury except in an immunosuppressed host. Maternal immunity appears to protect against intrauterine infection. Acute maternal toxoplasmosis is estimated to complicate 1 to 5 pregnancies per 1,000 (29). Approximately 40% to 50% of neonates born to mothers with acute toxoplasmosis show evidence of infection, and 10% of infected infants have severe disease. The severity of infection is worse with first trimester exposure, but the vertical transmission rate is higher with third trimester exposure. Ten percent of fetuses exposed in the first trimester have congenital infection, and 60% of neonates exposed in the third trimester have evidence of perinatal infection.

Manifestations of congenital toxoplasmosis include one or more components of the classic triad of hydrocephalus (or microcephaly), intracranial calcification, and chorioretinitis. Involvement of the central nervous system and ocular signs are the most important manifestations of disease, but one may also see extensive involvement of other organs including the liver, heart, and lungs (30). Infants infected with congenital toxoplasmosis can have fever, low birth weight, hepatosplenomegaly, icterus, and anemia. Some infants have primarily neurologic disease with seizures, intracranial calcifications, mental retardation, and hydrocephaly or microcephaly. Approximately 25% to 50% of symptomatic infants are delivered prematurely. About 75% of infants with congenital toxoplasmosis at birth are asymptomatic; however, one-third of all asymptomatic neonates who undergo detailed examinations are found to have abnormalities such as cerebrospinal fluid pleocytosis or elevated protein content (20%), chorioretinitis (15%), or intracranial calcifications (10%) (31). Weeks or months later, untreated asymptomatic infants go on to develop signs or symptoms of disease.

During the initial parasitemia, the placenta can become infected, then the infection can progress to the fetus. The lag time between placental and fetal infection is influenced by the virulence of the strain of *T. gondii,* its inoculum size, the developmental stage of the placenta, and maternal antibiotic administration. Unless the patient is immuno-compromised, congenital infection does not affect more than one pregnancy in a particular mother.

Prenatal Diagnosis

Ultrasound abnormalities are found in 30% to 40% of cases of congenital toxoplasmosis, the most common being ventriculomegaly (32). Ultrasound findings suggestive of infection include hydrocephalus, microcephaly, intracranial calcifications, ascites, hydrops, growth restriction, and placental thickening. Sonographic evidence of hydrocephaly appears to be associated with a poor prognosis.

PCR testing of amniotic fluid specimens can detect the presence of *T. gondii* DNA within 1 day. The sensitivity of this test appears to be good. In a study in which 34 of 339 infants at risk were found to have toxoplasmosis confirmed by serologic testing or autopsy, all amniotic fluid samples from affected pregnancies were positive by PCR (33). Before the advent of PCR testing of amniotic fluid, cordocentesis was used to detect *in utero* infection. The complication rate with cordocentesis (1%) is considerably higher than the complication rate with amniocentesis (0.5%). Cordocentesis is a more difficult procedure that requires considerable expertise and is available only in a few centers. Cordocentesis also fails to detect 10% of affected pregnancies. The superior sensitivity, safety, rapidity, and cost of PCR testing suggest that cordocentesis is no longer indicated for the prenatal diagnosis of fetal toxoplasmosis. Because the quality of PCR testing may vary among laboratories, mice inoculation with amniotic fluid may be used to confirm test results (27).

Management

Prenatal screening for toxoplasmosis has existed in France and Austria for many years (Fig. 33.5). Because 80% of French women are immune, this involves testing the 20% of the population that are susceptible to toxoplasmosis with monthly antibody measurements. Those who convert to seropositive during pregnancy, as demonstrated by the sudden presence of *Toxoplasma*-specific IgM or a fourfold increase in anti-*Toxoplasma* IgG, are offered amniocentesis to detect the presence of fetal infection. This system may be cost effective in France, where 80% of the population is immune, but this may not be so in the United States and the United Kingdom, where 80% of the population is susceptible and would require testing. However, the American College of Obstetricians and Gynecologists in 1993 did recommend preconceptional serologic screening (29). In 1992, a multidisciplinary committee of the Royal College

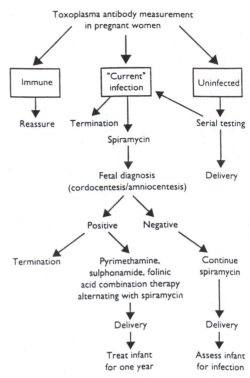

FIGURE 33.5. Simplified general model of prenatal screening for toxoplasmosis. (From Hall SM. Congenital toxoplasmosis. *BMJ* 1992;305:293, with permission.)

of Obstetricians and Gynaecologists recommended against instituting universal prenatal screening in the United Kingdom. When a *Toxoplasma*-susceptible woman is identified by preconceptional serologic screening, education about the following preventive measures should be given (27):

1. Wear gloves when gardening.
2. Avoid contact with cat feces, and preferably have someone else change the litter box. Otherwise, use gloves, empty the box daily, and wash hands immediately afterward.
3. Wash all fruits and vegetables before preparing or eating.
4. Cook meat thoroughly (150°F or 66°C, until juices are no longer pink). Meat that has been smoked or cured in brine is considered safe.
5. Avoid mucous membrane contact when handling uncooked meat, fruit, and vegetables, and wash hands thoroughly afterward.
6. Thoroughly clean all kitchen surfaces after contact with uncooked meat.
7. Prevent contamination of food by flies and cockroaches.
8. Avoid consumption of raw eggs or unpasteurized milk.

In healthy immunocompetent women, there is no maternal indication for treatment of toxoplasmosis because the disease is asymptomatic or self-limited and does not have sequelae. However, immunocompromised patients with toxoplasmosis should be treated with sulfadiazine (4 g oral loading dose initially, then 1 g four times daily) and pyrimethamine (50 to 100 mg orally, then 25 mg daily). Immunosuppressed patients may require extended courses of treatment to cure the infection (34).

Treatment of a pregnant woman with acute toxoplasmosis has clearly been shown to reduce the risk of congenital infection and to decrease late sequelae of infection (35). Women with acute infection as determined by serologic testing should be started immediately on spiramycin. Spiramycin is a macrolide antibiotic similar to erythromycin that is concentrated in the placenta, where the parasite is initially found. Although spiramycin has been used widely in Europe, it is available in the United States only through the Food and Drug Administration (301-443-4280) or though the manufacturer, Rhone-Poulenc Rorer, in Valley Forge, PA. Spiramycin is estimated to reduce the incidence of maternal-fetal transmission by as much as 60% (36), although it is ineffective in treating the already infected fetus because it does not cross the placenta well. It reduces the transmission of *T. gondii* from mother to fetus, but it does not alter fetal disease once infection has occurred. Spiramycin does not have any serious side effects, but it may cause gastrointestinal upset similar to erythromycin. It is administered as 1 g orally every 8 hours without food. If PCR testing of amniotic fluid is negative for *T. gondii*, spiramycin is continued for the remainder of the pregnancy. Because spiramycin is so difficult to acquire in the United States, other drugs such as azithromycin and clarithromycin are being investigated as alternative treatments to prevent *in utero* infection with *T. gondii*.

If amniotic fluid PCR testing for *T. gondii* is positive, the fetus will require treatment with pyrimethamine and either sulfadoxine or sulfadiazine to reduce the severity of congenital infection and to decrease the proportion of symptomatic infants at birth (37). Therapeutic abortion should also be discussed with these patients. In the absence of ultrasound abnormalities, neonatal outcome is usually good for treated infants; however, some fetuses with normal ultrasound findings have been found on termination of the pregnancy for first trimester infection to have severe brain damage and necrosis, so there is some risk of fetal brain damage even if ultrasound findings are normal (37). If a woman with an infected fetus and a normal ultrasound scan elects to continue her pregnancy, she should be treated with pyrimethamine and sulfadiazine for the remainder of the pregnancy. Pyrimethamine is a folic acid antagonist and is not recommended for use during the first trimester because of possible teratogenicity (folic acid is important for neural tube closure). Sulfonamides can be used alone in the first trimester, but single-agent therapy appears to be less effective than combination therapy (34). For treating the infected fetus, one commonly used regimen consists of 3-week courses of pyrimethamine (50 mg daily) and sulfadiazine (3 g daily in two divided doses), alternating with 3-week courses of spiramycin (3 g per day) until delivery. An alternate regimen is to give pyrimethamine (25 mg daily) and sulfadiazine (4 g daily) until delivery. Leucovorin (folinic

acid) (5 to 10 mg daily) is added during pyrimethamine and sulfadiazine administration to prevent bone marrow suppression (27). These regimens can cause anemia, granulocytopenia, and thrombocytopenia. A complete blood count and platelet count should be checked weekly, and treatment should be stopped if an abnormal result is found. For patients who cannot tolerate these drugs, trimethoprim-sulfamethoxazole with or without clindamycin has been effective in treating toxoplasmosis in nonpregnant patients, but its safety and efficacy for treating *in utero* infection are unknown (38).

Infants born with congenital toxoplasmosis should be treated aggressively with pyrimethamine, sulfadiazine, and leucovorin for 1 year (39). Early treatment reduces, but does not eliminate, the late sequelae of toxoplasmosis such as chorioretinitis.

PARVOVIRUS

The Parvoviridae family consist of small, single-stranded DNA viruses and are the smallest DNA viruses that infect mammalian cells. *Parvum* is Latin for small, and the parvoviruses are among the smallest viruses, usually 15 to 28 nm in diameter. The parvoviruses are common animal pathogens; however, parvovirus B19 is the only known pathogenic parvovirus in humans. Parvovirus B19 was discovered by accident in 1974 when investigators found a "serum parvovirus-like particle" while evaluating serum samples for hepatitis B surface antigen (40). The peculiar name of B19 came from the coding of that donor sample, as number 19 on plate B. The principal mode of B19 transmission is from person to person through direct contact with respiratory secretions, but the virus can also be transmitted parenterally by transfusion of blood or blood products and vertically from mother to fetus. Each virus particle consists of a protein icosahedron containing about 5,000 bases of single-stranded DNA. The absence of a lipid envelope contributes to the high heat stability of these viruses. The parvoviruses share a similar genomic organization with structural (capsid) proteins encoded by genes on the right and nonstructural proteins by genes on the left. *Termini*, or terminal repeat sequences, found at each end of the genome serve as the double-stranded matrix needed to initiate DNA synthesis and are required for viral propagation. The nonstructural proteins include proteins with nikase, helicase, and endonuclease activities. These proteins are required for parvovirus replication and RNA transcription.

Adult Disease

The newly discovered parvovirus was not associated with human disease until 1981, when it was detected in the sera of patients with sickle cell disease during acute aplastic crises (41). There was evidence of acute parvovirus infection (IgM or viral antigen) in the sera of Jamaican children living in

London who suffered from a complication of sickle cell disease called *transient aplastic crisis*. The virus affects erythroid precursor cells in the bone marrow and leads to anemia. Transient aplastic crisis occurs almost exclusively among patients with an underlying hemoglobinopathy.

In 1983, parvovirus was discovered to be the causative agent of *erythema infectiosum* (*fifth disease*) (42). This illness occurs in otherwise healthy children 5 to 14 years of age in elementary schools and day care centers in the late winter and early spring. The disease presents with a low-grade prodromal fever that precedes the development of a highly characteristic rash. This rash is pruritic and erythematous on the face ("slapped cheek" appearance) and is finely reticulated and erythematous on the trunk and extremities. Self-limited arthritis occurs in approximately 10% of children, but the incidence of this finding may exceed 50% in adults (43). Adults with the disease may present with fever, malaise, adenopathy, and polyarthritis affecting the hands, wrists, and knees. Adults usually do not develop the rash. Full recovery without sequelae is the usual outcome.

Fetal Disease

During investigation of a community outbreak of erythema infectiosum, it was discovered that parvovirus B19 is associated with *nonimmune fetal hydrops* and fetal death (44). Parvovirus B19 may be responsible for 10% to 15% of all cases of nonimmune hydrops (45). Hydrops appears to be caused primarily by viral infection of fetal erythroid stem cells, which leads to aplastic anemia and high-output congestive heart failure (Fig. 33.6). So just as parvovirus B19 causes transient aplastic crisis in children with underlying hemoglobinopathies by attacking erythroid precursor cells,

it can also attack erythroid precursor cells in the fetus and can lead to fetal hydrops. Because the fetus has a rapidly expanding red blood cell volume and a shortened red blood cell life span, if red blood cell production stops abruptly, the fetus will quickly become anemic (46). Fetal hydrops may also be partly the result of direct infection of myocardium by the virus. The risk of fetal infection is greatest when maternal illness occurs in the first trimester (47). When the time of exposure is between 1 and 12 weeks' gestation, 19% of fetuses are severely affected; between 13 and 20 weeks' gestation, 15% are severely affected; and at more than 20 weeks' gestation, 6% are severely affected. During an outbreak in Connecticut, the fetal loss rate was 5% in 39 infected women (48). In England, when 190 women acutely infected with parvovirus during pregnancy were followed prospectively, the transplacental infection rate was 33% (49). Midpregnancy infection was associated with 12% fetal loss, and the overall risk of fetal death was 9%. Early fetal death is usually not associated with hydrops, but hydrops is common in fetuses dying after midpregnancy (50). Parvovirus has not been shown to be teratogenic. Although some anecdotal reports have noted congenital anomalies in fetuses with acute parvovirus, there is no specific pattern of abnormalities, and this incidence does not exceed the expected frequency of congenital anomalies in the general population. Preterm labor, preterm delivery, and low birth weight are not increased among infants exposed to parvovirus.

Diagnosis of Maternal Infection

Women exposed to parvovirus during pregnancy should be screened serologically for specific IgG and IgM antibodies.

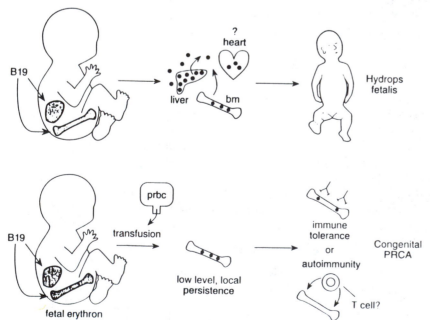

FIGURE 33.6. Pathogenesis of fetal diseases caused by B19 parvovirus. bm, bone marrow; prbc, packed red blood cells; PRCA, pure red cell aplasia. (From Young NS. B19 parvovirus. *Baillieres Clin Haematol* 1995;8:48, with permission.)

Antibody against parvovirus can be measured by enzyme-linked immunosorbent assay, radioimmunoassay, or Western blot. Anti-parvovirus IgM is usually positive by the third day after symptoms develop and may persist for up to 120 days. IgG is detectable by the seventh day of illness and persists for life (51). The presence of IgG antibody denotes immunity against the disease, and these patients can be reassured. Patients who are both IgG and IgM negative are susceptible to infection and should be cautioned to reduce their risk of exposure. During epidemics, infection rates for workers with close contact with elementary school-aged children are 20% to 30% (52). The risk that a susceptible mother will acquire infection from an infected household member is higher (50% to 90%) (53).

Parvovirus infection can also be diagnosed by culturing the virus from tissue culture of fresh bone marrow supplemented with erythropoietin, but it is rarely detected in acute infection because the period of viremia is so brief, usually lasting only 1 to 3 days (54). Infected cells show characteristic histologic changes such as eosinophilic inclusion bodies, marginated chromatin, and direct detection of viral particles by electron microscopy. Viral DNA may be detected in serum during the prodrome by DNA hybridization or PCR, but not after the rash develops.

Diagnosis of Fetal Infection

Mothers who are found to be IgM positive and IgG negative have acute parvovirus infection and should be closely monitored for the development of intrauterine fetal hydrops. The short viremic period and rapid elimination of parvovirus in the adult depend on a brisk antibody response that cannot be accomplished by the fetus until relatively late in gestation. This leads to the possibility that the incubation period may be much longer in the fetus. Because the incubation period of the virus may be longer in the fetus than in the child or adult, the patient should be followed with serial ultrasound examinations for up to 10 weeks after her acute illness (55). Hydrops usually occurs 4 to 6 weeks after infection. Although fetal infection can be diagnosed by detecting B19-specific IgM or DNA in umbilical cord blood, or finding B19 DNA in amniotic fluid, these tests are unreliable in predicting which fetuses will develop hydrops. The presence of B19 IgM depends on gestational age, and most infected fetuses are seronegative. Ultrasound is the most valuable test for diagnosis of fetal parvovirus infection because severely infected fetuses typically develop hydrops. Additional studies are unnecessary if the fetus is without hydrops. When a fetus does develop hydrops, cordocentesis with possible intrauterine transfusion may be done. Some investigators have described spontaneous resolution of hydrops after acute parvovirus infection (56), but because the criteria predictive of spontaneous resolution are not well established, fetuses found to be severely anemic should have an intrauterine transfusion (57). Possibly, younger fetuses at less than 20 weeks' gestation are more at risk, and older fetuses with a more mature immune system may be better able to tolerate the insult from a parvovirus infection.

Serial ultrasound studies have been found to be useful for the early detection of fetal hydrops, but maternal serum α-fetoprotein (MSAFP) testing is not of benefit. Several cases have been reported in which an elevated MSAFP preceded the development of hydrops by as long as 4 to 6 weeks (58), and some investigators have advocated MSAFP testing to predict those fetuses at highest risk. However, a normal MSAFP does not eliminate the need for serial ultrasound studies, and the MSAFP may be normal even when fetal disease is present (59). An elevated MSAFP in the absence of other evidence of B19 infection does not warrant B19-specific testing (60).

No antiviral agent or vaccine is currently available for treatment of parvovirus infection. Theoretically, because most of the adult population has been infected previously, administering intravenous Ig (IVIG) may be effective for postexposure prophylaxis (61). Administering IVIG worked in a canine model, but no reports have shown the usefulness of IVIG prophylaxis in humans. During endemic periods, the occupational risk of fetal death resulting from parvovirus B19 infection is so low (between 1 in 500 and 1 in 4,000) that screening and temporary reassignment of nonimmune employees to positions not involving child care are considered unjustified (62). Unfortunately, there is no good method to prevent acquiring infection from one's own school-aged children, the source of most maternal B19 infection. In view of the high prevalence of parvovirus B19, the low risk of ill effects to the fetus, and the finding that avoidance of child care or teaching can only reduce, not eliminate, the risk of infection, a policy of routinely excluding pregnant women from a workplace where erythema infectiosum is present is not recommended at this time (63).

Until recently, most authors had reported normal long-term development in infants surviving parvovirus infection during pregnancy. However, a 1993 study described persistent neurologic morbidity in three children after parvovirus infection that occurred at 21 to 24 weeks' gestation (64). A 1994 study described three infants with persistent severe anemia after intrauterine transfusion for parvovirus infection (65). Because of these few unfavorable cases, clinicians should be cautious in counseling parents regarding the long-term prognosis in affected infants.

GROUP B STREPTOCOCCUS

Streptococci have been characterized by the hemolytic reaction they produce on blood agar. On blood agar, the β-reaction is clear or complete hemolysis around the bacterial colony; the α-reaction is a greenish discoloration or partial hemolysis around the colony; and the γ-reaction refers to an absence of hemolysis around the colony. In 1933, Lancefield used serologic techniques to subdivide β-hemolytic streptococci into specific groups, which she named A, B, C, D, and E. Only groups A, B, and D have been linked to human disease.

Group A β-hemolytic streptococci (Streptococcus pyogenes) is rarely encountered today, but before the introduction of penicillin this organism was the major cause of puerperal sepsis and was responsible for 75% of maternal mortality resulting from infection. Group A streptococci can cause scarlet fever, erysipelas (an acute skin infection), and a toxic shock–like syndrome that can be fatal.

Group B β-hemolytic streptococci (Streptococcus agalactiae) are serologically classified into five serotypes on the basis of antigenic structure (types Ia, Ib, II, III, IV, V). Group B streptococci (GBS) were not linked to human disease until 1964, when they were found to cause infection in neonates and parturient women (66). Subsequently, an increasing number of reports documented concern about GBS infection in the neonate, and today GBS is the leading cause of neonatal sepsis, and it has replaced *Escherichia coli* as the most frequent microorganism associated with bacteremia or meningitis among infants during the first 2 months of life (67).

Maternal Infection

Approximately 20% of all women are asymptomatic carriers of GBS in their vagina and rectum. The Vaginal Infections and Prematurity Study Group reported that 15% to 20% of more than 8,000 pregnant women from 5 clinical centers had a lower genital tract culture positive for GBS done between 23 and 26 weeks' gestation (68). GBS is a major cause of chorioamnionitis, postpartum endometritis, and postcesarean wound infection. GBS-colonized patients who undergo cesarean delivery have a significantly enhanced risk of postpartum fever and endometritis. GBS is responsible for approximately 2% to 3% of urinary tract infections in pregnant women, but it usually does not cause pyelonephritis. Having a GBS urinary tract infection is a risk factor for premature rupture of membranes (PROM) and premature labor. In one study in which women at 27 to 31 weeks' gestation with streptococcal urinary tract infections were randomized to receive either penicillin or placebo, it was found that those treated with penicillin had a significant reduction in the frequency of both preterm PROM and premature labor (69). Women with preterm PROM who are colonized with GBS tend to have a shorter latent period and a higher frequency of chorioamnionitis and postpartum endometritis (70). GBS has been reported to cause postpartum maternal osteomyelitis, mastitis, pneumonia, and skin infections. GBS infections account for 10% to 20% of blood cultures isolated from women admitted to obstetric services (71). One-third of patients with GBS-induced endometritis or paraendometritis have bacteremia, and life-threatening complications of GBS bacteremia such as endo-

carditis, meningitis, and septicemia with multiorgan failure have been reported.

Neonatal Infection

Neonatal infection is divided into *early-onset infection* (occurs within 7 days of delivery) and *late-onset infection* (occurs from 7 days to 3 months after delivery). Approximately 80% of cases of neonatal GBS infection are of early onset, and these cases are almost always caused by vertical transmission from a colonized mother. The median age at onset of symptoms of early-onset GBS infection is 1 hour, and 90% of early-onset cases and almost all fatal cases occur within the first day of life. It appears that GBS infection is usually well established before birth. Signs of early-onset GBS disease include sepsis with or without signs of respiratory distress, apnea, and shock. Initially, early-onset GBS sepsis must be differentiated from idiopathic respiratory distress syndrome. Meningitis occurs in 5% to 10% of early-onset cases. In its most fulminant form, early-onset GBS infection presents as septic shock with respiratory distress leading to death within several hours after birth despite appropriate antibiotic therapy. Premature infants account for a disproportionately large number of cases of neonatal GBS disease (approximately 25%) (72). In preterm infants, the mortality from early-onset GBS infection is 25%. In term infants, the mortality is lower, averaging 5%. Major risk factors for early-onset GBS infection include the following: preterm labor, especially when complicated by PROM; intrapartum maternal fever (more than 38°C or 100.4°F); PROM of more than 18 hours' duration; and previous delivery of an infected infant (73). The incidence of GBS disease is higher among infants born to African-American mothers and to mothers less than 20 years of age (73). Women with heavy colonization of GBS in genital cultures (74), and those with low levels of anti-GBS capsular antibody (75), are also at increased risk of delivering an infant who has invasive GBS disease. The neonatal attack rate in colonized patients is 40% to 50% in the presence of a risk factor and 5% or less in the absence of a risk factor. Among GBS-infected infants, neonatal mortality approaches 30% to 35% when a maternal risk factor is present, but it is only 5% or less when all risk factors are absent (76). Of all infants born to colonized parturients, approximately 1% to 2% will develop early-onset invasive disease (67). A metaanalysis of 7 trials, which included studies of carriers with and without risk factors, estimated a 30-fold reduction in early-onset GBS disease with intrapartum chemoprophylaxis (77).

The 20% of cases of neonatal GBS infection that are of late onset occur as a result of both vertical and horizontal transmission. The median age at onset for late disease is 27 days, and maternal obstetric complications are uncommon among infants who later develop late-onset GBS infection (78). Meningitis is the predominant clinical manifestation among infants with late-onset GBS infection, but bacteremia and pneumonia may also occur. Although the mortality rate for late-onset GBS infection is lower (approximately 5% to 10% for both preterm and term infants), up to 50% of babies with meningitis subsequently demonstrate neurologic sequelae. Meningitis is related to the GBS serotype; 80% of cases of meningitis in early-onset GBS infections are caused by type III organisms, and 95% of cases of meningitis in late-onset disease are caused by type III (79). Prematurity is uncommon among infants with late-onset GBS infection, and unfortunately, obstetric interventions have proven ineffective in preventing late-onset neonatal infection.

Prevention

The current standard for diagnosing maternal asymptomatic genitourinary or gastrointestinal colonization with GBS is culture with a selective medium. The best medium for growing GBS is a selective broth medium, *Todd-Hewitt broth,* which contains gentamicin, polymyxin B, and nalidixic acid, which inhibit the growth of gram-negative Enterobacteriaceae and other genital tract flora that interfere with the recovery of GBS (80). Appropriate culture technique involves taking a simple cotton swab and rubbing it against the lower vagina (introitus) and perianal area before transfer to the selective broth media (73). The yield of GBS is lower from the cervix than from the introitus, and obtaining the culture does not require visualization of the cervix with a speculum. Culturing both the anorectum and the vaginal introitus increases the likelihood of GBS isolation by 5% to 27% over vaginal culture alone (81). Women colonized with GBS have an approximately 1 in 200 risk of having a neonate with early-onset GBS disease (67).

Because identification of GBS by culture usually takes 24 to 48 hours, intrapartum culture results are not available in time for intervention in most deliveries. In recent years, considerable research has been devoted to assessment of rapid diagnostic tests for the identification of GBS-colonized women. Although the rapid diagnostic tests have reasonable sensitivity in identifying heavily colonized patients, they have poor sensitivity in identifying lightly and moderately colonized patients, and this feature severely limits the usefulness of these tests in clinical practice (82).

Several different approaches to the problem of neonatal GBS infection have been advocated. In a prospective study of 18,738 neonates delivered during a 25-month period, one group received a single intramuscular dose of aqueous penicillin G after delivery, and the other group received only tetracycline ophthalmic ointment (83). In the group treated with penicillin, disease caused by penicillin-susceptible organisms was decreased, but there was an increase in the incidence of disease caused by penicillin-resistant organisms. This increase in penicillin-resistant neonatal infections makes universal penicillin prophylaxis a risky strategy.

In 1992, the American Academy of Pediatrics recommended universal screening of all pregnant women for GBS at 26 to 28 weeks' gestation and selective intrapartum treatment of colonized women with risk factors for GBS infection (84). Risk factors requiring intrapartum treatment included GBS carriers with rupture of membranes lasting more than 12 hours, onset of labor or rupture of membranes at less than 37 weeks, intrapartum fever, multiple gestation, and previous birth of an infant with GBS disease. One problem with this approach is that the presence of GBS at 26 to 28 weeks' gestation does not correlate perfectly with GBS presence at delivery. In one study, 7.4% of women with a negative culture at 26 to 28 weeks were found to carry GBS at delivery, and a single positive culture during pregnancy had a 67% predictive value at delivery (81). Therefore, treating patients at term based on a culture done at 26 to 28 weeks' gestation would lead to substantial overtreatment and undertreatment. Treating GBS carriers at 26 to 28 weeks has no effect on the presence of GBS at delivery. It is difficult to eradicate GBS from the rectum because of the presence of β-lactamase enzymes produced by Enterobacteriaceae that inactivate penicillin and ampicillin. Moreover, venereal transmission of GBS allows for reinfection. The high ratio of maternal and neonatal colonization to infection requires that 100 women and their sexual partners must be treated for each possible case of GBS infection (79).

Because of the high colonization rate (20%) and the low attack rate (1% to 2% of neonates born to colonized mothers develop early-onset disease), universal screening was not considered to be cost effective by the American College of Obstetricians and Gynecologists, which issued a statement in 1992 advocating intrapartum administration of ampicillin, penicillin G, or erythromycin based on the presence of risk factors instead of universal screening (73). Their risk factors included the following:

1. Preterm labor.
2. Preterm PROM.
3. Prolonged membrane rupture, defined as longer than 18 hours.
4. Sibling affected by symptomatic GBS infection.
5. Intrapartum maternal fever.

The criterion of more than 18 hours of rupture of membranes was selected on the basis of an observational study demonstrating a statistically significant increase in attack rate of GBS with rupture of membranes for more than 18 hours (81).

Through an elaborate theoretic decision analysis, one group of investigators came to the conclusion that universal antibiotic prophylaxis for all women in labor was the most cost-effective way to prevent neonatal GBS infection (85). Nineteen different strategies for the prevention of early-onset neonatal GBS sepsis were examined. These investigators concluded that the recommendations by the American

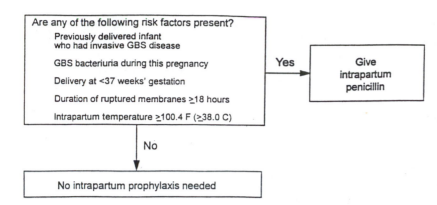

FIGURE 33.7. Prevention strategy for early-onset group B streptococci (GBS) disease using risk factors. (From Centers for Disease Control and Prevention. Prevention of perinatal group B streptococcal disease: a public health perspective. *MMWR Morb Mortal Wkly Rep* 1996;45:1–24, with permission.)

Academy of Pediatrics were among the least effective and most costly. Intrapartum treatment based solely on risk factors (the position of the American College of Obstetricians and Gynecologists) lowers the rate of neonatal sepsis to 31% of expected with an 18% maternal treatment rate and low total costs. Universal intrapartum maternal antibiotic treatment reduced early-onset neonatal GBS sepsis to 6% of expected and was the least costly. However, the benefit of GBS prevention must be weighed against the risk to the mother and fetus of maternal allergic reactions. Although the risk of fatal anaphylaxis has been estimated at 1 per 100,000, the risks of less severe anaphylactic or allergic reactions to the laboring mother and fetus are important (86). The risk of anaphylaxis is approximately 1 in 10,000, and the risk for a mild allergic reaction may be as high as 1 in 10. Administering intrapartum antimicrobial agents to all women who are GBS carriers could result in 10 deaths per year from anaphylaxis, assuming a GBS colonization rate of 25%, 4 million deliveries in the United States annually, and a rate of fatal anaphylaxis to penicillin of 0.001% (86).

The United States Centers for Disease Control and Pre-

vention convened a panel of obstetricians and pediatricians that decided on two equally acceptable alternatives for the prevention of perinatal GBS disease (87). The *risk-factor approach* involves giving intrapartum antibiotics based on risk factors as originally proposed by American College of Obstetricians and Gynecologists (Fig. 33.7). The *screening-based approach* calls for cultures to be done at 35 to 37 weeks with intrapartum penicillin G prophylaxis for all culture-positive women (Fig. 33.8). For intrapartum chemoprophylaxis, it was recommended to use intravenous penicillin G (5 million U initially then 2.5 million U every 4 hours) until delivery. Penicillin G is preferred because it has a narrow spectrum and is therefore less likely to select for antibiotic-resistant organisms. Ampicillin (2 g intravenous load, then 1 g intravenously every 4 hours until delivery) is an acceptable alternative to penicillin G. For penicillin-allergic women, clindamycin (900 mg intravenously every 8 hours until delivery) or erythromycin (500 mg intravenously every 6 hours until delivery) may be used, although the efficacy of these drugs for GBS prevention has not been assessed (73). Broader-spectrum antibiotics may be considered at the physician's discretion, based on clinical indica-

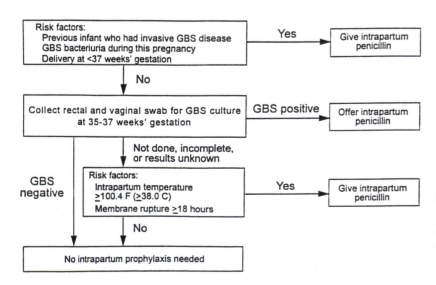

FIGURE 33.8. Prevention strategy for early-onset group B streptococci (GBS) disease using prenatal screening at 35 to 37 weeks' gestation. (From Centers for Disease Control and Prevention. Prevention of perinatal group B streptococcal disease: a public health perspective. *MMWR Morb Mortal Wkly Rep* 1996;45:1–24, with permission.)

tions. In either approach, if PROM occurs at less than 37 weeks' gestation and the mother is not in labor, a GBS culture should be taken and either (a) antibiotics should be administered until cultures are completed and the results are negative or (b) antibiotics should be begun only when positive cultures are available (87). Regardless of which approach is used, women with symptomatic or asymptomatic GBS bacteriuria during pregnancy should be treated at the time of diagnosis. Because women with GBS bacteriuria are heavily colonized by the pathogen, they should receive intrapartum chemoprophylaxis. For women who have previously given birth to an infant with GBS disease, prenatal screening is unnecessary because these women should receive intrapartum chemoprophylaxis regardless of a repeat culture result. Oral antibiotics should not be used to treat women who are found to be colonized with GBS during prenatal screening because treatment is not effective in eliminating carriage or in preventing neonatal disease (87). It is unlikely that a randomized prospective study will ever resolve which of these two approaches is the most effective against neonatal GBS infection because investigators have estimated that at least 100,000 pregnant women would need to be studied in each arm of the trial (88).

Because maternal antibody confers some protection against serious neonatal infection, maternal vaccination against GBS has been considered. Active maternal immunization with capsular polysaccharide antigen may prevent peripartum maternal and neonatal disease by transplacental transfer of protective IgG antibodies (89). Any vaccine would need to be polyvalent to cover all serotypes involved in early-onset sepsis. A GBS vaccine may be used to prevent disease in nonpregnant adults as well. However, the beneficial effects of a vaccine may be limited by reduced transplacental transport of protective antibody before 32 to 34 weeks, and some data suggest that preexisting type-specific antibodies may not protect against neonatal sepsis (90).

10 KEY POINTS

1. CMV is the most common cause of intrauterine infection, and as with other members of the Herpesviridae family, congenital infection may result from a maternal primary infection, reinfection, or reactivation of a latent infection.

2. Congenital CMV infection causes a syndrome that includes low birth weight, microcephaly, intracranial calcifications, chorioretinitis, mental and motor retardation, sensorineural deficits, hepatosplenomegaly, jaundice, hemolytic anemia, and thrombocytopenic purpura.

3. Because neither antiviral chemotherapy nor immunoprophylaxis is available to protect the fetus or neonate, routine prenatal screening for CMV infection is not recommended, and physicians should focus their attention on educating patients about preventive measures.

4. Toxoplasmosis can be transmitted by manual contact

with cat feces while gardening or handling cat litter boxes, by eating undercooked meat containing tissue cysts, by transfusion of infected blood or blood products, by heart or kidney transplants from seropositive donors to seronegative recipients, and by food contaminated by insect vectors.

5. Spiramycin, pyrimethamine, and sulfadiazine have been used to treat congenital toxoplasmosis diagnosed by PCR testing of amniotic fluid after maternal serologic study confirms an acute infection.

6. Parvovirus B19 causes erythema infectiosum (fifth disease) in children that is characterized by a "slapped cheek" rash, and in adults, it causes fever, malaise, adenopathy, and polyarthritis, but it can also lead to transient aplastic crisis in patients with underlying hemoglobinopathy.

7. Parvovirus B19 attacks erythroid precursor cells in the fetus and leads to hydrops, so once maternal infection is confirmed by serologic testing, serial ultrasound studies are done for approximately 10 weeks to watch for hydrops, which is treated by cordocentesis and transfusion.

8. Approximately 20% of all women are asymptomatic carriers of GBS, which is the leading cause of neonatal sepsis.

9. Early-onset GBS sepsis occurs within 7 days after birth, with the median age of onset being 1 hour after delivery, and risk factors include preterm labor, preterm PROM, intrapartum maternal fever (more than 38°C or 100.4°F), prolonged rupture of membranes for more than 18 hours, and previous delivery of an infected infant.

10. Strategies to decrease the incidence of early-onset GBS sepsis involve either culturing all patients at 35 to 37 weeks, and treating positive patients in labor, or not doing routine cultures and simply treating all patients with risk factors with intravenous penicillin G when they are in labor.

REFERENCES

1. Riley HD. History of the cytomegalovirus. *South Med J* 1997; 90:184–189.
2. Demmler G. Acquired cytomegalovirus infections. In: Feigin RD, Cherry JD, eds. *Textbook of pediatric infectious diseases,* 3rd ed. Philadelphia: WB Saunders, 1992:1532–1547.
3. Wilhelm JA, Malter L, Schopfer K. The risk of transmitting cytomegalovirus to patients receiving blood transfusions. *J Infect Dis* 1986;154:169.
4. Nelson CT, Demmler GJ. Cytomegalovirus infection in the pregnant mother, fetus, and newborn infant. *Clin Perinatol* 1997; 24:151–160.
5. Betts RF. Cytomegalovirus infection epidemiology and biology in adults. *Semin Perinatol* 1983;7:22.
6. Chandler SH, Alexander ER, Holmes HR. Epidemiology of cytomegalovirus infection in a heterogeneous population of pregnant women. *J Infect Dis* 1985;152:249.
7. Perlman JM, Argyle C. Lethal cytomegalovirus infection in preterm infants: clinical, radiological, and neuropathological findings. *Ann Neurol* 1992;330:901.
8. Stagno S, Pass RF, Dworsky ME, et al. Congenital cytomegalovirus infection. *N Engl J Med* 1982;306:945.
9. Fowler KB, Stagno S, Pass RF, et al. The outcome of congenital

cytomegalovirus infection in relation to maternal antibody status. *N Engl J Med* 1992;326:663.

10. Lange I, Rodeck CM, Morgan-Capner P, et al. Prenatal serological diagnosis of intrauterine cytomegalovirus infection. *BMJ* 1982;284:1673.

11. Hohlfeld P, Vial Y, Maillard-Brignon C, et al. Cytomegalovirus fetal infection: prenatal diagnosis. *Obstet Gynecol* 1991;78:615.

12. Lynch L, Daffos F, Emanuel D, et al. Prenatal diagnosis of fetal cytomegalovirus infection. *Am J Obstet Gynecol* 1991;165:714.

13. Donner C, Liesnard C, Content J, et al. Prenatal diagnosis of 52 pregnancies at risk for congenital cytomegalovirus infection. *Obstet Gynecol* 1993;82:481–486.

14. Suresh B, Boppana SB, Pass RF, et al. Symptomatic congenital cytomegalovirus infection: neonatal morbidity and mortality. *Pediatr Infect Dis J* 1992;11:93–99.

15. Lamy H, Mulongo K, Gadisseux JF, et al. Prenatal diagnosis of fetal cytomegalovirus infection. *Am J Obstet Gynecol* 1992;166:91–94.

16. Trang J, Kidd L, Gruber W, et al. Linear single-dose pharmacokinetics of ganciclovir in newborns with congenital cytomegalovirus infections. *Clin Pharmacol Ther* 1993;53:15.

17. Hocker J, Cook L, Adams G, et al. Ganciclovir therapy of congenital cytomegalovirus pneumonia. *Pediatr Infect Dis J* 1994;9:743.

18. Vallejo J, Englund J, Garcia-Prats J, et al. Ganciclovir treatment of steroid-associated cytomegalovirus disease in a congenitally infected neonate. *Pediatr Infect Dis J* 1994;13:239.

19. Adler SP, Finney JW, Manganello AM, et al. Prevention of child-to-mother transmission of cytomegalovirus by changing behaviors: a randomized controlled trial. *Pediatr Infect Dis J* 1996;15:240–246.

20. Beneson MW, Takafugi ET, Lemon SM, et al. Oocyst transmitted toxoplasmosis associated with ingestion of contaminated water. *N Engl J Med* 1982;307:666–669.

21. Freij BJ, Sever JL. What do we know about toxoplasmosis? *Contemp Obstet Gynecol* 1996;Feb:41–69.

22. Wong S-Y, Remington JS. Toxoplasmosis in pregnancy. *Clin Infect Dis* 1994;18:853.

23. Guerina NG, Hsu H-W, Meissner HC, et al. Neonatal serologic screening and early treatment for congenital *Toxoplasma gondii* infection. *N Engl J Med* 1994;330:1858.

24. Krick JA, Remington JS. Toxoplasmosis in the adult: an overview. *N Engl J Med* 1978;298:550.

25. Biedermann K, Flepp M, Fierz W, et al. Pregnancy, immunosuppression and reactivation of latent toxoplasmosis. *J Perinat Med* 1995;23:191–203.

26. Bobic B, Sibalic D, Djurkovic-Djakovic O. High levels of IgM antibodies specific for *Toxoplasma gondii* in pregnancy 12 years after primary *Toxoplasma* infection. *Gynecol Obstet Invest* 1991; 31:182.

27. Alger LS. Toxoplasmosis and parvovirus B19. *Infect Dis Clin North Am* 1997;11:55–75.

28. Guy EC, Joynson DHM. Potential of the polymerase chain reaction in the diagnosis of active *Toxoplasma* infection by detection of parasite in blood. *J Infect Dis* 1995;172:319.

29. American College of Obstetricians and Gynecologists. *Perinatal viral and parasitic infections.* Technical bulletin no. 177. American College of Obstetricians and Gynecologists, 1993.

30. Hall SM. Congenital toxoplasmosis. *BMJ* 1992;305:291–297.

31. Freij BJ, Sever JL. Toxoplasmosis. *Pediatr Rev* 1991;12:227.

32. Hohlfeld P, MacAleese J, Capella-Pavlovsky M, et al. Fetal toxoplasmosis: ultrasonographic signs. *Ultrasound Obstet Gynecol* 1991;1:241.

33. Hohlfeld P, Daffos F, Costa JM, et al. Prenatal diagnosis of congenital toxoplasmosis with a polymerase-chain reaction test on amniotic fluid. *N Engl J Med* 1994;331:695.

34. Duff P. Maternal and perinatal infection. In: Gabbe SG, Niebyl JR, Simpson JL, eds. *Obstetrics: normal and problem pregnancies,* 3rd ed. New York: Churchill Livingstone, 1996.

35. Daffos F, Forestier F, Capella-Pavlovsky M, et al. Prenatal management of 746 pregnancies at risk for congenital toxoplasmosis. *N Engl J Med* 1988;318:271–275.

36. Couvreur J, Desmonts G, Thulliez P. Prophylaxis of congenital toxoplasmosis: effects of spiramycin on placental infection. *J Antimicrob Chemother* 1988;22[Suppl B]:193.

37. Hohlfeld P, Daffos F, Thulliez P, et al. Fetal toxoplasmosis: outcome of pregnancy and infant follow-up after *in utero* treatment. *J Pediatr* 1989;115:765.

38. St. Georgiev V. Management of toxoplasmosis. *Drugs* 1994;48:179.

39. Guerina NG, Hsu HW, Meissner HC, et al. Neonatal serologic screening and early treatment for congenital *Toxoplasma gondii* infection. *N Engl J Med* 1994;330:1858.

40. Cossart YE, Field AM, Cant B, et al. Parvovirus-like particles in human sera. *Lancet* 1975;1:72.

41. Pattison JR, Jones SE, Hodgson J, et al. Parvovirus infections and hypoplastic crisis in sickle-cell anaemia [Letter]. *Lancet* 1981;1:664.

42. Anderson MR, Jones SE, Fisher-Hoch SP, et al. Human parvovirus, the cause of erythema infectiosum (fifth disease) [Letter]. *Lancet* 1983;1:1378.

43. Ware RE. Parvovirus infections. In: Krugman S, Katz SL, Gershon AA, et al., eds. *Infectious diseases of children,* 9th ed. St. Louis: CV Mosby, 1992:294.

44. Anderson LJ. Human parvovirus B19. *Pediatr Ann* 1990;19:509–513.

45. Brown KE, Young NS, Liu JM. Molecular, cellular and clinical aspects of parvovirus B19 infection. *Crit Rev Oncol Hematol* 1994;16:1.

46. Gray ES, Davidson RJC, Anand A. Human parvovirus and fetal anemia. *Lancet* 1987;1:1144.

47. Centers for Disease Control. Risks associated with human parvovirus B19 infection. *MMWR Morb Mortal Wkly Rep* 1989;38:81.

48. Rodis JF, Quinn, Gary GW Jr, et al. Management and outcomes of pregnancies complicated by human B19 parvovirus infection: a prospective study. *Am J Obstet Gynecol* 1990;163:1168.

49. Public Health Laboratory Service Working Party on Fifth Disease. Prospective study of human parvovirus (B19) infection in pregnancy. *BMJ* 1990;300:1166.

50. Wright C, Hinchliffe SA, Taylor C. Fetal pathology in intrauterine death due to parvovirus B19 infection. *Br J Obstet Gynaecol* 1996;103:133.

51. Kumar ML. Human parvovirus B19 and its associated diseases. *Clin Perinatol* 1991;18:209.

52. Gillespie SM, Cartter ML, Asch S, et al. Occupational risk of human parvovirus B19 infection for school and day-care personnel during an outbreak of erythema infectiosum. *JAMA* 1990; 263:2061.

53. Chorba T, Coccia P, Holman RC, et al. The role of parvovirus B19 in aplastic crisis and erythema infectiosum (fifth disease). *J Infect Dis* 1986;154:383.

54. Anderson MJ, Higgins PG, Davis LR, et al. Experimental parvoviral infection in humans. *J Infect Dis* 1985;152:257.

55. Duff P. Maternal and perinatal infection. In: Gabbe SG, Niebyl JR, Simpson JL, eds. *Obstetrics: normal and problem pregnancies,* 3rd ed. New York: Churchill Livingstone, 1996.

56. Fairley CK, Smoleniec JS, Caul OE, et al. Observational study of effect of intrauterine transfusions on outcome of fetal hydrops after parvovirus B19 infection. *Lancet* 1995;346:1335.

57. Sahakian V, Weiner CP, Naides SJ, et al. Intrauterine transfusion treatment of nonimmune hydrops fetalis secondary to human parvovirus B19 infection. *Am J Obstet Gynecol* 1991;164:1090.

58. Bernstein IM, Capeless EL. Elevated maternal serum alphafeto-

protein and hydrops fetalis in association with fetal parvovirus B19 infection. *Obstet Gynecol* 1989;74:456.

59. Sheikh AU, Ernest JM, O'Shea M. Long-term outcome in fetal hydrops from parvovirus B19 infection. *Am J Obstet Gynecol* 1992;167:337.

60. Johnson DR, Fisher RA, Helwick JJ, et al. Screening maternal serum alphafetoprotein levels and human parvovirus antibodies. *Prenat Diagn* 1994;14:455.

61. Schwarz F, Roggendorf M, Hottentrager B, et al. Immunoglobulins in the prophylaxis of parvovirus B19 infection. *J Infect Dis* 1990;162:1214.

62. Adler SP, Manganello AA, Koch WC, et al. Risk of human parvovirus B19 infections among school and hospital employees during endemic periods. *J Infect Dis* 1993;168:361.

63. American College of Obstetricians and Gynecologists. *Perinatal viral and parasitic infections.* Technical bulletin no. 177. American College of Obstetricians and Gynecologists, 1993.

64. Conry JA, Torok T, Andrews I. Perinatal encephalopathy secondary to *in utero* human parvovirus B-19 (HPV) infection. *Neurology* 1993;43:A346(abst).

65. Brown KE, Green SW, deMayolo JA, et al. Congenital anaemia after transplacental B19 parvovirus infection. *Lancet* 194;343:895.

66. Eickhoff TC, Klein JO, Daly AL, et al. Neonatal sepsis and other infections due to group B betahemolytic streptococci. *N Engl J Med* 1964;271:1221–1228.

67. Baker CJ, Edwards MS. Group B streptococcal infections. In: Remington JS, Klein JO, eds. *Infectious diseases of the fetus and newborn infant.* Philadelphia: WB Saunders, 1983.

68. Regan JA, Klebanoff MA, Nugent RP. The vaginal infections and prematurity study group: the epidemiology of group B streptococcal colonization in pregnancy. *Obstet Gynecol* 1991;77:875.

69. Thomsen AC, Morup L, Hansen KB. Antibiotic elimination of group-B streptococci in urine in prevention of preterm labor. *Lancet* 1987;1:591.

70. Newton ER, Clark M. Group B streptococcus and preterm rupture of membranes. *Obstet Gynecol* 1988;71:198.

71. Faro S. Group B beta-hemolytic streptococci and puerperal infections. *Am J Obstet Gynecol* 1981;140:686.

72. Zangwill KM, Schuchat A, Wenger JD. Group B streptococcal disease in the United States, 1990: report from a multistate active surveillance system. *MMWR CDC Surveill Summ* 1992;41:25–32.

73. American College of Obstetricians and Gynecologists. *Group B streptococcal infections in pregnancy.* Technical bulletin no. 170. American College of Obstetricians and Gynecologists, 1992.

74. Pass MA, Gray BM, Khare S, et al. Prospective studies of group B streptococcal infections in infants. *J Pediatr* 1979;95:431–443.

75. Baker CJ, Kasper DL. Correlation of maternal antibody deficiency with susceptibility to neonatal group B streptococcal infection. *N Engl J Med* 1976;294:753–756.

76. Boyer KM, Gotoff SP. Prevention of early-onset neonatal group B streptococcal disease with selective intrapartum chemoprophylaxis. *N Engl J Med* 1986;314:1665.

77. Allen UD, Navas L, King SM. Effectiveness of intrapartum penicillin prophylaxis in preventing early-onset group B streptococcal infection: results of a meta-analysis. *Can Med Assoc J* 1993;149:1659–1665.

78. Baker CJ. Group B streptococcal infections. *Clin Perinatol* 1997;24:59–47.

79. Gibbs RS, Sweet RL. Maternal and fetal infections: clinical disorders. In: Creasy RK, Resnik R, eds. *Maternal-fetal medicine: principles and practice,* 3rd ed. Philadelphia: WB Saunders, 1994:639–703.

80. Sweet RL, Gibbs RS. Group B streptococci. In: *Infectious diseases of the female genital tract,* 2nd ed. Baltimore: Williams & Wilkins, 1990:22–37.

81. Boyer KM, Gadzala CA, Kelly PD, et al. Selective intrapartum chemoprophylaxis of neonatal group B streptococcal early-onset disease. II. Predictive value of prenatal cultures. *J Infect Dis* 1983;148:802–809.

82. Yancey MK, Armer T, Clark P, et al. Assessment of rapid identification tests for genital carriage of group B streptococci. *Obstet Gynecol* 1992;80:1038.

83. Siegel JD, McCracken GH, Threlkeld N, et al. Single-dose penicillin prophylaxis against neonatal group B streptococcal infections. *N Engl J Med* 1980;303:769.

84. American Academy of Pediatrics Committee on Infectious Disease and Committee on Fetus and Newborn. Guidelines for prevention of group B streptococcal (GBS) infections by chemoprophylaxis. *Pediatrics* 1992;90:7775.

85. Rouse DJ, Goldenberg RL, Cliver SP, et al. Strategies for the prevention of early-onset neonatal group B streptococcal sepsis: a decision analysis. *Obstet Gynecol* 1994;83:483–494.

86. Schwartz B, Jackson L. Invasive group B streptococcal disease in adults. *JAMA* 1991;266:1112–1114.

87. Centers for Disease Control. Prevention of neonatal group B streptococcal disease: a public health perspective. *MMWR Morb Mortal Wkly Rep* 1996;45:1.

88. Landon MB, Harger J, McNellis D, et al. Prevention of neonatal group B streptococcal infection. *Obstet Gynecol* 1994;84:450–462.

89. Baker CJ, Rench MA, Edwards MS, et al. Immunization of pregnant women with a polysaccharide vaccine of group B streptococcus. *N Engl J Med* 1988;319:1180–1185.

90. Silver HM, Gibbs RS, Gray BM, et al. Risk factors for perinatal group B streptococcal disease after amniotic fluid colonization. *Am J Obstet Gynecol* 1990;163:19.

THE SPECTRUM OF HYPERTENSION IN LATE PREGNANCY

ROBIN L. PERRY
HARISH M. SEHDEV

One of the most common and deadly complications of pregnancy is *hypertension*. Pregnancy can both aggravate preexisting hypertension and induce hypertension in women who were previously normotensive. Despite extensive research, it still remains unclear how pregnancy aggravates or causes hypertension, and delivery remains the ultimate means of reversing the disease process. Untreated, hypertension increases both maternal and fetal morbidity and mortality. Pregnancies complicated by hypertensive disorders are at increased risk for such complications as abruptio placentae, intrauterine growth retardation, stillbirth, acute renal failure, hepatic dysfunction, coagulation disorders, and intracranial hemorrhage. Worldwide, it has been estimated that approximately 50,000 women die each year from preeclampsia (1), and in the United States, complications of pregnancy-induced hypertension are estimated to cause almost 18% of maternal deaths (2).

CLASSIFICATION

Classification and terminology describing hypertension in pregnancy are, according to the American College of Obstetricians and Gynecologists (ACOG), nonuniform, confusing, and steeped in tradition (3). The previously accepted classification scheme used four categories to describe hypertension in pregnancy (4,5). Important in any classification schema of hypertensive disorders in pregnancy is the identification and differentiation of hypertension that exists before pregnancy from hypertension that develops during pregnancy. Hypertension is generally defined as blood pressure equal to or greater than 140/90 mm Hg. The current classification scheme recommended by ACOG includes only chronic hypertension and pregnancy-induced hypertension and states that the "two conditions may coexist" (3).

Chronic Hypertension

Hypertension that antedates pregnancy, that is diagnosed before the twentieth week of gestation, or that persists for longer than 6 weeks post partum is defined as *chronic hypertension*. In normotensive and hypertensive gravidas, blood pressure decreases, owing to a decrease in systemic vascular resistance, in the second and early third trimester and then gradually returns to baseline. Therefore, the gravida with underlying hypertension who presents late in gestation with "normal" blood pressures may present a diagnostic dilemma when her blood pressure returns to its hypertensive levels in the third trimester. The prevalence of chronic hypertension in pregnancy varies among different populations, but it is estimated to represent between 1% and 5% of all pregnancies (6). Hypertension has multiple causes, and, as discussed later, preexisting hypertension poses its own risks and complications to the mother and fetus during pregnancy.

Pregnancy-Induced Hypertension

Pregnancy-induced hypertension is defined as hypertension (blood pressure greater than or equal to 140/90 mm Hg) that develops after the twentieth week of gestation, excluding pregnancies complicated by molar degeneration or hydatiform mole. Because Korotkoff phase IV cannot be reproduced accurately (7), in the United States it is usual practice to use Korotkoff phase V to measure diastolic blood pressure. In the past, criteria for diagnosing pregnancy-induced hypertension included a rise in blood pressure of 30 mm Hg systolic and 15 mm Hg diastolic on at least two occasions at least 6 hours apart. ACOG no longer considers this finding valid (3), because investigators have demonstrated that in normotensive pregnancies, almost 60% of primigravidas experience an increase in diastolic pressure of greater than 20 mm Hg, and more than 70% have an increase of more than 15 mm Hg (8,9). If hypertension is the only finding, it is considered nonproteinuric pregnancy-induced hypertension.

The second category within pregnancy-induced hypertension is *preeclampsia*. Traditionally, the diagnosis of preeclampsia included hypertension and the presence of new-onset proteinuria and generalized edema. *Edema* is such a common finding of late pregnancy that its presence or absence is not believed to validate or exclude the diagnosis of preeclampsia (5), and up to one-third of women with eclampsia may present without evidence of edema (10). In addition, the International Society for the Study of Hypertension in Pregnancy (11) and the Nelson classification system (12), used in the British Commonwealth, do not include edema in classifying preeclampsia. Nondependent edema, generally of the hands and face, and fluid retention manifested by rapid weight gain are signs of pathologic edema that should increase one's suspicion for preeclampsia.

Proteinuria is an important sign of preeclampsia, and without proteinuria, the diagnosis of preeclampsia should be questioned (13). New-onset proteinuria of greater than 300 mg in 24 hours or greater than 1+ on dipstick determinations at least 6 hours apart is diagnostic for preeclampsia. The level of proteinuria can vary during any 24-hour period, and thus, a single dipstick determination is not adequate to exclude the diagnosis. Proteinuria may be a late finding of preeclampsia, and 10% to 20% of eclamptic seizures develop before recognizable proteinuria occurs (10,13). Proteinuria in combination with hypertension greatly increases the risk of perinatal mortality and morbidity (14).

As discussed later, preeclampsia is further classified as either mild or severe. The distinctions are based on the degree of blood pressure elevation, on the degree of proteinuria, and on abnormal laboratory and clinical findings. The *HELLP syndrome* (hemolysis, elevated liver enzymes, and low platelets) is an additionally recognized entity that includes hematologic and hepatic abnormalities.

Finally, eclampsia is a further division of pregnancy-induced hypertension. *Eclampsia* is defined as the occurrence of seizures in a patient with pregnancy-induced hypertension without other identifiable causes. The seizures of eclampsia are grand mal, and they may occur before, during, and up to 10 to 14 days after labor and delivery (15,16).

Chronic Hypertension with Superimposed Preeclampsia

A woman may enter pregnancy with preexisting hypertension resulting from any of numerous causes. Pregnancy-induced hypertension may develop in as many as 20% to 50% of patients with chronic hypertension, and the prognosis for the patient and her fetus will be much worse than with either disease process alone. The diagnosis may be difficult to make, but it can be suspected by a rise in blood pressure of 30 mm Hg systolic or 15 mm Hg diastolic or a 20 mm Hg rise in mean arterial pressure (diastolic + [systolic − diastolic]/3) along with proteinuria (or worsening proteinuria in those with preexisting renal disease). Again, disease severity is classified as in pregnancy-induced hypertension.

Transient Hypertension

Transient hypertension, a category in previous classifications (4,5), is the development of new hypertension without proteinuria after the twentieth gestational week until 24 hours post partum. Any elevation of blood pressure should normalize within 10 days post partum. This diagnosis is made retrospectively. Again, because proteinuria is a late finding and because treatment of the gravid patient with increasing blood pressures does not differ even when transient hypertension is the ultimate diagnosis, this designation is no longer considered in the classification scheme recommended by ACOG.

PREGNANCY-INDUCED HYPERTENSION: INCIDENCE AND EPIDEMIOLOGY

The overall incidence of pregnancy-induced hypertension, a disease entity that is specific to human pregnancy, is between 5% and 10%, with variations depending on the population studied and the diagnostic criteria used. It is primarily a disease of young primigravidas. The incidence in primigravidas ranges between 10% and 4%, and it is between 5.7% and 7.3% in multiparous patients (9,17).

Several risk factors have been identified, and overall, pregnancy-induced hypertension has a higher incidence in primigravidas (18). Older gravidas, especially those older than 35 to 40 years of age, appear to be at a two- to threefold greater risk of experiencing pregnancy-induced hypertension (19,20), and in many cases, underlying chronic hypertension may play a role in the risk of disease. Patients entering pregnancy with chronic hypertension (21) and underlying renal disease (22) are also at greater risk for developing pregnancy-induced hypertension. Moreover, patients with diabetes mellitus (23) and the antiphospholipid syndrome (24) are reported to be at greater risk for developing pregnancy-induced hypertension.

Other risk factors for developing pregnancy-induced hypertension include African-American race (22), family history (25), and a history of pregnancy-induced hypertension with previous deliveries, especially if the complications arose remote from term (26). Patients with multiple gestations are also at greater risk of developing pregnancy-induced hypertension (27), and, compared with pregnancy-induced hypertension in singleton gestations, the disease process in patients with multiple gestations usually presents earlier and is more severe (28).

THEORIES FOR THE ETIOLOGY OF PREGNANCY-INDUCED HYPERTENSION

Multiple theories of the cause of pregnancy-induced hypertension have been proposed, and over time several have been dispelled. Several are still considered plausible, but the underlying mechanism and process that causes these disorders of pregnancy remain obscure.

Genetic Predisposition

In 1968, a study reported on the incidence of preeclampsia and eclampsia in daughters and daughters-in-law of women who themselves had eclampsia (29). The observed frequencies for hypertensive complications in this study agreed with calculated frequencies of hypertensive complications in daughters of women with eclampsia (30). From these studies and further observations of the sisters, daughters, daughters-in-law, and granddaughters of women with eclampsia, investigators concluded that preeclampsia-eclampsia was inheritable in a manner consistent with the single gene hypothesis (25). However, multifactorial inheritance could not be excluded.

More recent work has focused on single gene variants and the risk of developing pregnancy-induced hypertension. In one study, women with the angiotensinogen gene variant *T235* were shown to have a higher incidence of pregnancy-induced hypertension (31). This risk was further elevated when they were homozygous for this genetic variant; however, another study from a different population did not support these findings (32). Investigators have shown that women with preeclampsia have a higher incidence of the factor V Leiden mutation (33).

Immunologic Basis

The immunologic basis for developing pregnancy-induced hypertension is believed to be consistent with the findings that primigravidas are at greater risk for disease than multigravidas and the disease is more common in multiparous patients when they carry a pregnancy with a new partner (34,35). This theory purports that in the initial pregnancy with a new partner, the maternal immune response to paternal antigens in some way affects the placenta. With subsequent exposure to paternal antigens in later pregnancies, maternal antibodies are able to "block" these antigenic sites on the placenta and thereby to negate the maternal response that affects the process causing the development of pregnancy-induced hypertension. In this light, the increased incidence of disease in multiple gestations is supported by a relative imbalance of maternal antibodies to the number of antigenic sites (36). Other investigators have demonstrated that oral sex before pregnancy reduces the incidence of pregnancy-induced hypertension by providing prior exposure to paternal antigens that enable the women's immune system to develop the "blocking" antibodies to the antigenic sites that are responsible for affecting disease (37). However, data contradicting this "immunization" theory come from a study that shows only a minimal and nonsignificant decrease in the incidence of pregnancy-induced hypertension in primigravidas who had prior abortions of pregnancies with the same partner (38).

Dietary Influences

Several theories of the cause of pregnancy-induced hypertension have focused on *dietary deficiencies.* Underlying these theories is the tenet that pregnancy diminishes nutritional stores. This line of thinking would place multigravidas and, presumably, nonobese women at greater risk of developing pregnancy-induced hypertension. However, it is well documented that pregnancy-induced hypertension is more common in nulliparous patients, and investigators have shown that obesity and higher prepregnancy weight increase the risk of hypertensive disorders (39). Investigators have also demonstrated that levels of dietary protein are not related to the risk of developing pregnancy-induced hypertension (40).

Much attention has been focused on the role of calcium in the risk of pregnancy-induced hypertension. Several authors documented that women with preeclampsia and women with future hypertension had decreased urinary calcium excretion (41,42). Morever, calcium intake was shown to be inversely associated with maternal blood pressure. Investigators believed that calcium lowered blood pressure by altering plasma renin activity, and in pregnant women, calcium supplementation was shown to reduce vascular sensitivity to angiotensin II (43,44). Several studies also showed that calcium supplementation (2 g of elemental calcium after midgestation) seemed to reduce the risk of developing pregnancy-induced hypertension (44–46). Overall, at least nine trials on calcium supplementation have been conducted, and, unfortunately, there are many differences in the individual study designs and calcium doses used. In 1997, the results of a double-blind randomized trial evaluating calcium supplementation (2 g per day versus placebo beginning at 13 to 21 weeks' gestation) in healthy nulliparous patients was published (47). Overall, the study reported that calcium supplementation, in healthy primiparas, did not decrease the incidence of pregnancy-induced hypertension, preeclampsia, or adverse perinatal outcomes.

In addition to calcium deficiency, magnesium and zinc deficiency had also been reported to be associated with preeclampsia and poor pregnancy outcome (48,49). Separate randomized control trials involving zinc (50) and magnesium supplementation (51) versus placebo found no differences in incidence of pregnancy-induced hypertension, preterm delivery, or birth weight. In summary, the evidence does not support dietary supplementation with calcium, magnesium, or zinc for prevention of pregnancy-induced hypertension.

Vasoactive Mediators

Because of the belief that *vasospasm* plays a role in effecting maternal organ dysfunction from pregnancy-induced hypertension, attention has been paid to vasoactive compounds in the last decade. Endothelial cells synthesize a potent vasodilator, nitric oxide (formerly endothelium-derived relaxing factor) (52). Investigators have shown in humans and sheep that nitric oxide appears to play a role in maintaining the low-pressure vasodilated environment of the fetoplacental circulation (53,54). Although one author showed an increase in an endogenous nitric oxide synthesis inhibitor in patients with preeclampsia versus patients with nonproteinuric hypertension and normotensive pregnancies (55), another study evaluating levels of circulating nitrite and nitrate found no difference between normotensive control subjects and patients with severe preeclampsia (56). Furthermore, evidence suggests that decreased levels of nitric oxide in patients with pregnancy-induced hypertension do not occur before the onset of hypertension, a finding thereby suggesting that associated changes in nitric oxide levels are not the inciting event but are a result of pregnancy-induced hypertension (57). Another compound that has received attention is endothelin-1, a potent vasoconstrictor. Again, as with other theorized etiologic agents for pregnancy-induced hypertension, some studies have shown higher levels of endothelin-1 in patients with preeclampsia (58–60), while other studies have failed to confirm these findings (61,62).

Many investigators have tried to examine the role of prostanoids, lipid peroxides, and antioxidants in pregnancy. During pregnancy, production of prostanoids increases in both maternal and fetoplacental tissues. Most studies suggest that during normal pregnancy, both prostacyclin (a potent vasodilator) and thromboxane (a potent vasoconstrictor) production increases, and in normotensive pregnancies, the ratio favors prostacyclin to thromboxane (63). Overall studies suggest an imbalance in preeclampsia that distorts this ratio in favor of thromboxane (63,64), but for the most part, the data have been inconsistent. The inconsistencies in large part result from the method for assaying prostanoid levels that relies on measuring unstable metabolites. Another group further demonstrated an increase in the ratios of both prostacyclin to thromboxane and vitamin E to lipid peroxides (65). This group demonstrated that these ratios were reversed with preeclampsia (66). The data regarding an increase in lipid peroxides (67) and a decrease in serum antioxidant activity (66,68,69) in women with preeclampsia have been more consistent than the data on prostanoids, and these continue to be areas of aggressive investigation in trying to understand the causes of pregnancy-induced hypertension.

Two studies evaluating the complications of preeclampsia reported that smoking was associated with a decreased risk of pregnancy-induced hypertension (39,70). Smoking appears to decrease the activity of an enzyme that inhibits platelet-derived vasodilation and aggregation (71), thereby allowing normal vasodilation and inhibiting platelets from abnormal activation and aggregation.

PATHOPHYSIOLOGY OF PREGNANCY-INDUCED HYPERTENSION

Trophoblast Abnormalities and Endothelial Dysfunction

The model that has gained tremendous acceptance for explaining the pathophysiologic changes associated with pregnancy-induced hypertension is one that postulates *abnormal trophoblastic invasion of the uterine vessels*. In normal pregnancy, trophoblast invasion of the spiral arterioles causes degeneration of the muscular layer of these arteries that produces distention and results in the low pressure, low resistance, and high flow seen in the uteroplacental bed. This process appears to occur in two stages: the first stage (during the first trimester) involves invasion of the decidual portion of the spiral arteries, and in the second trimester, a second stage of invasion involves the myometrial segments (72). In pregnancies complicated by pregnancy-induced hypertension, this second stage of trophoblastic invasion appears to be hampered, and the myometrial segments of the spiral arterioles are left intact and are able to respond to vasoactive mediators.

These vascular abnormalities (a decrease in number of well-developed spiral arterioles and deficient muscular degeneration of the arteriolar walls) have been confirmed histologically (73). Placental bed biopsies confirmed these changes and also showed acute atherosclerotic changes in vessels of women with preeclampsia. Abnormal morphology of the spiral arterioles is not found in all the vessels of a placenta of a hypertensive pregnancy (74), and these findings are also noted in normotensive pregnancies complicated by growth retardation (75,76).

Overall, these vascular abnormalities result in poor perfusion of the fetoplacental unit, and this decreased perfusion is belived to result in the release of a factor that causes endothelial injury (77). Serum obtained from women with preeclampsia versus normotensive patients has been shown both to be cytotoxic to endothelial cells *in vitro* (78) and to cause an increase in prostacyclin production. Endothelial injury, ranging from swelling (with a decrease in the vascular lumen) to complete endothelial erosion with fibrin deposition, has been confirmed by electron microscopy in the placentas of pregnancies complicated by preeclampsia (79). This endothelial injury activates coagulation, increases vascular permeability, and increases vascular sensitivity to vasopressor agents causing the vasospasm that appears to be central to the pathophysiology of pregnancy-induced hypertension.

Vasospasm

The concept of *vasospasm* was proposed in 1918 from observations of small vessels in the fundi and nail beds (80), as well as from histologic changes seen in affected organs. The vasospasm causes development of hypertension as a result of arterial constriction, and further endothelial injury is postulated. These insults result in decreased perfusion and hypoxia that lead to hemorrhage and necrosis seen in organs affected by preeclampsia.

As stated earlier, abnormal trophoblastic invasion and endothelial injury seen with pregnancy-induced hypertension were postulated to result in increased vascular sensitivity to vasopressors. Evidence for this increased sensitivity to vasopressors in women with pregnancy-induced hypertension has been demonstrated with vasopressin (81), norepinephrine, and angiotensin II (82,83). In 1973, investigators showed that blood pressure response to angiotensin II infusion at 28 to 32 weeks' gestation could identify women destined to develop hypertensive disorders of pregnancy (84). Those at risk of hypertensive complications were more sensitive to angiotensin II infusion than those who remained normotensive and exhibited a minimal response to angiotensin II infusion. The mechanism for the normal insensitivity to angiotensin II is believed to be secondary to increased endothelial prostaglandins (85,86), an effect that is diminished with prostaglandin synthase inhibitors (87). Furthermore, women sensitive to angiotensin II infusion were also shown to demonstrate a rise in diastolic blood pressure when they changed from a lateral recumbent position to a supine position when they were tested at 28 to 32 weeks' gestation (88). The mechanism by which this "rollover test" causes an increase in blood pressure is not clearly understood, and various authors have found a wide range in sensitivity for this test in predicting preeclampsia.

Although vasospasm appears to play a major role in the pathogenesis of preeclampsia, the exact mechanism by which vasoactive substances (such as prostaglandins and nitric oxide) exert their effects remains unclear, as discussed earlier in more detail.

ORGAN SYSTEM CHANGES IN PREGNANCY-INDUCED HYPERTENSION

Cardiovascular Changes

Invasive techniques have been used by many authors to elucidate the cardiovascular changes associated with pregnancy-induced hypertension. Overall, findings for several parameters are variable. The variations in study results may result from many factors, including differences in definitions used for preeclampsia, the presence of underlying medical diseases in patients, the duration and severity of pregnancy-induced hypertensive disorders, and the interventions and treatments undertaken during and before measurements.

Studies of untreated patients with severe preeclampsia have demonstrated that both cardiac index and pulmonary capillary wedge pressures are both normal to low with increased vascular resistance and hyperdynamic left ventricular function (89–91). Treatment with magnesium sulfate and hydralazine lowers systemic vascular resistance (although it remains elevated compared with normotensive patients),

with persistent hyperdynamic left ventricular function (92,93). Treatment with large volumes of intravenous fluids appears to further lower vascular resistance but results in increased central pressures (pulmonary capillary wedge pressure) above normal and increased cardiac output (94,95). Another study has demonstrated that in women destined to develop hypertensive complications, elevated cardiac output appears early and increases progressively.

Overall, it appears that the increased blood volume of normal pregnancy (approximately 5,000 mL compared with 3,500 mL in the nonpregnant state) is diminished in patients with preeclampsia and eclampsia at the expense of an increased extracellular volume (96). Vasoconstriction and increased vascular permeability account for the decreased volume expansion and result in hemoconcentration. With recovery post partum, the vasculature dilates, and extravascular fluid returns to the vascular compartment, with resulting hemodilution that should be gradual. Acute changes in hemoglobin and hematocrit should raise concern for significant blood loss at delivery.

Hematologic Changes

In pregnancies complicated by pregnancy-induced hypertension, *thrombocytopenia* is the most frequent hematologic abnormality. If found, thrombocytopenia may worsen immediately after delivery, but it should begin to increase from the nadir after 48 hours. The cause of thrombocytopenia is unclear, but endothelial injury promotes platelet activation, microvasculature consumption of platelets, and increased clotting activity (97,98). Other investigators have postulated an immunologic role for thrombocytopenia. One study demonstrated increased levels of platelet-bound and circulating immunoglobulin capable of binding platelets in women with preeclampsia (99), and another study showed that the incidence of platelet-associated IgG was increased in patients with preeclampsia even when the platelet count remained normal (100).

The incidence of thrombocytopenia reported depends on the definitions used, the severity of disease, the presence of abruptio placentae, and the delay from time of disease onset to delivery. A study of 100 consecutive women with severe preeclampsia reported that 50% had a platelet count less than $150,000/mm^3$ and 36% had a platelet count less than $100,000/mL^3$ (101). Only 2 women had increased prothrombin and partial thromboplastin times, 13 had a fibrinogen level less than 300 mg/dL, and all these patients had thrombocytopenia. From this study, these authors conclude that only in those patients with thrombocytopenia less than $100,000/mm^3$ should prothrombin time, partial thromboplastin time, and fibrinogen levels be evaluated. Finally, thrombocytopenia secondary to severe preeclampsia or eclampsia is not associated with neonatal thrombocytopenia (102).

Other hematologic abnormalities have been associated

with preeclampsia, and, again, these abnormalities may be partially or completely associated with endothelial injury. In women with preeclampsia and chronic hypertension with superimposed preeclampsia, elevated fibronectin (secondary to endothelial injury), decreased antithrombin III (secondary to increased clotting), and lower levels of α-antiplasmin (secondary to fibrinolysis) have been reported (97). Other observed hematologic abnormalities noted include an increase in the D-dimer fragment of fibrin degradation (103), an increase in circulating thrombin-antithrombin III complexes, and decreased levels of protein C (104). Finally, plasma fibrinogen levels, which normally rise in pregnancy, are rarely decreased with preeclampsia in the absence of abruptio placentae.

Renal Changes

In normal pregnancy, serum creatinine, uric acid, and urea levels fall secondary to an increased glomerular filtration rate and increased renal plasma flow. With the vasospasm that accompanies preeclampsia, the glomerular filtration rate and renal perfusion decrease. Serum creatinine levels rarely increase, except in some cases of profound severe preeclampsia. Serum uric acid levels increase with preeclampsia, but elevations do not appear to correlate with or to predict adverse outcome (105). Moreover, diminished urinary excretion of calcium (secondary to increased tubular reabsorption) has been demonstrated in women with preeclampsia (106).

Patients with severe preeclampsia may develop *oliguria*. In patients with oliguria, normal left ventricular filling pressures have been noted (107). The vasospasm appears to mediate both the prerenal and intrinsic renal abnormalities that are responsible for oliguria. However, use of generous intravenous fluid therapy is not indicated in these patients, and treatment with renal vasodilators has been shown to increase urine output and fractional sodium excretion (108).

As discussed earlier, *proteinuria* is a major component in making the diagnosis of preeclampsia. Again, proteinuria is a late finding. In addition, levels of proteinuria can vary widely throughout the day, and therefore, proteinuria should be quantified by a 24-hour collection. Using a urinary dipstick value of 1+ or greater can predict 92% of patients with at least 300 mg protein per 24 hours, and values of 3+ or greater are predictive of only 36% of cases of severe preeclampsia (109). A negative dipstick evaluation for proteinuria has a negative predictive value of about one-third in patients with hypertension.

Preeclampsia causes glomerulonephropathy, and, as such, proteinuria involves increased albumin excretion as well as other larger proteins that are normally filtered at the glomerulus. Histologic changes in the kidneys of women with preeclampsia have been observed by both light and electron microscopy. Glomeruli are enlarged, with swollen endothelial cells, and subendothelial deposits are noted (glo-merular endotheliosis) (110,111). Capillary loops are also affected and can even be blocked by swollen endothelial cells. Renal tubular lesions are also seen. These lesions may represent cellular degeneration or reabsorbed protein from the filtrate. Obstruction of the collecting tubules may result from proteinaceous casts. Finally, tubular necrosis causing *acute renal failure* may occur in severe cases accompanied by significant hemorrhage either from delivery or abruption. Overall, renal abnormalities associated with preeclampsia resolve.

Liver Dysfunction and HELLP Syndrome

Preeclampsia does not primarily affect the liver, but liver abnormalities can be seen in up to 10% of women with severe preeclampsia (112). Liver abnormalities associated with preeclampsia include an elevation of liver enzymes but not bilirubin. The origin of liver enzyme elevations most likely involves periportal hemorrhagic necrosis associated with fibrin deposition. This abnormality has been diagnosed by liver biopsies, and the life-threatening complication of subcapsular hematoma formation with rupture can occur if there is bleeding in the areas of necrosis.

When one sees evidence of liver involvement as a result of pregnancy-induced hypertension, other systems often have evidence of derangements, including hemolysis, thrombocytopenia, and disturbances in renal function. This syndrome was labeled the *HELLP syndrome* in 1982 (112), and it is considered a variant of severe preeclampsia. Several opinions exist on how to define, diagnose, and manage this syndrome (113), the incidence of which ranges from 2% to 12% (114). It appears to be more common in whites, and it has a higher incidence in patients with preeclampsia who are managed conservatively.

Patients with this syndrome may not exhibit proteinuria or meet blood pressure criteria for severe or even mild preeclampsia. In one study, almost 15% of patients with HELLP syndrome had diastolic blood pressures less than 90 mm Hg (113). Patients often present with various symptoms that are not diagnostic of severe preeclampsia, and these patients are often misdiagnosed with other medical or surgical disorders including gastroenteritis, peptic ulcer disease, appendicitis, viral hepatitis, systemic lupus erythematosus, and other disorders. Although most cases develop ante partum, up to 30% may develop post partum (115). Maternal morbidity is common, and both perinatal morbidity and mortality are increased in pregnancies complicated by HELLP syndrome (113,115).

Microangiopathic hemolysis, believed to be secondary to platelet activation and vasospasm, is the cause of hemolysis in HELLP syndrome. Disseminated intravascular coagulation may develop in as many as 20% of patients with HELLP syndrome (115), with most cases occurring in pregnancies also complicated by abruptio placentae, significant hemorrhage with delivery, and subcapsular liver hematomas. Debate over the level of liver enzyme elevation and thrombocytopenia necessary for the diagnosis exists, and several studies do not even report the degree of liver enzyme abnormalities (114). One study demonstrated a strong association of HELLP syndrome with eclampsia, and the authors suggest that it may be a risk factor for developing eclampsia (116).

Central Nervous System Changes

How preeclampsia affects cerebral blood flow and the brain is not known. Vasospasm, which has been confirmed by angiography in a limited number of patients (117), may play a role, but it appears that loss of autoregulation of cerebral blood flow is an important mechanism for neurologic sequelae. As blood pressure exceeds 150 mm Hg, autoregulated vasoconstriction is normally impaired, and cerebral blood flow is increased. As blood flow increases, dilation and ischemia of the arterioles occur, and they become permeable, thus causing edema and compression of other vessels (118). This edema may be responsible for the neurologic findings of severe preeclampsia and may cause the seizures of eclampsia.

Eclamptic seizures usually occur ante partum, but up to 30% may occur post partum (10), usually within 48 hours. Up to 90% of patients with eclampsia have been shown to have abnormal electroencephalograms (EEGs) (119). The abnormalities seen are nonspecific, and although magnesium sulfate suppresses clinical seizure activity, some patients may still exhibit seizure activity on EEG recordings (120). Debate exists about the correlation of seizure activity on EEG and the level of blood pressure elevation (119,120), and most EEG abnormalities reverse after 12 weeks.

Pathologic abnormalities of the brain found at autopsy of women who died of eclampsia include edema, hemorrhage, and thrombosis. In a series from 1950, intracranial hemorrhage, ranging from petechial hemorrhages to gross bleeding, was discovered in more than 50% of autopsy specimens of women who had died of eclampsia (100). Histologic evaluation of vessel walls frequently reveals fibrinoid changes.

Several studies have reported on computed tomography (CT) findings in patients with eclampsia. Studies have shown that CT scans of the patient's head are abnormal in 30% to 40% of cases. Several abnormalities have been noted that range from hypodensities in cortical and subcortical areas (corresponding to petechial hemorrhages and infarction) to loss of normal cortical sulci, decreased ventricular size, intraventricular and parenchymal hemorrhage, and basal ganglia infarctions (118). Studies have also reported similar abnormalities seen using magnetic resonance imaging (MRI) (121,122). One study comparing CT and MRI in women with eclampsia found a higher rate of intracranial abnormalities with MRI (121). Overall, use of CT scans is considered safe in pregnancy, but MRI affords the benefits of not using ionizing radiation and can provide imaging in more planes than CT. Despite the abnormal

findings in women with eclampsia, management of a patient with eclampsia rarely changes based on radiographic findings (123).

Although patients with severe preeclampsia commonly report blurry vision (possibly from retinal artery vasospasm), blindness in patients with severe preeclampsia or eclampsia is rare. Radiologic findings in patients with blindness include extensive hypodensities in the occipital lobe. Blindness occurring in these patients persists for several hours up to 1 week (124). Rarely, patients with eclampsia may become comatose, and radiographic studies reveal more extensive cerebral edema.

PREVENTION OF HYPERTENSION

Many authors have examined the use of aspirin in the prevention of preeclampsia. Physiologically, preeclampsia is known to be associated with vasospasm and activation of the coagulation system. Platelet activation plays a role in this process and results in an abnormal thromboxane-to-prostacyclin ratio. Thromboxane is a vasoconstricting prostanoid, whereas prostacyclin is a potent vasodilator and platelet aggregation inhibitor.

Aspirin is known to inhibit prostaglandin synthesis by irreversibly inactivating cyclooxygenase. Platelet cyclooxygenase is more sensitive to inhibition by low-dose aspirin (less than 80 mg) than vascular endothelial cyclooxygenase. This difference could be used to alter the balance of thromboxane and prostacyclin by selectively suppressing platelet thromboxane synthesis and relatively sparing endothelial prostacyclin production (125,126). These observations have led to a series of studies evaluating the utility of low-dose aspirin in the prevention of preeclampsia in different populations.

Low-dose aspirin was shown to reduce intrauterine growth retardation and cesarean delivery in women at risk of pregnancy-induced hypertension in a metaanalysis of six controlled studies (127). In a large randomized study of normotensive nulliparous women, Sibai et al. compared 60 mg of aspirin with placebo. The treated group had a lower incidence of preeclampsia with no difference in perinatal morbidity. These investigators did, however, demonstrate a higher incidence of placental abruption in the treatment group (128). Other investigators have concluded that these abruptions are not clinically significant (129).

A large multinational randomized trial, the Collaborative Low-Dose Aspirin Study in Pregnancy (CLASP), evaluated low-dose aspirin for the prevention and treatment of preeclampsia and intrauterine growth retardation (130). In this randomized trial, 9,364 women were either assigned to receive 60 mg of aspirin or placebo. The two groups showed no difference in the incidences of preeclampsia, intrauterine growth retardation, abruptio placentae, or perinatal death. There was, however, a significant decrease in the incidence of preterm delivery.

These results suggest that low-dose aspirin, 60 to 80 mg, may be appropriate in women at high risk of pregnancy-induced hypertension. Use of aspirin is not, however, recommended for pregnancy-induced hypertension prophylaxis in low-risk, normotensive multiparous or nulliparous patients (3).

The role of calcium supplementation in the prevention of preeclampsia remains controversial. In one randomized prospective study of angiotensin-sensitive patients who received 2 g of oral calcium gluconate daily, a threefold decrease in preeclampsia was noted (131). Yet a large randomized study of 4,589 healthy nulliparous women failed to demonstrate a decrease in incidence or severity of preeclampsia or a delay in onset with 2 g of elemental calcium daily versus placebo (47). It appears that dietary supplementation with calcium has no proven benefit in the prevention of pregnancy-induced hypertension in the low-risk population.

CLINICAL EVALUATION

When evaluating the gravida with hypertension, a complete history should be obtained if possible. A sudden increase in weight, more than 2 lb in a week or 6 lb in any given month, is a significant historical fact supporting the diagnosis of preeclampsia. The presence of headache (significant frontal or occipital headache unrelieved by typical analgesics), visual disturbances (blurred vision, scotoma, or blindness), and epigastric or right upper quadrant pain will help to distinguish severe from mild disease. A history of preexisting hypertension or any underlying medical condition should be sought.

A complete physical examination needs to be performed. The patient's blood pressure should be obtained in an appropriate and reproducible manner. The cuff should be appropriately sized, and the nondependent arm should be held by the examiner at the level of the heart. Korotkoff phase V (disappearance of sound) should be used to represent the diastolic blood pressure because it has been shown to be more accurate than phase IV (muffling of sound) (7). With the patient in the lateral decubitus position, the lowest blood pressure is obtained, and patient positioning must be consistent on serial examinations. A baseline maternal weight should be recorded. The patient needs to be examined with special attention toward the presence of nondependent edema including periorbital edema, right upper quadrant or epigastric tenderness, and hyperreflexia.

Laboratory evaluation should be directed toward distinguishing mild from severe disease and identifying any effects of possible chronic hypertension. A complete blood count with platelets should be obtained while remembering that the hematocrit may be falsely elevated because of the hemoconcentration seen in preeclampsia. The presence of thrombocytopenia or clinical evidence of placental abruption warrants further coagulation studies. Fibrinogen levels, prothrombin time, and partial thromboplastin time need only

be obtained when the platelet count is less then 100,000/mm^3 (101). Renal function can be assessed with serum creatinine, blood urea nitrogen, and electrolytes. A serum uric acid level can be drawn; however, its clinical utility has been questioned by some investigators (105). Others have reported the presence of hyperuricemia in severe preeclampsia to be associated with a poor fetal prognosis regardless of maternal blood pressure (132,133). A random urine sample should be dipped for protein, and a 24-hour urine collection for protein and creatinine clearance should be initiated. The volume of maternal urine output should also be assessed over time. Laboratory evidence of HELLP syndrome should be sought with a peripheral blood smear, serum lactate dehydrogenase, and serum glutamic-oxaloacetic transaminase. In patients with long-standing severe chronic hypertension, an electrocardiogram and cardiac echocardiogram may be indicated.

Fetal well-being needs to be established with a nonstress test or biophysical profile. Fetal ultrasound imaging should be performed to rule out intrauterine growth restriction and oligohydramnios.

DIFFERENTIAL DIAGNOSIS

The major differential diagnosis when managing hypertension in pregnancy includes pregnancy-induced hypertension, chronic hypertension, and a combination of the two. Chronic hypertension, by definition, predates pregnancy, is diagnosed before 20 weeks' gestation, or persists past 6 weeks post partum. Most women with chronic hypertension have essential hypertension; however, many other possible causes do exist and should be considered.

Pregnancy-induced hypertension exists when hypertension develops after 20 weeks' gestation. The importance of accurate gestational dating and good prenatal care in establishing an appropriate diagnosis is self-evident. Preeclampsia is considered to exist when proteinuria, edema, or both are associated with hypertension in pregnancy. Preeclampsia can either be mild or severe.

Mild preeclampsia is diagnosed when the blood pressure is greater than 140/90 mm Hg on two occasions 6 hours apart and when proteinuria of greater than 300 mg in a 24-hour specimen or greater than 1+ on urine dipstick is detected on two occasions at least 6 hours apart. In mild preeclampsia, the diastolic blood pressure remains at less than 110 mm Hg.

The criteria for the diagnosis of severe preeclampsia are seen in Table 34.1. Patients with preeclampsia whose blood pressures are greater than 160/110 mm Hg on two occasions 6 hours apart on bed rest are considered to have *severe preeclampsia*. The presence of proteinuria greater than 5 g in a 24-hour urine specimen also indicates the presence of severe disease. Other conditions indicating severe disease include oliguria (less than 500 mL per 24 hours), elevated serum creatinine, headache, visual disturbances, epigastric

TABLE 34.1. SEVERE PREGNANCY-INDUCED HYPERTENSION (PIH): CLINICAL MANIFESTATIONS

Blood pressure > 160/110
Proteinuria > 5 g/24 hours
Hepatocellular dysfunction
Thrombocytopenia
Microangiopathic hemolysis
Elevated serum creatinine
Oliguria < 500 mL/24 hours
Grand mal seizures
Pulmonary edema
Unremitting headache
Visual disturbances
Epigastric or right upper quadrant pain
Intrauterine growth retardation
Oligohydramnios

From *ACOG Technical Bulletin* 1996;219, with permission.

or right upper quadrant pain, pulmonary edema, thrombocytopenia, microangiopathic hemolysis, hepatocellular dysfunction, intrauterine growth retardation, oligohydramnios, and grand mal seizures (3).

The *HELLP syndrome* can be considered a subset of severe preeclampsia and should be included in the differential diagnosis of hypertension in pregnancy. *Eclampsia,* grand mal seizures in patients with pregnancy-induced hypertension, is also a subset of severe disease.

Chronic hypertension with superimposed preeclampsia is an important clinical phenomenon. It can occur in 4.7% to 52% of patients with chronic hypertension, depending on the diagnostic criteria used and the severity of the underlying hypertension (134–136). The diagnosis of superimposed preeclampsia can at times be extremely difficult. In patients with no prenatal care who present late in pregnancy with hypertension and proteinuria, the distinction between preeclampsia and chronic hypertension with superimposed preeclampsia can be challenging. A second clinically challenging situation occurs when the gravida with chronic hypertension has undiagnosed underlying renal disease. Suggested diagnostic criteria include exacerbation of hypertension and the development of substantial proteinuria (greater than 1 g per 24 hours) or elevated serum uric acid levels. These patients tend to have an increased risk of placental abruption (47,137), fetal growth restriction, and midtrimester loss (138–140). The increased perinatal morbidity and mortality associated with superimposed disease make the diagnosis significant.

MANAGEMENT OF MILD PREECLAMPSIA

Once the diagnosis of preeclampsia has been made and the disease has been found to be mild, appropriate management depends on various clinical factors. The gestational age determines whether immediate delivery is warranted. The only definitive treatment for pregnancy-induced hypertension is delivery, and it is universally accepted that the patient with preeclampsia who has achieved term pregnancy (more than 37 weeks) should be delivered. Mode of delivery is vaginal through induction unless an obstetric contraindication exists. Again, an accurate knowledge of gestational age is essential for appropriate management. Should the cervix be unfavorable at term, it is reasonable to manage the patient conservatively as long as blood pressure, proteinuria, platelet count, hepatic function, and renal function are closely monitored and remain stable. Fetal well-being needs to be established and maintained throughout this period of conservative management. Pregnancy complicated by mild preeclampsia should not be allowed to continue past 40 weeks' gestation regardless of Bishop score.

In mild pregnancy-induced hypertension before term (less than 37 weeks), the initial approach should include hospitalization for patients with worsening blood pressures or proteinuria. During the hospital stay, the patient needs to be closely monitored for the development of severe disease. On a daily basis, the patient should be questioned regarding the presence of headache, visual changes, and epigastric or right upper quadrant pain. Daily maternal weights and urine dips for protein should be recorded. Blood pressures should be recorded every 4 hours during the day. Blood should be drawn to evaluate the hematocrit, liver and kidney function, and thrombocytopenia as frequently as is deemed clinically necessary. Fetal well-being needs to be established on a regular basis. Complete ultrasound assessment should be performed to rule out oligohydramnios and fetal growth restriction. This can be accomplished with serial ultrasound examinations every 3 to 4 weeks. During the hospital stay, the patient should have limited physical activity. Sodium and fluid intake does not need to be limited or forced.

The use of antihypertensive agents in patients with mild pregnancy-induced hypertension to prolong gestation and to reduce severity of disease has been the subject of studies. At least five randomized trials have been performed evaluating the utility of β-blockers versus placebo or no therapy in the treatment of mild preeclampsia before term (141–145). Four of the five studies showed no differences in perinatal outcome between the treatment and control groups. All the studies showed a decrease in progression to severe hypertension in the treatment group. Perinatal mortality could not be assessed in any study because of sample size. In the study by Sibai et al. using labetalol versus placebo, the incidence of intrauterine growth retardation was twice as high in the treatment group compared with the control group (141). Randomized placebo-controlled trials have also been performed to evaluate calcium channel blockers, nifedipine and israpidine for mild pregnancy-induced hypertension (146,147). In none of these studies were significant benefits of antihypertensive treatment demonstrated in mild pregnancy-induced hypertension remote from term.

Home management for patients with mild pregnancy-induced hypertension has become more popular as health care providers attempt to contain costs. Management at home was found by some investigators to be safe and cost effective in women with mild hypertension without protein-uria (148,149). Other investigators have supported early and prolonged hospitalizations for women with mild hypertension remote from term and have demonstrated reduced maternal morbidity and improved perinatal survival that make hospital-based management cost effective (23,141, 146,150). A compromise approach of monitored outpatient management was proposed by Barton et al. (151). Blood pressures were monitored four times daily. Maternal weight, proteinuria, and fetal movement were closely followed. This approach reduced days of maternal hospitalization while maintaining a similar maternal and perinatal outcome relative to inpatient management.

For outpatient management to be safe, certain factors need to be considered. The patient should be reliable. One should be reassured of fetal well-being. The patient's blood pressure needs to be stable, without significant proteinuria (less than 500 mg per 24 hours) or maternal symptoms (visual changes, headache, right upper quadrant or epigastric pain). These patients can then be instructed to rest at home, dip their urine daily for protein, and check their blood pressures (either by a visiting nurse or by themselves). They should be educated about preeclampsia and should be aware of the symptoms associated with severe disease. Maternal and fetal well-being should be established at least weekly in the office. If one notes worsening of disease or evidence of fetal compromise, the patient should be promptly admitted to the hospital.

MANAGEMENT OF SEVERE PREECLAMPSIA

When pregnancy-induced hypertension becomes severe, both maternal and perinatal morbidity and mortality significantly rise. In these patients, maternal risks must be weighed against perinatal risks for appropriate clinical management schemes to be developed. Delivery represents the cure of maternal disease, but it may end in neonatal loss in early-onset severe preeclampsia. Many studies have been undertaken to identify the gestational ages and clinical criteria that warrant immediate delivery and those that warrant conservative management.

Appropriate management of severe preeclampsia at term offers little challenge. These patients are delivered by induction, if possible, regardless of Bishop score. This approach is also considered appropriate for all patients after 34 weeks, or earlier if there is any evidence of maternal compromise or fetal distress (152).

Considerable disagreement exists regarding appropriate management of severe pregnancy-induced hypertension before 34 weeks' gestation. Some authors support delivery as definitive therapy regardless of gestational age. Others recommend conservative management and prolong pregnancy until 34 to 36 weeks, or until lung maturity, unless maternal or fetal distress intervenes (153–155).

In an attempt to clarify this confusing clinical situation, Sibai et al. performed a randomized study of 95 severe preeclamptics between 28 and 32 weeks' gestation (156). These women were randomly assigned to receive either aggressive management or expectant management. The expectant management group received bed rest and either nifedipine or labetalol by mouth. The aggressive management group received glucocorticoids and was delivered in 48 hours. In the expectant management group, pregnancy was prolonged significantly, and birth weights were significantly higher. No significant difference was noted in cesarean delivery rate, placental abruption, HELLP syndrome, or length of postpartum stay. The expectant management group had significantly fewer neonatal intensive care unit admissions and a shorter length of stay, with less respiratory distress syndrome and necrotizing enterocolitis. Indications for delivery in the expectant group included maternal reasons, fetal compromise, reaching 34 weeks' gestation, preterm labor, preterm rupture of the membranes, or vaginal bleeding. Maternal indications included thrombocytopenia, uncontrolled severe hypertension, persistent headache or blurred vision, epigastric pain, or severe ascites (156). These patients were kept under close observation in a tertiary care center.

Occasionally, severe preeclampsia occurs in the second trimester. When this does occur, the perinatal mortality rate can be extremely high. In one retrospective review of 60 cases managed conservatively (17 to 27 weeks), the perinatal mortality rate for severe preeclampsia was 87% (157). These patients were managed for the most part at level one hospitals.

Significant maternal complications, including pulmonary edema, pleural effusion, eclampsia, placental abruption, disseminated intravascular coagulation, and renal failure have also been reported with the conservative management of such cases (157,158). Sibai et al. proposed a management protocol for midtrimester severe preeclampsia (159). In this protocol, pregnancy termination was offered for all gestations presenting at 24 weeks or less. For those of more than 24 weeks' gestation, aggressive expectant management was suggested, with antihypertensive medications and daily evaluation for fetal and maternal well-being. Clearly, patients need to be carefully selected and closely monitored in a tertiary care center if conservative management in the second trimester is planned.

DELIVERY MANAGEMENT

Once the decision has been made to deliver the patient with preeclampsia, the goal is to stabilize the mother medically and to deliver the infant safely. Whenever possible, glucocorticoids should be administered to patients requiring delivery remote from term. It is commonly believed that the stress of preeclampsia accelerates fetal lung maturity; however, this has not been proven to be true in controlled studies (160). Control of hypertension and seizure prophylaxis are the cornerstones of delivery management. Preeclampsia alone is not an indication for cesarean section, and delivery should be accomplished by judicious use of oxytocin and vaginal delivery whenever possible.

Certain intravenous antihypertensive agents are available to control blood pressure when diastolic pressures exceed 110 mm Hg. Intravenous hydralazine has been demonstrated to be safe and effective (161). It can be used in 5- or 10-mg doses every 15 to 20 minutes until an appropriate response is achieved. The goal is to lower the diastolic blood pressure to 90 to 100 mm Hg; any further decrease may impede placental perfusion. A 5-mg test dose should always be used initially because response cannot be predicted by level of hypertension.

Labetalol, a β-blocker, can also be used as a parenteral antihypertensive agent in pregnancy. It compared favorably to hydralazine in the acute management of severe hypertension in pregnant women (162). Labetalol can be given as a 10-mg intravenous bolus. If within 10 minutes the blood pressure is not at a desirable level, 20 mg can be administered. This can be followed by a 40-mg dose 10 minutes later, then another 40 mg, and then 80 mg if necessary at 10-minute intervals. The total labetalol dose should not exceed 300 mg. Calcium channel blockers such as verapamil and nifedipine can also be used. Nifedipine has the benefit of being administered sublingually; however, it is so potent that it may cause significant hypotension.

Magnesium sulfate is used to prevent and to treat the seizures associated with severe preeclampsia. It is not used to treat hypertension. Any patient who meets criteria for preeclampsia should receive magnesium prophylaxis during labor and delivery and for the first 24 hours post partum. Magnesium sulfate can be administered intravenously or intramuscularly. The intravenous approach offers the benefit of being less painful and provides more precise control over blood levels. The initial loading dose ranges from 4 to 6 g, then 2 g per hour provide a maintenance dose. The therapeutic range for seizure prophylaxis is at a magnesium level of 4 to 7 mEq/L.

Magnesium circulates unbound to protein and is excreted in the urine. For this reason, urine output needs to be followed closely in these patients. A Foley catheter is often indicated. Because preeclampsia can significantly effect renal function and urine output, the patient must be closely monitored for evidence of magnesium toxicity. Deep tendon reflexes, maternal respiratory rate, and level of consciousness need to be evaluated frequently. At therapeutic levels, magnesium depresses central nervous system irritability and slows neuromuscular conduction. At toxic levels,

the patient can demonstrate somnolence, slurred speech, muscular paralysis, respiratory difficulty, or cardiac arrest (Table 34.2). In any patient receiving magnesium therapy, calcium gluconate should be kept at the bedside. If magnesium toxicity is diagnosed or suspected, magnesium sulfate should be discontinued. If respiratory depression occurs, 1 g (usually one ampule) of calcium gluconate should be administered intravenously over 3 minutes. In the case of respiratory arrest, mechanical ventilation may be appropriate.

Other antiepileptic agents have been evaluated for seizure prophylaxis in preeclampsia. Phenytoin sodium has been proposed as an alternative to magnesium for seizure prophylaxis in preeclampsia (163). Although phenytoin can be used as a seizure prophylactic and therapeutic agent, some evidence indicates that magnesium is superior in preventing preeclamptic seizures (164,165). Intravenous fluid management should be carefully monitored in these women. Lactated Ringer's solution with or without 5% dextrose can be infused at a rate of 50 to 125 mL per hour. Urine output and total intake should be assessed hourly. These patients are not only at risk of oliguria, but they can also develop significant pulmonary edema.

Providing adequate analgesia and anesthesia safely to the severe preeclamptic can be challenging. The constricted intravascular volume associated with pregnancy-induced hypertension makes these patients prone to hypotension with conduction anesthetics. If thrombocytopenia develops and is severe, conduction anesthesia will be relatively contraindicated.

Intravenous or intramuscular meperidine with or without promethazine can provide some relief of the discomforts of labor and the postpartum period. Another option would be a patient-controlled infusion pump. For delivery, local or pudendal analgesia is safe and usually effective. In the past, conduction analgesia was avoided because of concern about severe hypotension resulting from splanchnic blockade. Pressor agents or large volumes of intravenous fluids were then used in an attempt to correct the hypotension. Some studies have now shown that continuous conduction anesthesia, using an adequate preload, incremental blockade, and locally injected opiates, can be safely used in severe preeclampsia (166,167). General anesthesia can be associated with marked fluctuations in blood pressure during induction and awakening. These fluctuations may be dangerous in the patient with severe preeclampsia (168). These

TABLE 34.2. EFFECTS OF MAGNESIUM

Normal serum level	1.5 to 3 mEq/L
Therapeutic level for PIH	4 to 7 mEq/L
Loss of deep tendon reflexes	7 to 10 mEq/L
Respiratory paralysis	12 to 15 mEq/L
Cardiac arrest	>25 mEq/L

changes can be minimized with appropriate pharmacologic intervention.

HELLP SYNDROME

Controversy abounds regarding the definition, diagnostic criteria, incidence, origin, and appropriate management of this syndrome. Diagnostic criteria include *hemolysis,* defined as the presence of microangiopathic hemolytic anemia. This condition is considered the hallmark of the disease. The diagnosis of hemolysis can be made by an abnormal peripheral blood smear, an increased bilirubin level, and an increased lactic dehydrogenase level. *Elevated liver enzymes* can be documented by an elevated serum glutamic-oxaloacetic transaminase; how high this level should be is controversial. *Thrombocytopenia* is usually considered to be present when the platelet count is less than 100,000/mm³. The differential diagnosis of these patients includes thrombotic thrombocytopenic purpura, hemolytic uremic syndrome, and an exacerbation of systemic lupus erythematosus.

Little controversy exists about the association of HELLP syndrome with poor maternal and perinatal outcomes (113,115,169). Maternal mortality ranges from 0% to 24%. Maternal morbidity includes acute renal failure, pulmonary edema, hepatic rupture, placental abruption, and disseminated intravascular coagulation (115,170–173). Perinatal mortality can be significant and has been reported to range from 7.7% to 60%.

The reported incidence of HELLP syndrome ranges from 2% to 12% of patients with preeclampsia (114). It is more common in whites and in patients with severe preeclamsia who are managed conservatively. Patients usually present remote from term with epigastric or right upper quadrant pain, and some patients have nausea or vomiting. Most complain of malaise for a few days before presentation. Some may present with abnormal bleeding from significant thrombocytopenia. Hypertension and proteinuria, if present, may be only slight. Hypertension is not necessarily a frequent finding in HELLP syndrome (174,175).

The management of HELLP syndrome is also controversial. Numerous different approaches have been used in an attempt to prolong gestation in patients with this syndrome. Some of the therapies attempted include albumin (176), corticosteroids (169,177–179), aspirin and corticosteroids (180), and thromboxane synthesis inhibitors (181).

An acceptable approach to these patients is to stabilize the mother initially and then to assess fetal well-being with a nonstress test or biophysical profile. Based on the clinical presentation, either the patient should be immediately delivered or, if preterm, an amniocentesis and corticosteroids should be given in the hope of extending the pregnancy for 48 hours for the fetal benefit of steroids. If the fetal lungs are mature or if the patient has evidence of disseminated intravascular coagulation or severe epigastric or right upper quadrant pain suggestive of subcapsular hematoma, then delivery should be immediate. HELLP syndrome is not an indication for cesarean delivery; oxytocin induction and vaginal delivery may actually be superior.

Within 72 hours of delivery, most patients demonstrate resolution of their disease. If this does not occur and symptoms worsen, a trial of plasma exchange with fresh frozen plasma may be beneficial (182,183).

Subcapsular hematoma is a rare and potentially disastrous complication of HELLP syndrome. Patients with ruptured hematomas can present with severe epigastric pain, shoulder pain, shock, ascites, respiratory difficulty, and often intrauterine fetal demise. A ruptured hematoma is a surgical emergency. Resuscitation with massive transfusions of blood products, both for anemia and for the coagulopathy, followed by immediate laparotomy is indicated. Even with appropriate treatment, the maternal and fetal mortality rate can be more than 50%. Complications of the coagulopathy, such as exsanguination, adult respiratory distress syndrome, pulmonary edema, and acute renal failure contribute to the high mortality rate (115,173).

ECLAMPSIA

Eclampsia is defined as seizures occurring in a woman who meets the diagnostic criteria for preeclampsia and who has no other coincident neurologic disease, such as epilepsy, that could account for the seizure. These seizures can occur without severe preeclampsia. Eclampsia may occur even when few signs of preeclampsia exist (184).

The seizures associated with eclampsia can be generalized tonic-clonic or focal motor seizures. They can occur before, during, or after delivery, but most occur within 24 hours of delivery (10). Occasionally, eclampsia can occur as late as 1 week post partum. There are reports of eclamptic seizures occurring up to 26 days post partum (15,185,186).

The most common premonitory symptoms before eclampsia are headache, visual changes, right upper quadrant pain, and epigastric pain. In a series of 254 patients with eclampsia, edema was absent in 32% and proteinuria was absent in 19% (10).

Visual changes occur in many women with eclampsia. These changes can be caused by disease in the eye itself or in the visual cortex. Possible eye changes include retinal arteriolar dilatation, papilledema (187), angiospasm, and occlusion of the retinal artery (187,188). Edema, microhemorrhages, or microinfarctions can occur in the visual cortex and can result in cortical blindness (189). Visual changes usually resolve after delivery or control of the hypertension.

When a pregnant woman presents with a seizure, eclampsia must always be considered as a diagnosis. However, other causes of seizures need to be considered. Cerebrovascular compromise can occur from cerebral infarct or hemorrhage, subarachnoid hemorrhage, cerebral venous thrombosis, or cerebral edema and malignant hypertension. A mass lesion need also be considered. A vascular malformation, benign or malignant tumors, or cerebral abscess could also account for the presentation. Infectious diseases, toxic or metabolic disorders, and epilepsy are all part of the differential diagnosis (190).

If a cause other than eclampsia is clinically suspected or if the origin is uncertain, the use of CT or MRI can be safely considered. In uncomplicated eclampsia, changes can be seen with head imaging; however, these changes usually do not alter clinical management.

In managing a patient with eclampsia, certain precautions should be taken. The patient should be closely monitored. Guard rails on the bed should be padded and kept up, and a tongue blade and a syringe with 4 g of magnesium sulfate should be kept at the bedside. An ampule of calcium gluconate should also be kept at the bedside. A large-bore intravenous line should be started. Initial laboratory evaluation should include a complete blood count with platelets, liver function tests, electrolytes, creatinine, coagulation profile, and an arterial blood gas determination. A nonheparinized tube can be drawn for clot observation.

The seizures associated with eclampsia can be life-threatening. Each clinician needs to be familiar with an organized approach to this serious obstetric complication. When the convulsion, occurs the patient needs to be kept as safe from injury as possible. It is important to use the tongue blade and padded guard rails and to suction any secretions. The duration of an eclamptic seizure is usually 1 to 2 minutes, although it can seem longer. It is not necessary to shorten the initial seizure with diazepam. Oxygenation needs to be maintained. Any difficulty in keeping oxygen saturation at an appropriate level after a seizure suggests aspiration. A chest radiograph should then be obtained. Once the convulsion has ended, a large-bore intravenous line can be placed, and 6 g of magnesium sulfate can be administered over 15 to 20 minutes. A continuous drip of 2 g of magnesium sulfate per hour should then be started. Should the patient have a seizure again after the initial loading dose, another 2 g of magnesium sulfate should be administered over 3 to 5 minutes. Most patients with eclampsia do not have another seizure after a second bolus (96). No more than 8 g of magnesium sulfate should be given over a short period of time to control convulsions (96). Serial magnesium levels and deep tendon reflexes can be used to help avoid magnesium toxicity. If a patient continues to have seizures after receiving magnesium, a short-acting barbiturate can be used. Sodium amobarbital can be given in doses up to 250 mg intravenously over 3 to 5 minutes (191). Severe hypertension can be controlled with intravenous hydralazine or labetalol. Intravenous fluids should be limited, and urine output should be closely monitored. Maternal acidemia, if present, needs to be corrected. If the pH is below 7.1, sodium bicarbonate should be given.

Once the patient's condition is stabilized, induction of labor with oxytocin can be initiated. If the cervix is unfavorable and the pregnancy is at less than 30 weeks' gestation, then elective cesarean section should be considered. These patients have a high incidence of fetal distress, fetal growth restriction, and placental abruption (192).

CHRONIC HYPERTENSION

As stated earlier, *chronic hypertension* is diagnosed when a patient has hypertension (blood pressure greater than 140/90 mm Hg) that precedes the pregnancy, develops before 20 weeks' gestation, or persists beyond 6 weeks post partum. Again, as pregnancy progresses, blood pressure decreases from baseline values and then returns to prepregnancy levels in the third trimester. Because of this phenomenon, the hypertensive patient who presents late in gestation for prenatal care can pose a diagnostic dilemma when her blood pressure rises late in gestation. The causes of hypertension are many and include diabetes, hyperthyroidism, intrinsic renal disease, renal artery stenosis, connective tissue disorders, obesity, and essential hypertension, which accounts for over 90% of hypertension. In the gravida in whom the diagnosis is questionable, other clinical findings can be helpful, and these include an enlarged heart on chest radiograph, evidence of left ventricular hypertrophy on an electrocardiogram, retinal changes, or evidence of renal disease and decreased renal function.

The incidence of superimposed pregnancy-induced hypertension in the hypertensive gravida ranges from about 5% to 50% (134,135,136). Several factors account for this wide variation in incidence, including the severity of hypertension, the presence of impaired renal function (22), obesity (192), and the definitions used in the reports. Although the hypertensive gravida is already at increased risk of adverse pregnancy outcomes (including intrauterine growth retardation and abruptio placentae) and is at greater risk of maternal morbidity if her disease process is advanced, such as in cases of decreased cardiac function, the presence of superimposed pregnancy-induced hypertension increases the risk of adverse outcomes, both maternal and perinatal.

Chronic hypertension is defined as mild if systolic blood pressure is between 140 and 160 mm Hg and diastolic blood pressure is between 90 and 110 mm Hg. Severe chronic hypertension is defined as systolic pressure greater than 160 mm Hg or diastolic pressure greater than 110 mm Hg. Because of the increased risk of adverse outcomes, management of female patients with chronic hypertension ideally should begin before conception. This approach enables adequate diagnosis of the cause of the hypertension. Furthermore, the patient can be assessed for other medical diseases, such as diabetes, that in themselves can adversely affect pregnancy outcome and general maternal health. An important part of this survey includes assessment for the presence of renal disease, because this also increases the risks of superimposed pregnancy-induced hypertension and adverse pregnancy outcomes including preterm delivery, growth retardation, and perinatal loss (22,193). Pregnant women with significant renal disease are at risk of progression to end-stage renal disease. Furthermore, assessment of medication use for safety to the fetus must be considered, and changes must be made if needed.

Pregnant patients with chronic hypertension can occasionally present with significant life-threatening complications from elevated blood pressure. These complications include hypertensive encephalopathy, acute aortic dissection, and acute left ventricular failure. Again, the severity of underlying disease (significant cardiac and renal dysfunction) and the early onset of superimposed pregnancy-induced hypertension, with complications, place patients at greatest risk of these adverse events. These emergencies are usually the result of significant blood pressure elevations (194), and treatment involves intensive supportive management of the hypertensive crises.

Treatment

Although controlling hypertension is believed to be important in decreasing the risk of adverse cardiac and cerebrovascular outcomes in the nonpregnant patient, the question arises how to treat the pregnant patient who has underlying chronic hypertension. Overall, although few studies have been conducted on pregnancy outcome in patients with severe chronic hypertension, numerous studies have been done on outcomes in patients with mild chronic hypertension. Unfortunately, few of these studies have been randomized trials that evaluated consistent treatment regimens from an early gestational age. Six prospective controlled trials of pregnant patients with mild chronic hypertension have been conducted. Five studies compared methyldopa with placebo or no treatment (138,139,195–197), and one evaluated atenolol (198). Only one study randomized patients in the first trimester (138), and only two (197,198) were performed in a blinded placebo-controlled fashion (with small numbers in both). Overall, the sample sizes were too small to assess effects on perinatal outcome, and the only evident maternal benefit was a reduction in hypertension exacerbations. Furthermore, three studies have compared methyldopa and β-blockers (199–201). Again, all three were small studies with few patients enrolled in the first trimester. In these studies, the incidence of superimposed preeclampsia did not appear to be affected, and the small number of patients precludes any significant conclusion regarding benefits in perinatal death rates. Overall, these studies confirmed a worse prognosis for outcome when patients developed superimposed pregnancy-induced hypertension; however, it does not appear that the risk of this complication can be reduced with antihypertensive therapy.

Again, few studies have evaluated the effects of antihypertensive medications on pregnant patients with severe chronic hypertension. Most of the studies were retrospective evaluations before 1970, with high incidences of adverse outcomes. A study in 1986 evaluated 44 patients with blood pressure greater than 170/100 mm Hg before 11 weeks' gestation (137). All patients were treated with methyldopa and hydralazine to maintain diastolic blood pressure at less than 110 mm Hg. In the 23 patients who developed superimposed pregnancy-induced hypertension, all delivered preterm with 18 growth-restricted fetuses and 11 perinatal deaths. In the cohort without superimposed pregnancy-induced hypertension, 13 infants were delivered at term, and only 1 was small for gestational age.

As with any pregnancy, the goal of prenatal care is to minimize adverse outcomes. This is especially true of the gravida with chronic hypertension. From the previous discussion, treatment of the patient with mild hypertension does not seem to improve perinatal and maternal outcome, but it may reduce exacerbations of hypertension. Although the gravida with chronic hypertension does have an increased risk of preterm delivery, infants who are small for gestational age, and increased perinatal loss rate compared with normotensive control subjects, the greatest risk to maternal and perinatal outcome is the development of superimposed pregnancy-induced hypertension, a complication that is not averted with treatment.

The gravida with chronic hypertension requires more intensive prenatal care, manifested by a more intensive examination at screening. Initial evaluation consists of evaluating baseline renal function, assessment for cardiac disease, and evaluation for other medical conditions that can worsen pregnancy outcome, such as diabetes and lupus erythematosus. Subsequently, the gravida with chronic hypertension should be seen more frequently, should have renal function evaluation every trimester, and should undergo antepartum fetal surveillance, with nonstress tests in the third trimester. Patients with elevations of blood pressure require investigation for superimposed pregnancy-induced hypertension, and if the pregnancy is proceeding without complications, early induction of labor does not appear to be indicated.

As for treatment of blood pressure, many investigators advocate discontinuing medications at screening if the patient is normotensive. Several groups advocate treatment if blood pressure is elevated at the screening visit or rises during the gestation, to more than 150 to 160 mm Hg systolic or 100 to 110 mm Hg diastolic, or if there is longstanding hypertension with evidence of other end-organ dysfunction (cardiac or renal). Most advise initiating treatment with methyldopa. Methyldopa is the most commonly used drug in pregnancy (135,136), and it is the only drug the long-term maternal and fetal safety of which has been adequately evaluated. It is a mild antihypertensive that decreases vascular resistance. It can cause hemolytic anemia, liver function test abnormalities, and postural hypotension.

If maximal doses do not adequately control blood pressure, other medications can be added.

For the most part, other medications appear to be safe in pregnancy, except angiotensin-converting enzyme inhibitors. In human pregnancy, these drugs appear to cause fetal growth restriction, fetal renal failure, and neonatal death (202,203). Other drugs that appear safe in pregnancy include hydralazine and β-blockers. β-Blockers are commonly used outside the United States, and reports have noted that the use of these agents is associated with growth retardation, abnormal fetal heart rate tracings, neonatal hypoglycemia, and neonatal bradycardia (198,204,205); however, study design in several reports and possible effects of maternal disease bring these findings into question. The calcium channel blocker nifedipine has been used as a tocolytic and for treatment of hypertensive emergencies. There is limited experience with its use in pregnancy as a first-line agent, and the drug appears to pose no risk to the fetus. Overall, thiazide diuretics are commonly used in nonpregnant patients. Their use in pregnancy is associated with both maternal complications, such as hyperglycemia, hypokalemia and natremia, hyperlipidemia, and reduction in plasma volume (206), and fetal complications, such as thrombocytopenia, electrolyte imbalances, and growth restriction (207–209).

Finally, diagnosing superimposed pregnancy-induced hypertension can be difficult. Many gravidas with chronic hypertension may experience exacerbations of blood pressure elevation. Compared with patients who remain normotensive, patients with increases in blood pressure alone are not at increased risk of adverse outcome. The presence of new proteinuria is what increases the risk of adverse outcome, and therefore, it is usually recommended that superimposed pregnancy-induced hypertension be diagnosed if the patient has a concomitant increase in proteinuria (or new-onset proteinuria) with persistent blood pressure elevation.

10 KEY POINTS

1. Pregnancy-induced hypertension increases the risk of adverse maternal (approximately 18% of maternal deaths in the United States) and perinatal outcomes.

2. The current classification guidelines of the ACOG for hypertensive disorders includes chronic hypertension and pregnancy-induced hypertension (mild and severe preeclampsia, eclampsia, and all of these conditions superimposed on chronic hypertension).

3. Proteinuria, a key component in making the diagnosis of preeclampsia, is a late finding and should be diagnosed with a 24-hour urine collection.

4. Modifications in diet, including calcium, magnesium, and zinc supplementation, do not appear to decrease the risk of developing pregnancy-induced hypertension.

5. An accepted cause of the development of pregnancy-induced hypertension involves abnormal trophoblastic invasion of the myometrial segments of uterine spiral arterioles in the second trimester that ultimately induces endothelial injury, platelet activation and aggregation, and vasospasm.

6. Pregnancy-induced hypertension can cause significant, and usually transient, abnormalities in cardiovascular, renal, hepatic, and central nervous system function.

7. The only cure for pregnancy-induced hypertension is delivery, and conservative management is considered only when the risk to the neonate of immediate delivery is significant.

8. Magnesium sulfate is the ideal anticonvulsant for both treatment and prophylaxis of eclamptic seizures.

9. The HELLP syndrome is associated with significant fetal and maternal morbidity and mortality, and it can occur in the absence of maternal hypertension.

10. Methyldopa is the drug of choice for chronic hypertension during pregnancy.

REFERENCES

1. Duley L. Maternal mortality associated with hypertensive disorders of pregnancy in Africa, Asia, Latin America and the Caribbean. *Br J Obstet Gynaecol* 1992;99:547.
2. Berg CJ, Atrash HK, Koonin LM, et al. Pregnancy-related mortality in the United States, 1987–1990. *Obstet Gynecol* 1996;88:161.
3. American College of Obstetricians and Gynecologists. *Hypertension in pregnancy.* Technical bulletin no. 219. American College of Obstetricians and Gynecologists, 1996.
4. Hughes EC, ed. *Obstetric-gynecologic terminology.* Philadelphia: FA Davis, 1972.
5. National High Blood Pressure Education Program Working Group. Report on high blood pressure in pregnancy. *Am J Obstet Gynecol* 1990;163:169.
6. Chesley LC. *Hypertensive disorders in pregnancy.* New York: Appleton-Century-Crofts, 1978.
7. Shennan A, Gupta M, Halligan A, et al. Lack of reproducibility in pregnancy of Korotkoff phase IV as measured by mercury sphygmomanometry. *Lancet* 1996;347:139.
8. MacGillivray I, Rose GA, Rowe D. Blood pressure survey in pregnancy. *Clin Sci* 1969;37:395.
9. Villar MA, Sibai BM, Moretti ML, et al. The clinical significance of elevated mean arterial blood pressure in the second trimester and a threshold increase in systolic and diastolic blood pressures during the third trimester. *Am J Obstet Gynecol* 1989;160:419.
10. Sibai BM. Eclampsia. IV. Maternal-perinatal outcome in 254 consecutive cases. *Am J Obstet Gynecol* 1990;163:1045.
11. Davey DA, MacGillivray I. The classification and definition of the hypertensive disorders of pregnancy. *Am J Obstet Gynecol* 1988;158:892.
12. Nelson TR. A clinical study of preeclampsia. *J Obstet Gynaecol Br Emp* 1955;62:48.
13. Chesley LC. Diagnosis of preeclampsia. *Obstet Gynecol* 1985; 65:423.
14. Ferrazzani S, Caruso A, De Carolis S, et al. Proteinuria and outcome of 444 pregnancies complicated by hypertension. *Am J Obstet Gynecol* 1990;162:366.
15. Brown CEL, Cunningham FG, Pritchard JA. Convulsions in hypertensive, proteinuric primiparas more than 24 hours after

delivery: eclampsia or some other cause? *J Reprod Med* 1987; 32:499.

16. Lubarsky SL, Barton JR, Freidman SA, et al. Late postpartum eclampsia revisited. *Obstet Gynecol* 1994;83:502.

17. Long PA, Abell DA, Beischer NA. Parity and preeclampsia. *Aust N Z J Obstet Gynaecol* 1979;19:203.

18. Cunningham FG, Leveno KJ. Management of pregnancy-induced hypertension. In: Rubin PC, ed. *Handbook of hypertension: hypertension in pregnancy,* vol 10. Amsterdam: Elsevier Science, 1988:290.

19. Spellacy WN, Miller SJ, Winegar A. Pregnancy after 40 years of age. *Obstet Gynecol* 1986;68:452-454.

20. Hansen JP. Older maternal age and pregnancy outcome: a review of the literature. *Obstet Gynecol Surv* 1986;41:726.

21. Mabie WC, Pernoll ML, Biswas MK. Chronic hypertension in pregnancy. *Obstet Gynecol* 1986;67:197-205.

22. Cunningham FG, Cox SM, Harstad TW, et al. Chronic renal disease and pregnancy outcome. *Am J Obstet Gynecol* 1990; 163:453-459.

23. Siddiqi T, Rosen B, Mimouni F, et al. Hypertension during pregnancy in insulin-dependent diabetic women. *Obstet Gynecol* 1991;77:514-519.

24. Branch DW, Silver RM, Blackwell JL, et al. Outcome of treated pregnancies in women with antiphospholipid syndrome: an update on the Utah experience. *Obstet Gynecol* 1992;80:614-620.

25. Chesley LC, Cooper DW. Genetics of hypertension in pregnancy: possible single gene control of pre-eclampsia and eclampsia in the descendants of eclamptic women. *Br J Obstet Gynaecol* 1986;163:453-459.

26. Sibai BM, El-Nazer A, Gonzalez-Ruiz A. Severe preeclampsia-eclampsia in young primigravidas: subsequent pregnancy outcome and remote prognosis. *Am J Obstet Gynecol* 1986;155: 1011.

27. Thompson SA, Lyons TL, Makowski EL. Outcomes of twin gestations at the University of Colorado Health Sciences Center, 1973-1983. *J Reprod Med* 1987;32:328.

28. Long P, Oats J. Preeclampsia in twin pregnancy: severity and pathogenesis. *Aust N Z J Obstet Gynaecol* 1987;27:1.

29. Chesley LC, Annitto JE, Cosgrove RA. The familial factor in toxemia of pregnancy. *Obstet Gynecol* 1968;32:303.

30. Cooper DW, Liston WA. Genetic control of severe preeclampsia. *J Med Genet* 1979;16:409.

31. Ward K, Hata A, Jeunemaitre X, et al. A molecular variant of angiotensinogen associated with preeclampsia. *Nat Genet* 1993;4:59.

32. Morgan L, Baker P, Broughton Pipkin F, et al. Preeclampsia and the angiotensinogen gene. *Br J Obstet Gynaecol* 1995;102:489.

33. Dizon-Townsend D, Nelson L, Moline L, et al. Severe preeclampsia is associated with the factor V Leiden mutation. *Am J Obstet Gynecol* 1996;174:343.

34. Feeney JG, Scott JS. Preeclampsia and changed paternity. *Eur J Obstet Gynecol Reprod Biol* 1980;11:35.

35. Robillard PY, Hulsey TC, Perianin J, et al. Association of pregnancy-induced hypertension with duration of sexual cohabitation before conception. *Lancet* 1994;344:973.

36. Beer AE. Possible immunological basis of preeclampsia/eclampsia. *Semin Perinatol* 1978;2:39.

37. Dekker GA. Oral tolerization to paternal antigens and preeclampsia. *Am J Obstet Gynecol* 1996;174:450.

38. Strickland DM, Gouzick DS, Cox K, et al. The relationship between abortion in the first pregnancy and the development of pregnancy-induced hypertension in the subsequent pregnancy. *Am J Obstet Gynecol* 1986;154:146.

39. Sibai BM, Gordan T, Thom E, et al. National Institute of Child Health and Human Development Network of Maternal-Fetal Medicine Units: risk factors for preeclampsia in healthy nulliparous women—a prospective multicenter study. *Am J Obstet Gynecol* 1995;172:642.

40. Zlatnik FJ, Burmeister LF. Dietary protein and preeclampsia. *Am J Obstet Gynecol* 1983;147:345.

41. Sanchez-Ramos L, Jones DC, Cullen MT. Urinary calcium as an early marker for preeclampsia. *Obstet Gynecol* 1991;77:685.

42. August P, Marcaccio B, Gertner JM, et al. Abnormal 1,25-dihydroxy vitamin D metabolism in preeclampsia. *Am J Obstet Gynecol* 1992;166:1295.

43. Kawasaki N, Matsuri K, Nakamura T. Effect of calcium supplementation on vascular sensitivity to angiotensin II in pregnant women. *Am J Obstet Gynecol* 1985;153:576.

44. Sanchez-Ramos L, Briones DK, Kaunitz AM, et al. Prevention of pregnancy-induced hypertension by calcium supplementation in angiotensin II sensitive patients. *Obstet Gynecol* 1994; 84:349.

45. Belizan JM, Villar J, Gonzalez L, et al. Calcium supplementation to prevent hypertensive disorders of pregnancy. *N Engl J Med* 1991;325:1399.

46. Weigel RM, Yepez R. Calcium supplementation reduces the risk of pregnancy-induced hypertension in an Andes population. *Br J Obstet Gynaecol* 1989;96:648.

47. Levine RJ, Hauth JC, Curet LB, et al. Trial of calcium to prevent preeclampsia. *N Engl J Med* 1997;337:69.

48. Lazebnik N, Kuhnert BR, Kuhnert BM, et al. Zinc status, pregnancy complications and labor abnormalities. *Am J Obstet Gynecol* 1988;158:161.

49. Altura BM, Altura BT, Carella A. Magnesium deficiency induced spasm of umbilical vessels: relation to preeclampsia, hypertension, growth retardation. *Science* 1983;221:376.

50. Mohamed K, James DK, Golding J, et al. Zinc supplementation during pregnancy: a double-blind randomized controlled trial. *BMJ* 1989;299:826.

51. Sibai BM, Villar MA, Bray E. Magnesium supplementation during pregnancy: a double-blind randomized controlled clinical trial. *Am J Obstet Gynecol* 1989;161:115.

52. Palmer RMJ, Ashton DS, Moncada S. Vascular endothelial cells synthesize nitric oxide from L-arginine. *Nature* 1988;333:664.

53. Myatt L, Brewer AS, Langdon G, et al. Attenuation of the vasoconstrictor effects of thromboxane and endothelin by nitric oxide in the human fetal-placental circulation. *Am J Obstet Gynecol* 1992,166:224.

54. Chang JK, Roman C, Heymann MA. Effect of endothelium derived relaxing factor inhibition on umbilical-placental circulation in fetal lambs in utero. *Am J Obstet Gynecol* 1992;166:727.

55. Fickling SA, Williams D, Vallance P, et al. Plasma concentrations of an endogenous inhibitor of nitric oxide synthesis in normal pregnancy and preeclampsia. *Lancet* 1993;342:242.

56. Kupferminc M, Silver R, Russell T, et al. Evaluation of nitric oxide as a mediator in severe preeclampsia. *Am J Obstet Gynecol* 1996;174:451.

57. Morris NH, Eaton BM, Dekker G. Nitric oxide, the endothelin, pregnancy and preeclampsia. *Br J Obstet Gynaecol* 1996;103:4.

58. Nova A, Sibai BM, Barton JR, et al. Maternal plasma levels of endothelin is increased in preeclampsia. *Am J Obstet Gynecol* 1991;166:624.

59. Mastrogiannis DS, O'Brien WF, Krammer J, et al. Potential role of endothelin-1 in normal and hypertensive pregnancies. *Am J Obstet Gynecol* 1991;165:1711.

60. Schiff E, Ben-Baruch G, Feleg E, et al. Immunoreactive circulating endothelin-1 in normal and hypertensive pregnancies. *Am J Obstet Gynecol* 1992;166:624.

61. Otani S, Usuki S, Saitoh T, et al. Comparison of endothelin-1 concentrations in normal and complicated pregnancies. *J Cardiovasc Pharmacol* 1991;17:S308.

62. Benigni A, Orisio S, Gaspari F, et al. Evidence against a pathologic role for endothelin in pre-eclampsia. *Br J Obstet Gynaecol* 1992;99:798.

63. Friedman SA. Preeclampsia: a review of the role of prostaglandins. *Obstet Gynecol* 1988;71:122.

64. Walsh SW. Preeclampsia: an imbalance in placental prostacyclin and thromboxane production. *Am J Obstet Gynecol* 1985;152:335.

65. Wang Y, Walsh SW, Guo J, et al. Maternal levels of prostacyclin, thromboxane, vitamin E, and lipid peroxides throughout normal pregnancy. *Am J Obstet Gynecol* 1991;165:1990.

66. Wang Y, Walsh SW, Guo J, et al. The imbalance between thromboxane and prostacyclin in preeclampsia is associated with an imbalance between lipid peroxides and vitamin E in maternal blood. *Am J Obstet Gynecol* 1991;165:1695.

67. Walsh SW. Lipid peroxidation in pregnancy: hypertension in pregnancy. *Am J Obstet Gynecol* 1994;13:1.

68. Davidge ST, Hubel CA, Braden, RD, et al. Sera antioxidant activity in uncomplicated and preeclamptic pregnancies. *Obstet Gynecol* 1992;79:897.

69. Mikhail MS, Anyaegbunan A, Garfinkel D, et al. Preeclampsia and antioxidant nutrients: decreased plasma levels of reduced ascorbic acid, α-tocopherol, and beta-carotene in women with preeclampsia. *Am J Obstet Gynecol* 1994;171:150.

70. Klonoff-Cohen H, Edelstein S, Savitz D. Cigarette smoking and preeclampsia. *Obstet Gynecol* 1993;81:541.

71. Miyaura S, Eguchi H, Johnston JM. The effect of a cigarette smoke extract on the metabolism of the proinflammatory autocoid, platelet-activating factor. *Circ Res* 1992;70:341.

72. Brosens I. Morphological changes of the uteroplacental bed in pregnancy hypertension. *Clin Obstet Gynecol* 1977;4:583.

73. Frusca T, Morassi L, Pecorell S, et al. Histological features of uteroplacental vessels in normal and hypertensive patients in relation to birthweight. *Br J Obstet Gynaecol* 1989;96:835.

74. Meekins JW, Pijnenborg R, Hanssens M, et al. A study of placental bed spiral arteries and trophoblast invasion in normal and severe preeclamptic pregnancies. *Br J Obstet Gynaecol* 1994;101:669.

75. Kong TY, DeWolf F, Robertson WB, et al. Inadequate maternal vascular response to placentation in pregnancies complicated by preeclampsia and by small-for-gestational age infants. *Br J Obstet Gynaecol* 1986;96:835.

76. Sheppard BL, Bonnar J. An ultrastructural study of uteroplacental spiral arteries in hypertensive and normotensive pregnancy and fetal growth retardation. *Br J Obstet Gynaecol* 1981;88:695.

77. Roberts JM, Taylor RN, Musci TJ, et al. Preeclampsia: an endothelial cell disorder. *Am J Obstet Gynecol* 1989;161:1200.

78. Rodgers GM, Taylor RN, Roberts JM. Preeclampsia is associated with a serum factor cytotoxic to human endothelial cells. *Am J Obstet Gynecol* 1988;159:908.

79. Shalkin DR, Sibai BM. Ultrastructural aspects of preeclampsia. I. Placental bed and uterine boundary vessels. *Am J Obstet Gynecol* 1989;161:735.

80. Volhard F. *Die doppelseitigen haematogenen Nierenerkrankungen.* Berlin, Springer 1918.

81. Browne FJ. Sensitization of the vascular system in preeclamptic toxaemia and eclampsia. *Br J Obstet Gynaecol* 1946;53:510.

82. Raab W, Schroeder G, Wagner R, et al. Vascular reactivity and electrolytes in normal and toxemic pregnancy. *J Clin Endocrinol* 1956;16:1196.

83. Talledo OE, Chesley LC, Zuspan FP. Renin-angiotensin system in normal and toxemic pregnancies. III. Differential sensitivity to angiotensin II and norepinephrine in toxemia of pregnancy. *Am J Obstet Gynecol* 1968;100:218.

84. Gant NF, Daley GL, Chand S, et al. A study of angiotensin II pressor response throughout primigravid pregnancy. *J Clin Invest* 1973;52:2682.

85. Gant NF, Chand S, Whalley PJ, et al. The nature of pressor responsiveness to angiotensin II in human pregnancy. *Obstet Gynecol* 1974;43:854.

86. Cunningham FG, Cox K, Gant NF. Further observations on the nature of pressor repsonsivity to angiotensin II in human pregnancy. *Obstet Gynecol* 1975;146:581.

87. Everett RB, Worley RJ, MacDonald PC, et al. Effect of prostaglandin synthetase inhibitors on pressor response to angiotensin II in human pregnancy. *J Clin Endocrinol* Metab 1978;46:1007.

88. Gant NF, Chand S, Whalley PJ, et al. A clinical test useful for predicting the development of acute hypertension in pregnancy. *Am J Obstet Gynecol* 1974;120:1.

89. Wallenburg, HS. Hemodynamics in hypertensive pregnancy. In: Rubin PC, ed. *Handbook of hypertension: hypertension in pregnancy,* vol 10. Amsterdam: Elsevier Science, 1988:66.

90. Cotton DB, Lee W, Huhta JC, et al. Hemodynamic profile of severe pregnancy-induced hypertension. *Am J Obstet Gynecol* 1988;158:523.

91. Mabie WE, Ratts TE, Sibai BM. The hemodynamic profile of severe preeclamptic patients requiring delivery. *Am J Obstet Gynecol* 1989;161:1443.

92. Benedetti TJ, Cotton DB, Read JC, et al. Hemodynamic observations in severe preeclampsia with a flow-directed pulmonary artery catheter. *Am J Obstet Gynecol* 1980;136:465.

93. Hankins GDV, Cunningham FG. Severe preeclampsia and eclampsia: controversies in management. In: *Williams obstetrics,* 18th ed. Norwalk, CT: Appleton & Lange, 1991:Suppl 12.

94. Rafferty TD, Berkowitz RL. Hemodynamics in patients with severe toxemia during labor and delivery. *Am J Obstet Gynecol* 1980;138:263.

95. Phelan JP, Yurth DA. Severe preeclampsia. I. Peripartum hemodynamic observations. *Am J Obstet Gynecol* 1982;144:17.

96. Pritchard JA, Cunningham FG, Pritchard SA. The Parkland Memorial Hospital protocol for treatment of eclampsia: evaluation of 245 cases. *Am J Obstet Gynecol* 1987;69:292.

97. Saleh AA, Bottoms SF, Welch RA, et al. Preeclampsia, delivery, and the hemostatic system. *Am J Obstet Gynecol* 1987;157:331.

98. Saleh AA, Bottoms SF, Norman G, et al. Hemostasis in hypertensive disorders of pregnancy. *Obstet Gynecol* 1988;71:719.

99. Samuels P, Main EK, Tomaski A, et al. Abnormalities in platelet antiglobulin tests in preeclamptic mothers and their neonates. *Am J Obstet Gynecol* 1987;157:109.

100. Burrows RF, Hunter DJS, Andrew M, et al. A prospective study investigating the mechanism of thrombocytopenia in preeclampsia. *Obstet Gynecol* 1987;70:334.

101. Leduc L, Wheeler JM, Kirshon B, et al. Coagulation profile in severe preeclampsia. *Obstet Gynecol* 1992;79:14.

102. Pritchard JA, Cunningham FG, Pritchard SA, et al. How often does maternal preeclampsia-eclampsia incite thrombocytopenia in the fetus? *Obstet Gynecol* 1987;69:292.

103. Nolan TE, Smith RP, DeVoe LD. Maternal plasma D-dimer levels in normal and complicated pregnancies. *Obstet Gynecol* 1993;81:235.

104. DeBoer K, Tencate JW, Sturk A, et al. Enhanced thrombin generation in normal and hypertensive pregnancy. *Am J Obstet Gynecol* 1989;160:95.

105. Pritchard JA, Stone SR. Clinical and laboratory observations on eclampsia. *Am J Obstet Gynecol* 1967;99:754.

106. Taufield PA, Ales KL, Resnick LM, et al. Hypocalcuria in preeclampsia. *N Engl J Med* 1987;316:715.

107. Lee W, Gonik B, Cotton DB. Urinary diagnostic indices in preeclampsia-associated oliguria: correlation with invasive hemodynamic monitoring. *Am J Obstet Gynecol* 1987;156:100.

108. Kirshon B, Lee W, Mauer MB, et al. Effects of low dose

dopamine therapy in the oliguric patient with preeclampsia. *Am J Obstet Gynecol* 1985;66:299.

109. Meyer NL, Mercer BM, Friedman SA, et al. Urinary dipstick protein: a poor predictor of absent or severe proteinuria. *Am J Obstet Gynecol* 1994;170:328.

110. Sheehan HL. Pathological lesions in the hypertensive toxaemias of pregnancy. In: Hammond J, Browne FJ, Wolstenholme GEW, eds. *Toxaemias of pregnancy, human and veterinary.* Philadelphia: Blakiston, 1950.

111. Spargo B, McCartney CP, Winemiller R. Glomerular capillary endotheliosis in toxemia of pregnancy. *Arch Pathol* 1959;68:593.

112. Weinstein L. Syndrome of hemolysis, elevated liver enzymes, and low platelet count: a severe consequence of hypertension in pregnancy. *Am J Obstet Gynecol* 1982;142:159.

113. Siabi BM, Taslimi MM, El-Nazer A, et al. Maternal-perinatal outcome associated with the syndrome of hemolysis, elevated liver enzymes and low platelets in severe preeclampsia-eclampsia. *Am J Obstet Gynecol* 1986;155:501.

114. Sibai BM. The HELLP syndrome (hemolysis, elevated liver enzymes, and low platelets): much ado about nothing? *Am J Obstet Gynecol* 1990;162:311.

115. Sibai BM, Ramadan MK, Usta I, et al. Maternal morbidity and mortality in 442 pregnancies with hemolysis, elevated liver enzymes, and low platelets (HELLP syndrome). *Am J Obstet Gynecol* 1993;169:1000.

116. Miles JF Jr, Martin JN Jr, Blake PG, et al. Postpartum eclampsia: a recurring perinatal dilemma. *Obstet Gynecol* 1990;76:328.

117. Will AD, Lewis KL, Hinshaw DB Jr, et al. Cerebral vasoconstriction in toxemia. *Neurology* 1987;37:1555.

118. Barton JR, Sibai BM. Cerebral pathology in eclampsia. *Clin Perinatol* 1991;18:891.

119. Moodley J, Bobat SM, Hoffman M, et al. Electroencephalogram and computerized cerebral tomography findings in eclampsia. *Br J Obstet Gynaecol* 1993;100:984.

120. Sibai BM, Spinnato JA, Watson DL, et al. Eclampsia. IV. Neurological findings and future outcome. *Am J Obstet Gynecol* 1985;152:184.

121. Dahmus MA, Barton JR, Sibai BM. Cerebral imaging in eclampsia: magnetic resonance imaging versus computed tomography. *Am J Obstet Gynecol* 1992;167:935.

122. Digre KB, Varner MW, Osborn AG, et al. Cranial magnetic resonance imaging in severe preeclampsia vs. eclampsia. *Arch Neurol* 1993;50:399.

123. Brown CEL, Purdy PD, Cunningham FG. Head computed tomographic scans in women with eclampsia. *Am J Obstet Gynecol* 1988;159:915.

124. Cunningham FG, Fernandez CO, Hernandez C. Blindness associated with preeclampsia and eclampsia. *Am J Obstet Gynecol* 1995;172:1291.

125. Spitz B, Magness RR, Cox SM, et al. Low dose aspirin. I. Effect on angiotensin II pressor responses and blood prostaglandin concentration in pregnant women sensitive to angiotensin II. *Am J Obstet Gynecol* 1988;159:1035.

126. Brown CEL, Gant NF, Cox K, et al. Low-dose aspirin. II. Relationship of angiotensin II pressor responses, circulating eicosanoids, and pregnancy outcome. *Am J Obstet Gynecol* 1990;163:1863.

127. Imperiale TF, Petrulis AS. A meta-analysis of low-dose aspirin for the prevention of pregnancy-induced hypertensive disease. *JAMA* 1991;266:261.

128. Sibai BM, Caritis SN, Thom E, et al. Prevention of preeclampsia with low-dose aspirin in healthy, nulliparous pregnant women. *N Engl J Med* 1993;329:1213.

129. Hauth JC, Goldenberg RL, Parker CR Jr, et al. Low-dose aspirin: lack of association with an increase in abruptio placentae or perinatal mortality. *Obstet Gynecol* 1995;85:1055.

130. Collaborative Low-Dose Aspirin Study in Pregnancy Collaborative Group. CLASP: a randomized trial of low-dose aspirin for the prevention and treatment of preeclampsia among 9364 pregnant women. *Lancet* 1994;343:610.

131. Sanchez-Ramos L, Del Valle GO, Briones D, et al. Prevention of preeclampsia by calcium supplementation in angiotensin-sensitive patients. *Am J Obstet Gynecol* 1994;170:408.

132. Redman CWG, Beilin LJ, Bonner J. Plasma urate measurement in predicting fetal death in hypertensive pregnancies. *Lancet* 1976;1:1370.

133. Varma TR. Serum uric acid levels as an index of fetal prognosis in pregnancies complicated by preexisting hypertension and preeclampsia of pregnancy. *Int J Gynaecol Obstet* 1982;20:401.

134. Chesley LC, Annitto JE. Pregnancy in the patient with hypertensive disease. *Am J Obstet Gynecol* 1947;53:372.

135. Sibai BM, Abdella TN, Anderson GD. Pregnancy outcome in 211 patients with mild chronic hypertension. *Obstet Gynecol* 1983;61:571.

136. Sibai BM. Diagnosis and management of chronic hypertension in pregnancy. *Obstet Gynecol* 1991;78:451.

137. Sibai BM, Anderson GD. Pregnancy outcome of intensive therapy in severe hypertension in first trimester. *Obstet Gynecol* 1986;67:517.

138. Redman CWE, Beilin LJ, Bonnar J, et al. Fetal outcome in trial of antihypertensive treatment in pregnancy. *Lancet* 1976;2:753.

139. Leather HM, Humphreys DM, Baker PB, et al. A controlled trial of hypertensive agents in hypertension in pregnancy. *Lancet* 1968;1:488.

140. Silverstone A, Trudinger BJ, Lewis PJ, et al. Maternal hypertension and intrauterine fetal death in midpregnancy. *BMJ* 1966;87:457.

141. Sibai BM, Gonzalez AR, Mabie WC, et al. A comparison of labetalol plus hospitalization versus hospitalization alone in the management of preeclampsia remote from term. *Obstet Gynecol* 1987;70:323.

142. Pickles CJ, Symonds EM, Broughton Pipkin F. The fetal outcome in a randomized double-blind controlled trial of labetalol versus placebo in pregnancy-induced hypertension. *Br J Obstet Gynaecol* 1989;96:38.

143. Rubin PC, Clark DM, Sumner DJ, et al. Placebo-controlled trial of atenolol in treatment of pregnancy associated hypertension. *Lancet* 1983;1:431.

144. Plouin PF, Breart E, Llado J, et al. A randomized comparison of early bedrest with conservative antihypertensive drugs in the management of pregnancy-induced hypertension. *Br J Obstet Gynaecol* 1990;97:134.

145. Wichman K, Ryden E, Kalberg BE. A placebo controlled trial of metoprolol in the treatment of hypertension in pregnancy. *Scand J Clin Lab Invest* 1984;44:90.

146. Sibai BM, Barton JR, Akl S, et al. A randomized prospective comparison of nifedipine and bedrest versus bedrest alone in the management of preeclampsia remote from term. *Am J Obstet Gynecol* 1992;167:879.

147. Wide-Swensson DH, Ingemarsson I, Lunnell NO, et al. Calcium channel blockade (isradipine) in treatment of hypertension in pregnancy: a randomized placebo-controlled study. *Am J Obstet Gynecol* 1995;173:872.

148. Mathews DD. A randomized controlled trial of bed rest and sedation or normal activity and non-sedation in the management of nonalbuminuric hypertension in late pregnancy. *Br J Obstet Gynaecol* 1977;84:108.

149. Crawther CA, Boumeester AM, Ashwist HM. Does admission to hospital for bedrest prevent disease progression or improve

fetal outcome in pregnancy complicated by non-proteinuric hypertension? *Br J Obstet Gynaecol* 1992;99:13.

150. Gilstrap LC, Cunningham GR, Whalley PJ. Management of pregnancy-induced hypertension in the nulliparous patient remote from term. *Semin Perinatol* 1978;2:73.

151. Barton JR, Stanziano GJ, Sibai BM. Monitored outpatient management of mild gestational hypertension remote from term. *Am J Obstet Gynecol* 1994;170:765.

152. Schiff E, Friedman S, Sibai BM. Conservative management of severe preeclampsia remote from term. *Obstet Gynecol* 1994; 84:626.

153. Odendaal HJ, Pattinson RC, DuToit R. Fetal and neonatal outcome in patients with severe preeclampsia delivered before 34 weeks. *S Afr Med J* 1987;71:555.

154. Chua S, Redman CWG. Prognosis for preeclampsia complicated by 5 gm or more of proteinuria in 24 hours. *Eur J Obstet Gynecol Reprod Biol* 1992;43:9.

155. Olah KS, Redman CWG, Gee H. Management of severe early preeclampsia: is conservative management justified? *Eur J Obstet Gynecol Reprod Biol* 1993;51:175.

156. Sibai BM, Mercer BM, Schiff E, et al. Aggressive versus expectant management of severe preeclampsia at 28 to 32 weeks gestation: a randomized controlled trial. *Am J Obstet Gynecol* 1994;171:818.

157. Sibai BM, Taslimi M, Abdella TN, et al. Maternal and perinatal outcome of conservative management of severe preeclampsia in midtrimester. *Am J Obstet Gynecol* 1988;152:32.

158. Pattinson RC, Odendaal HJ, DuToit R. Conservative management of severe proteinuric hypertension before 28 weeks gestation. *S Afr Med J* 1988;73;516.

159. Sibai BM, Aki S, Fairlie F, et al. A proposal for managing severe preeclampsia in the second trimester. *Am J Obstet Gynecol* 1990;163:733.

160. Schiff E, Friedman SA, Mercer BM, et al. Fetal lung maturity is not accelerated in preeclamptic pregnancies. *Am J Obstet Gynecol* 1993;169:1096.

161. Patterson-Brown S, Robson SC, Redfern N, et al. Hydralazine boluses for the treatment of severe hypertension in pre-eclampsia. *Br J Obstet Gynaecol* 1994;101:409.

162. Mabie WC, Gonzalez AR, Sibai BM, et al. A comparative trial of labetalol and hydralazine in the acute management of severe hypertension complicating pregnancy. *Obstet Gynecol* 1987;70: 328.

163. Appleton MP, Kuehl TJ, Raebel MA, et al. Magnesium sulfate versus phenytoin for seizure prophylaxis in pregnancy-induced hypertension. *Am J Obstet Gynecol* 1991;165:907.

164. Eclampsia Trial Collaborative Group. Which anticonvulsant for women with eclampsia? Evidence from the Collaborative Eclampsia Trial. *Lancet* 1995;345:1455.

165. Lucas MJ, Leveno KJ, Cunningham FG. A comparison of magnesium sulfate with phenytoin for the prevention of eclampsia. *N Engl J Med* 1995;333:201.

166. Gutsche B. The experts opine: is epidural block for labor and delivery and for cesarean section a safe form of analgesia in severe preeclampsia or eclampsia? *Surv Anesth* 1986;30:304.

167. Jouppila P, Jouppila R, Hollmen A, et al. Lumbar epidural analgesia to improve intervillous blood flow during labor in severe preeclampsia. *Obstet Gynecol* 1982;59:158.

168. Hodgkinson R, Husain FJ, Hayashi RH. Systemic and pulmonary blood pressure during cesarean section in parturients with gestational hypertension. *Can Anaesth Soc J* 1980;27:389.

169. Magann EF, Perry KO Jr, Meydrech EF, et al. Postpartum corticosteroids: disease stablization in patients with the syndrome of hemolysis, elevated liver enzymes, and low platelets (HELLP). *Am J Obstet Gynecol* 1994;171:1154.

170. Van Dam PA, Reiner M, Baeklandt M, et al. Disseminated intravascular coagulation and the syndrome of hemolysis, elevated liver enzymes, and low platelets in severe preeclampsia. *Obstet Gynecol* 1989;73:97.

171. Sibai BM, Ramadan MK. Acute renal failure in pregnancies complicated by hemolysis, elevated liver enzymes, and low platelets. *Am J Obstet Gynecol* 1993;168:1682.

172. Woods JP, Blake PG, Perry KG Jr, et al. Ascites: a portent of cardiopulmonary complications in preeclamptic patients with the syndrome of hemolysis, elevated liver enzymes, and low platelets. *Obstet Gynecol* 1992;80:87.

173. Abroug F, Boujdaria R, Nouira S, et al. HELLP syndrome: incidence and maternal-fetal outcome: a prospective study. *Intensive Care Med* 1992;18:274.

174. Aarnoudse JG, Houthoff HF, Weits J, et al. A syndrome of liver damage and intravascular coagulation in the last trimester of normotensive pregnancy: a clinical and histopathological study. *Br J Obstet Gynaecol* 1986;93:145.

175. Schwartz ML, Brenner WE. Pregnancy-induced hypertension presenting with life-threatening thrombocytopenia. *Am J Obstet Gynecol* 1983;146:756.

176. Goodlin RC. Beware the great imitator: severe preeclampsia. *Contemp Obstet Gynecol* 1982;20:215.

177. Thiagarajah S, Bourgeois FJ, Harbert GM, et al. Thrombocytopenia in preeclampsia: associated abnormalities and management principles. *Am J Obstet Gynecol* 1984;150:1.

178. Clark SL, Phelan JR, Allen SH, et al. Antepartum reversal of hematologic abnormalities associated with the HELLP syndrome: a report of three cases. *J Reprod Med* 1986;31:70.

179. Magann EF, Bass D, Chauhan SP, et al. Antepartum corticosteroids: disease stablization in patients with the syndrome of hemolysis, elevated liver enzymes, and low platelets (HELLP). *Am J Obstet Gynecol* 1994;171:1148.

180. Heyborne KD, Burke MS, Porreco RP. Prolongation of premature gestation in women with hemolysis, elevated liver enzymes, and low platelets: a report of 5 cases. *J Reprod Med* 1990;35:53.

181. Van Assche FA, Spitz B. Thromboxane synthetase inhibition in pregnancy-induced hypertension. *Am J Obstet Gynecol* 1988; 159:1015.

182. Martin JN Jr, Blake PG, Lowry SL, et al. Pregnancy complicated by preeclampsia-eclampsia with the syndrome of hemolysis, elevated liver enzymes, and low platelet count: how rapid is postpartum recovery? *Obstet Gynecol* 1990;76:737.

183. Schwartz ML. Possible role for exchange plasmapheresis with fresh frozen plasma for maternal indications in selected cases of preeclampsia and eclampsia. *Obstet Gynecol* 1986;68:136.

184. Porapakkam S. An epidemiologic study of eclampsia. *Obstet Gynecol* 1979;54:26.

185. Sibai BM, Schneider JM, Morrison JC, et al. The late postpartum eclampsia controversy. *Obstet Gynecol* 1980;55:75.

186. Stander HJ, Bonsners RW, Stromme WB. Late postpartum eclampsia. *Am J Obstet Gynecol* 1946;52:765.

187. Hallum AV. Eye changes in hypertensive toxemia of pregnancy. *JAMA* 1936;106:1649.

188. Carpenter F, Kava HL, Plotkin D. The development of total blindness as a complication of pregnancy. *Am J Obstet Gynecol* 1953;66:641.

189. Sheehan HL, Lynch JB. *Pathology of toxaemia of pregnancy.* Baltimore: Williams & Wilkins, 1973.

190. Kaplan PW, Repke JT. Eclampsia. *Neurol Clin* 1994;12:565.

191. Sibai BM. Magnesium sulfate is the ideal anticonvulsant in preeclampsia-eclampsia. *Am J Obstet Gynecol* 1990;162:1141.

192. Sibai BM, Anderson GD, Abdella TN, et al. Eclampsia. III. Neonatal outcome, growth and development. *Am J Obstet Gynecol* 1983;146:307.

192. Rey E, Couturier A. The prognosis of pregnancy in women with chronic hypertension. *Am J Obstet Gynecol* 1994;171:410.

193. Abe S, Amagasaki Y, Konishi K, et al. The influence of antecedent renal disease on pregnancy. *Am J Obstet Gynecol* 1985; 153:508.

194. Barton JR, Sibai BM. Acute life-threatening emergencies in preeclampsia-eclampsia. *Clin J Obstet Gynecol* 1992;35:402.

195. Sibai BM, Mabie WC, Shamsa F, et al. A comparison of no medication versus methyldopa or labetalol in chronic hypertension in pregnancy. *Am J Obstet Gynecol* 1990;162:960.

196. Arias F, Zamora J. Antihypertensive treatment and pregnancy outcome in patients with mild chronic hypertension. *Obstet Gynecol* 1979;53:489.

197. Weitz C, Khouzami V, Maxwell K, et al. Treatment of hypertension in pregnancy with methyldopa, randomized double-blind study. *Int J Gynaecol Obstet* 1987;25:35.

198. Butters L, Kennedy S, Rubin PC. Atenolol in essential hypertension during pregnancy. *BMJ* 1990;301:587.

199. Gallery EDM, Saunders DM, Hunyor DN, et al. Randomised comparison of methyldopa and oxprenolol for treatment of hypertension in pregnancy. *BMJ* 1979;1:1591.

200. Fidler J, Smith V, Fayers P, et al. Randomized controlled comparative study of methyldopa and oxprenolol in treatment of hypertension in pregnancy. *BMJ* 1983;286:1927.

201. Plouin PF, Breart G, Maillard F, et al. The Labetalol Methyldopa Study Group: comparison of antihypertensive efficacy and perinatal safety of labetalol and methyldopa in treatment of hypertension in pregnancy—a randomized controlled trial. *Br J Obstet Gynaecol* 1988;95:868.

202. Rosa FW, Bosco LA, Graham CF, et al. Neonatal anuria with maternal angiotensin-converting enzyme inhibition. *Obstet Gynecol* 1989;74:371.

203. Lumbers ER, Burrell JH, Menzies RI. The effects of a converting enzyme inhibitor (captopril) and angiotensin II on fetal renal function. *Br J Pharmacol* 1993;110:821.

204. Rubin PC. Beta-blockers in pregnancy. *N Engl J Med* 1981; 305:1323.

205. Montan S, Ingemarsson I. Intrapartum fetal heart rate patterns in pregnancies complicated by hypertension. *Am J Obstet Gynecol* 1989;160:283.

206. Sibai BM, Grossman RA, Grossman HE. Effects of diuretics on plasma volume in pregnancies with long term hypertension. *Am J Obstet Gynecol* 1984;150:831.

207. Schoenfeld A, Segal J, Friedman S, et al. Adverse reactions to antihypertensive drugs in pregnancy. *Obstet Gynecol Surv* 1986; 41:67.

208. Sibai BM, Abdella TN, Anderson GD, et al. Plasma volume determination in pregnancies complicated by chronic hypertension and intrauterine fetal demise. *Obstet Gynecol* 1982;60:174.

209. McGillivray I. Sodium and water balance in pregnancy and hypertension: the role of diuretics. *Clin J Obstet Gynecol* 1977; 4:459.

SELECTED TECHNOLOGIES IN OBSTETRICS: DOPPLER, CORDOCENTESIS, TARGETED SONOGRAPHY, AND ANALYSIS OF FETAL CELLS IN MATERNAL CIRCULATION FOR PRENATAL DIAGNOSIS

JOSEPH P. BRUNER
AUDREY H. KANG
SANDRA R. SILVA

DOPPLER ULTRASOUND

Doppler ultrasonography is a noninvasive method used to assess characteristics of blood flow in the mother and fetus. First introduced in the 1980s, Doppler ultrasonography has now become an integral part of many comprehensive obstetric ultrasound examinations. The rapid incorporation of Doppler technology into clinical obstetrics results in large part from the unique advantages offered by this modality. First, whereas gray-scale ultrasonography evaluates form, Doppler ultrasonography reveals dynamic aspects of function. Second, whereas many testing modalities are limited to the late second and third trimesters of pregnancy, Doppler ultrasonography can be used as early as the beginning of the second trimester. The ability to assess placental perfusion early in pregnancy has allowed Doppler ultrasonography to occupy a unique niche among other methods of fetal surveillance.

Doppler ultrasonography is based on the principle of the *Doppler frequency shift*, first described by Christian Johann Doppler, an Austrian mathematician and physicist. The principle states that when energy is reflected from a moving interface, the returning echo undergoes a Doppler frequency shift. For example, if you are standing in the water at the edge of the ocean, the waves coming into the shore strike your feet at a given frequency. If you then walk briskly into the water, it appears that the waves strike your feet at a greater frequency. Of course, the tides have remained the same, but because you are wading into the water, you have become a moving interface, and a Doppler frequency shift has occurred. In medical imaging, sound waves striking blood cells moving through a blood vessel may produce a Doppler frequency shift.

The formula for calculating the Doppler frequency shift is $fd = 2fv\phi/c$, where fd is the Doppler frequency shift, f is the frequency of the transmitted sound energy, v is the velocity of the blood cells moving through the vessels, ϕ is the cosine of the angle of insonation or the angle at which the sound waves strike the blood cells, and c is a constant representing the velocity of sound in tissue (Fig. 35.1). By manipulating this formula [velocity = $(fd \times c)/(2f \times \phi)$], it is possible to calculate *true volume flow,* which is velocity multiplied by the cross-sectional area of the vessel (area = πr^2). True volume flow measurements, however, are fraught with technical difficulties. The radius of a vessel lumen cannot always be accurately measured, and as can be seen from the formula, any error in this calculation is squared. Estimates of the error in volume flow measurements ranging from 15% to 50% have been published. Because of these methodologic problems, true volume flow measurements are not commonly performed in clinical practice.

By contrast, Doppler frequency shifts are easily obtained from vessels of interest in obstetrics. Studies are most commonly performed with the aid of duplex Doppler ultrasonography, which incorporates the Doppler transducer into a real-time ultrasound transducer. After the vessel to be studied is identified, the Doppler gate (cursor) is placed over the target vessel lumen, and a sound beam is pulsed from the transducer. The computer within the ultrasound unit calculates the time required for the pulse to reach its target and to be reflected back to the transducer. When the transducer receives the anticipated echo, the information is captured for analysis. Using this technique, select information about blood flow in discrete vessels can be obtained. The raw signal is processed through a fast Fourier analyzer, and the resulting Doppler frequency shifts, which can be

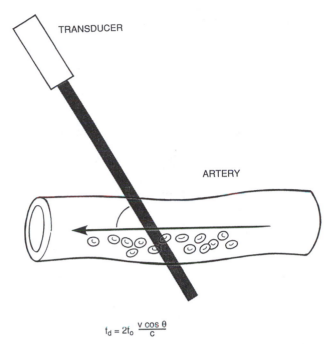

FIGURE 35.1. The formula for calculating the Doppler frequency shift is shown.

$$f_d = 2f_o \frac{v \cos \theta}{c}$$

heard in real time during signal capture, can also be displayed on a video monitor. When displayed visually, the frequency shifts are represented on the vertical axis with the horizontal axis scrolling over time (Fig. 35.2).

Because most blood vessels contain numerous blood cells, traveling in many different directions and at different velocities, a multitude of Doppler frequency shifts will be obtained. Not all this information is used in clinical practice. Only the maximum velocity envelope of the waveform is

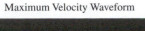

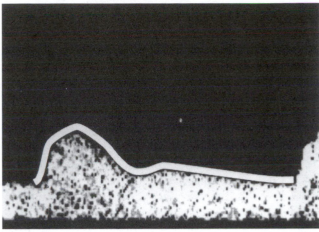

FIGURE 35.3. The maximum velocity envelope of the flow velocity waveform is highlighted.

used for analysis (Fig. 35.3). Commonly, one part of the waveform envelope is compared with another. By constructing such a ratio, the units of measurement cancel each other, and the result is a simple number. Several indices have been developed in this way. The simplest of these is the SD ratio, which compares the maximum systolic excursion to the minimum diastolic trough (Fig. 35.4). The resistance index (RI), also known as the Pourcelot index, measures the difference between systole and diastole divided by systole. Finally, the pulsatility index (PI) measures the difference between systole and diastole divided by the mean velocity measured throughout the cycle.

Any of these indices may be used in clinical practice, and correlation coefficients of Doppler indices are high (1).

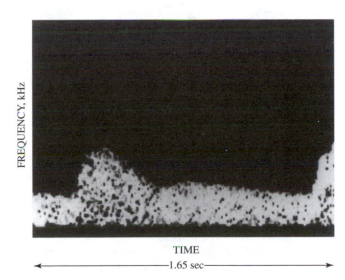

FIGURE 35.2. The Doppler flow velocity waveform. A uterine artery waveform is shown.

$$\frac{S}{D} = \text{S/D Ratio}$$

$$\frac{S-D}{S} = \text{Resistance Index (RI)}$$

$$\frac{S-D}{\text{Mean}} = \text{Pulsatility Index (PI)}$$

FIGURE 35.4. Doppler waveform indices compare one point on the maximum velocity envelope to another.

However, with extremely low diastolic blood flow, the SD ratio approaches infinity, and the RI approaches 1. In that situation, only the PI provides useful information. Fortunately, this is not a problem in most blood vessels studied in obstetrics because of the large amount of diastolic blood flow normally present. Therefore, the PI is usually reserved for gynecologic applications in which low blood flow is characteristic, whereas the SD ratio is usually preferred in obstetrics because of its ease of use.

Doppler flow velocity waveform (FVW) signals can be detected in the umbilical artery as early as 7 weeks' gestation (2). End-diastolic velocities are absent (AEDV) in the umbilical artery until approximately 12 weeks' gestation, and they are not consistently present in the umbilical circulation until after 15 weeks (2). Thereafter, diastolic blood flow demonstrates a steady increase with increasing gestational age. Therefore, values of the SD ratio, PI, and RI decrease with advancing gestation.

The primary determinant of umbilical artery waveform shape is placental impedance. In a study of 106 patients, placental microvascular anatomy was correlated with antenatal assessment of the umbilical circulation (3). Placental arterial resistance was quantitated by counting the number of small muscular arteries (the so-called *resistance vessels*) in the tertiary stem villi. The modal small arterial vessel count was shown to be significantly less among patients with a high SD ratio (1 to 2 arteries per field) than in control subjects (7 to 8 arteries per field). The authors of this study concluded that a specific microvascular lesion was present in the placenta, characterized by obliteration of small muscular arteries in the tertiary stem villi. This lesion has been termed *vascular sclerosis* (3).

In support of this theory, abnormal waveform changes have been induced in sheep fetuses by embolization of the resistance vessels of the placenta. The placentas of seven chronically catheterized sheep fetuses were progressively embolized from the fetal side with plastic microspheres (4). In all cases, the umbilical arterial waveform demonstrated a progression from normal end-diastolic velocities to AEDV with embolization. In six of seven animals, diastolic velocities eventually reversed in direction before fetal death (4). Finally, a mathematic model of the umbilical placental circulation has been used to examine the effect of different physiologic variables on the PI of the umbilical artery Doppler waveform (5). Using a model of progressive obliteration of the terminal branches of the arterial tree, placental resistance and the PI increased with vessel obliteration. The PI did not increase into the abnormal range, however, until more than 60% of the terminal branches were obliterated (5).

Umbilical artery waveform shape also varies according to the insonation site along the length of the cord. In general, resistance to umbilical artery blood flow is highest at the insertion of the umbilical cord into the fetal abdomen, and it is lowest at the placental cord insertion site. This umbilical artery Doppler ultrasonographic gradient may result in a decrease in measured values of the umbilical artery FVW SD ratio of up to 15%, a finding indicating the need for site-specific nomograms (6).

Because measured values of the umbilical artery Doppler indices decrease steadily with increasing gestation, gestational age–specific nomograms are also recommended for clinical use. Accurate determination of the gestational age is not always possible, however, prompting a need for age-independent assessments of placental function. One novel method of placental perfusion analysis using spectral Doppler signals is based on a comparison of umbilical artery with intraplacental waveforms (7). Because of the gradient described earlier (6), all intraplacental waveforms should demonstrate greater diastolic velocities than waveforms recorded at the placental cord insertion. Accordingly, the PI measured at the cord insertion to the placenta was compared with random recordings of the PI obtained from intraplacental signals in 83 pregnancies between 32 and 36 weeks of gestation. All 83 patients demonstrated umbilical artery Doppler indices within the normal limits for gestational age. The ratios between intraplacental and umbilical artery PI values were calculated. Nineteen patients with intraplacental-umbilical artery PI ratios greater than 1 (abnormal) had adverse pregnancy outcomes. Sixty-three percent of the fetuses were growth retarded, 37% of the mothers became preeclamptic, 68% of the labors were induced for reasons other than postdates, 42% of the infants were delivered by cesarean section for fetal distress, and 47% of the newborns were admitted to the neonatal intensive care unit. By contrast, only 1 of 64 pregnancies with an intraplacental-cord insertion PI ratio less than 1 (normal) was induced for reasons other than postdates, only 11% of the infants were delivered by cesarean section (none for fetal distress), and only 1 newborn was admitted to the neonatal intensive care unit (7).

In another study, intraplacental color Doppler flow patterns of villous arteries were examined in pregnancies with intrauterine growth retardation (IUGR) (8). A total of 192 uncomplicated pregnancies and 29 pregnancies with IUGR between 26 and 41 weeks' gestation were examined. Intraplacental color Doppler flow signals from 2 or more villous arteries were detected in all 192 normal pregnancies but were undetectable in 8 of 29 fetuses with IUGR. Absence of intraplacental color Doppler flow signals was associated with fetal distress in 6 of 8 cases (87.5%) and with perinatal death in 2 cases (25%), compared with 3 of 21 (14.2%; $p < .005$) and 0 of 21 (not significant) cases of IUGR with detectable intraplacental color Doppler flow. Failure to detect intraplacental color Doppler flow signals, therefore, was associated with IUGR and fetal distress (8).

Umbilical artery Doppler waveforms should be recorded, when possible, in the absence of fetal breathing movements. These movements can be detected by real-time gray scale imaging of the fetal diaphragm, or by Doppler insonation of the umbilical vein (9), and they are associated with an undulating umbilical venous pattern. When the fetus makes a breathing movement, blood return to the fetal heart is increased, causing a proportionate lengthening of the cardiac cycle. With a longer cardiac cycle, the diastolic downslope of the waveform is also longer, resulting in lower enddiastolic velocities. Shortening of the fetal cardiac cycle results in an increase in end-diastolic velocities. The resultant changes in FVW indices are small, however, and rarely cause a normal measurement to become abnormal, or *vice versa*. Similar concerns have been expressed about the need to correct umbilical artery Doppler waveform indices for the fetal heart rate (FHR). Such correction is unnecessary if the baseline heart rate is within normal limits (10).

Doppler Screening

One potential strategy for the clinical application of Doppler ultrasonography in obstetrics is as a screening test for high-risk pregnancies. One study reported on 92 consecutive women with various pregnancy complications who underwent Doppler ultrasonography of the umbilical artery in the second trimester (11). Values more than 2 standard deviations greater than the mean for gestational age correctly predicted 58% of women who became preeclamptic and 61% of infants who were small for gestational age. Of those fetuses with an abnormal test, 42% developed fetal distress, and 49% of newborns stayed in the hospital for more than 5 days or were admitted to the neonatal intensive care unit. All these values were significantly greater than those obtained in a control group of uncomplicated pregnancies or in a second control group of women with similar pregnancies but with normal umbilical artery waveforms (11). The sensitivity of umbilical artery Doppler velocimetry to detect fetuses that will eventually develop IUGR is 60% to 70% in various studies (12).

As with many screening tests in obstetrics, Doppler ultrasonography of the umbilical artery is associated with a high false-positive rate. One way to decrease false-positivity is to study selected populations. For example, in a study of 2,097 low-risk pregnancies in which Doppler testing was performed at 28, 34, and 38 weeks, the sensitivity of the test to detect IUGR was only 31% to 40% (13). By contrast, in a study of 2,178 high-risk pregnancies, more than half of the IUGR fetuses had an SD ratio greater than the ninety-fifth percentile (14). The odds ratio that a fetus with an elevated SD ratio would have a low birth weight was 5.9 (95% confidence interval, 4.7 to 7.3) (14).

Although the sensitivity of umbilical artery Doppler screening for detection of hypertension and IUGR in pregnancy is good, especially when the technique is used in a high-risk population, the true measure of the test is whether pregnancy outcome is improved by its use. The United States Preventive Services Task Force stated: "For routine ultrasonographic screening to be proven beneficial, evidence is needed that interventions in response to examination . . . lead to improved clinical outcome" (15). Umbilical artery Doppler availability was randomized, therefore, among pregnancies in a prospective trial (16). Fetal distress in labor, emergency cesarean sections, and time spent in the neonatal intensive care unit were all significantly reduced in pregnant women in whom Doppler testing was available. The availability of Doppler testing was not associated with an earlier delivery rate, and intervention rates were similar between study and control groups. The authors of this study concluded that the availability of Doppler ultrasonography during the pregnancy simply enabled caregivers to make better management decisions (16).

The most conclusive outcome data, however, come from a cumulative metaanalysis performed by Divon (17). Based on published and peer-reviewed randomized controlled trials using perinatal mortality as the primary outcome variable, the analysis consisted of 9 studies with 3,607 patients in the Doppler group and 3,698 patients in the control (non-Doppler) group. Cumulative metaanalysis revealed that the availability of umbilical artery Doppler studies significantly decreased perinatal mortality with a cumulative odds ratio of 0.44 and a 95% confidence interval of 0.31 to 0.78 ($p < .001$). Repeating the analysis after exclusion of malformed fetuses did not drastically change the results (17). Thus, ample data demonstrate that the availability of umbilical artery Doppler velocimetry in high-risk patients is associated with a significant decrease in perinatal mortality without a concomitant increase in maternal or neonatal morbidity. These results argue persuasively in favor of the incorporation of umbilical artery Doppler studies into the management protocols of high-risk pregnancies.

Doppler Categorization

In addition to early pregnancy screening, umbilical artery Doppler velocimetry can be used to categorize risk in obstetric patients already identified with a pregnancy complication. For example, pregnancies complicated by IUGR, defined as an estimated fetal weight lower than the tenth percentile for gestational age, are usually monitored with frequent clinic visits and antepartum fetal testing, often culminating in early induction of labor and an increased cesarean section rate. An estimated 10% of growth-retarded babies, however, have a genetic or chromosomal cause, and another 10% of cases of IUGR are estimated to result from early perinatal infection. In these cases, outcome usually cannot be improved either by increased levels of testing or by early delivery (18). A full 40% of fetuses that are small for gestational age are simply constitutionally small but have the same outcomes as other normal pregnancies. Any testing or intervention performed on these patients represents an expenditure of resources with no anticipated improvement of outcome (18). Therefore, attention should be focused on those 40% of cases of IUGR with a truly deprivational cause (18).

In an attempt to determine the clinical significance of IUGR associated with normal umbilical artery blood flow, a prospective comparative study of growth-retarded fetuses with normal and abnormal umbilical artery blood flow was performed in 179 women with singleton pregnancies in which the fetal abdominal circumference was less than the fifth centile for gestation (19). Significantly more babies with abnormal umbilical artery Doppler velocimetry were delivered preterm by emergency cesarean section for fetal distress. By contrast, when corrected for congenital anomalies, perinatal mortality among infants with normal Doppler studies was zero. The authors of this study concluded that IUGR associated with normal umbilical blood flow is a different and more benign entity than that associated with abnormal flow (19).

In a retrospective study of 81 patients with oligohydramnios in whom Doppler velocimetry of umbilical artery waveforms was performed, various measures of perinatal morbidity were correlated with the Doppler indices (20). Forty-six patients had normal SD ratios, whereas 30 had values greater than the ninety-fifth percentile adjusted for gestational age. Elevated umbilical artery SD ratios in patients with oligohydramnios identified an increased risk of perinatal morbidity, especially for a growth-retarded infant ($p <$ .001). Patients with abnormal Doppler waveforms were also significantly more likely to have newborns admitted to the neonatal intensive care unit, to experience fetal stress or distress in labor, and to undergo cesarean section. Patients with oligohydramnios and normal umbilical artery Doppler SD ratios were significantly ($p <$ .001) less likely to have poor perinatal outcome. Furthermore, 26% of patients with oligohydramnios and normal Doppler studies had labor induced preterm for no reason other than oligohydramnios. The authors of this study suggested that these may represent a subset of patients who could have avoided preterm delivery and its attendant complications if the low morbidity in this group when delivered at term had been taken into consideration (20).

Another commonly encountered situation in which risk categorization is useful is unexplained elevated maternal serum α-fetoprotein (MSAFP). When elevated MSAFP is detected by antepartum screening, obstetric ultrasonographic examination is indicated to rule out underestimated fetal age, multifetal gestation, fetal demise, and various anatomic malformations. If the ultrasonographic examination fails to identify any conditions commonly associated with abnormally elevated MSAFP concentrations, patients are categorized as having unexplained elevated MSAFP. Numerous studies (21) have shown that these women are at increased risk of various late pregnancy complications, including IUGR, preterm labor and delivery, placental abruption with intrauterine fetal death, perinatal death, and preeclampsia. All these complications are associated with poor placental function. Therefore, uterine and umbilical artery Doppler velocimetry was performed at the time of the scheduled ultrasound examination in 62 women with unexplained elevated MSAFP (Dellinger E, Bruner JP, unpublished data). Although the sensitivity of an abnormal test was only fair (50% to 100%), the negative predictive value was outstanding for the absence of IUGR (96%), fetal distress (93%), and preeclampsia (100%). When both uterine and umbilical artery Doppler velocimetry results were normal, none of the patients developed preeclampsia, and fetal distress or delivery of a growth retarded fetus was extremely rare. When women with unexplained elevated MSAFP have normal Doppler studies, the most likely explanation is that they are among the known 15% of women with a false-positive MSAFP test result.

Antepartum Fetal Surveillance

In contrast to its success as an early screening test and as a means of stratifying risk in patients with a known pregnancy complication, umbilical artery Doppler velocimetry has not proven efficacious as a strategy for routine antepartum testing. Devoe and co-workers examined 1,000 consecutive complicated pregnancies using the nonstress test, amniotic fluid volume measurements, and umbilical artery Doppler velocimetry (22). Clinical end points included perinatal mortality, intrapartum fetal distress, a 5-minute Apgar score of less than 7, and neonatal acidosis. Each testing method had specificity greater than 90%, but sensitivities ranged from 69% for the nonstress test to 21% for Doppler velocimetry. Negative predictive values of each method exceeded 85%, but positive predictive values ranged from 81% for the nonstress test to 42% for amniotic fluid measurements. Amniotic fluid measurements or Doppler velocimetry, when compared with the nonstress test, appeared to be less powerful "stand-alone" screening tests (22). In a similar study, Sarno and colleagues investigated the usefulness of umbilical artery Doppler velocimetry, amniotic fluid volume assessment, and FHR data in the early intrapartum period as predictors of subsequent fetal distress (23). The study included 109 patients seen in the latent phase of labor. Both an abnormal FHR and an amniotic fluid index less than or equal to 5.0 cm were associated with a significant increase in the incidence of intrapartum fetal distress. Conversely, an SD ratio greater than 3 by Doppler ultrasonography was not associated with increased fetal morbidity. Overall, the sensitivities, specificities, and positive predictive values of the FHR tracing and the amniotic fluid volume assessment were comparable. Doppler SD ratios showed poor sensitivity and positive predictive values (22).

The perceived failure of umbilical artery Doppler velocimetry as an accurate antepartum test arises in part from a misunderstanding of its assessment range. In the overall scheme of antepartum testing, electronic FHR monitoring and the biophysical profile are the most accurate tests commonly available for real-time determination of fetal status. By contrast, fetal growth and amniotic fluid volume assessments are more accurate determinants of the quality of the intrauterine environment over the preceding weeks to months; barring dramatic change, they allow general prognostication of perinatal outcome. Umbilical artery Doppler velocimetry, by virtue of its ability to determine the quality of placental function early in the second trimester, is a long-term predictor of pregnancy outcome; it can predict the onset of IUGR and hypertension long before clinical signs or symptoms appear and can be performed weeks before FHR monitoring or the biophysical profile are technically feasible. Doppler ultrasound does not accurately assess the presence of either hypoxia or acidosis in a fetus at any given time. In a report by Morrow and associates, prolonged hypoxia in fetal lambs did not alter umbilical artery waveform measurements (24). In another study, even acidosis in fetal lambs did not alter umbilical artery waveform indices (25).

One unique situation in which umbilical artery Doppler velocimetry does accurately identify current fetal condition is in the detection of AEDV or reversed end-diastolic velocities (REDV). Various studies of high-risk pregnancies report the incidence of AEDV as 2% to 8% (26). In 14 fetuses with AEDV evaluated by Reed and co-workers, 11 (78%) of the fetuses were growth retarded, and vaginal delivery was achieved in only 6 (43%). Only 1 of these babies was liveborn and underwent midforceps delivery for fetal distress. Cesarean sections were performed on 8 fetuses (57%), all for fetal distress. This group included 4 stillbirths (29%) with 2 neonatal deaths for a total perinatal mortality of 42% (27). In a review of 26 studies containing 785 patients with AEDV, 656 (84%) were diagnosed with IUGR (estimated fetal weight less than the tenth percentile) (25). In 16 studies of 524 patients with AEDV, 300 (57%) became hypertensive (25). A review of 31 studies of 940 fetuses with AEDV documented 337 perinatal deaths (36%) (25). Therefore, in the presence of AEDV or REDV, delivery should be considered if the gestational age is 34 weeks or greater. Between 30 and 34 weeks, amniocentesis should be considered for demonstration of fetal lung maturity.

In spite of almost universal recommendations for aggressive antepartum surveillance of fetuses with AEDV or REDV remote from term, current methods of antepartum testing do not guarantee a normal outcome in fetuses with markedly abnormal placentation. Hackett and co-workers studied 82 consecutive cases of IUGR managed by established inpatient criteria (28). Forty-six affected fetuses had abnormal umbilical artery Doppler velocimetry, whereas 26 had AEDV. All patients were managed at bed rest with intravenous hydration and treatment of any underlying medical or surgical disease. Daily nonstress testing was performed, and delivery was accomplished promptly in any patient with a nonreassuring test result. Those fetuses with AEDV had a much worse outcome than those with abnor-

mal Doppler velocimetry but measurable diastolic flow. In the first year of life, 35% of the AEDV group died, 27% had necrotizing enterocolitis, 42% had RDS, 31% had thrombocytopenia, 23% had pulmonary, gastrointestinal, or intraventricular hemorrhage, and 8% had renal failure. Only 15% of fetuses with AEDV developed no hemorrhagic complications as newborns (28). The explanation offered for such poor outcomes in spite of normal antepartum testing until the day of delivery is a weakness of the nonstress test. This test measures the interaction between the fetal heart and the brain. In the well-known head-sparing effect, the poorly perfused fetus redirects blood flow from the trunk to the heart and brain during periods of deprivation. Because of this, chronic ischemic damage can occur to organ vessel beds in spite of normal nonstress testing. A potentially more sensitive test for fetuses with AEDV or REDV may be umbilical venous velocimetry.

Three umbilical venous patterns have been identified (9) (Fig. 35.5). In the fetus at rest, umbilical venous blood flow is monotonous. In the presence of fetal breathing, umbilical venous waveforms are undulating and correspond with fetal inspiration. The third pattern, that of pulsations corresponding with the FHR, is an ominous finding. Umbilical venous pulsations identify the presence of venous pulses originating in the right atrium of the fetal heart and propagating down the vena cava, through the ductus venosus, and into the umbilical cord. The two most common causes of this abnormal finding are an anatomic defect on the right side of the heart and poor right ventricular function. Dameron and colleagues studied the relationship of umbilical artery SD ratios, umbilical venous pulsations, and late decelerations on FHR monitoring (29). Ten fetuses with AEDV and absent venous pulsations demonstrated no late decelerations during the contraction stress test. By contrast, nine of ten fetuses with AEDV but venous pulsations present demonstrated late decelerations in response to uterine contractions. In an appropriate context, the presence of venous pulsations may be a sensitive marker for fetal hypoxia or acidemia (29).

CORDOCENTESIS

Cordocentesis is an invasive technique that allows *in utero* diagnosis and therapy of a wide range of fetal disorders. Also known as *percutaneous umbilical blood sampling* (PUBS), cordocentesis consists of fine-needle aspiration of fetal blood using high-resolution ultrasound guidance. First described by Daffos in 1983, the procedure has now been successfully performed in thousands of pregnancies worldwide (30).

In 1990, the National PUBS Registry, which at the time consisted of 16 centers in the United States and Canada, reported a cumulative total of 5,280 procedures performed on 3,601 patients. Sixteen separate categories of maternal or fetal disease were listed as indications for performance

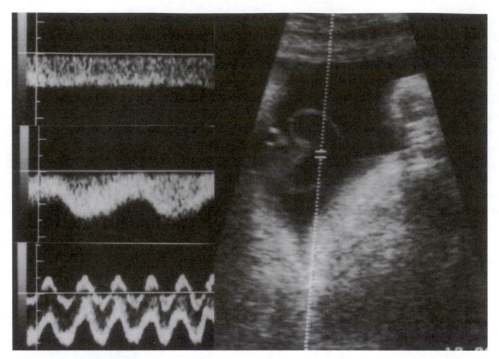

FIGURE 35.5. Three umbilical venous patterns have been identified.

of cordocentesis. Although the procedure was performed solely for diagnosis or treatment of serious disease, only 61 fetuses were lost as a direct result of the procedure, for a risk of 1.15% per procedure, or 1.69% per patient. Causes of the fetal losses were chorioamnionitis, rupture of membranes, bleeding from the cord puncture site, severe bradycardia, and umbilical cord thrombosis (Proceedings of the Fifth International Conference on Percutaneous Umbilical Blood Sampling, Philadelphia, 1990).

The basic steps involved in the performance of fetal blood sampling include careful ultrasonographic examination of the uterine contents to determine the most favorable entry site and pathway for the needle, preparation of a sterile field, readying of all equipment necessary for performance of the procedure, placement of the needle under real-time ultrasonographic guidance, aspiration of the specimen, and confirmation of the blood origin of the specimen.

The most common aspiration site is the placental cord insertion on an anterior or posterior placenta. When the cord insertion is on an anterior placenta, a transplacental approach to the umbilical vein can be used. Although this approach is extremely stable, because the needle is essentially invulnerable to fetal movement, lateral movement of the needle tip is limited, and a good aim is required. Furthermore, aspiration of amniotic fluid for additional studies requires a separate needle insertion. By contrast, crossing the amniotic cavity en route to the cord insertion on a posterior or lateral placenta enables the simultaneous collection of amniotic fluid during the same needle pass and allows for free manipulation of the needle tip as the target

is approached. When the placental cord insertion is covered by the fetal body, especially later in pregnancy when the fetus occupies relatively more space within the amniotic cavity, a free loop of cord, abdominal cord insertion, or intrahepatic umbilical vein may be used. Color Doppler sonography may be useful in identifying cord landmarks when visualization is difficult. Unfortunately, whenever the needle tip is passed through the amniotic cavity, the sudden and unexpected extension of a fetal limb or rolling movement of the fetus may result in displacement of the needle tip from the aspiration site and may lacerate the umbilical vessels.

All necessary equipment should be available before beginning cordocentesis. A sterile tray should contain enough heparinized needles and syringes to ensure satisfactory completion of the procedure. Ultrasound mapping of the uterine contents should be performed to determine the location of the placental cord insertion and the appropriate needle length before attempted aspiration. All anticipated medications should be measured and drawn into labeled sterile syringes.

When an active fetus is anticipated, pancuronium bromide (31,32) or vecuronium bromide (33), 0.1 mg/kg, may be injected directly into the umbilical vein to prevent fetal movement temporarily. The onset of action of these paralyzing agents is immediate, with a duration of 1 to 2 hours. If safe needle entry into the cord cannot be achieved, 0.2 mg/kg of the same medications may be injected intramuscularly into the fetal thigh or buttocks (34). Vecuronium bromide has the added advantage of a decreased incidence of fetal bradycardia and loss of FHR variability (33). By contrast, fetal analgesia is usually not administered for performance of cordocentesis. A fetal hormone stress response to invasive intrauterine procedures has been reported. Increased levels of fetal cortisol and β-endorphins have been measured in response to needle insertion into the fetal abdomen (35). The clinical effects of such a hormone response, however, are still unknown.

In most instances, the needle tip can be easily identified as it penetrates the target blood vessel. However, only 2 to 3 mm of the needle tip will actually enter the fetal blood vessel, which may be as small as 5 mm in diameter. Because the needle tip is being advanced in three-dimensional space, under the visual guidance of ultrasound, which is two-dimensional, one must be certain that the needle tip has been correctly inserted into the lumen of the vessel. When correct placement of the needle tip is suspected, the needle stylet is withdrawn and aspiration is attempted using a heparinized 1-mL tuberculin syringe. If nothing is aspirated, indicating placement in Wharton's jelly, or if amniotic fluid is aspirated, reinsertion of the needle tip is performed. If free-flowing blood is aspirated, the tip of the needle is likely positioned properly in the fetal blood vessel lumen. If the needle tip is in a free-floating loop of cord or the abdominal cord insertion site, there is no other possible source for the blood.

When the placental cord insertion is used, however, confirmation of fetal blood aspiration may be obtained by the rapid analysis of mean corpuscular volume in an automatic cell size analyzer, or Coulter counter, and compared with a maternal sample obtained on admission. A mean corpuscular volume range of 118 to 125 mL confirms fetal origin. Further confirmation of proper needle tip placement is easily and accurately obtained by injection of 0.5 to 1 mL of normal saline. If the needle tip is in the vein, streaming ultrasound turbulence is seen as the saline passes down the vein. Conversely, if the needle tip is in an artery, the turbulence of the infused saline may be seen moving in the opposite direction onto the surface of the placenta. If turbulence is seen in the amniotic fluid, the needle tip is in the amniotic cavity. If no turbulence is seen, the needle tip may be dislodged and embedded in Wharton's jelly. In this situation, further infusion should not be carried out because life-threatening umbilical vein compression may occur. Daffos reported that, in his experience, the duration of the procedure is less than 5 minutes in 70% of cases and less than 10 minutes in 90% of cases (36). He reported obtaining pure fetal blood on the first attempt in 97% of cases (36).

According to data collected by the National PUBS Registry, the top four indications for performance of cordocentesis account for almost 90% of recorded cases (Proceedings of the Fifth International Conference on Percutaneous Umbilical Blood Sampling, Philadelphia, 1990). These common indications are as follows: rapid karyotyping, 38%; fetal red cell isoimmunization, 29%; intrauterine fetal infection, 9%; and nonimmune hydrops fetalis, 5.5%.

Rapid Fetal Karyotype

Cytogenetic analysis of lymphocytes obtained from fetal blood yields a *fetal karyotype* in 2 days, compared with the 7 to 14 days required for analysis of amniocytes from the fluid. Direct preparation of fetal blood may even yield a karyotype within 24 hours. Because many anatomic malformations are associated with fetal aneuploidy, performance of cordocentesis for further evaluation of anomalies detected by ultrasound enables the physician to formulate optimal management strategies quickly.

For several years, percutaneous umbilical blood sampling was the most reliable means of obtaining a rapid fetal karyotype in those areas where the technique was readily available. More recently, promulgation of fluorescent *in situ* hybridization (FISH) technology has enabled many more centers to obtain a rapid fetal karyotype from amniocentesis. By using probes directed against known sites on various chromosomes, limited diagnosis of selected trisomies can be performed within 24 hours on amniocytes. A third technique for the rapid cytogenetic analysis of the fetus is transabdominal chorionic villous sampling. Unless the placenta is directly posterior, it is usually possible to pass a needle close to the chorionic plate and to obtain 5 mg or more of villi, an amount adequate for the direct preparation of a fetal karyotype within 24 hours.

Fetal Red Cell Isoimmunization

The use of cordocentesis for the diagnosis and treatment of *fetal red cell isoimmunization* has been a major advance in the management of women with Rhesus or atypical antibodies. Donor blood can be administered through the same needle used to perform diagnostic testing. When vascular access is obtained, a small amount of blood is withdrawn into heparinized 1-mL syringes, and the fetal packed cell volume (PCV) is immediately determined. Type 0 negative, leukocyte-poor, washed, and irradiated red blood cells are then transfused. A reasonable goal is to achieve a posttransfusion PCV of 40% to 45%.

After intravascular transfusion, the decline in the fetal hematocrit is primarily determined by the rate of fetal growth and the ratio of donor to fetal erythrocytes. Ongoing hemolysis is greatest between the first and second intravascular transfusions, when the ratio of fetal cells to donor cells is greatest. As a rule, after the first transfusion, the decline of the fetal hematocrit is about 1.5% per day, whereas after subsequent transfusions, the decline in fetal hematocrit is about 1.2% per day. Using intravascular transfusions for the management of severe fetal hemolysis, subsequent transfusions should be timed to maintain the PCV at more than 25%.

One-thousand five hundred sixty-eight intravascular transfusions were performed in 560 fetuses reported by the National PUBS Registry in 1990. Although 221 fetuses were hydropic before initiation of intrauterine intravascular transfusions, the overall survival rate was still 86% (Proceedings of the Fifth International Conference on Percutaneous Umbilical Blood Sampling, Philadelphia, 1990).

Until recently, fetal blood sampling in isoimmunized patients had several distinct advantages over other techniques. In the initial evaluation of an isoimmunized pregnancy, it is important to consider the possibility that the fetus may be antigen negative. In this case, no invasive testing is required. If a reasonable possibility exists that the father of the fetus is heterozygous, fetal blood sampling can be performed as early as 18 gestational weeks to determine the antigen status of the fetus. If the fetus proves to be antigen negative, the test will eliminate the need for multiple amniocenteses for optical density studies or multiple cordocenteses for determination of the PCV. When the maternal blood and fetal blood are incompatible, fetal blood sampling can establish the precise degree of hemolysis by evaluation of the fetal PCV, Coombs' test, and reticulocyte response. Today, however, determination of the fetal antigen status for most of the major erythrocyte antigens associated with hemolytic disease can be determined by polymerase chain reaction (PCR) evaluation of the DNA content of fetal amniocytes obtained by amniocentesis. Testing for the rhesus antigens Duffy, Kell, and Kidd are currently available.

Fetuses typically begin to develop signs of hydrops fetalis when the PCV drops to less than 15%. In such cases of severe fetal anemia, the PCV required to restore the blood count to normal exceeds even the ability of the fetus, with its low-resistance placental "sink," to absorb the excess volume. For example, Radunovic and colleagues reported a 37% loss rate within 72 hours of intravenous transfusion for anemia and hydrops (37). Hallak and co-workers reported that an increase in the measured umbilical venous pressure of at least 10 mm Hg identified 80% of fetuses who had died within 24 hours of transfusion (38). In an attempt to avoid circulatory overload in the severely anemic fetus, only a portion of the calculated transfusion volume should be given in one transfusion. The fetus should then be allowed to equilibrate its blood volume for 24 to 48 hours, and the transfusion can be completed after that time. If umbilical venous pressure is monitored during the procedure, the initial transfusion should be halted when the measured increase in pressure approaches 10 mm Hg (38). Otherwise, a fetal PCV of 25%, or a fourfold increase of the opening PCV, should not be exceeded (37).

If bank blood is unavailable for fetal transfusion, or if such blood is refused by the family, maternal blood can be safely used for fetal intravascular transfusion (39). Erythrocyte antibodies are located in maternal plasma, so most are removed or inactivated during the standard process of washing and irradiation as the unit is prepared for fetal transfusion. If maternal blood is to be used for fetal transfusion, the routine screening process used for any autologous donor should be followed. Prenatal vitamins, iron, and folate supplementation should be prescribed (39).

Today, clinicians may face a choice of performing serial amniocenteses for optical density measurements using the Liley curve, or direct fetal blood aspiration with measurement of the fetal PCV and reticulocyte count. For the Rh-sensitized patient in the third trimester, neither approach offers substantial benefit over the other (40). In practice, the management plan probably depends more on the availability of cordocentesis than on any other factor. In the second trimester of pregnancy, however, and in the presence of atypical antibodies, cordocentesis has been shown to be a more accurate test for the detection of the severely anemic fetus (41).

Intrauterine Fetal Infection

Many potentially serious *infections* in the fetus are best detected by direct analysis of fetal blood obtained at cordocentesis. In the United States, the most common infection leading to fetal testing with cordocentesis is parvovirus. Human *parvovirus B19* causes a mild viral illness known as erythema infectiosum or fifth disease. In otherwise healthy adults, parvovirus infection is characterized by a rash with a typical "slapped face" appearance, arthralgias, and lymphadenopathy. In most cases, the symptoms are so mild that they may not be noticed by the patient. In people with chronic hemolytic anemias, such as sickle cell disease, however, parvovirus B19 may precipitate an aplastic crisis because the virus infects and destroys erythroid precursor cells. Severe anemia may occur in the fetus after congenital infection by a similar mechanism. As in the adult, the virus has an affinity for erythroid cells. In addition, as in the adult with chronic hemolysis, erythrocytes in the fetus have a relatively short life span. Moreover, fetal erythropoiesis is already stressed by the physiologic expansion of the fetal red cell mass during the second trimester. For these reasons, impairment of fetal erythrogenesis by infection with human parvovirus B19 may result in severe fetal anemia with hydrops, especially if the infection occurs in the second trimester.

Fetal parvovirus infection typically occurs 4 to 6 weeks after maternal infection, although hydrops has been reported as late as 12 weeks (42). Therefore, after confirmation of maternal parvovirus infection by testing for specific immunoglobulin M (IgM), serial ultrasound scans should be performed weekly for 10 to 12 weeks. Invasive testing is not indicated for the nonhydropic fetus; cordocentesis should be reserved for cases with hydrops. When evidence of fetal decompensation is seen, cordocentesis should be performed for analysis of fetal blood. During the viremic episode, fetal laboratory findings include a negative direct Coombs' test, anemia, low reticulocyte count, and elevated total IgM (43). The primary method of fetal diagnosis, however, is direct detection of viral particles using PCR (44).

Because the fetal infection is transient, support of the anemic fetus by transfusion is the cornerstone of therapy. Once transfusions are begun, they should be continued until the reticulocyte count rises or the PCV becomes stable. In a review of ten hydropic fetuses with confirmed parvovirus infection, seven were transfused once, two were transfused twice, and one required three transfusions (42). As in red cell isoimmunization, resolution of the fetal hydrops may take several weeks after correction of the fetal anemia.

Other potentially serious perinatal infections that can be detected by fetal blood sampling include rubella and toxoplasmosis. *Rubella* has an incubation period of 14 to 21 days. In addition, the fetus is not immunocompetent until approximately 22 weeks' gestation. Therefore, serologic testing for rubella infection in the fetus should only be attempted at the end of the incubation interval and after 22 weeks' gestation. At that time, fetal blood can be tested for antirubella IgM (45). Anti-*Toxoplasma* IgM can be detected after 20 to 22 weeks (46), and *Toxoplasma* parasites can be detected by PCR (47).

Nonimmune Hydrops Fetalis

Analysis of fetal blood obtained at cordocentesis has been useful in the prenatal evaluation of *nonimmune hydrops*. The Latin term *hydrops fetalis* refers to pathologically increased fluid accumulation in serous cavities or edema of soft tissue in the fetus. Hydrops is characterized as "nonimmune" if there is no indication of fetal-maternal blood group incompatibility. Sonographically and grossly, nonimmune hydrops fetalis is indistinguishable from hydrops caused by isoimmunization.

In a series reported by Holzgreve, 64% of 128 fetuses with nonimmune hydrops had a lesion potentially identifiable with high-resolution ultrasound imaging (48). Even in this well-studied group, however, more than one-third of patients developed hydrops because of a chromosomal disorder, perinatal infection, or fetal hemoglobinopathy. Once noninvasive maternal studies, such as a complete blood count, Kleihauer-Betke test, TORCH (toxoplasmosis, rubella, cytomegalovirus, and herpes simplex) screen, and Venereal Disease Research Laboratory test, have been completed to rule out the common causes of nonimmune hydrops fetalis, careful anatomic ultrasound evaluation of the fetus should be performed to identify those recognizable malformations that can be considered etiologic (49). If further information is required for diagnosis or management, amniocentesis for performance of viral cultures and cordocentesis to obtain a rapid karyotype, fetal hematocrit, viral IgM antibodies, PCR, and plasma albumin may assist in identifying those specific fetal causes of the hydrops and may allow supportive treatment by means of red cell transfu-

sion or administration of medication (49). Nonimmune hydrops fetalis still has a reported mortality rate of 50% to 95% (48). Clearly, only early recognition and active perinatal intervention can improve this poor prognosis.

TARGETED ULTRASOUND

Ultrasound was first developed for navigation by sonar, in which submerged objects could be identified by underwater acoustic echoes. The use of sound waves exceeding 20,000 cycles per second was subsequently applied to medical imaging, including prenatal diagnosis. Both structural and functional characteristics of the fetus may now be readily detected using real-time imaging. In the United States, approximately 60% to 70% of women undergo ultrasonography at various times in gestation, although the clinical benefit of routine ultrasound screening has yet to be established (50).

In 1980, after the introduction of MSAFP screening into the United States, a two-tiered system of ultrasound examination was suggested for use in clinical obstetrics (51). A level I study was directed toward a general assessment of dates, growth, and detection of major anomalies; a level II study, triggered by an elevated MSAFP test, included more detailed views of the fetal heart and central nervous system. This approach was modified by the American College of Obstetricians and Gynecologists in 1988, when the two tiers were designated as basic and targeted (52). According to the recommended guidelines, a targeted scan is reserved for a patient in whom a physiologically or anatomically defective fetus is suspected, and this test should be performed by an experienced operator. Today, after several updates, guidelines developed by the American Institute of Ultrasound in Medicine and the American College of Radiology provide a minimum standard to improve detection of fetal anomalies (53). During the second and third trimesters, these guidelines include documentation of fetal life, number, presentation, biometry, estimated gestational age, weight, heart rate or rhythm, amniotic fluid volume, placental location, and abnormalities of the uterus and adnexae. A fetal anatomic survey should include, but is not limited to, views of the cerebral ventricles, four-chamber view of the heart, spine, stomach, bladder, abdominal umbilical cord insertion, and renal fossae. In spite of wide dissemination of the foregoing guidelines, however, many practitioners profess ignorance about which diagnoses "should" or "should not" be identified during a routine screening obstetric ultrasound evaluation.

In 1993, 52 physicians considered to be experts in the field of obstetric ultrasonography based on national reputation and published articles were asked to consider the probability of observing various fetal anomalies using the recommended guidelines of the American Institute of Ultrasound in Medicine and the American College of Radiology (54).

Fifteen anomalies from a list of 106 diagnoses were judged to be observable in virtually all instances. The only anomaly unanimously judged to be detectable in all cases was anencephaly. The other 14 anomalies included hydranencephaly, severe unilateral or bilateral hydronephrosis, marked ascites, alobar holoprosencephaly, omphalocele, bilateral renal agenesis, ectopia cordis, limb-body wall complex, proximal small bowel obstruction with polyhydramnios, cerebral ventriculomegaly exceeding 15 mm, large posterior fossa cysts, and hydrothorax with mediastinal shift. The authors of the study emphasized, however, that real-time observations or additional views may further modify the detection rate of the remaining anomalies. These 15 anomalies constitute a "short list" of diagnoses that should be identified during routine scanning, and they are the most likely reasons for performance of a targeted ultrasound.

Anencephaly

Anencephaly was the first congenital anomaly detected prenatally by ultrasound (55). A result of failure of the anterior neural tube to close, anencephaly is characterized by a varying degree of absence of the telencephalon and cranial vault. The remaining rhomboencephalon remains primarily intact. Other associated abnormalities include meningomyelocele, midline facial defects, talipes equinus, and omphalocele. Polyhydramnios may also be seen. Anencephaly occurs in 1 per 1,000 births, with a male-to-female ratio approximating 1:4. Multifactorial inheritance and environmental teratogens have been implicated. Although the recurrence risk for neural tube defects is 3% after a single affected pregnancy, periconceptual folate supplementation has been demonstrated to reduce this risk (56).

The sonographic diagnosis of anencephaly is made by failure to visualize the cranial vault, which is usually formed by 10 weeks. Because of foreshortening of the neural tube, the remaining facial and brainstem structures may resemble a frog. In addition to other associated anomalies, amniotic bands may occasionally be seen. Accurate diagnosis should exclude iniencephaly, exencephaly, and acrania, and this allows termination of pregnancy to be offered at any gestational age.

Hydranencephaly

Another severe brain anomaly is *hydranencephaly,* in which the cranium is filled with fluid and the cerebral hemispheres are absent. The brainstem and rhomboencephalon are usually intact. Although hydranencephaly is occasionally associated with chromosomal abnormalities such as trisomy 13, most of these lesions are thought to be the result of global infarction of the cerebral cortex from either vascular or infectious causes. Carotid and jugular occlusion in monkeys has been shown to result in hydranencephaly (57). Hydra-

nencephaly, therefore, may be considered an extreme version of porencephaly. Hydranencephaly is distinguished from hydrocephalus by the absence of a cortical lining, and holoprosencephaly may be excluded by the presence of frontal brain tissue and separate thalami. After diagnosis, other studies should include fetal karyotype and assessment for toxoplasmosis and cytomegalovirus infections. Termination of pregnancy may be offered, and cephalocentesis may be required for successful vaginal delivery.

Severe Unilateral or Bilateral Hydronephrosis

Dilation of the fetal renal collecting system is the most common anomaly diagnosed in the fetus by ultrasonography (Fig. 35.6). Occurring more often in males by a factor of 5:1, *hydronephrosis* is most frequently caused by ureteropelvic junction obstruction, although obstruction at any level of the genitourinary system may occur. In addition to assessment of the ureters, bladder, and contralateral kidney, a detailed anatomic survey should be performed, because other anomalies are also associated with this disorder. Up to 3.3% of fetuses with pyelectasis greater than 4 to 5 mm in the second trimester had trisomy 21 (58). Although no nomogram exists for renal pelvic size corrected for gestational age, the degree of dilation is a general guide to prognosis. When dilation of the renal pelvis is less than 10 mm without caliectasis, 94% to 97% of fetuses will have normal function after birth. By contrast, 39% of fetuses with 10- to 15-mm dilation without caliectasis will require surgery (59). Calyceal dilation frequently requires surgical treatment.

Renal obstruction is usually detectable by the second trimester, but serial evaluation by ultrasound is warranted, because other anomalies or problems may develop as the pregnancy progresses. Severe renal obstruction may result in dysplasia and irreversible renal dysfunction. Oligohydramnios usually develops only in cases of severe bilateral renal obstruction. Significant oligohydramnios may pose a serious risk for development of pulmonary hypoplasia, especially when it is seen before the third trimester. For this reason, oligohydramnios may be an indication for *in utero* intervention after assessment of remaining fetal renal function, or it may be an indication for early delivery.

Fetal Ascites

Marked *fetal ascites* is easily identified during ultrasonographic examination as hypoechoic areas surrounding the abdominal organs, omentum, and falciform ligament (Fig. 35.7). Smaller amounts of fluid may be difficult to distinguish from pseudoascites, an echogenic band around the fetal abdominal perimeter corresponding to periabdominal fat or abdominal wall musculature. A nonspecific finding,

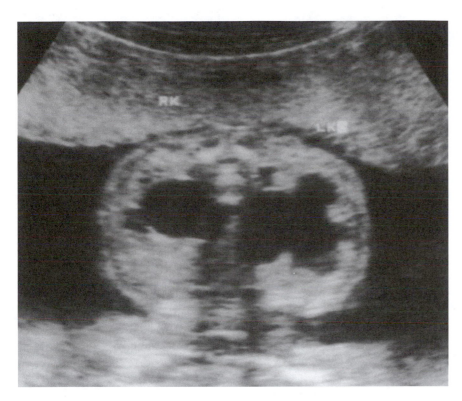

FIGURE 35.6. Severe bilateral hydronephrosis with normal amniotic fluid volume signals functional reserve in the fetal kidneys.

fetal ascites has diverse causes, including fetal gastrointestinal disorders, visceral perforations, or lymphatic disorders. Careful anatomic survey of the fetus is therefore necessary to look for potential causes. Furthermore, fetal ascites may be one of the initial signs of immune or nonimmune fetal hydrops, which may be caused by certain maternal, fetal, or placental factors. Some common causes include red blood cell isoimmunization, TORCH infections, cystic hygroma, fetal cardiac disorders, twin-twin transfusion, and chromosomal disorders. Therefore, amniocentesis to obtain fluid for determination of the fetal karyotype and for performance of viral cultures or PCR should be considered. The overall prognosis for fetuses with ascites ultimately depends on the cause. Women with severely hydropic fetuses and placentomegaly may develop preeclampsia, a phenomenon known as the *mirror syndrome* or *Ballantyne's syndrome* (60).

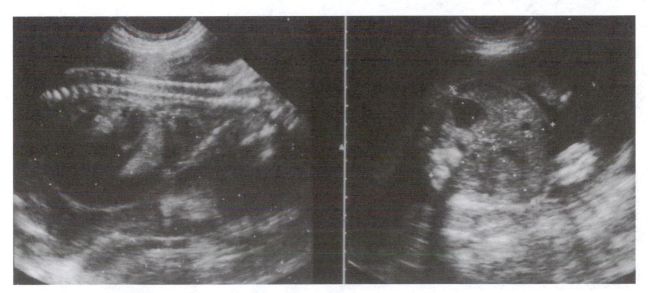

FIGURE 35.7. Marked ascites is seen in a fetus with nonimmune hydrops; sagittal view.

Alobar Holoprosencephaly

Holoprosencephaly results from the failure of cleavage of the prosencephalon that leads to midline abnormalities of the cerebral hemispheres and face (Fig. 35.8). A spectrum of disease is seen, based on the degree of division of the hemispheres and underlying structures. In increasing order of severity, these are termed lobar, semilobar, and alobar holoprosencephaly. The prognosis is directly related to the degree of separation (61). Although most cases are sporadic, holoprosencephaly is also seen in several multiple malformation syndromes and chromosomal disorders, including trisomy 13 and 18. During ultrasonographic examination, the alobar form is characterized by the finding of a single curved cerebral ventricle spanning the midline. A dorsal sac may also be seen, and the thalamus is fused to a varying degree. The interhemispheric fissure, corpus callosum, and cavum septum pellucidum are not present. Facial deformities may include cyclopia or extreme hypotelorism, a proboscis located above the orbits, and cleft lip or palate. A detailed anatomic survey should be performed, and the finding of other anomalies should prompt determination of the fetal

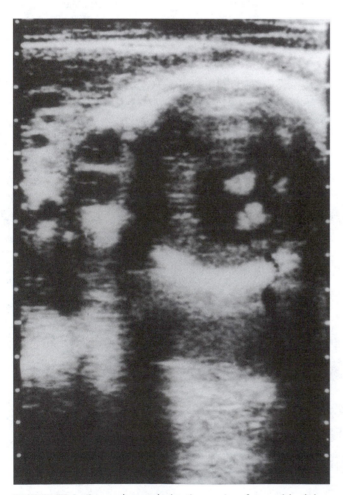

FIGURE 35.8. Severe hypotelorism is seen in a fetus with alobar holoprosencephaly.

karyotype. Infants with alobar holoprosencephaly invariably die in the first year of life. Termination of pregnancy may be considered, and cephalocentesis may be required to achieve successful vaginal delivery.

Omphalocele

Omphalocele results from the herniation of intraabdominal structures into the ventral insertion site of the umbilical cord (Fig. 35.9). More than half of all cases are associated with other anomalies, including chromosomal abnormalities such as trisomy 13 and 18, or as part of a multiple malformation syndrome such as Beckwith-Wiedemann syndrome, pentalogy of Cantrell, or cloacal extrophy. Although the condition is surgically correctable, the ultimate prognosis for omphalocele is primarily dependent on the presence and nature of other anomalies. Omphaloceles that contain only intestine are more often associated with chromosomal abnormalities than those containing liver (62). Omphaloceles are believed to represent an embryonic persistence of the body stalk. Fetal karyotyping should be considered in all cases of omphalocele after completion of a detailed anatomic survey. On ultrasonography, the diagnosis is made by the demonstration of liver, intestines, and occasionally ascites within a circumscribed mass at the insertion site of the umbilical cord. The abdominal contents are covered with peritoneum, and the umbilical cord can be seen inserting into the mass. Occasionally, omphaloceles may rupture, thus making them difficult to distinguish from gastroschisis. Omphaloceles are detectable as early as 11 to 12 weeks' gestation and should not be confused with the physiologic herniation of the intestines in the first trimester.

Bilateral Renal Agenesis

Renal agenesis is the absence of a kidney on one or both sides. Frequently associated with other anomalies, renal agenesis may also be part of multiple malformation syndromes such as VACTERL (vertebral, anal, cardiac, tracheal, esophageal, renal, and limb) syndrome. Isolated unilateral renal agenesis has no specific association with chromosomal abnormalities, but bilateral agenesis may be associated with trisomy 18. Unlike unilateral renal agenesis, which carries an excellent prognosis, bilateral renal agenesis is a lethal disorder. On ultrasonographic examination, severe oligohydramnios is noted, and the kidneys are nonvisualized. The adrenal glands are often enlarged in the second trimester and may sometimes be confused with the fetal kidneys. Color Doppler ultrasonography has greatly improved diagnostic accuracy, because the renal arteries are not present when the kidney is absent. Although the exact pathophysiology of renal agenesis is uncertain, the condition results from failure of the ureteral bud to develop. Because the fetal kidney normally begins to produce urine around the tenth week of gestation, bilateral renal agenesis soon

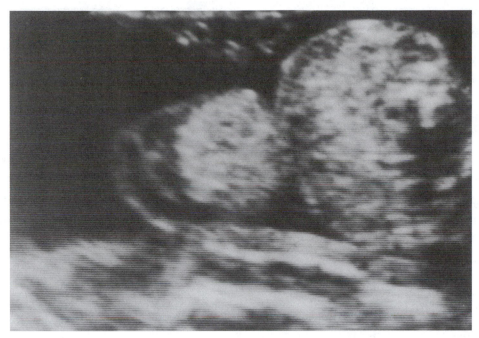

FIGURE 35.9. Omphalocele containing both bowel and liver. The umbilical cord inserts into the omphalocele sac.

leads to severe oligohydramnios. Fetal deformities resulting from prolonged oligohydramnios include severe pulmonary hypoplasia, limb contractures, and abnormal facies. This spectrum of findings is termed *Potter's syndrome* (63). Half of these infants will be stillborn, and the other half will die shortly after birth. Therefore, early accurate diagnosis may allow termination of pregnancy to be offered.

Ectopia Cordis

In *ectopia cordis,* the heart is located in an abnormal position outside the thorax. This extremely rare disorder is frequently associated with other anatomic defects, especially intracardiac anomalies. The prognosis for the fetus is generally dismal, but it may depend on the extent of the displacement and the presence of other anomalies. Ectopia cordis may also be seen as part of other constellations of anomalies such as the pentalogy of Cantrell and the amniotic band syndrome. Rare associations with chromosomal abnormalities such as trisomy 21 have been noted, so determination of the fetal karyotype should be considered. Both thoracic and thoracoabdominal locations of ectopia cordis have been described. In the former, the heart protrudes through a sternal defect, whereas in the latter, there is a partial sternal defect associated with a defect of the diaphragmatic pericardium.

Limb-Body Wall Complex

Also referred to as *body stalk anomaly, limb-body wall complex* is a severe defect stemming from early amnion disruption that interferes with development of the embryonic folds that normally obliterate the chorionic cavity. This leads to maldevelopment of the umbilical cord, skeletal deformities, and midline schisis; the fetus is characteristically fused to the placenta. The resulting spectrum of anomalies may include meningomyelocele, caudal regression, omphalocele, ectopia cordis, and missing limbs. Because of the absence of much of the abdominal musculature, severe scoliosis is the rule. The pattern of anomalies is inconsistent with any single chromosomal disorder and is usually sporadic. Limb-body wall complex is believed to be similar in pathogenesis to amniotic band syndrome, and it is a lethal anomaly. Therefore, termination of pregnancy may be considered.

Proximal Small Bowel Obstruction with Polyhydramnios

Bowel obstruction may occur at any level of the intestine, but it is seen about twice as often in small bowel than in large bowel. Obstruction may be mechanical, as is sometimes seen with meconium ileus or in the presence of ventral abdominal wall defects, but it often results from a congenital narrowing of the bowel lumen caused by atresia. Most isolated atresias are thought to be caused by vascular compromise resulting from volvulus, intussusception, or vascular malformation (64). One-half of cases will be associated with other gastrointestinal abnormalities, but anomalies in other systems and chromosomal disorders are rarer. When bowel obstruction presents as meconium ileus, the diagnosis of cystic fibrosis or other functional disorder should be strongly considered. Sonographically, multiple dilated loops of bowel are noted proximal to the obstruction. Although most commonly located in the proximal jejunum and distal ileum, the exact level of the atresia is often difficult to see, because large and small bowel may be similar in size in the fetus. Other cystic abdominal masses such as multicystic kidney, megaureter, mesenteric and ovarian cysts should be excluded. Polyhydramnios, rarely seen in large bowel atresias, poses a major risk in small bowel atresias because of resultant preterm labor. Serial decompression amniocenteses may be necessary to prolong gestation. Prognosis depends not only on gestational age and the presence of other anomalies, but also on the presence of meconium peritonitis, which occurs after bowel perforation and carries a 62% mortality rate (65).

Ventriculomegaly Exceeding 15 Millimeters

Hydrocephalus is the accumulation of cerebrospinal fluid in enlarged cerebral ventricles (Fig. 35.10). This is one of the most common congenital anomalies, and most cases are caused by obstruction to outflow of cerebrospinal fluid by intracranial processes. Aqueductal stenosis, obstruction to outflow between the third and fourth ventricles, has multiple causes, primarily infectious and vascular. Communicating hydrocephalus and Dandy-Walker malformations are also common. Extracranial anomalies are also frequent, especially meningomyelocele, which is associated with 90% of congenital hydrocephalus.

Ultrasonographic diagnosis relies on measuring the width of the atrium of the lateral ventricles, which should be less than 10 mm. Mild ventriculomegaly, between 10 and 15 mm, may indicate a chromosomal anomaly, most com-

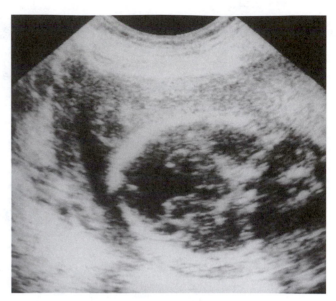

FIGURE 35.11. A large posterior fossa cyst, such as this Dandy-Walker malformation, carries a poor prognosis.

monly trisomy 21, and should be followed serially to rule out progression (66). Ventriculomegaly greater than 15 mm may be associated with an increase in head size or macrocrania (head circumference greater than the ninety-eighth percentile for gestational age). Severe cases may be confused with holoprosencephaly or hydranencephaly. If the head size is not enlarged in the presence of significant ventriculomegaly, Arnold-Chiari malformation should be considered. Whereas cortical mantle thickness has some relation to prognosis, eventual neurologic functioning is highly variable, depending primarily on the origin of the disorder and the nature of other anomalies. In the absence of macrocrania, vaginal delivery may be attempted, with prompt evaluation for shunt placement in the newborn. In cases of severe ventriculomegaly with macrocrania and other serious anomalies, vaginal delivery may be achieved with cephalocentesis, which carries a perinatal mortality rate in excess of 90% (67).

Large Posterior Fossa Cyst

Inside the fetal posterior fossa lie the cerebellum, cisterna magna, and the superior portion of the fourth ventricle. Large *cystic structures* in this area may have a dramatic impact on the fetus because of effects on these vital structures (Fig. 35.11). Differentiation of the origin of a cyst in this area may be difficult, even after delivery of the fetus, and ventriculomegaly is frequently seen. Dandy-Walker malformation consists of a defect in the cerebellar vermis through which a retrocerebellar cyst communicates with the fourth ventricle, with varying degrees of hydrocephalus. Dandy-Walker malformation is associated with aneuploidy in up to 30% of cases. Facial clefts and extracranial abnormalities are also frequently seen, and the condition is associated with multi-

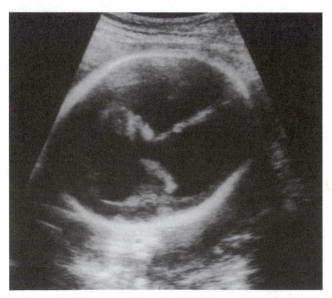

FIGURE 35.10. Massive accumulation of cerebrospinal fluid results in dilated lateral ventricles and possibly macrocrania.

ple malformation syndromes. Prognosis of Dandy-Walker malformation is poor, with fetal mortality in one-third and intellectual impairment in one-half of survivors. Enlargement of the cisterna magna exceeding 1 cm may be a variant of Dandy-Walker malformation, but it carries a better prognosis because the cerebellum is normally formed (68). Arachnoid cysts occurring in the posterior fossa are also associated with a normal-appearing cerebellum and a better prognosis. Less frequently, porencephalic cysts, resulting from a defect in cerebral cortical matter, often with a communication to the subarachnoid space, or cystic intracranial tumors may present in the posterior fossa. Prognosis, as described earlier, depends on the size of these lesions.

Hydrothorax with Mediastinal Shift

Many conditions can cause an accumulation of *fluid in the fetal thorax* as a consequence of obstruction of venous or lymphatic flow, and some of these conditions lead to nonimmune hydrops (Fig. 35.12). Processes associated with mediastinal shift, however, are primarily unilateral. This change in position of thoracic organs may lead not only to hydrops from impaired venous return and congestive failure, but also to pulmonary hypoplasia from compression of the contralateral lung. Esophageal compression may impair fetal swallowing and may lead to the development of polyhydramnios and preterm labor. Consequently, mediastinal shift is an ominous finding that may or may not be reversible with *in utero* intervention. One of the more common causes is congenital cystic adenomatoid malformation, which is a hamartoma of the lung in which the terminal bronchioles fail to form saccules for gas exchange. Usually unilateral, these lesions have three subtypes correlating to cystic size

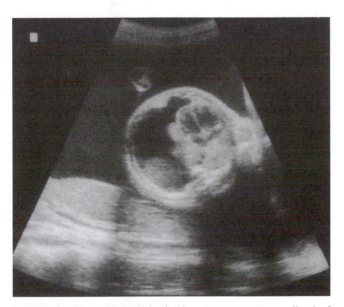

FIGURE 35.12. Unilateral hydrothorax may cause mediastinal shift, as in this fetus.

and prognosis. Other space-occupying lesions may include congenital chylothorax, a unilateral pleural effusion caused by accumulation of lymph and frequently seen in trisomy 21, or bronchopulmonary sequestration, in which a section of lung parenchyma has a separate systemic blood supply and no communication with pulmonary bronchioles. Both diagnoses can result in poor outcomes if hydrops results or pulmonary development is impaired. Persistent and life-threatening pleural effusions in the fetus have been successfully treated with continuous drainage by means of a pleuroamniotic shunt.

ANALYSIS OF FETAL CELLS IN MATERNAL CIRCULATION FOR PRENATAL DIAGNOSIS

The search for noninvasive methods of prenatal diagnosis, accessible to all pregnancies, has been one of the most challenging goals of medical genetics during the last 10 years. The peripheral maternal circulation, from which fetal nucleated cells are detected and isolated, potentially represents a risk-free source of fetal DNA, and although this approach is still in development, it is a promising method of prenatal screening or diagnosis for genetic diseases.

The observation of fetal cells in the maternal circulation was first reported as long ago as the 1950s. The idea of recovering fetal cells from maternal blood for prenatal diagnosis, however, was first suggested by Walknowska et al. in 1969 (69). Since then, many studies have been performed, and various fetal cells including trophoblasts, lymphocytes, and erythrocytes have been isolated from peripheral maternal blood, both in animals and humans (70). Fetal trophoblasts, for example, can be detected from as early as 6 weeks' gestation until term (71). Between 8 to 13 weeks, 80% of pregnancies have detectable amounts of diverse fetal cells in the peripheral maternal blood (72). However, the scarcity of fetal compared with maternal cells in a routine blood sample makes detection and isolation major obstacles to developing an accurate method for the screening or diagnosis of fetal disease. The ratio between fetal and maternal cells is estimated to be 1 in 475,000 to 600,000, depending on the gestational age when the sample is drawn and the technique employed for cell isolation (72). According to Bianchi et al., no more than 100 fetal cells can be found in any given 10-mL maternal blood sample (73). Exceptions to this rule are pregnancies in which invasive procedures, such as chorionic villus sampling, have been performed before the maternal blood analysis (74). Many techniques of enrichment and purification have been employed to improve the detection of fetal cells in maternal blood. However, all methods of fetal cell concentration are subject to significant levels of contamination with extraneous cell lines and thus are not yet suitable for routine clinical diagnosis. One study identified hematopoietic progenitor cells containing male DNA in blood samples of nonpregnant women who had previously delivered male fetuses from 6 months to 27 years before sampling (75). These results indicate long-term persistence of fetal cells such as hematopoietic stem cells, lymphoid-myeloid progenitors, and lymphocytes in the maternal circulation, and they highlight the need to understand the underlying biology to avoid misdiagnosis. Even when the pregnant patient has never delivered a male fetus, the possibility of a vanishing twin or maternal blood transfusion from a male donor must be considered (76). The prenatal detection of some aneuploidies, fetal sex, fetal rhesus blood type, and a few other conditions, however, is encouraging. On the basis of preliminary results, it seems likely that this noninvasive method will, in the future, became an important screening test incorporated into standard prenatal care (77–79).

Types and Characteristics of the Cells Identified

Three types of nucleated fetal cells have been detected in the peripheral maternal circulation and have been used experimentally for noninvasive prenatal diagnosis: trophoblasts, leukocytes, and erythroblasts (72,77,78). Fetal platelets can also be identified in the maternal circulation, but the absence of genomic DNA prevents the use of these cells for prenatal diagnosis (80).

Trophoblasts

The *trophoblastic invasion* of the uterus creates an intimate relationship between this organ and the trophoblastic cells. Desquamation of the chorionic villi into the maternal circulation allows trophoblastic cells access to the peripheral maternal blood (81). Trophoblasts were first detected by Ikle and Wagner at the level of the uterine vein, inferior vena cava, and pulmonary arteries during the 1960s (82,83). In 1984, Covone et al. described three different types of trophoblasts present in retroplacental blood: anucleated, mononucleated, and multinucleated cells (71). According to Gänshirt et al., about 100,000 of these trophoblasts are released daily into the maternal circulation (72). Only a fraction, however, reaches the peripheral circulation, probably because of obstruction to passage of the multinucleated syncytiotrophoblast cells through the maternal lungs, before reaching the peripheral blood (72). Even when fetal trophoblasts are successfully harvested from the maternal circulation, the presence of multiple nuclei among some syncytial cells complicates FISH analysis; and placental mosaicism, in which 1% of pregnancies have a placental karyotype different from the fetal karyotype, can be misleading (80). More than any other factor, however, the failure of most attempts to enrich and isolate trophoblasts from the peripheral maternal circulation in an adequate amount for diagnostic purposes suggests that this group of cells is poorly suited for prenatal assessment.

Lymphocytes

Lymphocytes were the first fetal cells sought in the maternal circulation, and their detection was based on maternal-fetal human leukocyte antigen (HLA) dissimilarities (77). The production of lymphocytes in fetuses starts after 20 weeks' gestation, when bone marrow blood formation begins. Thus, these cells only reach detectable levels in the peripheral maternal circulation late in the second trimester (72). The tendency of fetal lymphocytes to persist in maternal blood for many years postpartum is a major problem that could lead to misdiagnosis in multigravidas (80). As with trophoblastic cells, the number of maternal lymphocytes compared with fetal lymphocytes is large (72). Few researchers have succeeded in achieving prenatal diagnosis based on the isolation of fetal lymphocytes, and most studies currently focus on the detection of other cells.

Granulocytes are the least studied fetal cells for prenatal diagnosis, and the controversial results achieved with them are not encouraging.

Erythroblasts

Erythroblasts are mononuclear cells predominant early in the fetal circulation and detectable in maternal blood at anytime during the pregnancy, but they are rare in the normal adult circulation. These unique properties have made erythroblasts the subject of the most successful attempts to date at prenatal diagnosis using fetal cells. Using enriched nucleated red blood cells, the first successful diagnosis of fetal trisomy from analysis of maternal blood was accomplished in 1991 (74). The relatively short life span of erythroblasts (90 days) is an important characteristic of this group of cells. One major difficulty in the development of an accurate diagnostic method using fetal cells is the risk of isolating cells from previous pregnancies that have persisted in the maternal circulation. However, the use of erythroblasts, which have a short life span, dramatically reduces this risk. Some studies have detected decreased levels of fetal nucleated red blood cells after 16 weeks' gestation, a finding suggesting potential difficulty in the isolation of fetal erythrocytes beyond the midsecond trimester (80).

Methods of Fetal Cell Isolation from Maternal Blood

In spite of the promise offered by analysis of fetal cells in the maternal circulation, maternal cell cross-reaction is still significant; it decreases fetal cell yield and purity and complicates attempts at genetic diagnosis. Three major methods have been used for the isolation of fetal cells from maternal blood: fluorescence-activated cell sorting, magnetic-activated cell sorting, and immunomagnetic beads (84). All these methods have advantages as well as disadvantages, and it is still controversial whether any one technique is more accurate than the others. All the methods flow-sort target cells from the maternal circulation and use surface markers to distinguish fetal from maternal cells.

The most effective strategy to isolate the fetal cells consists of the employment of a monoclonal antibody that reacts uniquely with fetal antigens, thus reducing contamination with maternal cells. Unfortunately, the ideal antibody has not yet been identified. The most common antibodies used against trophoblasts include FD046B, 161G, 101X, QB, C3.3, and D31 (80). Monoclonal antibodies used to label fetal nucleated red cells include the transferrin receptor (CD71), thrombospondin receptor (CD36), glycophorin A (GPA), and FB3-2, H3-3, and 2-6B/6 (the last three recognize epitopes carried on cell surface proteins or glycoproteins) (85). Among the monoclonal antibodies, CD71 is the most commonly used label for fetal cell enrichment because of its high expression on nucleated red cells early in pregnancy. A study which employed flow cytometry, found that FB3-2, CD71, and 2-6B/6 are suitable antibodies for use during the first and early second trimesters. After 19 weeks' gestation, however, 2-6B/6 has more expression in fetal erythroblasts (60% of the cells) compared with the other two antibodies, which are expressed in just 50% of the fetal red cells. Both CD36 and GPA provide low fetal cell purity and are thus not strong candidates to label fetal erythroblasts in the maternal blood. Some evidence indicates that the availability of fetal cell antigens may be increased in fetuses with aneuploidies or multiple anomalies (85). Bianchi et al. reported a sixfold elevation of fetal cells in the maternal circulation when the fetus had Down's syndrome (76). Structural differences in placentas and the larger size of erythrocytes from aneuploid fetuses compared with cytogenetically normal fetuses may explain these findings (80).

Increased fetomaternal transfusion was also observed in other aneuploidies, and conditions such as pregnancy-induced hypertension, diabetes, multiple gestation, fetal-maternal blood group incompatibility, and vaginal bleeding are also likely to influence the number of circulating fetal cells (76,80). Holzgreve et al. demonstrated that the number of fetal erythroblasts is significantly elevated in the maternal circulation of patients with preeclampsia compared with levels in normotensive pregnant women (86). The abnormal cell traffic across the placental barrier in patients with preeclampsia elevated not only the number of fetal nucleated red blood cells, but lymphocytes and monocytes as well.

Techniques Employed for Fetal-DNA Sequence Amplification in Cells Isolated from Maternal Blood

Basically, two techniques have been used to isolate fetal DNA sequences from maternal blood samples: PCR and FISH.

Polymerase Chain Reaction

This technique has been used for Y-specific sequence DNA amplification, thus determining fetal sex (72–74,81). Bianchi et al. reported that male DNA could be detected in 99.3% of pregnant women carrying a male fetus, by using a single 16-mL blood sample (76). Some investigators have also employed PCR to study rhesus locus genes and paternally inherited HLA genes (72,87). Because of the low purity of fetal cells at this time, prenatal detection of diseases based on PCR is restricted to autosomal dominant disorders in which the father carries the mutation and autosomal recessive disorders in which the father and mother carry different mutations (72,77).

Fluorescence *In Situ* Hybridization

When used in association with chromosome-specific DNA probes, the FISH technique enables the detection of aneuploidies in interphase nuclei. Some investigators have already reported the use of FISH in the prenatal diagnosis of chromosomal abnormalities such as trisomies 21 and 18 and Klinefelter's syndrome (78). Accurate FISH analysis requires fetal cell purity of at least 20%. The low purity of fetal enriched cells currently attainable is the limiting factor preventing the application of this technique in all pregnancies (72).

10 KEY POINTS

1. Umbilical artery Doppler velocimetry measures impedance to blood flow in the placenta, as determined by the number of resistance vessels, or small muscular arteries in the tertiary villi. Obliteration of these resistance vessels is termed vascular sclerosis and is associated with development of IUGR, hypertension, and their sequelae.

2. Use of umbilical artery Doppler velocimetry as a screening test in high-risk patients is associated with a significant decrease in perinatal mortality without a concomitant increase in maternal or neonatal morbidity.

3. Umbilical artery Doppler velocimetry can be used to stratify risks in patients with a known obstetric complication, such as IUGR, oligohydramnios, or unexplained elevated MSAFP.

4. Umbilical venous pulsations identify the presence of poor right ventricular function, secondary to an anatomic defect or hypoxia in the fetus.

5. Cordocentesis or PUBS consists of fine-needle aspiration of fetal blood using high-resolution ultrasound guidance. In experienced hands, a pure specimen of fetal blood can be obtained in less than 10 minutes, with a fetal loss rate of about 1% per procedure.

6. Targeted ultrasound is performed on a patient in whom a physiologically or anatomically defective fetus is

suspected. Such examinations are usually performed by an experienced operator in a referral center.

7. Fetal anomalies that should be identified in virtually all instances in which a basic ultrasound examination is performed include anencephaly, hydranencephaly, severe unilateral or bilateral hydronephrosis, marked ascites, alobar holoprosencephaly, omphalocele, bilateral renal agenesis, ectopia cordis, limb-body wall complex, proximal small bowel obstruction with polyhydramnios, cerebral ventriculomegaly exceeding 15 mm, large posterior fossa cysts, and hydrothorax with mediastinal shift.

8. Various fetal cells including trophoblasts, lymphocytes, and erythrocytes have been isolated from peripheral maternal blood. Only a fraction of fetal cells released into the maternal circulation reaches the peripheral blood, however, mainly because of obstruction to passage through the maternal lungs. The scarcity of fetal cells in a routine maternal blood sample therefore makes detection and isolation major obstacles to developing an accurate method for the screening or diagnosis of fetal disease.

9. Erythroblasts are rare in the normal adult circulation and have a short life span (90 days), and fetal erythroblasts are detectable in maternal blood at any time during gestation. These unique properties have made erythroblasts the subject of the most successful attempts to date at prenatal diagnosis using fetal cells.

10. Analysis of fetal cells obtained from the maternal circulation has already resulted in the successful prenatal detection of fetal aneuploidies, sex, and rhesus blood type. An increased number of circulating fetal cells is likely to be observed in conditions such as fetal aneuploidy, preeclampsia, diabetes, multiple gestation, isoimmunization, and vaginal bleeding.

REFERENCES

1. Thompson RS, Trudinger BJ, Cook CM. A comparison of Doppler ultrasound waveform indices in the umbilical artery. I. Indices derived from the maximum velocity waveform. *Ultrasound Med Biol* 1986;12:835–844.
2. Den Ouden M, Cohen-Overbeck TE, Wladimiroff JW. Uterine and fetal umbilical artery flow velocity waveforms in normal first trimester pregnancies. *Br J Obstet Gynaecol* 1990;97:716–719.
3. Giles WB, Trudinger BJ, Baird PJ. Fetal umbilical artery flow velocity waveforms and placental resistance: pathological correlation. *Br J Obstet Gynaecol* 1985;92:31–38.
4. Morrow RJ, Adamson SL, Bull SB, et al. Effect of placental embolization on the umbilical arterial velocity waveform in fetal sheep. *Am J Obstet Gynecol* 1989;161:1055–1060.
5. Thompson RS, Trudinger BJ. Doppler waveform pulsatility index and resistance, pressure and flow in the umbilical placental circulation: an investigation using a mathematical model. *Ultrasound Med Biol* 1990;16:449–458.
6. Bruner JP, Sheppard CG, Reed GW, et al. The umbilical artery Doppler ultrasonographic gradient: confirmation, cause and comparison of continuous-wave and duplex ultrasonographic pulsed-wave measurements. *J Perinatol* 1994;14:386–392.
7. Haberman S, Friedman ZM. Intraplacental spectral Doppler scanning: fetal growth classification based on Doppler velocimetry. *Gynecol Obstet Invest* 1997;43:11–19.
8. Rotmensch S, Liberati M, Luo JS, et al. Color Doppler flow patterns and flow velocity waveforms of the intraplacental fetal circulation in growth-retarded fetuses. *Am J Obstet Gynecol* 1994; 171:1257–1264.
9. Bruner JP, Coggins T. Assessment of fetal breathing movements using three different ultrasound modalities. *J Clin Ultrasound* 1995;23:551–553.
10. Maulik D, Downing GJ, Yarlagadda P. Umbilical arterial Doppler indices in acute uteroplacental flow occlusion. *Echocardiography* 1990;7:619.
11. Bruner JP, Levy DW, Arger PH. Doppler ultrasonography of the umbilical cord in complicated pregnancies. *South Med J* 1993; 86:418–422.
12. Pollack RN, Divon MY. Intrauterine growth retardation: diagnosis. In: Copel JA, Reed KL, eds. *Doppler ultrasound in obstetrics and gynecology.* New York: Raven, 1995:171–177.
13. Beattie RB, Dornan JC. Antenatal screening for intrauterine growth retardation with umbilical artery Doppler ultrasonography. *BMJ* 1989;298:631–635.
14. Trudinger BJ, Cook CM, Giles WB, et al. Fetal umbilical artery velocity waveforms and subsequent neonatal outcome. *Br J Obstet Gynaecol* 1991;98:378–384.
15. U.S. Preventive Services Task Force. Screening ultrasonography in pregnancy. In: *U.S. Preventive Services Task Force: guide to clinical preventive services,* 2nd ed. Alexandria, VA: International Medical Publishing, 1996:407–417.
16. Trudinger BJ, Cook CM, Giles WB, et al. Umbilical artery flow velocity waveforms in high-risk pregnancy: randomised controlled trial. *Lancet* 1987;1:188–190.
17. Divon MY. Randomized controlled trials of umbilical artery Doppler velocimetry: how many are too many? *Ultrasound Obstet Gynecol* 1995;6:1–3.
18. Seeds JW, Cefalo RC. *Practical obstetrical ultrasound.* Rockville, MD: Aspen, 1986:70.
19. Burke G, Stuart B, Crowley P, et al. Is intrauterine growth retardation with normal umbilical artery blood flow a benign condition? *BMJ* 1990;300:1044–1045.
20. Carroll BC, Bruner JP. Umbilical artery Doppler velocimetry as a predictor of perinatal outcome in pregnancies complicated by oligohydramnios. (Submitted for publication.)
21. Trudinger BJ, Cook CM, Jones L, et al. A comparison of fetal heart rate monitoring and umbilical artery waveforms in the recognition of fetal compromise. *Br J Obstet Gynaecol* 1986;93: 171–175.
22. Devoe LD, Gardner P, Dear C, et al. The diagnostic values of concurrent nonstress testing, amniotic fluid measurement, and Doppler velocimetry in screening a general high-risk population. *Am J Obstet Gynecol* 1990;163:1040–1048.
23. Sarno AP, Ahn MO, Brar HS, et al. Intrapartum Doppler velocimetry, amniotic fluid volume, and fetal heart rate as predictors of subsequent fetal distress. I. An initial report. *Am J Obstet Gynecol* 1989;161:1508–1514.
24. Morrow RJ, Adamson SL, Bull SB, et al. Acute hypoxemia does not affect the umbilical artery flow velocity waveform in fetal sheep. *Obstet Gynecol* 1990;75:590–593.
25. Copel JA, Schlafer D, Wentworth R, et al. Does the umbilical artery systolic/diastolic ratio reflect flow or acidosis? An umbilical artery Doppler study of fetal sheep. *Am J Obstet Gynecol* 1990; 163:751–756.
26. Farine D, Kelly EN, Ryan G, et al. Absent and reversed umbilical artery end-diastolic velocity. In: Copel JA, Reed KL, eds. *Doppler ultrasound in obstetrics and gynecology.* New York: Raven, 1995:187–197.

27. Reed KL, Anderson CF, Shenker L. Changes in intracardiac Doppler blood flow velocities in fetuses with absent umbilical artery diastolic flow. *Am J Obstet Gynecol* 1987;157:774–779.

28. Hackett GA, Campbell S, Gamsu H, et al. Doppler studies in the growth retarded fetus and prediction of neonatal necrotising enterocolitis, haemorrhage, and neonatal morbidity. *BMJ Clin Res Ed* 1987;294:13–16.

29. Damron DP, Chaffin DG, Anderson CF, et al. Changes in umbilical arterial and venous blood flow velocity waveforms during late decelerations of the fetal heart rate. *Obstet Gynecol* 1994; 84:1038–1040.

30. Daffos F, Capella-Pavlovsky M, Forestier F. Fetal blood sampling via the umbilical cord using a needle guided by ultrasound: report of 66 cases. *Prenat Diagn* 1983;3:271–277.

31. de Crespigny L, Robinson HP, Quinn M, et al. Ultrasound-guided fetal blood transfusion for severe rhesus isoimmunization. *Obstet Gynecol* 1985;66:529–532.

32. Moise KJ Jr, Deter RI, Kirshon B, et al. Intravenous pancuronium bromide for fetal neuromuscular blockade during intrauterine transfusion for red cell alloimmunization. *Obstet Gynecol* 1989; 74:905–908.

33. Daffos F, Forestier F, MacAlesse J, et al. Fetal curarization for prenatal magnetic resonance imaging. *Prenat Diagn* 1988;8: 311–314.

34. Moise KJ Jr, Carpenter RJ Jr, Deter RL, et al. The use of fetal neuromuscular blockade during intrauterine procedures. *Am J Obstet Gynecol* 1987;157:874–879.

35. Giannakoulopoulos X, Sepulveda W, Kourtis P, et al. Fetal plasma cortisol and beta-endorphin response to intrauterine needling. *Lancet* 1994;344:77–81.

36. Daffos F. Fetal blood sampling. In: Harrison MR, Golbus MS, Filly RA, eds. *The unborn patient,* 2nd ed. Philadelphia: WB Saunders, 1991:75–81.

37. Radunovic N, Lockwood CJ, Alvarez M, et al. The severely anemic and hydropic isoimmune fetus: changes in fetal hematocrit associated with intrauterine death. *Obstet Gynecol* 1992; 79:390–393.

38. Hallak M, Moise KJ Jr, Hesketh DE, et al. Intravascular transfusion of fetuses with rhesus incompatibility: prediction of fetal outcome by changes in umbilical venous pressure. *Obstet Gynecol* 1992;80:286–290.

39. Gonsoulin WJ, Moise KJ Jr, Milam JD, et al. Serial maternal blood donations for intrauterine transfusion. *Obstet Gynecol* 1990;75:158–162.

40. American College of Obstetricians and Gynecologists. *Management of isoimmunization in pregnancy.* Educational bulletin no. 227. American College of Obstetricians and Gynecologists, 1996.

41. Nicolaides KH, Rodeck CH, Mibashan RS, et al. Have Liley charts outlived their usefulness? *Am J Obstet Gynecol* 1986;155: 90–94.

42. Moise KJ Jr, Schumacher B. Anaemia. In: Fisk NM, Moise KJ Jr, eds. *Fetal therapy.* Cambridge: Cambridge University Press, 1997:141–163.

43. Peters MT, Nicolaides KH. Cordocentesis for the diagnosis and treatment of human fetal parvovirus infection. *Obstet Gynecol* 1990;75:501–504.

44. Sheikh AU, Ernest JM, O'Shea M. Long-term outcome in fetal hydrops from parvovirus B19 infection. *Am J Obstet Gynecol* 1992;167:337–341.

45. Daffos F, Forestier F, Grangeot-Keros L, et al. Prenatal diagnosis of congenital rubella. *Lancet* 1984;2:1–3.

46. Daffos F, Forestier F, Cappella-Pavlovsky M, et al. Prenatal management of 746 pregnancies at risk for congenital toxoplasmosis. *N Engl J Med* 1988;318:271–275.

47. Dupouy-Camet J, Bougnoux ME, Lavareda de Souza S, et al. Comparative value of polymerase chain reaction and conventional biological tests for the prenatal diagnosis of congenital toxoplasmosis. *Ann Biol Clin (Paris)* 1992;50:315–319.

48. Holzgreve W. The fetus with nonimmune hydrops. In: Harrison MR, Golbus MS, Filly RA, eds. *The unborn patient,* 2nd ed. Philadelphia: WB Saunders, 1991:228–245.

49. Bruner JP, Fleischer AC, Jeanty P, et al. Sonography of nonimmune hydrops fetalis. In: Fleischer AC, Manning FA, Jeanty P, et al., eds. *Sonography in obstetrics and gynecology,* 5th ed. Stamford, CT: Appleton & Lange, 1996:565–581.

50. American College of Obstetricians and Gynecologists. *Practice patterns.* Educational bulletin no. 5. American College of Obstetricians and Gynecologists, 1997.

51. Haddow JE, Wald NJ, eds. Alpha-fetoprotein screening: the current issues. In: *Report of the third Scarborough conference.* Scarborough, ME: Foundation for Blood Research, 1981.

52. American College of Obstetricians and Gynecologists. *Ultrasound in pregnancy.* Technical bulletin no. 116. American College of Obstetricians and Gynecologists, 1988.

53. American Institute of Ultrasound in Medicine. *Guidelines for the performance of the antepartum obstetrical ultrasound examination.* Rockville, MD: American Institute of Ultrasound in Medicine, 1991.

54. Nelson NL, Filly RA, Goldstein RB, et al. The AIUM/ACR antepartum obstetrical sonographic guidelines: expectations for detection of anomalies. *J Ultrasound Med* 1993;4:189–196.

55. Campbell S, Johnstone FD, Holt EM, et al. Anencephaly: early ultrasonic diagnosis and active management. *Lancet* 1972;2:1226.

56. Centers for Disease Control and Prevention. Recommendations for use of folic acid to reduce number of spina bifida cases and other neural tube defects. *JAMA* 1993;269:1233, 1236–1238.

57. Myers RE. Brain pathology following fetal vascular occlusion: an experimental study. *Invest Ophthalmol* 1969;8:41.

58. Benacerraf BR, Mandell J, Estroff JA, et al. Fetal pyelectasis: a possible association with Down syndrome. *Obstet Gynecol* 1990; 76:58–60.

59. Grignon A, Filion R, Filiatrault D, et al. Urinary tract dilatation *in utero:* classification and clinical applications. *Radiology* 1986;160:645–647.

60. Van Selm M, Kanhai HH, Gravenhorst JB. Maternal hydrops syndrome: a review. *Obstet Gynecol Surv* 1991;46:785–788.

61. DeMyer W. Holoprosencephaly. In: Vinken PJ, Bruyn GW, eds. *Handbook of clinical neurology,* vol 30. Amsterdam: Elsevier, 1977:431–478.

62. Nyberg DA, Fitzsimmons J, Mack LA, et al. Chromosomal abnormalities in fetuses with omphalocele. *J Ultrasound Med* 1989; 8:299–308.

63. Potter EL. Bilateral absence of ureters and kidneys: report of fifty cases. *Obstet Gynecol* 1965;25:3–12.

64. Louw JH. Investigations into the etiology of congenital atresia of the colon. *Dis Colon Rectum* 1964;7:471.

65. Bergmans MGM, Merkus JMWM, Baars AM. Obstetrical and neonatological aspects of a child with atresia of the small bowel. *J Perinat Med* 1984;12:325.

66. Bromley B, Frigoletto FD, Benacerraf BR. Mild fetal lateral-cerebral ventriculomegaly: clinical course and outcome. *Am J Obstet Gynecol* 1991;164:863.

67. Chevenak FA, Berkowitz RL, Tortora M, et al. The management of fetal hydrocephalus. *Am J Obstet Gynecol* 1985;151:933.

68. Nyberg DA, Mahony BA, Hegge FN, et al. Enlarged cisterna magna and the Dandy-Walker malformation: factors associated with chromosome abnormalities. *Obstet Gynecol* 1991;77:436–442.

69. Walknowska J, Conte FA, Grumback MM. Practical and theoretical implications of fetal/maternal lymphocytes transfer. *Lancet* 1969;1:1119–1122.

70. Selypes A, Lorencz R. A noninvasive method for determination

of the sex and karyotype of the fetus from the maternal blood. *Hum Genet* 1988;79:357–359.

71. Covone AE, Mutton D, Johnson PM, et al. Throphoblast cells in peripheral blood from pregnant women. *Lancet* 1984;2:841–843.

72. Gänshirt D, Garritsen HSP, Holzgreve W. Fetal cells in maternal blood. *Curr Opin Obstet Gynecol* 1995;7:103–108.

73. Bianchi DW, Shuber AP, DeMaria MA, et al. Fetal cells in maternal blood: determination of purity and yield by quantitative polymerase chain reaction. *Am J Obstet Gynecol* 1994;171:922–926.

74. Price JO, Elias S, Wachtel SS, et al. Prenatal diagnosis with fetal cells isolated from maternal blood by multiparameter flow cytometry. *Am J Obstet Gynecol* 1991;165:1731–1737.

75. Bianchi DW, Zickwolf GK, Weil GJ, et al. Male fetal progenitor cells persist in maternal blood for as long as 27 years postpartum. *Proc Natl Acad Sci U S A* 1996;93:705–708.

76. Bianchi DW, Williams JM, Sullivan LM, et al. PCR quantification of fetal cells in maternal blood in normal and aneuploid pregnancies. *Am J Hum Genet* 1997;61:822–829.

77. Simpson JL. Preimplantation genetics and recovery of fetal cells from maternal blood. *Curr Opin Obstet Gynecol* 1992;4:295–301.

78. Pezzolo A, Santi F, Pistoia V, et al. Prenatal diagnosis of triploidy using fetal cells in the maternal circulation. *Prenat Diagn* 1997;17:389.

79. Holzgreve W. Will ultrasound-screening and ultrasound-guided procedures be replaced by non-invasive techniques for the diagnosis of fetal chromosome anomalies? *Ultrasound Obstet Gynecol* 1997;9:217–219.

80. Bianchi DW. Prenatal diagnosis by analysis of fetal cells in maternal blood. *J Pediatr* 1995;127:847–856.

81. Bruch JF, Metezeau P, Garcia-Fonknechten N, et al. Trophoblast-like cells sorted from peripheral maternal blood using flow cytometry: a multiparametric study involving transmission electron microscopy and fetal DNA amplification. *Prenat Diagn* 1991;11:787–798.

82. Ikle FA von. Dissemination von syncytiotrophoblastzellen im mütterlichen Blut whrend der Graviditt. *Bull Schweiz Akad Med Wiss* 1964;20:62–72.

83. Wagner D. Trophoblastic cells in the blood stream in normal and abnormal pregnancy. *Acta Cytol* 1968;12:137–139.

84. Bianchi DW, Klinger KW, Vadnais TJ, et al. Development of a model system to compare cell separation methods for the isolation of fetal cells from maternal blood. *Prenat Diagn* 1996;16:289–298.

85. Zheng Y-L, Zhen DK, DeMaria MA, et al. Search for the optimal fetal cell antibody: results of immunophenotyping studies using flow cytometry. *Hum Genet* 1997;100:35–42.

86. Holzgreve W, Ghezzi F, DiNaro E, et al. Disturbed feto-maternal cell traffic in preeclampsia. *Obstet Gynecol* 1998;61:669–672.

87. De la Cruz F, Shifrin H, Elias S, et al. Prenatal diagnosis by use of fetal cells isolated from maternal blood. *Am J Obstet Gynecol* 1995;173:1354–1355.

SUBJECT INDEX

Page numbers followed by *f* indicate figures; page numbers followed by *t* indicate tabular material.